TEXTBOOK OF
RADIOLOGY
AND IMAGING

SEVENTH EDITION

TEXTBOOK OF
RADIOLOGY
AND IMAGING

VOLUME 1

EDITED BY

DAVID SUTTON MD, FRCP, FRCR, DMRD, FCan.AR (Hon)

Consulting Radiologist
St Mary's Hospital and Medical School, London
Director, Radiological Department (1963-1984)
Consulting Radiologist, The National Hospital for Neurology
and Neurosurgery, London, UK.

ASSOCIATE EDITORS

Nuclear Medicine
PHILIP J.A. ROBINSON FRCP, FRCR

MRI
JEREMY P.R. JENKINS FRCP, DMRD, FRCR

CT
RICHARD W. WHITEHOUSE BSc, MB ChB, MD, FRCR

Ultrasound
PAUL L. ALLAN MSc, MBBS, DMRD, FRCR, FRCP(Ed)

Cardiac Radiology
PETER WILDE BSc, MRCP, FRCR

Neuroradiology
JOHN M. STEVENS MBBS, DRACR, FRCR

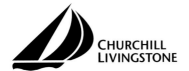

CHURCHILL
LIVINGSTONE

CHURCHILL LIVINGSTONE
An imprint of Elsevier Science Limited

First Edition 1969
Second Edition 1975
Third Edition 1980
Fourth Edition 1987
Fifth Edition 1993
Sixth Edition 1998

ISBN 0 443 071098
International Student Edition ISBN 0 443 07108X

British Library Cataloguing in Publication Data
A catalogue record for this book is available from the British Library

Library of Congress Cataloging in Publication Data
A catalog record from this book is available from the Library of Congress

Note
Medical knowledge is constantly changing. As new information becomes
available, changes in treatment, procedures, equipment and the use of drugs
become necessary. The editors, contributors and the publishers have, as far as
it is possible, taken care to ensure that the information given in this text is
accurate and up to date. However, readers are strongly advised to confirm that
the information, especially with regard to drug usage, complies with the latest
legislation and standards of practice.

The Publishers have made every effort to trace the copyright holders for
borrowed material. If they have inadvertently overlooked any, they will be
pleased to make the necessary arrangements at the first opportunity.

 your source for books,
journals and multimedia
in the health sciences
www.elsevierhealth.com

Commissioning Editor: Michael J. Houston
Project Development Manager: Martin Mellor
Project Manager: Nora Naughton (Aoibhe O'Shea)
Designer: Sarah Russell

The
publisher's
policy is to use
**paper manufactured
from sustainable forests**

Printed in China by RDC Group Limited

CONTENTS

Cover illustrations: Vol 1: *Front:* Figs. 2.09; 1.60; 1.61A,B; 15.139B *Back:* Figs. 25.144; 2.8; 15.144; 26.43C
Vol 2: *Front:* Figs. 59.26A; 59.39; 58.94A-D; 59.37 *Back:* Figs. 33.71B; 55.43C; 58.43C

SECTION **6**

Head and neck; CNS; recent technical advances

CONTRIBUTORS

Paul L. Allan MSc, MBBS, DMRD, FRCR, FRCP (Ed)
Honorary Consultant Radiologist
Royal Infirmary
Edinburgh, UK

Stefan Brew MB, ChB, MHB (Hons), MSc, FRANZCR, FRCR
Consultant Radiologist
National Hospital for Neurology and Neurosurgery
London, UK

Anne Boothroyd MBChB, FRCR
Consultant Radiologist
Royal Liverpool Children's Hospital
Liverpool, UK

Mark Callaway BM, MRCP, FRCR
Consultant Radiologist
Bristol Royal Infirmary
Bristol, UK

Otto Chan FRCS, FRCR
Consultant Radiologist
The Royal London Hospital
London, UK

Anthony H. A. Chapman FRCP, FRCR
Head of Clinical Radiology
Leeds NHS Trust
Consultant Radiologist
St James's University Hospital
Leeds, UK

Swarupsinh V. Chavda MBChB, DMRD, FRCR
Consultant Radiologist
St James's University Hospital
Leeds, UK

Graham R. Cherryman MBChB, FRCR
Professor of Radiology
University of Leicester
Honorary Consultant Radiologist
UHL NHS Trust
Leicester, UK

Roger Chisholm MA, MBBChir, MRCP, FRCR
Consultant Radiologist
Hope Hospital
Salford, UK

Mary Crofton FRCR, FRCP
Consultant Radiologist
Department of Radiology
St Mary's Hospital
London, UK

Mark Cobby MBChB, MRCP, FRCR
Consultant Radiologist
Frenchay Hospital
Bristol, UK

Keith Dewbury BSc, DMRD, FRCR
Consultant Radiologist
Southampton General Hospital
Southampton, UK

Robert Dick MB, BS(Syd), FRCAR, FRCR
Department of Radiology
Royal Free Hospital
London, UK

Paul Dubbins BSc, FRCR
Consultant Radiologist
Imaging Directorate
Derriford Hospital
Plymouth, UK

Stuart Field MA, MBBChir, DMRD, FRCR
Consultant Radiologist
Kent and Canterbury Hospital
Canterbury, UK

John A. Fielding MD, FRCP(Edin), FRCR
Consultant Radiologist
Royal Shrewsbury Hospital
Shrewsbury, UK

W. Gedroyc MRCP, FRCR
Consultant Radiologist
St Mary's Hospital
London, UK

Philip Gishen MB, BCh, DMRD, FRCR
Consultant Radiologist and Director of Imaging
Hammersmith Hospital
London, UK

Roger H. S. Gregson MSc, MB, FRCR, DMRD
Consultant Radiologist and Head of Training
University of Nottingham
Nottingham, UK

Ruth Green FRCR
Consultant Radiologist
Royal National Orthopaedic Hospital
Middlesex, UK

David Grier MBChB, MRCP, FRCR
Consultant Radiologist
Bristol Royal Hospital for Children
Bristol, UK

Leonie Gordon MD
Professor of Radiology and Nuclear Medicine
Medical University of South Carolina
Charleston,
South Carolina, USA

J. Ashley Guthrie BA, MRCP, FRCR
Consultant Radiologist
St James's University Hospital
Leeds, UK

Steve Halligan MBBS, MD, MRCP, FRCR
Consultant Radiologist
St Mark's Hospital
London, UK

Paul Hulse MRCP, FRCR
Consultant Radiologist
Christie Hospital
Manchester, UK

H. Rolf Jäger MD, FRCR
Consultant Radiologist
National Hospital for Neurology and Neurosurgery
London, UK

Jeremy P. R. Jenkins FRCP, DMRD, FRCR
Consultant Radiologist
Honorary Senior Clinical Lecturer
Manchester Royal Infirmary and University of Manchester
Manchester, UK

Andrew P. Jones MSc
Consultant Clinical Scientist
Head of MR Physics Group
Christie Hospital
Manchester, UK

Robert Jones BmedSci, BMBS, FRCS(Ed)
Urology Research Fellow
Bristol Royal Infirmary
Bristol, UK

John Karani MSc, MBBS, FRCR
Consultant Radiologist
King's College Hospital
London, UK

Julian Kabala MRCP, FRCR
Consultant Radiologist
Bristol Royal Infirmary
Bristol, UK

Brian E. Kendall FRCR, FRCP, FRCS
Consulting Radiologist
The National Hospital for Neurology and Neurosurgery
  and the Middlesex Hospital
London, UK

Chris Lawinksi BSc, MSc, MPhil
Consultant Physicist
King's College Hospital
London, UK

Richard Mason FRCS, MRCP, FRCR
Consulting Radiologist
Middlesex Hospital
University College of London Hospitals
London, UK

Michael J. Michell FRCR
Consultant Radiologist
King's College Hospital
London, UK

Katherine Mizkiel BM(Hons), MRCP, FRCR
Consultant Neuroradiologist
National Hospital for Neurology and Neurosurgery
London, UK

Bruno Morgan MA, MRCP, FRCR
Senior Lecturer and Honorary Consultant Radiologist
University Hospitals Leicester
Leicester, UK

Iain Morrison MB BS, MRCP, FRCR
Consultant Radiologist
Kent and Canterbury Hospital
Canterbury, UK

Janet Murfitt MB BS, MRCP, FRCR
Consultant Radiologist and Director of Diagnostic Imaging
St Bart's and The London NHS Trust
London, UK

Julie F.C. Olliff B Med Sci, BM BS, MRCP, FRCR
Consultant Radiologist
Honorary Senior Clinical Lecturer
University of Birmingham
Birmingham, UK

Catherine M. Owens BSc, MRCP, PFCR
Clinical Director Consultant Paediatric Radiologist
Department of Radiology
Great Ormond Street Hospital for Children
London, UK

Simon P.G. Padley MRCP, FRCR
Consultant Radiologist
Chelsea and Westminster Hospital
London, UK

Raj Persad ChM, FRCS, FRCS(Urol), FEBU
Consultant Urologist
Bristol Royal Infirmary
Bristol, UK

Peter D. Phelps MD, FRCS, FRCR
Former Consultant Radiologist
Royal National Orthopaedic Hospital and University
  College Hospital
Honorary Senior Lecturer
Institute of Orthopaedics
London, UK

Peter Renton FRCR, DMRD
Consultant Radiologist
Honorary Senior Lecturer
Royal National Orthopaedic Hospital
  and University College London Hospitals
London, UK

Philip J.A. Robinson FRCP, FRCR
Professor of Clinical Radiology
University of Leeds
Consultant Radiologist
Leeds Teaching Hospitals
Leeds, UK

M. I. Rothman MD
Assistant Professor of Radiology, Neurosurgery and
 Otolaryngology /Head and Neck Surgery,
Medical Director, Anna Gudelsky Magnetic Resonance Center
Baltimore,
Maryland, USA

Carl Roobottom MSc, MBChB(Hon), MRCP, FRCR
Consultant Radiologist
Derriford Hospital
Plymouth, UK

Michael B. Rubens MB, DMRD, FRCR
Consultant Radiologist and Director of Imaging
Royal Brompton Hospital
London, UK

Gary N. Sibley FRCS
Consultant Urologist
Department of Urology
Bristol Royal Infirmary
Bristol, UK

John A. Spencer MA, MD, MRCP, FRCR
Consultant Radiologist
St James's University Hospital
Leeds, UK

John M. Stevens MBBS, DRACR, FRCR
Consultant Radiologist
Department of Radiology
National Hospital for Neurology and Neurosurgery
London, UK

Nicola H. Strickland BM, BCh, MA(Hons)(Oxon), FRCP, FRCR
Consultant Radiologist
Hammersmith Hospital NHS Trust
London, UK

David Sutton MD, FRCP, FRCR, DMRD, FCan.AR (Hon)
Consulting Radiologist
St Mary's Hospital and Medical School, London
Director, Radiological Department (1963-1984)
Consulting Radiologist, The National Hospital for Neurology
 and Neurosurgery
London, UK

Will Teh MBChB, MRCP, FRCR
Consultant Radiologist
Northwick Park Hospital
Middlesex, UK

Karen E. Thomas MA, BM BCh, MRCP, FRCR
Consultant Paediatric Radiologist
Hospital for Sick Children
Toronto
Ontario, Canada

Sarah Vinnicombe BSc, MRCP, FRCR
Consultant Radiologist
Department of Diagnostic Imaging
St Bartholomew's Hospital
London, UK

Ioannis Vlahos MSc, MBBS, MRCP, FRCR
Research Fellow
Department of Diagnostic Imaging
St Bartholomew's Hospital
London, UK

Iain Watt FRCP, FRCR
Consultant Clinical Radiologist
Bristol Royal Infirmary
Bristol, UK

Anthony Watkinson Bmet, MSc, MBBS, FRCS, FRCR
Consultant and Senior Lecturer in Radiology
Royal Free Hospital
London, UK

Peter Wilde BSc, MRCP, FRCR
Consultant Cardiac Radiologist
Directorate of Clinical Radiology
Bristol Royal Infirmary
Bristol, UK

Richard W. Whitehouse BSc, MB ChB, MD, FRCR
Consultant Radiologist
Manchester Royal Infirmary
Manchester, UK

Tim Whittlestone MA, FRCS (Ebg), MD, FRCS(Urol)
Hunterian Professor of Surgery
Specialist Registrar in Urology
Bristol Royal Infirmary
Bristol, UK

Andrew R. Wright MA, MBBS, MRCP, FRCR
Consultant Radiologist
Honorary Senior Lecturer
St Mary's Hospital
Imperial College
London, UK

Jeremy W. R. Young MA, BM, BCh, FRCR
Professor and Chairman of Radiology, Medical University
 of South Carolina
Charleston
South Carolina, USA

Gregg Zoarski MD
Department of Diagnostic Radiology
University of Maryland Medical Center
Baltimore
Maryland, USA

PREFACE

The First Edition of this Textbook was conceived in the 1960s and published in 1969. I, like many of my contemporaries began my studies in Radiology at the end of the Second World War. My first post as an ex military service registrar was in the Radiology Department of the National Hospitals for Nervous Disease at Queen Square. It was pure serendipity that I should thus become associated with James Bull, the only British radiologist trained in Scandinavian neuroradiological techniques, including percutaneous angiography, and at that time representing the most advanced aspects of radiology.

My training in percutaneous cerebral angiography laid the foundation for other percutaneous techniques which I was able to apply when appointed to St. Mary's hospital in 1952. Here again pioneer work had already begun exploiting the potential for new methods in vascular surgery.

As a result of this background we were able to publish in 1962 the first personal monograph based on an experience of more than ten thousand cases. (See Ch. 15).

X-Rays were discovered by Roentgen in 1895, and though the importance of the discovery was immediately realised and widely discussed the impact on medical practice was surprisingly slow. The diagnosis and treatment of fractures and lesions of bones and joints was the first area to be thoroughly studied and surveyed. At the same time, the dangers and potential hazards of the new rays were becoming apparent for the first time, as was the therapeutic use of X-Rays.

In the Post war period, training and experience of a specialist radiologist was still a matter of considerable debate and concern. Broadly speaking, there were those who favoured a technical approach and training, usually pure scientists or physicists, and others who preferred a largely clinical approach with a minimum of technical training. Thus advanced training in medicine or surgery was regarded by many as essential for high quality radiology. The British Faculty of Radiologists was expanding rapidly and soon became the Royal College of Radiologists. The FRCR thus became the essential higher radiological qualification on a par with the MRCP or FRCS, and the DMRD was downgraded to a qualifying diploma.

At the time of this controversy, I took the opportunity to broaden my experience and expertise with the MD thesis, Membership of the Royal College of Physicians, London and Fellowship of the Faculty of Radiologists. This was undoubtedly the clinical, rather than technical approach to radiological expertise.

In 1955 I was appointed Editor to the Faculty Journal, and took the opportunity to persuade the Editorial Board to change its name to Clinical Radiology. Apart from showing where my own interest lay in the continual medico-political controversy between pure scientists (mainly physicists) and clinicians which many felt could adversely affect the future training and examination

syllabus for Specialist Radiologists, the change was highly successful from a purely practical point of view. Sales rose by 300% (from 1000 to 4000 copies per annum).

The first edition of this popular text-book was published in 1969 and this seventh edition in still growing strongly at the mature age of thirty three years. Review of the last five editions cover a period of exponential growth in radiological facilities and imaging. New fields were just beginning to open at the time of the first edition and these included ultrasound and nuclear medicine. Computer tomography began in the 1970s to be overtaken in the 1980s by magnetic resonance. It was generally felt that CT would soon be out-moded, but the last few years have seen a remarkable comeback from CT in the form of multi-slice spiral CT. As a result the versatility, speed and scope of CT examinations has been transformed.

In general, we hope this book reflects British Teaching Hospital Practice in the field of Imaging. The ISE edition remains very popular with non British readers and the 6th Edition has also been translated into two further languages, Greek and Portuguese. We believe that much of its success is due to the decision to concentrate on Clinical rather than Technical aspects of our rapidly expanding and evolving specialty.

Whilst each new edition has emphasised clinical rather then technical progress, the student must also be aware of, and absorb, the technical advances. The new edition therefore includes a chapter devoted to explaining this area. Other features of this new edition are the complete rewriting by mainly new authors of major sections of the text. These include the Cardiac, GU, Paediatric, Small and Large bowel, Major Abdominal Trauma and Interventional Neuroradiology chapters. Other chapters have been revised by deleting obsolete material or including new material. Recent clinical trends are also reflected in the revision. Thus imaging and staging of malignant tumours has been revised and updated in many areas, and the opportunity has been taken to integrate the latest version of the World Health Organisation (WHO) reclassification on a histopathological basis of primary cerebral tumours. The expansion of non invasive and minimally invasive angiography is monitored, and discussed. However, this is to some extent balanced by the increasing use of interventional techniques.

Radiology is a graphic subject, and images and illustrations are its vital tool. This edition contains no less then 5600 illustrations, some 2000 of which are new.

As in previous editions, we would remind the student that large textbooks, like large animals, have a longer period of gestation. It is therefore important to keep up with the current literature and attend up to date seminars.

David Sutton
2002

1

THE NORMAL CHEST: METHODS OF INVESTIGATION AND DIFFERENTIAL DIAGNOSIS

Janet Murfitt

with contributions from Philip J. A. Robinson, Richard W. Whitehouse, Andrew R. Wright and Jeremy P. R. Jenkins

METHODS OF INVESTIGATION

- Plain films:
  a PA, lateral
  b AP, decubitus, supine, oblique
  c Inspiratory–expiratory
  d Lordotic, apical, penetrated
  e Portable/mobile radiographs
- Tomography
- CT scanning
- Radionuclide studies
- Needle biopsy
- Ultrasound
- Fluoroscopy
- Bronchography
- Pulmonary angiography
- Bronchial arteriography
- MRI
- Digital radiography
- Lymphangiography.

The *plain postero-anterior (PA) chest film* is the most frequently requested radiological examination. Visualisation of the lungs is excellent because of the inherent contrast of the tissues of the thorax. Lateral films should not be undertaken routinely. Comparison of the current film with old films is valuable and should always be undertaken if the old films are available. A current film is mandatory before proceeding to more complex investigations.

Simple linear tomography remains a useful investigation when CT is unavailable. It is helpful for confirming that an abnormality suspected on a plain film is genuine and that it is intrapulmonary, although the high kilovoltage film has reduced the need for tomo-

graphy in these circumstances. In addition it is still used in some centres to assess a peripheral lung mass, the lung apices and the abnormal hilum.

However, *conventional CT scanning* is far superior for staging malignancy, detecting pulmonary metastases, and assessing chest wall and pleural lesions, the lung mass, the hilum and mediastinum. High-resolution CT scanning is of proven value in the diagnosis of diffuse lung disease, particularly in the early stages when the chest radiograph is normal, and for follow-up. In most centres high-resolution scanning is used for the detection of bronchiectasis, and surgery is undertaken without preoperative bronchography.

Radionuclide scanning is used as the first-line investigation of suspected pulmonary embolus in the majority of cases, with a normal scan excluding the presence of an embolus.

Pulmonary angiography remains the gold standard for the diagnosis of pulmonary embolism. It is usually undertaken in those patients with massive embolism when embolectomy or thrombolysis is contemplated. However, spiral CT angiography is showing sensitivity and specificity rates approaching those of conventional angiography in the diagnosis of pulmonary embolism, and can reliably demonstrate vessels down to the subsegmental level.

Ultrasound is of use for investigating chest wall and pleural lesions and lung lesions adjacent to the chest wall. It should be used for the localization of pleural fluid prior to a diagnostic tap or drainage to reduce the risk of a malpositioned catheter and pneumothorax. However, the acoustic mismatch between the chest wall and air-containing lung results in reflection of the ultrasound beam at the lung–pleura interface, so that normal lung cannot be demonstrated.

Biopsy of pulmonary lesions using a fine needle for aspiration has a high diagnostic yield for malignancy, excluding lymphoma, with a low incidence of complications. A cutting needle is associated with a higher complication rate but is more helpful in the diagnosis of lymphoma and benign lung conditions.

The value of *MRI* for diagnosing pulmonary disease is still in the assessment stage. No distinct advantage over high-resolution CT in the diagnosis of parenchymal disease has yet been shown but it is proven to be helpful in the diagnosis of hilar masses, lymphadenopathy and mediastinal lesions.

Diagnostic pneumothorax is an obsolete procedure which was once used to differentiate a pleural-based from a pulmonary lesion. The *barium/contrast swallow* has been supplanted by CT for assessing the non-oesophageal mediastinal mass but may be indicated in the investigation of conditions associated with pulmonary changes such as scleroderma, hiatus hernia and achalasia. It is used for demonstrating broncho-oesophageal fistulas, tracheal aspiration and vascular rings.

Chylous reflux with the formation of a chylothorax may be demonstrated by conventional *lymphangiography*.

THE PLAIN FILM

The PA view

By definition the patient faces the film chin up with the shoulders rotated forward to displace the scapulae from the lungs. Exposure is made on full inspiration for optimal visualisation of the lung bases, centring at T5. The breasts should be compressed against the film to prevent them obscuring the lung bases.

There is no general consensus regarding the kV used for chest radiography although the high kVp technique is widely used as a standard departmental film. High kVp, low kVp or intermediate kVp techniques are used with various film–screen combinations, grids or air-gap techniques.

Using a low kVp (60–80 kV) produces a high-contrast film (Fig. 1.1) with miliary shadowing and calcification being more clearly seen than on a high kV film. For large patients a grid reduces scatter. A FFD of 1.85 m (6 feet) reduces magnification and produces a sharper image. With high kilovoltages of 120–170 kVp the films are of lower contrast (Fig. 1.2A,B) with increased visualisation of the hidden areas of the lung due to better penetration of overlying structures. The bones and pulmonary calcification are less well seen. The exposure time is shorter so that movement blur due to cardiac pulsation is minimised. A grid or air gap is necessary to reduce scatter and improve contrast. An air gap of 15–25 cm between patient and film necessitates an increased FFD of 2.44 m (8 feet) to reduce magnification.

An automatic exposure system and dedicated automatic chest unit are desirable in a busy department.

The lateral view

A high kVp or normal kVp technique may be used with or without a grid. For sharpness the side of interest is nearest the film. With shoulders parallel to the film the arms are elevated, or displaced back if the anterior mediastinum is of interest.

Lesions obscured on the PA view are often clearly demonstrated on the lateral view. Examples of this are anterior mediastinal masses, encysted pleural fluid (Fig. 1.3) and posterior basal consolidation. By contrast, clear-cut abnormalities seen on the PA view may be difficult to identify on the lateral film because the two lungs are superimposed. An example of this is a left lung collapse (Fig. 1.4). This is particularly so with a large pleural effusion.

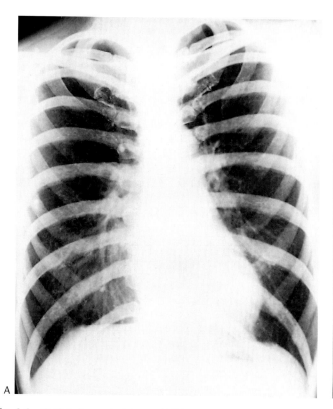
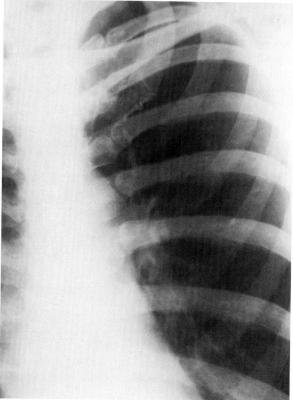

A

B

Fig. 1.1   (A,B) Radiographs taken at 60 kVp.

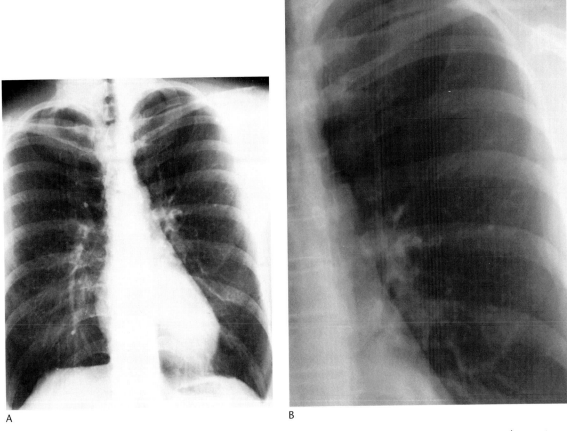

Fig. 1.2 (A,B) Radiographs of patient in Fig. 1.1 taken at 170 kVp. Note the improved visualisation of the main airways, vascular structures and the area behind the heart including the spine.

Other views

Although not frequently requested, additional plain films may assist with certain diagnostic problems before proceeding to the more complex and expensive techniques. *Oblique views* demonstrate the retrocardiac area, the posterior costophrenic angles and the chest wall, with pleural plaques being clearly demonstrated. In the AP position (as for patients unable to stand or portable radiographs) the ribs are projected over different areas of the lung from the PA view

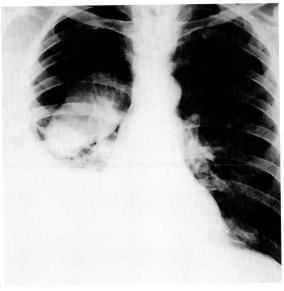

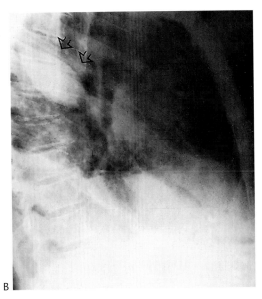

Fig. 1.3 Encysted pleural fluid. (A) PA film. A right pleural effusion with a large well-defined midzone mass. (B) Lateral film. Loculated fluid is demonstrated high in the oblique fissure.

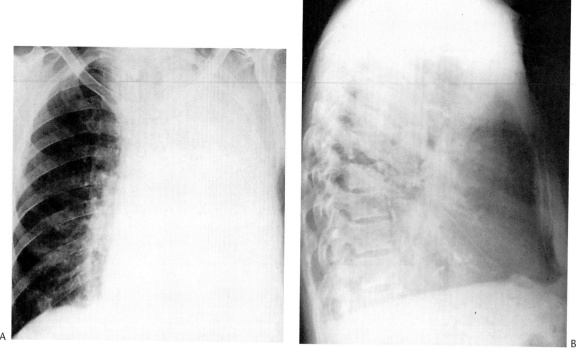

Fig. 1.4 Collapse of the left lung. (A) PA film. (B) Lateral film. Only the right hemidiaphragm is visible. The radiolucency of the lower vertebrae is decreased.

and the posterior chest is well shown. In contrast to the PA film the scapulae overlie the upper lungs and the clavicles are projected more cranially over the apices. The disc spaces of the lower cervical spine are more clearly seen, whereas in the PA film the neural arches are visualised. When a portable radiograph is undertaken, the shorter FFD results in magnification of the heart and the longer exposure time in increased movement blur.

Good visualisation of the apices requires projection of the clavicles upward, as in the *apical view* with the tube angled up 50–60°, or downward, as in the *lordotic view* with the patient in a lordotic PA position. In this view a middle lobe collapse shows clearly as a well-defined triangular shadow.

A subpulmonary effusion is frequently difficult to distinguish from an elevated diaphragm or consolidation. On the PA view the apex of the effusion has a more lateral position than that of a normal diaphragm. In the *supine* and *decubitus* positions (Fig. 1.5) free fluid becomes displaced. On the supine projection this results in the hemithorax becoming opaque with loss of the diaphragm

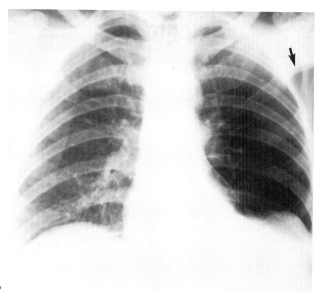
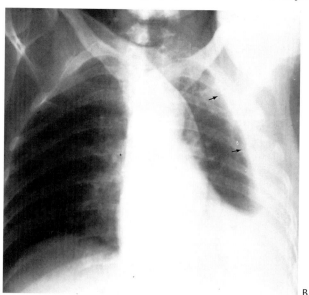

Fig. 1.5 Subpulmonary pleural fluid. (A) Erect PA radiograph. There is apparent elevation of the left hemidiaphragm. Increased translucency of the left lung is due to a left mastectomy. Note the abnormal axillary fold (arrow). (B) Left lateral decubitus film (with horizontal beam). Pleural fluid has moved to the most dependent part of the left hemithorax (arrows).

outline, an apical cap, blunting of the costophrenic angle and decreased visibility of the pulmonary markings.

The decubitus films shows fluid levels particularly well. Small amounts of pleural fluid may be shown with the affected side dependent.

Paired *inspiratory* and *expiratory* films demonstrate air trapping and diaphragm movement. Traditonally it has been taught that small pneumothoraces and interstitial shadowing may be more apparent on the expiratory film. However the inspiratory view is now considered to be as accurate as the expiratory view for diagnosing a pneumothorax. Paired views are very important in children with a possible diagnosis of an inhaled foreign body.

Viewing the PA film

Before a diagnosis can be made an abnormality, if present, must be identified. Knowledge of the normal appearance of a chest radiograph is essential. In addition the radiologist must develop a routine which ensures that all areas of the radiograph are scrutinised. Some prefer initially to view the film without studying the clinical information. Comparison of the current film with old films is important and often extremely helpful. A suggested scheme that examines each point in turn is shown in Box 1.1.

Technical aspects

Centring If the film is well centred the medial ends of the clavicles are equidistant from the vertebral spinous processes at the T4/5 level. Small degrees of rotation distort the mediastinal borders, and the lung nearest the film appears less translucent. Thoracic deformities, especially a scoliosis, negate the value of conventional centring. The orientation of the aortic arch, gastric bubble and heart should be determined to confirm normal situs and that the side markers are correct.

Box 1.1	Suggested scheme for viewing the PA film	
1.	Request form	Name, age, date, sex Clinical information
2.	Technical	Adequate inspiration Centring, patient position/rotation Side markers Exposure/adequate penetration Collimation
3.	Trachea	Position, outline
4.	Heart and mediastinum	Size, shape, displacement
5.	Diaphragms	Outline, shape Relative position
6.	Pleural spaces	Position of horizontal fissure Costophrenic, cardiophrenic angles
7.	Lungs	Local, generalised abnormality Comparison of the translucency and vascular markings of the lungs
8.	Hidden areas	Apices, posterior sulcus Mediastinum, hila, bones
9.	Hila	Density, position, shape
10.	Below diaphragms	Gas shadows, calcification
11.	Soft tissues	Mastectomy, gas, densities, etc.
12.	Bones	Destructive lesions, etc.

Penetration With a low kV film the vertebral bodies and disc spaces should be just visible down to the T8/9 level through the cardiac shadow. Underpenetration increases the likelihood of missing an abnormality overlain by another structure. Overpenetration results in loss of visibility of low-density lesions such as early consolidation, although a bright light may reveal the abnormality.

Degree of inspiration On full inspiration the anterior ends of the sixth ribs or posterior ends of the tenth are above the right hemidiaphragm although the degree of inspiration achieved varies with patient build. On expiration the heart shadow is larger and there is basal opacity due to crowding of the normal vascular markings. Pulmonary diseases such as fibrosing alveolitis are associated with reduced pulmonary compliance, which may result in reduced inflation with elevation of the diaphragms.

The trachea

The trachea should be examined for narrowing, displacement and intraluminal lesions. It is midline in its upper part, then deviates slightly to the right around the aortic knuckle. On expiration deviation to the right becomes more marked. In addition there is shortening on expiration so that an endotracheal tube situated just above the carina on inspiration may occlude the main bronchus on expiration.

Its calibre should be even, with translucency of the tracheal air column decreasing caudally. Normal maximum coronal diameter is 25 mm for males and 21 mm for females. The right tracheal margin, where the trachea is in contact with the lung, can be traced from the clavicles down to the right main bronchus. This border is the *right paratracheal stripe* and is seen in 60% of patients, normally measuring less than 5 mm. Widening of the stripe occurs most commonly with mediastinal lymphadenopathy but also with tracheal malignancy, mediastinal tumours, mediastinitis and pleural effusions. A left paratracheal line is not visualised because the left border of the trachea lies adjacent to the great vessels and not the lung.

The *azygos vein* lies in the angle between the right main bronchus and trachea. On the erect film it should be less than 10 mm in diameter. Its size decreases with the Valsalva manoeuvre and on inspiration. Enlargement occurs in the supine position but also with enlarged subcarinal nodes, pregnancy, portal hypertension, IVC and SVC obstruction, right heart failure and constrictive pericarditis.

Widening of the carina occurs on inspiration. The normal angle is 60–75°. Pathological causes of widening include an enlarged left atrium (Fig. 1.6) and enlarged carinal nodes.

The mediastinum and heart

The central dense shadow seen on the PA chest film comprises the mediastinum, heart, spine and sternum. With good centring two-thirds of the cardiac shadow lies to the left of midline and one-third to the right, although this is quite variable in normal subjects. The *transverse cardiac diameter* (normal for females less than 14.5 cm and for males less than 15.5 cm) and the *cardiothoracic ratio* are assessed. The normal cardiothoracic ratio is less than 50% on a PA film. Measurement in isolation is of less value than when previous figures are available. An increase in excess of 1.5 cm in the transverse diameter on comparable serial films is significant. However

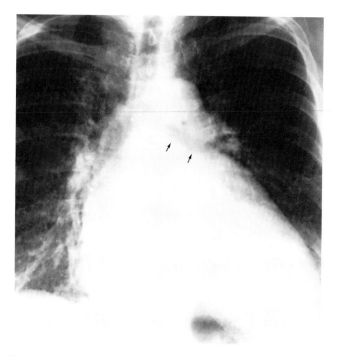

Fig. 1.6 Elevated left main bronchus (arrows) and widened carina. Patient with mitral valve disease and an enlarged left atrium.

the heart shadow is enlarged with a short FFD, on expiration, in the supine and AP projections and when the diaphragms are elevated. The normal AP value is less than 60%.

All borders of the heart and mediastinum are clearly defined except where the heart sits on the left hemidiaphragm. The right superior mediastinal shadow is formed by the SVC and innominate vessels; a dilated aorta may contribute to this border. On the left side the superior mediastinal border is less sharp. It is formed by the subclavian artery above the aortic knuckle.

Various junction lines may be visualised. These are formed by the pleura being outlined by the adjacent air-filled lung. The anterior junction line is formed by the lungs meeting anterior to the ascending aorta. It is only 1 mm thick and, overlying the tracheal translucency, runs downward from below the suprasternal notch, slightly curving from right to left. The posterior junction line, where the lungs meet posteriorly behind the oesophagus, is a straight or curved line convex to the left some 2 mm wide and extending from the lung apices to the aortic knuckle or below. The azygo-oesophageal interface is the shape of an inverted hockey stick and runs from the diaphragm on the left of midline up and to the right extending to the tracheobronchial angle where the azygos vein drains into the IVC. The curved pleuro-oesophageal stripe, formed by the lung and right wall of the oesophagus, extends from the lung apex to the azygos but is only visualised if the oesophagus contains air. The left wall of the oesophagus is not normally seen.

In young women the pulmonary trunk is frequently very prominent.

In babies and young children the normal *thymus* is a triangular sail-shaped structure with well-defined borders projecting from one or both sides of the mediastinum (Fig. 1.7). Both borders may be wavy in outline, the 'wave sign of Mulvey', as a consequence of indentation by the costal cartilages. The right border is straighter than

the left, which may be rounded. Thymic size decreases on inspiration and in response to stress and illness. The thymus is absent in DiGeorge's syndrome. Enlargement may occur following recovery from an illness. A large thymus is more commonly seen in boys.

Adjacent to the vertebral bodies run the *paraspinal lines*. On the left this is normally less than 10 mm wide; on the right less than 3 mm. The left paraspinal line is wider due to the descending thoracic aorta. Enlargement occurs with osteophytes, a tortuous aorta, vertebral and adjacent soft-tissue masses, a paravertebral haematoma and a dilated azygos system.

A search should be made for abnormal densities, fluid levels, mediastinal emphysema and calcification. Spinal abnormalities may accompany mediastinal masses; for example, hemivertebrae are associated with neuroenteric cysts.

The diaphragm

In most patients the right hemidiaphragm is higher than the left. This is due to the heart depressing the left side and not to the liver pushing up the right hemidiaphragm; in dextrocardia with normal abdominal situs the right hemidiaphragm is the lowest. The hemidiaphragms may lie at the same level, and in a small percentage of the population the left side is the higher; Felson (1973) reports an incidence of 3%. This is more likely to occur if the stomach or splenic flexure is distended with gas. A difference greater than 3 cm in height is considered significant.

On inspiration the domes of the diaphragms are at the level of the sixth rib anteriorly and at or below the tenth rib posteriorly. In the supine position the diaphragm is higher. Both domes have gentle curves which steepen toward the posterior angles. The upper borders are clearly seen except on the left side where the heart is in contact with the diaphragm, and in the cardiophrenic angles when there are prominent fat pads. Otherwise loss of outline indicates that the adjacent tissue does not contain air, for example in consolidation or pleural disease.

Free intraperitoneal gas outlines the undersurface of the diaphragm and shows it to be normally 2–3 mm thick (Fig. 1.8).

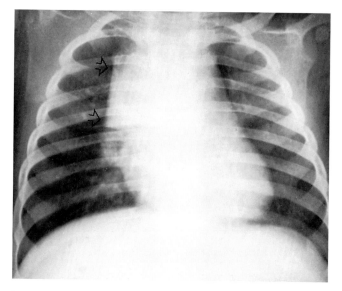

Fig. 1.7 Normal thymus in a child, projecting to the right of the mediastinum (arrows).

Congenital variations and other lesions of the diaphragm will be considered later.

The fissures

The main fissures

These fissures separate the lobes of the lung but are usually incomplete allowing collateral air drift to occur between adjacent lobes. They are visualised when the X-ray beam is tangential. The horizontal fissure is seen, often incompletely, on the PA film running from the hilum to the region of the sixth rib in the axillary line, and may be straight or have a slight downward curve. Occasionally it has a double appearance.

All fissures are clearly seen on the lateral film. The horizontal fissure runs anteriorly and often slightly downward. Both oblique fissures commence posteriorly at the level of T4 or T5, passing through the hilum. The left is steeper and finishes 5 cm behind the anterior costophrenic angle, whereas the right ends just behind the angle.

Accessory fissures

The *azygos* fissure is comma shaped with a triangular base peripherally and is nearly always right-sided (Fig. 1.9). It forms in the apex of the lung and consists of paired folds of parietal and visceral pleura plus the azygos vein which has failed to migrate normally. Enlargement occurs in the supine position. At postmortem the incidence is 1% but radiologically it is 0.4%. When left-sided, the fissure contains an accessory hemiazygos vein.

The *superior accessory fissure* separates the apical from the basal segments of the lower lobes. It is commoner on the right side and has an incidence of 5% at postmortem. On the PA film it resembles the horizontal fissure but on the lateral film it can be differentiated as it runs posteriorly from the hilum.

The *inferior accessory fissure* (Fig. 1.10) appears as an oblique line running cranially from the cardiophrenic angle toward the hilum and separating the medial basal from the other basal segments. It is commoner on the right side and has an incidence of 5–8% on the chest film.

The *left-sided horizontal fissure* (Fig. 1.11) separates the lingula from the other upper lobe segments. This is rare but in one study was found in 8% of postmortem specimens.

The costophrenic angles

The normal costophrenic angles are acute and well defined but become obliterated when the diaphragms are flat. Frequently the cardiophrenic angles contain low-density ill-defined opacity caused by fat pads.

The lungs

By comparing the lungs, areas of abnormal translucency or uneven distribution of lung markings are more easily detected. The size of the upper and lower zone vessels is assessed.

An abnormal opacity should be closely studied to ensure that it is not a composite opacity formed by superimposed normal structures such as vessels, bones or costal cartilage. The extent and location of the opacity is determined and specific features such as calcification or cavitation noted. A general survey is made to look for further lesions and displacement of the normal landmarks.

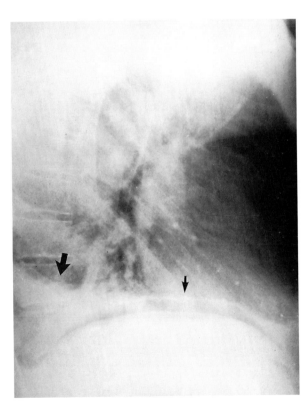

Fig. 1.8 Pneumoperitoneum after laparotomy. The thin right cupola (small arrow) is outlined by the adjacent aerated lung and the free abdominal gas. Posterior consolidation (large arrow) obscures the outline of the diaphragm posteriorly.

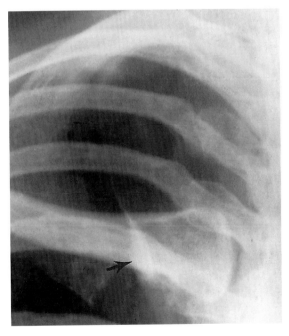

Fig. 1.9 Azygos fissure. The azygos vein is seen to lie at the lower end of the fissure (arrow).

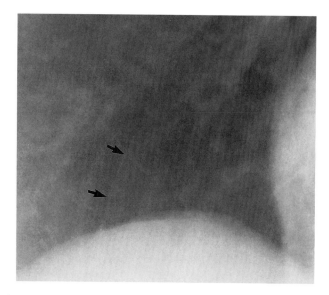

Fig. 1.10 Right inferior accessory fissure.

The hidden areas

The apices On the PA film the apices are partially obscured by ribs, costal cartilage, clavicles and soft tissues. Visualisation is very limited on the lateral view.

Mediastinum and hila Central lesions may be obscured by these structures or appear as a superimposed density. The abnormality is usually detectable on the lateral film.

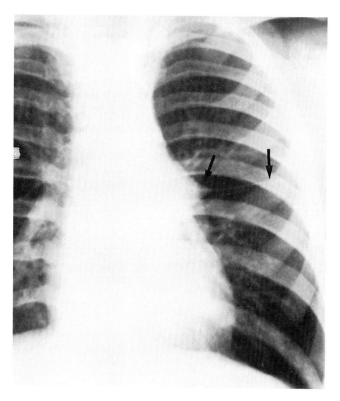

Fig. 1.11 Left-sided horizontal fissure.

Diaphragms The posterior and lateral basal segments of the lower lobes and the posterior sulcus are partially obscured by the downward curve of the posterior diaphragm. Visualisation is further diminished if the film is not taken on full inspiration.

Bones Costal cartilage or bone may obscure a lung lesion. In addition, determining whether a density is pulmonary or bony when overlying a rib may be difficult; AP, expiratory and oblique films may be helpful and preclude the need to proceed to CT.

The hila

In 97% of subjects the left hilum is higher than the right and in 3% they are at the same level. The hila should be of equal density and similar size with clearly defined concave lateral borders where the superior pulmonary vein meets the basal pulmonary artery. However there is a wide range of normal appearances. Any opacity which is not obviously vascular must be regarded with a high index of suspicion and investigated further. Old films for comparison are helpful in this situation.

Of all the structures in the hilum only the pulmonary arteries and upper lobe veins contribute significantly to the hilar shadows on the plain radiograph. Normal lymph nodes are not seen. Air can be identified within the proximal bronchi but normal bronchial walls are only seen end-on. The anterior segment bronchus of the upper lobe is seen as a ring adjacent to the upper hilum (Fig. 1.12), and is seen on the right side in 45% of cases and the left side in 50%. Normally there is less than 5 mm of soft tissue lateral to this bronchus. Thickening of the soft tissues suggests the presence of abnormal pathology such as malignancy.

The inferior pulmonary ligament

This is a double layer of pleura extending caudally from the lower margin of the inferior pulmonary vein in the hilum as a sheet which may or may not be attached to the diaphragm and which attaches the lower lobe to the mediastinum. It is rarely identified on a simple radiograph but is frequently seen at CT.

The pulmonary vessels

The left pulmonary artery lies above the left main bronchus before passing posteriorly, whereas on the right side the artery is anterior to the bronchus resulting in the right hilum being the lower. Hilar size is very variable. The maximum diameter of the descending branch of the pulmonary artery measured 1cm medial and 1cm lateral to the hilar point is 16 mm for males and 15 mm for females.

The upper lobe veins lie lateral to the arteries, which are separated from the mediastinum by approximately 1 cm of lung tissue. At the first intercostal space the normal vessels should not exceed 3 mm in diameter. The lower lobe vessels are larger than those of the upper lobes in the erect position, perfusion and aeration of the upper zones being reduced. In the supine position the vessels equalise. In the right paracardiac region the vessels are invariably prominent.

The peripheral lung markings are mainly vascular, veins and arteries having no distinguishing characteristics. There should be an even distribution throughout the lung fields.

Centrally the arteries and veins have different features. The arteries accompany the bronchi, lying posterosuperior, whereas veins do not follow the bronchi but drain via the interlobular septa eventually forming superior and basal veins which converge on the left atrium.

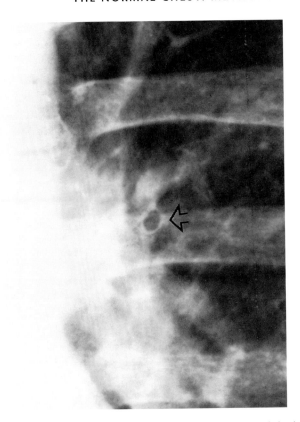

Fig. 1.12 Ring shadow of the anterior segment bronchus of the left upper lobe seen end-on.

This confluence of veins (Fig. 1.13) may be seen as a rounded structure to the right of midline superimposed on the heart, sometimes simulating an enlarged left atrium. It is visible in 5% of PA films according to Felson (1973). Pulmonary veins have fewer branches than arteries and are straighter, larger and less well defined.

The bronchial vessels

These are normally not visualised on the plain chest film. They arise from the ventral surface of the descending aorta at the T5/6 level. Their anatomy is variable. Usually there are two branches on the left and one on the right which often shares a common origin with an intercostal artery. On entering the hila the bronchial arteries accompany the bronchi. The veins drain into the pulmonary veins and to a lesser extent the azygos system.

Enlarged bronchial arteries appear as multiple small nodules around the hilum and as short lines in the proximal lung fields. Enlargement may occur with cyanotic heart disease, and focal enlargement with a local pulmonary lesion. Occasionally enlarged arteries indent the oesophagus.

Causes of enlarged bronchial arteries:
1. General—cyanotic congenital heart disease, e.g. pulmonary atresia, severe Fallot's tetralogy.
2. Local—bronchiectasis, bronchial carcinoma.

The pulmonary segments and bronchi

The pulmonary segments (Figs 1.14, 1.15) are served by segmental bronchi and arteries but unlike the lobes are not separated by pleura. Normal bronchi are not visualised in the peripheral lung fields.

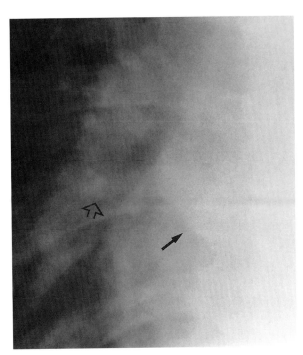

Fig. 1.13 Pulmonary vein (open arrow) draining into pulmonary confluence (closed arrow).

The right main bronchus is shorter, steeper and wider than the left, bifurcating earlier. The upper lobe bronchus arises 2.5 cm below the carina and is higher than the left upper lobe bronchus which arises after 5 cm. The bronchi divide between six and 20 times before becoming bronchioles with the terminal bronchioles measuring 0.2 mm in diameter. Each receives two or three respiratory bronchioles which connect with between two and 11 alveolar ducts. Each duct receives between two and six alveolar sacs which are connected to alveoli. The *acinus*, generally considered to be the functioning lung unit, is that portion of the lung arising from the terminal bronchiole (Fig. 1.16). When filled with fluid it is seen on a radiograph as a 5–6 mm shadow, and this comprises the basic unit seen in acinar (alveolar/air space) shadowing.

The primary lobule arises from the last respiratory bronchiole. The secondary lobule is between 1.0 and 2.5 cm in size and is the smallest discrete unit of lung tissue surrounded by connective tissue septa. When thickened these septa become Kerley B lines (Fig. 1.17).

Other connections exist between the air spaces allowing collateral air drift. These are the pores of Kohn, 3–13 μm in size, which connect the alveoli, and the canals of Lambert (30 μm) which exist between bronchioles and alveoli.

The lymphatic system

The lymphatics remove interstitial fluid and foreign particles. They run in the interlobular septa, connecting with subpleural lymphatics and draining via the deep lymphatics to the hilum, with valves controlling the direction of flow. Normal lymphatics are not seen but thickening of the lymphatics and surrounding connective tissue produces Kerley lines, which may be transient or persistent. Thickened connective tissues are the main contributors to the substance of these lines (Boxes 1.2, 1.3).

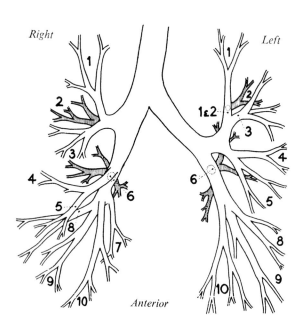

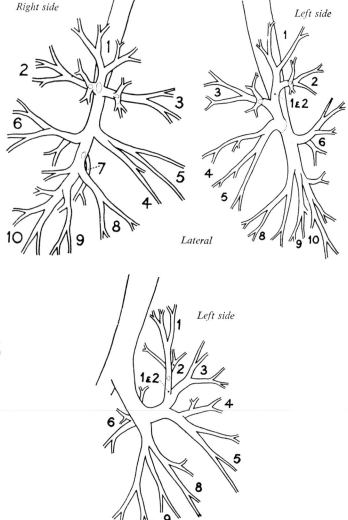

Fig. 1.14   The anatomy of the main bronchi and segmental divisions. Nomenclature approved by the Thoracic Society (reproduced by permission of the Editors of *Thorax*).

UPPER LOBE
1. Apical bronchus
2. Posterior bronchus
3. Anterior bronchus

Right

MIDDLE LOBE
4. Lateral bronchus
5. Medial bronchus

Left

LINGULA
4. Superior bronchus
5. Inferior bronchus

LOWER LOBE

6. Apical bronchus
7. Medial basal (cardiac)
8. Anterior basal bronchus
9. Lateral basal bronchus
10. Posterior basal bronchus

6. Apical bronchus
8. Anterior basal bronchus
9. Lateral basal bronchus
10. Posterior basal bronchus

The lymph nodes

The intrapulmonary lymphatics drain directly to the bronchopulmonary nodes and this group is the first to be involved by spread from a peripheral tumour. A small number of intrapulmonary nodes are present and can occasionally be seen at CT but never on the plain film. The node groups and their drainage are well described (Fig. 1.18). Extensive intercommunications exist between the groups but the pattern of nodal involvement can sometimes indicate the site of the primary tumour. Mediastinal nodes may be involved by tumours both above and below the diaphragm.

1. The *anterior mediastinal nodes* in the region of the aortic arch drain the thymus and right heart.
2. The *intrapulmonary nodes* lie along the main bronchi.
3. The *middle mediastinal nodes* drain the lungs, bronchi, left heart, the lower trachea and visceral pleura. There are four groups:
   a. Bronchopulmonary (hilar) nodes which drain into groups b and c. When enlarged they appear as lobulated hilar masses.

b. Carinal nodes.
c. Tracheobronchial nodes which lie adjacent to the azygos vein on the right side and near the recurrent laryngeal nerve on the left side.
d. Paratracheal nodes are more numerous on the right side. There is significant cross drainage from left to right.

4. The *posterior mediastinal nodes* drain the posterior diaphragm and lower oesophagus. They lie around the lower descending aorta and oesophagus.

5. The *parietal nodes* consist of anterior and posterior groups situated behind the sternum and posteriorly in the intercostal region, draining the soft tissues and parietal pleura.

Below the diaphragm

The lower lobes extend below the diaphragmatic outlines on the PA film. An erect chest film is preferred to an erect abdominal film for the diagnosis of a pneumoperitoneum. A search should be made for other abnormal gas shadows such as dilated bowel, abscesses, a displaced gastric bubble and intramural gas as well as calcified

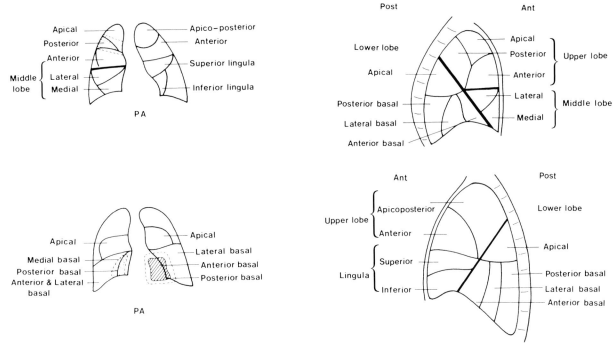

Fig. 1.15   The approximate positions of the pulmonary segments as they can be seen on the PA and lateral radiographs.

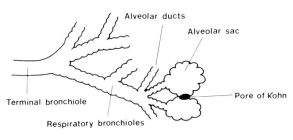

Fig. 1.16   Representation of the acinus.

lesions. Interposition of colon between liver and diaphragm, *Chilaiditi's syndrome* (Fig. 1.19), is a common and often transient finding particularly in the aged, the obvious haustral pattern distinguishing it from free gas. Subdiaphragmatic fat in the obese may be confused with free gas on a single film.

Soft tissues

A general survey of the soft tissues includes the chest wall, shoulders and lower neck.

It is important to confirm the presence or absence of breast shadows. The breasts may partially obscure the lung bases. Nipple shadows are variable in position, often asymmetrical, and frequently only one shadow is seen. Care is necessary to avoid misinterpretation as a neoplasm or vice versa. Nipple shadows are often well defined laterally and may have a lucent halo. Repeat films with nipple markers are necessary if there is any doubt.

Skin folds are often seen running vertically, particularly in the old and in babies. When overlying the lungs they can be confused with a pneumothorax. However, a skin fold if followed usually extends outside the lung field. The anterior axillary fold is a curvi-

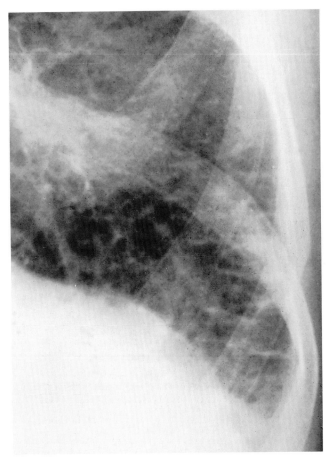

Fig. 1.17   Kerley B lines. Thickened interlobular septa in a patient with mitral valve disease.

Box 1.2   Kerley Lines

A lines
1–2 mm non-branching lines radiating from the hilum, 2–6 cm long
Thickened deep interlobular septa

B lines
Transverse non-branching 1–2 mm lines at the lung bases perpendicular to the pleura 1–3 cm long
Thickened interlobular septa

Box 1.3   Causes of Kerley lines

Pulmonary oedema	Pneumoconiosis
Infections (viral, mycoplasma)	Lymphangiectasia
Mitral valve disease	Lymphangitis carcinomatosis
Interstitial pulmonary fibrosis	Lymphatic obstruction
Congenital heart disease	Sarcoidosis
Alveolar cell carcinoma	Lymphangiomyomatosis
Pulmonary venous occlusive disease	Pulmonary haemorrhage
Lymphoma	Idiopathic (in the elderly)

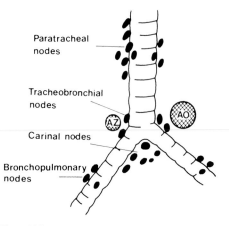

Fig. 1.18   The middle mediastinal nodes.

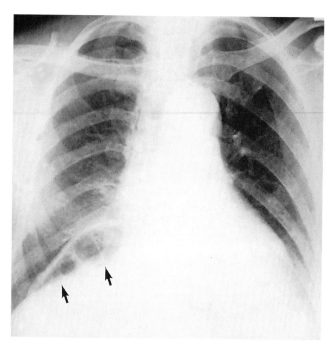

Fig. 1.19   Chilaiditi's syndrome. Interposition of colon between liver and diaphragm. Note the colonic haustral pattern.

linear shadow extending from the axilla onto the lung fields and frequently causing ill-defined shadowing which must be differentiated from consolidation.

At the apices the opacity of the sternocleidomastoid muscles curving down and slightly outward may simulate a cavity or bulla. The floor of the supraclavicular fossa often resembles a fluid level. A deep sternoclavicular fossa, commonly present in the elderly, appears as a translucency overlying the trachea and simulating a gas-filled diverticulum.

Subpleural thickening seen peripherally is often due to subpleural fat or prominent intercostal muscles rather than to pleural pathology.

Companion shadows are formed by the soft tissues adjacent to bony structures, are 2–3 mm thick, and are frequently seen running parallel to the upper borders of the clavicles and the inferior borders of the lower ribs.

Apical pleural thickening, 'the apical cap', has a reported incidence of 7% and occurs most commonly on the left side.

The bones

All the bones should be surveyed. On occasions identification of an abnormality in association with pulmonary pathology may help to narrow the differential diagnosis. Sometimes a normal bony structure appears to be a lung lesion and further films such as oblique, lateral, inspiratory and expiratory or CT may be necessary.

The sternum   The ossification centres are very variable in number, shape, position and growth rate. Usually there are single centres in the manubrium and xiphoid, with three or four centres in the body. Parasternal ossicles and, in infants, the ossification centres may be confused with lung masses.

The clavicles   The rhomboid fossa is an irregular notch at the site of attachment of the costoclavicular ligament. It lies up to 3 cm from the medial end of the clavicle inferiorly and has a well-corticated margin. It is unilateral in 6% of cases and should not be mistaken for a destructive lesion. Superior companion shadows are a usual finding. The medial epiphyses fuse at 25 years and on occasions may appear as lung nodules.

The scapulae   On the lateral film the inferior angle overlies the lungs and can simulate a lung mass. The spine of the scapula on the PA film casts a linear shadow which at first glance may seem to be pleural.

The ribs   Companion shadows are common on the upper ribs. Pathological rib notching, as seen with aortic coarctation, should not be confused with the normal notch on the inferior surface just lateral to the tubercle. The contours of the ribs are evaluated for destruction. However the inferior borders of the middle and lower ribs are usually indistinct.

The first costal cartilage calcifies early and is often very dense, partly obscuring the upper zone. Costal cartilage calcification is rare before the age of 20. Central homogeneous or spotty calcification occurs in females whereas there is curvilinear marginal calcification in males. On the lateral film the anterior end of the rib with its cartilage lying behind the sternum should not be confused with a mass.

The spine Routine evaluation is made for bone and disc destruction and spinal deformity. A scoliosis often results in apparent mediastinal widening, and oblique films may be necessary to fully visualise both lung fields. The ends of the transverse processes on the PA film may look like a lung nodule.

In the neonate the vertebral bodies have a sandwich appearance due to large venous sinuses. Residual grooves may persist in the adult.

Viewing the lateral film

Routinely the left side is adjacent to the film because more of the left lung than the right is obscured on the PA view, but if there is a specific lesion the side of interest is positioned adjacent to the film.

A routine similar to that used for the PA film should be employed. Important observations to make are described below (Fig. 1.20).

The clear spaces There are two clear spaces; these correspond to the sites where the lungs meet behind the sternum and the heart. Loss of translucency of these areas indicates local pathology. Obliteration of the retrosternal space occurs with anterior mediastinal masses such as a thymoma (Fig. 1.21), aneurysms of the ascending aorta and nodal masses. Normally this space is less than 3 cm deep maximum; widening occurs with emphysema.

Vertebral translucency The vertebral bodies become progressively more translucent caudally. Loss of this translucency may be the only sign of posterior basal consolidation.

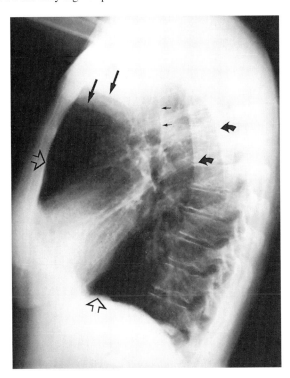

Fig. 1.20 Normal lateral film. Note the retrosternal and retrocardiac clear spaces (open arrows) and the increased translucency of the lower vertebrae. The axillary folds (straight black arrows) and scapulae (curved black arrows) overlie the lungs. The tracheal translucency is well seen (small black arrows)

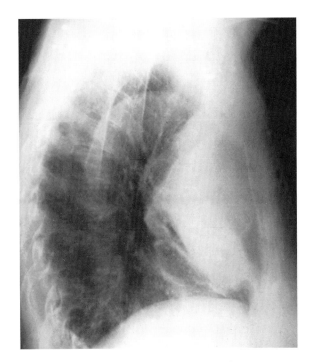

Fig. 1.21 Thymoma. Obliteration of the retrosternal space.

Diaphragm outline Both diaphragms are visible throughout their length, except the left anteriorly where it merges with the heart. A small segment of the right hemidiaphragm is effaced by the IVC. The posterior costophrenic angles are acute and small amounts of pleural fluid may be detected by blunting of these angles (Fig. 1.22).

The fissures The left greater fissure is steeper than the right and terminates 5 cm behind the anterior cardiophrenic angle. Loculated interlobar effusions are well shown and displacement or thickening of the fissures should be noted.

The trachea This passes down in a slightly posterior direction to the T6/7 level of the spine. It is partly overlapped by the scapulae and axillary folds. Anterior to the carina lies the right pulmonary artery. The left pulmonary artery is posterior and superior, and the veins are inferior. The venous confluence creates a bulge on the posterior cardiac border.

The normal posterior tracheal wall is invariably visible and measures less than 5 mm. This measurement includes both tracheal and oesophageal walls plus the pleura. Widening may occur with disease of all these structures. A branch of the aorta seen end-on may appear as a nodule overlying the trachea and above the aortic arch. The right upper lobe bronchus is seen end-on as a circular structure overlying the lower trachea. Lying inferiorly is the left upper lobe bronchus seen end-on with its artery superiorly and vein inferiorly.

Opacity seen in the region of the anterior cardiophrenic angle is thought to be due to *mediastinal fat* and the interface between the two lungs.

The sternum This should be studied carefully in known cases of malignancy or when there is a history of trauma.

INTERPRETATION OF THE ABNORMAL FILM

Helpful radiological signs

The silhouette sign

Described by Felson & Felson (1950), the 'silhouette sign' is the loss of an interface by adjacent disease and permits localisation of a lesion on a film by studying the diaphragm, cardiac and aortic outlines. These structures are normally seen because the adjacent lung is aerated and the difference in radiodensity is demonstrated. When air in the alveolar spaces is replaced by fluid or soft tissue, there is no longer a difference in radiodensity between that part of the lung and the adjacent structures. Therefore the silhoutte is lost and the 'silhoette sign' is present. Conversely if the border is retained and the abnormality is superimposed, the lesion must be lying either anterior or posterior. In 8–10% of people a short segment of the right heart border is obliterated by the fat pad or pulmonary vessels.

Obliteration of these borders may occur with pleural or mediastinal lesions as well as pulmonary pathology. The right middle lobe and lingula lie adjacent to the right and left cardiac borders, the apicoposterior segment of the left upper lobe lies adjacent to the aortic knuckle, the anterior segment of the right upper lobe and the middle lobe lie against the right aortic border, and the basal segments of the lower lobes lie adjacent to the hemidiaphragms. Pulmonary disease in these lobes and segments can obliterate the borders (Figs 1.23–1.25).

Using the same principle, a well-defined mass seen above the clavicles is always posterior whereas an anterior mass, being in contact with soft tissues rather than aerated lung, is ill defined. This is the *cervicothoracic sign*.

The *hilum overlay sign* helps distinguish a large heart from a mediastinal mass. With the latter the hilum is seen through the mass whereas with the former the hilum is displaced so that only its lateral border is visible.

The air bronchogram

Originally described by Fleischner (1941), and named by Felson (1973), the air bronchogram is an important sign showing that an opacity is intrapulmonary. The bronchus, if air filled but not fluid filled, becomes visible when air is displaced from the surrounding parenchyma. Frequently the air bronchogram is seen as scattered linear translucencies rather than continuous branching structures. It is most commonly seen within pneumonic consolidation and pulmonary oedema. An air bronchogram is not seen within pleural

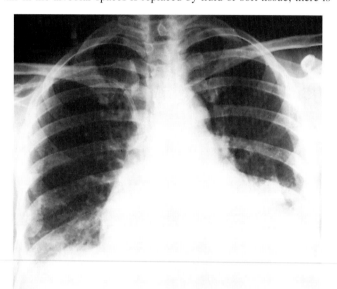

A

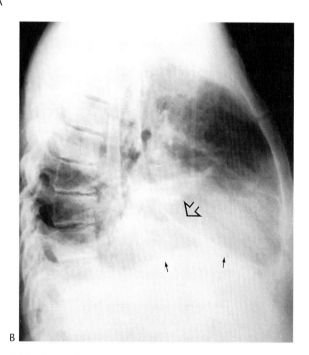

B

Fig. 1.22 (A) PA film. A moderate sized left pleural effusion and a small right effusion. (B) Lateral film. There is loss of translucency of the lower vertebrae, thickening of the oblique fissure (open arrow) and absence of the left hemidiaphragm, with loss of the right hemidiaphragm posteriorly (small arrows).

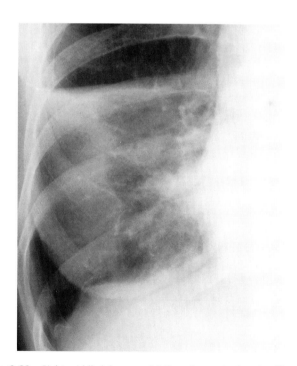

Fig. 1.23 Right middle lobe consolidation, demonstrating the silhouette sign with loss of outline of the right heart border.

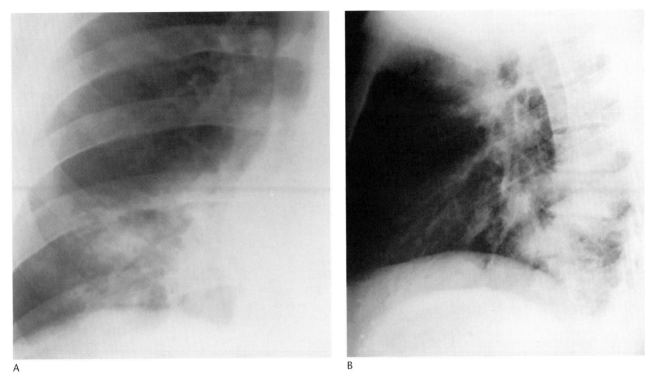

A   B

Fig. 1.24 Right lower lobe consolidation. (A) Shadowing at the right base but the cardiac border remains visible. (B) Lateral film. Consolidation in the posterior basal segment of the lower lobe with obliteration of the outline of the diaphragm posteriorly and loss of translucency of the lower vertebrae.

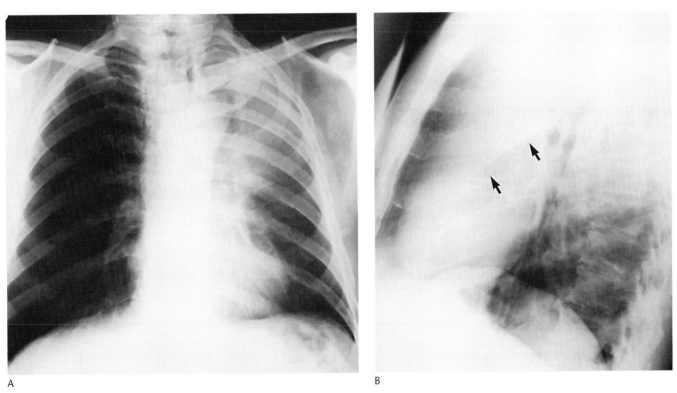

A   B

Fig. 1.25 Left upper lobe collapse. A carcinoma was present at the hilum. (A) Shadowing in the upper zone with loss of outline of the upper cardiac border. The aortic knuckle is outlined by compensatory hyperinflation of the superior segment of the lower lobe. There is tracheal deviation. (B) Anterior displacement of the collapsed lobe and greater fissure.

fluid and rarely within a tumour, with the exception of alveolar cell carcinoma and rarely lymphoma. It may be seen in consolidation distal to a malignancy if the bronchus remains patent (Fig. 1.26). An air bronchogram is usually a feature of air-space filling but is

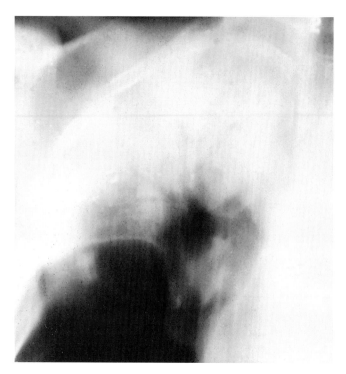

Fig. 1.26 Air bronchogram. An air bronchogram is clearly seen in the consolidated right upper lobe. A proximal carcinoma was present, although it is unusual for an air bronchogram to occur in the presence of a neoplasm.

described accompanying severe interstitial fibrosis such as may develop with sarcoidosis (Box 1.4).

Air-space (acinar/alveolar) pattern *(Box 1.5)*

Few disease processes truly only involve the interstitium or acinus on histological examination, but air-space shadowing on the chest radiograph has distinctive features . When the distal airways and alveoli are filled with fluid, whether it is transudate, exudate or blood, the acinus forms a nodular 4–8 mm shadow. These shadows coalesce into fluffy ill-defined round or irregular cotton-wool shadows, non-segmental, homogeneous or patchy, but frequently well defined adjacent to the fissures (Fig. 1.28). The acinar pattern is most evident on the edge of an area of consolidation. Vascular markings are usually obscured locally. The air bronchogram and silhouette sign are characteristic features. A ground-glass appearance or a generalised homogeneous haze may be seen with a bat's wing or butterfly perihilar distribution (Fig. 1.29), sparing the peripheral lungs which

---

Box 1.4   Causes of an air bronchogram

Common	Rare
Expiratory film	Lymphoma
Consolidation	Alveolar cell carcinoma
Pulmonary oedema	Sarcoidosis
Hyaline membrane disease	Fibrosing alveolitis
(Fig 1.27)	Alveolar proteinosis
	ARDS
	Radiation fibrosis

Box 1.5   Causes of air-space filling

Pulmonary oedema*
Cardiac
Non-cardiac
  Fluid overload
  Hypoalbumenaemia
  Uraemia
  Shock lung (ARDS)
  Fat embolus
  Amniotic fluid embolus
  Drowning
  Hanging
  High altitude
  Blast injury
  Oxygen toxicity
  Aspiration (Mendelson's syndrome)
  Malaria
  Inhalation of noxious gases
  Heroin overdose
  Drugs (e.g. nitrofurantoin)
  Raised intracranial pressure/head injury
Infections
Localised
Generalised, e.g. *Pneumocystis**, parasites, fungi
Neonatal
Hyaline membrane disease
Aspiration
Alveolar blood
Pulmonary haemorrhage, haematoma
Goodpasture's syndrome*
Pulmonary infarction
Tumours
Alveolar cell carcinoma*
Lymphoma, leukaemia
Metastatic adenocarcinoma
Miscellaneous
Alveolar proteinosis*
Alveolar microlithiasis
Radiation pneumonitis
Sarcoidosis
Eosinophilic lung
Polyarteritis nodosa
Mineral oil aspiration/ingestion
Drugs
Amyloidosis
Wegener's granulomatosis
Churg–Strauss syndrome
Allergic bronchopulmonary aspergillosis

* These are common causes of bats' wing shadowing

---

remain translucent. The distribution of opacity is frequently asymmetrical and may be unilateral, particularly with pulmonary oedema. When due to cardiac failure the opacity clears quickly with treatment. Other causes include *Pneumocystis* infection, alveolar proteinosis and non-cardiac causes of pulmonary oedema. Cavitation may occur.

Infective processes are usually localised, occasionally forming a round peripheral opacity which must be distinguished from a malignancy. If an infective process is bilateral and generalised it may well be due to an opportunistic infection. During resolution a mottled appearance can develop and this may give the impression that cavitation has occurred.

Air-space shadowing which rapidly resolves but reappears at the same site or elsewhere suggests pulmonary oedema, bronchopulmonary aspergillosis or eosinophilic pneumonia.

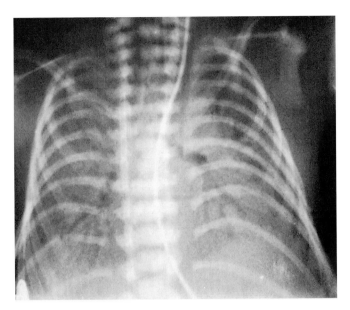

Fig. 1.27 Hyaline membrane disease. Extensive homogeneous consolidation with a prominent air bronchogram.

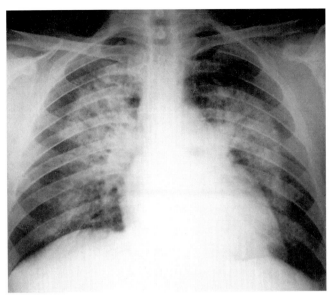

Fig. 1.29 Acute intra-alveolar pulmonary oedema with a bat's wing distribution.

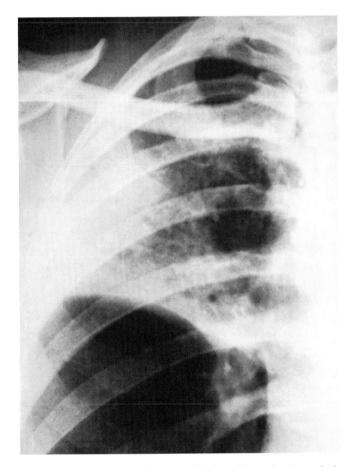

Fig. 1.28 Right upper lobe consolidation. Upper bowing of the horizontal fissure indicates some collapse. There is an acinar pattern with some confluence.

Consolidation in association with lobar expansion and bulging pleural fissures may be seen with bacterial pneumonia, in particular

Pneumococcus or Friedländer's bacillus, or in the presence of a central obstructing bronchial carcinoma.

Peripheral air-space shadows which are non-segmental are characteristic of chronic eosinophilic pneumonia.

Diffuse lung disease

Correlation between the plain film radiographic changes and the severity of the clinical respiratory symptoms is often poor, the plain film sometimes being normal in the presence of extensive interstitial disease. Earlier changes can be detected with high-resolution CT. A history of industrial dust exposure, bird fancying and disease processes such as rheumatoid arthritis is helpful.

Diffuse lung disease (Fig. 1.30) is non-homogeneous and includes various patterns such as linear, septal lines, miliary shadows, reticulonodular, nodular, honeycomb shadowing, cystic, peribronchial cuffing and the ground-glass pattern. Care is necessary to avoid mistaking normal vascular markings for early interstitial changes. Normal vessels are not seen in the periphery of the lung fields and unlike interstitial shadows vessels taper and branch. The presence of interstitial shadowing results in the normally visualised vessels becoming ill defined and then lost. The zonal distribution of the shadowing is helpful in determining the differential diagnosis, for example interstitial fibrosis following asbestos exposure typically affects the lung bases whereas sarcoidosis spares the lung bases; reticular upper zone opacity is typical of histiocytosis X whereas a unilateral distribution is characteristic of lymphangitis carcinomatosis. Loss of volume may occur due to fibrosis but lobar collapse is not a feature. Other helpful features include lymphadenopathy and pleural effusions.

The miliary pattern (Box 1.6) has widespread small discrete opacities of similar size 2–4 mm in diameter. This pattern is most often seen with tuberculosis (Fig. 1.31). Dense opacities occur with calcification and metallic dust disease (Fig. 1.32).

Ground-glass shadowing is a fine granular pattern which obscures the normal anatomical detail such as the vessels and

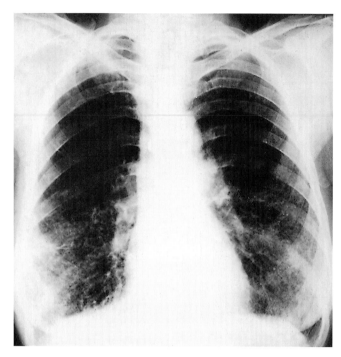

Fig. 1.30 Fibrosing alveolitis. Diffuse interstitial shadowing in the lower zones.

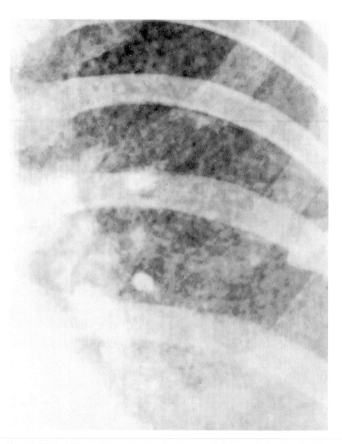

Fig. 1.31 Miliary tuberculosis. Widespread fine nodular shadowing without confluence.

Box 1.6   Causes of miliary shadowing

Infections:	Bronchiolitis obliterans
Tuberculosis	Alveolar microlithiasis
Coccidioidomycosis	Hyaline membrane disease
Blastomycosis	Metastases
Histoplasmosis	Histiocytosis X
Chickenpox	Haemosiderosis
Dust inhalation:	Sarcoidosis
Tin, barium	Secondary hyperparathyroidism
Beryllium, silicosis	Amyloidosis
Coal miner's pneumoconiosis	

diaphragms, and which may be seen with an interstitial or with an air-space pattern.

Reticulonodular shadowing is more common than reticular or nodular shadowing alone. The nodules are less than 1cm in diameter, ill defined and irregular in outline (Box 1.7).

Reticular/linear shadowing appears as a fine irregular network of lines surrounding air-filled lung.

Honeycomb shadowing is the result of parenchymal destruction leading to end-stage pulmonary fibrosis with the formation of thin-walled cysts, the wall being 2–3 mm thick and giving a coarse reticulonodular pattern. When these cysts are 5–10 mm in size the term honeycomb shadowing is used. This condition is associated with an increased risk of pneumothorax, often of the tension type.

Linear and band shadows

Normal structures such as the blood vessels and fissures form linear shadows within the lung fields. However, there are many disease processes which may result in linear shadows. Linear shadows are

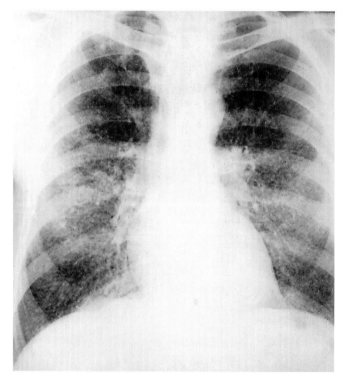

Fig. 1.32 Siderosis. Extensive dense miliary shadowing in an iron-foundry worker.

Box 1.7   Causes of diffuse bilateral reticulonodular shadowing

Infections (interstitial pneumonitis)	**Miscellaneous**
	Idiopathic interstitial fibrosis
Fungi	Extrinsis allergic alveolitis
Histoplasmosis	Drugs
Viruses	Chronic aspiration
Mycoplasma	Sarcoidosis
	Amyloidosis
Pneumoconiosis	Histiocytosis X
Coal miner's	Bronchiolitis obliterans
Silicosis	Lymphangiomyomatosis
Asbestosis	Neurofibromatosis
Berylliosis	Alveolar proteinosis
	Alveolar microlithiasis
Collagen diseases	Gaucher's disease
SLE	Lymphangitis carcinomatosis
Dermatomyositis	
Scleroderma	
Rheumatoid lung	
Cardiac	
Pulmonary oedema	
Haemosiderosis	

less than 5 mm wide, with band shadows defined as greater than 5 mm thick (Box 1.8).

Pulmonary infarcts These are variable in appearance. Occasionally they form irregular thick wedge-shaped lines with the base adjacent to the pleura, but more usually they are non-descript areas of peripheral consolidation at the lung bases. Accompanying features are splinting of the diaphragm and a pleural reaction. Resolution tends to be slow, in contrast to infections which often resolve quickly except in the elderly.

Plate atelectasis, described by Fleischner 1941, is often seen postoperatively and is thought to be due to underventilation with obstruction of medium-sized bronchi. These lines are several centimetres long, 1–3 mm thick, and run parallel to the diaphragms extending to the pleural surface. Resolution is usually rapid.

Mucus-filled bronchi Also known as bronchoceles, these are bronchi distended with mucus or pus beyond an obstructing lesion but with aeration of the distal lung from collateral air flow. Causes to consider include bronchopulmonary aspergillosis, malignancy, benign tumours, foreign-body aspiration and bronchial atresia. Typically the bronchus has a gloved finger branching pattern with the fingers several millimetres wide (Fig. 1.33).

Sentinel lines These are thought to be mucus-filled bronchi and appear as coarse lines lying peripherally in contact with the pleura

Box 1.8   Causes of linear and band shadows

Pulmonary infarcts
Sentinel lines
Thickened fissures
Pulmonary/pleural scars
Bronchial wall thickening
Curvilinear shadows (bullae, pneumatoceles)
Anomalous vessels
Artefacts
Fleischner lines (plate atelectasis)
Kerley lines
Resolving infection
Bronchoceles

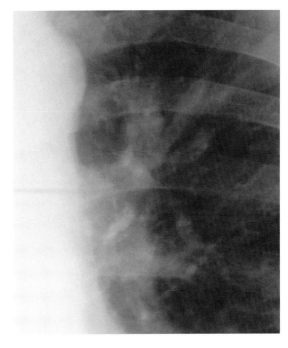

Fig. 1.33 Bronchocele with typical gloved-finger branching pattern.

and curving upward. They are often left-sided and associated with left lower lobe collapse. They may develop due to kinking of bronchi adjacent to the collapse.

Kerley B lines These have been described previously. Unilateral Kerley lines usually indicate lymphangitis carcinomatosa but may be seen with early cardiac failure.
   Normal and accessory fissures. These have been described.

Thickening of the fissures This is often seen accompanying cardiac failure. Bulging fissures indicate lobar expansion which may occur with an acute abscess (Fig. 1.34), infections—most commonly *Klebsiella* but also *Pneumococcus*, *Staphylococcus* and *tuberculosis*—and in the presence of large tumours.

Old pleural and pulmonary scars Scars are unchanged in appearance on serial films. Pulmonary scarring is a common end–result of infarction, appearing as a thin linear shadow often with associated pleural thickening and tenting of the diaphragm. Pleural scars extend to the pleural surface. Apical scarring is a common finding with healed tuberculosis, sarcoidosis and fungal disease (Fig. 1.35).

Curvilinear shadows These indicate the presence of bulles, pneumatoceles (Fig. 1.36) or cystic bronchiectasis.

Thickened bronchial walls These cast parallel tramline shadows which, when seen end-on, appear as ring shadows. They are a common finding in bronchiectasis, recurrent asthma, bronchopulmonary aspergillosis (Fig. 1.37), pulmonary oedema and lymphangitis carcinomatosis. If the peribronchial interstitial space becomes thickened by fluid or tumour, the walls are less clearly defined.

The single pulmonary nodule

Some 40% of solitary pulmonary nodules are malignant, with other common lesions being granulomas and benign tumours (Box 1.9).

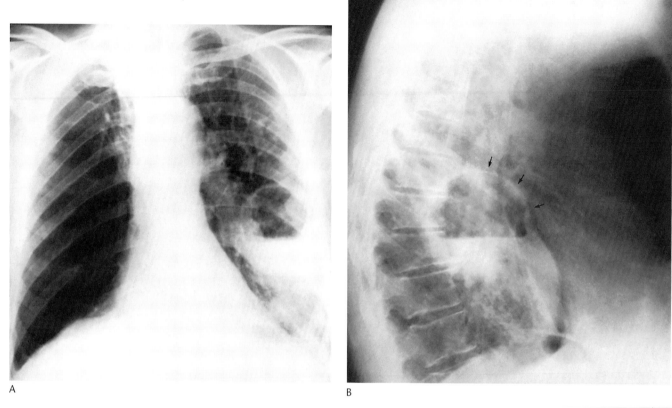

A   B

Fig. 1.34 (A) A large lung abscess witha fluid level distal to a hilar carcinoma. There is an old right upper lobe collapse with compensatory emphysema. (B) Note bulging of the oblique fissure adjacent to the abscess (arrows).

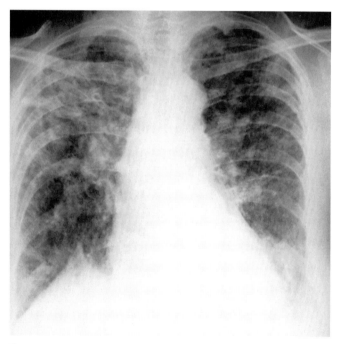

Fig. 1.35 Sarcoidosis. Fibrosis mainly affecting the upper zones with elevation of the hila and tenting of the right hemidiaphragm. A 55-year-old woman with a long history of sarcoidosis.

A lateral film is often necessary to confirm that a lesion is intrapulmonary before investigating further. Typically an intrapulmonary

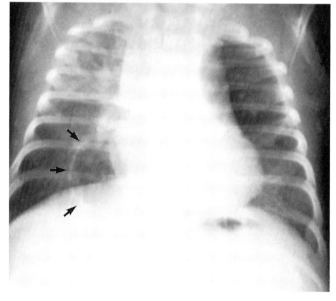

Fig. 1.36 Pneumatocele. Child with a staphylococcal pneumonia. Consolidation in the right upper lobe and a pneumatocele adjacent to the right heart border (arrows).

mass forms an acute angle with the lung edge whereas extrapleural and mediastinal masses form obtuse angles (Fig. 1.38).

A nodule is assessed for its size, shape and outline and for the presence of calcification or cavitation. A search is made for

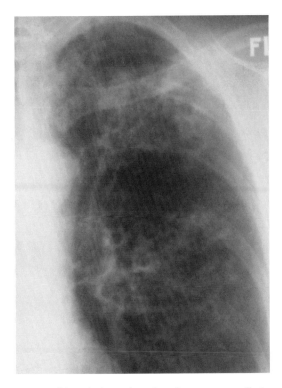

Fig. 1.37 Bronchiectasis due to bronchopulmonary aspergillosis.

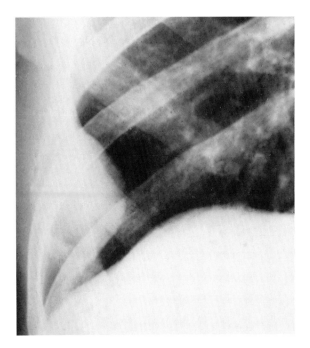

Fig. 1.38 Reticulum cell sarcoma of right lower rib with an extrapleural mass.

Box 1.9   Causes of a solitary pulmonary nodule

Malignant
  Primary nodule
  Secondary nodule
  Lymphoma
  Plasmacytoma
  Alveolar cell carcinoma
Benign
  Hamartoma
  Adenoma
  Connective tissue tumours
Granuloma
  Tuberculosis
  Histoplasmosis
  Paraffinoma
  Sarcoidosis
Infection
  Round pneumonia
  Abscess
  Hydatid
  Amoebic
  Fungi
  Parasites

Pulmonary infarct
Pulmonary haematoma
Collagen diseases
  Rheumatoid arthritis
  Wegener's granulomatosis
Congenital
  Bronchogenic cyst
  Sequestrated segment
  Congenital bronchial atresia
  AVM
Impacted mucus
Amyloidosis
Intrapulmonary lymph node
Pleural
  Fibroma
  Tumour
  Loculated fluid
Non-pulmonary
  Skin and chest wall lesions
  Artefacts

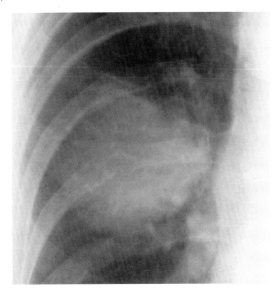

Fig. 1.39 Posteriorly positioned bronchial carcinoma with destruction of the adjacent rib.

associated abnormalities such as bone destruction (Fig. 1.39), effusions, lobar collapse, septal lines and lymphadenopathy. If previous films are available the doubling time can be assessed, that is the time taken for the volume of the mass to double. Usually malignant lesions have a doubling time of 1–6 months whereas masses are considered benign when they have not changed in size for 18 months. Malignant lesions may grow spasmodically however. Masses larger than 4 cm are predominantly primary malignancies, metastases or pleural fibromas although solitary metastases are rare. Tumours smaller than 10 mm cannot be seen clearly on a plain film and often appear as a 'smudge' shadow rather than a mass.

On occasions infective processes have a round appearance which is usually ill defined. Some change is seen at follow-up with simple consolidation after treatment.

Carcinomas often have irregular, spiculated or notched margins. Calcification favours a benign lesion although a carcinoma may arise coincidentally at the site of an old calcified focus. Popcorn calcification suggests a hamartoma (Fig. 1.40). Calcified metastases are rare, the primary tumour being usually an osteogenic or chondrosarcoma (Fig. 1.41).

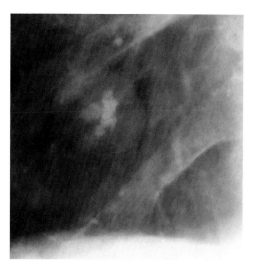

Fig. 1.40 Hamartoma with popcorn calcification.

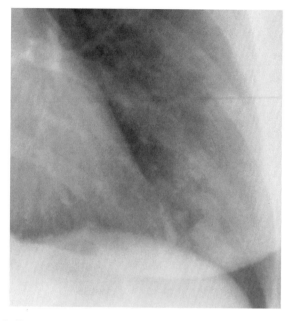

Fig. 1.42 Arteriovenous malformation with dilated feeding and draining vessels.

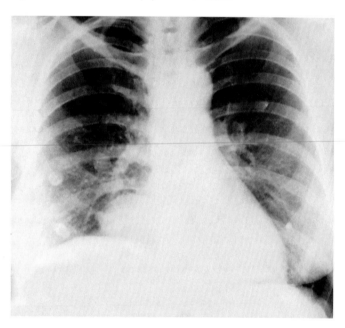

Fig. 1.41 Multiple calcified metastases from a chondrosarcoma of the right tenth rib.

Box 1.10   Causes of multiple pulmonary nodules

Tumours
  Benign—hamartoma, laryngeal papillomatosis
  Malignant—metastases, lymphoma
Infection
  Granuloma—tuberculosis, histoplasmosis, fungi
  Round pneumonia
  Abscesses
  Hydatid cysts
Inflammatory
  Caplan's syndrome
  Wegener's granulomatosis
  Sarcoidosis
  Drugs
Vascular
  Arteriovenous malformations
  Haematomas
  Infarcts
Miscellaneous
  Mucus impaction
  Amyloidosis

Granulomas frequently calcify and are usually well defined and lobulated. Multiple lesions tend to be similar in size, whereas metastases are frequently of variable size but are well defined. *Arteriovenous malformations* (AVM) characteristically have dilated feeding arteries and draining veins (Fig. 1.42); they are multiple in 30% of cases. Most *bronchogenic cysts* are mediastinal but some 20–30% are intrapulmonary and usually arise in the lower zones.

Multiple pulmonary nodules

Multiple small nodules 2–4 mm are called miliary shadows (see previously). In the majority of cases multiple nodules are metastases or tuberculous granulomas. Calcified nodules are generally benign except for metastases from bone or cartilaginous tumours. The doubling time of metastases is highly variable, with a range of a few days to in excess of 2 years. It is well documented that thyroid metastases can persist unchanged for many years (Box 1.10).

Cavitating lesions and cysts

A cavity is a gas-filled space surrounded by a complete wall which is 3 mm or greater in thickness. Thinner walled cavities are called cysts or ring shadows. Cavitation occurs when an area of necrosis communicates with a patent airway. Particular features of importance are the location of the cavity, its outline, wall thickness, the presence of a fluid level, contents of the cavity, satellite lesions, the appearance of the surrounding lung and multiplicity of lesions. CT often provides additional helpful information. Fluid within a cavity can be demonstrated only when using a horizontal beam.

Common cavitating processes are tuberculosis, staphylococcal infections (Fig. 1.43) and carcinoma. The tumour mass itself or the distal lung may cavitate (Box 1.11).

The site Tuberculous cavities are usually upper zone, in the posterior segments of the upper lobes or apical segments of the

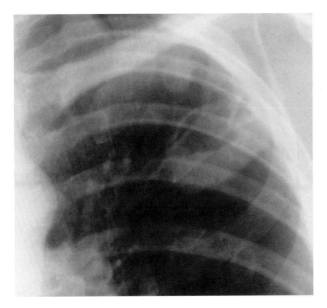

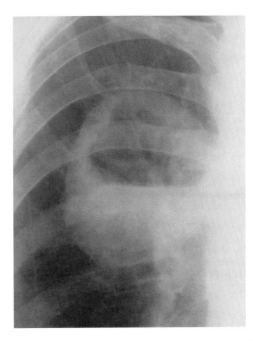

Fig. 1.43 Staphylococcal abscesses. Multiple cavitating abscesses in a young male heroin addict. Bilateral effusions also present.

Fig. 1.44 Large irregular thick-walled cavitating neoplasm with air–fluid level.

Box 1.11	**Cavitating pulmonary lesions**
Infections	Pulmonary infarct
Staphylococcus	Pulmonary haematoma
Klebsiella	Pneumoconiosis
Tuberculosis	Pulmonary massive fibrosis
Histoplasmosis	Caplan's syndrome
Amoebic	Collagen diseases
Hydatid	Rheumatoid nodules
Paragonimiasis	Wegener's granulomatosis
Fungal	Developmental
Malignant	Sequestrated segment
Primary	Bronchogenic cyst
Secondary	Congenital cystic adenomatoid malformation
Lymphoma	Sarcoidosis
Abscess	Bulles, blebs
Aspiration	Traumatic lung cyst
Blood-borne	Pneumatocele

lower lobes. The site of lung abscesses following aspiration depends on patient position at the time but they are most often right-sided and lower zone. Traumatic lung cysts are often subpleural. Amoebic abscesses are nearly always at the right base, the infection extending from the liver. Pulmonary infarcts are usually lower zone and sequestrated segments are left-sided.

The wall of the cavity Thick-walled cavitating lesions (Fig. 1.44) include acute abscesses, most neoplasms (usually squamous cell), lymphoma, most metastases, Wegener's granulomas and rheumatoid nodules. Thin-walled lesions or ring shadows are usually benign and may be bulles (Fig. 1.45), pneumatoceles, cystic bronchiectasis, hydatid cysts, traumatic lung cysts, chronic inactive tuberculous cavities and neoplasms. Pneumatoceles often develop in children after a staphylococcal pneumonia, and a rapid change in size is a feature. In adults they develop following *Pneumocystis* pneumonia. In addition they frequently form following pulmonary contusion and hydrocarbon ingestion.

Satellite lesions are a common feature of benign lesions, usually tuberculous. Multiple ring shadows, 5–10 mm in diameter, are seen with honeycomb shadowing.

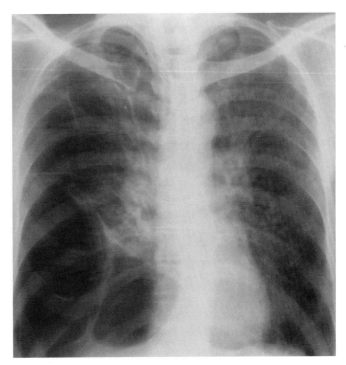

Fig. 1.45 Bullous emphysema with curvilinear shadows in the right lung and an associated paucity of vascular markings.

Fluid levels

Fluid levels are common in primary tumours, and irregular masses of blood clot or necrotic tumour may be present. Fluid levels are uncommon in cavitating metastases and tuberculous cavities (Box 1.12).

The *air crescent (meniscus) sign* is seen when an intracavitory body is surrounded by a crescent of air. It is commonly described with fungus balls such as an aspergilloma (Fig. 1.46). There is movement of the ball with change in the patient's position.

Box 1.12   Fluid levels on a chest radiograph

Intrapulmonary
Hydropneumothorax
  Trauma, surgery
  Bronchopleural fistula
Oesophageal
  Pharyngeal pouch, diverticula
  Obstruction—tumours, achalasia
  Oesophagectomy—bowel interposition
Mediastinal
  Infections
  Oesophageal perforation
Pneumopericardium
  Trauma, surgery, iatrogenic
Chest wall
  Plombage with lucite balls (Fig. 1.47)
  Infections
Diaphragm
  Hernias, eventration, rupture

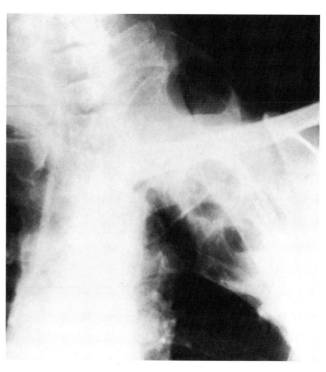

Fig. 1.47 Apical plombage. Hollow lucite spheres with fluid levels which have formed because of leakage of the walls of the spheres.

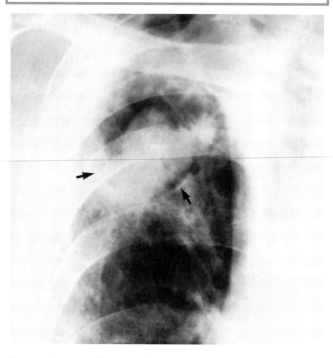

Fig. 1.46 Aspergillus mycetoma. A large mycetoma within an old tuberculous cavity in a fibrotic upper lobe. The mycetoma is surrounded by an air crescent.

Ruptured hydatid cysts may have daughter cysts floating within the cavity, the *waterlily sign*. Other intracavitory lesions include inspissated pus, blood clot and cavernoliths. Blood clot may form within cavitating neoplasms, tuberculosis and pulmonary infarcts.

Calcification *(Box 1.13)*

Calcification is most easily recognised with low kVp films. In the elderly calcification of the tracheal and bronchial cartilage is common. Calcification of the bronchioles, *osteopathia racemosa*, is of no significance.

Tuberculosis is the commonest calcifying pulmonary process with small scattered foci of various sizes, usually upper zone (Fig. 1.48). Chickenpox foci are smaller (1–3 mm), regular in size and widely distributed (Fig. 1.49). Characteristically the foci of *histoplasmosis* are surrounded by small halos.

Box 1.13   Calcification on the chest radiograph

Intrapulmonary	**Lymph nodes**
Granuloma, infection	Tuberculosis
Tuberculosis	Histoplasmosis
Histoplasmosis	Sarcoidosis
Chickenpox	Silicosis
Coccidioidomycosis	Lymphoma postirradiation
Actinomycosis	**Pleural**
Hydatid cyst	Tuberculosis
Chronic abscess	Silicosis
Tumours	Asbestosis
Metastases	Old haemothorax, empyema
Osteogenic sarcoma, chondrosarcoma	**Mediastinal**
Cystadenocarcinoma	*Cardiac*
Benign	Valvular
Arteriovenous malformation	Infarcted muscle
Hamartoma, carcinoid	Pericardial
Primary	Aneurysms
Miscellaneous	Tumours
Haematoma	*Vascular*
Infarction	Tumours
Mitral valve disease	**Pulmonary artery**
Broncholith (tuberculosis)	Pulmonary hypertension
Alveolar microlithiasis	Aneurysm
Idiopathic	Thrombus
Rare	**Chest wall**
Metabolic—hypercalcaemia	Costal cartilage
Silicosis	Breast tumours, fat necrosis
Sarcoidosis	Bones tumours, callus
Rheumatoid arthritis	Soft-tissue parasites,
Amyloid	tumours, etc
Osteopathia racemosa	

Alveolar microlithiasis appears as tiny sand-like densities in the mid and lower zones, due to calcium phosphate deposits in the alveoli. Punctate calcification may develop within the pulmonary nodules of silicosis. Popcorn calcification is often present in hamar-

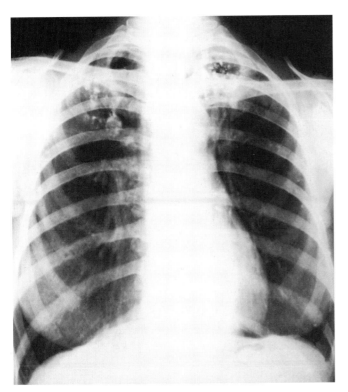

Fig. 1.48 Pulmonary tuberculosis. Numerous calcified foci in both upper zones with left upper lobe fibrosis.

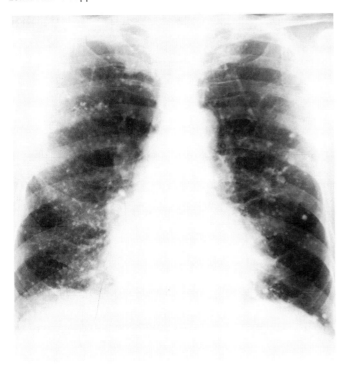

Fig. 1.49 Chickenpox. Widespread small calcified opacities following a previous chickenpox pneumonia.

tomas. Occasionally phleboliths are present in arteriovenous malformations. Very rarely a fine rim of calcification forms in the wall of a hydatid cyst.

Pleural plaques may be irregularly calcified.

Lymph node calcification occurs in a number of conditions. An 'eggshell' pattern is characteristic of sarcoidosis and silicosis.

Calcification may be seen within metastases particularly with osteogenic sarcoma. Calcification is not a feature of a primary lung malignancy, although 6–7% of lung primaries contain calcification on CT. However a carcinoma may develop coincidentally adjacent to a calcified granuloma and therefore an area of eccentric calcification should not be presumed to exclude malignancy.

Apical shadowing *(Box 1.14)*

Apical pleural thickening, the 'pleural cap', has a reported incidence of 7% and is more commonly left sided. It is crescent shaped, frequently irregular, and if bilateral is usually asymmetrical. The significance is uncertain but it may represent old pleural thickening. If the thickening is irregular or markedly asymmetrical or unduly prominent or convex, the underlying rib must be assessed for destruction as the possibility of a Pancoast (superior sulcus) tumour must be considered; this usually presents as a mass but in a quarter of cases it presents as a pleural cap (Fig. 1.50).

The lung apex is a common site for tuberculosis and fungal diseases including *histoplasmosis, coccidioidomycosis, blastomycosis* and *aspergillosis*. Assessment of active disease is difficult in the presence of fibrotic changes. Previous films for comparison are invaluable.

Extrinsic shadows should be excluded (Fig. 1.51). Invariably in these cases the edge of the lesion is seen to extend beyond the limits of the lung and pleura into the soft tissues.

Box 1.14 Common causes of apical shadows
Pleural caps
Pleural fluid
Bullae
Pancoast tumour
Pneumothorax
Infections—tuberculosis
Soft tissue, e.g. companion shadows, hair, sternocleidomastoid muscles

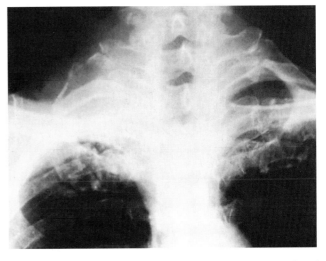

Fig. 1.50 Pancoast tumour. There is apical shadowing on the right side simulating pleural thickening. Note destruction of the first rib.

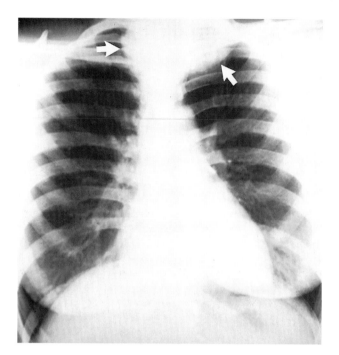

Fig. 1.51 A woman with her hair in a plait overlying the upper mediastinum and simulating mediastinal widening.

Signs of loss of volume

In the majority of cases loss of volume, or collapse, is caused by obstruction of a bronchus by tumour, mucus or foreign body, or extrinsic compression by nodes. More rarely it is due to broncho-stenosis following trauma. The signs of lobar or pulmonary collapse can be divided into direct and indirect. The direct signs are: (i) opacity of the affected lobe(s); (ii) crowding of the vessels and bronchi within the collapsed area, and (iii) displacement or bowing of the fissures (Fig 1.52). Indirect signs are: (i) compensatory hyperinflation of the normal lung or lobes resulting in an increase in transradiancy with separation of the vascular marking; (ii) displacement of the mediastinal structures toward the affected side (Fig. 1.53); (iii) displacement of the ipsilateral hilum which changes shape;

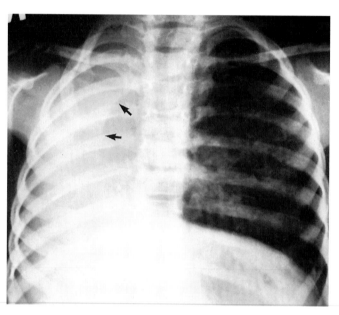

Fig. 1.53 Pulmonary agenesis. The right lung is absent. The heart and mediastinum are displaced to the right. Note herniation of the left lung across the midline (arrows). The rib spaces are narrowed on the right.

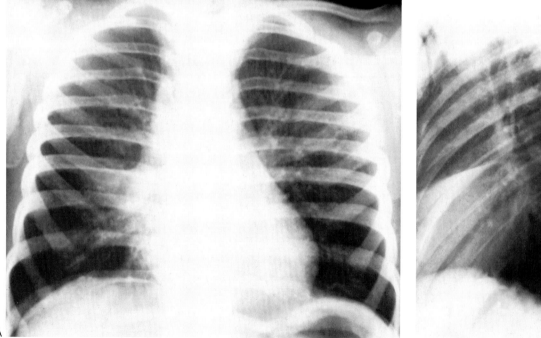
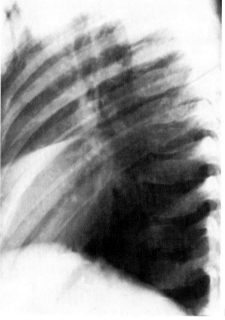

A

B

Fig. 1.52 Right middle lobe collapse. (A) Loss of definition of the right heart border with adjacent shadowing. (B) Lobar collapse with displacement of the fissures clearly shown.

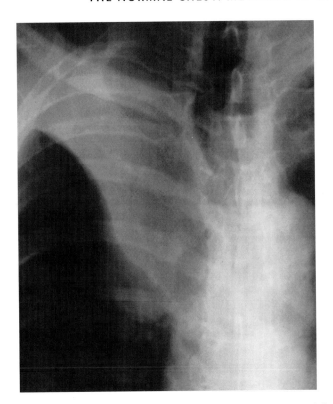

Fig. 1.54 'Golden S sign.' Collapsed right upper lobe with mass at right hilum.

(iv) elevation of the ipsilateral hemidiaphragm; and (v) crowding of the ribs on the affected side, particularly common in children.

With major collapse there is herniation of the contralateral lung with displacement of the anterior mediastinal line. Obliteration of the bronchus at the site of the obstruction may be evident but this is more clearly seen at CT. The presence of a hilar mass with collapse can be identified by the 'Golden S sign' (Fig. 1.54). The central mass gives a convexity to the concave displaced fissure (as described by Golden) forming the shape of an S.

Hilar enlargement

The normal pulmonary hilum has a very variable appearance. It is difficult to detect minor degrees of pathological enlargement and to distinguish a prominent pulmonary artery from a small mass lesion, although branch vessels can often be traced back to an enlarged artery. A hilum should be assessed for its position, size and density, with a comparison of the two hila. Any possible abnormality can be assessed further with contrast-enhanced CT or flexible bronchoscopy.

Bilateral hilar enlargement is commonly due to enlarged lymph nodes, which appear as lobulated masses, or to vascular enlargement. The adjacent bronchi may be slightly narrowed. Unilateral enlargement is most commonly due to a neoplasm or vascular dilatation but is also seen with infections such as tuberculosis and whooping cough (Box 1.15). Nodes affected by lymphoma are often asymmetrically involved (Fig. 1.55). Bilateral involvement occurs with sarcoidosis, silicosis and leukaemia. Tuberculous lymphadenopathy without an identifiable peripheral pulmonary lesion is a common finding in the Asian population.

Small hila are usually the result of congenital cyanotic heart disease (Box 1.16).

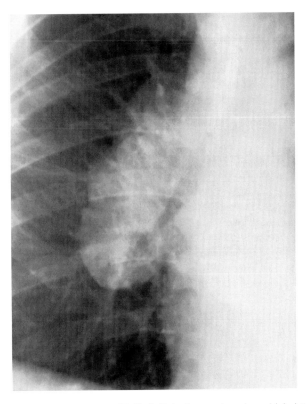

Fig. 1.55 A young man with Hodgkin's disease. An enlarged lobulated right hilum typical of bronchopulmonary glandular enlargement.

Unilateral hypertranslucency

Comparison of the lungs should reveal any focal or generalized abnormality of transradiancy. Increased transradiancy may be accompanied by signs of obstructive or compensatory emphysema such as splaying of the ribs, separation of the vascular markings, mediastinal displacement and depression of the hemidiaphragm.

Patient rotation and scoliosis are the commonest causes of increased transradiancy (Box 1.17). With rotation to the left, the left

---

Box 1.16   Causes of a small hilum

Unilateral
    Apparent: Rotation, scoliosis
    Normal: especially the left side
    Lobar collapse, lobectomy
    Hypoplastic pulmonary artery
    Macleod's syndrome
    Unilateral pulmonary embolus
Bilateral
    Cyanotic congenital heart disease
    Central pulmonary embolus

Box 1.17   Causes of unilateral hypertranslucency

Normal
    Increased density of contralateral lung, e.g. pleural effusion/thickening,
        consolidation
Technical
    Rotation, scoliosis
Soft tissue
    Mastectomy
    Congenital absence of pectoralis muscle
    Poliomyelitis
Emphysema
    Compensatory: lobar collapse, lobectomy
    Obstructive: foreign body, tumour, Macleod's syndrome, congenital
        lobar emphysema
    Bullous
Vascular
    Absent/hypoplastic pulmonary artery
    Obstructed pulmonary artery, e.g. by tumour, embolus
    Macleod's syndrome
Pneumothorax

Box 1.18   Causes of an opaque hemithorax

Technical
    Rotation, scoliosis
Pleural
    Hydrothorax, large effusion
    Thickening, mesothelioma
Surgical
    Pneumonectomy, thoracoplasty
Congenital
    Pulmonary agenesis
Mediastinal
    Gross cardiomegaly, tumours
Pulmonary
    Collapse, consolidation, fibrosis
Diaphragmatic hernias

---

side becomes more radiolucent. Mastectomy is another important cause. An abnormal axillary fold is seen following a radical mastectomy. However, the less extensive breast surgery favoured currently is difficult to detect on the chest film.

With conditions such as *Macleod's syndrome*, congenital lobar emphysema and an inhaled foreign body, an expiratory film will demonstrate obstructive emphysema (Fig. 1.56). There is displacement of the mediastinum away from the affected side with depression of the ipsilateral diaphragm. Congenital lobar emphysema

usually affects the right upper or middle lobes. A small pulmonary artery is a feature of Macleod's syndrome and congenital hypoplasia or absence of the artery.

The commonest causes of increased translucency of both lungs are asthma, emphysema and reduced pulmonary perfusion.

The opaque hemithorax *(Box 1.18)*

All the causes described of unilateral hypertranslucency may be responsible for an apparent contralateral increase in density. Penetrated and lateral films are usually helpful. Signs of collapse, fluid levels, mediastinal displacement and rib abnormalities are important findings. Pulmonary agenesis is associated with hypoplastic ribs and is invariably left sided.

The chest film of the elderly person

With age the thorax changes shape and the AP diameter increases. A kyphosis develops so that the chin overlies the lung apex. Frequently only an AP film in the sitting position can be obtained, usually with a limited degree of inspiration so that the lung bases are poorly visualised.

Bone demineralisation increases, with vertebral body compression and rib fractures being common. Bony margins become irregular. Costal cartilage and vascular calcification is prominent. Often there is calcification of the cartilaginous rings of the trachea and bronchi.

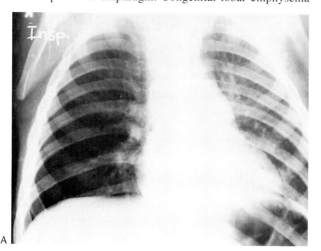 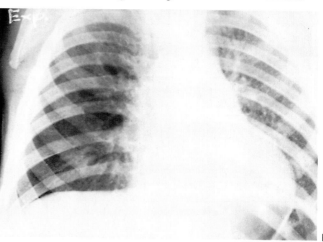

Fig. 1.56   Obstructive emphysema. This child inhaled a peanut. (A) Inspiratory film shows a hypertransradiant right lung. (B) Expiratory film. There is air trapping on the right side with further shift of the mediastinum to the left.

The major blood vessels become unfolded. On a lateral film the aorta is visualised throughout its length. Unfolding of the innominate and subclavian vessels results in widening of the upper mediastinum. Prominent hilar vessels accompany obstructive airways disease and the peripheral vessels become more obvious.

There may be changes due to old pathology with linear scars, pleural thickening, tenting of the diaphragm and calcified foci. Blunted costophrenic angles and flattened diaphragms are common findings in the elderly.

Limitations of the plain chest film

First, the radiologist may fail to spot a lesion. Felson reported that 20–30% of significant information on a chest film may be overlooked by a trained radiologist.

Second, a disease process may fail to appear as a visible abnormality on a plain film. Examples include miliary shadowing, metastases, infective processes such as tuberculosis, histoplasmosis and *Pneumocystis*, bronchiectasis and small pleural effusions. Such lesions are demonstrated earlier using high-resolution CT. Inflamed bronchi are not easily seen and obstructive airways disease may be associated with a normal chest film. Small pulmonary emboli without infarction cannot be diagnosed.

Finally, the shadow patterns themselves are rarely specific to a single disease process. For example, consolidation due to infection or following infarction may have identical appearances.

OTHER METHODS OF INVESTIGATION

TOMOGRAPHY

Tomography is performed:
1. to improve visualisation of a lesion
2. to localise a lesion and to confirm it is intrapulmonary
3. to evaluate the hilum and proximal airways
4. to search for a suspected lesion, e.g. metastases
5. to evaluate the mediastinum and chest wall.

Technique
A recent chest film is mandatory. The examination should be closely supervised by the radiologist with particular attention to the radiographic technique, ensuring that the area of interest is included on the films taken. Linear tomography is usually adequate although more complex movements may be used. Cuts are routinely made at 1-cm intervals.

AP tomography, supplemented with lateral tomography, is satisfactory for peripheral lesions. The hilum is best visualised in the 55° posterior oblique position with the side of interest dependent (Fig. 1.57). On this view the bronchi are projected in profile. A penetrated view to show the carina is routinely obtained.

The peripheral mass
Features of diagnostic importance include calcification, cavitation, the outline of the mass, bronchial narrowing and the presence of an air bronchogram (Fig. 1.58). Spiculation is a strong indicator of malignancy.

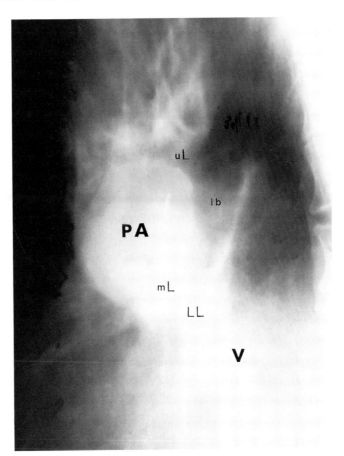

Fig. 1.57 Right posterior oblique (55°) tomogram of right hilum. PA = pulmonary artery; V = pulmonary vein; uL = upper lobe bronchus; ib = intermediate bronchus; mL = middle lobe bronchus; LL = lower lobe bronchus.

The hilum
Hilar tomograms are difficult to interpret. It is helpful to remember that normal sized nodes are not usually seen, and that enlarged nodes are well defined. The vessels, unlike a mass lesion, branch and taper. If a mass is identified the adjacent bronchi should be assessed for narrowing or occlusion.

FLUOROSCOPY

Fluoroscopy is of value for assessing chest wall and diaphragm motion, and for demonstrating mediastinal shift in cases of air trapping. It is helpful in uncooperative children when the radiograph is non-diagnostic due to movement and poor inspiration.

Screening may be used to differentiate pulmonary from pleural lesions by rotating the patient and noting movement of the lesion with respect to the sternum and spine. Pulsation is often a misleading sign; it may be transmitted to a mass lying adjacent to a vascular structure. Masses of vascular origin change size with the Valsalva manoeuvre and with patient position. Pulmonary lesions move with respiration whereas mediastinal lesions do not.

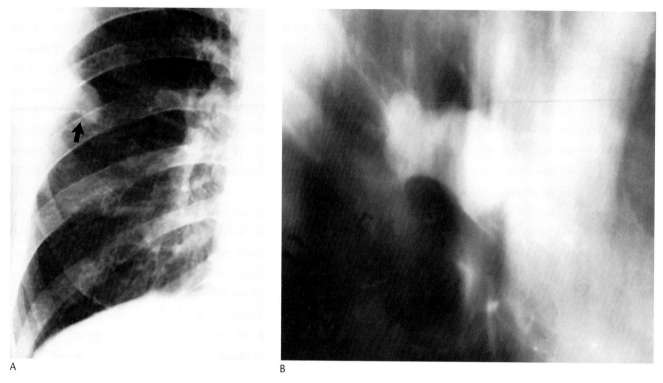

Fig. 1.58   Oat cell carcinoma. (A) Peripheral mass adjacent to the ribs. (B) Oblique tomogram shows an irregular mass with thin strands extending into the surrounding lung.

CT SCANNING OF THE LUNGS

Richard W. Whitehouse and Andrew R. Wright

Technical considerations

Computed tomography of the thorax is a relatively high radiation dose examination, capable of giving an effective dose 50–500 times higher than a conventional chest radiograph. The wide dose range is largely due to variations in technique between different operators. Appropriate patient selection and choice of scan parameters is therefore paramount in thoracic CT scanning.

The development of spiral CT scanning technology has been of great benefit in the imaging of the thorax. Spiral scanning involves continuous rotation of the X-ray tube and smooth passage of the patient through the scanner aperture. This enables the whole thorax to be covered rapidly within the time of a single breath-hold. Breathing artefact and misregistration of adjacent slices, a common problem with conventional single-section CT, are abolished. The speed of scanning also means that intravenous contrast agents can be deployed very accurately to maximise their effectiveness.

A recent refinement of spiral scanning is to replace the single bank of X-ray detectors with multiple rows of detectors, allowing several interlaced data helices to be acquired simultaneously. Multidetector or multislice CT allows larger volumes to be scanned with thinner sections, and yet shorter scan times. The speed of scanning makes multislice CT well suited to the demonstration of thoracic vasculature, including pulmonary arteries, and permits a shorter contrast medium injection, thus reducing contrast usage (Fig. 1.59). The datasets produced are well suited to image post-processing, for example multiplanar reformats (MPR) in various

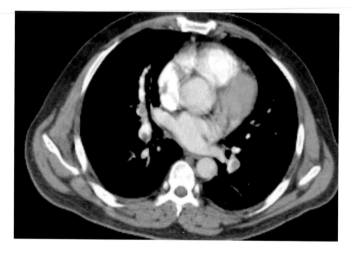

Fig. 1.59   Extensive pulmonary embolism within both lower lobe arteries and right middle lobe artery.

planes, surface-rendered and maximum intensity projection (MIP) reconstructions, volume-rendered images and 'virtual endoscopy' views (Figs 1.60, 1.61).

The thorax contains tissues with CT numbers ranging from −1000 for air through lung parenchyma, fat and soft tissue, to cortical bone with a CT number of over 1500. Comprehensive evaluation of these tissues therefore requires interrogation of the greyscale image at a variety of window levels and widths. Wide window widths are necessary for bone and lung parenchyma, with a higher window level for bone, whilst a narrow window is necessary to demonstrate the smaller density differences that may be present between soft-tissue structures.

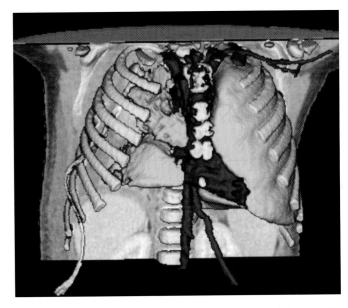

Fig. 1.60 3D surface-rendered image from segmented dataset of a paediatric chest scan. The umbilical vein (visible due to an in situ catheter) and abdominal aorta are both depicted in red below the diaphragm, a right-sided chest drain is also present.

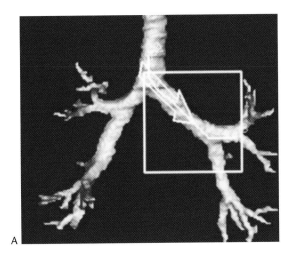

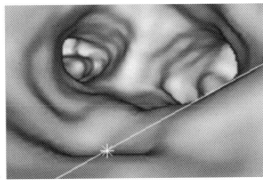

Fig. 1.61 'Virtual bronchoscopic' view from multislice CT dataset. (A) Surface-rendered 3D reconstruction of the trachea and bronchial tree used to demonstrate the direction of view of surface-rendered 3D reconstruction of the bronchial walls (B) viewed from within the left main bronchus looking towards the upper and lower lobe orifices.

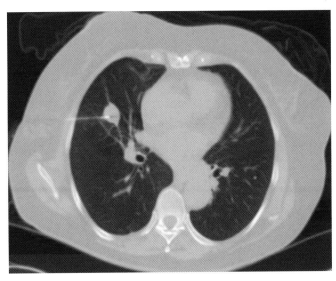

Fig. 1.62 Cutting needle biopsy of right mid-zone mass under CT control (carcinoid). The low-attenuation artefact shows the precise position of the needle tip.

CT is a useful technique for guiding thoracic biopsy, both pulmonary fine needle aspiration and larger cutting needle biopsies of pulmonary, pleural and mediastinal masses (Fig. 1.62). *CT fluoroscopy*, a continuously updated near real-time CT image, can be used to facilitate rapid and accurate CT-guided interventional techniques but can expose both the patient and operator to significant radiation doses.

Anatomical considerations

Both the pulmonary arteries and the bronchi branch out from the hila to the lung periphery. Similarly the pulmonary veins radiate from the venous confluence and left atrium. CT through the upper or lower chest passes through these structures obliquely or in cross-section, resulting in a ring appearance for bronchi and filled circles or ovals for vessels. CT through the midpart of the thorax will demonstrate greater lengths of each individual structure as they arborise within the scan

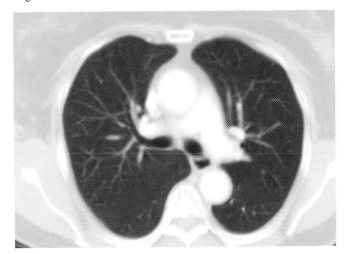

Fig. 1.63 Conventional 7-mm-thick section through the mid chest, viewed on a lung window. Note the branching pulmonary vessels and the paucity of vessels at the sites of fissures.

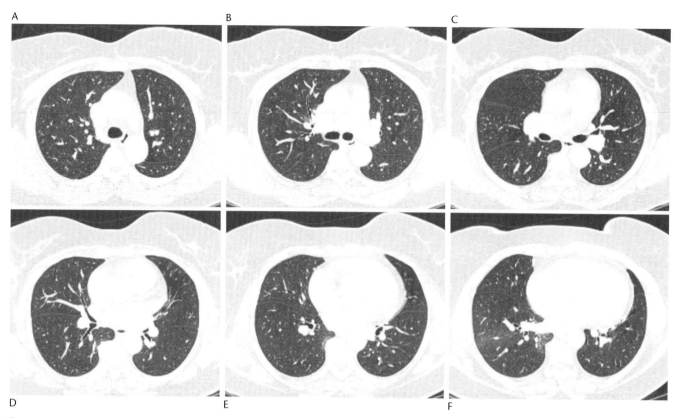

Fig. 1.64 High-resolution sections through the thorax demonstrate the segmental bronchi. (A) Upper section; upper lobe segmental bronchi are seen passing perpendicular to the plane of the slice. (B) At the level of origin of right upper lobe bronchus. The proximal upper lobe segmental bronchi are well seen. (C) At the level of origin of left upper lobe bronchus. The oblique and horizontal fissures are shown. (D) On each side the apical segment lower lobe bronchi are seen posteriorly, as well as the middle lobe bronchus and parts of the lingular bronchi anteriorly. (E) The lower lobe bronchi are dividing on each side into segmental bronchi. (F) The right lower lobe bronchus has divided into medial, anterior, lateral and posterior basal segmental bronchi. The left lower lobe bronchus has divided into anterior, lateral and posterior basal segmental bronchi.

plane (Fig. 1.63). Careful reference to adjacent sections is therefore necessary to trace vessels and bronchi out from the hila to the apices and bases in order to demonstrate the continuity of these structures and to confirm whether small opacities in the pulmonary periphery are normal vessels or pulmonary nodules.

The location of the pulmonary fissures on thick-section (7-mm) CT scans can usually be inferred by a paucity of vessels in that region, whilst the fissures can usually be directly identified on thin-section high-resolution CT (compare Figs 1.63 and 1.64). The azygos fissure, when present, is clearly seen as it is perpendicular to the plane of section (Fig. 1.65). Careful interrogation of adjacent sections in both directions from the hila will usually allow

identification of the segmental bronchi and often the subsegmental bronchi beyond this (Fig. 1.64).

Toward the lung bases, the apex of the right hemidiaphragm will usually appear centrally first, resulting in increased density in the middle of the lung image.

Physiological considerations

Respiratory phase The density of the pulmonary parenchyma is strongly dependent upon the respiratory phase. In expiration there is a striking increase in density, particularly in the dependent part of the lung. This is likely to be due to reduced alveolar inflation

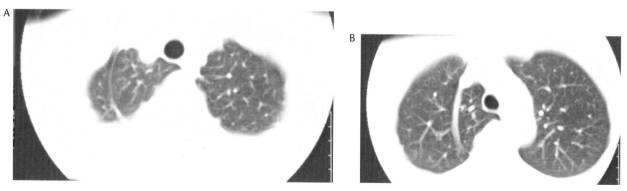

Fig. 1.65 (A,B) The azygos fissure is clearly seen on CT.

with consequent crowding of the alveolar walls and pulmonary vasculature but may also have a contribution from altered perfusion. Lung parenchyma is best assessed by scanning in suspended full inspiration.

Posture The influence of gravity on pulmonary vessel calibre is well demonstrated by CT. Dependent vessels are notably larger. Slightly increased parenchymal density, probably due to hypostatic parenchymal oedema, may also be seen in the dependent part of the lungs on CT. This can be cleared by placing the patient prone and repeating the scan after a few minutes (Fig. 1.66). Scanning of the thorax with the patient in the decubitus position results in compression of the dependent lung, which is most noticeable during expiration, whilst the uppermost lung is in a state of relative inspiratory apnoea and oligaemia. Mediastinal structures may also move considerably under the influence of posture, particularly in patients with emphysema (Fig. 1.66).

ROLE OF CT IN DISEASES OF THE LUNG AND PLEURA

The chest radiograph usually reveals the anatomical distribution of lobar or segmental disease and can demonstrate generalised or diffuse pulmonary parenchymal abnormalities as an alteration in the pattern of pulmonary markings. High-resolution CT can confirm the location and extent of disease and can further characterise the location and pattern of disease (Fig. 1.67). Mediastinal or chest wall involvement by pulmonary pathology may also be demonstrated by CT (Fig. 1.68). Ascertaining the solitary nature of a pulmonary nodule or detection of other unsuspected nodules, determination of the probability of malignancy, contribution to staging prior to treatment and monitoring of response to treatment are all important roles for CT.

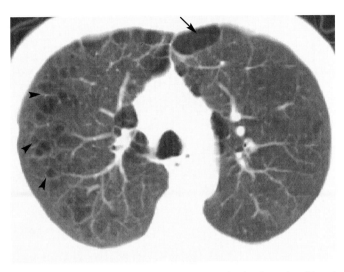

Fig. 1.67 Large areas of reduced pulmonary density (arrowheads) and bulla (arrow) in emphysema.

High-resolution CT (HRCT)

The use of thin sections (1–3 mm) combined with a high spatial resolution reconstruction algorithm (e.g. the 'bone' algorithm) and targeting the scan to the lungs (i.e. using a field of view just large enough to encompass the region of interest) results in clear depiction of the distribution and higher definition of the appearance of pulmonary parenchymal disease. In-plane spatial resolution of around 300 μm can be achieved using this technique. This has proved valuable in the demonstration and differential diagnosis of diverse interstitial pulmonary diseases. The severity and extent of bronchiectasis can be demonstrated (Figs 1.69, 1.70). The technique can identify regions most suitable for biopsy at a time when

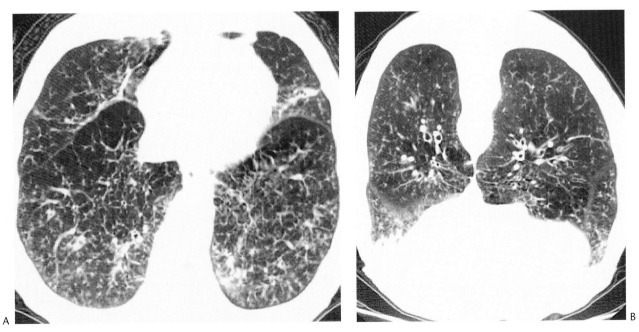

Fig. 1.66 (A) Supine scan in chronic airways disease. The lungs are overinflated and postural increase in pulmonary density is evident posteriorly. (B) Prone scan at the same level. The posterior increased density seen in (A) has cleared. Note the marked mobility of the mediastinum with the heart now flattened against the anterior chest wall.

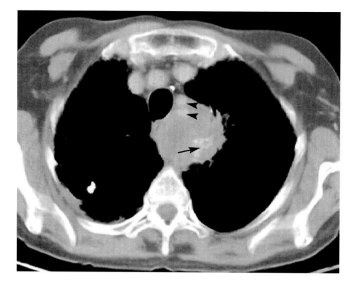

Fig. 1.68 Carcinoma of the lung incorporating calcification (arrow) from previous tuberculous granuloma. The tumour is extending into the mediastinum to encase the left common carotid and subclavian arteries (arrowheads).

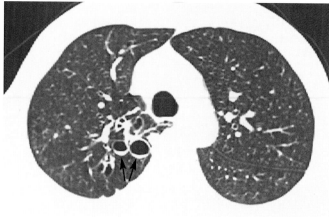

Fig. 1.70 Saccular bronchiectasis (arrows).

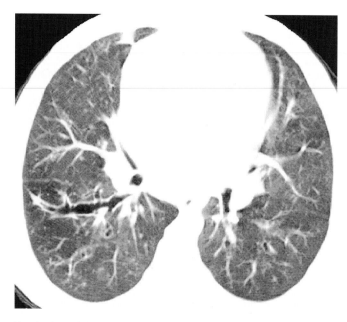

Fig. 1.69 Tubular bronchiectasis in a patient with cystic fibrosis.

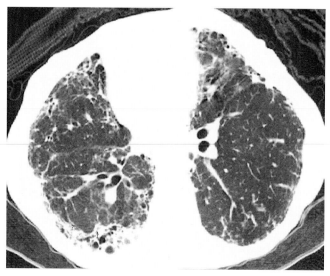

Fig. 1.71 HRCT 3-mm section. Fibrosing alveolitis. Note the predominantly peripheral involvement. (Courtesy of Dr P. M. Taylor.)

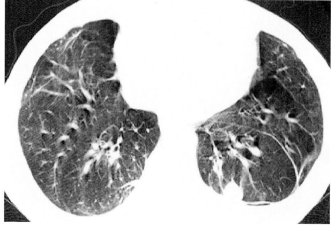

Fig. 1.72 HRCT asbestosis. Early subpleural increase in density on a prone scan. (Courtesy of Dr P. M. Taylor.)

the chest radiograph is normal. Scans taken in the expiratory phase can be useful in the diagnosis of small airways disease, where they may show evidence of air trapping.

Interstitial diseases

In *fibrosing alveolitis* and *systemic sclerosis*, CT demonstrates a typical peripheral distribution of disease involving the outer third of the lungs. This starts as a posterior basal subpleural crescent of increased attenuation, progressing to peripheral 'honeycombing'. The pleural and mediastinal interfaces may become irregular with a 'saw-tooth' margin (Fig. 1.71). In *asbestosis* HRCT may demonstrate subpleural curvilinear opacities, parenchymal bands, thickened inter- and intra-lobular lines, increased subpleural attenuation and honeycombing (Figs 1.72, 1.73). Pleural thickening and calcification will also be demonstrated in cases of asbestos-related pleural disease (Fig. 1.74). HRCT has a 100% positive-predictive value in asbestosis with pleural thickening. *Rounded atelectasis*, a fibrosing condition most commonly associated with asbestosis, is also clearly demonstrated on CT, the 'comet tail' of incurving vessels being characteristic (Fig. 1.75); other features include adjacent pleural thickening and an air bronchogram within the lesion. Recognition of these features may prevent unnecessary pulmonary resection for a supposed carcinoma but biopsy may be necessary as both *pulmonary carcinoma* and *pleural mesothelioma* are commoner in this group of patients. Irregular thickening of the interlobular septa, producing a reticular pattern, can be appreciated on HRCT in *lymphangitis carcinomatosa* before it is apparent on the chest radiograph (Fig. 1.76). In chronic *sarcoidosis* nodules at

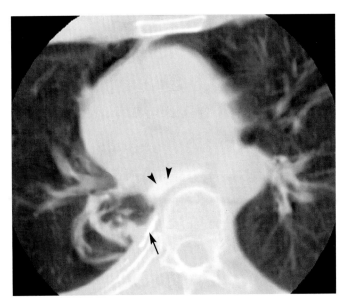

Fig. 1.75 Rounded atelectasis with 'comet tail' of vessels running into the mass which is adherent to the pleura. Adjacent calcified pleural plaque is evident (arrow). There is also oral contrast medium in the oesophagus (arrowheads).

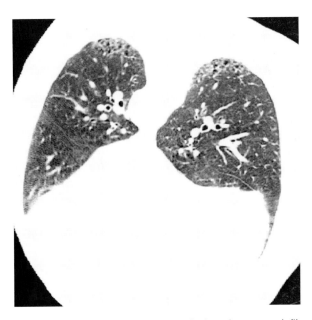

Fig. 1.73 HRCT asbestosis. Note the thickened septa and fibrous parenchymal and subpleural bands. (Courtesy of Dr P. M. Taylor.)

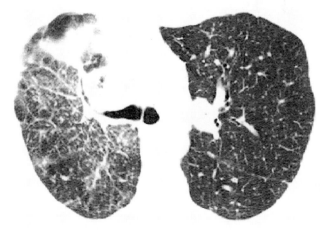

Fig. 1.76 HRCT lymphangitis carcinomatosa from carcinoma of the breast. Note the thickened interlobular septa. (Courtesy of Dr P. M. Taylor.)

branchpoints of pulmonary vessels and bronchi may be seen, and beading of the bronchi is typical (Figs 1.77, 1.78). Air-space opacification and thickening of the interlobular septa produces a characteristic 'crazy-paving' effect in *alveolar proteinosis*. *Lymphangioleiomyomatosis* is a condition only occurring in women of reproductive age; the CT appearance is of multiple cystic spaces replacing the lung parenchyma. *Acute alveolar disease* is clearly demonstrated from whatever cause (Figs 1.79, 1.80), as is *miliary nodularity* (Fig. 1.81).

Pulmonary nodules and carcinoma

CT is the most sensitive imaging modality available for the identification of pulmonary nodules of 3 mm or greater in diame-

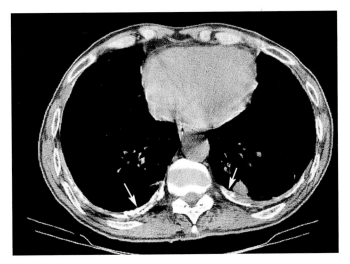

Fig. 1.74 HRCT soft-tissue window demonstrates asbestos-related pleural disease with posteromedial calcified pleural plaques (arrows).

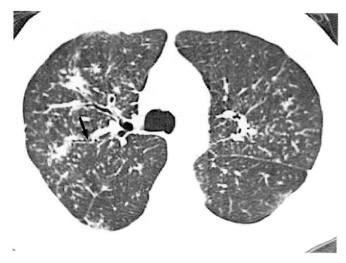

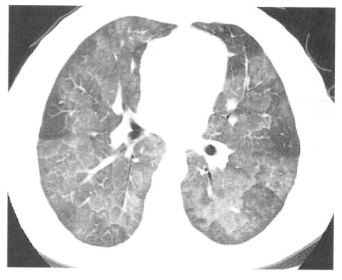

Fig. 1.77 HRCT sarcoidosis with beading of the segmental bronchial walls (arrow). (Courtesy of Dr P. M. Taylor.)

Fig. 1.79 HRCT diffuse alveolar disease in extrinsic allergic alveolitis. (Courtesy of Dr P. M. Taylor.)

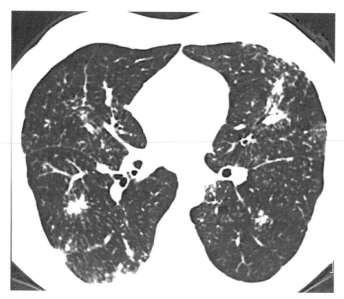

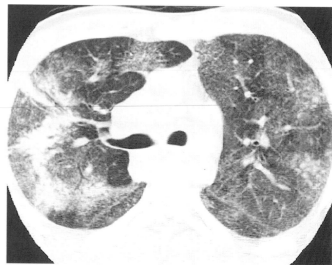

Fig. 1.78 HRCT sarcoidosis with patchy peribronchial shadowing.

Fig. 1.80 HRCT acute sarcoidosis with widespread alveolar shadowing.

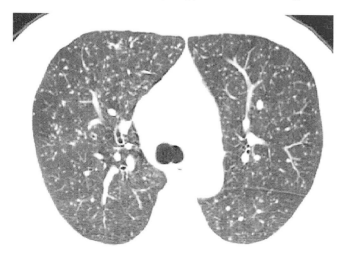

Fig. 1.81 HRCT miliary tuberculosis.

ter, but is relatively insensitive to smaller nodules. The specificity for small nodules is also poor, with up to 60% of small nodules in patients with malignant disease being unrelated granulomas indistinguishable from metastases on CT. Most pulmonary metastases are found in the outer third of the lungs, more commonly toward the bases, and the majority of them are subpleural (Fig. 1.82). Spiral scanning has improved the detection rate for pulmonary nodules but has not improved specificity. Assessment of the margins of pulmonary nodules is unreliable in differentiating benign from malignant disease. The presence of definite calcification in a pulmonary nodule suggests a granuloma and thus benign disease. However, scar carcinomas can arise in old tuberculous lesions (Fig. 1.68) and up to 14% of carcinomas demonstrate histological calcification. Thus, to suggest benignity, the amount of calcification should represent over 10% of the nodule, the calcification should not be stippled and the lesion should not be greater than 3 cm in diameter. Unequivocal demonstration of fat density within a pulmonary nodule is almost diag-

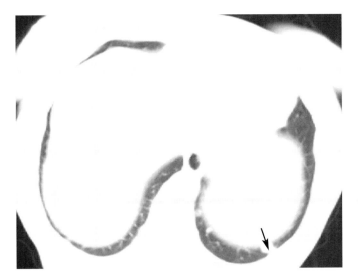

Fig. 1.82 Occult metastasis in the posterior costophrenic sulcus (arrow).

nostic of an *hamartoma*. Lack of growth of a nodule over a 2-year period is also indicative of benignity. Cavitation can be demonstrated early by CT but does not necessarily indicate malignancy (Fig. 1.83). In pulmonary malignancy CT can demonstrate spread to the hilum, mediastinum (Fig. 1.68), pleura or chest wall and also allows assessment of mediastinal lymph nodes and the adrenal glands (common sites for metastatic spread). CT can guide biopsy of pulmonary lesions where required (Fig. 1.62).

HRCT should not be used for the detection of pulmonary nodules as non-contiguous sections are commonly performed in this technique. The use of multislice spiral CT for screening patients at risk of bronchial carcinoma is gaining popularity, particularly in Japan

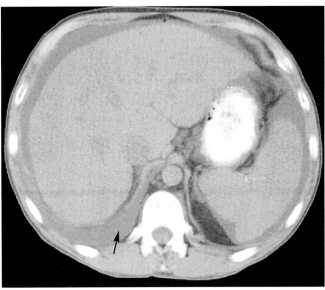

Fig. 1.84 Pleural effusion and ascites—note the relationship of the fluid to the right diaphragmatic crus with pleural fluid lying posterior to (and therefore above) the crus (arrow). Ascitic fluid is evident around the spleen and anterolateral to the liver.

and the USA. 'Ultra-low dose' techniques are being investigated to reduce the relatively high radiation exposure associated with conventional CT of the chest.

Pleural disease

Differentiation of pulmonary from pleural disease is possible using CT. The distinction of a pleural effusion from subdiaphragmatic fluid is achieved by recognising the relationship of the fluid to the diaphragm or its crura (Fig. 1.84). Pleural plaques in asbestos-related pleural disease are commonly discrete lesions arising over the diaphragmatic and posterolateral parietal pleura and may show characteristic calcification (Fig. 1.74). Pleural tumours (mesothelioma, metastatic adenocarcinoma, spread from thymic tumours) characteristically encase the lung, reducing its volume (Figs 1.85, 1.86).

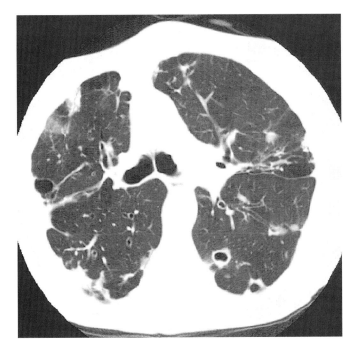

Fig. 1.83 HRCT rheumatoid lung with cavitating nodules, bronchiectasis and emphysema.

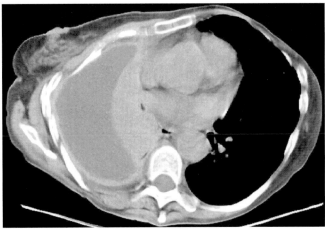

Fig. 1.85 Pleural metastatic tumour from carcinoma of the breast, encasing the lung with consequent volume loss, crowding of the ribs and a malignant effusion. Note the contralateral mastectomy.

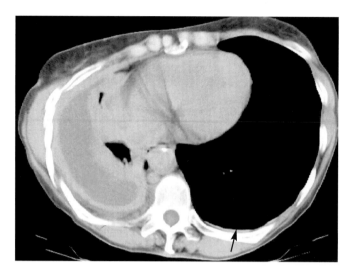

Fig. 1.86 Pleural mesothelioma. Similar characteristics to Fig. 1.85. Note the contralateral posterior pleural plaque indicating previous asbestos exposure (arrow).

MRI IN CHEST DISEASES

Jeremy P. R. Jenkins

The role of MRI and its relation to other imaging techniques in chest diseases has yet to be defined and is still evolving. The main advantages of MRI include a multiplanar facility and a high intrinsic soft-tissue contrast discrimination, allowing vascular structures and lesions in the mediastinal and hilar regions to be defined separately from other tissues, in particular the aortopulmonary window and subcarinal space, without the need for contrast-medium administration. Disadvantages of MRI include respiratory and cardiac motion artefacts and an inability to visualise small branching pulmonary vessels and bronchi, and lung parenchyma. These structures, however, are better depicted on CT. The introduction of faster MR scan times, enabling images to be obtained within a single breath-hold, combined with a good signal-to-noise ratio (SNR), may alleviate some of these problems, as can the use of ECG- and respiratory-gated techniques. At present, MRI is unable to provide the same anatomical detail and spatial resolution in the lung as HRCT. The ease of performance and wider availability of CT makes it the procedure of choice in the assessment of most lesions in the thorax, including lung metastases and pulmonary emboli. MRI can be useful in certain situations, for example in the separation of mediastinal masses from normal or abnormal vessels, the illustration of the craniocaudal extent of large lesions and lesions at the lung apex, lung base and chest wall, in the evaluation of diaphragmatic hernia, in the assessment of pathology affecting major vessels and the brachial plexus (see Ch. 2), and can be used in patients with suspected pulmonary embolism who are allergic to iodinated contrast medium.

Anatomical detail of *lung parenchyma* is limited on MRI due to respiratory and cardiac motion artefacts, an intrinsically low SNR from the lung air spaces, a poorer spatial resolution than conventional radiography and CT, and difficulty in precise localisation of disease due to lack of normal anatomical landmarks. Normal lobar fissures and small peripheral pulmonary vessels and bronchi are not visualised, and alveolar and interstitial changes within the lung cannot be distinguished. Failure to visualise aerated lung is due to the magnetic

susceptibility effects between air and soft tissue, creating magnetic field gradients at each of the million alveolar wall interfaces. This effect is quite marked leading to shortening of the T_2 relaxation time of aerated lung to approximately 7 ms, compared with a T_2 of 80 ms for collapsed non-aerated lung. The use of minimum echo times (TE 7 ms) has been used with the T_1-weighted spin echo sequence to compensate for this T_2 effect, and provides a 3.5-fold increase in the SNR from the lung compared with conventional TE values of 20 ms. MRI is unable to compete with thin-section high-resolution CT in the assessment or detection of small peripheral lung carcinomas, metastases or calcifications. CT is the imaging method of choice in the detection and evaluation of lung nodules, including metastases. MRI can be useful, however, in differentiating lung nodules from vessels, particularly in the hilar region.

The ability to image in the sagittal and coronal planes allows the integrity of the diaphragm to be assessed. On T_1- and T_2-weighted images the diaphragm, although not usually visualised as a separate structure, abuts onto the bright signal from the adjacent pleural fat, with any encroachment and loss of this fat plane indicating tumour infiltration or penetration by abdominal or pulmonary lesions (e.g. diaphragmatic hernias) (see Fig. 4.49).

Cystic lesions of the lung (e.g. bronchogenic cysts and bronchial atresia with mucocele formation secondary to mucoid impaction) can be clearly demonstrated as areas of high signal on T_2-weighted images. Vascular lesions (e.g. scimitar syndrome and pulmonary A/V fistulas) may be missed on MRI due to lack of contrast from the low signal or signal void from flowing blood within the vessel and the surrounding air space. This problem can be overcome by the use of phase-sensitive flow sequences, which provide increased signal from coherently flowing blood.

There is considerable overlap in the MRI characteristics of parenchymal consolidation, which may be due to a variety of causes. In the experimental situation it has been possible to separate cardiogenic from non-cardiogenic pulmonary oedema, although the clinical utility is unclear. MRI may be of value in assessing activity of interstitial lung disease by the demonstration of excess water in active pathology. Granulation tissue and compressed lung enhance markedly following intravenous administration of gadolinium–chelate, with chronic inactive disease and tumour enhancing also, but to a lesser degree.

RADIONUCLIDE IMAGING

Philip J. A. Robinson

Technetium-labelled agents or radioactive gases are used to investigate regional ventilation (V) and perfusion (Q) in the lung (VQ imaging). Positron emission tomography (PET) imaging (see below and Ch. 58) is increasingly being used for staging of lung tumours and the detection of residual or recurrent disease after treatment. Radionuclide techniques for localising infection and single photon tumour imaging agents (e.g. labelled white cells, gallium and octreotide) also have applications in the investigation of chest disease.

VQ imaging—rationale

VQ imaging is used to investigate suspected acute pulmonary embolism and also to assess regional lung function in patients with other types of focal disease. Most lung pathologies cause reduced parenchymal perfusion but it is primarily in acute pulmonary embolism that there is a distinct discrepancy in the affected areas of lung between perfusion—which is absent or severely impaired—and ventilation which is normal or only a little reduced. In infection, perfusion is also reduced but ventilation is more severely impaired than perfusion, or may be absent if the lung is consolidated. Destructive lesions such as emphysema cause equal loss of both perfusion and ventilation. Hilar tumours typically impair both perfusion and ventilation, but occasionally may shut down perfusion completely to one side of the chest at an early stage when the chest radiograph may be relatively normal.

Major indications for VQ imaging are:

1. Suspected pulmonary embolism.
2. Assessment of regional lung function in patients with focal lung disease who may be candidates for surgery, for example lung tumours, bullous emphysema, bronchiectasis, congenital heart disease.

Perfusion scintigraphy

This method demonstrates the distribution of lung perfusion using a technetium-labelled albumin tracer in the form of small particles. The particles are of such a size (about 15–70 μm) that they will be trapped in the precapillary arterioles of the lung in their first passage after intravenous injection. To ensure uniform mixing, the adult dose includes 40 000–200 000 particles which have about the same density as red cells. After trapping in the lung, the particles are removed by the reticuloendothelial system over several hours.

The healthy adult lung contains about 3×10^8 arterioles so the injected particles occlude less than 0.1% of the vascular bed. However, in patients with advanced destructive disease of the lung, typically manifest as severe pulmonary hypertension, there is a potential risk of worsening heart failure, so the injection must be given with caution. Similarly, in patients with a right to left cardiac shunt there is a potential risk of systemic embolisation. In either of these circumstances, the number of particles should be reduced towards the lower end of the diagnostic range.

Ventilation scintigraphy

The aim is to demonstrate the distribution of lung ventilation using an inhaled tracer. Numerous methods have been described, of which three are still in routine use. krypton-81m (^{81m}Kr) is a radioactive gas with gamma emissions suitable for gamma camera imaging and a half-life of about 14 seconds, which can be continuously generated from a source of rubidium-81. Because of the short half-life, re-breathing apparatus is not required and the radiation dose is extremely small. Distribution of ^{81m}Kr in the lung is proportional to the regional ventilation, because the short half-life does not allow time for equilibration, and only a small proportion of the inhaled tracer is expired. ^{81m}Kr is also insoluble in blood so there is no vascular contamination of the ventilation images. Because its gamma emission energy is distinct from that of technetium-99m (^{99m}Tc), perfusion and ventilation can be measured sequentially, or simultaneously if a dual energy acquisition system is used. Rubidium-81 itself has a half-life of 4.7 hours, and this limits the availability of the ^{81m}Kr technique.

^{99m}Tc-labelled ventilation agents include aerosols (e.g. ^{99m}Tc-DTPA in solution) and 'smoke'—^{99m}Tc-labelled carbon particles produced by combustion of a carbon crucible containing pertechnetate solution. With both methods, the labelled particles produced need to be small enough to reach the terminal bronchioles, and a rebreathing apparatus or expiratory filter is needed. In patients with severe airways disease there is a tendency for particles to be deposited in the more proximal bronchi. Because ^{99m}Tc is the label also used for perfusion imaging, ventilation imaging should be performed first so that at least some of the activity will clear from the lungs by the time perfusion imaging is done.

Some centres still employ the older technique using xenon-133 (^{133}Xe). Because its half-life is 5.3 days, rebreathing of xenon for a few minutes results in a stable distribution of gas throughout the lung, so that the regional count rate is proportional to lung volume rather than to ventilation. An indication of ventilation can be obtained by obtaining a wash-out phase in which the inflow of xenon is replaced by room air, whilst the exhaled gas is collected in the rebreathing system. The rate of replacement of xenon in each area of the lung is then proportional to the local ventilation. Single-breath inhalation of ^{133}Xe may also be used as an indicator of regional ventilation, but the count rate obtained with this approach is much smaller than that available with the ^{81m}Kr or ^{99m}Tc techniques. The main advantage of ^{133}Xe is its longer half-life which allows ready availability for urgent usage. One major disadvantage is that because most of the ventilation data is obtained during the wash-out phase, it is technically cumbersome, time consuming and costly to obtain multiple projections, so basic technique includes only a single view.

Perfusion imaging and ventilation using ^{81m}Kr or ^{99m}Tc requires anterior, posterior and posterior oblique images, which are preferred to lateral views in order to avoid small defects in one lung being obscured by counts shining through from the opposite lung.

Interpretation

Normal lung shows convex chest wall margins, flat or concave margins at the diaphragmatic surface, and a cardiac impression of varying size (Fig. 1.87A). Ventilation images will also show the trachea and main bronchi (Fig. 1.87B). Interpretation requires the availability of a concurrent chest radiograph, not only to confirm suspicions of anatomical abnormalities (e.g. cardiomegaly, kyphoscoliosis, elevated hemidiaphragm, etc.), but also to improve the specificity of diagnosis. Almost all lung pathologies cause reduction in perfusion whilst ventilation is affected by obstructive airways disease and also by any condition in which alveolar air is replaced by fluid or tumour. Characteristically, pulmonary embolism results in severe reduction or total loss of perfusion to the areas of lung supplied by the affected arteries, whilst ventilation remains unchanged or shows only a minor

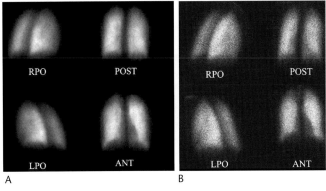

Fig. 1.87   Normal lung perfusion (A) and ventilation (B) images.

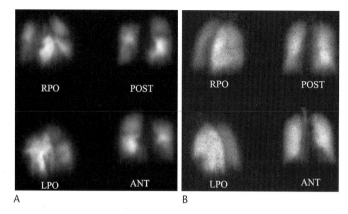

Fig. 1.88 Pulmonary embolism. Perfusion images (A) show multiple segmental perfusion defects while ventilation images (B) are normal.

reduction (Fig. 1.88). Destruction of lung tissue (e.g. emphysema) results in patchy loss of both perfusion and ventilation, but the abnormalities are usually well matched. In infective consolidation, ventilation is usually severely affected whereas perfusion is reduced to a lesser degree (reverse mismatch). In the normal lung, perfusion is gravity dependent, with the lower lobes receiving about three-quarters of the cardiac output. With left heart failure, this gradient is lost or reversed owing to vasoconstriction in basal pulmonary arterioles.

Scintigraphy in the diagnosis of pulmonary embolism

Pulmonary embolism is common, but difficult to diagnose accurately. In some cases, pulmonary embolism (PE) produces no clinical signs or symptoms, and in most other cases the clinical features are non-specific, i.e. the same signs and symptoms may be produced by other conditions. Although the chest radiographic appearances may be suggestive, they cannot be relied on either to diagnose or exclude embolism. Characteristic ECG changes occur only when there is obstruction of a substantial proportion of the pulmonary circulation, i.e. enough to cause right ventricular strain. Scintigraphy shows only the distribution of perfusion and ventilation—not the responsible pathology. However, in large numbers of cases, pulmonary arteriography has been compared with lung scintigraphy in patients both with and without PE, so the predictive value of the scintigraphic findings has been validated. The usual approach is to use a system of high, medium and low probabilities using criteria for diagnosis, which are based on these comparative studies of VQ scintigraphy and arteriography. Although the probability system appears not to give a clear-cut diagnostic result, its objective is to reduce the degree of uncertainty about each individual patient. The scan result can then be compounded with clinical data to give a likelihood of PE. Box 1.19 illustrates such a probability system. A number of additional points need to be noted when interpreting lung scintigraphy:

1. Image artefacts may result from clumping of inhaled particles in some patients with severe airways disease, or in cases where errors occurred in the preparation or administration of the particles, for example by allowing blood to mix in the syringe at the time of injection (Fig. 1.89).

2. The rate of recovery of the lung circulation following PE is approximately exponential—most of the improvement takes place

---

Box 1.19 A scheme for the interpretation of VQ scintigraphy

1. **Normal**—no perfusion defects; perfusion outlines the shape of the lung as shown on chest X-ray (CXR). Normal lung perfusion **excludes pulmonary embolism**, i.e. arteriograms never show emboli of segmental or larger size in patients with **good quality** normal perfusion scintigraphy, unless there has been a new inicident

2. **High probability**—2 or more large (>75% of a segment) mismatched perfusion defects with no **corresponding** CXR abnormalities
   or 1 large and ≥2 moderate sized (25–75% of a segment) mismatched perfusion defects with no **corresponding** CXR abnormalities
   or 4 or more moderate-sized mismatches with no **corresponding** CXR

   NB: the CXR doesn't have to be normal

3. **Low probability**—multiple matched VQ defects, regardless of size, with normal CXR
   or triple matched (i.e. matched VQ defect plus CXR lesion in same area) in **upper or mid zone**
   or perfusion defects surrounded by normally perfused lung (**stripe sign**)
   or matched VQ defect with **large** effusion
   or any perfusion defect with a **substantially larger** CXR abnormality
   or **non-segmental** defects—e.g. cardiomegaly, aortic impression, enlarged hila

4. **Intermediate probability**—a mixture of matched and unmatched defects
   or single **moderate-sized** mismatch with normal CXR
   or triple match in **lower** zone
   or matched VQ defect with **small** effusion
   or 1 moderate to <2 large mismatches with no **corresponding** CXR abnormalities
   or doesn't fit into normal, low or high probability categories

---

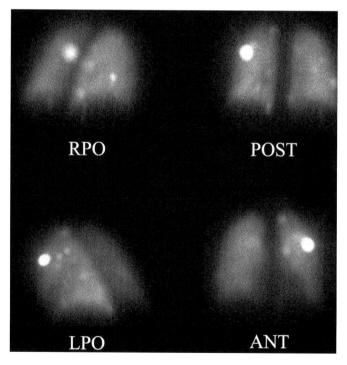

Fig. 1.89 Artefacts on perfusion images produced by clumping of albumin particles in the syringe at the time of injection.

within days or even hours of the embolic event—so it is helpful to obtain investigations as soon as possible after the onset of symptoms or of clinical suspicion.

3. Errors will arise if diagnosis is made from the scintigraphy without reference to a concurrent chest radiograph. Careful review of both together will minimise the proportion of indeterminate results.

4. The left and right posterior oblique views display each lung with the segments approximately orientated as radiating wedge-shaped areas with the hilum at the centre. Segmental perfusion defects may appear as wedge shaped, but may also present as local concavities in the outer contour of the lung, particularly with emboli which partly occlude a segmental artery.

5. Matched defects of ventilation and perfusion occur in areas of parenchymal lung disease and may also result from airways' obstruction (Fig. 1.90). Because the resolution of the ventilation image is less good than that of the perfusion image, ventilation defects may appear smaller and less well defined that the corresponding perfusion defect. Very small subsegmental lesions causing peripheral perfusion defects may not be visible at all on the ventilation image.

6. Pulmonary emboli usually produce segmental or lobar defects in the acute phase, but if the patient survives the initial episode the emboli usually break up and become more peripheral in distribution. At this stage the segmental origin of the perfusion defects becomes much less obvious and the defects themselves are smaller. Loss of perfusion to an entire lung can result from carcinoma at the hilum of the lung, congenital hypoplasia of the lung, hypoplasia or aplasia of the pulmonary artery, ventricular septal defect and some other congenital heart anomalies. Unilateral PE is recognised but not common—the majority of patients with PE have multiple lesions.

7. Reversed mismatches (loss of ventilation with perfusion preserved or less severely reduced) are typical of infective consolidation or atelectasis (Fig. 1.91).

8. Visible renal uptake indicates a right to left shunt or faulty radiopharmaceutical preparation (Fig. 1.92). Thyroid activity usually indicates the presence of unbound pertechnetate in the injected dose.

In assessing the likelihood of PE, the scintigraphic result must be considered together with the level of clinical suspicion before the test, based on history, examination and in particular the presence of established risk factors (immobility, recent surgery, concurrent or previous deep vein thrombosis (DVT), and previous PE). A suggested diagnostic strategy might then be as follows:

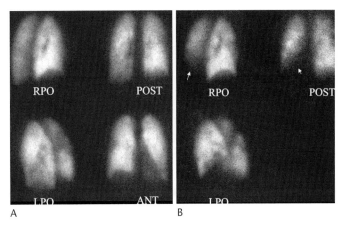

Fig. 1.91 Infective consolidation. Perfusion (A) is reduced at the left base, but ventilation (B) is totally lost (arrows), producing a 'reverse mismatch'.

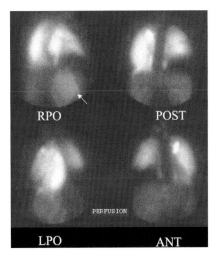

Fig. 1.92 Systemic shunting. In the presence of a right to left shunt, some of the tracer escapes into the systemic circulation; uptake in right kidney is arrowed.

- Lung VQ first—if normal, seek other explanations for the symptoms.
- If V/Q high probability, with strong clinical suspicion—treat for PE.
- If V/Q low probability with low clinical suspicion—seek other pathologies.
- If V/Q low probability with high clinical suspicion or high probability with low clinical suspicion, or indeterminate V/Q result—further tests will be required, either a DVT study (usually sonovenography of the legs) or pulmonary CT angiography.

OTHER RADIONUCLIDE TECHNIQUES FOR THE LUNG

Regional lung function in emphysema

When surgery is being considered for diffuse lung disease, assessment of regional lung function becomes critical. Perfusion imaging with single photon emission tomography (SPECT) allows a three-dimensional demonstration of regional lung function which

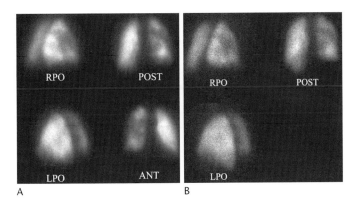

Fig. 1.90 Obstructive airways disease. Both perfusion (A) and ventilation (B) images show multiple peripheral defects which are matched.

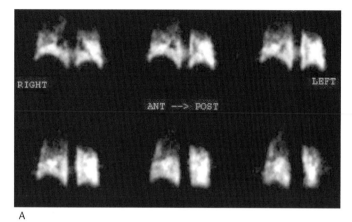

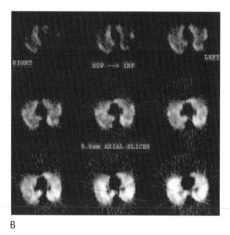

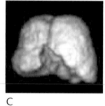

Fig. 1.93   Bullous emphysema. SPECT images showing multiple areas of reduced perfusion particularly affecting lung apices, as shown on coronal (A) and axial (B) slices, and truncated apices shown on 3D volume-rendered image (C). (Courtesy of Dr R. Robertson).

can be correlated with CT appearances to optimise the planning of volume reduction surgery, which may be helpful in cases of severe bullous emphysema (Fig. 1.93).

Lung tumours

In addition to the use of PET for detecting mediastinal lymph node metastases in lung cancer (see below), metabolically active metastases are also shown using specifically targeted radionuclides. Whole-body imaging with iodine-123 is used to find metastases from functioning thyroid tumours after removal of the primary from the neck. Metastases from malignant adrenal tumours (phaeochromocytoma and neuroblastoma) can be detected in the chest and elsewhere using whole-body imaging with metaiodobenzylguanidine (mIBG), whilst somatostatin receptor scintigraphy (SRS) using indium-111-labelled octreotide is used to stage carcinoids, pancreatic islet cell tumours, and other metabolically active malignancies of gastrointestinal origin (Fig. 1.94). A new somatostatin analogue, ^{99m}Tc-labelled depreotide, has recently become available for the differential diagnosis of benign (low uptake) from malignant (high uptake) lesions in the lung. Multicentre clinical studies have indicated both high sensitivity and high specificity in the characterisation of solitary lung

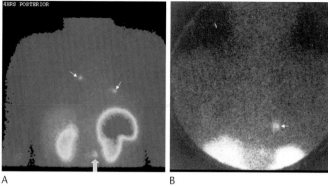

Fig. 1.94   Unsuspected lung metastases shown by somatostatin receptor scintigraphy. (A) Primary pancreatic islet cell tumour (large arrow) with small lung lesions (small white arrows). (B) An occult lung metastasis in a patient with abdominal carcinoid.

nodules. Further studies should clarify whether depreotide has a broader role in the management of lung cancer.

Gallium imaging

Gallium is a trivalent heavy metal which is bound to lactoferrin and transferrin in the blood and which has an affinity for chronic inflammatory tissue and some tumours (Fig. 1.95). Gallium has little or no role in detecting intrathoracic disease but may be used like PET to discriminate between areas of metabolically active disease, and areas of inactive fibrosis. The change in uptake of gallium can also be used as an indicator of response to treatment, but clearly in such applications it is necessary to obtain a pretreatment study to act as a baseline against which future imaging can be compared.

This technique may be used in patients with chronic lung disease associated with cystic fibrosis, sarcoidosis, and other fibrotic conditions of the lung and mediastinum. Detection of residual disease in treated lymphoma is also useful in cases where fibrous tissue remains and anatomical imaging is inconclusive.

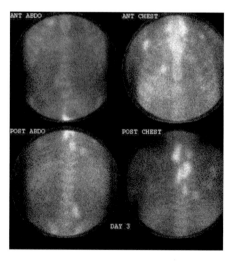

Fig. 1.95   Gallium imaging in lymphoma. Delayed images of chest and abdomen show multiple foci of active disease in mediastinal, para-aortic and right axillary nodes.

Function of the 'mucociliary escalator'

This can be investigated by measuring the rate of removal of labelled solid particles which are inhaled as an aerosol but not absorbed through the mucosal surface. This technique may be useful in assessing the severity of the functional deficit in cystic fibrosis, bronchiectasis and chronic bronchitis, and can be used to monitor the results of treatment of these conditions.

Permeability of lung capillaries

Lung capillary permeability can be assessed by measuring the rate of clearance of inhaled ^{99m}Tc-DTPA in aerosol form. This method may be used as an indicator of the severity of lung injury in adult respiratory distress syndrome (ARDS) and in other disorders involving oedema or inflammatory reaction at capillary level in the lung.

These last two techniques are mainly applied in pathophysiological research and in the assessment of new types of treatment, so they do not have a major role in diagnosis.

POSITRON EMISSION TOMOGRAPHY

The physical principles and general applications of positron emission tomography (PET) are described in Chapter 58. The current applications of PET in lung disease arise from the ability of this technique to demonstrate the level of metabolic activity in abnormal tissues. Intravenously administered deoxyglucose labelled with fluorine-18 (FDG) accumulates in metabolically active cells as FDG-6-phosphate, but does not enter the citric acid cycle, so the distribution remains relatively stable for long enough to acquire whole-body images. FDG uptake correlates with the level of glycolytic activity in the cell, and this is itself an indicator of the rate of cell growth and the degree of malignancy of tumours. Although there is no absolute cut-off point, the majority of malignant tumours show a distinctly greater uptake of FDG than benign or inactive lesions.

Lung cancer

PET is now the most accurate imaging technique for the staging of primary lung tumours. All metastases start out as small deposits, and the major difficulty in staging primary lung cancer by CT or MRI arises from the inability of anatomical techniques to detect the presence of metastasis in nodes of normal size. In addition, patients with lung cancer frequently have uninvolved nodes which are enlarged through reactive change. The hyper-

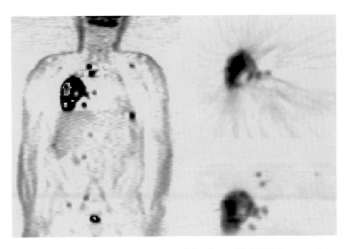

Fig. 1.97 Unresectable carcinoma of the lung. FDG-PET images show large primary tumour but also multiple metastases in lymph nodes, bone and right adrenal. (Courtesy of the Clinical PET Centre, Guy's and St Thomas's Hospitals, London.)

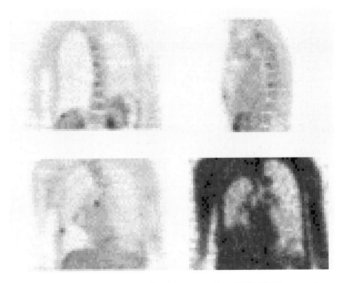

Fig. 1.98 Recurrent tumour after lung resection. FDG-PET images show active deposits in right lung, mediastinum, liver and bone. (Courtesy of the Clinical PET Centre, Guy's and St Thomas's Hospitals, London.)

active metabolism of malignant deposits is shown by PET irrespective of the size of the involved nodes, allowing a significant improvement in the accuracy of preoperative staging compared with CT alone (Figs 1.96, 1.97). Areas of residual scarring often develop after radiotherapy or chemotherapy and mediastinal anatomy may be difficult to interpret after surgery. The detection of residual or recurrent disease in these circumstances is particularly difficult, and again, the intensity of FDG uptake as shown by PET will often distinguish recurrent malignancy from fibrosis (Fig. 1.98).

Solitary lung nodules

Although some solitary lung nodules have CT features pointing strongly towards a specific pathology, many remain indeterminate. PET is used to identify those which are distinctly benign

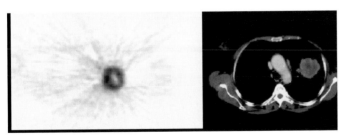

Fig. 1.96 Resectable carcinoma of the lung. FDG-PET (A) and CT (B) images show primary tumour but no mediastinal lesions; correct staging was confirmed at surgery and histology. (Courtesy of the Clinical PET Centre, Guy's and St Thomas's Hospitals, London.)

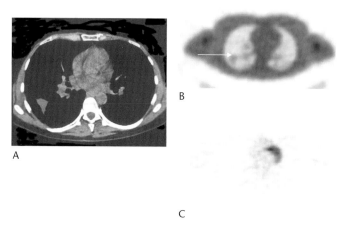

Fig. 1.99 Benign solitary lung nodule. The lesion shown on CT (A) and on the PET transmission image (B) is inactive on the FDG-PET image (C). (Reproduced with permission from Maisey et al.)

(low uptake of FDG; Fig. 1.99) and those which have a high probability of being malignant (high uptake of FDG). Using PET in this way, the number of thoracotomies for benign disease is reduced, and biopsy can be avoided in a substantial proportion of cases.

LUNG BIOPSY

The following techniques are employed:

1. *Open biopsy* is obtained at surgery and entails the risks of a thoracotomy and general anaesthetic, although an adequate specimen is obtained. With the increased use of percutaneous and endoscopic techniques, open biopsy is undertaken less often.

2. During *flexible bronchoscopy* biopsy can be made of central lesions. Brushings, washings and bacterial samples may be obtained. The success rate is high and the complication rate low.

3. *Catheter biopsy* is made with a French 7 or 8 catheter inserted via the cricothyroid membrane and screened into the relevant bronchus. Central masses can be biopsied.

4. *Percutaneous biopsy* has become a routine procedure in many centres. It may be performed with a fine needle (22–23 gauge) for aspiration or with a cutting needle using fluoroscopy, CT and, when appropriate, ultrasound.

The procedure is contraindicated in patients on anticoagulants or with a bleeding diathesis, or if the mass is thought to be vascular. It is inadvisable in patients with multiple bulles, in those with pulmonary hypertension, and in patients who have had a pneumonectomy. Patient cooperation is essential and uncontrolled coughing a contraindication. Biopsy of a suspected hydatid cyst is inadvisable because of the theoretical risk of anaphylaxis.

Using aspiration fine needle cytology the diagnostic yield is high for non-lymphomatous malignancy, in the region of 95% for a lesion exceeding 5 mm, but lower for benign lesions, around 75%. Fine needle aspiration (FNA) has the disadvantage that the tumour cell type cannot be determined and it is important to be able to distinguish between small cell and non-small cell tumours as the treatment is different. FNA has a yield of 70% in the diagnosis of pulmonary infective processes. In addition there is a low complication rate. In some centres FNA is the preferred initial technique for a suspected malignancy reverting to core biopsy if the result is non-diagnostic.

Large-bore cutting needles (18–20 gauge) are used for pleural-based and intrapulmonary masses. Up to six passes are made. The specificity is reported as 100% and the sensitivity 90%. There is a higher associated incidence of pneumothorax.

The site of the lesion must be determined. Biopsy is performed using biplanar screening or CT. Ultrasound can be used for pleural and chest wall lesions as well as peripheral lung masses. The shortest route is determined for passage of the needle avoiding vascular structures, the fissures and bulles. The puncture site is marked and anaesthetised before inserting the needle on suspended respiration. Ideally the biopsy is taken from the periphery of a mass to avoid central necrotic tissue and to increase the likelihood of a positive biopsy. Some resistance is often experienced on entering the mass. Once its position is confirmed the biopsy is taken. With a fine needle suction is applied with a syringe and several passes are made with the needle. Ideally a cytologist should be at hand to prepare the slides.

Following the biopsy, a CT image or a chest film are taken to exclude a pneumothorax (Fig. 1.100). This has a reported incidence of some 20%, although only one-fifth of these will require tube drainage. Initially the pneumothorax can be aspirated and drainage is only necessary if the pneumothorax recurs. The incidence is higher with smaller lesions and those further away from the chest wall. The patient should lie biopsy side down for 4 hours to reduce the risk of a pneumothorax, with a film taken after this time prior to discharge.

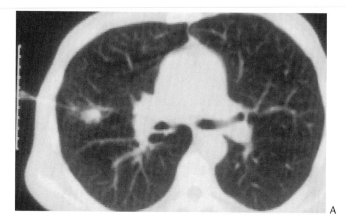

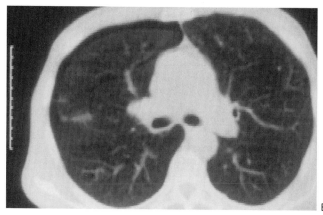

Fig. 1.100 (A) CT percutaneous biopsy right lung mass (carcinoma). (B) Small right pneumothorax.

Complications reported include:

1. pneumothorax
2. haemoptysis—incidence 10%, usually transient
3. intraparenchymal bleeding (5%)
4. haemothorax
5. empyema
6. subcutaneous emphysema, pneumomediastinum
7. seeding of malignant cells along the needle track
8. air embolism (very rare)
9. death (reported rate of 1 : 5–10 000).

BRONCHOGRAPHY

Until recently bronchography was the definitive investigation for the diagnosis of bronchiectasis (Fig. 1.101) and for assessing the extent of the disease. High-resolution CT is now widely preferred (Fig. 1.102). Occasionally bronchography is used to investigate recurrent haemoptysis when all other investigations are negative and to demonstrate bronchopleural fistulas and congenital lesions such as sequestration and agenesis. Rarely it is used to elucidate the nature of a lesion by assessing bronchial distortion and displacement.

Severe or partial impairment of pulmonary function, massive haemoptysis, recent pneumonia, active tuberculosis and a history of allergy are recognised contraindications. A limited examination is performed if pulmonary function is reduced.

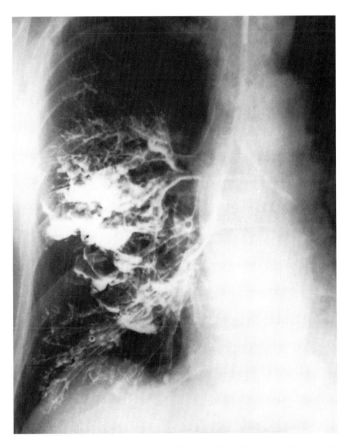

Fig. 1.101 Bronchogram. Patient with cystic bronchiectasis. The majority of the bronchi outlined with contrast medium are dilated.

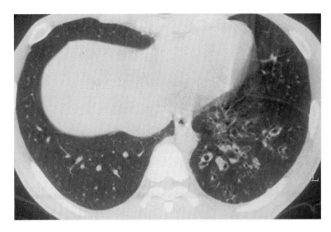

Fig. 1.102 High-resolution CT. Left lower lobe bronchiectasis.

The technique is well described elsewhere. Approaches include cricothyroid puncture, nasal or transoral drip, and tracheal intubation under local or general anaesthesia. Bronchography by contrast inhalation is not widely performed. Physiotherapy before and after the procedure, and atropine to reduce the secretions are essential. Films taken include AP, lateral, obliques and, if necessary, tomograms. Delayed films demonstrate distal filling. Cinebronchography has its exponents.

All the bronchi should be surveyed for evidence of narrowing, occlusion, intraluminal filling defects and dilated mucosal glands, as seen with bronchitis and bronchiectasis.

ULTRASOUND

The acoustic mismatch between the chest wall and the adjacent aerated lung results in almost total reflection of the ultrasonic beam. Therefore ultrasound is useful only for assessing superficial pulmonary, pleural-based and chest wall lesions. It is helpful in the diagnosis and localisation of pleural effusions and collections and their drainage percutaneously, for subphrenic collections, in differentiating fluid from a mass lesion, and for studying diaphragm movement. Biopsy of the pleura and chest wall lesions may be performed with ultrasound guidance using a cutting needle or fine needle.

A 3.5 or 5.0 mHz transducer is preferred. Scanning can be performed with the patient sitting upright or supine. On supine scanning the right diaphragm and surrounding areas are clearly seen through the liver (Fig. 1.103). However, on the left side visualisation is hampered by intervening bowel. Filling the stomach with water to use as an acoustic window and scanning obliquely improves visualisation.

Pleural fluid appears as an echofree area outlining the pleural space (Fig. 1.104). Internal echoes may be due to blood or pus, with septa indicating loculation and a thick wall suggesting an empyema, within which gas may be occasionally identified.

Pleural-based masses are usually of low echogenicity and pleural thickening is easily identified. If consolidation is visualised fluid-filled or air-filled bronchi may be seen within it.

Percutaneous drainage of fluid collections
Persistent large parapneumonic and malignant effusions and empyema can be drained percutaneously with ultrasound or CT

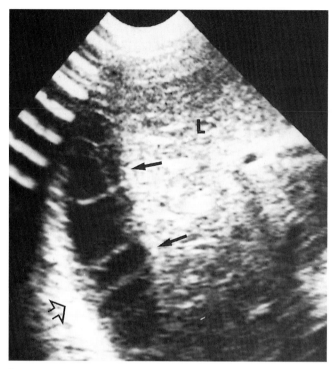

Fig. 1.103 Ultrasound scan of subphrenic abscess. There is a transonic area (arrows) between the liver (L) and diaphragm (open arrow). Strands crossing this area indicate loculation.

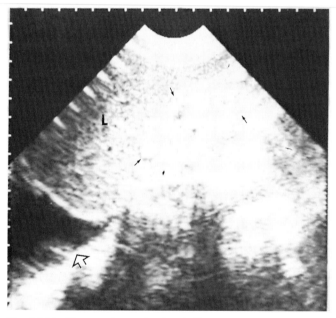

Fig. 1.104 Ultrasound scan of a pleural effusion. A patient in renal failure with acute glomerulonephritis. There is a moderate sized effusion (open arrow) seen as a transonic area in the posterior sulcus above the diaphragm. Note the highly echogenic kidney (small arrows).

guidance to ensure appropriate positioning of the drainage catheter within the collection. 7–14 French catheters have been shown to be as effective as larger bore catheters. Failure of the catheter to drain satisfactorily may be due to occlusion by thick or fibrinous fluid, to malpositioning of the catheter outside the thorax or within the

fissures, or to kinking of the catheter. Frequent flushing of the catheter with normal saline may prevent occlusion.

If the collection is multiloculated or septated, multiple drainage catheters may be necessary and intrapleural fibrinolytics such as streptokinase increase drainage success by reducing intrapleural adhesions. With malignant pleural effusions, over 90% will re-accumulate within 1 month or sooner. The recurrence rate is reduced to below 50% by the use of intrapleural agents such as tetracycline, talc and bleomycin to produce a chemical pleurodesis.

PULMONARY ANGIOGRAPHY

The main indications are:

1. diagnosis of pulmonary embolism
2. evaluation of pulmonary hypertension
3. diagnosis of vascular lesions, e.g. pulmonary hypoplasia, arteriovenous malformations, pulmonary artery aneurysms
4. embolisation of pulmonary arteriovenous malformations.

In the majority of cases embolism is excluded by a normal radionuclide perfusion scan. However for a definitive diagnosis, particularly if surgery is anticipated, angiography or contrast-enhanced spiral CT is performed. In cases of pulmonary hypertension lower doses of contrast are used because of the increased risk of cardiogenic shock.

The right heart may be approached from the basilic vein after cutdown or via the femoral vein, provided femoral, iliac and IVC thrombus has been excluded by ascending phlebography or Doppler ultrasound examination in order to prevent dislodging a large clot.

All procedures require ECG monitoring and pressure studies including right heart and pulmonary wedge pressures. A fairly rapid injection of a large bolus of contrast (50–60 ml at 20–25 ml/s) is necessary with a rapid film sequence (Fig. 1.105).

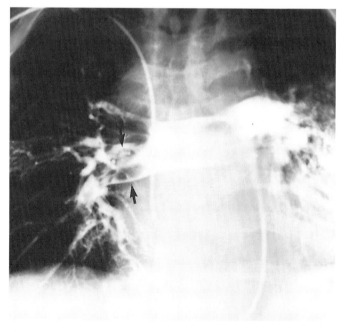

Fig. 1.105 Pulmonary angiogram. A 55-year-old man 4 days after a thoracotomy developed a DVT and pulmonary embolism. There are large thrombi (arrows) in the main arteries and peripheral perfusion is poor.

Improved arterial visualisation is achieved with selective right and left artery injections, particularly if the peripheral vessels are of interest, but the main pulmonary artery only is injected if searching for a saddle embolus.

Magnification views help in the diagnosis of small peripheral emboli, as do occlusive balloons. DSA allows the use of smaller contrast volumes but disadvantages are the relatively poor resolution and artefacts due to chest motion affecting the quality of subtraction.

Embolisation of pulmonary arteriovenous malformations is now considered the first-line treatment for these patients who are at risk from paradoxical embolism and chronic hypoxaemia. Most of these patients have hereditary haemorrhagic telangiectasia. Without treatment there is a reported mortality rate of 40% due to catastrophic haemorrhage and cerebral incidents including cerebral abscess. Embolisation is performed with metal coils or balloons.

BRONCHIAL ARTERIOGRAPHY

Angiography followed by embolisation of bronchial and intercostal branches is a recognised treatment for life-threatening or recurrent severe haemoptysis, usually due to bronchiectasis or a mycetoma, when surgery is contraindicated. Its value is limited in the investigation of pulmonary abnormalities, malignant and benign lesions often having similar vascular patterns.

The anatomy of the bronchial arteries is very variable, the spinal branches often arising from the intercostal arteries or intercostal-bronchial trunks, in which case embolisation should not be performed because of the risk of spinal cord infarction.

Success rates of up to 90% have been reported for control of bleeding in the short term, but rebleeding occurs within 6 months in around one quarter of patients, and in up to 50% in the long term.

THE CHEST WALL

The bones

The clavicles

Old healed fractures are frequent findings. Erosion of the outer ends of the clavicles is associated with rheumatoid arthritis and hyperparathyroidism. Hypoplastic clavicles may be seen with the Holt–Oram syndrome and cleidocranial dysostosis.

Sternum

Developmental abnormalities such as perforation, fissures and agenesis are rare. Several sternal abnormalities are associated with congenital heart disease; examples include sternal agenesis, premature obliteration of the ossification centres and pigeon chest which are found with ventricular septal defects, and depressed sternum, associated with atrial septal defects and Marfan's syndrome. Delayed epiphyseal fusion is a feature of cretinism, and double ossification centres in the manubrium commonly occur in Down's syndrome.

A *depressed sternum* (pectus excavatum) results in the anterior ribs being more vertical and the posterior ribs more horizontal than normal (Fig. 1.106). The heart is displaced to the left and posteriorly and appears enlarged with a straight left border and indistinct right border, with prominent lung markings and

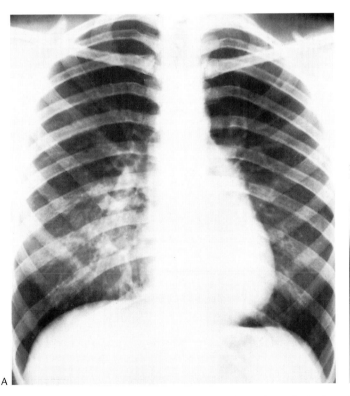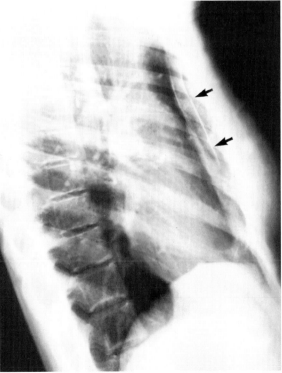

Fig. 1.106 Pectus excavatum (depressed sternum). (A) Prominent shadowing adjacent to the right heart border. The heart is displaced to the left and has a straight left border. (B) Note the posteriorly displaced sternum (arrows).

ill-defined shadowing in the right cardiophrenic angle. This should not be confused with middle lobe consolidation. The lower thoracic spine is clearly seen through the heart.

Erosion of the sternum may occur with adjacent anterior mediastinal lymphadenopathy or tumours, aortic aneurysms and infective processes.

Primary *tumours* are rare and usually cartilaginous. The sternum may be the site of metastases, lymphoma and myeloma.

Sternal fractures are often due to a steering wheel injury, with injury of the thoracic spine being commonly associated.

The ribs

Rib notching may affect the superior or inferior surface of the rib and be unilateral or bilateral.

Superior notching (Fig. 1.107) may be a normal finding in the elderly but has been reported in patients with rheumatoid arthritis, SLE, hyperparathyroidism, Marfan's syndrome, neurofibromatosis and in paraplegics and polio victims.

Inferior notching (Fig. 1.108) develops as a result of hypertrophy of the intercostal vessels or with neurogenic tumours (Box 1.20). Obstruction of the aorta results in reversed blood flow through the intercostal and internal mammary arteries. With coarctation the first

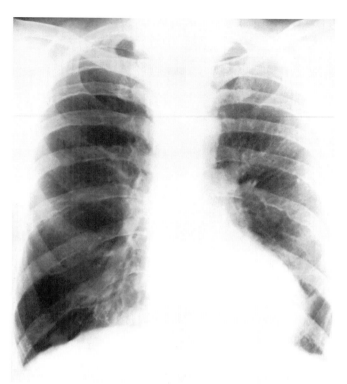

Fig. 1.108 Inferior rib notching. An elderly man who presented with hypertension. Coarctation of the aorta with rib notching most prominent in the fourth to eighth ribs.

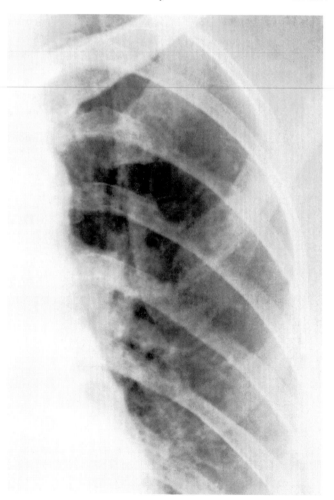

Fig. 1.107 Superior rib notching in a patient with a long history of paralysis following poliomyelitis.

Box 1.20 Causes of inferior rib notching

Unilateral
 Blalock–Taussig operation
 Subclavian artery occlusion
 Aortic coarctation involving left subclavian artery or anomalous right subclavian artery
Bilateral
 Aorta—coarcation, occlusion, aortitis
 Subclavian—Takayasu's disease, atheroma
 Pulmonary oligaemia—Fallot's tetralogy; pulmonary atresia, stenosis; truncus type IV
 Venous—SVC, IVC obstruction
 Shunts—intercostal–pulmonary fistula; pulmonary–intercostal arteriovenous fistula
 Others—hyperparathyroidism; neurogenic; idiopathic

---

and second intercostal arteries and ribs are not affected because they arise proximally from the costocervical trunk. The lower ribs are not affected unless the lower abdominal aorta is also involved. A preductal coarctation does not produce rib notching.

Congenital rib anomalies such as hypoplasia, bridging and bifid ribs are common. Hypoplastic first ribs, arising from T1, are distinguished from cervical ribs (Fig. 1.109) which arise from C7 by the transverse processes of C1 pointing caudally whereas the transverse processes of D1 are cranially inclined. Cervical ribs have an incidence of 1–2% and are usually bilateral but frequently asymmetrical.

With *Down's syndrome* there are often only 11 pairs of ribs.

An *intrathoracic rib* is uncommon. It appears as a ribbon-like shadow near to the spine attached by one or both ends.

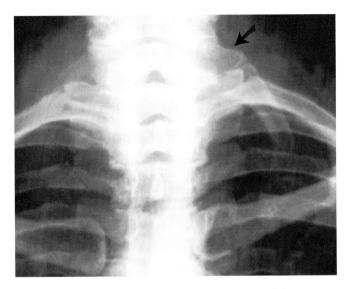

Fig. 1.109 Cervical ribs. Note the downward direction of the transverse process of C7 (arrow).

In *Tietze's syndrome* the anterior ends of the ribs are usually normal but are occasionally enlarged or have a spotty appearance.

At *surgery* a rib may be removed (Fig. 1.110) or partially amputated. Periosteal stripping results in irregularity.

Soft-tissue masses such as a lipoma or neurofibroma may displace adjacent ribs and create a defect from pressure erosion.

Crowding of the ribs occurs with a scoliosis and major pulmonary collapse, particularly in children. It is an early sign of a mesothelioma. Hyperinflation results in the ribs having a horizontal lie.

Fractures are often difficult to spot on the high kVp film. There may be an accompanying extrapleural haematoma, a pneumothorax or surgical emphysema. Callus may simulate a lung mass. The sixth to

ninth ribs in the axillary line are the common sites for *cough fractures*. *Stress fractures* usually affect the first ribs. *Pathological fractures* may be due to a local rib lesion or to a generalised reduction in bone mass as occurs with senile osteoporosis, myeloma, Cushing's disease and other endocrine disorders, steroid therapy and diffuse metastases. Cushing's disease is associated with abundant callus formation.

The *Looser's zones*, or pseudofractures, of osteomalacia represent areas of uncalcified osteoid and the resulting rib deformity creates a bell-shaped thorax.

Rib *sclerosis* occurs with generalised disorders such as osteopetrosis, myelofibrosis, fluorosis and metastases, or with localised lesions such as Paget's disease (Fig. 1.111), in which bony enlargement is characteristic. *Postirradiation necrosis* results in un-united rib fractures, bony sclerosis or an abnormal trabecular pattern and soft-tissue calcification, and is often associated with a mastectomy.

Localized *rib expansion* occurs with fibrous dysplasia, myeloma, Gaucher's disease and benign tumours such as eosinophilic granuloma, haemangioma, chondroma, the brown tumours of hyperparathyroidism and aneurysmal bone cyst. In Hurler's syndrome there is generalised expansion of the ribs, sparing the proximal ends, whereas in thalassaemia expansion is most marked proximally and the trabecular pattern abnormal. Widening of the ribs is seen with rickets (Fig. 1.112) and scurvy. *Rib destruction* due to an infection or tumour of the soft tissues, lung or pleura is usually accompanied by an extrapleural mass. Characteristically actinomycosis infection is associated with a wavy periostitis of the ribs. Many malignant processes including metastases, lymphoma and myeloma commonly destroy the ribs.

Thoracic spine

A survey is made to check for abnormal curvature or alignment, bone and disc destruction, sclerosis, paravertebral soft-tissue masses and

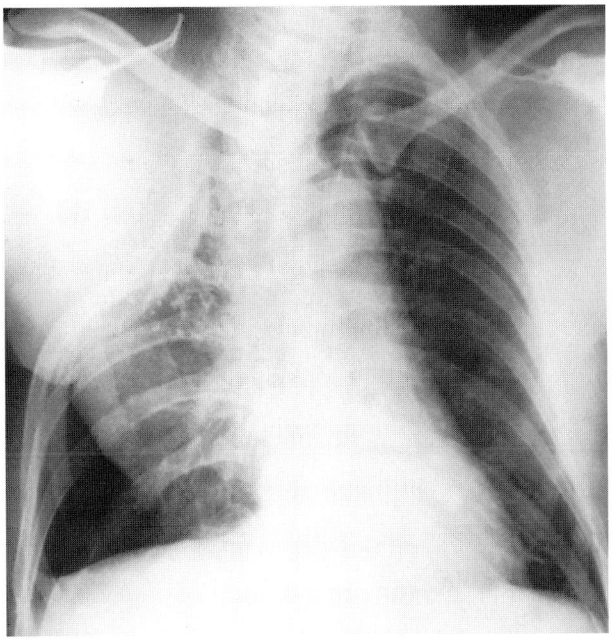

Fig. 1.110 Right thoracoplasty for tuberculosis. Removal of the upper ribs with collapse of the upper lobe.

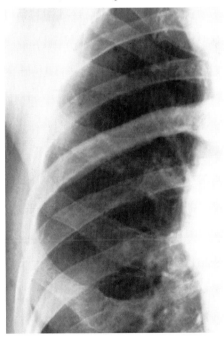

Fig. 1.111 Paget's disease. An enlarged sixth rib with a coarse trabecular pattern and of increased density.

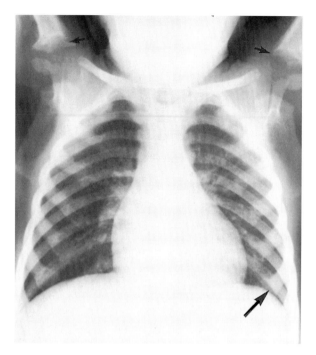

Fig. 1.112 Rickets. Enlargement and cupping of the anterior ends of the ribs (large arrow). Note the metaphyseal changes in the humeri (small arrow).

congenital lesions such as butterfly vertebrae. Scoliosis and Klippel–Feil syndrome are associated with an increased incidence of congenital heart disease. With a severe scoliosis, when the curve exceeds 60°, cardiorespiratory complications are common in adults.

With the *straight back syndrome* the normal kyphosis is reduced so that the sternum and spine are virtually parallel, resulting in compression of the mediastinum. Characteristically on the PA film the heart appears enlarged, is displaced to the left of midline and has a prominent left atrial appendage and aorta. On auscultation there is an ejection systolic murmur with accentuation on expiration.

Anterior erosion of the vertebral bodies sparing the disc spaces may occur with aneurysms of the descending aorta, vascular tumours, gross left atrial enlargement and neurofibromatosis, which may also cause posterior scalloping of the vertebral bodies and enlarged intervertebral foramina.

Destruction of a pedicle is typical of metastatic disease. A single dense vertebra, the ivory vertebra, is the classical appearance of lymphoma but is also seen with other conditions such as Paget's disease and metastases. Destruction of the disc with adjacent bony involvement is characteristic of an infective process.

Disc calcification may be idiopathic or post-traumatic and occurs in ochronosis and ankylosing spondylitis.

Soft tissues

Artefacts

Hair plaits and fasteners, buttons, clothing and jewellery, etc., overlying the lungs may simulate a lung lesion. Tracing the edges of a lesion will show whether it extends beyond the lung margins, in which case the lesion is non-pulmonary. The suprasternal fossa, particularly in the elderly, may appear as a large translucency over-lying the supraclavicular spine and should not be mistaken for a pharyngeal pouch.

Skin lesions

Skin lesions including naevi and lipomas may simulate lung tumours. Multiple nodules occur with neurofibromatosis (Fig. 1.113). Pedunculated lesions have well-defined edges, being surrounded by air, and lung markings should be visible through the lesion. It is most helpful to examine the patient.

The breast

Mastectomy is one of the commonest causes of a translucent hemithorax. With a simple mastectomy the axillary fold is normal, but following a radical mastectomy the normal downward curve of the axillary fold is replaced by a dense ascending line due to absence of pectoralis major (Fig. 1.114). In addition there may be a congenital absence of pectoralis major and minor, sometimes associated with syndactyly and rib abnormalities (*Poland's syndrome*).

Surgical emphysema

This often accompanies a pneumothorax (Fig. 1.115) and pneumo-mediastinum. After surgery an increase in the amount of emphy-

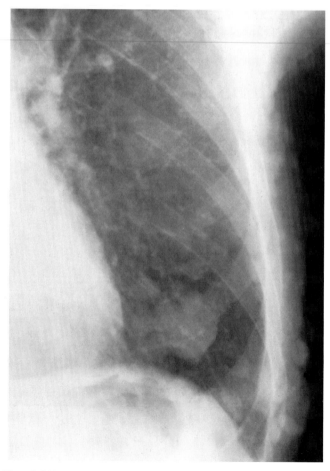

Fig. 1.113 Neurofibromatosis. Multiple soft-tissue lesions, those overlying the lung fields simulating intrapulmonary nodules.

racic duct in the left upper zone where the duct drains into the innominate vein and there may be transient miliary shadowing in the lung fields due to oil emboli. Occasionally in patients who have undergone myelography with Myodil (Pantopaque) there is tracking of the residual Myodil along the intercostal nerves to give a bizarre appearance. This contrast medium is no longer in use.

The diaphragm

The normal appearances of the diaphragm have already been described.

Normal variants

Scalloping *(Fig. 1.116)* Short curves of diaphragm convex upward are seen and this occurs predominantly on the right side.

Muscle slips *(Fig. 1.116)* These are most commonly seen in tall, thin patients and in those with emphysema. They appear as small curved lines, concave upward, and are more common on the right side.

Diaphragm humps and dromedary diaphragm *(Fig. 1.116)* These variants are probably mild forms of eventration with incomplete muscularisation of the hemidiaphragm but no muscle defect. They arise anteriorly and are usually right-sided, containing liver. There is no diaphragm defect. On the PA film the hump appears as a shadow in the right cardiophrenic angle and must

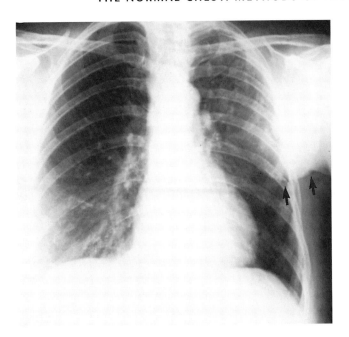

Fig. 1.114 Left mastectomy. Note the abnormal left axillary fold passing cranially (arrows). The left lung is hypertransradiant at its base. Note radiation necrosis of the upper ribs and soft-tissue calcification.

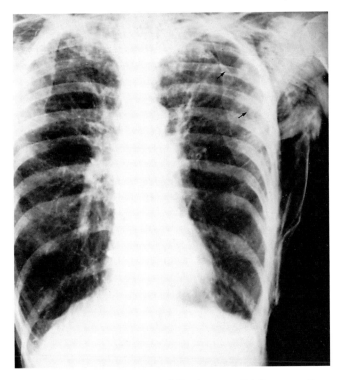

Fig. 1.115 Surgical emphysema following a small left pneumothorax (arrows) in a man with chronic obstructive airways' disease.

sema on serial films suggests the development of a bronchopleural fistula.

Miscellaneous

Calcified nodes and parasites such as cysticercosis may overlie the lung fields. After lymphography contrast may be seen in the tho-

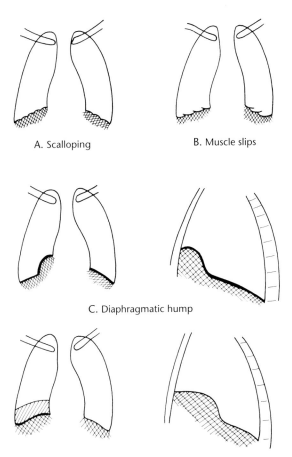

Fig. 1.116 (A–C) Normal variants of the diaphragm.

be distinguished from a fat pad, lipoma, pericardial cyst and Morgagni hernia. On the lateral film the hump overlies the cardiac shadow and should not be confused with middle lobe consolidation. The dromedary diaphragm is a more severe form of diaphragm hump appearing as a double contour on the PA view.

Eventration *(Fig. 1.117)* This is nearly always left sided, the hemidiaphragm being considerably elevated with characteristically marked mediastinal displacement to the right, a feature rarely seen with paralysis of the diaphragm. The muscle is thin and weak with movement reduced, paradoxical or absent on fluoroscopy. There may be an associated gastric volvulus with rotation along its long axis resulting in the greater curve being uppermost. Eventration must be distinguished from absence and rupture of the diaphragm as well as paralysis.

Accessory diaphragm This rare condition is asymptomatic and usually right sided. The hemithorax is partitioned by the accessory diaphragm running parallel to the oblique fissure and resembling a thickened fissure. Its blood supply is often anomalous. Reported associations are other congenital lesions of the lungs such as anomalous venous drainage and lobar hypoplasia.

Diaphragm movement

Respiratory excursion is easily assessed at fluoroscopy. Normally the left side moves slightly more than the right with an excursion of between 3 cm and 6 cm. Paradoxical movement occurs when the pressure exerted by the abdomen exceeds that of the weak diaphragm so that on inspiration or sniffing movement is upward. This occurs with diaphragm paralysis, eventration and subdiaphragmatic infection. However paradoxical movement is also seen in a small number of normal subjects. Reduced excursion of the diaphragm

frequently occurs with inflammatory processes either above or below the diaphragm; examples are subphrenic abscess and basal pneumonia.

The elevated diaphragm *(Box 1.21)*

Frequently no cause can be found to explain an elevated hemidiaphragm. The clinical history is important. It is essential to exclude an active lesion, particularly malignancy, by carefully assessing the lung fields, hila and mediastinum. Eventration is associated with marked cardiac displacement. Pleural thickening

Box 1.21 Causes of elevation of the diaphragm	
Bilateral	Pulmonary
Reduced pulmonary compliance	Pulmonary and lobar collapse
e.g., fibrosing alveolitis,	Pulmonary hypoplasia
lymphangitis, carcinomatosis	Pneumonectomy
Technical	Pulmonary embolism
Supine film, expiratory film	Basal pneumonia
Postoperative pain	Pleural
Subdiaphragmatic	Thickening
Ascites, obesity	Pleurisy
Abdominal mass, pregnancy	Subpulmonary effusion
Bowel distension	Bony
Unilateral	Scoliosis
Paralysis	Rib fractures
Surgery and trauma	Subdiaphragmatic
Idiopathic	Gas-distended viscus
Radiotherapy	Subphrenic abscess
Neoplastic	Pancreatitis
Diabetes mellitus	Abdominal mass
Infections, TB glands, herpes zoster	Hepatomegaly
Congenital	Splenomegaly
Eventration and humps	

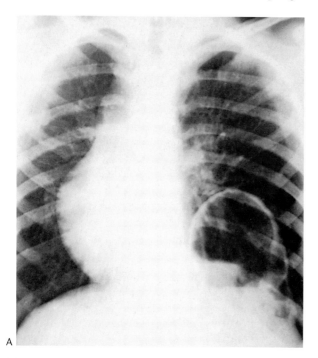

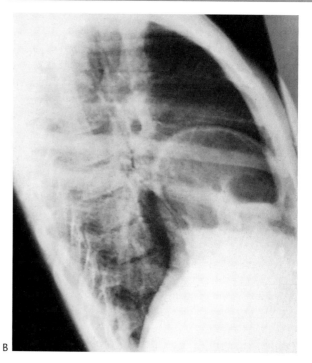

Fig. 1.117 Eventration. (A) The left cupola is elevated and the heart displaced to the right. (B) The lateral film shows the elevated left cupola with a distended stomach and a normal right cupola.

is often accompanied by tenting of the diaphragm, with loss of definition and obliteration or blunting of the costophrenic angles and thickened fissures. Subpulmonary fluid may be difficult to distinguish from an elevated diaphragm. Typically it has a straighter upper border and will change shape with patient position if it is not loculated. Loculated subpulmonary effusions are very difficult to distinguish from a high diaphragm on plain films. Ultrasound is the definitive diagnostic investigation.

Splinting of the diaphragm occurs with upper abdominal inflammatory processes, basal pneumonia and embolism.

Determining whether diaphragm elevation is due to paralysis or an abdominal mass elevating the diaphragm may be difficult on the plain film. The position of the liver edge should be noted. If the liver edge is low then there is probably a mass within or between the liver and diaphragm, whereas a normally positioned or high liver edge favours paralysis as a cause. On the left side the gastric bubble is assessed using the same principles.

A depressed diaphragm is seen with pulmonary hyperinflation and large pleural effusions.

Subphrenic abscess

These are often associated with recent surgery or sepsis. A subphrenic abscess is more common on the right than the left side. Ultrasound and CT are the investigations of choice with percutaneous drainage if appropriate.

Plain film signs of a subphrenic abscess include:

1. Ipsilateral basal atelectasis and pleural effusion.
2. Elevated hemidiaphragm with paradoxical or decreased movement.
3. Abnormal gas shadow beneath the diaphragm due to infection with gas-forming organisms (Fig. 1.118); hori-

zontal beam films improve visualisation of the abscess cavity.

4. Depression of the liver edge or gastric fundus.

The thickness of the diaphragm

The normal diaphragm is 2–3 mm thick. On the left side where the gastric bubble lies beneath the diaphragm, the stomach wall and diaphragm form a linear density 5–8 mm thick. However on the right side thickness cannot be assessed unless the inferior surface is outlined by free intraperitoneal gas. Thickening may be a normal variant but occurs with tumours of the diaphragm, stomach and pleura, subpulmonary fluid, diaphragm humps, and abdominal lesions including subphrenic abscess, hepatomegaly and splenomegaly.

Tumours of the diaphragm

Tumours of the diaphragm are rare. Benign lesions include lipomas, neurofibromas, fibromas and cysts. Sarcomas commonly present with a pleural effusion. Diaphragm tumours may appear as smooth or lobulated masses and need to be differentiated from lung and liver masses, hernias and diaphragm humps. CT is the most helpful investigation.

Hernias of the diaphragm

The classic appearance of a *hiatus hernia*, with a fluid level superimposed on the cardiac shadow on the PA film, is well known (Fig. 1.119). A *Bochdalek hernia* arises posterolaterally through the pleuroperitoneal canal and is usually congenital, presenting at birth as respiratory distress. Ninety per cent are left sided. The hernia may contain omentum, fat, spleen, kidney and bowel, in which case a gas shadow is seen within the mass. The ipsilateral lung is invariably hypoplastic with deviation of the mediastinum away from the side of the hernia. In the neonate this condition needs to be distinguished from cystic adenomatoid malformation of the lung.

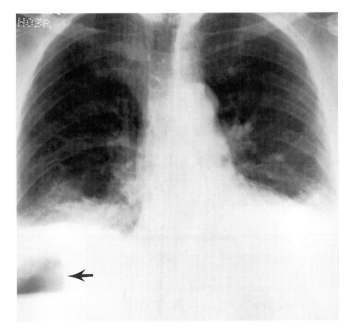

Fig. 1.118 Right subphrenic abscess following cholecystectomy. A large gas shadow with an air–fluid level is seen below the right hemidiaphragm (arrow). There are bilateral effusions with patchy shadowing at the right base.

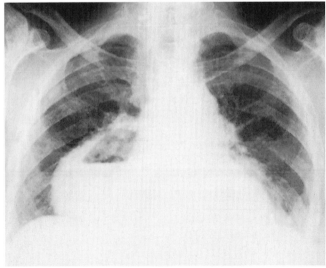

Fig. 1.119 Hiatus hernia. An elderly symptomatic patient. A large fluid level superimposed on the cardiac shadow: a typical appearance of a hiatus hernia.

The *Morgagni hernia* is usually asymptomatic, presenting in adults as an incidental finding on a chest film. It is right sided and anterior, appearing as an homogeneous shadow in the cardiophrenic angle. The hernia contains fat or occasionally bowel (Fig. 1.120).

Rupture of the diaphragm

This usually results from trauma but may be idiopathic or related to previous surgery. Presentation is commonly acute but may be delayed, in which case bowel strangulation may occur. Some 80% of cases are left sided. Herniation of the stomach with gastric obstruction is common and must be distinguished from a pneumothorax and eventration. The gastric wall rarely abuts all the borders of the thoracic cage but if there is a diagnostic problem passage of a nasogastric tube or oral contrast should be helpful. Herniation of colon, spleen and kidney is less common. Appearances on the PA film may be normal if there is rupture without herniation, or the diaphragm may be elevated with an abnormal outline. CT and ultrasound may be helpful.

REFERENCES AND SUGGESTIONS FOR FURTHER READING

Alexander, G. (1966) Diaphragmatic movement and the diagnosis of diaphragmatic paralysis. *Clinical Radiology*, **17**, 79–83.
Armstrong, P., Wilson, A. G., Dee, P., Hansel, D. M. (2000) *Imaging of Diseases of the Chest*, 3rd edn. St Louis: Mosby.
Bergin, C. J., Muller, N. L. (1985) CT in the diagnosis of interstitial lung disease. *American Journal of Roentgenology*, **145**, 505–510.
Boone, M. L., Swenson, B. E., Felson, B. (1964) Rib notching: its many causes. *American Journal of Roentgenology*, **91**, 1075–1088.
Campbell, J. A. (1963) The diaphragm in roentgenology of the chest. *Radiologic Clinics of North America*, **1**, 394–410.
Felson, B. (1967) The roentgen diagnosis of disseminated pulmonary alveolar diseases. *Seminars in Radiology*, **2**, 3–21.
Felson, B. (1973) *Chest Roentgenology*. Philadelphia: W. B. Saunders.
Felson, B. (1979) A new look at pattern recognition of diffuse pulmonary disease. *American Journal of Roentgenology*, **133**, 183–189.
Felson, B., Felson, H. (1950) Localisation of intrathoracic lesions in the PA roentgenogram. *Radiology* **55**: 363–374.
Fleischner, F. G. (1941) Linear shadows in the lung. *American Journal of Roentgenology*, **46**, 610–618.
Fraser, R. G., Pare, J. A. P., Fraser, R. S., Genereux, G. P. (1991) *Diagnosis of Diseases of the Chest*, 4th edn. Philadelphia: W. B. Saunders.
Freeman, L. M., Blaufox, M. D. (1980) Radionuclide studies of the lung. *Seminars in Nuclear Medicine*, **x**, 198–310.
Godwin, J. D., Tarver, R. D. (1985) Accessory fissures of the lung. *American Journal of Roentgenology*, **144**, 39–47.
Golden, R. (1925) The effect of bronchostenosis upon the roentgen-ray shadows in carcinoma of the bronchus. *American Journal of Roentgenology*, **13**, 21–30.
Goralnik, C. H., O'Connell, D. M., El Yousef, S. J., Haage, J. R. (1988) CT-guided cutting-needle biopsies of selected chest lesions. *American Journal of Roentgenology*, **151**, 903–907.
Greene, R., McCloud, T. C., Stark, P. (1977) Pneumothorax. *Seminars in Roentgenology*, **12**, 313–325.
Huston, J., Muhm, J. R. (1987). Solitary pulmonary opacities: plain tomography. *Radiology*, **163**, 481–485.
Jereb, M. (1980) The usefulness of needle biopsy in chest lesions of different sizes and locations. *Radiology*, **134**, 13–15.
Keats, T. E. (1979) *An Atlas of Normal Roentgen Variants that may Simulate Disease*, 2nd edn, pp. 427–500. Chicago: Year Book Medical Publishers.
Kerr, I. H. (1984) Interstitial lung disease: the role of the radiologist. *Clinical Radiology*, **35**, 1–7.
Khouri, N. F., Stitik, F. P., Erozan, Y. S., et al (1985) Transthoracic needle aspiration biopsy of benign and malignant lung lesions. *American Journal of Roentgenology*, **144**, 281–288.
Lavender, J. P. (1982) Radioisotope lung scanning and the chest radiograph in pulmonary disease. In: Steiner, R. E., Lodge, E. (eds) *Recent Advances in Radiology 6*. Edinburgh: Churchill Livingstone.
Milne, E. N. C. (1973) Correlation of physiologic findings with chest radiology. *Radiologic Clinics of North America*, **11**, 17–47.
Proto, A. V., Tocino, I. (1980) Radiographic manifestations of lobar collapse. *Seminars in Roentgenology*, **15**, 117–173.
Reed, J. C., Madewell, J. E. (1975) The air bronchogram in interstitial disease of the lungs. *Radiology*, **116**, 1–9.
Remy, J., Armand, A., Fardon, H. (1977) Treatment of haemoptysis by embolisation of bronchial arteries. *Radiology*, **122**, 33–37.
Ruskin, J. A., Gurney, J. W., Thorsen, M. K., Goodman, L. R. (1987) Detection of pleural effusions on supine chest radiographs. *American Journal of Roentgenology*, **148**, 681–683.
Sandler, M. S., Velchick, M. G., Alavi, A. (1988) Ventilation abnormalities associated with pulmonary embolism. *Clinics in Nuclear Medicine*, **13**, 450–458.
Savoca, C. J., Austin, J. H. M., Goldberg, H. I. (1977) The right paratracheal stripe. *Radiology*, **122**, 295–301.
Simon, G. (1975) The anterior view chest radiograph—criteria for normality derived from a basic analysis of the shadows. *Clinical Radiology*, **26**, 429–437.

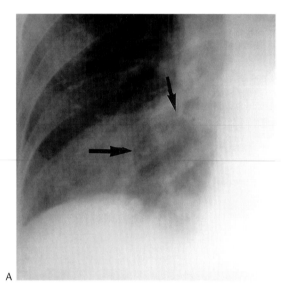

A

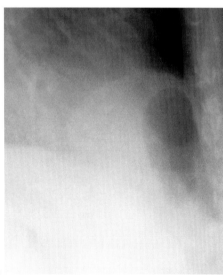

B

Fig. 1.120 Morgagni hernia. (A) Soft-tissue mass in the right cardiophrenic angle with an associated gas shadow (arrowed). (B) Hernia containing loop of bowel lying anteriorly in lateral view.

Simon, G. (1978) *Principles of Chest X-ray Diagnosis*, 4th edn. London: Butterworths.

Simon, G., Bonnell, J., Kazantzis, G., Waller, R. E. (1969) Some radiological observations on the range of movement of the diaphragm. *Clinical Radiology*, **20**, 231–233.

Strickland, B. (1976) Sentinel lines—an unusual sign of lower lobe contraction. *Thorax*, **31**, 517–521.

Tattersall, D. J., Traill, Z. C, Gleeson, F. V. (2000) Chest drains: does size matter? *Clinical Radiology*, **55**, 415–421.

Trapnell, D. (1973) The differential diagnosis of linear shadows in chest radiographs. *Radiologic Clinics of North America*, **11**, 77–92.

Vix, V. A., Klatte, E. C. (1970) The lateral chest radiograph in the diagnosis of hilar and mediastinal masses. *Radiology*, **96**, 307–316.

CT of the lungs

Council, The Royal College of Radiologists (1994) *The Use of Computed Tomography in the Initial Investigation of Common Malignancies*, pp.15–16. London: Royal College of Radiologists.

Dalrymple-Hay, M. J. R., Drury, N. E. (2001) Screening for lung cancer. *Journal of the Royal Society of Medicine, * **94**, 2–5.

Irie,T. et al (2001) Biopsy of lung nodules with use of I-I device under intermittent CT fluoroscopic guidance: preliminary clinical study. *Journal of Vascular and Interventional Radiology*, **12**, 215–219

Muller, N. L. (ed.) (1991) Imaging of diffuse lung diseases. *Radiologic Clinics of North America*, **29**, 1043–1094.

Padley, S.P.G. (2001) Thoracic radiology. *Clinical Radiology*, **56**, 191–192.

Remy-Jardine, M., Remy, J., Farre, I., Marquette, C. H. (1992) Computed tomographic evaluation of silicosis and coal workers pneumoconiosis. *Radiologic Clinics of North America*, **30**, 1155–1176.

Rubboli, A. and Euler, D. E. (2000) Current perspectives. The diagnosis of acute pulmonary embolism. A review of the literature and current clinical practice. *Italian Heart Journal*, **1**, 585–594.

Rydberg, J., et al (2000) Multisection CT: scanning techniques and clinical applications. *Radiographics*, **20**, 1787–1806.

Staples, C. A. (1992) Computed tomography in the evaluation of benign asbestos-related disorders. *Radiologic Clinics of North America*, **30**, 1191–1208.

Tockman, M. S., Mulshine, J. L. (2000) The early detection of occult lung cancer. *Chest Surgery Clinics of North America*, **10**, 737–749.

Wegener, O. H. (1992) The lungs. In: *Whole Body Computed Tomography*, pp.182–222. Massachusetts: Blackwell Scientific.

Woodring, J. H. (ed.) (1990) Lung cancer. *Radiologic Clinics of North America*, **28**, 511–646.

MRI

Edelman, R. R., Hesselink, J. R., Zlatkin, M. B. (eds) (1996) *Clinical Magnetic Resonance Imaging*, 2nd edn. Philadelphia: W.B. Saunders.

Mayo, J. R. (1994) Magnetic resonance imaging of the chest: where we stand. *Radiologic Clinics of North America*, **32**, 795–809.

Moller, T. B., Reif, E. R. (eds) (2000) *Pocket Atlas of Sectional Anatomy: Computed Tomography and Magnetic Resonance Imaging*, vol 2. *Thorax, Abdomen, Pelvis*, 2nd edn. Thieme Publishing Group.

Naidich, D. P., Webb, R., Mueller, N. L., Krinsky, G. A., Zerhouni, E. A., Siegelman, S. S. (eds) (2000) *Computed Tomography and Magnetic Resonance of the Thorax*, 3rd edn. New York: Lippincott Williams & Wilkins.

Radionuclide imaging

Blum, J., Handmaker, H., Lister-James, J., Rinne, N. (2000) A multicentre trial with a somatostatin analogue (99m)Tc depreotide in the evaluation of solitary pulmonary nodules. *Chest*, **117**, 1232–1238.

Coleman, R. E. (1999) PET in lung cancer. *Journal of Nuclear Medicine*, **40**, 814–820.

Maisey, M. N., Wahl, R. W., Barrington, S. F. (1999) *Atlas of Clinical Positron Emission Tomography*. Springer.

O'Doherty, M. J. (1998) Other pulmonary applications. In: Maisey, M. N., Britton, K. E., Collier, B. D. (eds) *Clinical Nuclear Medicine*. London: Chapman and Hall, pp. 237–244.

Royal, H. D. (1998) Pulmonary embolism. In: Maisey, M. N., Britton, K. E. Collier, B. D. (eds) *Clinical Nuclear Medicine*, pp. 215–230. London: Chapman and Hall.

Schuster, D. P. (1998) The evaluation of lung function with PET. *Seminars in Nuclear Medicine*, **28**, 341–351.

Suga, K., Matsuoka, T., Tanaka, T. et al (1998) Lung volume reduction surgery for pulmonary emphysema using dynamic xenon-133 and Tc99m-MAA SPECT images. *Annals of Thoracic and Cardiovascular Surgery*, **4**, 149–153.

2

THE MEDIASTINUM

Roger H. S. Gregson
with contributions from Richard W. Whitehouse, Andrew R. Wright and Jeremy P. R. Jenkins

Mediastinal disease is usually initially demonstrated on a chest radiograph and appears as a mediastinal soft-tissue mass, widening of the mediastinum or a pneumomediastinum. However the chest radiograph may appear normal in the presence of mediastinal disease, which is subsequently clearly demonstrated by CT or MRI.

The commonest mediastinal abnormalities seen on a chest radiograph in adults are undoubtedly lymph node enlargement, vascular abnormalities and a hiatus hernia, but in infants and children the commonest abnormality is the normal thymus gland. Mediastinal tumours, cysts and lymph node masses tend to predominate in surgically treated patients with about 20% thymic tumours, 20% neurogenic tumours, 20% benign foregut cysts, 15% lymphoma, 10% germ cell tumours, 5% thyroid masses and 5% mesenchymal and other tumours occurring in most series.

The typical sites of the common and rare mediastinal masses are shown in Figure 2.1 and Table 2.1, and although it is initially helpful to localise a mediastinal mass into one of the anatomical compartments of the mediastinum it is important to remember that they can involve adjacent compartments.

ANATOMY

The mediastinum is situated between the lungs in the centre of the thorax. It extends from the thoracic inlet above to the central tendon of the diaphragm below with the sternum anteriorly, the thoracic spine posteriorly and the parietal pleura laterally.

It is useful to divide up the mediastinum into three parts from a radiological point of view, because the differential diagnosis of a mediastinal mass is dependent upon its anatomical location. The anterior division lies in front of the anterior pericardium and trachea, the middle division within the pericardial cavity but including the trachea, and the posterior division lies behind the posterior pericardium and trachea. Some structures such as the thoracic aorta and the mediastinal lymph nodes are present in all three divisions.

The anatomical structures that produce the outline of the mediastinum on a chest radiograph are discussed in Chapter 1, but by using a high kV technique (120–150 kVp) the various mediastinal lines such as the anterior and posterior junctional lines, the right

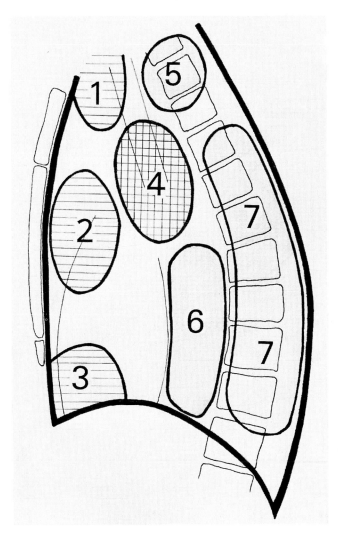

Fig. 2.1 Typical sites of the common and rare mediastinal masses listed in Table 2.1.

Table 2.1 The anatomical location of mediastinal masses

Position in mediastinum	Common lesions	Rare lesions
Anterior division	1. Tortuous innominate artery Lymph node enlargement Retrosternal goitre Fat deposition	Aneurysm of innominate artery Parathyroid adenoma Lymphangioma
	2. Lymph node enlargement Aneurysm of ascending aorta Thymoma Germ cell tumour	Sternal mass Lipoma Haemangioma
	3. Epicardial fat pad Diaphragmatic hump Pleuropericardial cyst	Morgagni's hernia
Middle division	4. Lymph node enlargement Aneurysm of aortic arch Enlarged pulmonary artery Dilatation of superior vena cava Bronchogenic cyst	Tracheal lesion Cardiac tumour
Posterior division	5. Neurogenic tumour Pharyngo-oesophageal pouch	
	6. Hiatus hernia Aneurysm of descending aorta Oesophageal dilatation Dilatation of azygos vein	Neurenteric cyst Pancreatic pseudocyst Sequestrated lung segment
	7. Neurogenic tumour Paravertebral mass	Bochdalek's hernia Extramedullary haemopoiesis

paratracheal stripe, the azygo-oesophageal line, the descending thoracic aortic line and the right and left paraspinal lines are often demonstrated. CT shows how the lines are formed by the X-ray beam passing tangential to the pleural-covered surfaces of these mediastinal structures adjacent to the lungs.

All the anatomical structures within the mediastinum are surrounded by fatty connective tissue and are well demonstrated by CT, including the phrenic nerves. The anatomy is illustrated diagrammatically at various levels through the mediastinum in Figure 2.2 and is discussed below.

RADIOLOGICAL INVESTIGATION

Patients with mediastinal disease may be completely asymptomatic or present with symptoms and signs suggesting intrathoracic pathology. Symptoms such as a cough, chest pain and weight loss are quite non-specific, but dysphagia, stridor and superior vena caval obstruction are helpful in localising the mediastinal disease process to an anatomical site. Patients with myasthenia gravis may

have an occult thymoma and it is important to assess the anterior mediastinum with CT in these cases.

A mediastinal abnormality is detected by observing a change in the normal mediastinal radiographic anatomy on a chest radiograph. The mediastinal mass usually has a sharp well-defined outline, may displace or compress mediastinal structures and produces an obtuse angle with the adjacent lung.

A variety of imaging modalities are available for investigating the mediastinum, but CT and MRI are undoubtedly the most versatile radiological investigations for evaluating an abnormality demonstrated on the high kV chest radiograph. The indications for their use include:

1. the investigation of an obvious mediastinal mass
2. the investigation of the wide mediastinum
3. the investigation of the abnormal hilum
4. the staging of malignant disease
5. the investigation of a suspected vascular abnormality
6. the detection of occult mediastinal disease.

The chest radiograph may be the only radiological investigation required to confirm the cause of a mediastinal abnormality such as a hiatus hernia, but CT and MRI are used to demonstrate the size and position of a mediastinal mass and to assess its relationship to the surrounding structures as well as its attenuation value or signal intensity. Even with CT a histological diagnosis cannot necessarily be made as many of the mediastinal lesions have similar appearances.

Calcification is well demonstrated by CT (but not MRI) and occurs in a number of mediastinal lesions, as shown in Box 2.1. The presence of fat in a mediastinal mass is a more helpful diagnostic feature as it only occurs in germ cell tumours, a mediastinal hernia, a thymolipoma, and a lipoma or a liposarcoma. The demonstration of fluid, which has an attenuation value of 0 to +20 HU, indicates a mediastinal cyst, but if this contains either mucoid or haemorrhagic material the attenuation value may reach +50 HU and the mass can then be mistaken for a solid tumour. Necrosis and cystic degeneration within a solid tumour produce an attenuation valve lower than soft tissue.

CT can distinguish between lymphadenopathy, fat deposition and haemorrhage when there is mediastinal widening on a chest radiograph and can differentiate between a solid mass and a pulmonary vessel when there is an abnormal hilum. CT is used in the staging of malignant disease to demonstrate mediastinal lymph node enlargement, pulmonary and bone metastases in the chest, and hepatic and adrenal metastases in the abdomen. CT is also used to detect occult disease in the mediastinum, such as a thymoma or enlarged lymph nodes, when the chest radiograph appears normal. A mediastinal lymph node is regarded as normal if it has a short axis diameter of less than 10 mm, and as enlarged if it has a short axis diameter of more than 15 mm. CT (or MRI) cannot however distinguish between reactive hyperplasia, and inflammatory or neoplastic causes of lymph node enlargement. The superior pericardial recesses and vascular anomalies also mimic enlarged nodes.

CT and MRI can both confirm the diagnosis of an aortic aneurysm, aortic dissection and pulmonary emboli, but MRI does not necessarily require contrast medium and can also produce direct coronal, sagittal and oblique images, whereas CT needs a reconstruction to produce these other planar projections. MRI should therefore be used in patients with a contraindication to intravenous non-ionic contrast medium but can also be used in patients with a

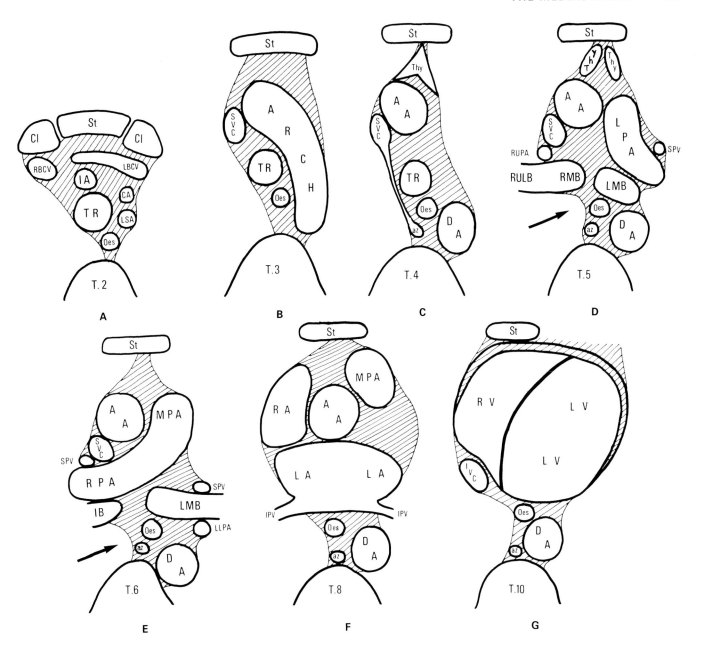

Fig. 2.2 Normal mediastinal anatomy at various levels through the thorax and features which can be identified by CT. (A) Above the aortic arch through the sternoclavicular joints. (B) Arch of aorta. (C) Below the aortic arch through the aortopulmonary window. (D) Left pulmonary artery. (E) Main and right pulmonary arteries. (F) Left and right atria. (G) Left and right ventricles. Arch = arch of aorta; AA = ascending aorta; DA = descending aorta; IA = innominate artery; CA = left common carotid artery; LSA = left subclavian artery; MPA = main pulmonary artery; RPA = right pulmonary artery; LPA = left pulmonary artery; RUPA = right upper lobe pulmonary artery; LLPA = left lower lobe pulmonary artery; SPV = superior pulmonary vein; IPV = inferior pulmonary vein; SVC = superior vena cava; IVC = inferior vena cava; a. = azygos vein; RBCV and LBCV = right and left brachiocephalic or innominate veins; TR = trachea; RMB = right main bronchus; LMB = left main bronchus; IB = intermediate bronchus; RULB = right upper lobe bronchus; LV = left ventricle; RV = right ventricle; LA = left atrium; RA = right atrium; Oes = oesophagus; St = sternum; Cl = clavicle; Thy = thymus gland; → = azygo-oesophageal recess.

posterior mediastinal mass because it demonstrates involvement of the spinal canal so well.

Fine needle biopsy of mediastinal mass lesions is being increasingly used to produce a pathological diagnosis instead of mediastinoscopy or a surgical exploration. Aspiration of mediastinal cysts can also be performed. These procedures are carried out under local anaesthetic using an 18–22 gauge needle with CT guidance (see Fig. 2.15), although fluoroscopy and ultrasound can also be used.

They produce a histological diagnosis in about 80% of patients but in the remainder a specific diagnosis cannot be made because the small samples of tissue obtained in comparison to a surgical biopsy, limit the pathological interpretation, especially in the diagnosis of lymphoma and thymoma. The complications of these procedures include a minor pneumothorax in 15% of patients, a major pneumothorax requiring treatment in 3% of patients, haemoptysis, mediastinal haematoma and haemorrhage into the pleura or pericardium.

Box 2.1 The causes of calcification in a mediastinal mass

Anterior mediastinum
Aneurysm of ascending aorta
Retrosternal goitre
Thymoma
Germ cell tumour
Lymphoma after radiotherapy
Haemangioma

Middle mediastinum
Lymph node enlargement
  Tuberculosis
  Histoplasmosis
  Lymphoma after radiotherapy
  Sarcoidosis
  Silicosis
  Amyloidosis
  Mucin-secreting adenocarcinoma

Aneurysm of aortic arch
Bronchogenic cyst

Posterior mediastinum
Aneurysm of descending aorta
Neurogenic tumour
  Neuroblastoma
  Neurofibrosarcoma
  Ganglioneuroma
Neurenteric cyst
Abscess
Haematoma
Leiomyoma of oesophagus

Barium studies, radionuclide imaging, ultrasound and angiography are still occasionally used to confirm a particular diagnosis in mediastinal disease.

CT OF THE MEDIASTINUM

Richard W. Whitehouse and Andrew R. Wright

Technical considerations

The greater proportion of the mediastinal volume is occupied by the heart and blood vessels and their contents. Adequate evaluation of the mediastinum therefore requires understanding and demonstration of the vascular anatomy. Spiral CT scanning with the use of intravenous contrast enhancement is ideal for CT demonstration of the mediastinum. Multislice CT allows more rapid data acquisition with thinner slices (typically 2.5–5 mm), giving improved in-plane resolution and better multiplanar and 3D reconstructions.

Normal appearances

If adequate mediastinal fat is present, the major vascular structures of the mediastinum, the trachea and the oesophagus can be accurately identified (Fig. 2.2) and abnormal masses distinguished. At the level of the sternoclavicular joints, an axial CT section will demonstrate the trachea as an air-filled round or horseshoe-shaped structure lying centrally. Surrounding it in a clockwise direction from the right anterolateral position round to a posterior position lie the brachiocephalic trunk ('innominate artery'), the left common carotid artery, the left subclavian artery and the oesophagus. Anterior to this ring of structures lie the right and left brachiocephalic veins. The right vein is rounded in cross-section, reflecting its vertical orientation, whilst the left vein is oval or tadpole shaped as it courses obliquely from left to right across the anterior mediastinum (Fig. 2.3A). On lower sections these veins join to form the superior vena cava, lying to the right of the ascending aorta (Fig. 2.3B,C). Dense intravenous contrast medium may cause significant artefacts from these veins; lower density contrast may be appropriate (200 mg I/ml) if dynamic contrast-enhanced scanning of the upper mediastinum or neck is performed.

A CT section at the level of the manubrio-sternal junction will demonstrate the arch of the aorta curving round to the left of the trachea with the superior vena cava and oesophagus to the right of the anterior and posterior parts respectively (Fig. 2.3B). Sections below this will demonstrate the ascending and descending aortic limbs. The thymus lies anterior to the ascending aorta and may be seen as an arrowhead-shaped structure in the anterior mediastinal fat. The azygos vein appears posterolaterally to the right of the oesophagus and passes forward to join the superior vena cava over the top of the junction between the right main bronchus and right upper lobe bronchus (Fig. 2.3C), seen on the adjacent section (Fig. 2.3D). The division of the trachea into right and left main bronchi occurs at around the level of the fifth thoracic vertebra. The left pulmonary artery appears on this section as it passes over the top of the left main bronchus whilst the main pulmonary trunk and right pulmonary artery appear on lower sections (Fig. 2.3E), coursing from the left, adjacent to the ascending aorta, to the right, anterior to the bronchus intermedius, through the middle of the mediastinum. On sections below the carina, the left atrium appears anterior to the oesophagus and descending aorta (Fig. 2.3F). The superior vena cava blends into the right atrium, becoming larger and less rounded in shape. The pulmonary trunk passes anterior to the aortic root to arise from the right ventricle (Fig. 2.3G). Posterior to the ascending aorta, the superior pericardial recess may cause a water density mass which should not be mistaken for a lymph node. At the level of the ventricles, the interventricular septum may be identified on contrast-enhanced scans as a soft-tissue density

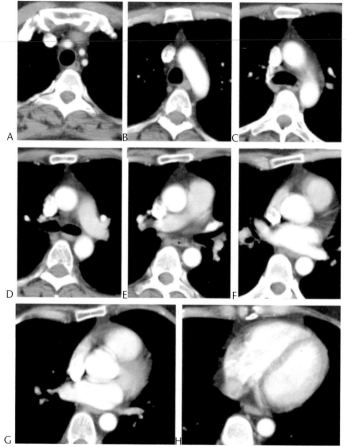

Fig. 2.3 (A–H) Contrast-enhanced sections illustrating the vascular anatomy of the mediastinum.

band between the denser contrast-laden blood in the ventricles (Fig. 2.3H). The diaphragmatic crura are clearly seen on lower sections, surrounding the aortic hiatus as curvilinear soft-tissue bands. The right crus is commonly longer and thicker than the left and can mimic a para-aortic mass on upper abdominal sections. The retrocrural space contains fat, the aorta, the azygos vein, thoracic duct and lymph nodes; the latter should not be greater than 6 mm in diameter.

The tissue planes contributing to the lines, edges and stripes identified on conventional chest radiographs can be directly identified and evaluated, thus the right paratracheal stripe is formed by the interface between the right upper lobe and the right lateral wall of the trachea. The *azygo-oesophageal recess* is part of the right lower lobe, bounded by the posterior wall of the right main bronchus, the oesophagus and the azygos vein. Carinal node enlargement expands into this space at an early stage. The *aortopulmonary window* is occupied by part of the left lower lobe, bounded by the descending aorta and the left pulmonary artery; nodal enlargement can again expand into this space, being detectable on both conventional chest radiography and on CT.

CLINICAL APPLICATIONS

Mediastinal masses

CT demonstrates the size, site, extent and contour of mediastinal masses. It will differentiate vascular from neoplastic masses and is particularly useful for evaluating regions poorly demonstrated on conventional radiographs, for example the retrocrural, retrosternal or subcarinal areas (Fig. 2.4). Characteristic fat or calcium densities may be demonstrated in dermoids or lipomas. Homogeneous water density and alteration in shape with posture may indicate a fluid-filled lesion and may also demonstrate a consistent relationship with a normal structure such as the pericardium in the case of a pericardial cyst (Fig. 2.5). Thymic masses (Fig. 2.6) and diffuse thymic enlargement can be demonstrated. Diffuse mediastinal involvement by infiltrating malignant disease or fibrosis can also be demonstrated. CT is suitable for guidance of biopsy procedures (Fig. 2.7).

Hilar masses

Hilar adenopathy can be distinguished from prominent vessels, particularly if dynamic contrast enhancement is used. Subtle masses in the azygo-oesophageal recess or aortopulmonary window can be demonstrated.

Paraspinal masses

Paraspinal masses are clearly demonstrated on CT (Fig. 2.8). Appropriate section thickness and imaging on lung, bone and soft-tissue windows is imperative to assess the relationship of a lesion to the vertebrae, exit foramina, pleura, lung and associated tissues.

Vascular abnormalities

Dynamic contrast-enhanced spiral CT is an excellent method of demonstrating vascular pathology in the mediastinum. The entire length of the thoracic aorta can be imaged during peak contrast

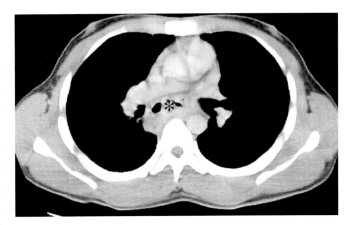

Fig. 2.4 Cavitating subcarinal mass (*), due to tuberculous adenopathy with oesophageal erosion.

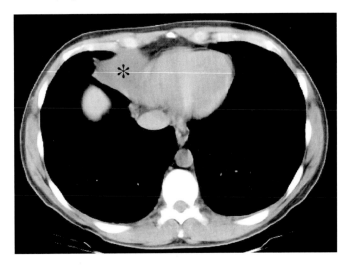

Fig. 2.5 Pericardial springwater cyst (*).

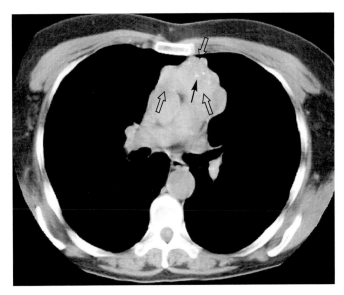

Fig. 2.6 Calcification (arrow) in a thymoma (open arrows).

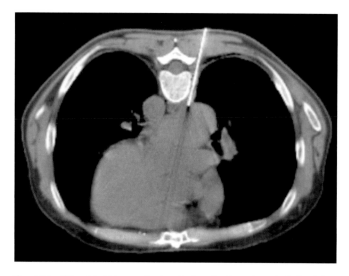

Fig. 2.7 CT-guided biopsy of subcarinal nodes (lymphoma). Saline injection has been used to widen the extrapleural space, thus avoiding transgression of the pleura.

enhancement for the demonstration of aortic dissection or aneurysm (Figs 2.9–2.11). The central pulmonary artery and first to fourth order pulmonary artery branch thrombus can also be demonstrated by this technique in pulmonary thromboembolic disease. The sensitivity and specificity of multislice CT pulmonary angiography for pulmonary embolus approaches that of conventional pulmonary angiography. CT is being increasingly used as a first-line modality in suspected pulmonary embolism, particularly when the chest radiograph is abnormal, and a V/Q scan is therefore more likely to be indeterminate. Major vessel anomalies may be evident with or without intravenous contrast enhancement (Figs 2.12, 2.13).

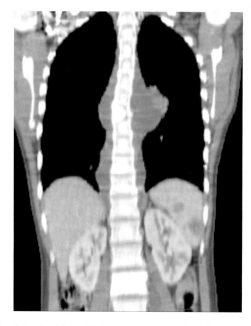

Fig. 2.8 Extensive bilateral tuberculous paravertebral abscesses with spine involvement. Coronal reconstruction from multislice contrast-enhanced CT dataset. Note the involvement of L3 with a left psoas abscess in addition to the mid thoracic disease.

Tracheobronchial pathology

CT allows the cross-sectional area and shape of the trachea and larger bronchi to be assessed. The use of spiral CT and subsequent image manipulation on a workstation can be used to produce 3D surface-rendered, reformatted or minimum-intensity projection images of the airways. This is valuable for the assessment of bronchial strictures or obstruction from tumours, after surgery, endotracheal tube removal or stenting procedures, and also in diseases such as relapsing polychondritis, tracheobronchomalacia (Fig. 2.14) and the sleep apnoea syndrome.

THYROID MASSES

Thyroid disease is common and enlargement of the thyroid gland can be due to a number of causes including a non-toxic multinodular enlargement of the gland, thyrotoxicosis, thyroid adenoma, thyroid carcinoma, lymphoma and Hashimoto's thyroiditis. Less than 5% of enlarged thyroid glands in the neck extend into the mediastinum to produce a retrosternal goitre, but this is usually due to a non-toxic multinodular enlargement of the gland. A mass developing within a heterotopic thyroid gland in the mediastinum is rare.

A retrosternal goitre is usually seen as an incidental mediastinal mass on a chest radiograph in an adult female patient. The goitre

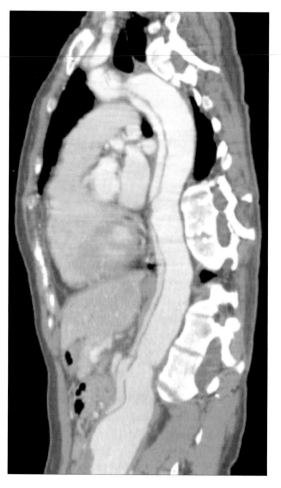

Fig. 2.9 Chronic aortic dissection in Marfan's syndrome. Curved-plane reconstruction.

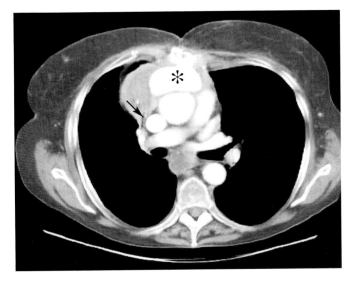

Fig. 2.10 False aneurysm of the ascending aorta (*), secondary to chronic osteomyelitis of the sternum from previous aortic valve replacement surgery. Note the bronchus entering the posterior aspect of the mass of thrombus (arrow)—the patient presented with haemoptysis.

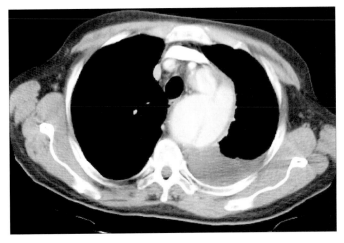

Fig. 2.11 Acute aortic dissection; note the haematoma over the left lung apex.

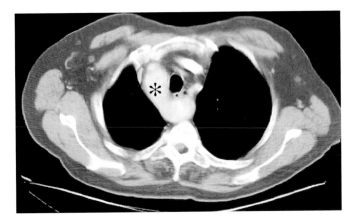

Fig. 2.12 Right-sided aortic arch (*).

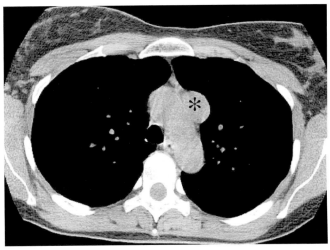

Fig. 2.13 Left-sided superior vena cava (*).

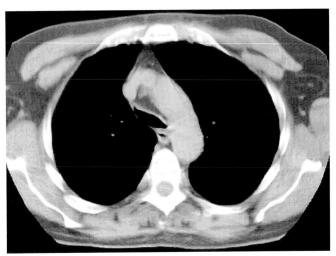

Fig. 2.14 Abnormal shape to the trachea due to distortion of the tracheal cartilage in tracheobronchomalacia.

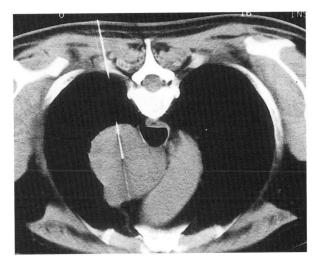

Fig. 2.15 A CT-guided biopsy from a right paratracheal lymph node mass in the middle mediastinum using a 20G needle in a 62-year-old man following a left nephrectomy for renal cell carcinoma 14 years previously. Histology showed metastatic disease from the original primary tumour.

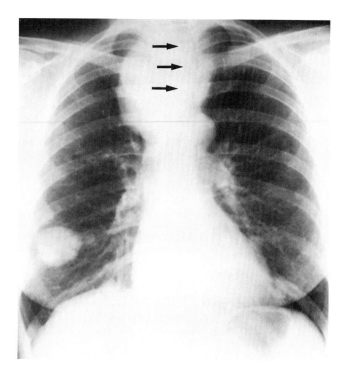

Fig. 2.16 Carcinoma of the thyroid. 53-year-old woman presenting with a painful goitre and dysphagia. PA film shows an oval mass in the superior part of the anterior mediastinum with displacement of the trachea (arrows) to the left and multiple pulmonary metastases.

is often asymptomatic but can produce dysphagia, dyspnoea and stridor. The development of pain in the goitre, vocal cord paralysis or superior vena caval obstruction suggests the presence of malignancy.

A retrosternal goitre appears as a well-defined round or oval soft-tissue mass in the superior part of the anterior or middle mediastinum, which fades off into the neck. The soft-tissue mass often contains central nodular, linear or crescentic patterns of calcification and produces lateral displacement and compression of the trachea in the thoracic inlet (Fig. 2.16). About 25% of goitres are retrotracheal and displace the oesophagus posteriorly and the trachea anteriorly (Fig. 2.17). Rapid increase in the size of the mass indicates internal haemorrhage into a cyst.

The diagnosis is confirmed by CT (or MRI), which shows a mass of mixed soft-tissue attenuation which enhances after intravenous contrast medium and extends into the mediastinum from the lower pole of one of the lobes of the thyroid gland in the neck down towards the aortic arch. The mass may have a higher attenuation than muscle due to its iodine content and contain foci of calcification or lesions of low attenuation due to cystic degeneration (Fig. 2.17). MRI shows a mass of intermediate signal intensity on T_1-weighted images.

The diagnosis can also be confirmed by a radionuclide scan using ^{123}I-sodium iodide or ^{99m}Tc-sodium pertechnetate, which shows an area of increased activity extending below the sternal notch into the mediastinum.

THYMIC TUMOURS

A normal thymus gland is the commonest cause of a mediastinal abnormality in infants and is usually seen as a triangular soft-tissue

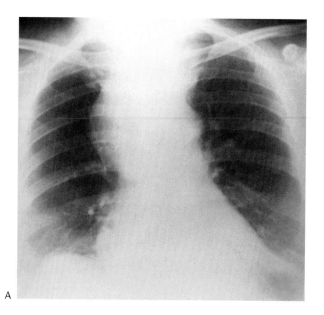

A

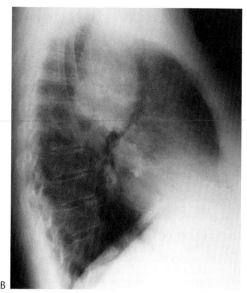

B

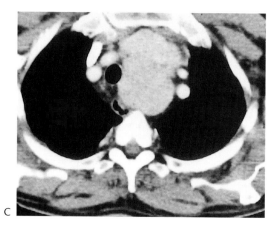

C

Fig. 2.17 Thyroid adenoma. 67-year-old woman presenting with a goitre. PA (A) and lateral (B) films show an oval mass in the superior part of the middle mediastinum with displacement of the trachea forward and to the right. Diagnosis confirmed by surgery.

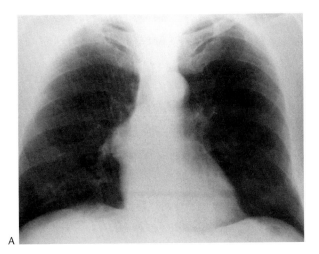

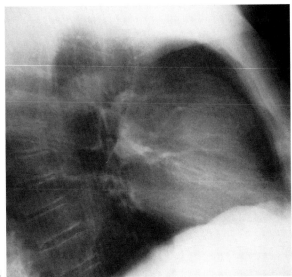

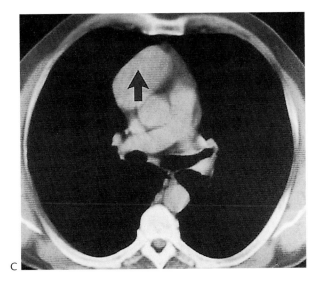

Fig. 2.18 Thymoma. 55-year-old man presenting with hypertension due to a phaeochromocytoma. PA (A) and lateral (B) films show a round mass in the anterior mediastinum overlying the right hilum. CT scan with contrast enhancement (L +50, W 500) (C) at the level of the tracheal bifurcation shows an oval mass of soft-tissue density (arrow), 7 cm in size, in the anterior mediastinum. Diagnosis confirmed by surgery.

mass which projects to one side of the mediastinum, often the right on a chest radiograph. The thymus gland disappears during severe neonatal infection or after major surgery or corticosteroid treatment, but may re-appear following recovery from illness. The thymus gland is also completely absent in DiGeorge's syndrome, an immune deficiency disease involving the T lymphocytes. The normal thymus gland is seen as a triangular arrowhead or bilobed structure in children and young adult patients on CT, but undergoes fatty involution in elderly adult patients.

Enlargement of the thymus gland can be due to a number of causes including thymoma, hyperplasia of the gland, thymic carcinoma, lymphoma, carcinoid and germ cell tumours, thymic cysts and thymolipoma. Thymomas are the commonest of the thymic tumours in adults and 30% are invasive or malignant. The staging of a thymoma is done by CT or MRI and at surgery:

Stage 1	no capsular invasion
Stage 2	capsular invasion
Stage 3	invasion of the mediastinal structures or lung
Stage 4A	disseminated tumour within the thorax
Stage 4B	distant metastases.

Thymoma

A thymoma is usually seen as an anterior mediastinal mass on a chest radiograph in an adult patient. The thymoma is often asymptomatic but can also present with myasthenia gravis, red cell aplasia or hypogammaglobulinaemia, as well as many other conditions. About 10–25% of patients with myasthenia have a thymoma and about 25–50% of patients with a thymoma have myasthenia. In patients with a thymoma, about 25–50% have red cell aplasia and 10% have hypogammaglobulinaemia and more than 50% of patients with myasthenia have thymic hyperplasia.

Thymic hyperplasia also occurs in association with thyrotoxicosis, Addison's disease, acromegaly, systemic lupus erythematosus, rheumatoid arthritis and after stress atrophy, where the thymus gland initially atrophies in patients on chemotherapy or corticosteroid treatment and then enlarges once the treatment is stopped. This is called rebound thymic hyperplasia and should not be confused with recurrent malignant disease in patients with lymphoma. Thymic carcinoid tumours can present with Cushing's syndrome, hyperparathyroidism and inappropriate antidiuretic hormone secretion.

A thymoma appears as a well-defined round or oval soft-tissue mass which projects to one side of the anterior mediastinum when large, but may be undetectable on the chest radiograph when small, indicating the need for CT (Fig. 2.18). The soft-tissue mass may also contain curvilinear or nodular calcification. The presence of vascular encasement or pleural metastases indicates an invasive thymoma (Fig. 2.19) and a very large soft-tissue mass with less radiographic density than expected for its size, which alters in shape on respiration, indicates a thymolipoma.

The diagnosis of a thymoma is confirmed by CT (or MRI), which shows a mass of soft-tissue attenuation which may contain areas of low attenuation due to cystic degeneration (Fig. 2.19). MRI shows a mass of intermediate signal intensity on T_1-weighted images and high signal intensity on T_2-weighted images. CT also demonstrates an enlarged but normal-shaped gland in thymic hyperplasia, a cystic mass containing fluid in a thymic cyst or a fat-containing mass in a thymolipoma.

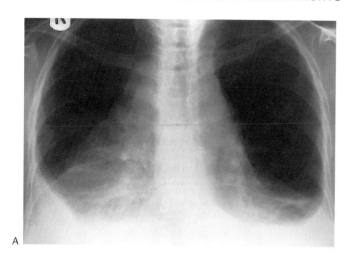

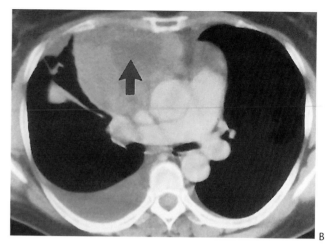

Fig. 2.19 Invasive thymoma. 43-year-old woman presenting with chest pain and dyspnoea. PA film (A) shows widening of the mediastinum on the right with bilateral pleural effusions. CT scan with contrast soft-tissue enhancement (L +50, W 500) (B) at the level of the tracheal bifurcation shows an oval mass of mixed density (arrow), 9 cm in size, in the anterior mediastinum with a small pleural mass anteriorly on the right. Diagnosis confirmed by needle biopsy and surgery.

GERM CELL OR TERATODERMOID TUMOURS

The germ cell tumours of the mediastinum arise from primitive germ cell rests that have been left in the anterior mediastinum during their embryological migration to the urogenital ridge. The majority of germ cell tumours are benign and include the dermoid cyst and benign teratoma, but 30% are malignant tumours such as seminoma, embryonal cell carcinoma, choriocarcinoma and endodermal sinus or yolk sac tumour. The dermoid cyst consists mainly of ectodermal tissues, whereas the solid teratoma usually contains tissues of ectodermal, mesodermal and endodermal origin.

Germ cell tumours are usually seen as an incidental anterior mediastinal mass on a chest radiograph in a young adult male patient. The tumour is often asymptomatic but can produce cough, chest pain and dyspnoea. Rarely these cystic tumours can become infected and rupture into the mediastinum or bronchial tree and haemorrhage into the tumour can also occur. The striking diagnostic symptom of trichoptysis is rare.

A dermoid cyst or benign teratoma appears as a well-defined round or oval soft-tissue mass, which usually projects to only one side of the anterior mediastinum (Fig. 2.20). The soft-tissue mass may also contain a peripheral rim or central nodules of calcification, a fat–fluid level or even a rudimentary tooth, which is of course a diagnostic radiological sign. Rapid increase in the size of the mass indicates internal haemorrhage or the development of malignancy. An air–fluid level is present after rupture of an infected cyst into the bronchial tree with atelectasis or consolidation in the adjacent lung. A malignant germ cell tumour appears as a lobulated soft-tissue mass, which projects on both sides of the anterior mediastinum.

The diagnosis is confirmed by CT (or MRI), which shows a cystic mass containing fluid, soft tissue, fat, calcification or bone (Fig. 2.20). MRI shows a mass of variable high signal intensity on T_1-weighted images if it contains fat, protein or blood. The malignant germ cell tumours also produce tumour markers such as human chorionic gonadotrophin (HCG) and alphafetoprotein (AFP).

FAT DEPOSITION/MEDIASTINAL LIPOMATOSIS

The excessive deposition of fat in the mediastinum is usually seen as an incidental finding on a chest radiograph in an asymptomatic obese adult patient, but it can also occur in patients with Cushing's syndrome and in patients receiving long-term high-dose corticosteroid treatment. Steroids cause mobilisation of body fat with its subsequent redistribution in the anterior mediastinum, cardiophrenic angles and paravertebral regions. This produces smooth widening of the superior mediastinum without tracheal displacement, large epicardial fat pads and lateral displacement of the paraspinal lines on the chest radiograph. The widening of the mediastinum can be difficult to differentiate from mediastinal haemorrhage or generalised lymphadenopathy, but the diagnosis is easily confirmed by CT (or MRI), which shows the excess mediastinal fat with its typical low CT number of −70 to −130 HU (Fig. 2.21). MRI shows the mediastinal fat as high signal intensity on T_1-weighted images and low signal intensity on a fat-suppression STIR sequence.

PLEUROPERICARDIAL CYST

A pleuropericardial cyst is a thin-walled cyst lined by mesothelial cells, which contains clear fluid and is attached to the parietal pericardium. A pleuropericardial cyst is usually seen as an incidental anterior mediastinal mass on a chest radiograph in an adult patient. The cyst is usually asymptomatic but can produce chest pain, cough and dyspnoea.

The majority of pleuropericardial cysts occur in the right anterior cardiophrenic angle (Fig. 2.22), but they can occur in the left anterior cardiophrenic angle or in the middle mediastinum. They appear as a well-defined round, oval or triangular soft-tissue mass, which can alter in shape on respiration. This can be difficult to differentiate from other causes of a soft-tissue mass in the right anterior cardiophrenic angle and the differential diagnosis includes a large epicardial fat pad, a Morgagni's hernia, epicardial lymphadenopathy due to lymphoma or metastatic disease, a pleural tumour or a right middle lobe mass.

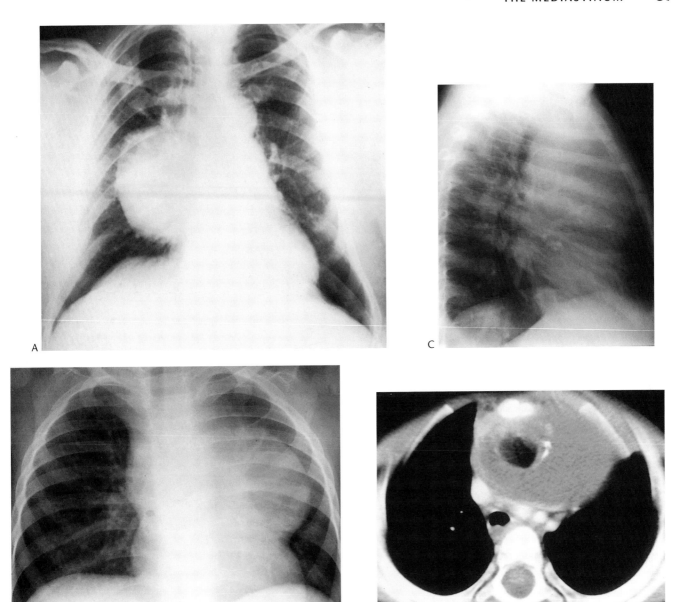

Fig. 2.20 (A) Benign teratoma. 65-year-old man presenting with chest pain. PA film shows a large round mass in the anterior mediastinum overlying the right hilum. Germ cell tumour. 2-year-old child presenting with a cough. AP (B) and lateral (C) films show an oval mass in the anterior mediastinum overlying the left hilum. CT scan with contrast enhancement (L +50, W 350) (D) above the aortic arch shows an oval mass of soft-tissue density, 7 cm in size, containing fat and calcification in the anterior mediastrinum. Diagnosis confirmed by surgery.

The diagnosis is confirmed by ultrasound, which shows a transonic cystic mass adjacent to the pericardium, or by CT (or MRI), which shows a thin-walled cyst containing fluid of low attenuation (0–20 HU) (Fig. 2.22). MRI shows a water-containing mass with a low signal intensity on T_1-weighted images and a high signal intensity on T_2-weighted images. Direct needle puncture of a pleuropericardial cyst with aspiration of its fluid contents can be performed under CT or ultrasound guidance.

MORGAGNI'S HERNIA

The foramen of Morgagni is a persistent developmental defect in the diaphragm anteriorly, between the septum transversum and the right and left costal origins of the diaphragm. A hernia through the foramen of Morgagni is usually seen as an anterior mediastinal mass on a chest radiograph in an adult patient. The hernia is usually asymptomatic, but can produce retrosternal chest pain, epigastric pain and dyspnoea. Strangulation of the contents of the hernial sac is rare.

More than 90% of Morgagni's hernias are situated in the right anterior cardiophrenic angle (Fig. 2.23), due to the protective effect of the pericardium on the left. The smaller hernias contain omentum, which appears as a well-defined round or oval soft-tissue mass and has a lower radiographic density than would be expected for its size. This can be difficult to differentiate from an epicardial fat pad or a pleuropericardial cyst, although occasionally the properitoneal fat line can be seen continuing upwards from the anterior abdominal wall around the hernial sac on a lateral chest

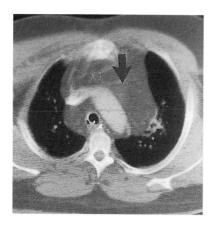

Fig. 2.21 Fat deposition. 40-year-old man presenting with chest pain after a road traffic accident and a widened mediastinum on a chest film. CT scan with contrast enhancement (L +50, W 750) above the tracheal bifurcation shows excess deposition of fat throughout the mediastinum, particularly anteriorly (arrow).

film. The larger hernias usually contain transverse colon, which appears as a gas-filled loop of bowel within the soft-tissue mass, but can also contain liver, stomach and small intestine.

The diagnosis is confirmed by CT, which shows the omental fat (−70 to −130 HU) and gas-containing colon above the diaphragm (Fig. 2.23). The diagnosis can also be confirmed by a barium follow-through examination or a barium enema, which show either upward tenting of the transverse colon towards the hernia or a loop of transverse colon above the diaphragm.

PARATHYROID ADENOMA

An adenoma in an ectopic parathyroid gland is occasionally demonstrated in the chest in an adult patient with hyperparathyroidism. An ectopic parathyroid adenoma is not usually seen in the mediastinum on a chest radiograph, because of its small size at presentation. It is a rare tumour, which occurs in the superior, anterior or posterior mediastinum. It appears as a small mass which enhances after intravenous contrast medium within the mediastinal fat on CT, but can be difficult to differentiate from mediastinal lymph nodes.

The diagnosis is confirmed by MRI, which shows the ectopic adenoma as a lesion with a very high signal intensity on a fat-suppression STIR sequence. The diagnosis can also be confirmed by a radionuclide scan using ^{201}Tl-thallium chloride or ^{99m}Tc-technetium sestamibi (Fig. 2.24) and by selective arteriography.

LYMPHANGIOMA/CYSTIC HYGROMA

A lymphangioma is a congenital malformation of the lymphatic system that produces a soft-tissue swelling in the neck that also extends down into the mediastinum. A lymphangioma is usually seen as an incidental mediastinal mass on a chest radiograph in a child. It is a rare mesenchymal tumour, which occurs in the superior, anterior or posterior mediastinum. It appears as a round or oval soft-tissue mass on the chest radiograph, can alter in shape on respiration and extends up into the neck. A chylothorax may also occur.

The diagnosis is confirmed by ultrasound, which shows a multilocular transonic cystic mass in the neck and mediastinum, or by CT (or MRI), which shows a thin-walled cyst containing septae and fluid of low attenuation (0–20 HU).

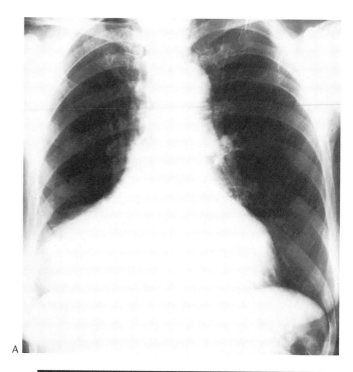

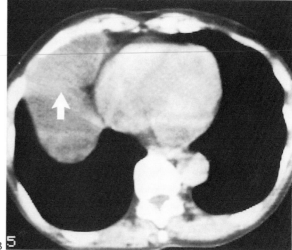

Fig. 2.22 Pleuropericardial cyst. 72-year-old woman presenting with dyspnoea. PA film (A) shows a large oval mass in the right cardiophrenic angle and CT scan (L +40, W 512) (B) below the tracheal bifurcation shows an oval mass (arrow), 10 cm in size, separate from the heart in the anterior and middle mediastinum. The density of the mass (average +9 HU) is typical of cyst fluid.

LIPOMA/LIPOSARCOMA

A lipoma or liposarcoma is usually seen as an incidental mediastinal mass on a chest radiograph in an asymptomatic adult patient. It is a rare mesenchymal tumour, which occurs in the anterior or posterior mediastinum. It appears as a well-defined round or oval soft-tissue mass on the chest radiograph, has a lower radiographic density than would be expected for its size and can alter in shape on respiration (Fig. 2.25).

The diagnosis is confirmed by CT, which shows a solid mass of fat attenuation (−70 to −130 HU) containing strands of soft tissue.

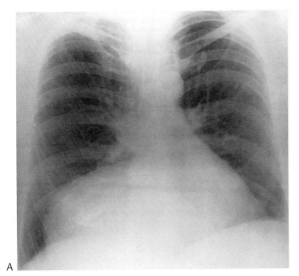

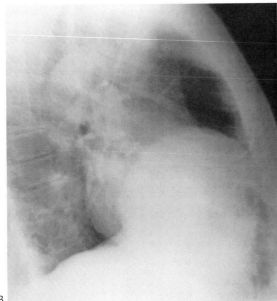

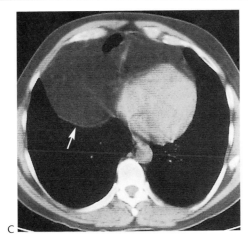

Fig. 2.23 Morgagni's hernia. Asymptomatic 49-year-old man. PA (A) and lateral (B) films show a large round mass in the right cardiophrenic angle. CT scan (L +50, W 500) (C) below the tracheal bifurcation shows an oval mass of fat density (arrow), 18 cm in size, which contains transverse colon in the anterior mediastinum.

HAEMANGIOMA/HAEMANGIOENDOTHELIOMA

A haemangioma or haemangioendothelioma is a vascular malformation of the capillaries or veins, which is usually seen as an incidental mediastinal mass on a chest radiograph in an asymptomatic adult patient. It is a rare mesenchymal tumour, which occurs in the anterior or posterior mediastinum. It appears as a round or oval soft-tissue mass on the chest radiograph, which may also show phleboliths in the mediastinum.

The diagnosis is confirmed by CT, which shows a mass of soft-tissue attenuation containing calcification and phleboliths, which enhances after intravenous contrast medium.

OTHER RARE MEDIASTINAL LESIONS

Other tumours of mesenchymal origin, such as fibroma, fibrosarcoma, soft-tissue osteosarcoma and haemangiopericytoma, can also occur in the anterior or posterior mediastinum.

The small tumours are usually asymptomatic, whereas the larger tumours tend to produce symptoms depending upon their anatomical location such as retrosternal chest pain, back pain or dysphagia. They appear as a round or oval soft-tissue mass on the chest radiograph.

Tumours involving bone, such as a plasmacytoma of the sternum, a chondrosarcoma of a rib or a chordoma of the thoracic spine may also produce a mass that involves the anterior or posterior mediastinum. A desmoid tumour of the chest wall may involve the mediastinum and a cyst of the thoracic duct may produce a posterior mediastinal mass.

MEDIASTINAL LYMPHADENOPATHY

Lymph nodes occur throughout the mediastinum but are found predominantly in its middle division where the paratracheal,

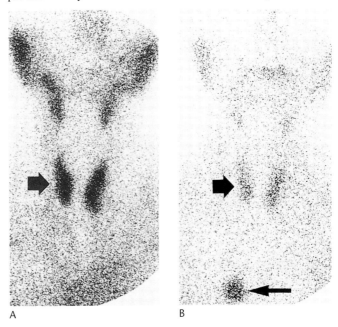

Fig. 2.24 Parathyroid adenoma. 64-year-old woman presenting with hypercalcaemia. Radionuclide scans with ^{99m}Tc (A) and ^{201}Tl (B) show activity in the salivary glands and thyroid gland ($\rightarrow$) (larger arrows) and in the parathyroid adenoma in the mediastinum ($\leftarrow$) (smaller arrow). The latter is shown only on the thallium scan, even without computerised subtraction of scan A from scan B.

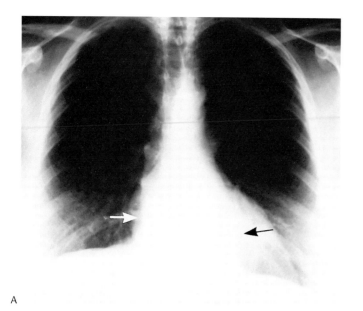

A

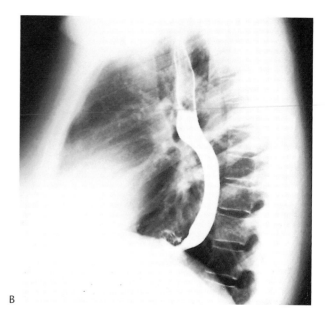

B

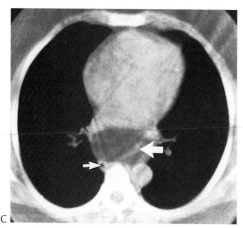

C

Fig. 2.25 Lipoma. Asymptomatic 42-year-old woman. PA film (A) and barium swallow (B) show an oval mass with less density than expected for its size, particularly in the lateral view, behind the heart. (C) CT scan (L –150, W 800) below the tracheal bifurcation shows an oval mass of fat density (←), 8 cm in size, in the posterior mediastinum, with displacement of the oesophagus (→) to the right. (A and B courtesy of Dr P. Ho; C courtesy of Dr T.J. Bloomberg.)

tracheobronchial, subcarinal and bronchopulmonary or hilar groups are situated (Fig. 2.15).

Mediastinal lymphadenopathy is common and can be due to many causes including metastatic disease, lymphoma, leukaemia, sarcoidosis, tuberculosis, histoplasmosis, other infections and inflammatory conditions.

Mediastinal lymphadenopathy is usually seen as either a middle mediastinal mass or multiple mediastinal masses on a chest radiograph in a child or adult patient. The enlarged lymph nodes are often asymptomatic, but can produce cough, dyspnoea and weight loss and may be associated with generalised lymphadenopathy.

Mediastinal lymphadenopathy appears as widening of the right paratracheal stripe, a bulge in the aorto-pulmonary window, lateral displacement of the azygo-oesophageal line, lobulated widening of the mediastinum and unilateral or bilateral lobulated hilar soft-tissue masses depending on which lymph node groups are enlarged (Figs 2.26, 2.27). Calcification in the mediastinal lymph nodes can be due to many causes including tuberculosis, sarcoidosis, silicosis,

histoplasmosis, Hodgkin's disease following irradiation, metastases from mucin-secreting adenocarcinoma, amyloidosis, Castleman's disease and *Pneumocystis carinii* pneumonia in AIDS.

The diagnosis is confirmed by CT, which shows multiple masses of soft-tissue attenuation in the mediastinum (Fig. 2.28), or MRI, which shows multiple masses of intermediate signal intensity on T_1-weighted images which stand out against the signal void from the flowing blood in the vessels and the air in the trachea and main bronchi. CT is more sensitive than plain films in the detection of mediastinal lymph node calcification (Fig. 2.29), which is not seen on MRI at all. CT may also show enlarged lymph nodes with low attenuation centres due to necrosis in tuberculosis, histoplasmosis, *Mycobacterium avium intracellulare*, Hodgkin's disease and metastases from testicular tumours (Fig. 2.30). Enhancement of the enlarged lymph nodes after intravenous contrast medium occurs in both inflammatory and neoplastic conditions, particularly in vascular metastases from renal cell carcinoma, thyroid carcinoma, carcinoid tumours, melanoma and leiomyosarcoma.

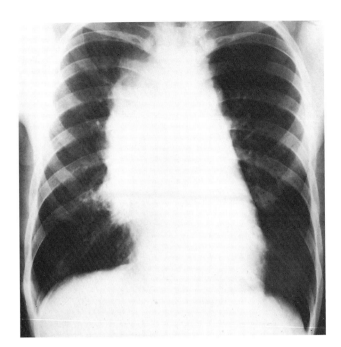

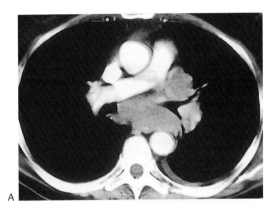

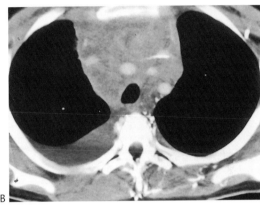

Fig. 2.26 Hodgkin's disease. 18-year-old man presenting with cervical lymphadenopathy. PA film shows asymmetrical lobulated widening of the mediastinum, due to involvement of the middle and anterior mediastinal lymph nodes, particularly on the right.

Metastatic disease can produce enlargement of any of the lymph node groups within the mediastinum. A bronchial carcinoma is the commonest tumour to metastasise to the mediastinal lymph nodes, but other primary intrathoracic tumours, such as oesophageal carcinoma as well as extrathoracic tumours such as breast carcinoma, renal, adrenal and testicular tumours, thyroid carcinoma, melanoma and head and neck tumours can also produce mediastinal lymph node metastases. Associated pulmonary metastases, lymphangitis and pleural effusions are also frequently present.

Fig. 2.28 (A) Carcinoma of the bronchus. 67-year-old woman presenting with haemoptysis and a left hilar mass on a chest film. CT scan with contrast enhancement (L +35, W 325) below the tracheal bifurcation shows a left hilar mass and subcarinal lymphadenopathy. Diagnosis confirmed at bronchoscopy. (B) Non-Hodgkin's lymphoma. 18-year-old man presenting with superior vena caval compression, a widened mediastinum and a right pleural effusion on a chest film. CT scan with contrast enhancement (L +35, W 325) above the aortic arch shows a round mass of mixed soft-tissue density, 10 cm in size, in the anterior and middle mediastinum with compression of the left brachiocephalic vein and contrast medium filling collateral veins in the left chest wall. Diagnosis confirmed by CT-guided needle biopsy.

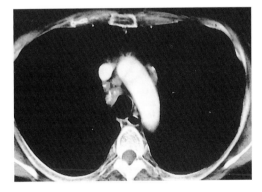

Fig. 2.29 Sarcoidosis. 67-year-old woman presenting with a cough and bilateral hilar and paratracheal lymphadenopathy on a chest film. CT scan with contrast enhancement (L +35, W 325) above the tracheal bifurcation shows enlarged mediastinal lymph nodes containing calcification. Diagnosis confirmed by high-resolution CT scan.

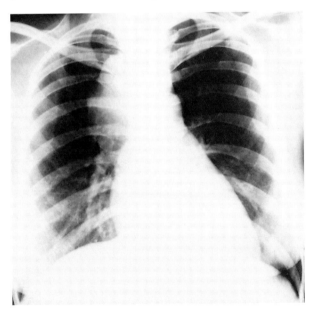

Fig. 2.27 Tuberculosis. Asymptomatic 29-year-old woman with chronic renal disease treated with immunosuppressive drugs. PA film shows a right paratracheal mass of enlarged lymph nodes in the middle mediastinum.

Hodgkin's disease, the non-Hodgkin's lymphomas and the lymphatic leukaemias produce middle mediastinal lymphadenopathy which is often unilateral, but the lymphomas, particularly Hodgkin's

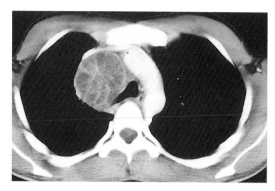

Fig. 2.30   Tuberculosis. 22-year-old man presenting with weight loss and a right paratracheal mass on a chest film. CT scan with contrast enhancement (L +35, W 325) at the tracheal bifurcation shows a round mass of low soft-tissue density, 6 cm in size, in the middle mediastinum. Diagnosis confirmed by CT-guided needle biopsy.

disease, also frequently involve the anterior mediastinum, to produce a lobulated soft-tissue mass due to indentation by the anterior ribs (Fig. 2.26). Parenchymal involvement of the lungs also occurs and calcification occasionally develops in Hodgkin's disease after irradiation.

Mediastinal radiotherapy may produce a chronic mediastinitis with fibrosis extending into the lungs. This is quite characteristic and appears as a straight line, widening the mediastinum on both sides and corresponding to the treatment field (Fig. 2.31). This fibrosis is more likely to develop in patients who are also receiving cytotoxic chemotherapy, particularly cyclophosphamide.

Castleman's disease is an unusual form of benign lymph node hyperplasia. This disease produces large mediastinal lymph node masses, which enhance after intravenous contrast medium, and may contain calcification.

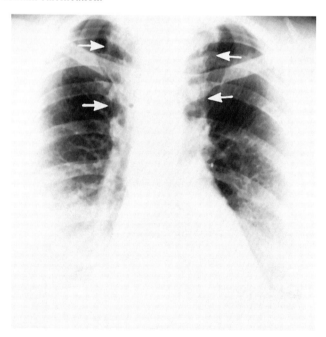

Fig. 2.31   Radiotherapy to the mediastinum. Asymptomatic 40-year-old woman with Hodgkin's disease in remission treated with mediastinal radiotherapy several years previously. PA film shows widening of the superior part of the mediastinum due to radiation fibrosis extending into the lungs (arrows).

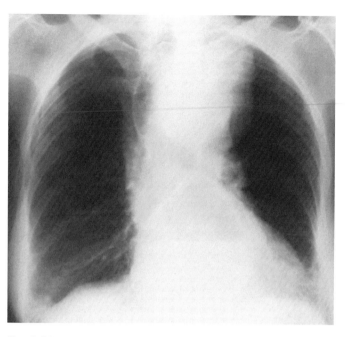

Fig. 2.32   Aneurysm of arch of aorta and hiatus hernia. 83-year-old woman presenting with dyspnoea and hypertension. PA film shows a large round mass, which has some calcification in its wall, in the middle mediastinum, with displacement of the trachea to the right, and another large round mass containing an air–fluid level behind the heart in the posterior mediastinum.

Sarcoidosis produces enlargement of the bronchopulmonary and paratracheal lymph nodes, which is usually bilateral. Parenchymal involvement of the lungs also occurs and peripheral egg shell calcification may develop in the lymph nodes.

Primary tuberculosis produces an area of consolidation in one lobe with unilateral enlargement of the bronchopulmonary, paratracheal and subcarinal lymph nodes. A pleural effusion also occurs and complete calcification of the lymph nodes may develop as healing occurs. Tuberculosis can also produce unilateral mediastinal lymphadenopathy without pulmonary involvement in immuno-suppressed patients (Fig. 2.27).

Fungal infections such as histoplasmosis, coccidioidomycosis and blastomycosis produce hilar or paratracheal mediastinal lymphadenopathy with or without pulmonary involvement. Calcification of the lymph nodes may also develop as healing occurs, especially in histoplasmosis. Actinomycosis also produces enlarged mediastinal lymph nodes.

There are many other infective and inflammatory causes of enlarged mediastinal lymph nodes including infectious mononucleosis, measles, whooping cough, mycoplasma, adenoviruses and lung abscess. Peripheral egg shell calcification occurs in the enlarged lymph nodes in silicosis and amyloidosis.

Patients with AIDS may have enlarged mediastinal lymph nodes due to tuberculosis, *Mycobacterium avium intracellulare*, fungal infections, *Pneumocystis carinii* infection, Kaposi's sarcoma and lymphoma. Patients with cystic fibrosis may have enlarged hilar shadows due to enlarged lymph nodes or cor pulmonale.

THORACIC AORTIC ANEURYSM

Vascular disease is common and aneurysmal dilatation of the thoracic aorta can be due to a number of causes including athero-

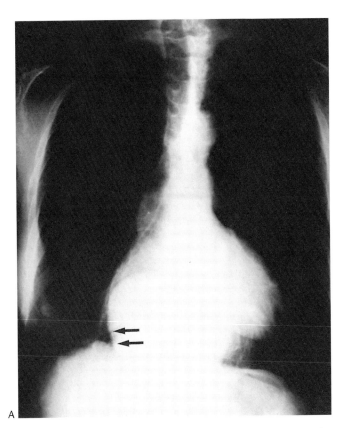
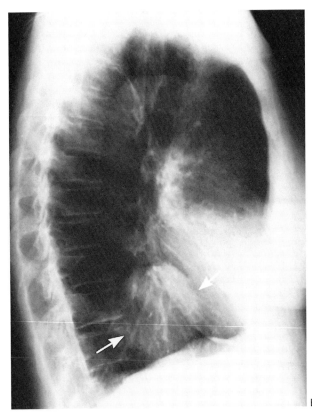

A   B

Fig. 2.33 Aneurysm of descending aorta. 59-year-old woman presenting with haematemesis from a benign gastric ulcer. PA (A) and lateral (B) films show a large round mass, which has some peripheral calcification in its wall (arrows) in the posterior mediastinum behind the heart. Diagnosis confirmed by ultrasound, using the liver as a window into the mediastinum.

sclerosis, hypertension, blunt chest trauma, mycotic dissection, cystic medial necrosis in Marfan's syndrome and Ehlers–Danlos syndrome, aortitis in tertiary syphilis and Takayasu's disease and congenital anomalies such as an aneurysm of the sinus of Valsalva or coarctation of the aorta.

A thoracic aortic aneurysm is usually seen as an incidental mediastinal abnormality on a chest radiograph in an elderly adult patient. The aneurysm is often asymptomatic but can produce chest pain, back pain and aortic incompetence, as well as a hoarse voice, dysphagia and left lower lobe infections, due to compression of the left recurrent laryngeal nerve, the oesophagus or the left lower lobe bronchus respectively.

A thoracic aortic aneurysm appears as either widening of the mediastinum or as a well-defined round or oval soft-tissue mass in any part of the mediastinum, often with curvilinear calcification in its wall (Figs 2.32, 2.33). Calcification in an ascending thoracic aortic aneurysm can be due to either syphilitic aortitis or atherosclerosis, but is now commoner in the atheromatous aneurysms. Displacement of the peripheral rim of calcification away from the wall of the thoracic aorta indicates an aortic dissection, which may also produce a left pleural effusion. A thoracic aortic aneurysm can also produce pressure erosion defects in the sternum or vertebral bodies of the thoracic spine. Thoracic aortic aneurysms appear as pulsatile masses on fluoroscopy, but this sign does not differentiate them from other mediastinal masses adjacent to the aorta, which show a transmitted pulsation.

The diagnosis is confirmed by CT (or MRI), which shows the dilated aorta measuring more than 4 cm in diameter and containing

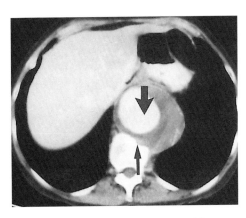

Fig. 2.34 Aneurysm of descending aorta. 45-year-old woman presenting with back pain. CT scan with contrast enhancement (L +50, W 500) below the tracheal bifurcation shows an aneurysm of the descending aorta (↓), 8 cm in size, which contains thrombus, has calcification in its wall, and is eroding the adjacent lower thoracic vertebral body (↑).

contrast-enhanced blood in its lumen with surrounding mural thrombus of lower attenuation and calcification in its wall (Fig. 2.34). MRI shows the aneurysm in an oblique projection with no signal from the flowing blood on T_1-weighted images. Arch aortography will also confirm the diagnosis.

The diagnosis of aortic dissection is confirmed by demonstrating an intimal flap between the true and false aortic lumen by CT, MRI, transoesophageal echocardiography or angiography. The extent of the dissection is used to classify dissecting aneurysms into Type A, which involve the ascending aorta (and may involve the arch and descending aorta), and Type B, which may involve the descending aorta (see Ch. 15). Type A dissections (previously classified as De Bakey type 1 and 2) are treated surgically and Type B dissections (previously classified as De Bakey type 3) are treated medically by controlling the hypertension. An intramural haematoma is classed as a type of aortic dissection without an intimal flap in the aortic lumen and is demonstrated on unenhanced CT as a high attenuation lesion in the thickened aortic wall. A penetrating aortic ulcer is also classed as a type of aortic dissection in the descending thoracic aorta and is demonstrated on contrast-enhanced CT as a projection through the aortic wall.

A tortuous innominate artery produces widening of the superior mediastinum on the right and an aneurysm of the innominate or subclavian arteries produces a superior mediastinal mass. The very common tortuous descending thoracic aorta produces widening of the mediastinum on the left, often at the level of the left hilum simulating a hilar mass.

Dilatation of the main pulmonary artery due to pulmonary arterial hypertension, pulmonary valve stenosis with a poststenotic dilatation or a pulmonary artery aneurysm also produces an apparent left hilar mass.

Coarctation of the aorta and kinking of the aorta (pseudo-coarctation) produce an abnormal mediastinal configuration on the left and a right-sided aortic arch produces an abnormal mediastinal configuration on the right. The diagnosis of these arterial abnormalities is confirmed by CT, MRI or angiography.

MEDIASTINAL VENOUS ABNORMALITIES

A dilated superior vena cava produces slight widening of the mediastinum on the right on a chest radiograph. This is usually caused by a raised central venous pressure, which occurs in patients with congestive cardiac failure, tricuspid valve disease, constrictive pericarditis and partial anomalous pulmonary venous drainage to a right-sided superior vena cava.

A persistent left-sided superior vena cava produces slight widening of the mediastinum on the left and the supracardiac form of total anomalous pulmonary venous drainage produces widening of the mediastinum on both sides. Complete transposition of the great vessels produces a narrow mediastinal configuration and a left superior intercostal vein is occasionally seen as a nipple-like projection from the aortic knuckle.

In patients with superior vena caval obstruction due to carcinoma of the bronchus, mediastinal lymph node metastases, lymphoma or a mediastinal tumour, the mediastinal abnormality is produced by the mass of tumour (Fig. 2.28). Mediastinal fibrosis and central venous catheter-induced thrombosis of the superior vena cava also produce superior vena caval obstruction.

A dilated azygos vein produces an oval soft-tissue mass in the right tracheobronchial angle on a chest radiograph. This is usually caused by a raised central venous pressure, superior or inferior vena caval obstruction, portal hypertension and the congenital azygos continuation of the inferior vena cava. A dilated azygos vein can be difficult to differentiate from enlarged azygos lymph nodes, but the azygos vein decreases in size in the erect position, on deep inspiration and during a Valsalva manoeuvre. Oesophageal varices may also produce a mass in the posterior mediastinum behind the heart.

The diagnosis of these venous abnormalities is confirmed by CT, MRI, angiography or phlebography.

BRONCHOGENIC CYST

A bronchogenic cyst is a thin-walled foregut cyst lined by ciliated columnar epithelial cells of respiratory origin, which contains viscid mucoid material. A bronchogenic cyst is usually seen as an incidental middle mediastinal mass on a chest radiograph in a young adult patient. The cyst is usually asymptomatic, but may produce cough, chest pain and dyspnoea in adult patients and stridor in infants. Rarely the cyst can become infected in children and rupture into the bronchial tree and haemorrhage into the cyst can also occur.

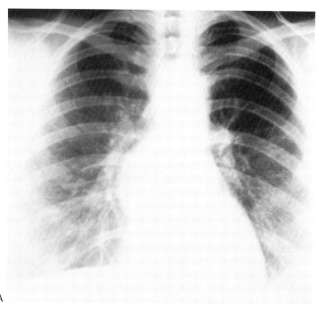

A

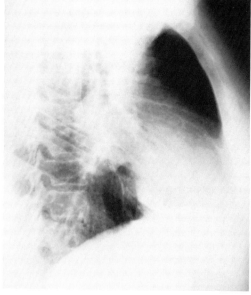

B

Fig. 2.35 Bronchogenic cyst. Asymptomatic 21-year-old woman. PA (A) and lateral (B) films show an oval mass in the middle mediastinum below the carina on the right. Diagnosis confirmed by surgery.

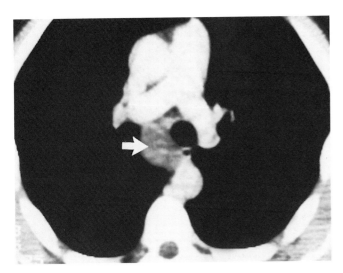

Fig. 2.36 Bronchogenic cyst. 25-year-old man presenting with cough. CT scan with contrast enhancement (L +40, W 512) at the level of the tracheal bifurcation shows a round mass (arrow), 3 cm in size, in the middle mediastinum. The density of the mass (average +45 HU) is typical of mucoid material.

The majority of bronchogenic cysts occur around the carina in the subcarinal region of the middle mediastinum (Fig. 2.35), but they can occur in the right paratracheal region or in the posterior mediastinum. They appear as a well-defined round or oval soft-tissue mass, which can alter in shape on respiration. Rapid increase in the size of the mass indicates haemorrhage into the cyst and an air–fluid level is present after rupture of an infected thick-walled cyst into the bronchial tree.

The diagnosis is confirmed by CT (or MRI), which shows a thin-walled cyst containing fluid of either low attenuation (0–20 HU) or soft-tissue attenuation (20–50 HU) (Fig. 2.36), if it contains mucinous material. Calcification can occasionally occur in the wall of the cyst. MRI shows a water-containing mass with a low signal intensity on T_1-weighted images and high signal intensity on T_2-weighted images or a high signal intensity on T_1- and T_2-weighted images if it contains protein or blood.

Direct needle puncture of a bronchogenic cyst with aspiration of its fluid contents can also be performed under CT guidance, unless the cyst is treated surgically.

TRACHEAL LESIONS

Lesions in the trachea usually present with either cough or dyspnoea due to recurrent chest infections or stridor in children and adult patients. Tracheal lesions can produce narrowing or widening of the trachea or a mass within its lumen on the chest radiograph.

Malignant tracheal tumours such as squamous cell carcinoma and adenoid cystic carcinoma or cylindroma, benign tracheal tumours such as hamartoma and chondroma and other lesions such as tracheobronchial papillomatosis and amyloidosis can produce a soft-tissue mass in the trachea.

Widening of the trachea is seen in tracheobronchiomegaly or the Mounier–Kuhn syndrome, which is associated with the Ehlers–Danlos syndrome. Narrowing of the trachea is seen in the sabre sheath trachea of chronic obstructive pulmonary disease, relapsing polychondritis, Wegener's granuloma, sarcoidosis, tuberculosis, trauma, tracheopathia osteochondroplastica and tracheomalacia. The diagnosis of all tracheal lesions is confirmed by CT which shows the narrowed

or widened trachea, intraluminal soft-tissue masses, a thick-walled trachea or extrinsic mediastinal disease. Tracheal lesions are discussed in more detail in Chapter 16 (see also Figure 1.61).

NEUROGENIC TUMOURS

The neurogenic tumours of the mediastinum develop from either the peripheral nerves, the thoracic sympathetic chain ganglia or the paraganglionic nerve tissue and are therefore divided into three groups. The first group are known as nerve sheath tumours and include the neurofibroma, the schwannoma or neurilemmoma; the neurofibrosarcoma and the malignant schwannoma and are the commonest of the neurogenic tumours in the mediastinum in adults. The second group are known as ganglion cell tumours and include the ganglioneuroma; the ganglioneuroblastoma and the neuroblastoma and are the commonest of the neurogenic tumours in the mediastinum in children. The third group include chemodectomas and phaeochromocytomas and are the rarest of the neurogenic tumours in the mediastinum. The majority of the neurogenic tumours are benign, but 30% are malignant.

Neurogenic tumours are usually seen as an incidental posterior mediastinal mass on a chest radiograph in a child or young adult patient. The tumour is often asymptomatic, but can produce back pain or spinal cord compression if it extends through an intervertebral foramen into the spinal canal producing a 'dumb-bell' tumour, which is usually a neurofibroma. These tumours can be multiple in patients with neurofibromatosis and can also arise in the vagus and phrenic nerves, but a mediastinal mass in a patient with this neurocutaneous syndrome can also be due to a lateral thoracic meningocoele.

A neurogenic tumour appears as a well-defined round or oval soft-tissue mass in the paravertebral gutter, which usually projects to only one side of the posterior mediastinum (Fig. 2.37). The nerve sheath tumours are usually circular in shape, whereas the ganglion cell tumours are more elongated.

The ganglion cell tumours, particularly the neuroblastoma, may contain central spicules or nodules of calcification, which is rare in the nerve sheath tumours. Neurogenic tumours may also involve adjacent bones to produce splaying of several thin posterior ribs, a localised pressure erosion defect of a vertebral body, enlargement of an intervertebral foramen, rib notching and scoliosis. Rapid increase in the size of the mass in association with bony destruction and a pleural effusion indicates the development of malignancy.

The diagnosis is confirmed by MRI (or CT), which shows a mass of intermediate signal intensity on T_1-weighted images and high signal intensity on T_2-weighted images with enhancement after gadolinium. MRI also demonstrates any intraspinal extension or cystic degeneration, but not the presence of calcification. CT shows a mass of soft-tissue attenuation which enhances after intravenous contrast medium and may contain calcification. Computer-assisted myelography also demonstrates intraspinal extension.

HIATUS HERNIA

A fixed or irreducible hiatus hernia is one of the commonest causes of a mediastinal abnormality and is usually seen as an incidental posterior mediastinal mass on a chest radiograph in an elderly patient. The hernia is often asymptomatic, but can produce dyspnoea, retrosternal chest pain, epigastric discomfort and iron deficiency anaemia. Incarceration of the stomach is uncommon.

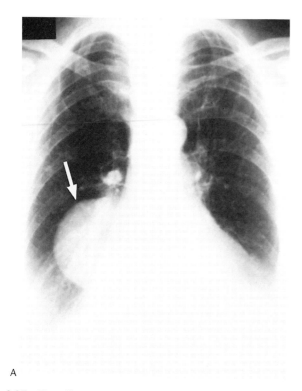

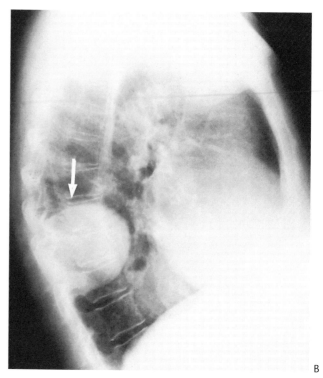

A   B

Fig. 2.37   Neurofibroma. Asymptomatic 57-year-old woman. PA (A) and lateral (B) films show a round mass in the posterior mediastinum behind the heart on the right. Lateral tomogram showed enlargement of the intervertebral foramen.

A hiatus hernia appears as a round soft-tissue mass often containing either gas or an air–fluid level behind the heart, and usually lies to the left of the midline in the posterior mediastinum (Fig. 2.32). The larger hernias can also contain small intestine, colon and liver.

The diagnosis is readily confirmed by a lateral film, or a barium meal, which shows the stomach above the diaphragm (see Fig. 18.60). The diagnosis is also often confirmed by CT which shows the contrast medium-filled stomach above the diaphragm with surrounding fatty tissue.

OESOPHAGEAL LESIONS

Lesions in the oesophagus usually present with dysphagia in an adult patient, but can also produce a cough and dyspnoea due to aspiration pneumonitis, from spillover of the oesophageal contents into the trachea and main bronchi. Oesophageal lesions can cause a number of different abnormalities in the posterior mediastinum on the chest radiograph.

A pharyngo-oesophageal pouch or Zenker's diverticulum is produced by herniation of the pharyngo-oesophageal mucosa through Killihan's dehiscence, usually on the left, between the muscle fibres of the inferior constrictor muscle. The mediastinum appears normal on a chest radiograph if the pouch is small, but a large pouch appears as a round mass containing an air–fluid level in the superior part of the posterior mediastinum. The pouch lies in the midline and displaces the trachea forwards.

A leiomyoma or a leiomyosarcoma and occasionally even a carcinoma of the oesophagus may become large enough to produce a soft-tissue mass in the posterior mediastinum and a large diverticulum of the lower oesophagus occasionally produces a

round mass containing an air–fluid level behind the heart. Achalasia of the cardia, a benign oesophageal stricture, a carcinoma of the oesophagus, systemic sclerosis and South American trypanosomiasis or Chagas disease can all cause a dilated or mega-oesophagus. The oesophagus dilates proximal to the longstanding obstruction or due to the degeneration of Auerbach's plexus in its wall. A mega-oesophagus produces widening of the posterior medi-

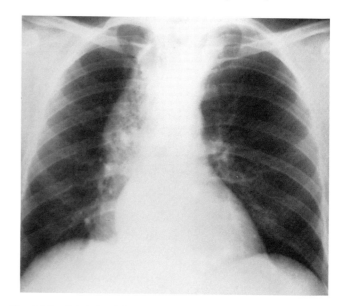

Fig. 2.38   Achalasia of the cardia. 31-year-old man presenting with dysphagia. PA film shows a dilated oesophagus containing food behind the heart on the right, with absence of air in the gastric fundus. Diagnosis confirmed by barium swallow.

astinum on the right from the thoracic inlet to the diaphragm by displacing the azygo-oesophageal line laterally (Fig. 2.38). The dilated oesophagus displaces the trachea forwards and contains an air–fluid level with the non-homogeneous mottled appearance of food mixed with air beneath it. There may also be patchy pneumonic consolidation, bronchiectasis or occasionally even pulmonary fibrosis in both lower lobes on the chest radiograph due to the recurrent aspiration pneumonitis.

The diagnosis of all oesophageal lesions is confirmed by a barium swallow or CT which shows the dilated oesophagus, large pouches or diverticula, soft-tissue masses or a thick-walled oesophagus. Oesophageal lesions are discussed in more detail in Chapter 18.

PARAVERTEBRAL LESIONS

Paravertebral lesions of the dorsal spine usually present with back pain in an adult patient and produce a bilateral abnormality in the posterior mediastinum on the chest radiograph.

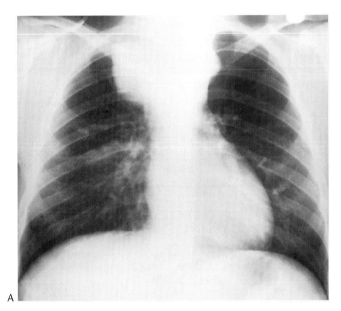

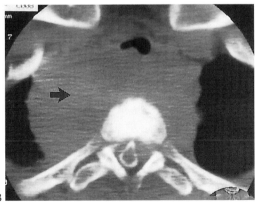

Fig. 2.39 Metastatic Ewing's sarcoma paravertebral mass. 22-year-old man presenting with spastic paraparesis. (A) PA film shows an asymmetrical paravertebral mass in the posterior mediastinum. (B) CT scan after myelography (L +175, W 1400) shows an osteoblastic bone metastasis of the upper thoracic vertebral body of T2 with an associated paravertebral soft-tissue mass (arrow) which is compressing the trachea and the spinal canal.

The differential diagnosis of a paravertebral mass includes a traumatic wedge compression fracture of a vertebral body with paraspinal haematoma formation, a pyogenic or tuberculous paraspinal abscess, metastatic carcinoma, lymphoma and multiple myeloma as well as neurofibromatosis which has been discussed above and extramedullary haemopoiesis which will be discussed below.

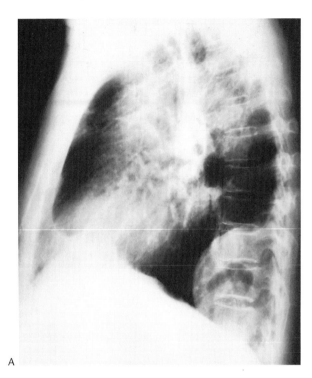

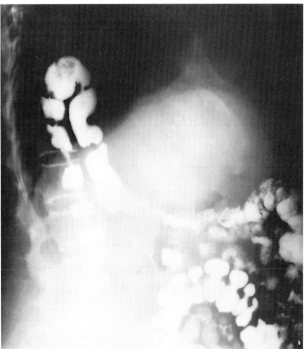

Fig. 2.40 Bochdalek's hernia. Asymptomatic 65-year-old man. (A) The lateral film shows an oval mass, which contains a loop of bowel, in the left posterior costophrenic angle. (B) Barium meal and follow-through showed the splenic flexure of the colon within the hernia.

A paravertebral mass appears as a smooth fusiform bilateral soft-tissue mass in association with abnormalities of the intervertebral disc space or vertebral body (Fig. 2.39). Narrowing of the disc space with involvement of the vertebral end-plate is a feature of an infective lesion and bone destruction with a pathological fracture of the vertebral body is a feature of a neoplastic lesion.

The diagnosis is confirmed by CT or MRI (Fig. 2.39) and needle aspiration or biopsy under fluoroscopic or CT guidance can be very useful in establishing the exact cause of an inflammatory or neoplastic mass.

BOCHDALEK'S HERNIA

The foramen of Bochdalek is a persistent developmental defect in the diaphragm posteriorly, produced by a failure of the pleuro-peritoneal canal membrane to fuse with the dorsal oesophageal mesentery medially and the body wall laterally. A hernia through the foramen of Bochdalek is usually seen as a posterior mediastinal mass in an elderly adult patient, but can present with acute respiratory distress in the neonatal period. The hernia is usually asymptomatic in an adult patients, but can produce abdominal discomfort. Strangulation of the herniating bowel is rare in neonates.

The majority of Bochdalek's hernias occur in the left hemi-diaphragm (Fig. 2.40), due to the protective effect of the liver on the right, but they can occur in the right hemidiaphragm or bilaterally. The smaller hernias usually contain retroperitoneal fat, kidney or spleen, which appears as a smooth round bulge on the posterior aspect of the diaphragm. The smaller hernias can also contain the splenic flexure of the colon, which appears as a gas-filled loop of bowel in the posterior costophrenic angle (Fig. 2.40).

The large congenital hernias contain stomach, small intestine and colon, which appears as multiple gas-filled ring shadows in the left hemithorax. The air-filled loops of bowel in the chest produce displacement of the heart and mediastinum into the contralateral hemithorax and a compressed hypoplastic lung in the ipsilateral hemithorax. The larger hernias can also contain liver.

The diagnosis is confirmed by CT, which shows the retroperitoneal fat (-70 to -130 HU) and kidney above a defect in the diaphragm. The diagnosis can also be confirmed by a barium follow-through examination or a barium enema, which show a loop of colon above the diaphragm (Fig. 2.40). Thirteen pairs of ribs may occur in association with a Bochdalek's hernia.

NEURENTERIC CYSTS

The developmental anomalies produced by partial or complete persistence of the neurenteric canal or its incomplete resorption include gastrointestinal reduplications, enteric cysts, neurenteric cysts, anterior meningocoeles and cysts of the cord. These rare developmental cysts are closely related not only to the oesophagus, to which there may be fibrous attachments, but also to the thoracic spine, in which there may be congenital bony abnormalities such as block vertebra, hemivertebra, butterfly vertebra and spina bifida (hence the split notochord syndrome).

A neurenteric cyst is a thin-walled foregut cyst lined by stratified squamous or ciliated columnar epithelial cells of both gastro-intestinal and notochordal or neural origin, which contains fluid material. A neurenteric cyst usually presents with either respiratory distress or feeding difficulties in infants. An anterior meningocoele is usually asymptomatic, but an oesophageal duplication cyst can produce dysphagia or chest pain in a child or young adult patient. Rarely haemorrhage into the cyst can occur or the cyst can become infected and rupture into the oesophagus. These cysts appear as a well-defined round or oval soft-tissue mass in the posterior mediastinum.

The diagnosis of an anterior meningocoele is confirmed by computer-assisted myelography, which shows the contrast medium entering the meningocoele in the prone position.

The diagnosis of an oesophageal duplication cyst is occasionally confirmed by a barium swallow, if the contrast medium actually enters the cyst, but is more likely to show extrinsic compression of the oesophagus. The diagnosis of a neurenteric cyst is confirmed by ultrasound which shows a transonic cystic mass, or CT which shows a mass of either low or soft-tissue attenuation, or MRI which shows a mass with variable signal intensity on T_1- and T_2-weighted images.

PANCREATIC PSEUDOCYST

A pseudocyst of the pancreas extending through the oesophageal or aortic hiatus into the chest is a rare complication of acute pancreatitis. A mediastinal pseudocyst can produce dysphagia, dyspnoea and chest pain and is seen in the posterior mediastinum on a chest radiograph in an adult patient.

The pseudocyst appears as a round or oval soft-tissue mass behind the heart often in association with a left pleural effusion and atelectasis in the lower lobes on the chest radiograph.

The diagnosis is confirmed by CT, which shows a thin-walled cystic mass containing fluid in the posterior mediastinum behind the heart in continuity with a similar thin-walled cystic mass in the lesser sac, adjacent to the pancreas (Fig. 2.41).

EXTRAMEDULLARY HAEMOPOIESIS

Extramedullary haemopoiesis in the chest is a rare manifestation of the chronic haemolytic anaemias, such as thalassaemia major and sickle cell disease, but can also occur in myelofibrosis. Extramedullary haemopoiesis is usually seen as an incidental posterior

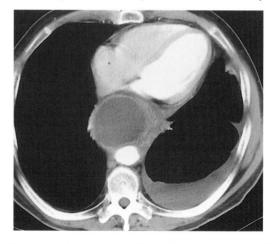

Fig. 2.41 Pancreatic pseudocyst. 65-year-old man presenting with acute pancreatitis and a left pleural effusion on a chest film. CT scan with contrast enhancement (L +35, W 325) above the diaphragm shows a round cystic mass, 8 cm in size, behind the heart in the posterior mediastinum.

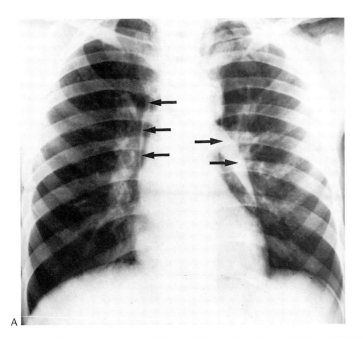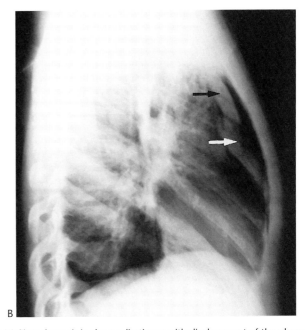

Fig. 2.42 Pneumomediastinum. 12-year-old boy with asthma. PA (A) and lateral (B) films show air in the mediastinum with displacement of the pleura (←) and demonstration of the thymus gland (→).

mediastinal mass on a chest radiograph in children or young adult patients with a chronic haemolytic anaemia. It appears as bilateral lobulated paravertebral soft-tissue masses behind the heart. The diagnosis is confirmed by CT (or MRI) which shows the haemopoietic tissue as high signal intensity on T_1- and T_2-weighted images.

PNEUMOMEDIASTINUM

Air in the mediastinum is usually seen as an incidental finding on a chest radiograph in an asymptomatic child or adult patient due to spontaneous rupture of the alveoli in the lungs. A spontaneous pneumomediastinum is caused by asthma, prolonged coughing as in whooping cough, exercise, prolonged vomiting as in diabetic ketoacidosis, childbirth and intermittent positive-pressure ventilation especially in neonates. A pneumomediastinum can also occur following perforation of the oesophagus due to endoscopy or treatment of an oesophageal stricture, rupture of the oesophagus due to repeated vomiting in Boerhaave's syndrome, after median sternotomy or mediastinoscopy, rupture of the trachea or main bronchi in chest trauma and pneumoperitoneum from any cause.

Air in the mediastinum appears as translucent streaks of gas outlining the blood vessels and other structures with lateral displacement of the parietal layer of the pleura on the chest radiograph. A large volume of air tracks throughout the mediastinum and up into the neck to produce surgical emphysema on the PA film, but a small volume of air is only seen behind the sternum or heart on a lateral film (Fig. 2.42).

The presence of chest pain and fever in a patient with air in the mediastinum indicates acute mediastinitis, which is usually due to perforation of the pharynx or oesophagus. Acute mediastinitis produces widening of the mediastinum which contains translucent streaks of gas with a round or oval soft-tissue mass containing bubbles of gas or an air–fluid level if an abscess develops

(Fig. 2.43). The diagnosis of a pneumomediastinum, acute mediastinitis or a mediastinal abscess is confirmed by CT, which readily demonstrates the presence of gas in the mediastinal tissues.

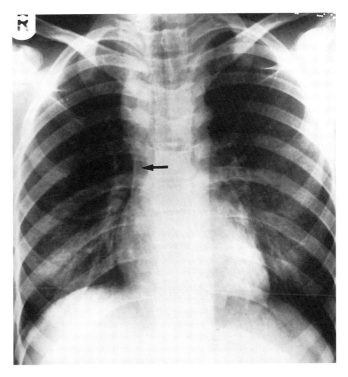

Fig. 2.43 Abscess. 15-year-old girl with a short history of pyrexia several days after a pharyngo-oesophageal tear produced by an explosion of a well-known soda pop into her mouth as she opened the bottle with her teeth. PA film shows a right paratracheal mass in the middle mediastinum and traces of the resolving mediastinal gas (arrow).

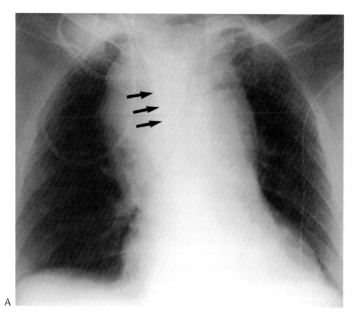
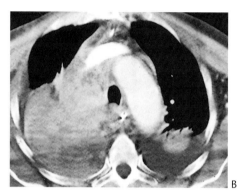

Fig. 2.44 Haemorrhage. 75-year-old man with chest pain following the insertion of a central venous catheter in theatre. AP film (A) shows widening of the mediastinum and the catheter (arrows) whose tip was in the innominate artery. CT scan with contrast enhancement (L +50, W 350) (B) above the tracheal bifurcation shows haemorrhage throughout the mediastinum with a left pleural effusion and consolidation.

MEDIASTINAL FIBROSIS

Mediastinal fibrosis is usually seen as a mediastinal abnormality on a chest radiograph in an adult patient who has had radiotherapy or a chronic inflammatory mediastinitis due to tuberculosis, histoplasmosis or coccidioidomycosis. It can also occur in patients with idiopathic retroperitoneal fibrosis or Riedel's thyroiditis and in patients on treatment with methysergide.

Mediastinal fibrosis is often asymptomatic but can produce superior vena caval obstruction or compression of other mediastinal structures. The mediastinal fibrosis produces widening of the mediastinum, which may contain calcified lymph nodes (Fig. 2.31). The diagnosis is confirmed by CT (or MRI), which shows the fibrous tissue as streaky soft-tissue attenuation and calcification within the mediastinal fat. MRI shows the mediastinal fibrosis as low signal intensity on T_1- and T_2-weighted images. The diagnosis can also be confirmed by phlebography, which shows smooth narrowing or complete occlusion of the brachiocephalic veins and superior vena cava (see Fig. 15.92).

MEDIASTINAL HAEMORRHAGE

Mediastinal haemorrhage is usually seen as a mediastinal abnormality on a chest radiograph in an adult patient who has sustained either blunt or penetrating chest trauma, but it can also occur in patients with an aortic dissection, a leaking thoracic aneurysm or a bleeding disorder and in patients receiving anticoagulant or thrombolytic treatment. The blood may be initially localised within the mediastinum but gradually tracks throughout it. This produces widening of the mediastinum with tracheal displacement, a mediastinal soft-tissue mass or lateral displacement of the paraspinal lines on the chest radiograph. The widening of the mediastinum can be difficult to differentiate from mediastinal lipomatosis, but in a patient with a history of trauma the diagnosis is easily confirmed by CT (or MRI), which shows the blood as patchy or diffuse soft-tissue attenuation within the mediastinal fat with its typical higher CT number than soft tissue (Fig. 2.44). MRI shows the mediastinal haemorrhage as low signal intensity on T_1-weighted images and high signal intensity on T_2-weighted images in the presence of fresh thrombus, but its appearance changes as the thrombus matures. CT may show the cause of the mediastinal haemorrhage as a spinal fracture or aortic rupture with false aneurysm formation in patients following a road traffic accident, but if there has been a high-speed deceleration injury then arch aortography is essential to confirm the diagnosis of aortic rupture in the haemodynamically stable patient (see Fig. 15.32).

MRI OF THE MEDIASTINUM

Jeremy P. R. Jenkins

MRI can stage certain mediastinal lesions more accurately than CT. The advantages of MRI include the differentiation of solid lesions from vessels, the direct visualisation of the spinal canal and its neural contents, and the differentiation between chronic fibrosis (low signal) and recurrent lymphoma or tumour (intermediate signal). In children MRI may be the preferred technique, obviating the need for intravenous contrast enhancement, but in adults CT is more often used in conjunction with MRI. MRI is particularly indicated when the administration of intravenous contrast medium is contraindicated or when vascular opacification is suboptimal. Surgical clips can produce significant streak artefacts on CT, whereas on MRI only a localised signal void is produced. In the postoperative patient, where residual or recurrent tumour is suspected, distortion of the hilar and mediastinal anatomy can be more easily assessed on MRI because of its multiplanar capability and greater intrinsic soft-tissue and vascular contrast discrimination.

ANTERIOR MEDIASTINUM

Mediastinal thyroid

This is the commonest mass lesion in the thoracic inlet. Sagittal and transverse T_1-weighted scans demonstrate its extent and relationship to adjacent major vessels. The thyroid gland gives a signal intensity slightly greater than muscle on T_1-weighted images and a much more intense signal on T_2-weighted scans. Thyroid masses have longer relaxation times than normal thyroid and thus are of lower and higher signal on T_1- and T_2-weighted images respectively. Measurement of relaxation times is unhelpful in separating this lesion from other tumours. Haemorrhage within cysts can be shown but calcification is better demonstrated by CT. The internal architecture of this tumour, including cystic and necrotic changes, can be shown on T_2-weighted scans but better assessed using intravenous gadolinium-chelate.

Thymus

The *normal thymus* has a non-specific long T_1 and T_2 and appears of low signal, contrasting well with the high signal from surrounding fat on T_1-weighted scans but remaining isointense with fat on T_2-weighted images. The superior soft-tissue contrast resolution of MRI allowed the correct diagnosis to be made in a patient with an ectopic thymus in the posterior mediastinum because of its similarity in signal intensity characteristics to the normally positioned thymus. With increasing age, fat deposition within the normal thymus shortens its T_1 value, thereby reducing its contrast with adjacent fat.

The majority (90%) of *thymomas* are located in the anterior mediastinum and cannot be differentiated from other solid mediastinal tumours. Inhomogeneities in the tumour can occur due to cyst formation, necrosis or haemorrhage, and may be better delineated by the administration of gadolinium-chelate. A disadvantage of gadolinium-chelate enhancement in T_1-weighted images is the loss of contrast between fat and enhancing tumour, although this can be obviated by the use of frequency-offset fat-suppression technique. *Malignant thymomas* cannot be differentiated from benign tumours on signal intensity appearances or on relaxation time measurements, but can be recognised by evidence of invasion of adjacent structures.

Cystic mediastinal masses

MRI can demonstrate the cystic nature of lesions in the mediastinum when this is difficult to ascertain by other imaging techniques, including CT. *Simple cysts* typically have a very long T_1 and T_2, with a signal intensity similar to that of cerebrospinal fluid or urine. The actual signal intensity within the cyst does, however, depend upon its contents (Fig. 2.45). It is important, therefore, to appreciate that the MR appearance may be ambiguous and, in the presence of haemorrhage or an increase in the proteinaceous material within the cyst, may suggest a solid mass. The use of intravenous gadolinium-chelate is helpful in confirming a solid mass lesion which demonstrates enhancement compared with a non-enhancing central cyst. A uniformly high signal intensity on T_1-weighted images, due to the presence of altered haemorrhage, is a typical feature of a benign cyst. In the assessment of *teratodermoids*,

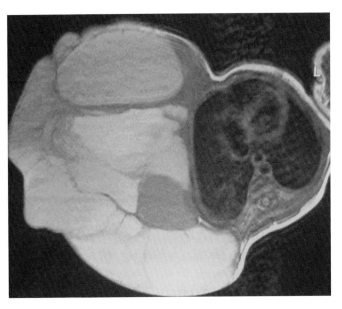

Fig. 2.45 Extrathoracic cystic hygroma (lymphangioma) in a 3-day-old neonate showing high signal due to dilated lymphatic spaces on a T_1-weighted spin-echo image.

CT is superior to MRI because of its ability to detect calcification. Lipid is well shown by both techniques.

MIDDLE MEDIASTINUM

Nodal disease

There is debate as to the relative merits of ECG-gated or rapid-acquisition non-gated T_1-weighted images in the demonstration of mediastinal and hilar nodes. Both techniques provide equivalent morphological detail and reduce cardiac and respiratory motion artefacts, but the rapid-acquisition non-gated scans are more heavily T_1-weighted, providing greater soft-tissue contrast between lymph nodes and fat. It is generally agreed that MRI is slightly superior to CT in the detection of lymph node enlargement of the hilum but equivalent in the general assessment of enlarged nodes in the mediastinum. As hilar nodes are closely related to vessels, the superior contrast and multiplanar capability of MRI more than compensates for its slightly inferior spatial resolution. MRI can be of value in evaluating the *aortopulmonary window* and *subcarinal spaces* (Fig. 2.46)—areas that are difficult to delineate using the transverse plane of CT. MRI, however, has poorer spatial resolution and may not resolve small adjacent but separate nodes. *Calcification* within nodes, which may be useful as an estimate of benignity, is not easily detected. In patients with little mediastinal fat, small nodes can be difficult to define.

The diagnosis of nodal disease depends on the same *size* criteria as for CT. There is current debate as to the precise size criteria to be applied in different nodal areas, and also which dimension of the node (short or long axis) should be used for measurement. Generally, nodes greater than 10 mm are considered to be enlarged and involved by tumour. It should be recognised, however, that not all enlarged nodes are tumorous and that metastases can occur in normal-sized nodes. It is not possible from measured relaxation time values or other MRI criteria to distinguish between tumour-

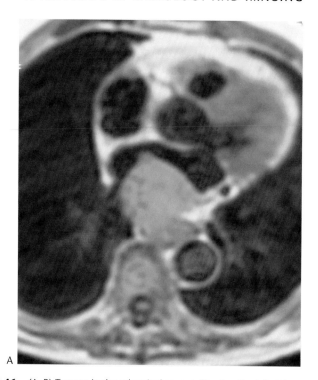

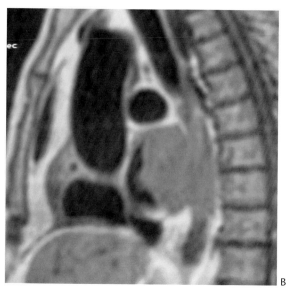

Fig. 2.46 (A, B) Tumour in the subcarinal space infiltrating the left atrium on transverse and sagittal ECG-gated T_1-weighted spin echo images.

involved nodes and reactive hyperplastic nodes. An in vitro study of freshly removed lymph nodes from patients with lung cancer has shown significant ($P < 0.05$) differences in the mean T_1 values of tumorous (640 ms) and non-tumorous (566 ms) nodes. There was, however, too much overlap between the two groups for this to be of clinical relevance.

Although relaxation time values in themselves have limited value in the differentiation of pathology, the use of more sophisticated image analysis techniques, including texture analysis, may have great potential in detecting changes between tumour and non-tumour tissue which may not be demonstrable on visual inspection alone.

A new MRI lymphographic contrast agent, using an ultrasmall (<10 nm diameter) superparamagnetic iron oxide preparation, is available for imaging the lymphatic system (see Ch. 59). Following intravenous administration the ultrasmall iron oxide compound is able to bypass the mononuclear phagocytic system of the liver and spleen, cross capillary walls and achieve widespread tissue distribution, including lymph nodes and bone marrow. The particles accumulate in normal lymph nodes markedly reducing their signal intensity, producing a single void, by a superparamagnetic effect. Malignant tissue is spared, and metastatic nodes, therefore, appear more intense than normal nodes. The use of such an agent could enable visualisation of normal nodal anatomy and thus enhance the detection of nodal disease irrespective of size or anatomical distribution.

Lymphoma

MRI is not able to characterise tissue reliably. Most malignancies have a non-specific long T_1 and T_2, and their enhancement characteristics using gadolinium-chelate are similar. Lymphoma usually has a homogeneous intermediate signal intensity on T_1-weighted images and appears isointense with fat on T_2-weighted scans.

Nodular sclerosing Hodgkin's disease can appear heterogeneous, with low signal areas which are presumed to be due to a high fibrous content in this tumour type.

In the early post-treatment phase (8–12 weeks), responding lymphomas demonstrate heterogeneity in signal intensity, with a decrease in the T_2-weighted signal, associated with reduction in tumour size. Inactive residual masses assume a homogeneous low signal intensity pattern. Recurrent disease may be detected as an increase in signal intensity on the T_2-weighted images prior to evidence of a clinical relapse. Problems in interpretation, however, may result from intermixing of surrounding fat with an inactive mass. Postradiation or reactive inflammatory changes may also simulate active disease. A low signal from *fibrosis* is a more reliable indicator of tissue type than a high signal intensity which is not specific for tumour. MRI, nevertheless, has a role in the assessment of response to treatment and in the detection of recurrent mediastinal disease.

Great vessels

Mediastinal disease can involve the mediastinal great vessels. Vascular abnormalities can be assessed with MRI without the need for the administration of intravenous contrast medium. The high intrinsic soft-tissue contrast, due to the low signal from flowing blood compared with the intermediate signal from the vessel wall and high signal from adjacent fat, gives MRI significant advantages over CT. Flow artefacts with signal within vessels during different phases of the cardiac cycle using conventional pulse sequences need to be recognised and correctly interpreted. MRI has been shown to be useful in the evaluation of central pulmonary embolism and pulmonary arterial hypertension. Peripheral emboli are poorly shown due to the intrinsic low signal from inflated lung.

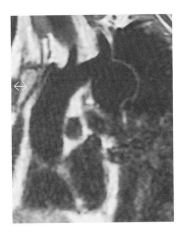

Fig. 2.47 Aneurysm at the site of a previous coarctation repair on a sagittal-oblique T_1-weighted ECG-gated spin echo image.

Aorta

Both acquired and congenital lesions of the thoracic aorta can be shown to advantage with MRI, which has significant advantages over CT and angiography, particularly in the evaluation of *aortic aneurysms* and *coarctation* (Fig. 2.47) (see Ch. 15). The dimensions and extent of an aneurysm, the differentiation of a patent lumen from thrombus formation and the delineation of vessel wall from surrounding mediastinal fat can all be assessed. The use of multiplanar imaging allows the aortic valve and proximal origin of the great vessels to be demonstrated.

The origin and extent of *aortic dissection*, involvement of the arch and the dissecting flap can be well shown on MRI (Fig. 2.48). The distinction between slow-flowing blood and thrombus may be difficult on conventional pulse sequences and does require a more flow-sensitive sequence (phase-sensitive or gradient-echo even-echo rephasing). The ability to measure blood flow velocity in vivo

using flow-sensitive sequences enables a clear separation between the true and false lumens to be made, together with an assessment of the re-entry site in aortic dissection (see Ch. 15). Three-dimensional gadolinium-enhanced MR angiography can provide a comprehensive mapping of the entire thoracic aorta and its major branches within a breath-hold. In this technique an intravenous infusion of gadolinium-chelate is used to shorten the T_1 relaxation time of blood, making it possible to outline the aorta on a heavily T_1-weighted sequence without depending on the time-of-flight effect. This method uses a standard three-dimensional gradient-echo pulse sequence and the conventional body, or preferably a phased-array coil. A particular advantage of this technique is that the images are acquired without the need for ECG-gating useful in patients with arrhythmias. Also, the data set can be reformatted in any imaging plane by postprocessing. The main disadvantage is the requirement of a contrast injection, as most thoracic aorta pathologies can be diagnosed on conventional sequences without the use of gadolinium-chelate.

Mediastinal veins

Superior vena caval infiltration or obstruction secondary to thoracic tumour can be well shown on transverse and coronal T_1-weighted images (Fig. 2.49). The same flow void phenomenon is observed in veins as in arteries, but signals within veins due to slow flow can be difficult to interpret. The distinction between slow flow and thrombus may require the use of phase-sensitive or gradient-rephasing sequences. Gadolinium-chelate can be useful in showing intraluminal tumour infiltration, which enhances compared with intraluminal thrombus (which shows no change in signal intensity). Gadolinium-chelate can also enhance slow-flowing venous blood, producing an increase in intraluminal signal, but this is usually more pronounced than that from tumour enhancement.

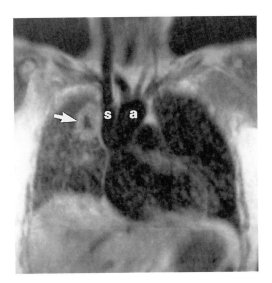

Fig. 2.49 Recurrent malignant fibrous histocytoma of the right lung (arrow) following previous lobectomy on coronal spin echo (1100/26) image. The tumour is attached to and involves the lateral wall of the superior vena cava(s). a = aortic arch. (Reproduced with permission from Jenkins, J. P. R., Isherwood, I. (1987) Magnetic resonance of the heart: a review. In: Rowlands, D. J. (ed.) *Recent Advances in Cardiology 10*. Edinburgh: Churchill Livingstone.)

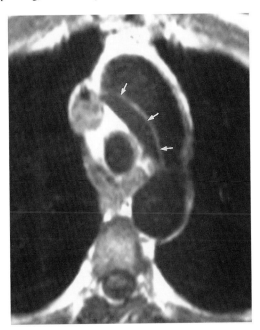

Fig. 2.48 Dissection flap (arrow) in the aortic arch on an ECG-gated T_1-weighted spin echo (700/20) image.

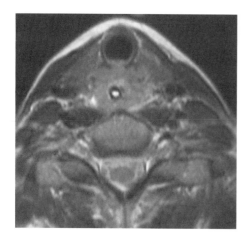

Fig. 2.50 Postcricoid carcinoma infiltrating the posterior wall of the trachea on a T$_2$-weighted spin echo image. A nasogastric tube is in situ.

Tracheal tumours

The reduced spatial resolution of MRI compared with CT accounts for the lower accuracy in the detection of 319 normal and 79 diseased bronchi confirmed bronchoscopically—40% normal and 70% diseased bronchi were visualised on MRI and 98% for both groups on CT. MRI and CT are considered equivalent in the visualization of larger airways (Fig. 2.50), but MRI has the possible advantage of imaging the whole trachea and major bronchi in a single oblique plane or by using a volume scanning technique. CT is superior, however, to MRI in the detection of endotracheal and endobronchial lesions.

POSTERIOR MEDIASTINUM

Neurogenic tumours

MRI is superior to CT in the detection and evaluation of neurogenic tumours within the posterior mediastinum (Figs 2.51 and

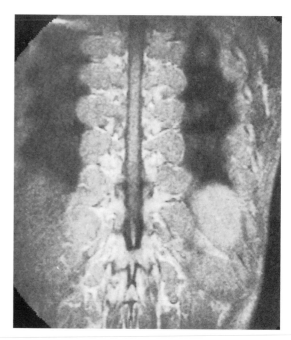

Fig. 2.51 Multiple paraspinal, intercostal and intra-abdominal neurofibromas in a patient with neurofibromatosis, on a coronal T$_1$-weighted (spin echo 700/40) image through the thorax.

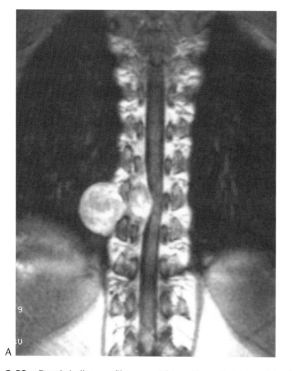

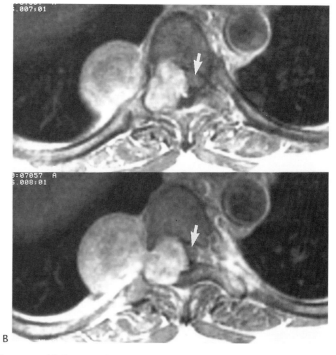

Fig. 2.52 Dumb-bell neurofibroma within a thoracic intervertebral foramen with intra- and extraspinal extensions on coronal (A) and transverse (B) T$_1$-weighted gradient-echo (300/14/90°) postgadolinium-chelate injection. Note the displacement of the adjacent thoracic cord (arrowed).

2.52). This is due to the higher soft-tissue contrast discrimination, allowing direct visualisation of the spine, spinal canal and cord (including nerve roots) without the need for intrathecal contrast medium, together with the multiplanar imaging facility. Calcification, which is common in neuroblastoma, is better shown by CT.

Oesophageal lesions

Smooth muscle has similar values of relaxation time to skeletal muscle. There is therefore greater soft-tissue contrast between oesophageal tumour (high signal) and muscle (low signal) on T_2-weighted images. Conventional T_2-weighted images of the mediastinum are, however, prone to significant motion artefacts and have a much lower signal-to-noise ratio than T_1-weighted images. The advent of faster scanning techniques (by use of digital RF) has overcome some of these problems, improving image appearance. On T_1-weighted images there is reduced tumour-to-muscle contrast. The use of MRI affords no advantages over CT in the assessment of oesophageal tumour, as MRI is unable to demonstrate small intraluminal and intramural tumours. Infiltration of the oesophageal wall cannot be detected, and difficulty does occur in separating tumour from intraluminal contents in stenotic lesions. Tumour enhancement may be achieved by the use of gadolinium-chelate. Equivalent assessment of mediastinal infiltration can be demonstrated on both CT and MRI.

Extramedullary haematopoiesis

Extramedullary haematopoiesis has similar signal intensity characteristics to the spleen (long T_1/long T_2). The appearances are non-specific and indistinguishable from other mediastinal tumours. Similar morphological criteria to those applied to CT can be used with MRI.

Diaphragmatic hernias

Coronal and sagittal plane imaging are particularly useful in delineating the diaphragm, which has a low signal. The relationship of intrathoracic masses to the diaphragm can be well visualised, as can the contents of the hernial sac, which determine the signal intensity.

Fibrosing mediastinitis

CT is superior to MRI in the detection of calcification invisible on chest radiographs, a feature which is important in suggesting the diagnosis of fibrosing mediastinitis. A low signal on both T_1- and T_2-weighted images, due to the presence of fibrosis, is very often sufficiently different from that from tumour to suggest the correct diagnosis.

REFERENCES AND SUGGESTIONS FOR FURTHER READING

Adler, O. B., Rosenberger, A., Peleg, H. (1983) Fine needle aspiration biopsy of mediastinal masses. *American Journal of Roentgenology*, **140**, 893–896.

Baron, R. L., Levitt, R. G., Sagel, S. S., Stanley, R. J. (1981) Computed tomography in the evaluation of mediastinal widening. *Radiology*, **138**, 107–113.

Baron, R. L., Lee, J. K. T., Sagel, S. S., Peterson, R. R. (1982) Computed tomography of the normal thymus. *American Journal of Roentgenology*, **142**, 121–125.

Cohen, A. M., Creviston, S., Li Puma, J. P., Lieberman, J., Haaga, J. R., Alfidi, R. J. (1983) Nuclear magnetic resonance imaging of the mediastinum and hili. *American Journal of Roentgenology*, **141**, 1163–1169.

Crowe, J. K., Brown, L. R., Muhm, J. R. (1978) Computed tomography of the mediastinum. *Radiology*, **128**, 75–87.

Day, D. L., Gedgaudas, E. (1984) The thymus. *Radiologic Clinics of North America*, **22**, 519–538.

Egan, T. J., Neiman, H. L., Herman, R. J., Malave, S. R., Sanders, J. H. (1980) Computed tomography in the diagnosis of aortic aneurysm dissection or traumatic injury. *Radiology*, **136**, 141–146.

Fon, G. T., Bein, M. E., Mancuso, A. A., Keesey, J. C., Lupetin, A. R., Wong, W. S. (1982) Computed tomography of the anterior mediastinum in myasthenia gravis. *Radiology*, **142**, 135–141.

Gamsu, G., Webb, W. R., Sheldon, P., Kaufman, L. Crooks, L. E., Birnberg, F. A., Goodman, P., Hincliffe, W. A., Hedgecock, M. (1983) Nuclear magnetic resonance imaging of the thorax. *Radiology*, **147**, 473–480.

Glazer, H. S. (1989) Differential diagnosis of mediastinal pathology. *CT Review*, **1**, 41–51.

Heitzman, E. R., Goldwin, R. L., Proto, A. V. (1977) Radiological analysis of the mediastinum utilizing computed tomography. *Radiologic Clinics of North America*, **15**, 309–329.

Husband, J. E. S. (1989) Thymic masses and hyperplasia. *CT Review*, **1**, 53–63.

Kirks, D. R., Korobkin, M. (1981) Computed tomography of the chest in infants and children: techniques and mediastinal evaluation. *Radiologic Clinics of North America*, **19**, 409–419.

Lyons, H. A., Calvey, G. L., Sammons, B. P. (1959) The diagnosis and classification of mediastinal masses: a study of 782 cases. *Annals of Internal Medicine*, **51**, 897–932.

McLoud, T. C., Meyer, J. E. (1982) Mediastinal metastases. *Radiologic Clinics of North America*, **20**, 453–468.

Morrison, I. M. (1958) Tumors and cysts of the mediastinum. *Thorax*, **13**, 294–307.

Oudkerk, M., Overbosch, E., Dee, P. (1983) CT recognition of acute aortic dissection. *American Journal of Roentgenology*, **141**, 671–676.

Pugatch, R. D., Faling, L. J., Robbins, A. H., Spira, R. (1980) CT diagnosis of benign mediastinal abnormalities. *American Journal of Roentgenology*, **134**, 685–694.

Siegal, M. J., Sagel, S. S., Reed, K. (1982) The value of computed tomography in the diagnosis and management of pediatric mediastinal abnormalities. *Radiology*, **142**, 149–155.

Von Schulthess, G. K., McMurdo, K., Tscholakoff, D., De Geer, G., Gamsu, G., Higgins, C.B. (1986) Mediastinal masses: MR imaging. *Radiology*, **158**, 289–296.

Westcott, J. L. (1981) Percutaneous needle aspiration of hilar and mediastinal masses. *Radiology*, **141**, 323–329.

Wychulis, A. R., Payne, W. S., Clagett, O. T., Woolner, L. B. (1971) Surgical treatment of mediastinal tumours: a 40-year experience. *Journal of Thoracic and Cardiovascular Surgery*, **62**, 379–392.

MRI of the mediastinum

Armstrong, P. (2000) Mediastinal and hilar disorders. In: Armstrong, P., Wilson, A. G., Dee,P., Hansell, D. M. (eds) *Imaging of Diseases of the Chest*, 3rd edn, ch. 15, pp. 789–892. C. V. Mosby.

Herold, C. J., Zerhouni, E. A. (1992) The mediastinum and lungs. In: Higgins, C. B., Hricak, H., Helms, C. A. (eds) *Magnetic Resonance Imaging of the Body*, 2nd edn, ch. 22, pp. 461–523. New York: Raven Press.

Husband, J. E. S., Resnek, R. (eds) (1998) *Imaging in Oncology*. Oxford: ISIS Medical Media.

Lesko, N. M., Link, K. M. (1999) Mediastinum and lung. In: Stark, D. D., Bradley, W.G. (eds) *Magnetic Resonance Imaging*, 3rd edn, ch. 18, pp. 355–371. St Louis: C.V. Mosby.

Link, K. M. (1992) Great vessels. In: Stark, D. D., Bradley, W. G. (eds) *Magnetic Resonance Imaging*, 2nd edn, ch. 46, pp. 1490–1530. St Louis: C. V. Mosby.

Matsumoto, A. H., Tegtmeyer, C. J. (1995) Contemporary diagnostic approaches to acute pulmonary emboli. *Radiologic Clinics of North America*, **33**, 167–183.

Naidich, D. P., Webb, R., Mueller, N. L., Krinsky, G. A., Zerhouni, E. A., Siegelman, S. S. (eds) (2000) *Computed Tomography and Magnetic Resonance of the Thorax*, 3rd edn. New York: Lippincott Williams & Wilkins.

Prince, M. R., Narasimham, D. L. Jacoby, W. T., Williams, D. M., Cho, K. J., Marx, M. V., Deeb, G. M. (1996) Three-dimensional gadolinium-enhanced MR angiography of the thoracic aorta. *American Journal of Roentgenology*, **166**, 1387–1397.

Scott, S. (1995) Basic concepts of magnetic resonance angiography. *Radiologic Clinics of North America*, **33**, 91–113.

Weissleder, R., Elizondo, G., Wittenberg, L., Lee, A. S., Josephson, L., Brady, T. (1990) Ultrasmall superparamagnetic iron oxide; an intravenous contrast agent for assessing lymph nodes with MR imaging. *Radiology*, **175**, 494–498.

White, C. S. (ed.) (2000) MR imaging of the thorax. *MRI Clinics of North America*, **8**, 1–224.

Zerhouni, E. A., Herold, C. J., Hahn, D. (1992) Mediastinum and lung. In: Stark, D. D., Bradley, W. G. (eds) *Magnetic Resonance Imaging*, 2nd edn, ch. 45, pp. 1429–1489. St Louis: C. V. Mosby.

CT of the mediastinum

Costello, P. (1995) Thoracic imaging with spiral CT. In: Fishman, E. K., Jeffrey, R. B. (eds) *Spiral CT: Principles, Techniques and Clinical Applications*, pp. 109–130. New York: Raven Press.

Prokop, M. (2000) Multislice CT angiography. *European Journal of Radiology*, **36**, 86–96.

Rydberg, J., Buckwalter, K. A., Caldemeyer, K. S., Phillips, M. D., Conces, D. J., Aisen, A. M., Persohn, S. A., Kopecky, K. K. (2000) Multisection CT: scanning techniques and clinical applications. *Radiographics*, **20**, 1787–1806.

Wegener, O. H. (1992) The mediastinum. In: *Whole Body Computed Tomography*, pp. 137–170. Massachusetts: Blackwell Scientific.

3

THE PLEURA

Michael B. Rubens and Simon P. G. Padley

Basic anatomy

The pleura is a serous membrane which covers the surface of the lung and lines the inner surface of the chest wall. The visceral pleura, over the lung, and the parietal pleura, over the chest wall, are continuous at the hilum, where a fold of pleura extends inferiorly to form the inferior pulmonary ligament. The two layers of pleura are closely applied to each other, being separated by a thin layer of lubricating pleural fluid. The parietal pleura, and the visceral pleura over the periphery of the lung are not normally visible radiographically. However, where the visceral pleura lines the interlobar fissures of the lung it is often visible, there being two layers of pleura outlined by aerated lung. The horizontal fissure of the right lung is often seen on a frontal chest film, and the oblique fissures will usually be seen on the lateral views. Some patients have one or more accessory fissures, the most common being the azygos fissure and the inferior accessory fissure of the right lower lobe. Occasionally anterior or posterior junction lines are seen in the frontal chest film, where the left and right lungs come into contact in the mediastinum.

Some physiological considerations

The normal anatomy of the lungs is maintained by a balance between different elastic forces of the chest wall and lungs. The lung has a natural tendency to collapse toward its hilum, and this is opposed by forces of similar magnitude in the chest wall tending to expand outward. The visceral and parietal layers of pleura are thus kept in close apposition. If increased fluid or air collects in the pleural space, the effect of the outward forces on the underlying lung is diminished, and the lung tends to retract toward its hilum. Therefore, in an erect patient a small pleural effusion which has gravitated to the base of the lung causes retraction of the lower part of the lung, but has comparatively little effect at the apex. Conversely, a small pneumothorax will collect at the apex and have little effect at the lung base. Obviously, large intrapleural collections will affect the entire lung. These basic patterns may be altered by the state of the underlying lung and the presence of pleural adhesions. Fibrotic, emphysematous or consolidated lung may not be able to retract and adhesions may prevent the usual distribution of air or fluid.

DISEASES OF THE PLEURA

PLEURAL FLUID

Fluid will accumulate in the pleural space if the rate of its production exceeds its rate of resorption. This may be due to: (i) increased microvascular pressure in the lungs (e.g. in heart failure); (ii) reduced plasma oncotic pressure (e.g. in hypoproteinaemia); (iii) increased microvascular permeability (e.g. in pleurisy); (iv) reduced lymphatic drainage from the pleural space (e.g. in lymphangitis); or (v) passage of peritoneal fluid across defects in the diaphragm.

Fluid which accumulates in the pleural space may be transudate, exudate, pus, blood or chyle. Radiographically these produce similar shadows and are therefore indistinguishable. However, there may be clinical data to point to the aetiology, or the chest film may show other abnormalities, such as evidence of heart failure or trauma, which indicate the cause. Sometimes the definitive diagnosis is only made after thoracentesis or pleural biopsy; not infrequently it remains obscure.

Transudates Transudates contain less than 3 g/dl of protein, and are usually clear or faintly yellow, watery fluids. A pleural transudate may be called a hydrothorax. They are often bilateral. The commonest cause is *cardiac failure*, when the effusion usually accumulates first on the right, before becoming bilateral. Other causes are *hypoproteinaemia* (especially the nephrotic syndrome, hepatic cirrhosis and anaemia), *constrictive pericarditis, Meigs' syndrome* and *myxoedema*.

Exudates Exudates contain in excess of 3 g/dl of protein, and vary from amber, slightly cloudy fluid, which often clots on standing, to frank pus. A purulent pleural effusion is termed an empyema. The commonest causes of pleural exudate are *bacterial pneumonia, pulmonary tuberculosis, carcinoma of the lung, metastatic malignancy* and *pulmonary infarction*. Less common causes are *subphrenic infection, connective tissue disorders* (especially systemic lupus erythematosus and rheumatoid disease) and *non-bacterial* pneumonias. Unusual causes include *postmyocardial infarction syndrome, acute pancreatitis* and *primary neoplasia* of the pleura.

Haemothorax Bleeding into the pleural space is almost always secondary to open or closed trauma to the chest. Rarely, it is due to *haemophilia* or excessive *anticoagulation*. The effusions associated with pulmonary infarction and carcinoma of the lung are frequently blood stained but rarely pure blood.

Chylothorax Chyle is a milky fluid high in neutral fat and fatty acids. Chylothorax may develop secondary to damage or obstruction of the thoracic lymphatic vessels. The commonest cause is chest *trauma*, usually surgical. Other causes include *carcinoma of the lung, lymphoma* and *filariasis. Lymphangiomyomatosis* is a rare cause.

Radiological appearances of pleural fluid

Free fluid Pleural fluid casts a shadow of the density of water or soft tissue on the chest radiograph. In the absence of pleural adhesions, the position and morphology of this shadow will depend upon the amount of fluid, the state of the underlying lung and the position of the patient. The most dependent recess of the pleura is the posterior costophrenic angle. A *small effusion* will, therefore, tend to collect posteriorly and in most patients 100–200 ml of fluid are required to fill this recess before fluid will be seen above the dome of the diaphragm on the frontal view (Fig. 3.1). Small effusions may thus be seen earlier on a lateral film than on a frontal film, but it is possible to identify effusions of only a few millilitres using decubitus views with a horizontal beam (Fig. 3.2), ultrasound or CT (Fig. 3.3). As more fluid accumulates, the costophrenic angle on the frontal view fills, and with increasing fluid a homogeneous opacity spreads upward, obscuring the lung base. Typically this opacity has a fairly well defined, concave upper edge, is higher laterally than medially and obscures the diaphragmatic shadow (Fig. 3.4). Frequently fluid will track into the pleural fissures. If the film is sufficiently penetrated, pulmonary vessels in the lung masked by the effusion will be seen. A *massive effusion* may cause

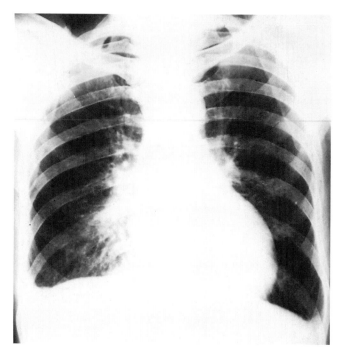

Fig. 3.1 Small bilateral pleural effusions. Man aged 58 with ischaemic heart disease. The left costophrenic angle is blunted by a small effusion. The right pleural effusion is larger, and fluid is beginning to extend up the chest wall.

complete radiopacity of a hemithorax. The underlying lung will have retracted toward its hilum, and the space-occupying effect of the effusion will push the mediastinum toward the opposite side (Fig. 3.5). In the presence of a large effusion, lack of displacement of the mediastinum suggests that the underlying lung is completely collapsed and when the effusion is of moderate size mediastinal

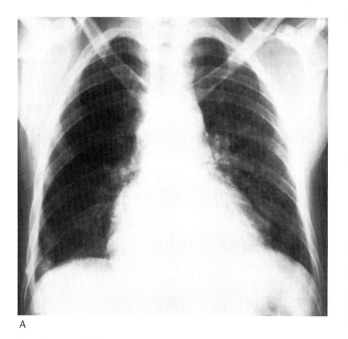

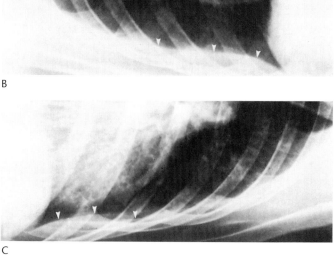

Fig. 3.2 Small bilateral pleural effusions. Man aged 34, renal transplant patient with cytomegalovirus pneumonia. The effusions probably relate to renal failure rather than the pneumonia. (A) PA film shows subtle filling in of both costophrenic angles. (B, C) Horizontal-beam right and left lateral decubitus films show obvious free pleural effusions collecting along the dependent lateral costal margins (arrowheads).

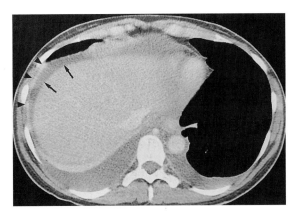

Fig. 3.3 CT scan through the dome of the right diaphragm. There are small pleural effusions in the posterior costophrenic recesses bilaterally. There is also a small volume of abdominal ascites (arrows) between the anterior surface of the liver and the undersurface of the diaphragm (arrowheads).

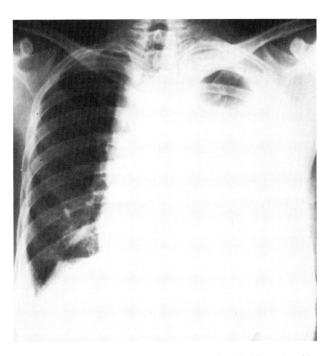

Fig. 3.5 Large pleural effusion. Man of 28 with well-differentiated lymphocytic lymphoma. PA film shows a large left pleural effusion extending over apex of lung and pushing the mediastinum to the right. A small right pleural effusion is also present, and right paratracheal shadowing represents lymphadenopathy.

The contour of the 'diaphragm' is altered, its apex being more lateral than usual, and there may be some blunting of the costophrenic angle or tracking of fluid into fissures (Fig. 3.7). On the left side increased distance between the gastric air bubble and lung base may be apparent. A subpulmonary effusion in a free pleural space will move with changes of posture, as can be demonstrated by horizontal-beam lateral decubitus or supine films. A large right pleural effusion may collect in the azygo-oesophageal recess and mimic a

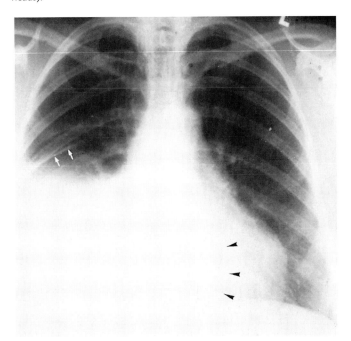

Fig. 3.4 Moderate-size pleural effusion in a woman of 56. Effusions of unknown aetiology. PA film demonstrates typical pleural opacity with concave upper border, slightly higher laterally, and obscuring the diaphragm and underlying lung. Fluid is extending into the fissure (arrows) and also into the azygo-oesophageal recess, producing a retrocardiac opacity (arrowheads).

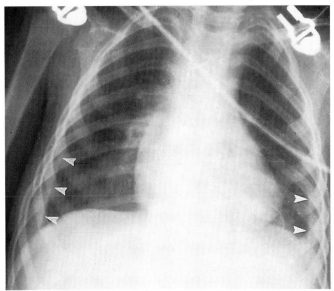

Fig. 3.6 Lamellar pleural effusions, postcardiac surgery. Erect AP film shows fluid filling both costophrenic angles and extending up the lateral chest wall (arrowheads).

shift toward the side of collapse may occur. This is likely to be due to carcinoma of the bronchus. In the presence of pleural disease the ipsilateral hemidiaphragm is usually elevated. However, the weight of a large effusion may cause inversion of the diaphragm, and this sign is probably best demonstrated by ultrasound.

Atypical distribution of pleural fluid is quite common. *Lamellar effusions* are shallow collections between the lung surface and the visceral pleura (Fig. 3.6), sometimes sparing the costophrenic angle. Strictly, lamellar effusions represent interstitial pulmonary fluid. Occasionally quite large effusions accumulate between the diaphragm and undersurface of a lung, mimicking elevation of that hemidiaphragm. This is the so-called *subpulmonary pleural effusion.*

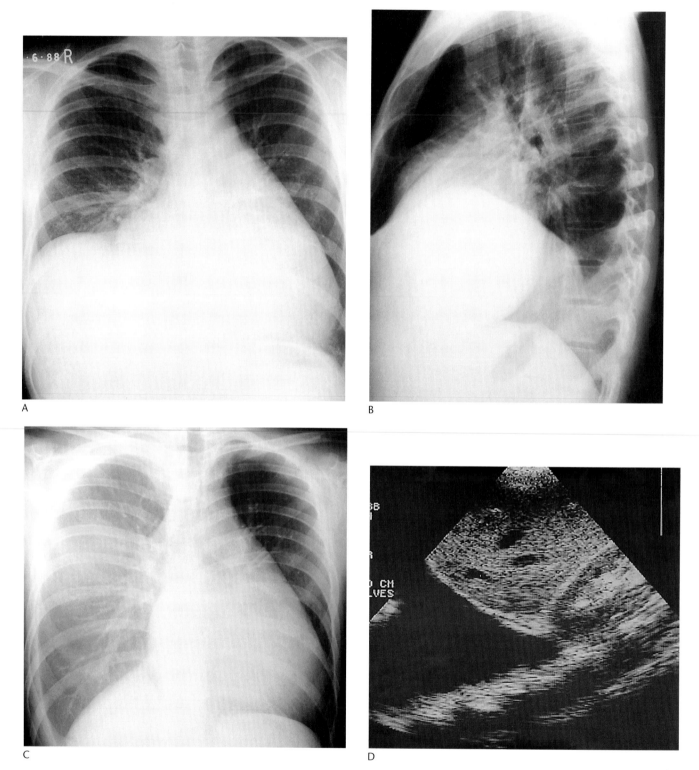

Fig. 3.7 Fifteen-year-old male with adriamycin-induced cardiomyopathy and recently increasing shortness of breath. (A) Erect PA film shows a large heart and apparent elevation of the right hemidiaphragm due to a large subpulmonic effusion. (B) Lateral film shows fluid tracking up the posterior chest wall and blunting the posterior costophrenic recess. (C) Supine chest radiograph obtained shortly afterwards showing redistribution of pleural fluid. The appearances are now typical of a large supine pleural effusion with increased density of the right hemithorax. (D) Ultrasound of the right lung base reveals a large anechoic space consistent with an uncomplicated pleural effusion.

retrocardiac mass (Figs 3.4, 3.8). The reasons for atypical distribution of pleural fluid are often unclear, but it may be associated with abnormality of the underlying lung.

Loculated fluid The pleural space may be partially obliterated by pleural disease, causing fusion of the parietal and visceral layers. Encapsulated and free pleural fluid can be distinguished by gravitational methods. Encapsulated fluid, however, may be difficult to differentiate from an extrapleural opacity, parenchymal lung disease or mediastinal mass, but there are some useful diagnostic points.

An encysted effusion is often associated with free pleural fluid or other pleural shadowing, and may extend into a fissure (Fig. 3.9). Loculated effusions tend to have comparatively little depth, but considerable width, rather like a biconvex lens. Their appearance, therefore, depends on whether they are viewed en face, in profile or obliquely. Fluoroscopy is often helpful in determining the best projection for radiographic demonstration. Extrapleural opacities tend to have a much sharper outline, with tapered, sometimes concave edges where they meet the chest wall. Peripheral pleurally based lung lesions may show an air bronchogram that will distinguish them from true pleural disease (Fig. 3.10). The differentiation between pleural thickening or mass and loculated pleural fluid may be difficult on plain films, and CT and ultrasound are particularly useful in this context (Fig. 3.11).

Fluid may become loculated in one or more of the interlobar fissures. This is an uncommon occurrence and is most often seen in heart failure. The appearances depend upon which fissure is affected and the quantity of fluid. Fluid collecting in the horizontal fissure produces a lenticular, oval or round shadow, with well-demarcated edges. Fluid extending into the adjacent parts of the fissure may make it appear thickened. In both frontal and lateral projections the shadow appears rounded. Loculated fluid in an oblique fissure may be poorly defined on a frontal radiograph, but a lateral film is usually diagnostic since the fissure is seen tangentially, and the typical lenticular configuration of the effusion is demonstrated (Fig. 3.12).

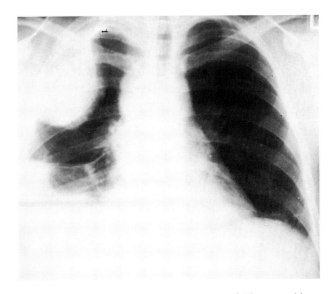

Fig. 3.9 Loculated pleural effusion in a man of 19 years with non-Hodgkin's lymphoma. Erect PA film shows well-circumscribed convex opacity adjacent to right upper costal margin and extending around apex of lung. Right paratracheal shadowing is partly due to lymph-node enlargement, and partly due to loculated pleural fluid. Pleural fluid is also present at the right base extending into the horizontal fissure.

Loculated interlobar effusions can appear rounded on two views. Following treatment they may disappear rapidly, and are hence known as 'pseudo-' or 'vanishing' tumours. They may recur in subsequent episodes of heart failure.

Empyema This may be suspected on a plain film by the spontaneous appearance of a fluid level in a pleural effusion, but is best diagnosed by CT or ultrasound (Figs 3.13, 3.14). On CT an empyema usually has a lenticular shape and may compress the underlying lung. Fluid, with or without gas, may be present in the

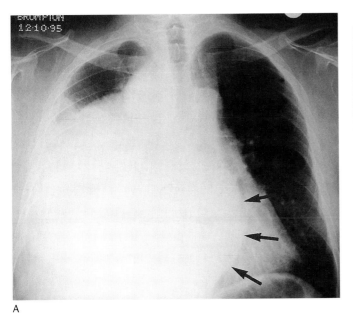

A

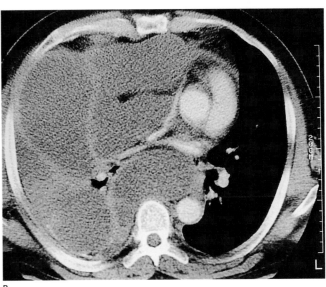

B

Fig. 3.8 Fifty-five-year-old male with adenocarcinoma of the pleura from an unknown primary site. (A) PA chest radiograph reveals extensive opacification of the right hemithorax with a lobulated upper margin. There is shift of the azygo-oesophageal line to the opposite side (arrows). (B) Enhanced CT scan at the level of the main pulmonary artery showing mediastinal displacement due to the large loculated pleural fluid collection.

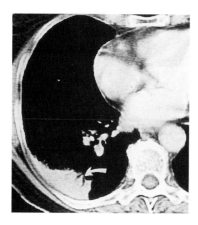

Fig. 3.10 Peripheral consolidation demonstrating the presence of an air bronchogram (arrow) in a patient with organising pneumonia.

pleura and both layers of the pleura may be thickened. Because the likelihood of successful small bore catheter drainage decreases with time and the development of a pleural rind, rapid diagnosis and treatment should be the aim. If a complicated effusion becomes chronic, *thickening* of the visceral or parietal pleura may occur. The former may prevent re-expansion of the lung, and surgical decortication may be necessary if respiratory function is significantly impaired.

Multiple septations within an infected or reactive pleural collection may be broken down by the instillation of *fibrinolytic agents* such as *urokinase* (Fig. 3.15). Typically 100 000 IU of urokinase are instilled in 50 ml of normal saline. The drain is then clamped for 1 hour, after which free drainage or low-pressure suction is reinstituted. This treatment, which may be repeated daily for up to 5 days, significantly increases the success rate of radiologically guided closed drainage and reduces the need for large bore drain insertion or surgical intervention. Regular (8-hourly) flushing of narrow bore catheters with 10 ml of

normal saline will help to prevent the lumen becoming occluded with fibrinous debris.

Ultrasound appearance of pleural fluid *(Fig. 3.14)* Ultrasound is an excellent method for locating loculated pleural fluid prior to diagnostic or therapeutic aspiration. The fluid may be anechoic or contain particulate material. It is possible to visualise septations in loculated collections and also to identify pleural thickening and masses. Transudates are almost always anechoic but exudates may or may not contain reflective material. The presence of pleural masses in association with an effusion is highly suggestive of malignant disease (Fig. 3.11B).

CT and pleural fluid CT may be complimentary to the chest X-ray and ultrasound scan in investigating some cases of pleural disease. CT is more sensitive than the plain chest X-ray in detecting small pleural effusions, and is better than ultrasound in defining the total extent of a pleural abnormality. CT can also identify and characterise associated abnormalities in the underlying lung. On CT, pleural fluid usually shows lower attenuation than pleural thickening or consolidated or fibrotic lung, although haemothorax may show increased attenuation. When both pleural fluid and pleural thickening are present the effusion is likely to be an exudate.

Differentiation between pleural and ascitic fluid on CT scans is sometimes a problem, and may be resolved by a number of signs, which are describe below.

Displaced crus sign Pleural fluid may collect posterior to the diaphragmatic crus and therefore displace the crus anteriorly, whereas ascites collects anterior to the crus and may cause posterior displacement (Fig. 3.16A).

Diaphragm sign As an extension of the displaced crus sign, any fluid that is on the exterior of the dome of the diaphragm is in the pleura, whereas any that is within the dome is ascites (Fig. 3.16A).

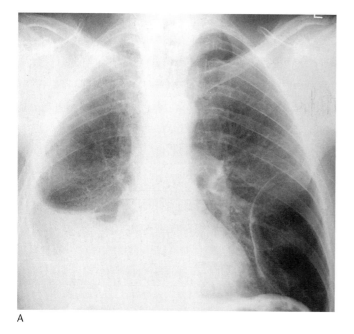
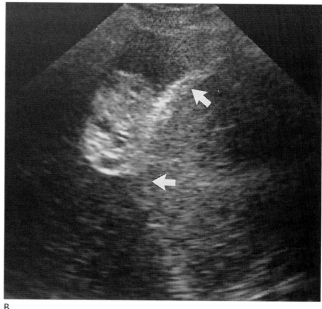

A   B

Fig. 3.11 (A) PA radiograph of a 55-year-old male patient with disseminated adenocarcinoma. The right hemidiaphragm is obscured by what appears to be a simple pleural effusion. (There is a large bulla at the left lung base.) (B) Ultrasound of the right lung base reveals a tumour nodule on the dome of the diaphragm (arrows) surrounded by pleural fluid.

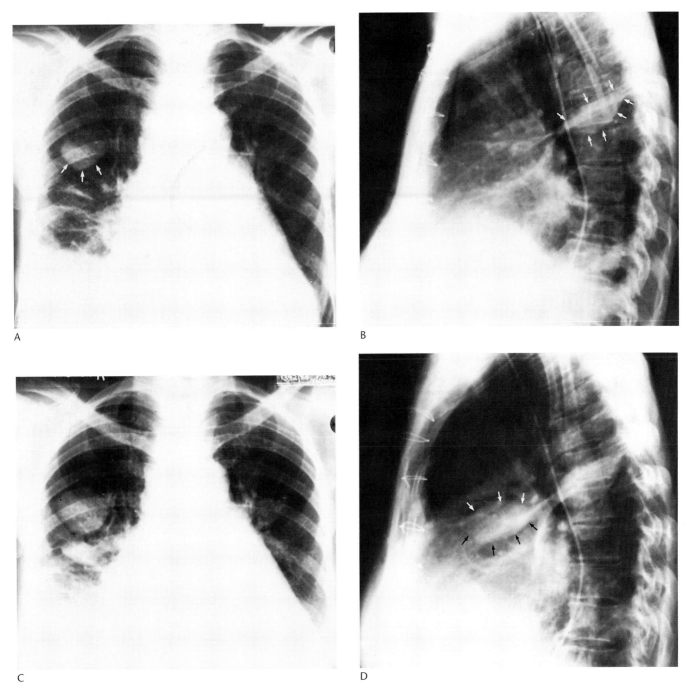

A

B

C

D

Fig. 3.12 Loculated interlobar pleural effusions in a woman of 60 after replacement of the aortic root. (A) Nineteen days postoperatively a right mid-zone opacity appears (arrows), with a sharp lower margin and an indistinct upper margin. The right costophrenic angle has also filled in. (B) Lateral projection demonstrates typical lenticular configuration of fluid loculated in the oblique fissure (arrows). (C) Seven days later a second round opacity has appeared below the first. This opacity is well circumscribed. (D) Lateral projection confirms that this is fluid loculated in the horizontal fissure (arrows).

Interface sign The interface between the liver or spleen and pleural fluid is said to be less sharp than that between the liver or spleen and ascites (Fig. 3.16B).

Bare area sign The peritoneal coronary ligament prevents ascitic fluid from extending over the entire posterior surface of the liver, whereas in a free pleural space, pleural fluid may extend over the entire posterior costophrenic recess behind the liver (Fig. 3.16B).

PNEUMOTHORAX

Pneumothorax is the presence of air in the pleural cavity. Air enters this cavity through a defect in either the parietal or the visceral pleura. Such defects are the result of lung pathology, trauma or deliberate introduction of air, respectively, giving rise to spontaneous, traumatic or artificial pneumothoraces. If pleural adhesions are present the pneumothorax may be localised, otherwise it is generalised. If air can move freely in and out of the pleural space during respiration it is an

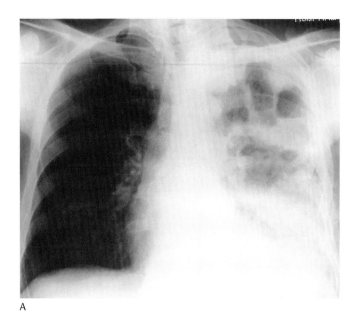

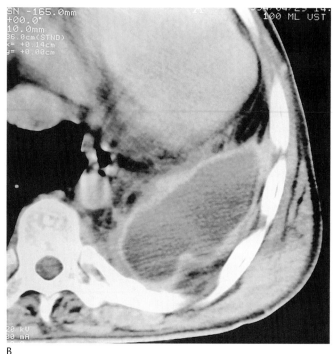

A

B

Fig. 3.13 Two patients with empyema. (A) PA chest radiograph showing multiple fluid levels in a patient with a heavily loculated empyema complicating attempted pleurodesis. (B) CT scan through the lower thorax in a patient with a right basal empyema collection. There is associated pleural thickening and compression of the adjacent lung parenchyma.

open pneumothorax, if no movement of air occurs it is closed, and if air enters the pleural space on inspiration, but does not leave on expiration, it is valvular. As intrapleural pressure increases in a valvular pneumothorax a tension pneumothorax develops.

Aetiology
Spontaneous pneumothorax is the commonest type, and typically occurs in young men, due to rupture of a congenital pleural bleb. Such blebs are usually in the lung apex and may be bilateral.

In older patients chronic bronchitis and emphysema are common factors. Rarer causes include bronchial asthma, rupture of a tension cyst in staphylococcal pneumonia, rupture of a subpleural tuberculous focus, rupture of a subpleural tension cyst in carcinoma of the bronchus and rupture of a cavitating subpleural metastasis. Other associations include many of the causes of interstitial pulmonary fibrosis (cystic fibrosis, histiocytosis, tuberous sclerosis, sarcoidosis and some of the pneumoconioses).

Traumatic pneumothorax may be the result of a penetrating chest wound, closed chest trauma (particularly rupture of a bronchus in a road accident), rib fracture, pleural aspiration or biopsy, lung biopsy, bronchoscopy, oesophagoscopy and positive-pressure ventilation. The pleura may also be violated during mediastinal surgery and nephrectomy.

Artificial pneumothorax as treatment for pulmonary tuberculosis is now of historical interest only, as is diagnostic pneumothorax.

Radiological appearances
A small pneumothorax in a free pleural space in an erect patient collects at the apex. The lung apex retracts towards the hilum and on a frontal chest film the sharp white line of the visceral pleura will be visible, separated from the chest wall by the radiolucent pleural space, which is devoid of lung markings (Fig. 3.17). This should not be confused with the appearances of a skin fold, in which there is no discrete pleural line (Fig. 3.18). The affected lung usually remains aerated: however perfusion is reduced in proportion to ventilation and therefore the radiodensity of the partially collapsed lung remains normal. A small pneumothorax may easily go unseen and it may be necessary to examine the film with a bright light. An expiratory film will make a closed pneumothorax easier to see, as on full expiration the lung volume is at its smallest, while the volume of pleural air is unchanged. Generally, expiratory radiographs are not routinely required. A lateral decubitus film with the affected side uppermost is occasionally helpful, as the pleural air can be seen along the lateral chest wall. This view is particularly useful in infants, because small pneumothoraces are difficult to see in supine AP films, as the air tends to collect anteriorly and medially (Fig. 3.19). Alternatively, a horizontal beam 'shoot-through' lateral film may identify anterior pneumothoraces in the supine patient.

A large pneumothorax may lead to complete relaxation and retraction of the lung, with some mediastinal shift toward the normal side, which increases on expiration.

Tension pneumothorax (Figs 3.19, 3.20A, 3.21) may lead to massive displacement of the mediastinum, kinking of the great veins and acute cardiac and respiratory embarrassment. Radiologically the ipsilateral lung may be squashed against the mediastinum, or herniate across the midline, and the ipsilateral hemidiaphragm may be depressed. On fluoroscopy the mediastinal shift to the contralateral side is greatest in inspiration, an observation that distinguishes a tension pneumothorax from a large pneumothorax not under strain.

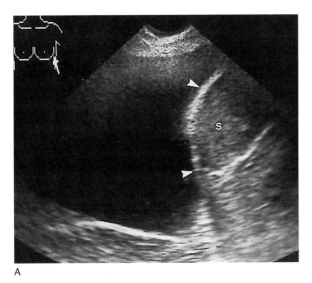

A

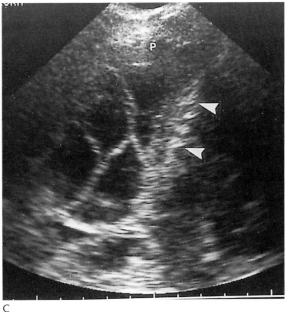

C

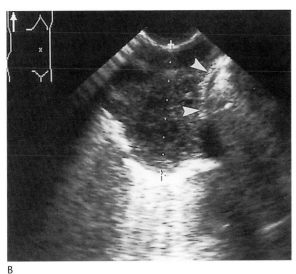

B

Fig. 3.14 (A) Large left pleural effusion due to carcinoma of bronchus. There is a large echo-free effusion above the left hemidiaphragm (arrowheads) and spleen(s). (B) Empyema following right lower lobectomy. A poorly echogenic collection is seen above the diaphragm (arrowheads). (C) Loculated pleural effusion due to tuberculosis. Ultrasound demonstrates thickening of the parietal pleura (P) and multiseptated fluid collection above the diaphragm (arrowheads).

Complications of pneumothorax

Pleural adhesions may limit the distribution of a pneumothorax and result in a *loculated* or *encysted pneumothorax*. The usual appearance is an ovoid air collection adjacent to the chest wall, and it may be radiographically indistinguishable from a thin-walled subpleural pulmonary cavity, cyst or bulla. *Pleural adhesions* are occasionally seen as line shadows stretching between the two pleural layers, preventing relaxation of the underlying lung (Fig. 3.20). Rupture of an adhesion may produce a *haemopneumothorax*, or discharge of an underlying infected subpleural lesion, leading to a *pyopneumothorax*. Collapse or consolidation of a lobe or lung in association with a pneumothorax are important complications which may delay re-expansion of the lung.

Because the normal pleural space contains a small volume of fluid, blunting of the costophrenic angle by a short fluid level is commonly seen in a pneumothorax (Fig. 3.22). In a small pneumothorax this fluid level may be the most obvious radiological sign. A larger fluid collection usually signifies a complication and represents exudate, pus or blood, depending on the aetiology of the pneumothorax.

The usual radiological appearance of a *hydropneumothorax* is that of a pneumothorax containing a horizontal fluid level which separates opaque fluid below from lucent air above. This demonstration requires a horizontal beam film (Fig. 3.23), so that if the patient is not fit enough for an upright film a lateral decubitus film or 'shoot-through' lateral film may be indicated.

Occasionally, rapid re-expansion of a lung following drainage of a large pneumothorax may be associated with so-called *re-expansion pulmonary oedema*. This may also complicate rapid drainage of a large pleural effusion, and is characterised by the development of extensive consolidation throughout the ipsilateral lung, which usually resolves within a day or two.

BRONCHOPLEURAL FISTULA

Bronchopleural fistula is a communication between the airway and the pleural space. It is most frequently a complication of complete or partial *pneumonectomy*, and is discussed under postoperative complications in Chapter 8. Other causes include *carcinoma of the bronchus* and *ruptured lung abscess*. The radiological appearance is that of a hydro- or pyo-pneumothorax.

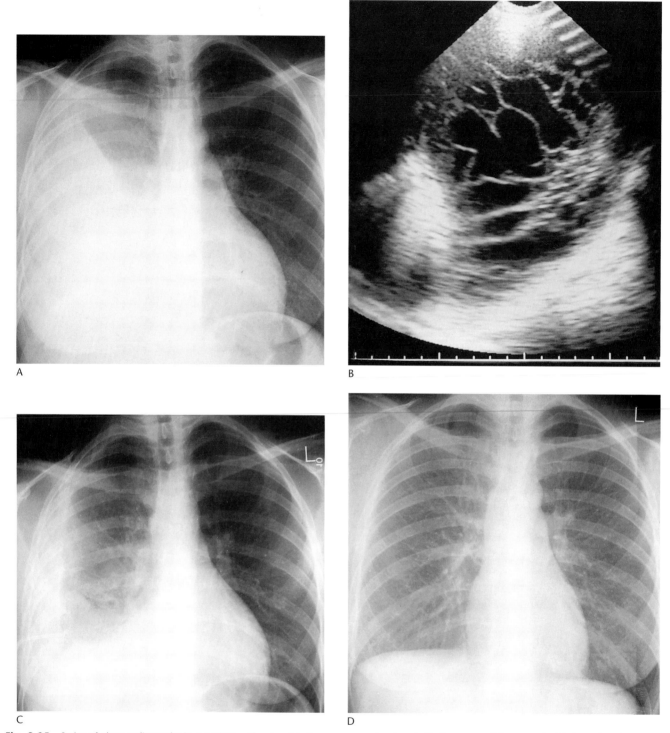

Fig. 3.15 Series of chest radiographs in a patient with a loculated parapneumonic pleural effusion successfully treated with intrapleural urokinase. (A) The initial chest radiograph demonstrates a large right pleural effusion which an ultrasound scan (B) shows to be heavily loculated. (C) PA radiograph 24 hours after fine-bore catheter insertion and instillation of streptokinase. (D) PA chest radiograph 5 months later.

PLEURAL THICKENING

Blunting of a costophrenic angle is a frequent incidental finding on a chest X-ray. It is due to localised pleural thickening and usually results from a previous episode of pleuritis, although a previous history of chest disease is often lacking. In the asymptomatic patient

and in the absence of other radiological abnormality it is of no other significance. It may mimic a small pleural effusion, and if a previous film is not available for comparison a lateral decubitus film or ultrasound scan will exclude free pleural fluid. Localised pleural thickening extending into the inferior end of an oblique fissure may produce so-called tenting of the diaphragm, and is of similar significance. This

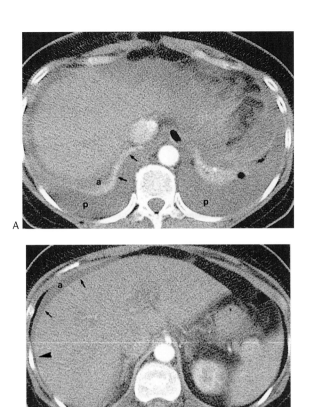

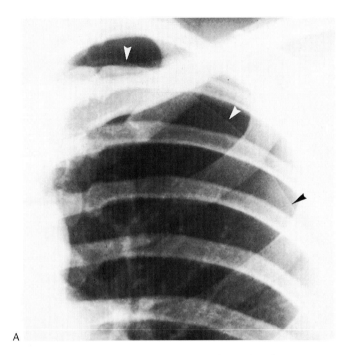

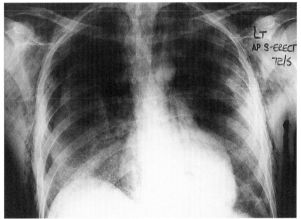

Fig. 3.16 CT signs which may differentiate pleural effusion and ascites. Scans through lower thorax/upper abdomen in patient with bilateral pleural effusions and ascites. (A) *Displaced crus sign:* The right pleural effusion collects posterior to the right crus of the diaphragm (arrows) and displaces it anteriorly. *Diaphragm sign:* The pleural fluid (p) is over the outer surface of the dome of the diaphragm, whereas the ascitic fluid (a) is within the dome. (B) *Interface sign:* The interface (arrows) between the liver and ascites is usually sharper than between liver and pleural fluid. *Bare area sign:* Peritoneal reflections prevent ascitic fluid from extending over the entire posterior surface of the liver (arrowhead), in contrast to pleural fluid in the posterior costophrenic recess.

latter appearance may also result from basal intrapulmonary scarring, due to previous pulmonary infection or infarction.

Bilateral apical pleural thickening is also a fairly common finding. It is more frequent in elderly patients, and is not due to tuberculosis. Its aetiology is uncertain, but ischaemia is probably a factor. Such apical shadowing is usually symmetrical (Fig. 3.24). Asymmetrical or *unilateral apical pleural thickening*, however, may be of pathological significance, especially if associated with pain. If asymmetrical, apical pleural shadowing may represent a *Pancoast tumour*, and it is important to visualise the adjacent ribs and spine (Fig. 3.25). Penetrated films and tomography may be indicated, because evidence of bone involvement will almost certainly indicate a carcinoma.

More *extensive unilateral pleural thickening* is usually the result of a previous thoracotomy or pleural effusion. Empyema and haemothorax are especially likely to resolve with *pleural fibrosis*. Chronic pneumothorax is a rarer cause. These causes of pleural fibrosis all involve the visceral layer and the thickened pleura may calcify. If the entire lung is surrounded by fibrotic pleura, this is termed a *fibrothorax*. The pleural peel may be a few centimetres thick, and may cause reduced ventilation of the surrounded lung

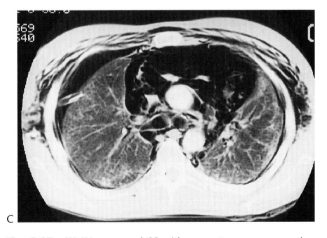

Fig. 3.17 (A) Woman aged 22 with a spontaneous pneumothorax. PA film showing apical pneumothorax. The visceral pleural (arrowheads) separates aerated lung from the radiolucent pleural space. AP chest radiograph (B) and CT scan (C) in a patient with *Pneumocystis carinii* pneumonia complicated by bilateral pneumothoraces and extensive mediastinal and surgical emphysema.

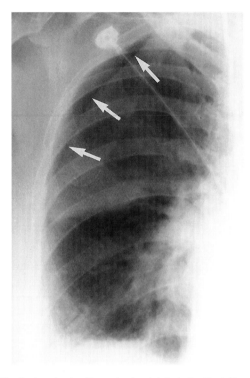

Fig. 3.18 Supine chest radiograph of an intubated patient. There is a skin fold projected over the right lung apex simulating a pneumothorax (arrows). Close inspection reveals lung markings extending beyond the skin fold, and no fine pleural line that should be visible with a genuine pneumothorax (cf. Fig. 3.17A).

and subsequent decrease in volume of that hemithorax. If the chest X-ray shows that the vascularity of the affected lung is decreased relative to the other lung, then significant ventilatory restriction is likely and surgical decortication may be necessary.

Bilateral pleural plaques are a common manifestation of asbestos exposure, and occasionally more diffuse pleural thickening is seen.

PLEURAL CALCIFICATION

Pleural calcification has the same causes as pleural thickening. Unilateral pleural calcification is, therefore, likely to be the result of previous empyema, haemothorax or pleurisy, and bilateral calcification occurs after asbestos exposure and in some other pneumoconioses, or occasionally after bilateral effusions. As with the incidental finding of pleural thickening, pleural calcification may be discovered in a patient who is not aware of previous or current chest disease.

The calcification associated with previous pleurisy, empyema or haemothorax occurs in the visceral pleura; associated pleural thickening is almost always present, and separates the calcium from the ribs. The calcium may be in a continuous sheet or in discrete plaques, usually producing dense, coarse, irregular shadows, often sharply demarcated laterally (Fig. 3.26). If a plaque is viewed en face it may cast a less well defined shadow and mimic a pulmonary infiltrate. However, a lateral view will often demonstrate the calcified plaque over the anterior or posterior pleura but it may be necessary to fluoroscope the patient to obtain the best tangential projection for demonstration of the plaque.

The calcification associated with asbestos exposure is usually more delicate and bilateral (Fig. 3.27). It is frequently visible over the diaphragm and adjacent to the axillae. Tangential views show it to be situated immediately deep to the ribs, and it is in fact located in the parietal pleura (Fig. 3.28). The most sensitive method

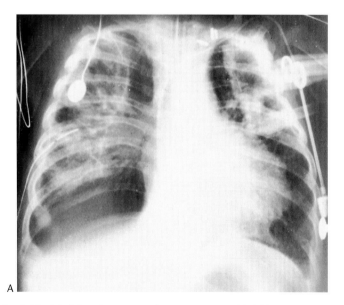

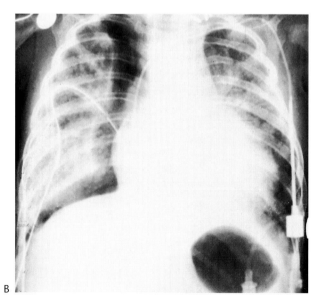

Fig. 3.19 Medial tension pneumothorax in a 1-year-old-child on a ventilator following closure of patent ductus arteriosus and resection of coarctation of aorta. (A) Supine AP film demonstrates a right pneumothorax, the intrapleural air collecting anteriorly and medially, and the lung collapsing posteriorly and laterally. The pleural tube is situated laterally and is therefore not decompressing the pneumothorax. The right hemidiaphragm is depressed, and the mediastinum is displaced to the left, indicating a tension pneumothorax. (B) Following insertion of another pleural tube more medially, the pneumothorax is smaller and the right hemidiaphragm and mediastinum have returned to their normal positions.

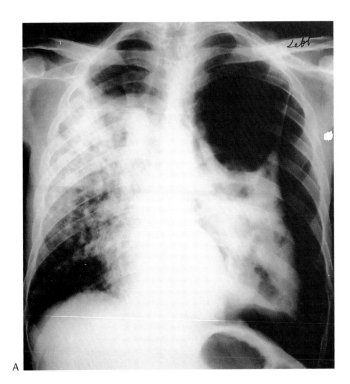

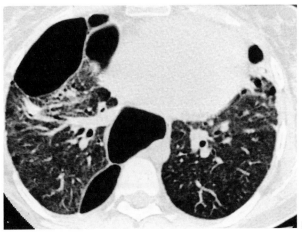

Fig. 3.20 (A) Tension pneumothorax with a pleural adhesion. Elderly man with spontaneous pneumothorax secondary to extensive cavitating pulmonary tuberculosis. The left lung is prevented from collapsing completely by the extensive consolidation, and by tethering of an adhesion. The mediastinum is displaced to the right. (B) Non-tension pneumothoraces in a 26-year-old female patient demonstrating multiple pleural adhesions causing loculation of air.

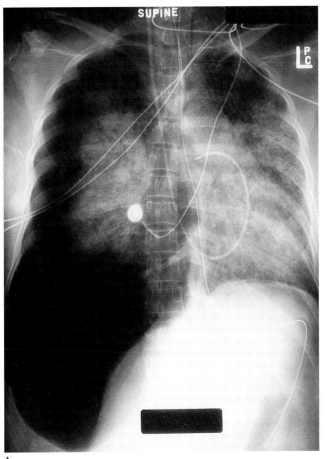

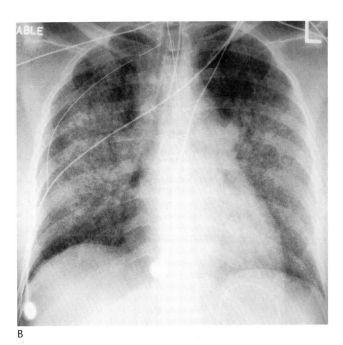

Fig. 3.21 (A) Tension pneumothorax following a transbronchial lung biopsy. There is inversion of the right hemidiaphragm, and deviation of the mediastinum to the opposite side. (B) Following insertion of a right-sided chest drain the diaphragm and mediastinum have returned to a normal position. The diffuse bilateral infiltrate is due to pre-existing pulmonary haemorrhage.

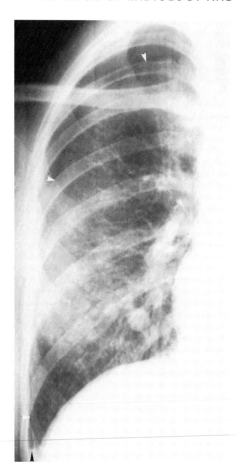

Fig. 3.22 Shallow hydropneumothorax in a man of 18 years. Spontaneous pneumothorax, probably due to rupture of subpleural cavitating metastatic osteogenic sarcoma. The primary tumour was in the right scapula, which has been removed, and pulmonary metastases are seen in the right lower zone. The visceral pleura is faintly seen (white arrowheads) and a short fluid level (black arrowhead) is present just above the right costophrenic angle.

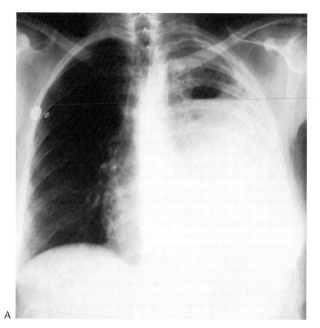

A

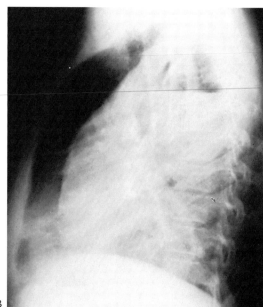

B

Fig. 3.23 Loculated pyo-pneumothorax in a woman of 45 following gunshot wound to chest. (A) Erect PA film shows a fluid level in the left upper zone, and pleural thickening over the apex. (B) Lateral film shows that the fluid level is situated posteriorly. The differential diagnosis lies between a pyopneumothorax and a lung abscess.

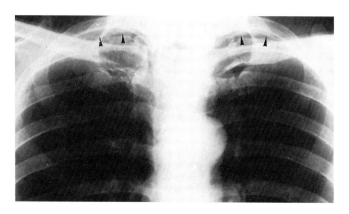

Fig. 3.24 Bilateral apical pleural thickening. An incidental finding in a 67-year-old man with ischaemic heart disease. The apical pleural shadowing (arrowheads) is symmetrical, although the edge is better seen on the left.

for demonstrating a pleural plaque is high-resolution CT (HRCT) (Fig. 3.29), and ultrasound can be helpful in differentiating a plaque from loculated fluid.

PLEURAL TUMOURS

Primary neoplasms of the pleura are rare. Benign tumours of the pleura include localised fibrous tumours (or fibroma) and lipoma. The commonest malignant disease of the pleura is metastatic (Fig. 3.30), the most frequent primary tumours being of the

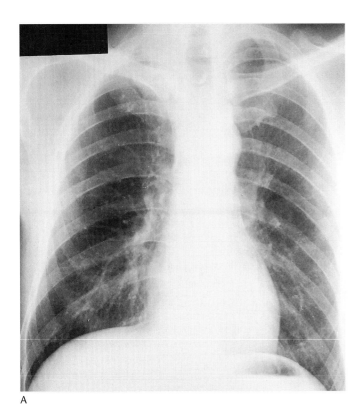

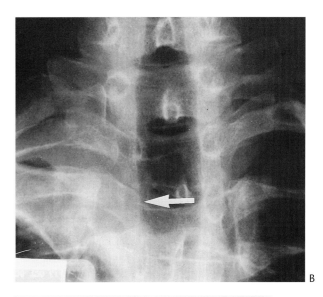

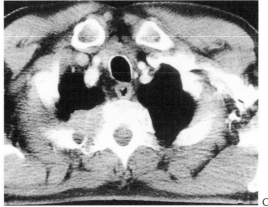

Fig. 3.25 Unilateral apical pleural thickening. Man aged 46 with pain in the right side of the neck and right arm. (A) Dense pleural shadowing is present at the right apex. The left apex is clear. (B) An AP view of the cervical spine demonstrates absence of the right pedicle of T3 (arrow). Histology: anaplastic carcinoma. (C) CT demonstrates a right apical mass infiltrating the third thoracic vertebra.

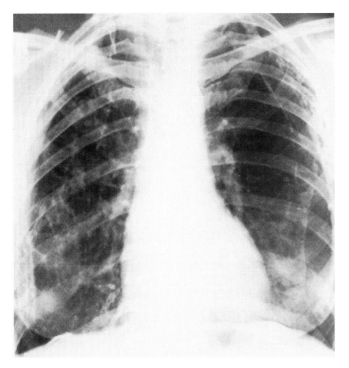

Fig. 3.26 Pleural calcification in a middle-aged woman with a history of recurrent episodes of pleurisy, presumed to be tuberculous. Extensive plaques of pleural calcification surround both lungs.

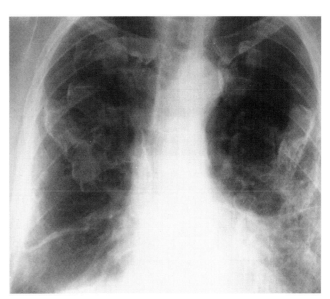

Fig. 3.27 Bilateral calcified pleural plaques seen en face over both lungs due to exposure to asbestos.

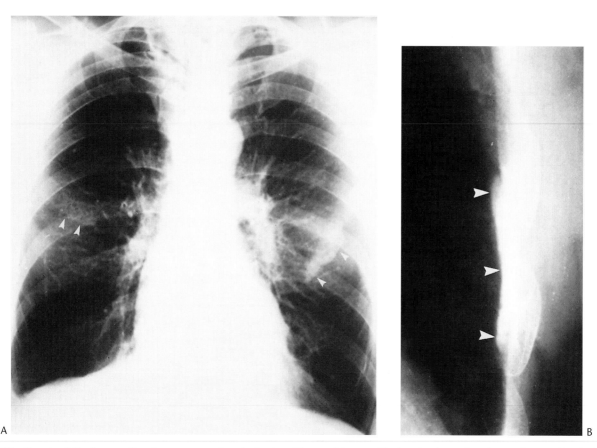

Fig. 3.28   Pleural calcification resulting from exposure to asbestos in a 51-year-old man with chronic obstructive airways disease. (A) The lungs are hyperinflated. Calcified pleural plaques are present in both mid zones (arrowheads). (B) An oblique film, aided by fluoroscopy, shows the left-sided plaque tangentially (arrowheads); it is situated in the parietal pleura, immediately deep to the ribs.

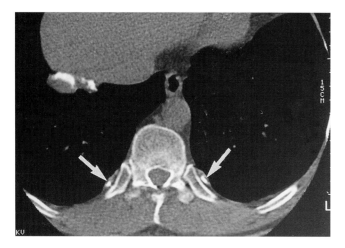

Fig. 3.29   CT demonstration of pleural abnormalities due to asbestos exposure in a middle-aged man. There are small calcified pleural plaques in the paraspinal gutters (arrows) and calcified pleural plaques over the right hemidiaphragm.

bronchus and breast. Primary malignancy of the pleura (malignant mesothelioma) is usually associated with asbestos exposure.

Localised fibrous tumours of the pleura are often asymptomatic presenting as an incidental finding on a chest X-ray. However, they may present with finger clubbing and joint pains due to hyper-

trophic osteoarthropathy, or with hypoglycaemia. They tend to grow slowly and are usually benign, but some show malignant features. The radiographic appearance is of a well-defined lobulated mass adjacent to the chest wall, mediastinum, diaphragm or a pleural fissure (Fig. 3.31). The mass may be small or occupy most of the hemithorax (Fig. 3.32). On CT large tumours may show areas of differential enhancement, and also areas of low attenuation due to necrosis. In the presence of osteoarthropathy, the diagnosis is almost certain, but if necessary, percutaneous needle biopsy is probably the investigation of choice.

Subpleural lipomas appear as well-defined rounded masses. They may change shape with respiration, being soft tumours, and if large enough may erode adjacent ribs. Because they comprise fat the CT appearance is diagnostic (Fig. 3.33). The characterstic features on MRI are high signal on T_1-weighted images and intermediate signal on T_2-weighted images.

Malignant mesothelioma is usually due to prolonged exposure to asbestos dust, particularly crocidolite. The latent period between first exposure to asbestos and development of mesothelioma is typically 20–40 years. The usual appearance is nodular pleural thickening around all or part of a lung (Fig. 3.34). A haemorrhagic pleural effusion may be present but the lung changes of asbestosis may be absent. The effusion may obscure the pleural masses. Often the mediastinum is central, despite the presence of a large effusion, and this is thought to result from volume loss of the underlying lung secondary to either

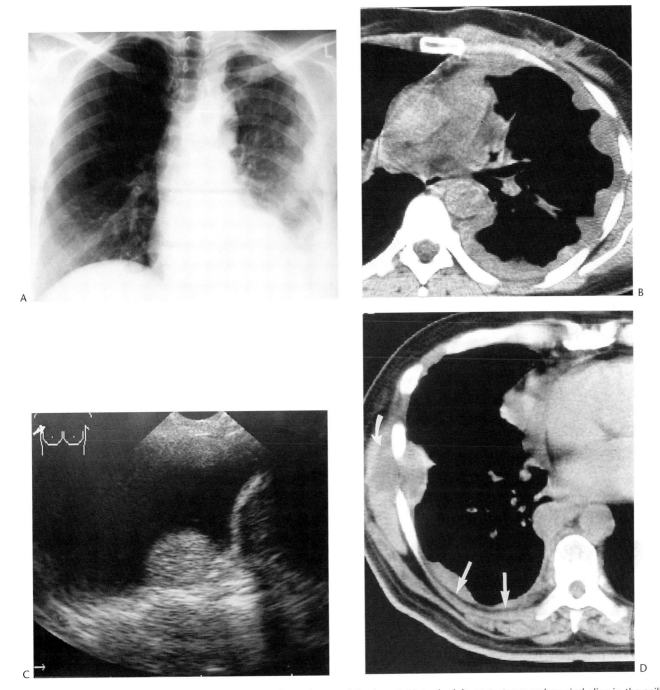

Fig. 3.30 (A) Nodular pleural thickening due to metastatic carcinoma of the breast. Note the left mastectomy and surgical clips in the axilla. (B) Same patient as (A). CT demonstration of pleural deposits. The whole lung is encased by pleural tumour. (C) Metastatic pleural tumour nodule in a patient with carcinoma of the ovary demonstrated by ultrasound. (D) Pleural tumour deposits from adenocarcinoma of the oesophagus. The largest nodule has crossed the pleural fat stripe, which is still visible elsewhere (arrows), and is invading the chest wall musculature (curved arrow).

ventilatory restriction by the surrounding tumour, or bronchial stenosis by tumour compression at the hilum. Rib involvement may occur with malignant mesothelioma, but the presence of a pleural mass and adjacent rib destruction is more likely to be due to metastatic bone tumour, or possibly a primary bone tumour.

The extent of malignant mesothelioma is best assessed by CT or MRI. Features which suggest that pleural thickening is malignant rather than benign are: thickening that is nodular rather than smooth, pleural thickening that extends into fissures or over the mediastinal surface, encasement of the lung and loss of volume of the ipsilateral lung. MRI is probably superior to CT in assessing involvement of the mediastinum and chest wall. Typically with MRI, signal intensity from a mesothelioma is slightly greater than muscle on both T_1- and T_2-weighted images. A tissue diagnosis may be obtained by *percutaneous needle biopsy*. Occasionally malignant mesothelioma is complicated by tumour seeding along biopsy or chest drain tracts (Fig. 3.35).

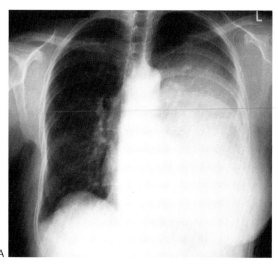

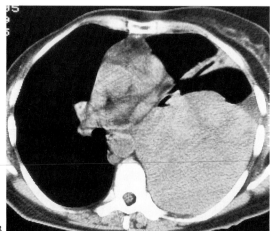

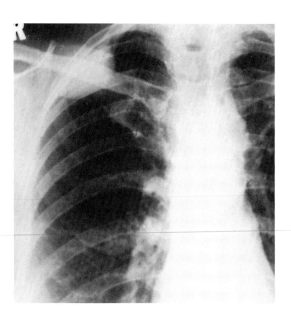

Fig. 3.31 Pleural fibroma or benign mesothelioma. Incidental finding in a 48-year-old woman with a past history of left apical tuberculosis. A sharply demarcated peripheral upper zone opacity is present, making an obtuse angle with the adjacent chest wall, and without other pleural abnormality. It was removed. Histology: benign fibrous mesothelioma.

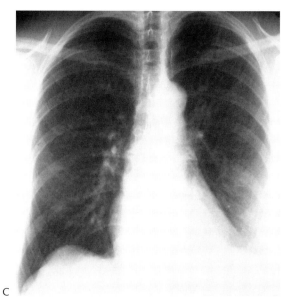

Fig. 3.32 (A) Giant pleural fibroma in a patient with a distant history of a right mastectomy for carcinoma. (B) CT scan in the same patient shows a large heterogeneous mass occupying most of the left hemithorax and associated with a small pleural effusion. There is no radiological evidence of chest wall invasion. (C) Appearances immediately following surgery. The tumour was completely resected and there was no invasion of adjacent structures.

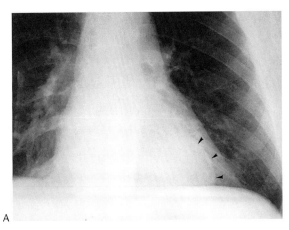

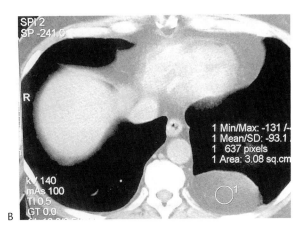

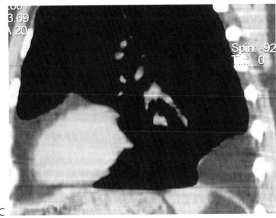

Fig. 3.33 Pleural lipoma. (A) Chest radiograph of an asymptomatic patient shows a well-circumscribed, round capacity (arrowheads) projected over the heart. (B) CT scan shows it to be a pleural mass of entirely fat density. (C) Parasagittal reconstruction of the multislice CT scan shows the mass lying above the diaphragm within the posterior costophrenic recess.

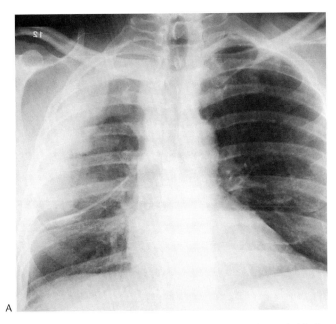

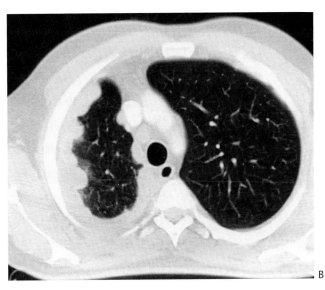

Fig. 3.34 Malignant mesothelioma. Abnormal chest radiograph (A) shows lobulated left pleural opacities. (B) CT scan through the mid thorax demonstrates encasement of the right lung by nodular pleural tumour. Calcified pleural plaques were evident on other sections.

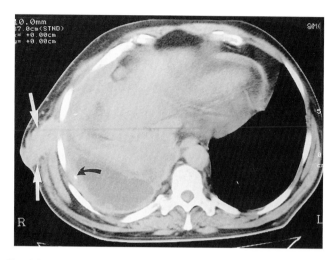

Fig. 3.35   CT scan through the lower thorax of a patient with malignant mesothelioma. There is metastatic tumour seeding along the biopsy tract (arrows). Note the fleck of pleural calcification (curved arrow).

REFERENCES AND SUGGESTIONS FOR FURTHER READING

Armstrong, P., Wilson, A. G., Dee, P., Hansell, D. M. (2000) *Imaging of Diseases of the Chest*, 3rd edn. St Louis: Mosby.

Felson, B. (1973) *Chest Roentgenology*. Philadelphia: W.B. Saunders.

Fraser, R. S., Muller, N. L., Colman, N., Pare, P. D. (1999) *Fraser and Pare's Diagnosis of Diseases of the Chest*, 4th edn. Philadelphia: W. B. Saunders.

Simon, G. (1978) *Principles of Chest X-ray Diagnosis*, 4th edn. London: Butterworths.

The pleura

Albelda, S. M., Epstein, D. M., Gefter, W. B., Miller, W. T. (1982) Pleural thickening: its significance and relationship to asbestos dust exposure. *American Review of Respiratory Disease*, **126**, 621–624.

Bury, T. H., Paulus, P., Dowlati, A. et al (1997) Evaluation of pleural disease with FDG–PET imaging: preliminary report. *Thorax*, **52**, 187–189.

Desser, T. S., Stark, P. (1998) Pictorial essay: solitary fibrous tumor of the pleura. *Journal of Thoracic Imaging*, **13**, 27–35.

Henschke, C. I., Davis, S. D., Romano, P. M., Yankelvitz, D. F. (1989) The pathogenesis, radiological evaluation and therapy of pleural effusions. *Radiologic Clinics of North America*, **27**, 1241–1255.

Hillerdal, G. (1983) Malignant mesothelioma 1982: review of 4710 published cases. *British Journal of Diseases of the Chest*, **71**, 321–343.

Kawashima, A., Libshitz, H. I. (1990) Malignant pleural mesothelioma: CT manifestations in 50 cases. *American Journal of Roentgenology*, **155**, 965–969.

Leung, A. N., Müller, N. L., Miller, R. R. (1990) CT in differential diagnosis of diffuse pleural disease. *American Journal of Roentgenology*, **154**, 487–492.

McLeod, T. C., Flower, C. D. R. (1991) Imaging the pleura: sonography, CT and MR imaging. *American Journal of Roentgenology*, **156**, 1145–1153.

McLeod, T. C., Isler, R. J., Novelline, R. A., Putman, C. E., Simeone, J., Stark, P. (1981) The apical cap. *American Journal of Roentgenology*, **137**, 299–306.

McLeod, T. C. (1998) CT & MR in pleural disease. *Clinics in Chest Medicine*, **192**, 261–276.

Miller, B. H., Rosado-de-Christenson, M. L., Mason, A. C., et al (1996) From the archives of the AFIP: malignant pleural mesothelioma: radiological–pathological correlation. *Radiographic*, **16**, 613–644.

Moskowitz, P. S., Griscom, N. T. (1976) The medial pneumothorax. *Radiology*, **120**, 143–147.

Müller, N. L. (1993) Imaging of the pleura. *Radiology*, **186**, 297–309.

Rasch, B. N., Carsky, E. W., Lane, E. T., Callaghan, J. P. O., Heitzman, E. R. (1982) Pleural effusion: explanation of some atypical appearances. *American Journal of Roentgenology*, **139**, 899–904.

Stark, D. D., Federle, M. P., Goodman, P. C., Padrasky, A. E., Webb, W. R. (1983) Differentiating lung abscess and empyema: radiography and computed tomography. *American Journal of Roentgenology*, **141**, 163–167.

Stuart, G., Silverman, M. D., Saini, S., Mueller, P. R. (1989) Pleural interventions. *Radiologic Clinics of North America*, **27**, 1257–1267.

Woodring, J. H. (1984) Recognition of pleural effusion on supine radiographs: how much fluid is required? *American Journal of Roentgenology*, **142**, 59–64.

Wright, F. W. (1976) Spontaneous pneumothorax and pulmonary malignant disease—a syndrome sometimes associated with cavitating tumours. *Clinical Radiology*, **27**, 211–222.

Yang, P-C., Luh, K-T., Chang, D-B., Wu, H-D., Yu, C-J., Kuo, S-H. (1992) Value of sonography in determining the nature of pleural effusion: analysis of 320 cases. *American Journal of Roentgenology*, **159**, 29–33.

4

TUMOURS OF THE LUNG

Michael B. Rubens and Simon P. G. Padley
with a contribution from Jeremy P. R. Jenkins

A wide variety of neoplasms may arise in the lungs. While many lung tumours are overtly malignant and others are definitely benign, some fall both histologically and in their clinical behaviour between these two extremes. Pulmonary tumours may be classified histologically or according to their presumed tissue of origin. However, it should be borne in mind that histopathologists do not always agree on the classification of an individual tumour. Carcinoma of the bronchus is by far the commonest and most important primary tumour of the lung.

CARCINOMA OF THE BRONCHUS

Carcinoma of the bronchus is the commonest fatal malignancy in adult males in the western world. It is commoner in men than in women, but the incidence in women is rising. Most cases occur between 40 and 70 years, and it is unusual below 30 years of age. The most important single aetiological factor is cigarette smoking. This is dose related, the risk being proportional to the number of cigarettes smoked. Other factors include atmospheric pollution and certain occupations. Smokers who are exposed to asbestos have an increased risk of lung cancer when compared to smokers without such exposure. Exposure to radioactivity and some industrial chemicals has caused increased mortality from lung cancer in some occupations. These include the mining of uranium, haematite and pitchblende, as well as working with gas retorts, chromates, nickel and arsenic.

PATHOLOGY

Most carcinomas of the lung fall into one of four types:

1. *Squamous cell (or epidermoid) carcinoma*, which account for 30–35% of cases of primary lung cancer
2. *Adenocarcinoma* (including alveolar cell carcinoma), accounting for 30–35% of cases
3. *Large cell undifferentiated*, accounting for 15–20% of cases
4. *Small (oat) cell carcinoma*, accounting for 20–25% of cases.

Some lung cancers do not fall neatly into one of these categories, and may have components that resemble more than one type, for

example *adenosquamous carcinomas*. Other rarer tumours are classified separately, for example *clear cell carcinoma*, *basal cell carcinoma* and *carcinosarcoma*.

Approximately 50% of lung cancers arise centrally, i.e. in or proximal to segmental bronchi (Fig. 4.1). The tumour arises in the bronchial mucosa and invades the bronchial wall. Tumour may grow around the bronchus and also into the bronchial lumen. Obstruction of the lumen leads to collapse, and often infection, in the lung distal to the tumour. Tumours that arise peripherally appear as soft-tissue nodules or irregular masses (Fig. 4.2), and invade the adjacent tissues. Signs of collapse or consolidation may occur, but are less obvious than with central tumours. Both central and peripheral tumours may be associated with hilar or mediastinal lymph node enlargement, and this is also a potential cause of central

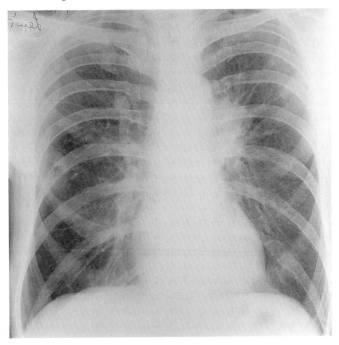

Fig. 4.1 Carcinoma of bronchus. The primary tumour is at the left hilum. Soft-tissue nodules in both lungs are metastases, and there is a lytic metastasis in the right eighth rib.

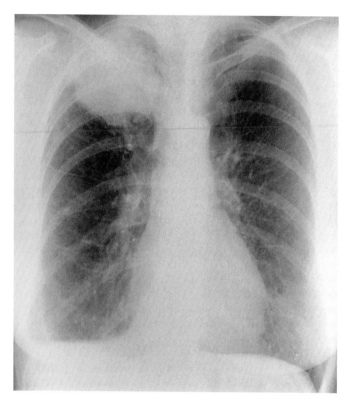

Fig. 4.2 Carcinoma of bronchus. A large, round soft-tissue mass is present at the right apex. Blunting of the right costophrenic angle is due to a small pleural effusion.

airway obstruction (Fig. 4.3). The tumour may also undergo central necrosis leading to cavitation. Peripheral tumours sometimes arise in pulmonary scars, and there is evidence that pulmonary fibrosis predisposes to neoplastic change. Although lung cancer usually presents as a single primary tumour, synchronous tumours are not rare (Fig. 4.4). Metastases from lung cancer may occur anywhere in the body, but hilar, mediastinal and supraclavicular lymph nodes are the commonest sites, followed by the liver, bones, brain, adrenal glands and skin. Lung cancer is a common cause of *lymphangitis carcinomatosa*.

The different cell types of lung cancer tend to show differences in behaviour. *Squamous cell cancers* tend to arise centrally, grow relatively slowly and cavitate more often than other cell types. *Adenocarcinomas* usually arise peripherally, sometimes in fibrotic lung, and cavitate less often. *Small cell tumours* have the fastest rate of growth and are usually disseminated at the time of presentation. They are usually central and are typically associated with mediastinal and hilar adenopathy, but rarely cavitate.

CLINICAL PRESENTATION

Respiratory symptoms such as cough, wheeze, sputum production, breathlessness, chest discomfort and haemoptysis are the commonest presenting symptoms in patients with lung cancer, although approximately 20% of patients are asymptomatic at presentation. Other presentations include finger clubbing, superior vena caval obstruction, Horner's syndrome, chest wall pain, dysphagia and signs of pericardial tamponade. An abnormal chest X-ray is a common presentation in patients who are symptom free or who have non-specific symptoms. Patients may also present with symptoms of metastatic disease such as bone pain or signs of an intracranial tumour or general debility. Pneumonia, particularly if it does not respond to treatment, may be due to an underlying neoplasm. A small number of patients present with paraneoplastic syndromes such as hypertrophic osteoarthropathy, endocrine disturbance (e.g. inappropriate ADH secretion, Cushing's syndrome, hypercalcaemia), peripheral neuropathy and recurrent peripheral venous thrombosis.

RADIOLOGICAL FEATURES

The radiological features of lung cancer are a reflection of the pathology, and depend upon the size and site of the tumour and its histology.

Hilar enlargement

This is a common radiographic manifestation of lung cancer. If the primary tumour is central this represents the tumour itself (Fig. 4.1). If the tumour is peripheral, it represents metastasis to bronchopulmonary lymph nodes (Fig. 4.5), and the primary tumour may or may not be visible. Occasionally, hilar involvement is subtle and presents as increased density of the hilum rather than as enlargement (Fig. 4.6). The true extent of nodal disease is best demonstrated by CT (Fig. 4.7C,D) or MRI. Extensive hilar and mediastinal lymphadenopathy is frequently seen with small cell tumours.

Airway obstruction

Bronchial narrowing due to tumour growth eventually causes collapse of the lung distal to the tumour. Depending on the location of the tumour, segmental or lobar collapse (Fig. 4.3) or, less often, collapse of an entire lung (Fig. 4.8) may be seen. Prior to collapse of a lobe or segment, infection may develop distal to the bronchial obstruction. Consequently, segmental or lobar consolidation may be a manifestation of lung cancer, and as this is secondary to bronchial occlusion an air bronchogram is usually absent. As the primary tumour may be obscured by surrounding consolidation, the possibility of an underlying endobronchial lesion should always be considered in cases of segmental or lobar pneumonia which do not resolve despite appropriate treatment. Occasionally a tumour arising in a segmental or subsegmental bronchus will lead to mucoid impaction and the development of a bronchocele or mucocele (Fig. 4.9).

Peripheral mass

A peripheral pulmonary mass on the chest X-ray is a common presentation of lung cancer (Figs 4.2, 4.3). If other features are present, such as hilar enlargement or bony metastases, then the malignant nature of the mass is easily appreciated (Fig. 4.1). Frequently, however, a mass is the only apparent abnormality and then the differential diagnosis is more difficult. There are no radiological features that can reliably differentiate between a benign and a malignant pulmonary nodule or mass. However, malignant tumours are usually larger than benign lesions at the time of presentation. Furthermore, peripheral lung cancers tend to have poorly defined, lobulated or umbilicated margins, or may appear spiculated (Fig. 4.10). *Satellite opacities* around the main lesion are more frequently seen with benign masses, but may be associated with

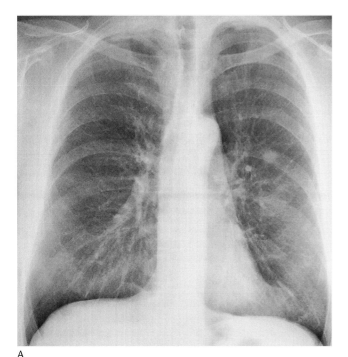

A

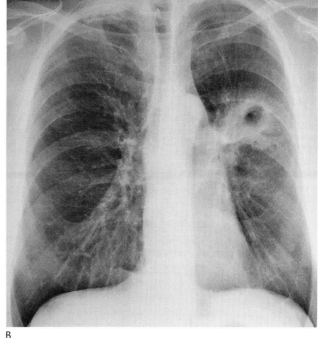

B

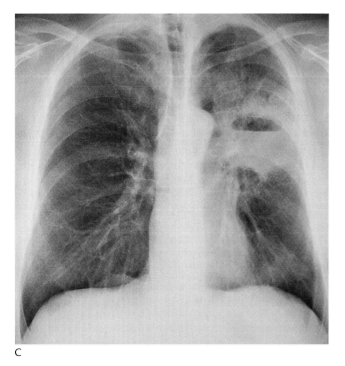

C

Fig. 4.3 Squamous cell carcinoma of bronchus—natural history over 3 years in a patient who declined treatment. (A) A small soft-tissue nodule is present in the left midzone. (B) Eighteen months later the tumour has enlarged and cavitated, and there is bulging of the aortopulmonary window, indicating lymph node enlargement. (C) A further 6 months later, the tumour has further enlarged, and a fluid level is present in the cavity. Patchy consolidation is present in the left upper lobe.

carcinomas (Fig. 4.10). Diffuse or central *calcification* in a peripheral pulmonary mass is very suggestive of a benign lesion, but occasionally a calcified granuloma will have been engulfed by a malignant tumour. Bronchial carcinomas usually have a *doubling time* of between 1 and 18 months. Therefore, comparison with previous X-rays can be very helpful, and any mass or nodule that has not changed in appearance over a 2-year period is almost certainly benign.

Cavitation is visible in about 10–15% of peripheral lung cancers on plain X-rays (Figs 4.3, 4.11) and is better demonstrated by CT (Fig. 4.12). It is due to either central necrosis of the tumour or abscess formation secondary to bronchial obstruction, and a fluid level may be present within the cavity. Typically, malignant cavities are thick walled with an irregular, nodular inner margin, but some may appear thin walled. Because lung cancers tend to be associated with bronchial occlusion they virtually never show an air bronchogram on the plain X-ray. However, it is not unusual to see an air bronchogram on the CT of an adenocarcinoma, and it is a common finding in alveolar cell carcinoma.

Bronchial carcinomas arising at the lung apex were formerly regarded as an entity distinct from other lung cancers and were known as *Pancoast* or *superior sulcus tumours*. Histologically they are similar to other primary carcinomas of the lung. However,

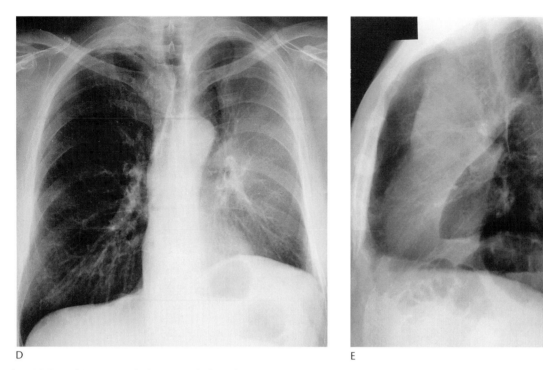

D   E

Fig. 4.3 (contd.)   (D, E) A further 3 months later there is now complete collapse of the left upper lobe, and the left hemidiaphragm is elevated due to phrenic nerve involvement.

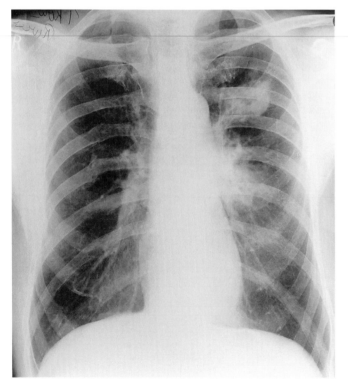

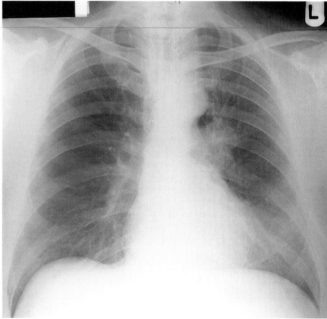

Fig. 4.5   Carcinoma of bronchus. The left hilum is enlarged by lymphadenopathy due to adenocarcinoma. The primary tumour is not visible.

Fig. 4.4   Synchronous bronchial carcinomas. The soft-tissue mass overlying the left hilum was an adenocarcinoma in the apical segment of left lower lobe, and the mass in the left upper zone was an upper lobe squamous cell carcinoma.

because of their location they have a tendency to invade ribs, the spine, the brachial plexus and the inferior cervical sympathetic ganglia. The plain film may show an obvious mass with associated

bone destruction (Fig. 4.13), but frequently only asymmetrical apical pleural thickening is visible, and the full extent of the tumour is best demonstrated by CT or MRI (Fig. 4.14). Bone involvement is often best shown by CT, but MRI can produce images in the coronal and sagittal planes which are ideal for demonstrating the relationship of the tumour to the brachial plexus and subclavian vessels, and for showing involvement of the extrapleural fat over

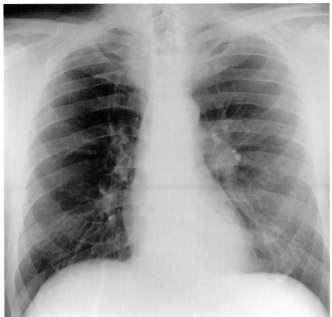

Fig. 4.6 Carcinoma of bronchus. Chest X-ray shows a dense left hilum, but no definite mass. Bronchoscopy showed a squamous carcinoma in the left main bronchus.

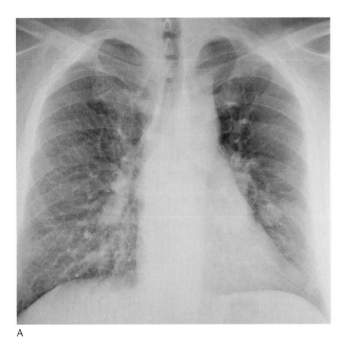

A

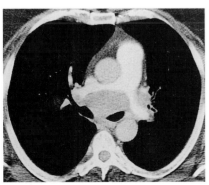

C

the lung apex (Fig. 4.15). However, for the purpose of percutaneous biopsy, these tumours are often most conveniently visualised by ultrasound scanning from the supraclavicular fossa (Fig. 4.14C).

Mediastinal involvement

Enlargement of mediastinal lymph nodes is a typical feature of small cell tumours, but occurs with other bronchial carcinomas. The mediastinum appears widened and may have a lobulated outline (Fig. 4.16). In non-small cell tumours lymph node involvement is less florid, and since its full extent may not be appreciated on the chest X-ray it is best assessed non-invasively by CT or MRI (Fig. 4.17).

Enlarged mediastinal lymph nodes or central tumours may distort the *oesophagus*. Barium swallow may, therefore, be used to assess the mediastinum, and is essential in patients with dysphagia (Fig. 4.18). In these patients oesophageal compression or invasion may be demonstrated. Mediastinal invasion may involve the *phrenic nerve*, and in patients with lung cancer elevation of a hemidiaphragm suggests this complication or may be due to pulmonary collapse or subphrenic disease. Fluoroscopy or ultrasound scan of the diaphragm may be used to determine if an elevated dome moves paradoxically and is paralysed.

Mediastinal spread of tumour may also cause *superior vena caval obstruction*, and this may be confirmed by superior vena

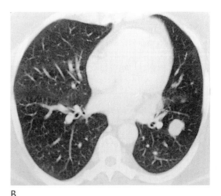

B

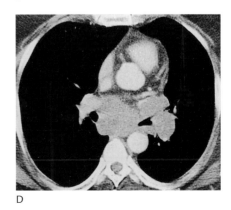

D

Fig. 4.7 Carcinoma of bronchus. (A) Chest X-ray shows a soft-tissue nodule in the left midzone and prominence of the left hilum. (B) Contrast-enhanced CT on lung window confirms left lower lobe mass, which proved to be an adenocarcinoma. (C, D) CT on mediastinal windows shows left hilar lymphadenopathy, but more importantly there is very extensive mediastinal adenopathy surrounding the pulmonary arteries and extending into the subcarinal region and down into the azygo-oesophageal recess.

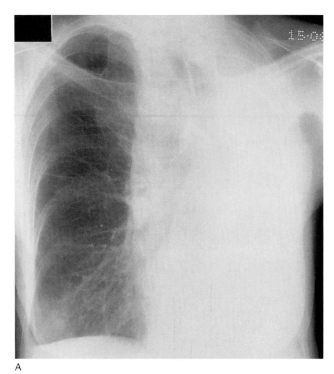

A

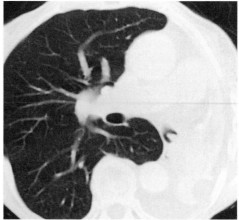

B

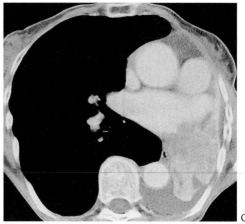

C

Fig. 4.8   Carcinoma of bronchus. (A) Chest X-ray shows collapse of left lung. (B) Contrast-enhanced CT on lung window confirms collapsed left lung, shows small pleural effusion and demonstrates tumour extending into the left main bronchus. (C) CT on mediastinal window demonstrates tumour invading posterior wall of left atrium (confirmed at surgery).

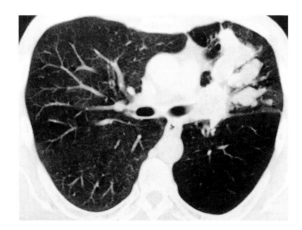

Fig. 4.9   Bronchocele due to carcinoma of bronchus. CT shows dilated, fluid-filled bronchi in lingula, secondary to carcinoma at left hilum.

cavography, dynamically enhanced CT or MRI. Invasion of the pericardium by metastatic lymph nodes or the primary tumour itself may result in pericarditis and pericardial effusion (Fig. 4.16).

Pleural involvement

Pleural effusion may be due to direct spread of the tumour but may also be the result of lymphatic obstruction or be secondary to an obstructive pneumonitis. Pleural effusion also occurs as a sympathetic response to the tumour, in which case there is no cytological or histological evidence of pleural malignancy. Rarely,

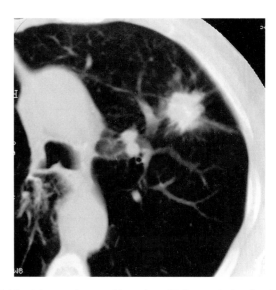

Fig. 4.10   Adenocarcinoma of bronchus. CT shows spiculated, soft-tissue mass with strands of tissue extending into the adjacent lung parenchyma.

a cavitating subpleural tumour will cause a spontaneous pneumothorax.

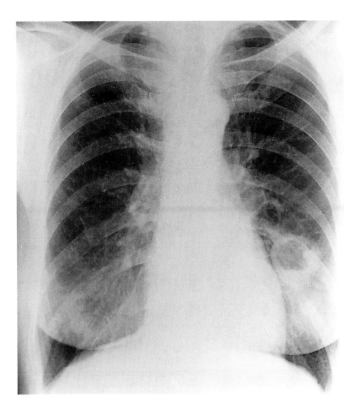

Fig. 4.11 Squamous cell carcinoma of bronchus. Chest X-ray shows a cavitating mass with a fluid level in the left mid zone.

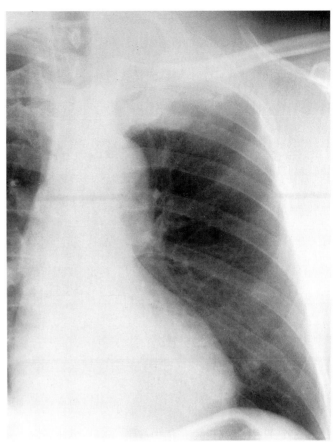

Fig. 4.13 Pancoast tumour. Chest X-ray shows a left apical mass with destruction of the second and third ribs posteriorly.

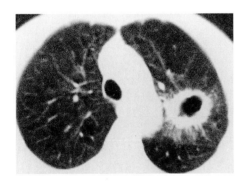

Fig. 4.12 Squamous cell carcinoma of bronchus. CT shows a thick-walled cavitating mass with a spiculated outer surface and nodular inner surface.

DIAGNOSTIC IMAGING AND THE MANAGEMENT OF CARCINOMA OF THE BRONCHUS

Imaging makes an important contribution to three aspects of the management of lung cancer. These are:

1. Making the diagnosis
2. Staging the tumour
3. Assessing treatment.

Making the diagnosis

The prognosis and treatment of lung cancer depends upon the general condition of the patient and on the histology of the tumour and its extent at the time of presentation. Currently there are trials under way in both the USA and Europe assessing the efficacy of low-dose spiral CT in screening for lung cancer. Small cell tumours metastasise early and are usually disseminated at the time of presentation. Non-small cell tumours metastasise later, the natural history of squamous cell carcinoma being longer than that of adenocarcinoma and undifferentiated large cell carcinoma. Moreover, small cell tumours are more sensitive to chemotherapy than non-small cell tumours. Therefore, when planning treatment it is important to know the histology of the tumour. Sputum cytology and bronchoscopic biopsies or washings usually provide the cell type of

Bone involvement

Peripheral carcinomas may invade the ribs or spine directly (Figs 4.13–4.15). Haematogenous metastases from lung to bone are usually osteolytic (Fig. 4.1). They are often painful, and are identified earliest by isotope bone scan. Bone pain, particularly in the wrists, hands, ankles and feet, may also be due to hypertrophic osteoarthropathy. On plain films the affected bones show well-defined periosteal new bone formation. Isotope bone scan may be positive before radiographic changes are visible.

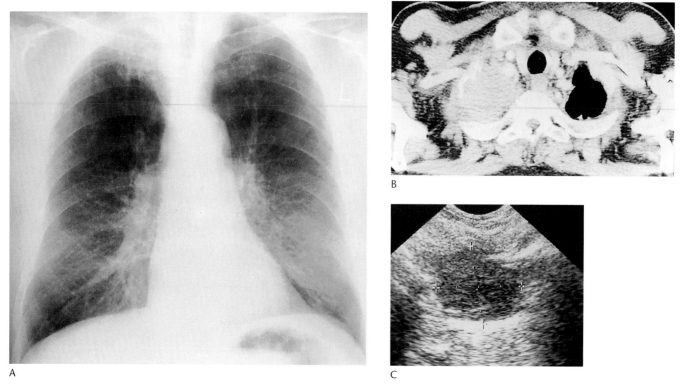

Fig. 4.14 Pancoast tumour. (A) Chest X-ray shows asymmetrical right apical pleural thickening. (B) CT shows large right apical soft-tissue mass extending through chest wall into apex of right axilla. (C) Ultrasound scan from right supraclavicular fossa shows apical pulmonary mass of relatively low echogenicity, and demonstrates the easiest route of access for percutaneous biopsy.

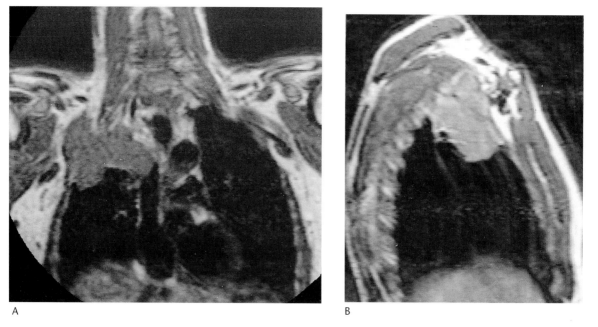

Fig. 4.15 Pancoast tumour. T_1-weighted coronal (A) and sagittal (B) MRI shows precise extent of right apical mass with obliteration of the extrapleural fat where the mass invades the chest wall and enters the root of the neck.

central tumours, but peripheral tumours may require percutaneous biopsy. This may be done with fluoroscopic, CT or ultrasound guidance (Fig. 4.19). Depending on the needle used the specimens may be suitable for cytological or histological evaluation, but in either case it is important to have available a pathologist skilled in examining small specimens.

Management of a *solitary pulmonary nodule* in an asymptomatic patient in the cancer age group is not a rare problem. Obviously the differential diagnosis will be influenced by other clinical data such as a background of cancer or rheumatoid disease. Comparison with previous imaging is invaluable, as a nodule that has not changed on the chest radiograph over 2 years is likely to be benign. There may be features that confidently allow a diagnosis of benign disease on the chest radiograph or CT, for example a classical appearance of infolded lung, or diffuse calcification within the nodule. Recently developed strategies to differentiate benign from malignant tumours include CT densitometry and positron emission tomography (PET) using ^{18}F-fluorodeoxyglucose (FDG). Compared to benign nodules, malignant nodules show a greater degree of enhancement following intravenous injection of iodinated contrast medium, such that an increase in attenuation on CT scanning of greater than 20 Hounsfield units is very suggestive of malignancy. For nodules 2 cm in diameter or greater, PET with FDG appears to be highly specific and sensitive in identifying malignant lesions. However, if the possibility of lung cancer remains the nodule should be closely monitored, biopsied or excised.

Staging the tumour

Without treatment only about 1% of patients with lung cancer will survive 3 years from the time of diagnosis. Currently the main hopes for curative treatment lie with surgery for non-small cell cancer, and chemotherapy for small cell tumours. The main purposes of accurate staging of lung cancer are:

1. To identify those patients with non-small cell tumours who will benefit from surgery
2. To avoid surgery in those who will not benefit, and
3. To provide accurate data for assessing and comparing different methods of treatment.

The TNM system (Box 4.1), where T describes the primary tumour, N the regional lymph nodes and M distant metastases, is widely used. The International Staging System (Table 4.1) based on the TNM system is designed to be used by thoracic surgeons considering tumour resection and by radiotherapists and oncologists treating more extensive disease.

Stage I indicates a T1 or T2 tumour without associated lymphadenopathy or distant metastases; such a tumour is likely to be amenable to surgical resection. Stage II tumours are similar primary tumours, but have associated ipsilateral hilar adenopathy; they are also potentially surgically curable, but the prognosis is less favourable. Stage IIIA tumours have extensive local intrathoracic disease which may be amenable to surgical resection; Stage IIIB tumours have local intrathoracic disease that is too extensive for resection, but may be treatable with radical radiotherapy. Stage IV tumours have distant metastases.

Thus, a tumour is likely to be inoperable if it extends directly into parietal pleura, chest wall, diaphragm or mediastinum, or is within 2.0 cm of the main carina. In addition, metastasis to contralateral hilar nodes, mediastinal nodes or more distantly precludes surgical cure. The plain chest film should be carefully scrutinised for evidence of spread of tumour. If the tumour appears localised and appears operable on bronchoscopy, *isotope bone scan* and *liver ultrasound* may be performed and, if the tumour still appears operable, the mediastinum should be assessed by CT or MRI (Fig. 4.20). Any node over 2 cm in diameter is likely to be involved, and nodes of 1 cm or less are usually regarded as normal. Nodes between 1 and 2 cm present a diagnostic problem, and the ability of CT to predict involvement by tumour is limited. However if the enlarged nodes are those that most directly drain the lung tumour, and other mediastinal lymph nodes are normal in size, the likelihood of malignant involvement is increased. In equivocal cases *mediastinoscopy* is indicated prior to subjecting the patient to thoracotomy. PET using ^{18}F-FDG is proving to be a more sensitive and specific method than either CT or MRI for identifying intrathoracic lymph node involvement, and also more distant disease (Fig. 4.21).

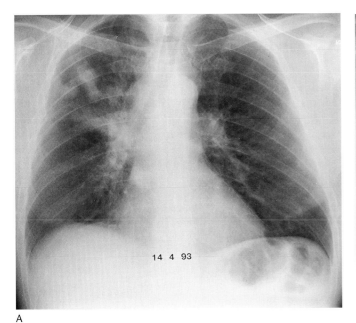

A

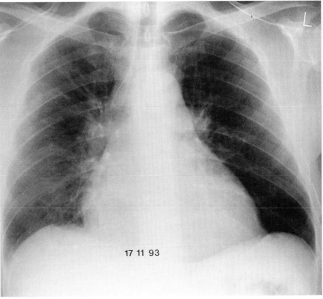

B

Fig. 4.16 Small cell carcinoma of bronchus. (A) Chest X-ray shows right upper lobe masses and extensive right paratracheal and right hilar lymphadenopathy. Five months later, following chemotherapy the disease was in remission and the X-ray was normal. (B) A further 2 months later the tumour has recurred with enlargement of the heart shadow due to pericardial effusion (confirmed by echocardiography).

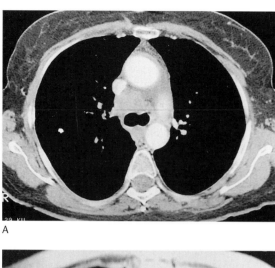

A

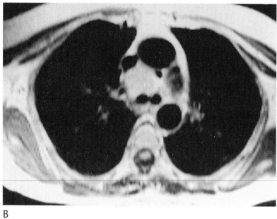

B

Fig. 4.17 Carcinoma of bronchus. Contrast-enhanced CT scan (A) and T₁-weighted MRI scan (B). Axial scans at level of carina show similar anatomical detail, with retrocaval lymphadenopathy. In general, CT provides better spatial resolution, but MRI has better natural contrast.

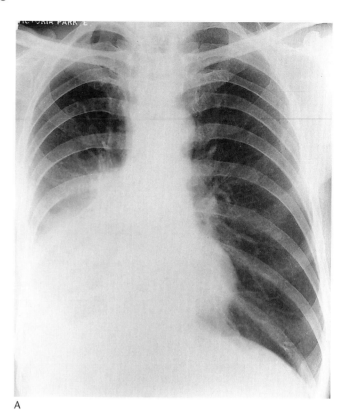

A

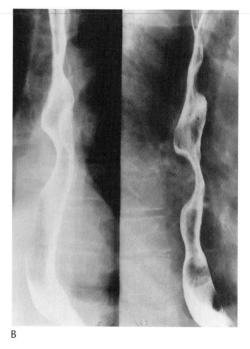

B

Fig. 4.18 Carcinoma of bronchus. (A) Chest X-ray shows collapse and consolidation of right lower lobe. (B) Barium swallow performed to investigate dysphagia shows extrinsic compression of mid oesophagus by enlarged subcarinal lymph nodes.

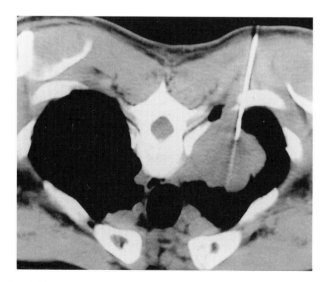

Fig. 4.19 Carcinoma of bronchus. CT of prone patient during percutaneous biopsy. The end of the biopsy needle is in the tumour.

Assessing treatment

Following chemotherapy for small cell cancer, bulky mediastinal and hilar nodes and peripheral lesions may show complete regression (Fig. 4.16). Follow-up chest X-rays are required to detect local recurrence, although recurrent disease is often extrathoracic. These patients are also prone to opportunistic infections. Following radiotherapy radiation pneumonitis and pulmonary fibrosis may occur, and radiation oesophagitis may be a consequence of mediastinal irradiation. Postoperative appearances are discussed in Chapter 8.

ALVEOLAR CELL CARCINOMA

Alveolar cell carcinoma is also known as bronchiolar or bronchioloalveolar carcinoma, and is a subtype of adenocarcinoma with certain special features. It arises more peripherally than typical lung cancer, probably from type II pneumocytes. It accounts for 2–5% of all lung cancers, usually occurring between the ages of 50 and 70 years with an equal sex incidence. It is not associated with smoking but may be associated with diffuse pulmonary fibrosis and pulmonary scars.

Box 4.1 TNM descriptions of non-small cell bronchial carcinoma. (From Mountain 1997.)

Primary tumour (T)

TX Primary tumour cannot be assessed, or tumour proven by the presence of malignant cells in sputum or bronchial washings but not visualised by imaging or bronchoscopy

T0 No evidence of primary tumour

Tis Carcinoma in situ

T1 Tumour <3 cm in greatest dimension surrounded by lung or visceral pleura, without bronchoscopic evidence of invasion more proximal than the lobar bronchus (i.e. not in the main bronchus)

T2 Tumour with any of the following features of size or extent: >3 cm in greatest dimension; involves main bronchus >2 cm distal to the carina; invades the visceral pleura; associated with atelectasis or obstructive pneumonitis that extends to the hilar region but does not involve the entire lung

T3 Tumour of any size that directly invades any of the following: chest wall (including superior sulcus tumours), diaphragm, mediastinal pleura, parietal pericardium; or tumour in the main bronchus <2 cm distal to the carina, but without involvement of the carina; or associated atelectasis or obstructive pneumonitis of the entire lung

T4 Tumour of any size that invades any of the following: mediastinum, heart, great vessels, trachea, oesophagus, vertebral body, carina; or tumour with a malignant pleural or pericardial effusion, or with satellite tumour nodule(s) within the ipsilateral primary tumour lobe of the lung

Regional lymph nodes (N)

NX Regional lymph nodes cannot be assessed

N0 No regional lymph node metastasis

N1 Metastasis to ipsilateral peribronchial and/or ipsilateral hilar lymph nodes and intrapulmonary nodes involved by direct extension of the primary tumour

N2 Metastasis to ipsilateral mediastinal and/or subcarinal lymph node(s)

N3 Metastasis to contralateral mediastinal, contralateral hilar, ipsilateral or contralateral scalene, or supraclavicular lymph node(s)

Distant metastasis (M)

MX Distant metastasis cannot be assessed

M0 No distant metastasis

M1 Distant metastasis present

Table 4.1 Stages for International Staging System for lung Cancer. (From Mountain 1986.)

Stage	Definition*
I	T1, N0, M0
	T2, N0, M0
II	T1, N1, M0
	T2, N1, M0
IIIA	T3, N0, M0
	T3, N1, M0
	T1-3, N2, M0
IIIB	Any T, N3, M0
	T4; any N, M0
IV	Any T; any N, M1

*See Box 4.1.

These tumours arise within alveoli and produce areas of consolidation. It is uncertain whether they originate multicentrically or focally; clinically two patterns are seen. The focal form arises as a solitary peripheral mass (Fig. 4.22) in which, unlike other forms of lung cancer, an air bronchogram is often visible. The diffuse form manifests itself as multiple acinar shadows throughout the lungs, often with areas of confluence, and the appearance may resemble pulmonary oedema or bronchopneumonia. These features are elegantly demonstrated by CT which may show any combination of ground-glass opacification, small nodular opacities, frank consolidation and thickened interlobular septa (Fig. 4.23). The focal form may spread via the airways and progress to the diffuse pattern (Fig. 4.22).

METASTATIC LUNG DISEASE

Metastases most commonly reach the lung haematogenously via the systemic veins and pulmonary arteries. They may originate at any site, but primary tumours of the breast, skeleton and urogenital system account for approximately 80% of pulmonary metastases. Lymphatic spread is less common and endobronchial spread is rare, usually being a manifestation of alveolar cell carcinoma.

Approximately 3% of asymptomatic pulmonary nodules are metastases. The commonest primary tumours producing solitary pulmonary metastases are carcinomas of the *colon, kidney* and *breast, testicular tumours, bone sarcomas* and *malignant melanoma*. In about 75% of cases metastatic lung disease presents as multiple pulmonary nodules. Metastases to the lung are usually bilateral, affecting both lungs equally, with a basal predominance (Fig. 4.24). They are often peripheral and may be subpleural (Fig. 4.25).

Pulmonary metastases vary in size from a few millimetres in diameter (Fig. 4.26) to several centimetres. They tend to be spherical with a well-defined margin. An ill-defined margin may signify haemorrhage. *Cavitation* may occur in metastases from any primary site, but is more common in squamous carcinomas (Fig. 4.27) and sarcomas. Cavitation of a subpleural metastasis is a recognised cause of spontaneous pneumothorax. *Calcification* is unusual in pulmonary metastases, being seen most often in osteogenic sarcoma (Fig. 4.28), and rarely in chondrosarcoma and mucinous adenocarcinoma.

Endobronchial metastases are rare, the commonest primary tumours being carcinoma of kidney, breast and large bowel. They may occlude the airway and cause segmental or lobar collapse.

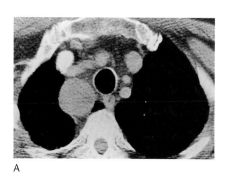
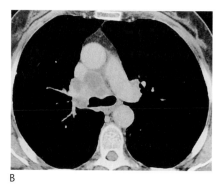
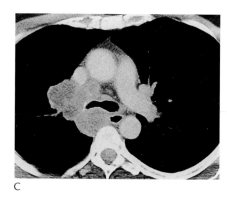

Fig. 4.20   Carcinoma of bronchus. Contrast-enhanced CT demonstration of mediastinal lymphadenopathy in three different patients. (A) An enlarged right paratracheal node. (B) Retrocaval and right hilar adenopathy. Ring enhancement of the glands indicates central necrosis. (C) Retrocaval, subcarinal and right hilar adenopathy.

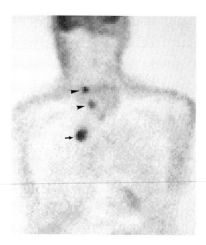

Fig. 4.21   PET scan showing abnormal uptake of FDG in primary lung cancer in right upper lobe (arrow) and in two superior mediastinal lymph nodes (arrowheads). A contemporary CT scan (not shown) demonstrated the primary tumour, but did not show any lymphadenopathy.

Lymphangitis carcinomatosa results from haematogenous metastases invading and occluding peripheral pulmonary lymphatics. The commonest primary sites are carcinoma of the lung, breast, stomach, pancreas, cervix and prostate. Lymphangitis carcinomatosa is usually bilateral, but lung and breast cancer may cause unilateral lymphangitis (Fig. 4.29). The chest X-ray shows coarse, linear, reticular and nodular basal shadowing, often with pleural effusions and hilar lymphadenopathy (Fig. 4.30). In the early stages of lung involvement the chest X-ray may suggest lymphangitis, but may not be diagnostic. In these cases a high-resolution CT scan may be undertaken to establish the diagnosis, when the typical appearance is nodular thickening of the interlobular septa and thickening of the centrilobular bronchovascular bundles (Fig. 4.31).

INTRATHORACIC LYMPHOMA AND LEUKAEMIA

HODGKIN'S DISEASE

Hodgkin's disease is the commonest lymphoma. It is distinguished from other lymphomas by the presence of Reed–Sternberg cells. It

is the commonest neoplasm of young adults with a peak incidence at 25–29 years of age, and a second, smaller peak at 70–74 years. The disease usually arises in lymph nodes, and hilar or mediastinal lymph node enlargement is seen on the chest X-ray at the time of presentation in about 50% of cases. The lymphadenopathy is frequently bilateral but, unlike in sarcoidosis, it is often asymmetrical and involves anterior mediastinal glands (Fig. 4.32). These retrosternal nodes may erode the sternum. CT may identify nodal disease not apparent on the chest X-ray, particularly in the retrosternal and paraspinal regions. Following treatment by radiotherapy or chemotherapy, lymph node calcification may occur (Fig. 4.33).

Involvement of lung parenchyma is seen in about 30% of cases. It is usually due to spread of disease from hilar lymph nodes along the peribronchial connective tissue space. The resulting pulmonary infiltrate may resemble lymphangitis carcinomatosa. Pulmonary involvement may also occur, usually by direct extension from mediastinal lymph nodes across the pleura (Fig. 4.34). Lung involvement in the absence of lymphadenopathy is rare if the patient has not already been treated. The pulmonary infiltrate may also appear as solitary areas of consolidation, larger confluent areas or miliary nodules. The pulmonary opacities may have an air bronchogram, and may cavitate. Involvement of the bronchial wall may lead to areas of collapse and consolidation in the peripheral lung.

Pleural effusion occurs in approximately 30% of cases and is usually due to lymphatic obstruction. Pleural involvement by the disease itself is less common, but is a cause of pleural plaques and effusion.

NON-HODGKIN'S LYMPHOMA

Malignant proliferation of a specific lymphoreticular cell line will give rise to a B-cell, T-cell or histiocytic lymphoma. Classification of these tumours is constantly being revised. Current clinical classifications are based on grading systems that relate the morphology of the tumour to prognosis (i.e. going from less to more aggressive: low grade, intermediate grade and high grade) and tumour architecture (i.e. follicular (or nodular) and diffuse lymphomas). Although the large majority of lymphomas arise within lymph glands (or the thymus), mucosa-associated lymphoid tissue (MALT) within the lung may also give rise to primary non-Hodgkin's lymphoma. These are usually low-grade B-cell lymphomas and manifest as one or more areas of pulmonary consolidation (Fig. 4.35), with or without associated adenopathy.

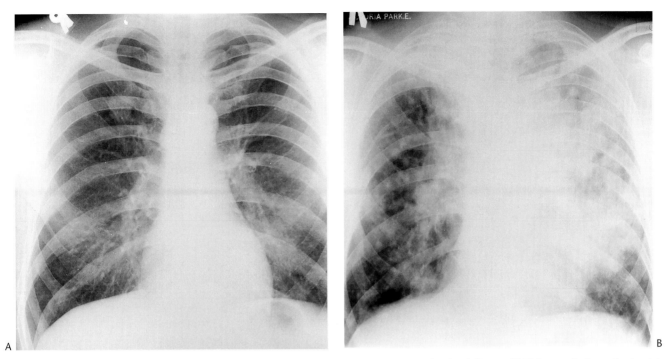

Fig. 4.22 Alveolar cell carcinoma. (A) Chest X-ray shows solitary right upper zone mass suggesting focal disease. (B) Eight months later, despite right upper lobectomy (note excised sixth rib), the disease has rapidly progressed to the diffuse pattern with widespread nodules and consolidation.

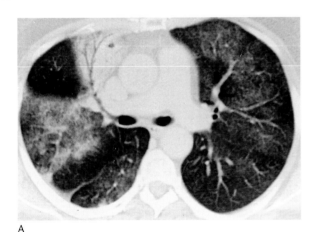

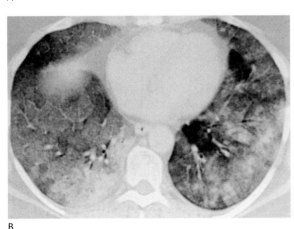

Fig. 4.23 Alveolar cell carcinoma. (A, B) CT shows diffuse, small, nodular shadows, widespread ground-glass opacification and dense consolidation with an air bronchogram in the anterior segment of the right upper lobe.

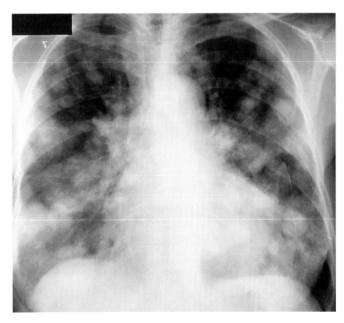

Fig. 4.24 Pulmonary metastases. Adenocarcinoma from unknown primary. Multiple, well-defined round opacities are present throughout both lungs.

In general, the radiographic manifestations of non-Hodgkin's and Hodgkin's lymphomas are similar (Fig. 4.36). However, the progression of disease in the non-Hodgkin's group is less orderly with pulmonary and pleural involvement often preceding mediastinal disease. There is also a greater tendency for the pulmonary infiltrates to traverse fissures and involve the pleura (Fig. 4.37).

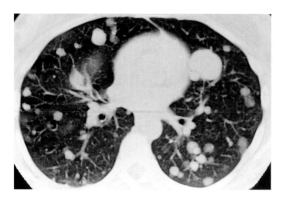

Fig. 4.25 Pulmonary metastases. Soft-tissue sarcoma. CT shows subpleural location of several of the metastases.

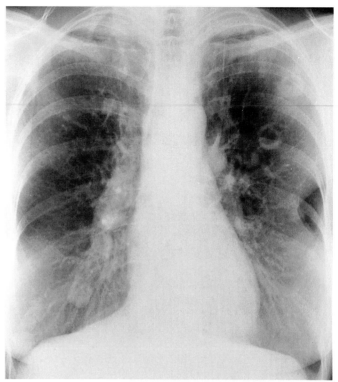

Fig. 4.27 Pulmonary metastases. Carcinoma of cervix. Multiple cavitating masses are present in both lungs.

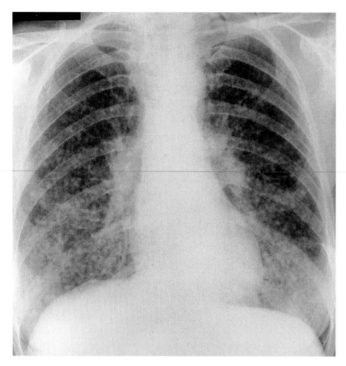

Fig. 4.26 Pulmonary metastases. Adenocarcinoma from unknown primary. Multiple small nodules are present throughout both lungs.

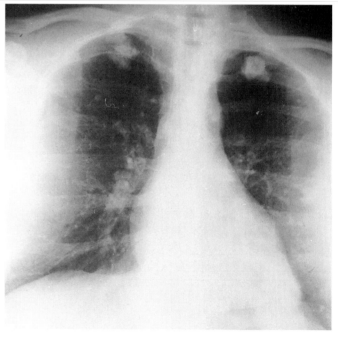

Fig. 4.28 Pulmonary metastases. Osteogenic sarcoma. Densely calcified masses are present in both lungs.

OTHER LYMPHOID DISORDERS

Pseudolymphoma

This is a rare tumour-like condition characterised by solitary or multiple areas of pulmonary consolidation (Fig. 4.38), which are predominantly due to aggregations of mature lymphocytes and variable numbers of plasma cells. Recent work suggests that cases previously described as this entity may in fact be MALT lymphomas. An air bronchogram is often visible and cavitation may occur. Lymphadenopathy and pleural effusion are rarely present. It usually behaves benignly, and the patients are often asymptomatic. However, there have been cases in which it appears to have undergone malignant transformation to pulmonary lymphoma.

Lymphocytic interstitial pneumonitis (LIP)

This condition is microscopically similar to pseudolymphoma, but instead of being a focal abnormality it is characterised by a more

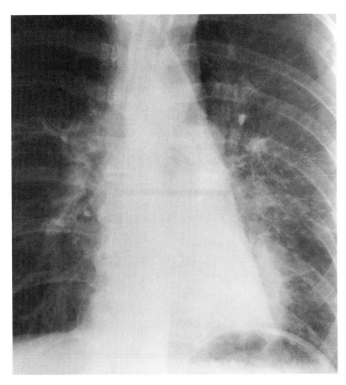

Fig. 4.29 Unilateral lymphangitis carcinomatosa. Carcinoma of the left lower lobe. There are several horizontal septal lines in the periphery of the left lung.

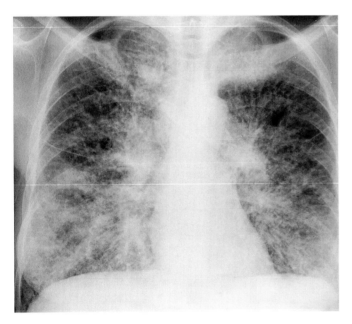

Fig. 4.30 Lymphangitis carcinomatosa. Carcinoma of cervix. Coarse reticular shadowing is present throughout both lungs, and there is bilateral hilar lymphadenopathy.

diffuse interstitial infiltrate, and it may proceed to pulmonary fibrosis. It may develop as a solitary abnormality, or in association with a variety of autoimmune conditions such as Sjögren's syndrome, but particularly in children there is an association with AIDS. Radiologically there is bilateral reticulonodular shadowing, sometimes with areas of consolidation, and there may be progres-

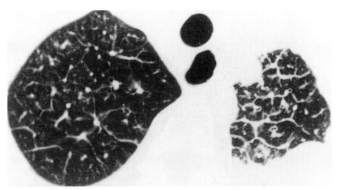

Fig. 4.31 Lymphangitis carcinomatosa. Breast cancer. High resolution CT (HRCT) shows marked nodular thickening of the interlobular septa and thickening of the centrilobular bronchovascular bundles in the left upper lobe, and early similar changes in the right upper lobe.

sion to honeycomb shadowing. Pleural effusions may occur, but lymphadenopathy is usually absent unless lymphomatous change occurs.

Lymphomatoid granulomatosis

This has been defined as 'an angiocentric, angiodestructive lymphoreticular, proliferative and granulomatous disease involving predominantly the lungs'. Hence, it was formerly thought of as a vasculitis, but is now regarded as being a T-cell non-Hodgkin's lymphoma. Radiologically it usually appears as multiple ill-defined pulmonary nodules, often resembling metastases, although an air bronchogram is often seen (Fig. 4.39). Cavitation occurs in about 10% of cases, but lymphadenopathy and pleural effusion are unusual.

LEUKAEMIA

Radiographic abnormalities of the chest in leukaemia are more commonly a manifestation of a complication of the disease rather than due to the disease itself. These complications include pneumonia, opportunistic infection, heart failure, pulmonary haemorrhage and reactions to therapy (drugs, transfusions and radiotherapy).

Mediastinal lymph node enlargement and pleural effusion are the commonest radiographic abnormalities due to leukaemia. Mediastinal lymphadenopathy is unusual without evidence of lymphadenopathy elsewhere. It occurs most frequently in lymphatic and monocytic leukaemias, but is rare in myeloid leukaemia. Leukaemic infiltrates in the lung are often a terminal event and are commoner in lymphatic leukaemia than myeloid leukaemia. The chest X-ray shows either bilateral streaky or reticular shadows similar to lymphangitis carcinomatosa or patchy consolidation.

PULMONARY SARCOMA

Although the lungs are a common site for metastatic sarcoma, primary sarcoma of the lung is rare. Prior to the AIDS epidemic *Kaposi's sarcoma* occurred mostly as a tumour of skin; however, there are now increasing numbers of cases of pulmonary Kaposi's

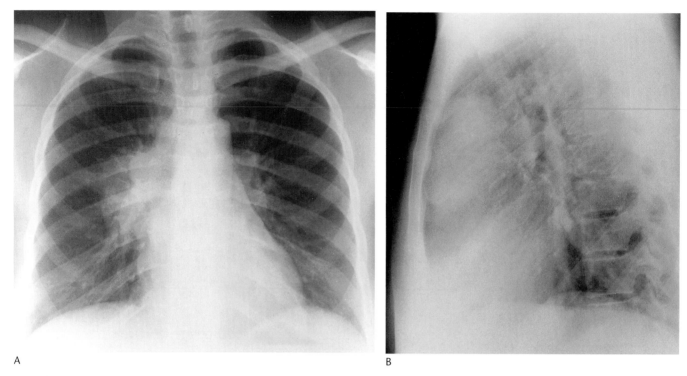

A   B

Fig. 4.32   Hodgkin's disease. Chest X-ray (A) shows right hilar lymphadenopathy and the lateral film (B) shows a large anterior mediastinal lymph node mass.

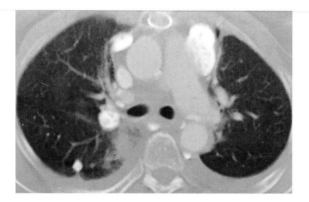

Fig. 4.33   Hodgkin's disease. CT shows extensive calcification in mediastinal lymph nodes in a patient previously treated for Hodgkin's disease.

sarcoma complicating AIDS. A localised form appears as segmental or lobar consolidation, but more commonly it is widespread with multiple nodular and linear opacities and areas of consolidation in both lungs. In addition, pleural effusions and hilar and mediastinal lymphadenopathy may be present.

Other primary pulmonary sarcomas may arise from any of the mesenchymal tissues in the lung. The most common are *fibrosarcoma*, *leiomyosarcoma* and *pulmonary artery angiosarcoma*; others include carcinosarcoma, pulmonary blastoma and malignant haemangiopericytoma. They most often present as a solitary pulmonary mass, radiographically indistinguishable from a carcinoma of the lung. Angiosarcoma of the pulmonary artery may present as a hilar mass and signs of pulmonary embolism and pulmonary arterial hypertension.

SALIVARY GLAND TYPE TUMOURS

These are mostly *adenoid cystic carcinomas*, which usually arise in the trachea or major bronchi. They grow beneath the bronchial epithelium in a tubular fashion and extend outward into the tracheal or bronchial wall (Fig. 4.40). Local invasion is common. They present radiologically as a tumour mass with or without airway obstruction. *Mucoepidermoid tumours* are also locally invasive. *Bronchial cystadenomas* are small polypoidal tumours that project into the bronchial lumen and may, therefore, cause areas of atelectasis and infection, though they themselves are truly benign.

BRONCHIAL CARCINOID

Carcinoids are neuroendocrine tumours and are derived from bronchial APUD (amino precursor uptake decarboxylation) cells. These are the same cells which give rise to small cell carcinoma. Bronchial carcinoids are described as either typical or atypical. Approximately 90% are typical and these tend to behave benignly, growing slowly and metastasising infrequently. Atypical carcinoids have histological and clinical features that lie between those of typical carcinoids and small cell carcinoma, and approximately 50% will eventually metastasise.

Approximately 80% of carcinoids arise in lobar or main segmental bronchi (Fig. 4.41). Growth of tumour into the lumen may cause bronchial obstruction and collapse of the lung peripheral to the tumour. Lesser degrees of bronchial obstruction may result in recurrent segmental pneumonia, bronchiectasis or abscess formation, or

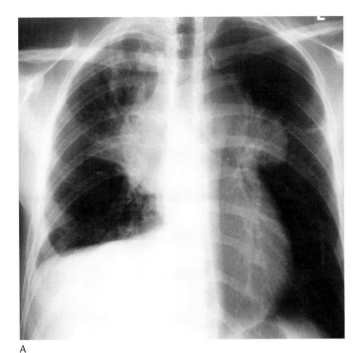

A

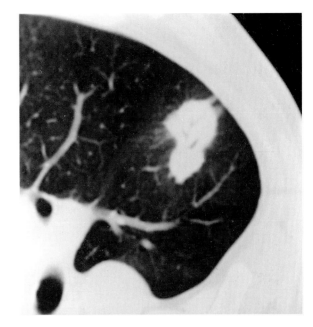

Fig. 4.35 Pulmonary lymphoma. CT shows an irregular soft-tissue mass with an air bronchogram.

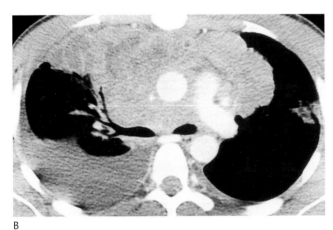

B

Fig. 4.34 Hodgkin's disease. (A) Chest X-ray shows bilateral hilar adenopathy, mediastinal adenopathy, right upper lobe pulmonary shadowing and a right pleural effusion. (B) Contrast-enhanced CT shows massive anterior mediastinal adenopathy, with direct infiltration of the right upper lobe and a large pleural effusion.

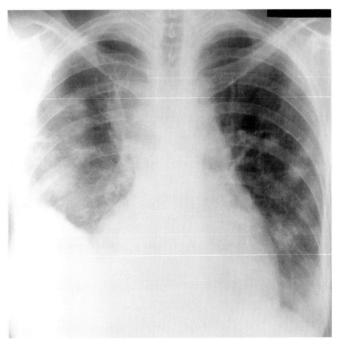

Fig. 4.36 Histiocytic lymphoma. Chest X-ray shows mediastinal adenopathy, multiple ill-defined pulmonary nodules and a right pleural effusion.

air trapping in the lung distal to the tumour. If the tumour extends extrabronchially, lung infiltration may occur.

Peripheral carcinoids appear as well-circumscribed, round or ovoid solitary nodules (Fig. 4.42). On CT calcification they may be seen within the tumour, and many show obvious enhancement following intravenous contrast medium.

Carcinoids may produce a variety of hormones. These include serotonin, kallikrein, histamine, ACTH, insulin and substances similar to antidiuretic hormone and gastrin. Rarely, production of these hormones may lead to clinical syndromes such as the carcinoid syndrome. Carcinoid syndrome due to a lung primary usually indicates hepatic metastases. Skeletal metastases from bronchial carcinoids may be osteoblastic.

PULMONARY HAMARTOMA

A hamartoma is a tumour which consists of an abnormal arrangement of the tissues normally found in the organ concerned. Most pulmonary hamartomas have a large cartilaginous component, and there may also be an appreciable fatty component. They are rarely seen in childhood and most often present as a solitary pulmonary

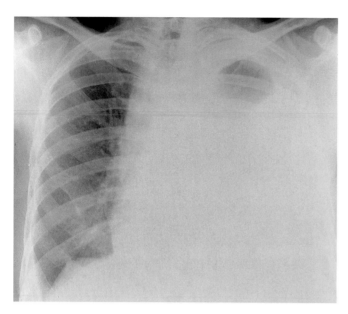

Fig. 4.37   Lymphocytic lymphoma. Chest X-ray shows a large left pleural effusion, a small right pleural effusion and right paratracheal adenopathy.

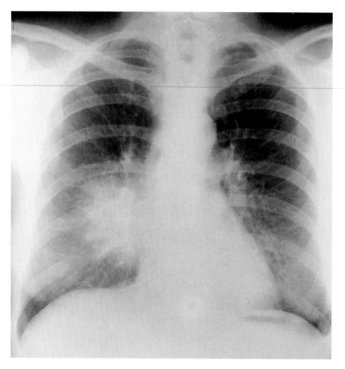

Fig. 4.38   Pseudolymphoma. Consolidation in the right middle lobe obscures the right hilum and heart border.

nodule in an asymptomatic adult. Unlike bronchial carcinoids, most pulmonary hamartomas are peripheral. They appear as well-circumscribed nodules varying in diameter from a few millimetres to several centimetres (Fig. 4.43). They do not cavitate, and any low density within them represents fat. On the chest X-ray approximately 30% show calcification, often with a characteristic 'popcorn' appearance (Fig. 4.44). On serial films they may be seen to grow slowly. CT may demonstrate or confirm the presence of fat or calcification within the nodule, allowing a precise diagnosis to be

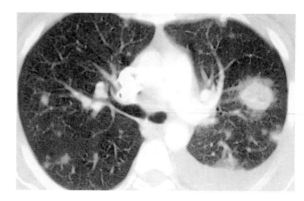

Fig. 4.39   Lymphomatoid granulomatosis. CT scan demonstrates multiple pulmonary nodules and a larger mass in the left upper node which shows an air bronchogram. Subcarinal lymph node enlargement and a left pleural effusion are also present.

made. Rarely they arise endobronchially and may then present with signs of bronchial obstruction.

OTHER BENIGN PULMONARY TUMOURS

This heading covers many rarities including *bronchial chondroma, pulmonary fibroma, pulmonary myxoma, plasma cell granuloma (also known as histiocytoma, sclerosing granuloma or inflammatory pseudotumour), bronchial lipoma, myoblastoma of the bronchus (or granular-cell tumour), bronchial papilloma* and *benign clear cell tumour.* They are often asymptomatic, presenting as a solitary pulmonary nodule, although some may be multiple. Some may cause bronchial obstruction and therefore present with signs of lobar or segmental collapse or consolidation. In general, apart from lipomas, none of these tumours have features that allow a confident diagnosis based upon imaging alone.

MRI IN TUMOURS OF THE LUNG

Jeremy P. R. Jenkins

CT is an established technique in the staging of lung carcinoma, with MRI currently used in a problem-solving role. Both CT and MRI are equally good at assessing tumour size. CT is more accurate in the demonstration of small nodules, except for those located

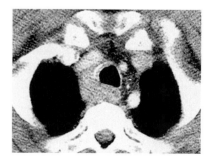

Fig. 4.40   Adenoid cystic carcinoma of trachea. CT scan shows tumour arising in right posterolateral wall of trachea and infiltrating the adjacent mediastinal tissues.

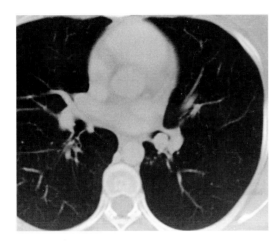

Fig. 4.41 Bronchial carcinoid. CT shows soft-tissue tumour in wall of left main bronchus, causing severe narrowing of the bronchial lumen.

close to hilar vessels, where MRI has the advantage. MRI has been shown to be more accurate than CT in evaluating mediastinal and vascular tumour invasion, and in the demonstration of apical (superior sulcus) tumours. MR images of the lungs have a low signal-to-noise ratio (SNR). Contrast between tumour and lung is essentially independent of pulse sequence, due to the inherently low proton density and magnetic susceptibility between air and soft tissue with aerated lung. Contrast and detail can be improved by enhancement of the mass with gadolinium-chelate. A major disadvantage of MRI compared with CT is that peripheral pulmonary vessels and lobar fissures are not visualised, making it difficult to demonstrate the position of a lung mass with respect to a lobe or segment.

Superior sulcus tumours can be better visualised by MRI than by CT, due to improved anatomical display on coronal and sagittal plane images (Figs 4.45, 4.46), aiding radiation treatment planning. In a study of 31 patients with a superior sulcus tumour, the accuracy of MRI in the evaluation of tumour invasion of adjacent structures was 94%, compared with 63% by CT. T_1-weighted images showed the tumour as intermediate signal in contrast with the high signal from surrounding fat, enabling better delineation of chest wall invasion, adjacent vessels, brachial plexus and spinal structures. If motion artefacts obscure detail then the combination of gadolinium-chelate injection with a T_1-weighted fat-suppressed sequence can be helpful in demonstrating the extent of the tumour. The use of this technique aids the delineation of tumour extension into the spinal canal by more clearly separating tumour from CSF compared with T_2-weighted images.

In a small series of patients with proximal lung carcinoma and distal lobar collapse, evaluated by dynamic contrast-enhanced CT and MRI, CT was more successful than MRI in differentiating tumour mass from collapsed lung (Fig. 4.47). Dynamic contrast-enhanced CT was able to differentiate tumour from collapsed lung in eight of 10 patients, whereas MRI demonstrated signal intensity differences in only half those patients. It should be noted that in two patients in whom differentiation between tumour and collapsed lung was not achieved by contrast-enhanced CT, MRI showed separation, suggesting a possible complementary role for the techniques. T_2-weighted sequences were most useful in demonstrating a higher signal (longer T_2) from the collapsed lung than from the tumour. It is likely that the use of gadolinium-chelate would improve the accuracy of MRI. MRI can identify any underlying mass lesions in a completely opacified hemithorax.

The *normal pleural space* cannot be resolved by MRI but adjacent *fat* is well shown. Early *chest wall invasion* by tumour is better demonstrated on MRI than CT. T_1-weighted images provide good morphological detail and contrast discrimination between tumour (intermediate signal) and fat (high signal). The presence of a high signal within chest wall muscle on T_2-weighted images suggests more extensive invasion. The changes however are non-specific. Similar increased signal intensity can occur with inflammatory disease. *Rib destruction* is not well shown on MRI. Although cortical bone is better shown by CT, the extension of tumour into the marrow space is better identified on MRI (Fig. 4.48). CT and MRI are unreliable in demonstrating mediastinal pleural infiltration, although the better contrast resolution of MRI has the greater

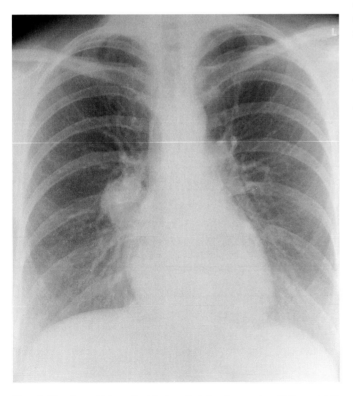

Fig. 4.42 Bronchial carcinoid. A well-defined, round, soft-tissue mass overlies the right hilum.

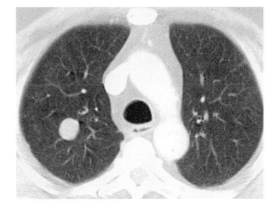

Fig. 4.43 Pulmonary hamartoma. CT scan shows a well-circumscribed right upper lobe soft-tissue-density mass.

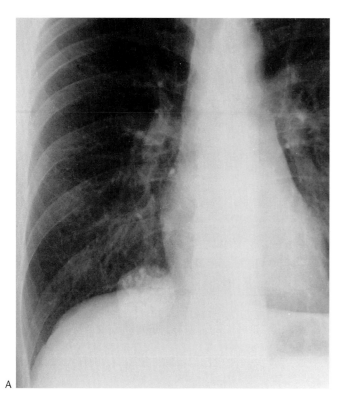
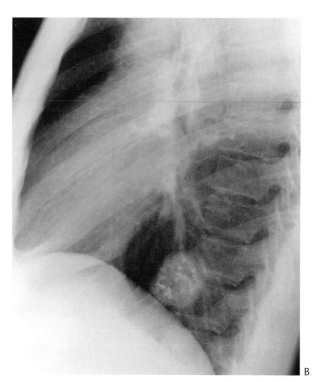

Fig. 4.44   Pulmonary hamartoma. (A, B) A well-defined, round soft-tissue mass with extensive, central 'popcorn' calcification is present in the right lower lobe.

potential. Microscopic invasion of the mediastinum by tumour without bulk change cannot be detected. Invasion can be assumed if interdigitation of tumour into the mediastinum or chest wall is present. The differentiation of pleural thickening can be further aided by the use of gadolinium-chelate injection. Interruption of the normal low signal intensity line of the pericardium, which is less than 2 mm thick and best delineated on coronal and transverse ECG-gated T_1-weighted images, suggests *pericardial invasion.*

Similarly, interruption of the low intensity line of the diaphragm adjacent to a mass, on sagittal and coronal images, suggests infiltration (Fig. 4.49). *Lymph node* assessment is discussed elsewhere (see Ch. 2). Vascular invasion by tumour is more clearly demonstrated by MRI than by CT while CT is more sensitive in the detection of pleural effusions. On MRI, effusions are more clearly shown on T_2- or proton-density-weighted images as a high signal, compared with a low signal on T_1-weighted scans. MRI is helpful in differentiating pleural from parenchymal disease and has the potential to elucidate complex effusions. It is complementary to CT in the evaluation of pleural abnormalities, and can be used for the further assessment of focal non-calcified pleural lesions for which the level of confidence of CT in offering a diagnosis is low. In these cases signal iso- or hypo-intensity (with respect to intercostal muscle) on T_2-weighted scans from the focal pleural lesion is a reliable predictor of benign (fibrotic) pleural disease. Lymphangitis carcinomatosa has the distinctive appearance of a hilar or mediastinal mass with peripherally dilated pulmonary lymphatics.

In the evaluation of distant metastases from carcinoma of the lung, MRI has the potential for characterising some adrenal masses. On T_2-weighted images adrenal metastases have a high signal intensity, whereas benign non-functioning adenomas give a low signal similar to surrounding liver. There is, however, some overlap, which limits its clinical value. MRI combined with contrast administration is a more sensitive technique than CT in the detection of CNS and liver metastases.

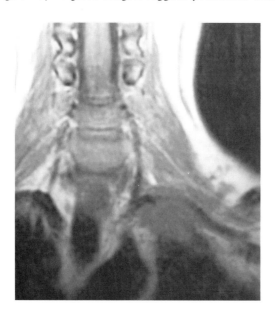

Fig. 4.45   Pancoast tumour infiltrating the left brachial plexus and subclavian artery on a coronal T_1-weighted spin-echo image.

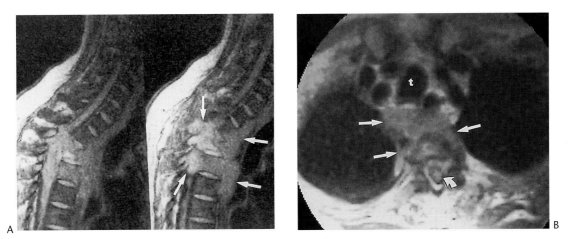

Fig. 4.46 Posterior mediastinal carcinoma (straight arrows) infiltrating two adjacent thoracic vertebral bodies with partial collapse and extradural extension, on T$_1$-weighted sagittal (A) (spin-echo 740/40) and transverse (B) (partial saturation recovery 500/18) scans. Note low signal from dural sac (curved arrow); t = trachea.

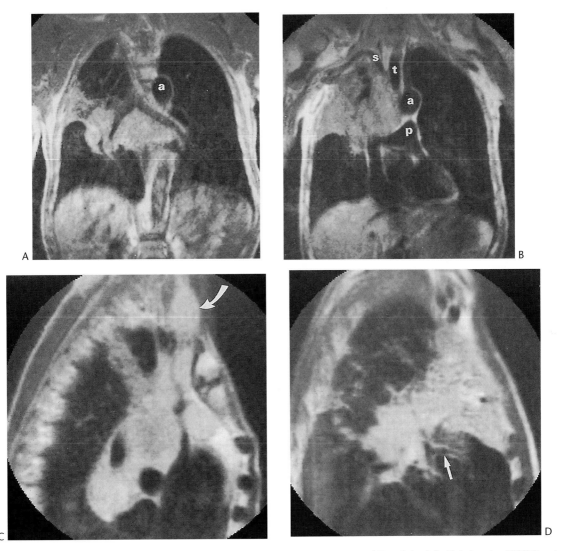

Fig 4.47 Carcinoma of the lung with lymphadenopathy and distal collapse/consolidation on coronal T$_1$-weighted (A, B) (spin-echo 560/26) and parasagittal intermediate-weighted (C,D) (spin-echo 1200/60) images. The collapse/consolidation in the anterior and posterior segments of the right upper lobe shows heterogeneity and higher signal than the more uniform intensity of the central tumour, but clear separation is difficult. Nodal disease in the neck (curved arrow) is demonstrated in (C). Straight arrow in D = middle lobe bronchus; a = aortic arch; p = left pulmonary artery; s = subclavian artery; t = trachea.

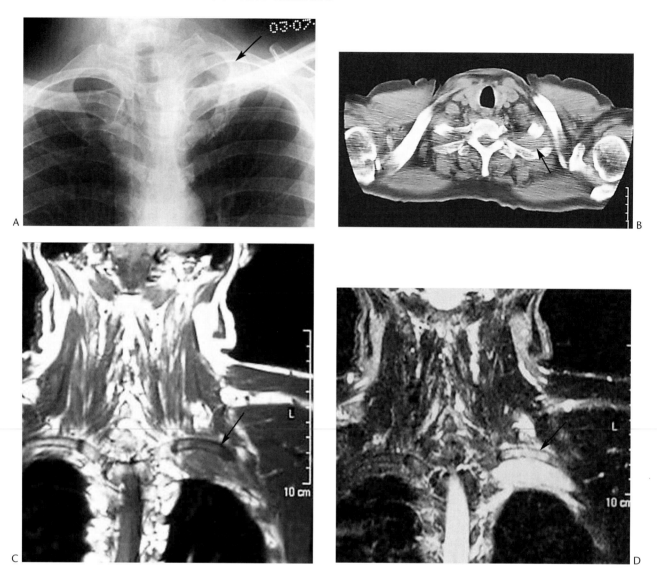

Fig. 4.48 Indeterminate soft-tissue pleural mass (arrow) in the left apex without evidence of any rib destruction on frontal chest radiograph (A) and CT examination (B). MR examination with coronal T_1-weighted (C) and T_2-weighted (D) spin-echo images shows low and high signal from the pleural mass together with marrow oedema within the adjacent first rib (arrow) confirming this to be a Pancoast tumour, which was subsequently confirmed on biopsy.

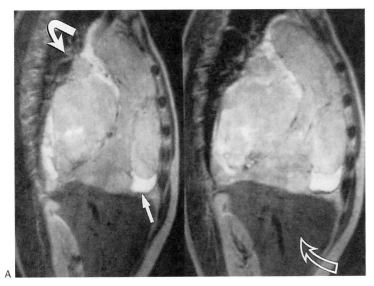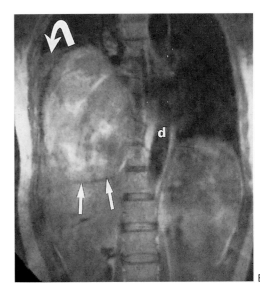

Fig. 4.49 Large pleural fibrosarcoma compressing lung (curved closed arrow) and displacing liver (curved open arrow) on two contiguous sagittal T_2-weighted (A) (spin-echo 1660/80) and a coronal T_1-weighted (B) (spin-echo 560/26) images. The liver is not directly infiltrated and neither is the anterior chest wall. The diaphragm can be seen as a low-intensity line (straight arrows), most clearly beneath a small anterior pleural effusion in (A) d = descending aorta. (Reproduced with permission from: Jenkins, J.P.R. (1990) Magnetic resonance imaging in oncology. In: Johnson, R. J., Eddleston, B., Hunter, R. D. (eds) *Radiology in the Management of Cancer.* Edinburgh: Churchill Livingstone.)

REFERENCES AND SUGGESTIONS FOR FURTHER READING

Adler, B., Padley, S., Miller, R., et al (1992) High-resolution CT of bronchoalveolar carcinoma. *American Journal of Roentgenology*, **159**, 275–277.

Altman, R. L., Miller, W. E., Carr, D. T., et al (1973) Radiographic appearances of bronchial carcinoid. *Thorax*, **28**, 433–434.

Armstrong, P. (2000) Neoplasms of the lungs, airways and pleura. In: Armstrong, P., et al (eds) *Imaging Diseases of the Chest*, pp. 305–465, St. Louis, Mosby Yearbook.

Arnold, A. M., Williams, C. J. (1979) Small cell lung cancer: a curable disease? *British Journal of Diseases of the Chest*, **73**, 327–348.

Aronchick, J. M., Wexler, J. A., Christen, B., et al (1986) Computed tomography of bronchial carcinoid. *Journal of Computer Assisted Tomography*, **10**, 71–74.

Au, V., Leung, A. N. (1997) Radiologic manifestations of lymphoma in the thorax. *American Journal of Roentgenology*, **168**, 93–98.

Balikian, J. P., Herman, P. G. (1979) Non-Hodgkin's lymphoma of the lungs. *Radiology*, **132**, 569–576.

Bateson, E. M. (1965) An analysis of 155 solitary lung lesions illustrating the differential diagnosis of mixed tumours of the lung. *Clinical Radiology*, **16**, 51–59.

Batra, P., Brown, K., Collins, J. D., et al (1988) Evaluation of intrathoracic extent of lung cancer by plain chest radiography, computed tomography and magnetic resonance imaging. *American Review of Respiratory Diseases*, **137**, 1456–1462.

Blank, N., Castellino, R. A. (1987) The mediastinum in Hodgkin's and non-Hodgkin's lymphomas. *Journal of Thoracic Imaging*, **2** (1), 66–71.

Bower, S. L., Choplin, R. H., Muss, H. B. (1983) Multiple primary carcinomas of the lung. *American Journal of Roentgenology*, **140**, 253–258.

Bragg, D. G. (1978) The clinical, pathological and radiographic spectrum of the intrathoracic lymphomas. *Investigative Radiology*, **13**, 2–11.

Bragg, D. G. (1987) Radiology of the lymphomas. *Current Problems in Diagnostic Radiology*, **16**, 183–206.

Bragg, D. G., Colby, T. V., Ward, J. H. (1986) New concepts in the non-Hodgkin lymphomas: radiologic implications. *Radiology*, **159**, 291–304.

Buy, J. N., Ghossain, M. A., Poirson, F. (1988) Computed tomography of mediastinal lymph nodes in non-small cell lung cancer: a new approach based on the lymphatic pathway of tumour spread. *Journal of Computer Assisted Tomography*, **12**, 545–552.

Cabanillas, F., Fuller, L. M. (1990) The radiological assessment of the lymphoma patient from the standpoint of the clinician. *Radiologic Clinics of North America*, **28**, 683–695.

Castellino, R. A. (1986) Hodgkin disease: practical concepts for the diagnostic radiologist. *Radiology*, **159**, 305–310.

Castellino, R. A. (1991) The non-Hodgkin's lymphomas: practical concepts for the diagnostic radiologist. *Radiology*, **178**, 315–321.

Chiles, C., Ravin, C. E. (1985) Intrathoracic metastases from an extrathoracic malignancy; radiographic approach to patient evaluation. *Radiologic Clinics of North America*, **23**, 427–438.

Cho, S. R., Henry, D. A., Beachley, M. C., Brooks, J. W. (1981) Round (helical) atelectasis. *British Journal of Radiology*, **54**, 643–650.

Choplin, R. H., Rawamoto, E. H., Dyer, R. B., et al (1986) Atypical carcinoid of the lung: radiographic features. *American Journal of Roentgenology*, **146**, 665–668.

Coppage, L., Shaw, C., Curtis, A. M. (1987) Metastatic disease to the chest in patients with extrathoracic malignancy. *Journal of Thoracic Imaging*, **2**(4): 24–37.

Corrin, B., Liebow, A. A., Friedman, P. J. (1975) Pulmonary lymphangiomyomatosis. *American Journal of Pathology*, **79**, 348–383.

Daly, B. D. T., Faling, L. J., Gunars Bite, P. A. C. (1987) Mediastinal lymph node evaluation by computed tomography in lung cancer: an analysis of 345 patients grouped by TNM staging, tumor size and tumor location. *Journal of Thoracic and Cardiovascular Surgery*, **94**, 644–672.

Davis, S. D., Zirn, J. R., Govoni, A. F. (1990) Peripheral carcinoid tumor of the lung: CT diagnosis. *American Journal of Roentgenology*, **155**, 1185–1187.

Dee, P. M., Arora, N. S., Innes, D. I. (1982) The pulmonary manifestations of lymphomatoid granulomatosis. *Radiology*, **143**, 613–618.

Epstein, D. M. (1990) Bronchioloalveolar carcinoma. *Seminars in Roentgenology*, **25**, 105–111.

Falaschi, F., Battolla, L., Mascalchi, M., et al (1996) Usefulness of MR signal intensity in distinguishing benign from malignant pleural disease. *American Journal of Roentgenology*, **166**, 963–968.

Feigin, D. S., Siegelman, S. S., Theros, E. G., et al (1977) Non-malignant lymphoid disorders of the chest. *American Journal of Roentgenology*, **129**, 221–228.

Forster, B. B., Müller, N. L., Miller, R. R., et al (1989) Neuroendocrine carcinomas of the lung: clinical, radiologic and pathologic correlation. *Radiology*, **170**, 441–445.

Gefter, W. B. (1990) Magnetic resonance imaging in the evaluation of lung cancer. *Seminars in Roentgenology*, **25**, 73–84.

Gibson, M., Hansell, D. M. (1998) Lymphocytic disorders of the chest: pathology and imaging. *Clinical Radiology*, **53**, 469–480

Heath, D., Reid, R. (1985) Invasive pulmonary haemangiomatosis. *British Journal of Diseases of the Chest*, **79**, 284–294.

Heelan, R. T., Demas, B. E., Caravelli, J. F., et al (1989) Superior sulcus tumors: CT and MR imaging. *Radiology*, **170**, 637–641.

Heitzman, E. R., Markarian, B., DeLise, C. T. (1975) Lymphoproliferative disorders of the thorax. *Seminars in Roentgenology*, **10**, 73–81.

Henschke, C. I., Davis, S. D., Romano, P. M., Yankelevitz, D. F. (1989) The pathogenesis, radiologic evaluation, and therapy of pleural effusions. *Radiologic Clinics of North America*, **27**, 1241–1255.

Herbert, A., Wright, D. H., Isaacson, P. G., Smith, J. L. (1984) Primary malignant lymphoma of the lung: histopathologic and immunologic evaluation of nine cases. *Human Pathology*, **15**, 415–422.

King, L. J., Padley, S. P., Nicholson, A. G. (1998) Primary pulmonary lymphoma of MALT origin: imaging findings in 22 patients. *Radiology*, **209**(P), 376.

Lahde, S., Paivansalo, M., Rainio, P. (1991) CT for predicting the resectability of lung cancer: a prospective study. *Acta Radiologica*, **32**, 449–454.

Lewis, E. R., Caskey, C. I., Fishman, E. K. (1991) Lymphoma of the lung: CT findings in 31 patients. *American Journal of Roentgenology*, **156**, 711–714.

Libshitz, H. I. (1989) Imaging and staging of lung cancer. *Current Opinion in Radiology*, **1**, 21–24.

Libshitz, H. I. (1990) Computed tomography in bronchogenic carcinoma. *Seminars in Roentgenology*, **25**, 64–72.

Lillington, G. A., Stevens, G. M. (1976) The solitary nodule. The other side of the coin. *Chest*, **70**, 322–323.

McLoud, T. C., Bourgouin, P. M., Greenberg, R. W., et al (1992) Bronchogenic carcinoma: analysis of staging in the mediastinum with CT by correlative lymph node mapping and sampling. *Radiology*, **182**, 319–323.

Madewell, J. E., Feigin, D. S. (1977) Benign tumours of the lung. *Seminars in Roentgenology*, **12**, 175–186.

Maile, C. W., Moore, A. V., Ulreich, S., et al (1983) Chest radiographic–pathologic correlation in adult leukemia patients. *Investigative Radiology*, **18**, 495–499.

Mayo, J. R. (1994) Magnetic resonance imaging of the chest: where we stand. *Radiologic Clinics of North America*, **32**, 795–809.

Mountain, C. F. (1986) A new international staging system for lung cancer. *Chest*, **89** (Suppl), 225S–233S.

Mountain, C. F. (1997) Revisions in the international system for staging lung cancer. *Chest*, **111**, 1710–1717.

Müller, N. L., Miller, R. R. (1990) Neuroendocrine carcinomas of the lung. *Seminars in Roentgenology*, **25**, 96–104.

Munk, P. L., Müller, N. L., Miller, R. R., et al (1988) Pulmonary lymphangitic carcinomatosis: CT and pathologic findings. *Radiology*, **166**, 705–709.

Naidich, D. P. (1990) CT/MR correlation in the evaluation of tracheobronchial neoplasia. *Radiologic Clinics of North America*, **28**, 555–571.

Nessi, R., Ricci, P. B., Ricci, S. B., et al (1991) Bronchial carcinoid tumors: radiologic observations in 49 cases. *Journal of Thoracic Imaging*, **6**(2), 47–53.

North, L. B., Libshitz, H. I., Lorigan, J. G. (1990) Thoracic lymphoma. *Radiologic Clinics of North America*, **28**, 745–762.

Padovani, B., Mouroux, J., Seksik, L., et al (1993) Chest wall invasion by bronchogenic carcinoma: evaluation with MR imaging. *Radiology*, **187**, 33–38.

Pancoast, H. K. (1932) Superior sulcus tumor: tumor characterized by pain, Horner's syndrome, destruction of bone and atrophy of hand muscles. *Journal of the American Medical Association*, **99**, 1391–1396.

Patz, E. F., Goodman, P. C. (1994) Positron emission tomography imaging of the thorax. *Radiologic Clinics of North America*, **32**, 811–823.

Ray, J. F., Lawton, B. R., Magnin, G. E., et al (1976) The coin lesion story: update 1976. *Chest*, **70**, 332–336.

Rigler, L. G. (1955) The roentgen signs of carcinoma of the lung. *American Journal of Roentgenology*, **74**, 415–428.

Romney, B. M., Austin, J. H. M. (1990) Plain film evaluation of carcinoma of the lung. *Seminars in Roentgenology*, **25**, 45–63.

Schiepers, C. (1999) Positron emission tomography: a new tool in diagnosing, staging and treatment monitoring of lung cancer. In: Van Houtte, P., Klatersky, J., Rocmans, P. (eds) *Progress and Perspective in the Treatment of Lung Cancer*, pp. 39–46. Berlin: Springer.

Siegelman, S. S., Khouri, N. F., Scott, W. W., et al (1986) Pulmonary hamartoma: CT findings. *Radiology*, **160**, 313–317.

Templeton, P. A., Zerhouni, E. A. (1990) MR imaging in the management of thoracic malignancies. *Radiologic Clinics of North America*, **27**, 1099–1111.

Templeton, P. A., Caskey, C. I., Zerhouni, E. A. (1990) Current uses of CT and MR imaging in the staging of lung cancer. *Radiologic Clinics of North America*, **28**: 631–646.

Various authors (1977) Pulmonary neoplasms. *Seminars in Roentgenology*, **12**, 161–246.

Webb, W. R., Gatsonis, C., Zerhouni, E. A., et al (1991) CT and MR imaging in staging non-small cell bronchogenic carcinoma: report of the Radiologic Diagnostic Oncologic Group. *Radiology*, **178**, 705–713.

Woodring, J. H. (1990) Unusual radiographic manifestations of lung cancer. *Radiologic Clinics of North America*, **28**, 599–618.

MRI

Armstrong, P. (2000) Neoplasms of the lung, airways and pleura. In: Armstrong, P., Wilson, A. G., Dee, P., Hansell, D. M. (eds) *Imaging of Diseases of the Chest,* 3rd edn, ch. 7, pp. 305–465. St. Louis, Mosby–Year Book

Husband, J. E. S., Resnek, R. (eds) (1998) *Imaging in Oncology*. Oxford: ISIS Medical Media.

Lesko, N. M., Link, K. M. (1999) Mediastinum and lung. In: Stark, D. D., Bradley, W. G. (eds) *Magnetic Resonance Imaging*, 3rd edn, ch. 18, pp. 355–371. St Louis: CV Mosby.

Naidich, D. P., Webb, R., Mueller, N. L., Krinsky, G. A., Zerhouni, E. A., Siegelman, S. S. (eds) (2000) *Computed Tomography and Magnetic Resonance of the Thorax*, 3rd edn. New York: Lippincott/Williams & Wilkins.

Thompson, B. H., Stanford, W. (2000) MR imaging of pulmonary and mediastinal malignancies. *MRI Clinics of North America*, **8**, 729–739.

White, C. S. (e.) (2000) MR imaging of the thorax. *MRI Clinics of North America*, **8**, 1–224.

5

PULMONARY INFECTIONS

Simon P. G. Padley and Michael B. Rubens

Inflammatory disease of the lung may be referred to as either pneumonia or pneumonitis. Although these terms are interchangeable, *pneumonia* usually implies an infection by pathogenic organisms resulting in consolidation of lung, whereas *pneumonitis* tends to refer to those inflammatory processes that primarily involve the alveolar wall, for example fibrosing alveolitis in the UK or usual interstitial pneumonia (UIP) in the USA. Pneumonias may be classified on the basis of morphology or aetiology.

ACUTE PNEUMONIA

A causative organism is only likely to be found in 50% of cases, usually because of prior treatment with antibiotics or an inability to provide a satisfactory sputum specimen. Of these organisms there will be approximately a third each of bacterial, non-bacterial and viral. Of the bacterial causes the *pneumococcus* (*Streptococcus pneumoniae*) is most common, with much smaller numbers of *Staphylococcus aureus*, *Haemophilus influenzae*, *Klebsiella pneumoniae* and *Legionella pneumophila*.

Of the non-bacterial causes *Mycoplasma pneumoniae* is most common. In fact, it is the most common proven cause of primary pneumonia in the UK at the present time. Other non-bacterial causes found in small numbers are *Chlamydia psittaci* (psittacosis) and *Coxiella burnetii* (Q fever). The viruses are almost all *influenza* and *cold viruses*. Mixed infections are found in approximately 10% of cases.

Lobar pneumonia commences as a localised infection of terminal air spaces. Inflammatory oedema spreads to adjacent lung via the terminal airways and pores of Kohn, and causes uniform consolidation of all or part of a lobe.

In lobar pneumonia the usual homogeneous lung opacification is limited by fissures and affected lobes retain normal volume and often show air bronchograms. The onset may be so acute that opacification is often at its maximum on the initial radiograph. However, consolidation may not be obvious on the initial radiograph. *Streptococcus pneumoniae* classically causes lobar pneumonia. The classical appearance of lobar pneumonia is increasingly uncommon, partly because early antibiotic treatment aborts the progression of disease. Consolidation may not spread uniformly throughout the lobe. From the initial focus of infection inflammatory oedema spreads via the air passages and the pores of Kohn, and as a result consolidation may conform to segmental boundaries.

Occasionally rounded lesions with ill-defined margins appear, especially in children, producing a so-called 'round pneumonia'. Kerley B lines may appear in the affected area from a temporary overloading of lymphatics and oedema of interlobular septa. The distribution of the inflammatory exudate can be influenced to some degree by the effect of gravity, best seen in the immobile patient. Resolution is accompanied by diminution of the density of the opacity as air returns to the lobe, and it is usually complete, with the lung architecture being restored to normal.

Bronchopneumonia is a multifocal process which commences in the terminal and respiratory bronchioles and tends to spread segmentally. It may also be called lobular pneumonia, and produces patchy consolidation. The commonest causes are *S. aureus* and Gram-negative organisms.

In clinical practice the most useful classification is according to the causative organism, as this is what influences the management and outcome of the infection. Unfortunately, it is not possible to diagnose the organism from radiology alone. However, radiology is important in confirming the presence and location of pneumonia, as well as following its course. Moreover, the chest radiograph may indicate complications of a pneumonia such as pleural effusion, empyema, pneumothorax, atelectasis, abscess formation and scarring.

BACTERIAL PNEUMONIAS

Streptococcus pneumoniae

This is a common cause of pneumonia in all age groups, and particularly in young adults. Typically it produces lobar consolidation (Fig. 5.1), which is often basal but may occur anywhere in the lung. The volume of the consolidated lung is normal, and an air bronchogram may be visible. Occasionally oedema of the interlobular septa causes septal lines. Pleural effusion, empyema and cavitation are unusual if the infection is treated promptly, but may be seen in debilitated patients. Resolution is usually complete.

Staphylococcus aureus

This is a common cause of pneumonia in debilitated patients. It may also cause superinfection in influenza (Fig. 5.2). Haematogenous infection of the lungs may occur in septicaemia, and is a common complication of intravenous drug abuse; when dissemination is haematogenous the typical appearance is of multiple poorly

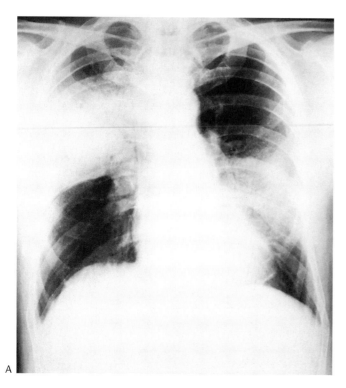
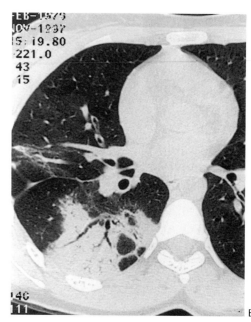

Fig. 5.1 (A) Pneumococcal pneumonia. Lingular and right upper lobe consolidation with sparing of the apex. (B) CT image from a different patient demonstrating air bronchograms in an area of peripheral consolidation due to an organising pneumonia.

defined rounded nodules that develop rapidly over a few days (Fig. 5.3). Usually cavitation is evident, especially on later examinations. When pneumonia occurs as a complication of intravenous drug abuse echocardiography should be undertaken since in most of these patients the source of septic emboli is an infective endocarditis on the tricuspid valve.

Infection may also be the result of inhalation, typically causing a bronchopneumonia with multiple, patchy areas of consolidation (Fig. 5.4). Confluence of these areas may develop. Again cavitation is common, and in children pneumatoceles may develop. Pleural effusion, empyema and areas of atelectasis are common complications.

Klebsiella pneumonia

This is due to *Friedländer's bacillus* and typically occurs in elderly debilitated men. There is usually lobar consolidation (Fig. 5.5), more often right sided, and frequently upper lobe. The volume of the affected lung is maintained, or may be increased causing bulging of the fissures. Cavitation is common (Fig. 5.6) and if there is healing with fibrosis then cavities may become permanent and mimic TB. A bronchopneumonic pattern may also occur (Fig. 5.7).

Legionnaire's disease

In 1976 an explosive epidemic of severe respiratory illness occurred at an American Legionnaires' convention in Philadelphia. It was a rapidly extending pneumonia complicated by shock, mental confusion, respiratory and renal failure, unresponsive to the usual antibiotics, with a case fatality of 16%. A previously unknown Gram-negative bacillus was eventually isolated and given the name *Legionella pneumophila*. The organism is ubiquitous in water, multiplying in water coolers, air conditioners and showers, and infec-

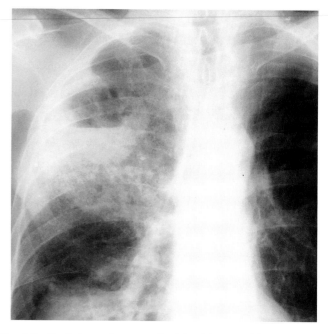

Fig. 5.2 Staphylococcal pneumonia of the right upper lobe with abscess formation.

tion takes place from inhalation of an aerosol mist. It is prone to attack smokers and the debilitated. Radiographically there is spreading consolidation, and although it may be confined to one lobe initially it soon extends to others and to the opposite lung (Fig. 5.8). Another characteristic feature is the slow resolution over several weeks, but this is usually complete. Small *pleural effusions* are common; abscess and pneumatocele formation are rare.

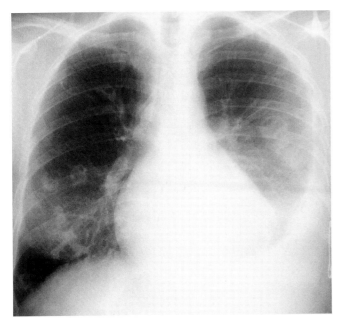

A

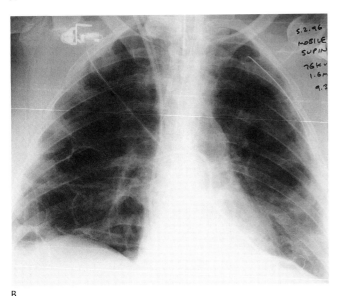

B

Fig. 5.3 (A) Haematogenous staphylococcal abscess formation in an intravenous drug abuser. There are multiple thin-walled cavities and an associated left pleural effusion. (B) Multiple large thin-walled pneumatoceles in a different intravenous drug abuser with staphylococcal tricuspid endocarditis.

Haemophilus influenzae

This is a commensal of the upper respiratory tract, but as it is sometimes found in large numbers in the sputum in association with chronic lung diseases and treatment aimed at its eradication is often followed by clinical improvement, it is accorded a potentially pathogenic role. It is a secondary invader found in chronic bronchitis, cystic fibrosis and debilitated states. It is also found in influenza and other virus infections. Any pulmonary opacities found in *Haemophilus* infection are disseminated and bronchopneumonic; there are no characteristic radiographic appearances (Fig. 5.9).

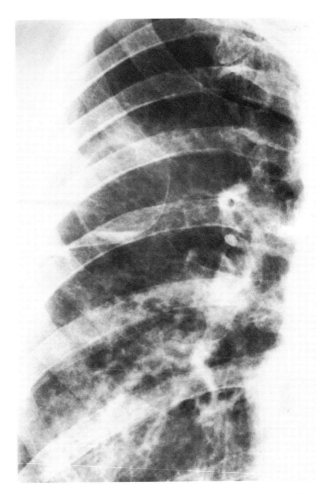

Fig. 5.4 Staphylococcal bronchopneumonia. A pneumatocele has developed in the right upper lobe. The radiograph eventually returned to normal.

OTHER GRAM-NEGATIVE PNEUMONIAS

Pseudomonas aeruginosa and Escherichia coli

These are two of the many Gram-negative organisms which normally inhabit the upper respiratory tract and gastrointestinal tract and may cause pneumonia or other infections in debilitated and hospitalised patients. Pneumonia in these patients is more likely to occur due to a number of factors. Normal commensals may be replaced by pathogens of increased virulence. This is often coupled with decreased clearance of upper pharyngeal secretions due to sedation or drowsiness, or endotracheal or nasogastric intubation. Infections also tend to occur following major surgery and in patients who have received long-term broad-spectrum antibiotics. Thus they are particularly prone to colonise patients on long-term mechanical ventilation. Pneumonia normally results from inhalation, but may also be haematogenous in origin. The radiographic appearances are of a bronchopneumonia which is often basal. Gram-negative organisms are also likely to be pathogenic in patients with chronic lung disease such as cystic fibrosis, as well as in patients who are immunosuppressed or have diabetes.

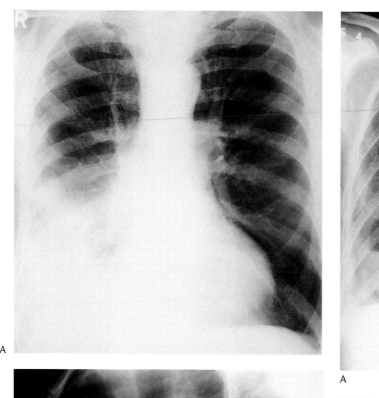

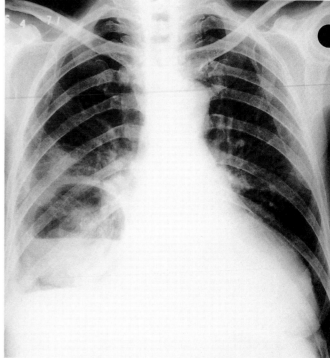

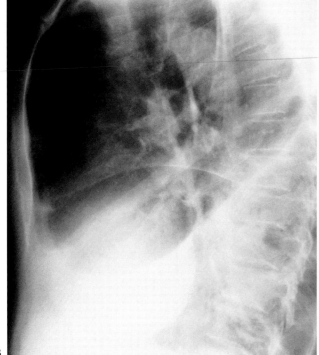

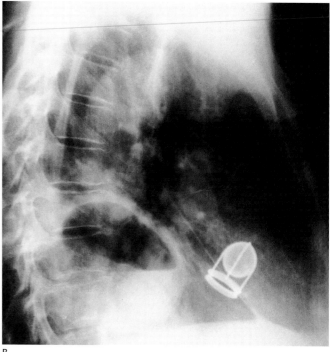

Fig. 5.5 (A, B) *Klebsiella* pneumonia. There is consolidation in the right lower lobe with associated loss of volume evident on the lateral view.

Melioidosis

Melioidosis, a disease of tropical countries of the East, is caused by *Pseudomonas pseudomallei*. It may manifest years after the patient has left an endemic area. There are two pulmonary forms: a septicaemic disseminate infection with necrotising lesions, and a chronic apical pneumonia which breaks down to form a thin-walled cavity.

Fig. 5.6 (A, B) *Klebsiella* pneumonia. There is a large cavity in the right lower lobe following cavitation of pneumonic consolidation. An aortic valve replacement is present.

Tularaemia

Discovered in Tulare, California, infection with *Francisella tularensis* is endemic amongst small mammals and is spread by ticks. Humans acquire the infection either by inoculation or inhalation. Remarkably

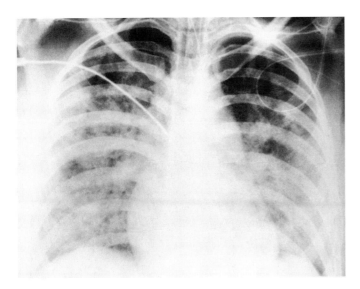

Fig. 5.7 *Klebsiella* septicaemia. There is diffuse patchy alveolar shadowing with air bronchograms.

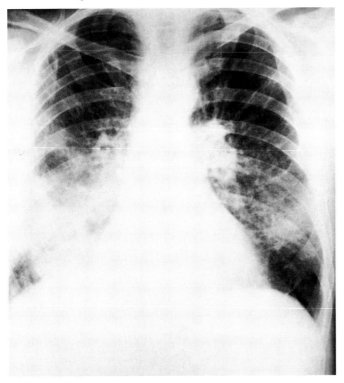

Fig. 5.8 Legionnaire's disease. There is bilateral consolidation, more marked on the right.

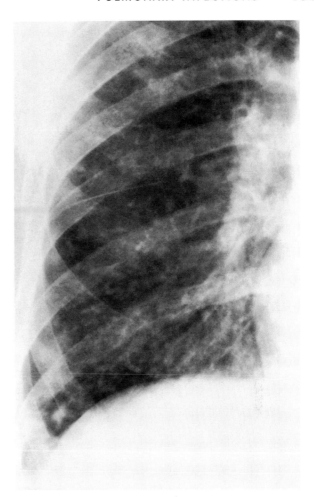

Fig. 5.9 *Haemophilus* infection. Widespread small nodular opacities are evident.

few organisms are required to cause illness. In the bacteraemic form there are small oval pulmonary lesions and hilar adenopathy (Fig. 5.10). Inhalation infection causes one or more areas of consolidation, also with hilar adenopathy. Untreated the consolidated lung cavitates and fibroses and may then mimic tuberculosis.

ATYPICAL PNEUMONIAS

This term was originally used to describe an acute febrile illness characterised by acute inflammatory changes centred within the alveolar walls and interstitium. 'Atypical' denotes the lack of the alveolar exudate evident in most pneumonic infections. Because of this feature the term interstitial pneumonia has been suggested as a preferred alternative. A variety of organisms may be responsible, the most important being *Mycoplasma pneumoniae*, but also including viruses, especially influenza viruses types A and B, respiratory syncytial virus and adenovirus, *Chlamydia psittaci* (psittacosis) and *Coxiella burnetti* (Q fever). The illness often manifests with systemic symptoms overshadowing those due to the pneumonia, and the course of disease may be less dramatic but more prolonged than with a typical pneumonia.

Mycoplasma pneumoniae

This is the only member of the mycoplasma group that is commonly pathogenic in man. Although classed as bacteria these organisms are unlike other common bacterial species, being smaller and lacking rigid cell walls containing peptidoglycan. As a result they are not susceptible to antibiotics that act on cell wall synthesis such as the penicillins. *Mycoplasma* is most frequently encountered in young adults and is the commonest isolate from primary pneumonias in the UK, accounting for 10–20% of cases, but only in a small proportion does it cause a major respiratory illness.

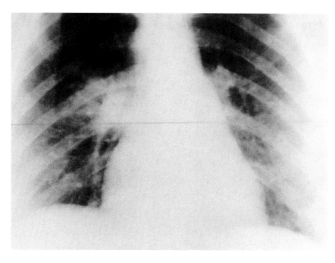

Fig. 5.10 Tularaemia. There is right hilar nodal involvement and perihilar consolidation.

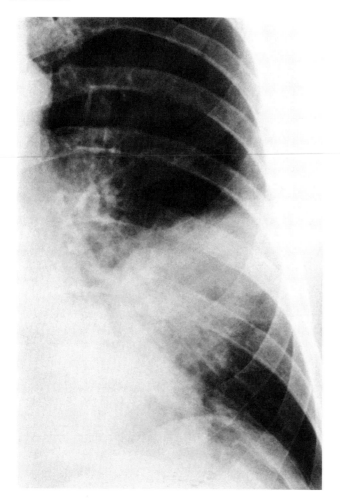

Fig. 5.11 Mycoplasma pneumonia. There is a patch of left mid zone consolidation obscuring the left heart border.

The earliest radiographic signs are fine reticular or nodular shadows followed by the appearance of consolidation, which may be segmental or lobar, and is usually unilateral (Fig. 5.11). Lymph node enlargement and pleural effusion are uncommon and cavitation is rare.

VIRAL PNEUMONIAS

Viral pneumonia usually commences in distal bronchi and bronchioles as an interstitial process with destruction of the epithelium, oedema and lymphocytic infiltration. There may also be focal inflammation of the terminal bronchioles and alveoli and progression to haemorrhagic pulmonary oedema.

The radiological appearances of a viral pneumonia are very varied, but often include:

1. Peribronchial shadowing (Fig. 5.12)
2. Reticulonodular shadowing (Fig. 5.13)
3. Patchy or extensive consolidation (Fig. 5.14).

Viral pneumonia is uncommon in adults, unless the patient is immunocompromised. Most pneumonias that complicate viral infections in adults are due to bacterial superinfection. However, viral pneumonias are not rare in infants and children.

Influenza virus

Pneumonia as a complication of influenza is normally due to secondary bacterial infection, often *Staphylococcus aureus*, *Streptococcus pneumoniae* or *Haemophilus*. However, the very young, the elderly and debilitated patients may develop a primary viral pneumonia with patchy consolidation. Occasionally, especially during influenza epidemics, a fulminating haemorrhagic pneumonia may be seen with widespread consolidation indistinguishable from non-cardiogenic pulmonary oedema or adult respiratory distress syndrome (Fig. 5.14). If the patient survives, extensive pulmonary fibrosis may develop.

Herpes varicella zoster

Varicella pneumonia occurs more often in adults than in children. In the acute phase of infection the chest radiograph may show widespread nodular shadows up to 1 cm in diameter, and clinically the pneumonia will be concurrent with the typical skin rash (Fig. 5.15). Following recovery a small proportion of these nodules calcify and, if multiple, may produce a characteristic radiographic appearance (Fig. 5.16). These patients are often able to give a history of severe chickenpox as an adult.

Measles giant cell pneumonia

In addition to the common secondary respiratory infections associated with measles, there is a specific pulmonary viral infection characterised by multinucleate giant cells with cytoplasmic inclusions in the respiratory epithelium. Although a disease of childhood, it has been recorded in adults. The mediastinal and hilar nodes are commonly enlarged but other radiographic abnormalities are variable and include streaky basal linear shadows, widespread reticular shadows and diffuse ill-defined nodular opacities (Fig. 5.17). Remarkably swift resolution can take place, over the course of a few days.

Infectious mononucleosis

Less than 10% of cases have intrathoracic manifestations during the disease. The commonest abnormality on the chest X-ray is lymph node enlargement, and the lungs may show an isolated opacity or reticulonodular shadows.

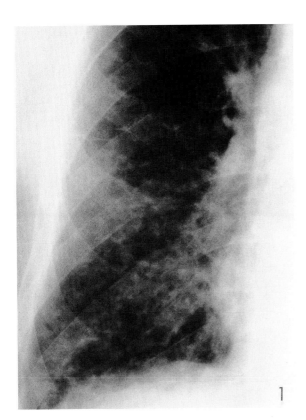

Fig. 5.12 Adenovirus chest infection. There is reticulonodular infiltrate, most marked in a bronchovascular distribution at the right base.

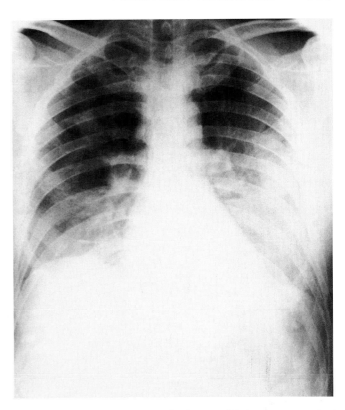

Fig. 5.14 Influenza A. Haemorrhagic consolidation was present at postmortem.

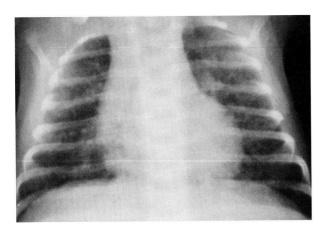

Fig. 5.13 CMV pneumonia in a $2\frac{1}{2}$-month-old child. There is reticular nodular shadowing throughout both lungs.

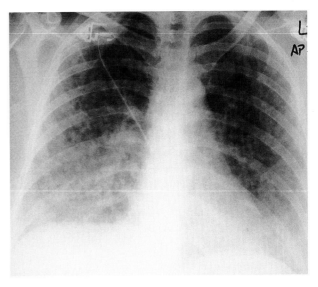

Fig. 5.15 Chickenpox pneumonia occurring during pregnancy. There is widespread, predominantly nodular shadowing throughout both lungs. The patient made a complete recovery.

CHLAMYDIAL AND RICKETTSIAL PNEUMONIAS

Psittacosis and ornithosis

Usually acquired by contact with sick parrots or domestic fowl, this infection is due to *Chlamydia psittaci*. The pneumonia usually presents as patchy or lobar consolidation, although nodular shadows may be seen. There is often hilar lymphadenopathy. The radiographic changes may take several weeks to resolve.

Q fever

This is usually acquired by contact with cattle or sheep and is due to *Coxiella burnetii*. The pneumonia typically presents as rounded areas of consolidation, up to 10 cm in diameter, in both lungs, lobar consolidation, or linear densities due to atelectasis. Lymph node enlargement is unusual. The radiographic changes may take a month or more to resolve, during which time the ill-defined opac-

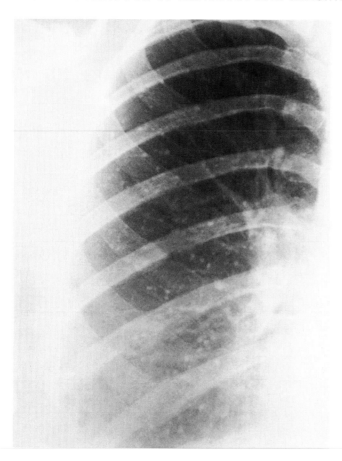

Fig. 5.16   Multiple calcified varicella scars.

ities become more sharply defined, smaller and denser. Rarely Q fever produces an endocarditis, meningoencephalitis or hepatitis.

Rocky Mountain spotted fever

This tick-borne disease is endemic to the southern USA as well as the Rocky Mountains. It may cause patchy consolidation, pleural effusions, and be complicated by secondary bacterial pneumonia. Overall there is a 5% mortality.

Scrub typhus

This rickettsial disease is endemic in the countries of the Pacific basin, and causes pulmonary abnormalities in approximately 10% of cases. The radiographic pattern is diverse and takes the form of interstitial, lobar or widespread pulmonary opacities. The latter presentation resembles adult respiratory distress syndrome both clinically and radiographically, but it clears rapidly with appropriate treatment.

LUNG ABSCESS

Suppuration and necrosis of pulmonary tissue may be due to tuberculosis, fungal infection, malignant tumour and infected cysts. However, the term lung abscess usually refers to a cavitating lesion secondary to infection by pyogenic bacteria. This is most frequently due to aspiration of infected material from the upper respiratory

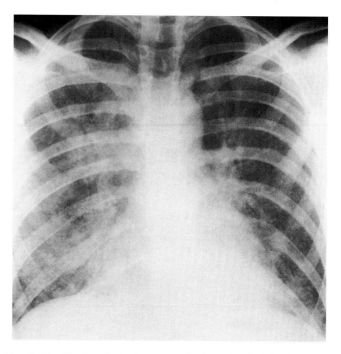

Fig. 5.17   Measles giant cell pneumonia. Extensive ill-defined opacities with air bronchograms. The changes are more marked on the right than the left.

tract, and is often associated with poor dentition and periodontal infection (Fig. 5.18). A variety of organisms may be responsible, and anaerobic bacteria are frequently found in the sputum. Occasionally there is a history of loss of consciousness and presumed aspiration. Other causes of lung abscess include staphylococcal (Fig. 5.19) and *Klebsiella* pneumonia, septic pulmonary emboli (Fig. 5.3) and trauma.

Radiographically an abscess may or may not be surrounded by consolidation. Appearance of an air–fluid level indicates that a communication with the airways has developed. The wall of the abscess may be thick at first, but with further necrosis and coughing up of infected material it becomes thinner (Fig. 5.18).

ASPIRATION AND INHALATION

The effects of aspiration of particulate or liquid foreign material into the lungs are twofold: those due to mechanical bronchial obstruction and those due to the irritant properties of the aspirate. When the cough reflex is suppressed by stupor, alcohol or drugs, aspiration of food from the stomach during vomiting is likely to occur. The inflammatory response excited by vegetable matter is intense and commonly followed by secondary infection with commensals and anaerobic organisms. Aspiration of infected material from nasal and oral sepsis is a common cause of lung abscess. The radiological patterns are therefore those of atelectasis or suppurative bronchitis and pneumonia. Metallic or inorganic particles may excite little response, the mechanical effects of uncomplicated atelectasis or obstructive emphysema predominating, and they may remain undetected for long periods.

Aspiration of mineral oils results in *lipoid pneumonia* (Fig. 5.20). The prolonged use of liquid paraffin for constipation is the usual cause and a precipitating factor is chronic oesophageal obstruction. The oil floats to the top of any residue in the oesophagus, the

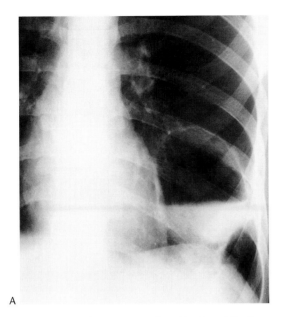
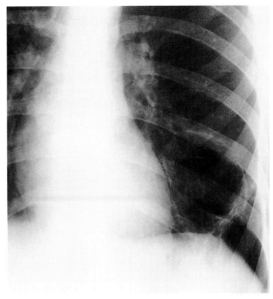

Fig. 5.18 (A) Lung abscess. There was poor dental hygiene. Mixed anaerobic growth. (B) Several weeks later a thin-walled pneumatocele remains.

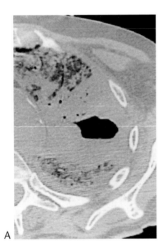

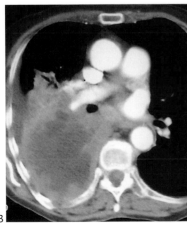

Fig. 5.19 (A) Staphylococcal abscess in a patient with adult respiratory distress syndrome. A cavity with a fluid level is present within a dense area of consolidation. (B) Lung abscess in a different patient developing in a large necrotic adenocarcinoma. Percutaneous aspiration revealed a mixed growth of *Haemophilus* and *Streptococcus*.

optimal position for aspiration. The oil is almost inert and the reaction is indolent, granulomatous and fibrotic; any lung damage is permanent. Radiographically there are dense well-defined tumour-like masses or an extensive bilateral opacity spreading outward from the hilar regions. Vegetable oils and animal fats such as milk induce a greater inflammatory response and the opacities are ill defined and bronchopneumonic. Influenced by gravity, the lesions of aspiration and inhalation are found predominantly in the posterior parts of the lungs. Small aspirates are common in the aged from incompetence of the closing mechanism of the larynx. These recurrent aspirations produce coarse peribronchial thickening, small patches of pneumonia and eventually fibrosis and bronchiectasis.

Mendelson's syndrome

This is a chemical pneumonia caused by aspiration of acid gastric contents during anaesthesia. An intense bronchospasm is rapidly followed by a flood of oedema throughout the lungs, resulting in hypoxia and requiring high ventilation pressures. The radiographic appearance of massive pulmonary oedema taken together with the clinical presentation is pathognomonic (Fig. 5.21).

In cases of *near drowning* the lungs show widespread, ill-defined alveolar opacities due to pulmonary oedema. The effects of salt water are less severe and of shorter duration than those due to hypotonic fresh water.

Inhalation of irritant gases

Inhalation of gases such as ammonia, chlorine and nitrogen dioxide produces an acute focal or diffuse pulmonary oedema followed by functional derangements indicative of bronchiolar and alveolar damage. It is a cause of *bronchiolitis obliterans*. Widespread tubular bronchiectasis and severe emphysema have been reported as sequels to accidental smoke inhalation.

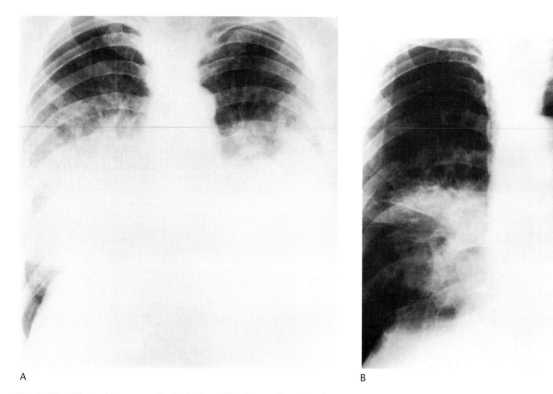

A   B

Fig. 5.20 (A) Lipoid pneumonia. Aspiration of liquid paraffin. (B) Eight years later there has been significant clearing but severe residual fibrosis is now present.

PULMONARY TUBERCULOSIS

Mycobacterium tuberculosis is responsible for most cases of tuberculosis; fewer than 5% of cases are caused by atypical mycobacteria. Infection from milk is now rare where pasteurised milk is available. Infection is usually by inhalation of organisms from open cases of the disease. Transmission is by droplet inhalation, and the dose of viable organisms received is critical. Children, the immunocompromised, especially HIV-positive patients, and some immigrant groups

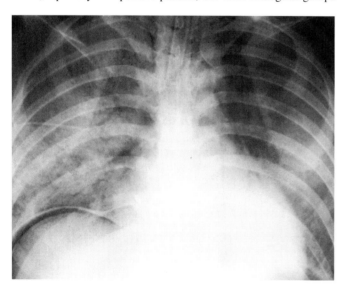

Fig. 5.21 Mendelson's syndrome. Postoperative aspiration of gastric contents. Note the subdiaphragmatic air following laparotomy.

are particularly susceptible. All these factors are reflected in the recommendations current in the UK concerning isolation of patients, treatment of contacts and general control measures. A chest radiograph is part of these control measures, and follow-up of contacts for 2 years may be judged necessary.

The occupational risk of hospital personnel is, in general, minimal and only a pre-employment chest radiograph is needed. Annual chest radiographs are not required. Those judged to be at higher risk should be offered an annual chest radiographic examination. Staff in any institution who will be in regular contact with children should have a chest radiograph as part of a pre-employment check, but routine periodic radiography is not necessary.

There are racial differences in the incidence of tuberculosis; in Britain it is 30 times more common in immigrants from the Indian subcontinent than in the indigenous population. Other factors that predispose to infection are old age, poor nutrition, alcoholism, silicosis, diabetes, pregnancy, malignant disease and immunosuppression, especially by HIV infection.

Previous infection or BCG vaccination render most patients hypersensitive to tuberculoprotein. Possession of such hypersensitivity influences the course of the disease, and it is traditional to classify tuberculosis as *primary*, if the patient is not sensitised, and *post-primary* if the patient is. Most cases of post-primary infection are due to reactivation of previous infected foci, often many years after first infection. Occasionally, a primary infection progresses to the post-primary phase without an intervening latent period.

Primary pulmonary tuberculosis

Most cases of primary pulmonary tuberculosis are subclinical, although there may be fever, respiratory symptoms or erythema nodosum. Organisms settle and multiply in an alveolus anywhere in the lungs, but most commonly in a subpleural site in the well-ventilated lower lobes. There is an area of peripheral consolidation (the Ghon focus), and spread from this along the draining lymphatics may lead to enlargement of regional lymph nodes. This combination is referred to as a primary complex. Subpleural infection may cause a serous effusion. Activation of the immune system usually leads to resolution, healing and fibrosis at this stage. Usually a fibrous capsule walls off the lesion and dystrophic calcification may occur. If the response to infection is weak the disease may progress and there is little difference between lesions of primary and post-primary evolution. This may manifest as further consolidation, possibly with cavitation, and bronchogenic spread of infection. Rupture of a cavity into the pleura may cause *pneumothorax*, *pleural effusion* or *empyema*, and erosion into a pulmonary vessel may lead to haematogenous spread and *miliary infection*.

Lymphadenopathy is a common feature of primary infection, but is rare in post-primary tuberculosis except in the HIV-positive population. Enlarged lymph nodes may press on adjacent airways and cause pulmonary collapse or air trapping with hyperinflation. Caseating nodes may also erode into airways, causing bronchopneumonia, and into vessels causing miliary infection.

Post-primary pulmonary tuberculosis

This follows the primary infection after a latent interval, however short or long, and is due to either reactivation or reinfection. It is now generally accepted that almost all post-primary tuberculosis is due to reinfection.

The lesions usually start in the subapical parts of the upper lobes or in the apical segment of the lower lobes as small areas of exudative inflammation. These extend, coalesce, caseate and cavitate. Typically there is a large cavity with several smaller satellite cavities, often bilateral but more advanced on one side. Cavity walls are lined by tuberculous granulation tissue and traversed by fibrotic remnants of bronchi and vessels. A vessel which has not been totally obliterated may dilate—a Rasmussen aneurysm.

Dispersal of infection from the cavities to other parts of the lungs takes place as in the primary form, and results in numerous small areas of caseous pneumonia, often in the lower lobes. Massive dispersal may lead to caseation of a whole lobe.

Adhesions usually limit pleural spread but sometimes the lung becomes encased in a thick coating of caseous material, fibrosis and hyaline connective tissue. Small cavities that heal leave radiating fibrotic strands puckering the lung. Large cavities become lined by columnar or squamous epithelium and are prone to secondary infection or fungal colonisation.

RADIOLOGY OF PULMONARY TUBERCULOSIS

Consolidation in primary infection

This may involve any part of the lung, and the appearance is non-specific unless there is coincidental lymphadenopathy. The area involved may be small or affect an entire lobe, and an air bronchogram may be visible (Figs 5.22, 5.23). Occasionally consolidation appears as a well-defined nodule or nodules. Healing is often complete without any sequelae on the chest radiograph although fibrosis and calcification may occur (Fig. 5.24).

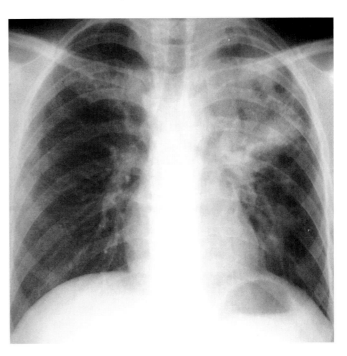

Fig. 5.22 Tuberculous pneumonia. Air bronchograms are present in the left upper lobe consolidation. Less marked right upper lobe consolidation is also present.

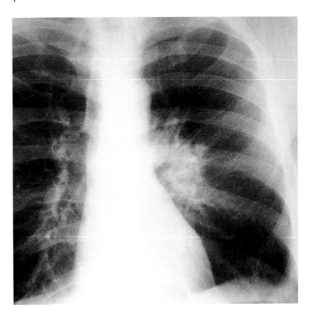

Fig. 5.23 Tuberculosis. There is left hilar enlargement and perihilar consolidation.

Consolidation in post-primary infection

This usually appears in the apex of an upper or lower lobe, and almost never in the anterior segments of the upper lobes. The consolidation is often patchy and nodular and may be bilateral (Fig. 5.25). A minimal apical lesion can easily be overlooked because of overlapping shadows of ribs and clavicle (Fig. 5.26). Comparison with the opposite side is then helpful, looking for asymmetries of density. The apical projection was designed to overcome this difficulty, but is rarely useful. Progressive

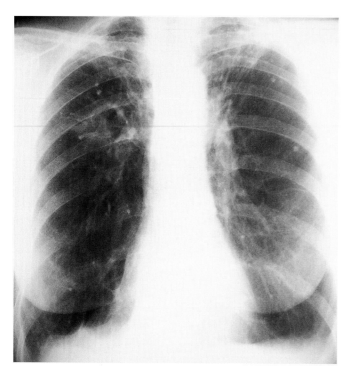

Fig. 5.24 Healed tuberculosis. There is bilateral upper lobe fibrosis with elevation of both hila. Basal emphysema has developed. There are multiple calcified granulomas in the mid and upper zones.

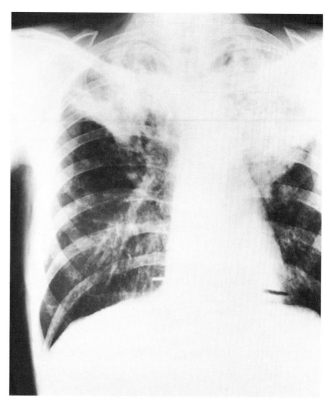

Fig. 5.25 Tuberculosis. Dense non-homogeneous opacities. Contracted right upper lobe.

infection is indicated by extension and coalescence of the areas of consolidation, and the development of cavities (Fig. 5.27).

Simultaneously there may be fibrosis and volume loss indicating healing (Fig. 5.24). Cavities may be single or multiple, large or small and thin or thick walled. Fluid levels are sometimes visible within cavities. With fibrosis there is often obliteration of cavities; however, larger cavities may persist and areas of bronchiectasis and emphysema may develop. Healed lesions often calcify. Because the upper lobes are predominantly involved, the effects of fibrotic contraction are seen as the trachea being pulled away from the midline, elevation of the hila and distortion of the lung parenchyma (Fig. 5.28). Chronic cavities are often colonised by *Aspergillus* and other fungi, and mycetomas may develop (Fig. 5.29). Disease activity is monitored by periodic radiographs, the appearance of new lesions or the extension of old ones indicating continued activity, whereas contraction indicates that the balance has been tilted in favour of healing. Once the radiographic signs have stabilised, any subsequent change in size or density must be regarded as suspicious of reactivation, fungal colonisation or complication by neoplasm.

Tuberculous bronchopneumonia

This may occur in both primary and post-primary infection, causing patchy, often nodular, areas of consolidation (Figs 5.27B, 5.30).

Miliary tuberculosis

This is due to haematogenous spread of infection and may be seen in both primary and post-primary disease. In the former the patient is often a child, and in the latter case the patients are often elderly, debilitated or immunocompromised. At first the chest radiograph may be

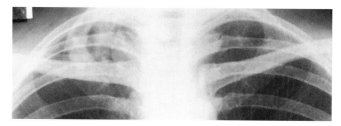

Fig. 5.26 Tuberculosis. Minimal right apical lesion.

normal, but then small, discrete nodules, 1–2 mm in diameter, become apparent, evenly distributed throughout both lungs (Fig. 5.31). These nodules may enlarge and coalesce, but with adequate treatment they slowly resolve. Occasionally, some may calcify.

Tuberculoma

This is a localised granuloma due to either primary or post-primary infection. It usually presents as a solitary well-defined nodule, up to 5 cm in diameter. Calcification is common but cavitation is unusual (Fig. 5.32).

Lymphadenopathy

Hilar and mediastinal lymphadenopathy is a common feature of primary infection and may be seen in the presence or absence of peripheral consolidation. Following healing, involved nodes may calcify. Lymphadenopathy is usually unilateral but may be bilateral,

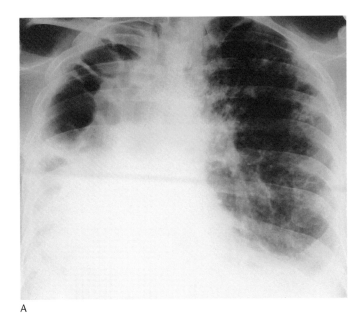

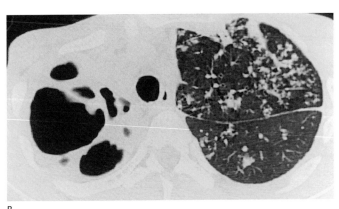

Fig. 5.27 Tuberculosis. (A, B) Chest radiograph and CT scan demonstrating almost complete destruction of the right lung due to pulmonary tuberculosis. The CT reveals bronchopneumonic spread to the opposite lung.

in which case the differential diagnosis includes lymphoma and sarcoidosis. It is often more pronounced in children (Fig. 5.33).

Pleural changes

Pleural effusion complicating primary infection is usually unilateral and due to subpleural infection. Pulmonary consolidation and/or lymphadenopathy may or may not be apparent. At presentation the effusion may be large and relatively asymptomatic. These effusions usually resolve without complication. Pleural effusion in post-primary infection, however, often progresses to empyema. Healing is then complicated by pleural thickening and often calcification (Fig. 5.34). Uncommon complications of tuberculous empyema are bronchopleural fistula, osteitis of a rib, pleurocutaneous fistula and secondary infection. Previous thoracoplasty may also complicate the appearances.

Pleural thickening over the apex of the lung often accompanies the fibrosis of healing apical tuberculosis.

Pneumothorax may complicate subpleural cavitatory disease.

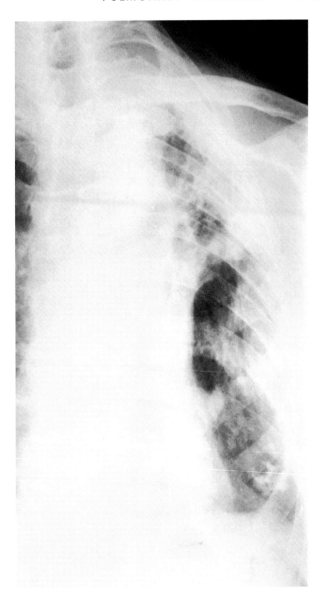

Fig. 5.28 Tuberculosis. There is fibrotic shrinkage of the left upper lobe with mediastinal and hilar displacement and apical pleural thickening.

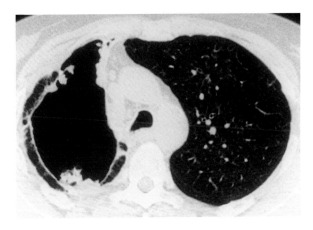

Fig. 5.29 Right apical aspergilloma in a patient with previous TB. Note the mycetoma material lying free in the dependent part of the cavity as well as the nodules adherent to the cavity walls anteriorly.

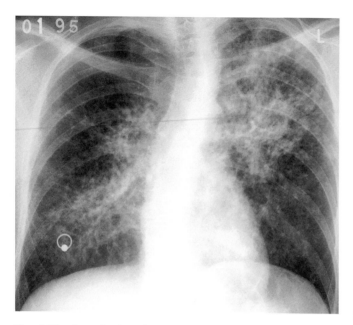

Fig. 5.30 Extensive bronchopneumonic spread of tuberculosis in an HIV-positive patient.

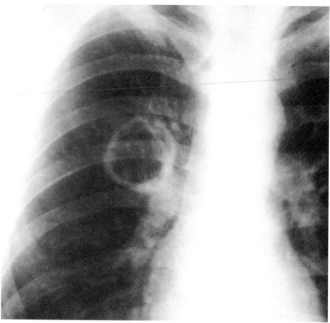

Fig. 5.32 Tuberculoma. A well-defined cavity is projected adjacent to the right hilum.

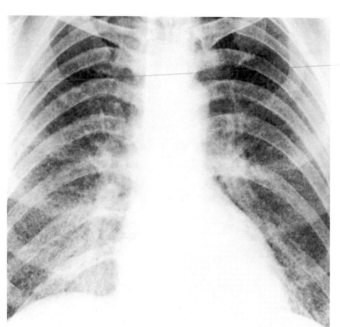

Fig. 5.31 Miliary tuberculosis. There are innumerable well-defined nodules present.

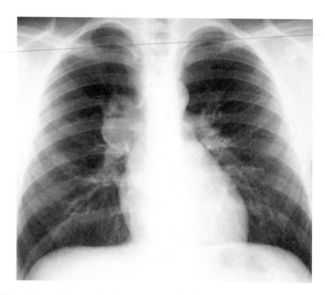

Fig. 5.33 Tuberculosis. There is right hilar lymph node enlargement.

Airway involvement

This may be secondary to lymphadenopathy or endobronchial infection and may therefore complicate both primary and post-primary disease. Compression of central airways by enlarged nodes may cause pulmonary collapse or air trapping (Fig. 5.35). Healing of endobronchial infection with fibrosis may also result in broncho-stenosis. The lung distal to bronchial narrowing may develop bronchiectasis.

OTHER MYCOBACTERIAL PULMONARY INFECTIONS

There are a number of related bacilli with morphology and staining properties very similar to those of the tubercle bacillus. Of these atypical mycobacteria, those most frequently the cause of human disease are *Mycobacterium xenopi*, *M. kansasii* and *M. battei*. Their infectivity is low but their sensitivities to drugs differ from that of *M. tuberculosis*. In general they cause less fibrosis and are less prone to spread but more prone to cavitate than *M. tuberculosis* infections. A common pattern is of a cluster of small opacities

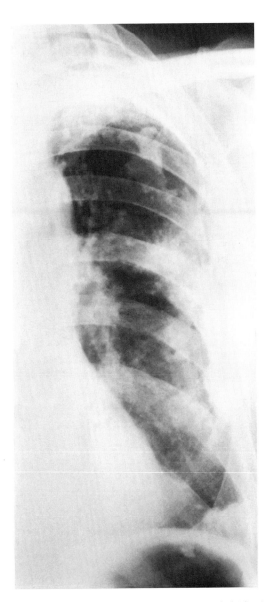

Fig. 5.34 Tuberculosis. There is generalised pleural thickening with extensive pleural calcification.

grouped around a central lucency. The cavities are thin-walled. Pleural disease, miliary disease and node enlargement are rare. These differences are not however sufficient, in an individual case, to differentiate them from *M. tuberculosis* infections.

BRANCHING BACTERIA

Actinomycosis

Actinomyces israelii is a commensal of the oropharynx and may rarely cause pulmonary infection by aspiration or direct extension from oesophagus or mediastinum. Classically it causes abscess formation, pleural invasion, osteomyelitis of ribs and sinuses to the chest wall. Apical disease may mimic tuberculosis, and occasionally a patchy pneumonia may develop. Presentation nowadays is most often as a mass-like area of consolidation which may resemble lung cancer (Fig. 5.36).

Nocardiosis

Nocardia asteroides is a saprophyte found worldwide in soil. Infection usually occurs as a result of inhalation by debilitated individuals. Most commonly there is non-segmental, cavitating pneumonia, often with pleural effusion or empyema. It may also present as a solitary pulmonary nodule, with or without cavitation, and occasionally with hilar lymphadenopathy (Figs 5.37, 5.38).

FUNGAL INFECTIONS

Histoplasmosis

Infection with *Histoplasma capsulatum* is usually due to inhalation of soil or dust contaminated by bat or bird excreta. Although widespread it rarely causes chest infection, except in the eastern USA. Infection is usually subclinical and heals spontaneously, sometimes leaving small, calcified pulmonary nodules (Fig. 5.39) or calcified hilar or mediastinal nodes. When many nodules are scattered throughout the lungs they closely resemble the scars of miliary tuberculosis or varicella pneumonia except that they tend to be rather more variable in size (Fig. 5.40). Rarely a calcified node may erode and obstruct a bronchus.

Progression of one or more of these foci leads to larger nodules. Hilar node enlargement is common and may be the only visible manifestation. Locally progressive disease may also take the form of consolidation, acute or chronic, the latter associated with fibrosis and cavitation (Fig. 5.41). The presence of cavitation within an area of lung distorted by fibrosis produces an appearance similar to tuberculosis.

When massive inhalation of organisms occurs the presentation may be one of wheezing, dyspnoea, a dry cough and fever. The chest radiograph shows diffuse small nodular shadows (Fig. 5.42) which, following resolution, may calcify (Fig. 5.40). A histoplasmoma may resemble a tuberculoma, being round, usually well circumscribed and often calcified. Pleural disease and haematogenous spread are rare.

An uncommon late manifestation of histoplasmosis is a *fibrosing mediastinitis* which can cause stenosis of the venae cavae, oesophagus, trachea, bronchi or central pulmonary vessels (Fig. 5.43). The chest radiograph will then show a widened mediastinum. Large hilar shadows with opacities extending into the lungs and Kerley B lines may appear.

Coccidioidomycosis

Coccidioides immitis causes endemic disease in parts of the south west USA. Some 60% of infections are asymptomatic and the commonest radiographic finding is a nodule which calcifies as it heals. However *C. immitis* may cause a pneumonic illness, and the chest radiograph may show patchy consolidation which may cavitate and be associated with pleural effusion or hilar or mediastinal adenopathy. Alternatively single or multiple pulmonary nodules may develop, up to 3 cm in diameter, and these have a tendency to form thin-walled cavities (Fig. 5.44). The fungus may also cause isolated mediastinal or hilar adenopathy and so raise the possibility of lymphoma or sarcoidosis in the differential diagnosis. Rarer manifestations are progressive upper lobe consolidation with fibrosis and cavitation, similar to tuberculosis, and miliary disease.

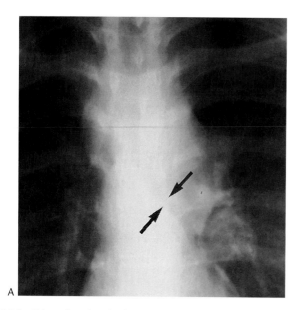

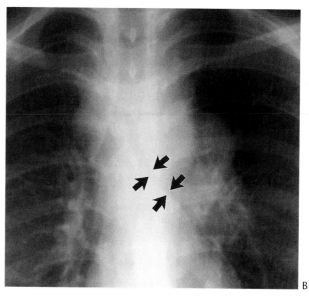

Fig. 5.35 Tuberculous lymphadenopathy. (A) There is mediastinal and left hilar lymph node enlargement causing some narrowing of the left main bronchus. (B) One month later appearances have significantly progressed with enlargement of the hilar and mediastinal nodes and increased left main bronchial narrowing.

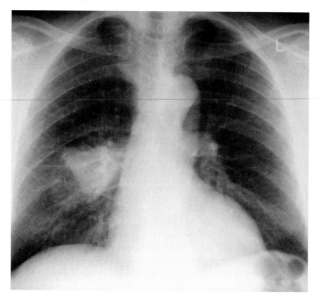

Fig. 5.36 Actinomycosis. There is a dense mass-like area of consolidation in the right mid zone.

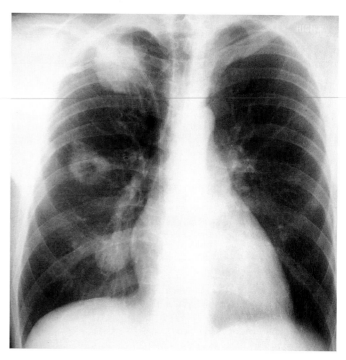

Fig. 5.37 *Nocardia asteroides* pneumonia. There are multiple cavities within the right lung, one of which has cavitated.

Blastomycosis

Blastomyces dermatitidis is found in parts of the south east USA, and may cause infection similar to other fungi. Hence presentations include an asymptomatic solitary nodule, a pneumonic illness with chronic consolidation, lymphadenopathy, fibronodular disease or miliary disease. Cavitation is occasionally seen, but calcification is rare. Unlike histoplasmosis and coccidioidomycosis, fibrosis is uncommon, and once lesions have healed, scars are frequently inconspicuous.

Cryptococcosis (torulosis)

Cryptococcus neoformans is a yeast form of fungus found world-wide. Infection is mostly subclinical, but may be important in debil-

itated patients. It may present with a pleural-based mass (torulosis), possibly cavitating, that may be indistinguishable radiographically from lung cancer (Fig. 5.45). Nodal enlargement and cavitation are unusual. However other presentations include segmental or lobar consolidation and miliary nodules. As with most fungal infections almost any radiographic pattern may occur.

Candidiasis

Candida albicans is a normal mouth commensal which, when conditions are favourable, causes moniliasis (thrush), a superficial

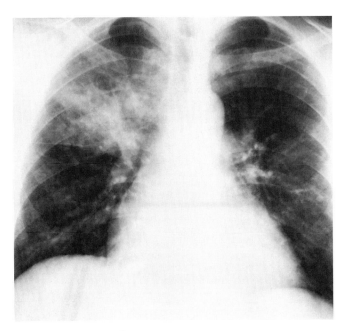

Fig. 5.38 Nocardiosis. There is non-homogeneous consolidation in the right upper lobe.

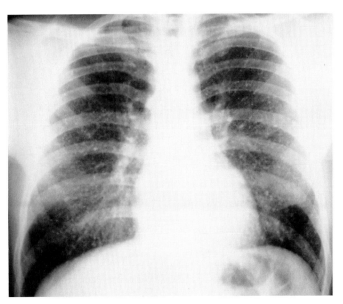

Fig. 5.40 Histoplasmosis. Incidental finding of multiple calcified pulmonary nodules.

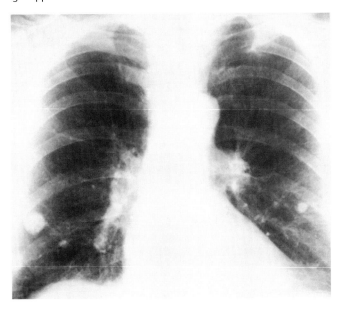

Fig. 5.39 Histoplasmosis. Calcified nodules of varying size are present in both lungs. Calcified hilar nodes are also present.

surface infection. It is rarely invasive unless the patient is immuno-compromised. Lung infection, when it occurs, is probably from haematogenous spread. The pulmonary lesion is a chronic pneumonia which breaks down with the formation of an abscess. A mycetoma may develop in the abscess, which is then indistinguishable from aspergilloma.

Mucormycosis

The *Mucorales* group of fungi are best known as causes of a spreading destructive infection of the face and sinuses in diabetics or the immunosuppressed. Lung infection is a rapidly progressive, dense, cavitating bronchopneumonia.

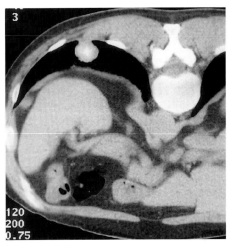

Fig. 5.41 Histoplasmosis. CT examination through a right lower lobe histoplasmoma that demonstrates central calcification. Patient is being examined in the prone position prior to percutaneous needle biopsy.

Aspergillosis

Aspergillus fumigatus is widespread in the atmosphere and it is inevitable that man inhales the spores from time to time. It is capable of multiplying in air passages when the conditions are favourable. The pulmonary manifestations are grouped into three categories.

1. Aspergilloma

Any chronic pulmonary cavity may be colonised by fungus. Such cavities are mostly secondary to tuberculosis, histoplasmosis or sarcoidosis, and are, therefore, usually in the upper lobes. The fungal hyphae form a ball or mycetoma which lies free in the cavity.

The *chest radiograph* may show a density surrounded by air within a cavity, but this is best shown by tomography (Fig. 5.29) or CT. By altering the position of the patient the ball is seen to be mobile. There is almost always pleural thickening related to the

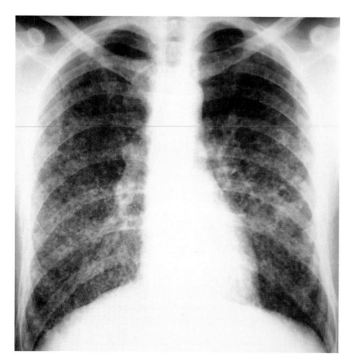

Fig. 5.42   Acute histoplasmosis following massive exposure whilst visiting a bat-infested cave. There are widespread bilateral well-defined 3–5-mm nodules.

mycetoma. The differential diagnosis of a mycetoma in a cavity includes *blood clot, cavitating tumour, lung abscess* and *hydatid cyst*.

Mycetomas are associated with development of vascular granulation tissue in the cavity wall, which may bleed. Life-threatening haemoptysis may be difficult to treat surgically, and may be better managed by *bronchial* or *intercostal artery embolisation*.

2. Invasive aspergillosis

In immunocompromised individuals *Aspergillus* may cause primary infection of the lung. This may be a bronchopneumonia, lobar consolidation or multiple nodules (Fig. 5.46). On high-resolution CT scanning a halo of increased attenuation in the surrounding lung may be seen (Fig. 5.47). Histologically this corresponds to surrounding haemorrhagic inflammation, and although this finding on CT scanning is not completely diagnostic, it is highly suggestive. Cavitation is common, and following bone marrow transplantation often occurs when the white-cell count recovers. The appearances may then mimic an intracavitary mycetoma (Fig. 5.48) although, in contrast to aspergilloma formation in the immunocompetent patient, in the immunosuppressed patient this will occur in an area of previously normal lung.

3. Allergic bronchopulmonary aspergillosis

Aspergillus is the commonest cause of pulmonary eosinophilia in the UK; the patient is usually an asthmatic in whom the fungus has colonised the lobar and segmental bronchi, where it produces a Type III reaction. Patients present with a cough and wheeze and often expectorate mucus plugs which contain fungi.

In the acute phase the chest radiograph shows patchy consolidation, often in the upper zones. Mucus plugging may cause lobar collapse (Fig. 5.49), and dilated mucus-filled bronchi may be visible as finger-like, tubular shadows (Fig. 5.50). Appearances may return

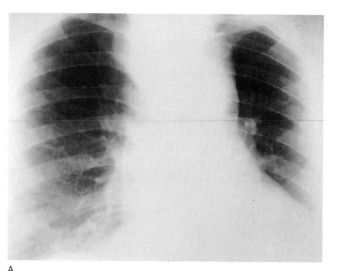

A

B

Fig. 5.43   Fibrosing mediastinitis following histoplasmosis. (A) Chest X-ray shows widening of the upper mediastinum. (B) Right arm phlebogram demonstrating compression of the right innominate vein. There is also a degree of tracheal narrowing.

completely to normal with appropriate treatment. However, with repeated attacks there may be pulmonary fibrosis and bronchiectasis. Fibrotic changes tend to occur in the upper zones. Bronchiectasis may produce ring shadows and tramline shadows. Unlike other causes of bronchiectasis, allergic bronchopulmonary aspergillosis may produce changes that are more severe in the central airways than peripherally (Fig. 5.51).

The condition pursues an intermittent course over many years and the frequency of chronic changes increases with the number of acute episodes. Within areas previously the site of transient opacities, the bronchi dilate and contain plugs of tough, stringy mucus mixed with small numbers of the aspergillus. Mucoid impaction is a dilated bronchus packed tightly with this material. Because of their thickened walls, bronchi may be visible as tubes, rings or cavities or, if impacted, as bulbous 'gloved-finger' or branching opacities. Air may return to impacted bronchi if the material is coughed up. Plugging of central bronchi can lead to collapse of lobes or whole lungs. Continued damage and repair by fibrosis will lead to focal emphysema, perma-

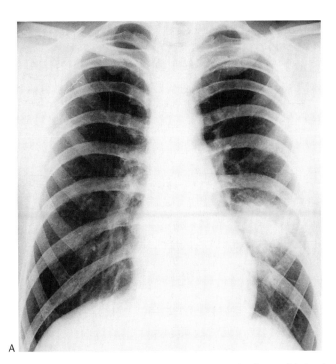
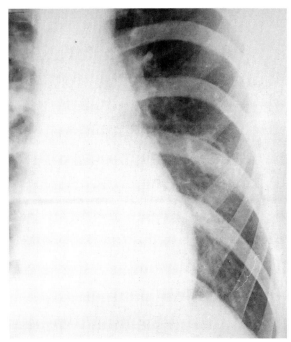

Fig. 5.44 Coccidioidomycosis. (A) A non-specific patch of consolidation is present in the left lower lobe. (B) One year later a thin-walled cavity is evident.

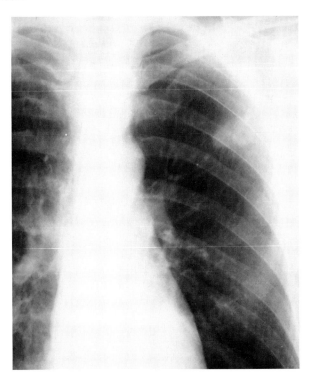

Fig. 5.45 Cryptococcus. A pleurally based mass-like area of consolidation in the left upper lobe is present in a patient who also had cryptococcal meningitis.

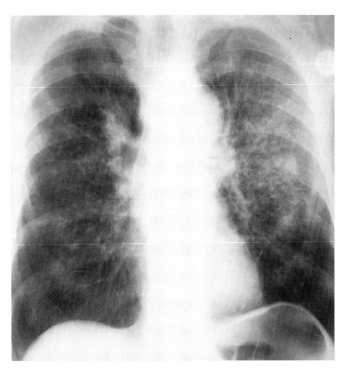

Fig. 5.46 Invasive aspergillosis. There is widespread bronchopneumonic change in a patient receiving chemotherapy for oat cell carcinoma.

nent shrinkage and eventually end-stage upper lobe fibrosis. Thus, although pulmonary opacities are transient, in only a minority of cases does the chest radiograph become completely normal between acute episodes. A mycetoma may form, not always in the upper lobes.

PROTOZOAL INFECTIONS

Pneumocystis

This is discussed under 'Acquired immune deficiency syndrome' (see p. 155).

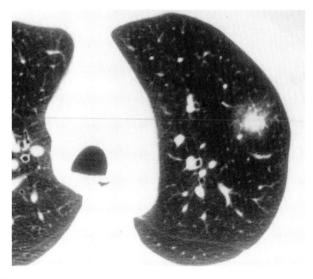

Fig. 5.47 Invasive aspergillosis. HRCT through a left upper lobe nodule demonstrating a halo of increased attenuation. Pathologically this correlates with a surrounding zone of haemorrhagic necrosis.

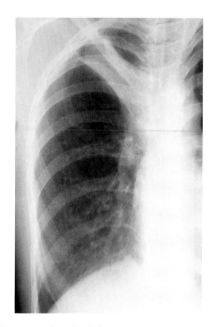

Fig. 5.49 Asthmatic with allergic bronchopulmonary aspergillosis. Mucus plugging has resulted in collapse of the right upper lobe. Complete resolution followed treatment.

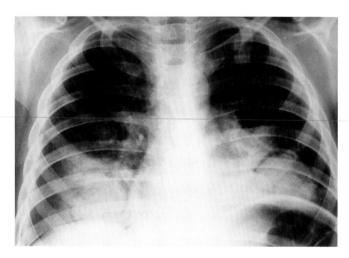

Fig. 5.48 Invasive aspergillosis in a patient with acute lymphoblastic leukaemia. A necrotising pneumonia in both lower zones has cavitated, mimicking the formation of fungus balls.

Toxoplasmosis

This is a protozoal disease widespread in mammals and birds; human acquisition is from cats or uncooked meat.

Although *toxoplasmosis* rarely involves the lungs, it may on occasion be responsible for an interstitial pneumonia, in which case the chest radiograph may show patchy consolidation and mediastinal lymphadenopathy.

Entamoeba histolytica

This protozoon is also found worldwide although amoebiasis tends to occur in the tropics and subtropics. Involvement of the chest is usually secondary to hepatic infection and is therefore usually right sided. A hepatic amoebic abscess may erode the diaphragm and cause diaphragmatic elevation, pleural effusion, basal consolidation and lower lobe cavitation. *Ultrasound* scan may reveal liver abscesses, and allows assessment of the diaphragm and pleural spaces.

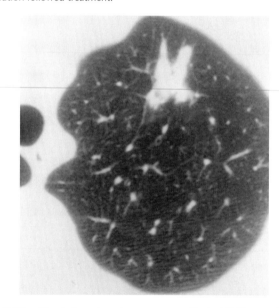

Fig. 5.50 Allergic bronchopulmonary aspergillosis. HRCT scan demonstrating finger-like opacities due to dilated mucus-filled bronchi.

METAZOAN INFECTIONS

Loeffler's syndrome

This may be caused by many parasitic worms, including *Ascaris*, *Taenia*, *Ankylostoma* and *Strongyloides*, all of which may lodge in or migrate through the lungs at some stage of their life cycles. The term *Loeffler's syndrome* is now applied to almost any transient pulmonary opacities of a predominantly eosinophilic histology associated with a blood eosinophilia. The heavier the infestation the more profuse are the pulmonary lesions. *Strongyloides stercoralis* in particular is capable of causing widespread opacities and a serious

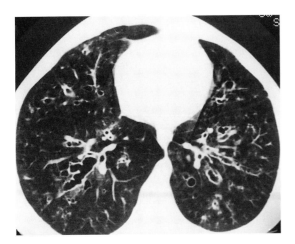

Fig. 5.51 Allergic bronchopulmonary aspergillosis. HRCT demonstrating widespread bronchiectasis of the medium and large airways.

pulmonary illness. Such *hyperinfection* can be activated by immuno-suppression.

Schistosomiasis

Schistosomiasis may cause pulmonary eosinophilia. If the eggs lodge in pulmonary arteries of less than 100 μm, the lesions they cause are small granulomas like miliary tuberculosis or sarcoidosis, but if they lodge in arteries a larger size the irritation causes vascular necrosis and fibrotic occlusion. The latter results in pulmonary hypertension if sufficient vessels are occluded. A third type of reaction results in diffuse interstitial fibrosis.

Paragonimiasis

Infestation is usually acquired in the tropics from eating infected shellfish. The commonest reactions in the lung are formation of multiple 1–2-cm-diameter cysts and bronchopneumonic shadowing, which may resemble tuberculosis. The dead flukes may calcify.

Armillifer armillatus

This is usually acquired by eating infected snakes. The larvae may migrate to the lungs where they encyst, die and calcify. The typical radiographic appearance is of multiple thin-walled cysts in a subpleural distribution. Dead larvae may calcify and be visible within the cysts as coils, targets or signet ring shapes.

Hydatid disease

This is caused by *Echinococcus granulosus*. Dogs are the principal reservoir of the adult worm, and most mammals serve as intermediate host for the larvae (echinococci). The hydatid is a parasitic echinococcal cyst consisting of three layers: an adventitia formed of compressed host tissue, a middle layer of friable ectocyst and an inner germinal layer from which is produced large numbers of scolices which are the heads of developing worms. Daughter cysts are formed if the viability is threatened but in the lung the cyst is unilocular (Fig. 5.52). Cysts mainly occur in the lungs and liver. Approximately 20% of the pulmonary cysts are bilateral, and about

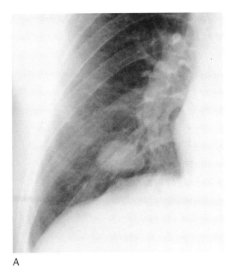

A

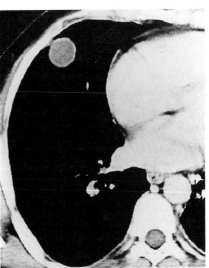

B

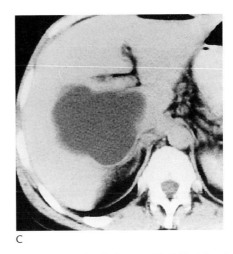

C

Fig. 5.52 Pulmonary hydatid disease. (A) Well-defined right basal pulmonary mass. (B) The CT scan reveals the well-defined wall and cystic contents. (C) This patient also had a large hepatic hydatid cyst.

10% are associated with hepatic cysts. Uncomplicated pulmonary hydatid cysts appear as well-circumscribed, round or oval, homogeneous masses, which may be up to 10 cm in diameter. Calcification is rare. Cysts may rupture into the pleura or bronchi. Following rupture into a bronchus an air–fluid level may appear or the ectocyst may separate from the adventitia so that a double-walled cyst may be seen. The choice of treatment of pulmonary hydatid disease lies between medical therapy (albendazole) or surgery, when the cyst must be removed intact.

CONGENITAL ABNORMALITIES THAT PREDISPOSE TO PULMONARY INFECTION

Cystic fibrosis

This is an autosomal recessive condition that occurs in 1 in 2000 live births and produces a generalised disease of exocrine glands and mucous glands. The latter produce abnormally viscous mucus which impairs mucociliary function and in the chest predisposes to frequent chest infections and development of bronchiectasis. It is now relatively common for patients to survive into adulthood, but overall the prognosis remains poor, with most deaths being a direct result of respiratory complications. *Pseudomonas aeruginosa, Staphylococcus aureus, Haemophilus influenzae* and *Klebsiella* species are frequent causes. The early radiographic changes may be limited to hyperexpansion, but eventually after repeated episodes of infection, a combination of bronchial wall thickening and dilatation and scarring produces a characteristic pattern. Clusters of ring shadows, some containing air–fluid levels, may be visible, together with evidence of air trapping, lobar or segmental collapse or consolidation. The latter usually indicates superadded infection. As respiratory failure progresses cor pulmonale may develop, as may repeated episodes of haemoptysis which may be life threatening. Repeated pneumothoraces, often resistant to tube drainage, are a further potentially fatal complication (see Ch. 6).

Hypogammaglobulinaemia

This predisposes to bacterial infections with resultant bronchiectasis in long-term survivors.

Chronic granulomatous disease

Only in rare instances do patients with this condition survive to adult life. Phagocytosis is normal but the polymorphs are incapable of destroying the ingested bacteria at a normal rate. Children suffer from recurrent pneumonias, but with increasing age these become less frequent. The lungs usually show bilateral interstitial fibrosis. Other thoracic complications are bronchiectasis and granulomatous mediastinitis.

Impaired neutrophil chemotaxis

Phagocytic cells are attracted to sites of bacterial infection by chemotactic substances released by the organisms or locally produced by the host. Activated complement is one such host substance. Instances have been found of impaired neutrophil chemotactic responses which have an adverse effect on the frequency and severity of infections. Abscesses and skin sepsis are the common manifestations and recurrent staphylococcal pneumonias are not infrequent.

Congenital dyskinetic ciliary syndromes

The 'immotile cilia syndrome' was the term originally applied to this group of conditions, but this is too restrictive because it is now known that there can be abnormalities of synchrony as well as total immotility. This collective term encompasses a heterogeneous mixture of structural and functional abnormalities of cilia. It is now postulated that the beating of embryonic cilia determines organ situs; if the beat is abnormal the situs will be randomly allocated and 50% will have situs inversus. Sperm tails are also cilia, and males with the condition will be infertile, hence explaining the combination of bronchiectasis, situs inversus and male infertility in *Kartagener's syndrome.*

Impairment of mucociliary clearance renders the lungs more susceptible to bronchopulmonary infections, but this is only a serious problem if the infections are repeated and severe. The radiographic signs are those of bronchiectasis, atelectasis and chronic obstructive airways disease.

Young's syndrome

This is a combination of obstructive azoospermia, sinusitis and chronic pulmonary infections. The latter begin in childhood and eventually most patients develop bronchiectasis. There is no structural abnormality of cilia but mucociliary transport is impaired. Spermatogenesis is normal, but the infertility of these men is due to a progressive obstruction of the epididymis by inspissated secretions.

Congenital pulmonary sequestration

This is an abnormality in which some lung tissue develops separated from the normal airways and pulmonary vessels. The blood supply is derived from the descending aorta. Sequestrated segments are situated basally in contact with the diaphragm, and appear solid when uncomplicated. They may become infected and develop a communication with the bronchial tree, following which they may cavitate and show a fluid level (Fig. 5.53).

ACQUIRED CONDITIONS THAT PREDISPOSE TO PULMONARY INFECTION

Systemic conditions that are associated with decreased immunity include old age, poor nutrition, diabetes, alcoholism, connective tissue disorders, many malignant diseases and AIDS.

Pulmonary abnormalities that predispose to chest infections include bronchiectasis and chronic bronchitis. In addition general anaesthesia, especially if prolonged, may be associated with pneumonia.

Iatrogenic causes include cancer chemotherapy, steroids, immunosuppression following organ transplantation, and radiotherapy.

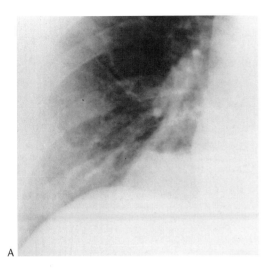

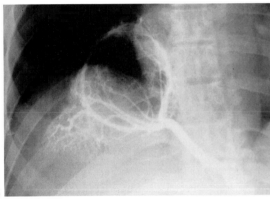

Fig. 5.53 Pulmonary sequestration. (A) The chest radiograph demonstrates a cavitating mass-like lesion in the right lower lobe. Note the preservation of the heart border and diaphragm. (B) Angiogram demonstrating the typical blood supply from a side branch of the subdiaphragmatic aorta.

Chronic infection of the paranasal sinuses and *oesophageal obstruction* may cause pneumonia or lung abscesses due to aspiration.

PULMONARY INFECTIONS IN IMMUNOCOMPROMISED PATIENTS—NON-AIDS

Pulmonary opportunistic infections are a common complication in immunocompromised patients. The radiographic appearances are often non-specific, and despite the high morbidity and mortality associated with chest infection in these patients a definitive diagnosis may be difficult to reach. In order for the radiologist to have a meaningful input into the assessment of the immunocompromised patient with acute chest symptoms, the underlying cause of immunodeficiency, type of immunosuppressive therapy, white blood cell count and overall medical status of the patient must be known. Whilst the role of the radiologist in these patients has primarily been one of detection and monitoring of pulmonary abnormalities, the introduction of high-resolution CT (HRCT) now makes it possible to offer earlier and more specific diagnostic infor-

mation. Furthermore HRCT allows prediction of the relative chances of obtaining a positive diagnosis from transbronchial versus percutaneous biopsy, particularly when other techniques have proved non-diagnostic.

Immunodeficiency may occur as a result of impaired cell-mediated immunity (T cells), for example in patients with lymphoma, patients who have undergone bone marrow transplantation or who are immunosuppressed following solid organ transplantation. Reduced humoral immunity (B cells) is most commonly seen in patients with myeloma, non-Hodgkin's lymphoma and lymphoblastic leukaemia. Reduced granulocyte number and/or function is encountered in patients with leukaemia and in those undergoing immunosuppressive therapy following transplantation.

Bacterial pneumonias

These are the most frequent pulmonary infections in the immunocompromised patient and rapid progression may occur. In addition to the common pathogens, debilitated patients—including diabetics and patients on steroid therapy—are also prone to the legionella group of bacteria. When tuberculosis occurs in this patient group it is usually due to reactivation. *Nocardia asteroides* has a predilection for immunosuppressed patients.

Invasive aspergillosis

This may occur in patients following solid organ or bone marrow transplantation. Diagnosis may be difficult, and CT should be considered early in the investigation of the immunocompromised patient with clinical evidence of chest infection but a normal chest radiograph. The radiographic pattern is discussed elsewhere.

Candida albicans pneumonia

This may occur in severely immunosuppressed patients with leukaemia or lymphoma, and lung disease usually develops as part of hematogenous dissemination, often as a preterminal event (Fig. 5.54). As a result there is frequently evidence of oral, cutaneous or hepatic disease. The radiographic changes are non-specific, with widespread interstitial or alveolar disease or lobar segmental consolidation. Occasionally, multiple nodules occur. Other fungi may cause disease in immunocompromised patients, as discussed above (Figs 5.55, 5.56).

ACQUIRED IMMUNE DEFICIENCY SYNDROME

AIDS is due to infection by the human immunodeficiency virus (HIV), and classically exposes the patient to infections normally resisted by cell-mediated immunity. The syndrome comprises opportunistic infections and certain rare malignancies, and in the UK is most often seen in homosexual males, drug addicts and haemophiliacs. Although a wide variety of infectious and non-infectious pulmonary diseases occur in AIDS, the commonest remains opportunistic infection.

PNEUMOCYSTIS CARINII PNEUMONIA (PCP)

This protozoal infection occurs in all groups of immuno-compromised patients with reduced cell-mediated immunity. It is particularly common in the AIDS population and remains the most common opportunistic infection. In older series approximately 60–80% of all patients with AIDS would suffer from at least one episode of PCP during the course of their illness. Approximately 40% of patients will have recurrent episodes of PCP, and PCP was the initial AIDS-defining illness in 50% of patients. The incidence of PCP has changed considerably in the west in recent years, with

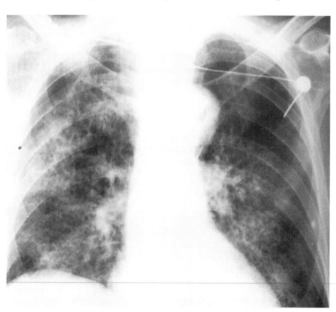

Fig. 5.54 *Candida albicans* bronchopneumonia. Mixed infection with Gram-negative organisms. Chronic alcoholic. Postmortem confirmation.

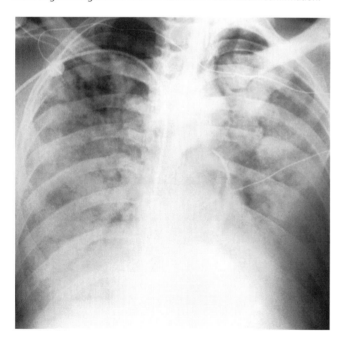

Fig. 5.55 Mucormycosis. The patient was an alcoholic. Fungal infection followed Rocky Mountain spotted fever. Mixed infection with Gram-negative organisms. Postmortem confirmation.

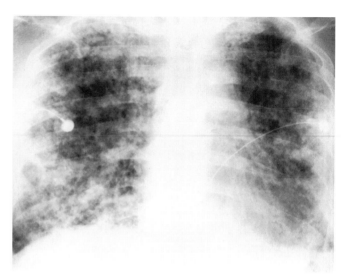

Fig. 5.56 Disseminated cryptococcosis. Mixed infection with Gram-negative organisms. Patient on steroids for systemic lupus.

PCP becoming rather less common due to early use of antibiotic prophylaxis and wide availability and uptake of retroviral therapy. Symptomatically, patients present with dry cough and shortness of breath, frequently accompanied by a pyrexia. Whilst the radiographic appearances may be normal early in the disease in up to 10% of patients and the degree of dyspnoea may be in advance of the radiographic changes, most patients will develop perihilar and mid and lower zone bilateral interstitial or ground-glass infiltrate (Fig. 5.57). This may rapidly progress to involve the entire lung (Fig. 5.58). On HRCT scanning the characteristic appearances are of a ground-glass infiltrate extending from the hilar regions into the surrounding lung, occasionally demonstrating a geographical pattern. Cavities, usually thin walled, but occasionally with a wall up to several millimetres in thickness, may develop (Fig. 5.59).

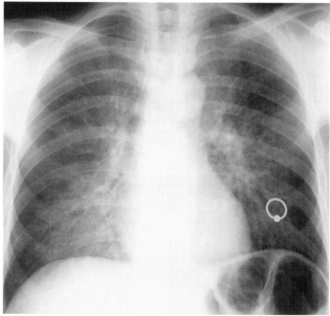

Fig. 5.57 *Pneumocystis carinii* pneumonia. There is widespread bilateral mid and lower zone ground-glass infiltrate.

Although appearances may return entirely to normal, some residual scarring and cyst formation is not uncommon. Pneumothorax is a well-recognised complication of PCP, usually in association with cystic change (Fig. 5.60). When pneumothorax occurs later in the course of disease, tube drainage may be ineffective and pleurodesis may be required. Extensive mediastinal and surgical emphysema may develop, and this combination of clinical features has a poor outlook (Fig. 5.61). Many less common manifestations of PCP are well recognised and include miliary disease, discrete pulmonary nodules, pleural effusions and mediastinal lymphadenopathy. Mediastinal lymph nodes may become calcified and are particularly well seen on CT scanning. Many AIDS patients in the west will take prophylactic antibiotics, and for those unable to tolerate sulphonamides, aerosolised pentamidine may be preferred. These patients are more likely to develop atypical patterns of disease with an apical distribution of involvement (Figs 5.62, 5.63). Other unusual manifestations of *P. carinii* infection include calcified hilar and abdominal nodes and viscera, and pulmonary cystic disease. PCP may present with unilateral disease and occasionally may mimic a bacterial pneumonia, with focal or lobar consolidation. Miliary disease is occasionally encountered (Fig. 5.64).

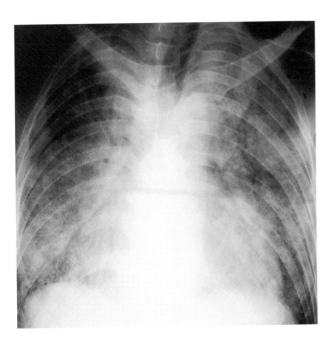

Fig. 5.58 *Pneumocystis carinii* pneumonia. Extensive bilateral consolidation.

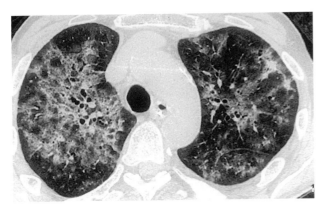

Fig. 5.59 *Pneumocystis carinii* pneumonia. HRCT image through the upper lung zones demonstrating bronchocentric ground-glass infiltrate with a degree of asymmetry.

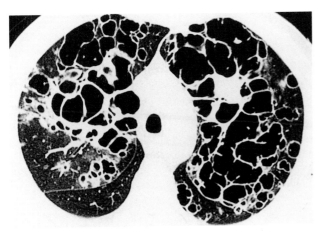

Fig. 5.60 HRCT scan through the lungs demonstrating multiple areas of cystic destruction following repeated *Pneumocystis* infection. (Courtesy of C. D. R. Flower, Addenbrooke's Hospital, Cambridge.)

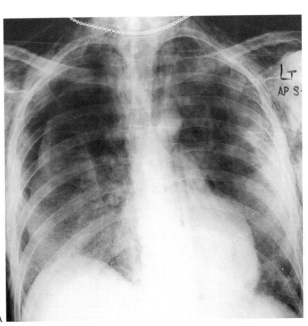

A

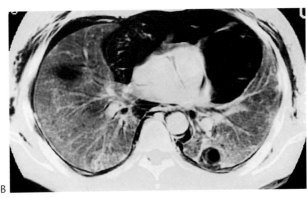

B

Fig. 5.61 *Pneumocystis carinii* pneumonia. Chest radiograph (A) and CT scan (B) demonstrating extensive mediastinal and surgical emphysema with bilateral pneumothoraces.

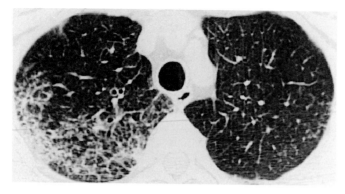

Fig. 5.62 *Pneumocystis carinii* pneumonia. Asymmetrical interstitial infiltrate in the right apex, barely visible on the chest radiograph, in a patient on aerosolised pentamidine.

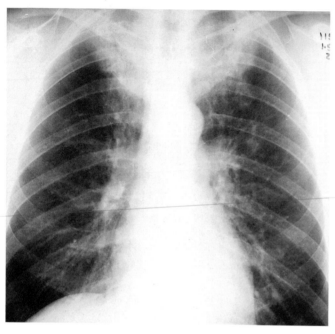

Fig. 5.63 *Pneumocystis carinii* pneumonia. Chest radiograph demonstrating bilateral apical infiltrates in a patient on aerosolised pentamidine prophylaxis.

Whilst the radiographic changes may be highly suggestive of PCP the diagnosis is usually made on examination of induced sputum, which has a yield of approximately 80–90%. When induced sputum examination is negative in patients with clinical and radiological features of PCP, including desaturation on exercise, a trial of therapy may be commenced. It is usual to reserve bronchoscopy for patients who subsequently fail to respond to a trial of therapy.

BACTERIAL PNEUMONIA

Although the major immune deficiency in AIDS patients relates to T-cell function, B-cell function and antibody production are also affected thus increasing susceptibility to pyogenic organisms. Bacterial pneumonias tend to occur throughout the course of HIV illness, becoming increasingly common with a falling CD4+ count. Because they often occur at relatively high CD4+ counts, bacterial infections tend to be the first pneumonic process to occur prior to the onset of full-blown AIDS.

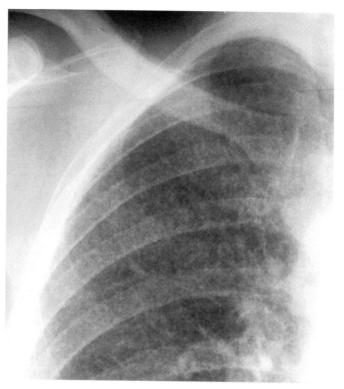

Fig. 5.64 *Pneumocystis carinii* pneumonia causing miliary shadowing. Appearances resolved on appropriate treatment.

AIDS patients are prone to community-acquired pneumonias such as *Streptococcus pneumoniae*, *Staphylococcus aureus* and *Pseudomonas aeruginosa*. Whilst disease progression may be unusually rapid and severe in this patient group, with cavitation and pleural effusions being more frequent than in non-immunocompromised patients, most commonly the pattern of disease is the same as in the normal population.

MYCOBACTERIAL INFECTION

Mycobacterial infection is also common in the AIDS population; equally, AIDS is commonly detected underlying a new case of TB. Indeed the HIV-positive rate in patients with active TB in the USA is between 4 and 40%, depending on the population centre.

Mycobacterium tuberculosis (MTB)

Radiological manifestations of MTB depend on the degree of immunosuppression. In the early stages of HIV infection appearances are similar to those of reactivation TB in the normal population. When the CD4+ count falls in the later stages of HIV disease, appearances become more in keeping with primary TB. Cavitation becomes less common and mediastinal nodal enlargement typically shows marked central low-density change with a rim of enhancing tissue (Fig. 5.65). Lung changes include non-specific areas of pulmonary consolidation and the presence of round or branching pulmonary nodules. Occasionally a miliary pattern is seen.

Mycobacterium avium intracellulare (MAI)

MAI is frequently isolated in the AIDS population and is a common postmortem finding. Despite this there is frequently no clinical

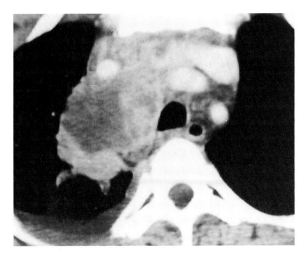

Fig. 5.65 Tuberculous lymph node enlargement in a patient with AIDS. There is a central low-density area surrounded by a rim of enhancing nodal material.

evidence of infection prior to death. Although in the immuno-competent population MAI is usually confined to the chest, in the HIV-positive group the infection is almost always disseminated and may be identified from a bone marrow aspirate or blood culture. Within the chest appearances are similar to MTB, although pleural effusions are more common with MAI and miliary disease is particularly uncommon.

Atypical mycobacterial infections

These occur with a similar frequency in the AIDS population as in the general population. However miliary disease is considerably more common in the AIDS population.

Multiple drug-resistant TB (MDRTB)

This is considerably more common in the AIDS population and is becoming an increasingly major problem.

Cytomegalovirus (CMV)

Although CMV inclusion bodies are a frequent finding in lung material from AIDS patients, CMV rarely causes clinical infection; when identified in patients with acute pulmonary disease it is often in association with other pathogenic organisms (Fig. 5.66).

TOXOPLASMOSIS

There is a high prevalence of previous exposure in the HIV-positive adult population. However genuine pulmonary involvement is distinctly unusual, despite the frequent occurrence of CNS toxoplasmosis. The chest radiographic appearances are non-specific.

FUNGAL INFECTION

Fungal infections are encountered in AIDS patients but are uncommon in comparison with other infective disorders since the host defence mechanisms rely more on phagocytic cells than on

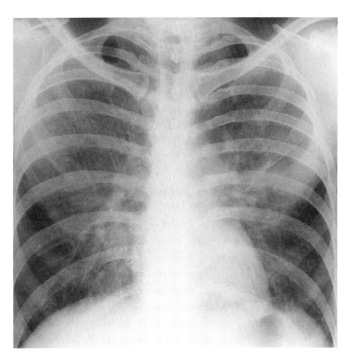

Fig. 5.66 Cytomegalovirus in AIDS. Although CMV is rarely a cause of pneumonia in isolation, on occasion other organisms are not identified.

T-cell-mediated mechanisms. The relative frequency of different varieties of fungal pathogens is largely dependent on the endemic rate in the local population.

Histoplasma capsulatum infection occurs in patients who have visited or reside in areas where the organism is endemic, such as the central USA and Central and South America. The disease is usually widely disseminated, and when pulmonary abnormalities are evident they normally take the form of a diffuse non-specific interstitial infiltrate or bilateral discrete non-calcified nodules. Lymphadenopathy occurs more frequently than in PCP. The diagnosis is usually made from bone marrow aspirate and culture.

Coccidioides immitis is also widespread in the central USA and occasionally causes coccidioidomycosis in exposed AIDS patients. The radiographic features are non-specific with a bilateral nodular or reticulonodular infiltrate, usually without mediastinal and hilar lymph node enlargement. Occasionally, solitary pulmonary nodules occur with this infection.

Cryptococcus neoformans When *Cryptococcus* causes clinical disease in the HIV population it is usually due to infection of the brain or meninges, and when pulmonary disease occurs it is usually in association with CNS disease. Radiographic changes are non-specific and include single or multiple nodules, consolidation with or without cavitation, interstitial infiltrates and enlargement of mediastinal lymph nodes.

Aspergillus fumigatus infection is being increasingly encountered as patients with profound immunosuppression are surviving for longer in the latter stages of HIV infection. A number of forms of infection have been described, usually in series based on chest radiographic appearances. CT most commonly demonstrates thick-walled cavities or lung abscess formation. In keeping with other groups of immunocompromised patients, these appearances are due pathologically to haemorrhagic infarction as a result of angio-invasion (Fig. 5.67).

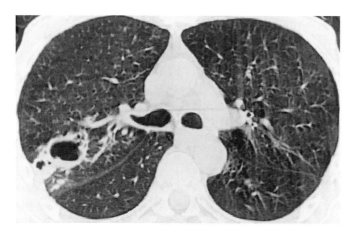

Fig. 5.67 Right upper lobe cavity colonised by aspergillus in an AIDS patient.

NON-INFECTIOUS PULMONARY DISEASE IN AIDS

Kaposi's sarcoma

Kaposi's sarcoma is the most common AIDS-associated malignancy in western countries and Africa. The incidence now appears to be falling due to the widespread use of antiherpes virus drugs and combination antiretroviral therapy. A virus from the herpes family has been identified as the causal agent for Kaposi's sarcoma and is referred to as Kaposi's sarcoma associated herpes virus (KSHV) or human herpes virus 8. Almost all cases of Kaposi's sarcoma (KS) have been documented in either homosexual or bisexual men and their partners.

Pulmonary KS occurs in up to 47% of patients with known cutaneous KS, and can affect the lung parenchyma, pleura or tracheobronchial tree. Pulmonary KS is rare in the absence of cutaneous or visceral involvement. When there is pulmonary involvement, disease is usually evident bronchoscopically as distinctive raised erythematous plaques within the airways. If these plaques become sufficiently enlarged they may occlude segmental bronchi resulting in atelectasis. The commonest reported CT findings are ill-defined parenchymal nodules, which may be surrounded by a small area of ground-glass density. Bilateral perihilar pulmonary infiltrates are seen in the majority of patients, which extend into the pulmonary parenchyma along the bronchovascular bundles (Fig. 5.68). Associated findings include thickening of the interlobular septa and nodularity of the fissures. Pleural effusions, pericardial effusions and mediastinal lymphadenopathy are also recognised features and chest wall disease involving the sternum, ribs, thoracic spine and subcutaneous tissues has been reported.

A variety of *lymphoproliferative disorders* are associated with AIDS including *lymphocytic interstitial pneumonitis* (LIP), seen most frequently in the non-AIDS population in association with Sjögren's syndrome and Systemic lupus erythematosus (SLE). When occurring in the AIDS population it is most frequent in children although adult cases are regularly encountered. The radiological appearances are most commonly a mid and lower zone

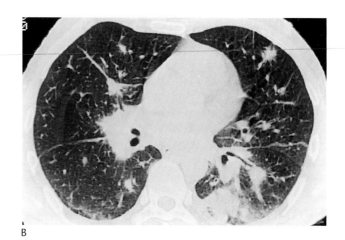

B

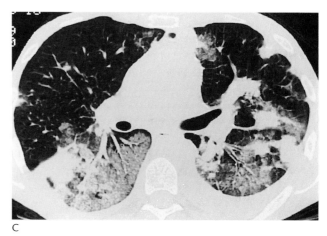

A

C

Fig. 5.68 Kaposi's sarcoma. (A) Multiple poorly defined pulmonary nodules are present bilaterally in a patient with bronchial and cutaneous Kaposi's sarcoma. (B, C). CT scans of two different patients demonstrating multiple poorly defined pulmonary nodules with a mid and lower zone and peribronchovascular predominance.

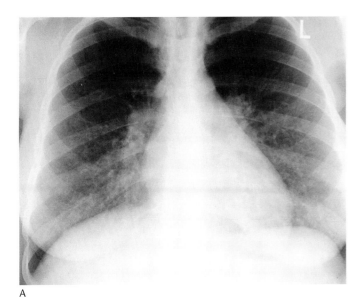

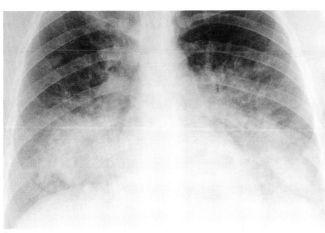

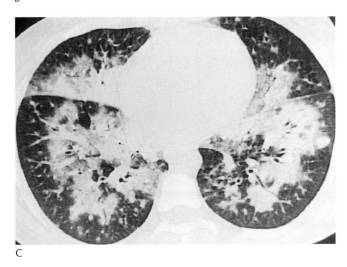

Fig. 5.69 Lymphocytic interstitial pneumonitis. (A) Chest X-ray demonstrating bilateral mid and lower zone 2–5-mm nodules. (B) Three years later there is an extensive mid and lower zone pulmonary infiltrate. (C) HRCT scan demonstrating the bronchovascular distribution of confluent infiltrate with more peripheral discrete nodules. Transbronchial biopsy confirmed the diagnosis of lymphocytic interstitial pneumonitis.

reticular or reticulonodular infiltrate. Although it is radiographically indistinguishable from opportunistic infection, slow progression of radiological change is suggestive of the diagnosis (Fig. 5.69). Neither pleural nor lymph node enlargement is associated with LIP, and if present should prompt a search for an alternative diagnosis. Bronchiectasis may occasionally occur. Features of LIP may regress as the degree of immunocompromise progresses.

Non-specific pneumonitis

This is a relatively poorly defined condition that occurs in the immunosuppressed patient with or without AIDS. It has been attributed to a variety of causes including unidentified viral infection, drug therapy and irradiation. Symptoms in patients with histological confirmation of the diagnosis are variable although reduction of the diffusing capacity of the lungs appears to be a more constant feature. The chest radiographic appearances are non-specific. Appearances may be normal or there may be alveolar or interstitial infiltrate; differentiation from other opportunistic infection is therefore not possible. Bronchiectasis has been observed to develop in a number of cases (Fig. 5.70). Failure to respond to treatment for infective causes and a relatively indolent course should raise the possibility of this diagnosis in a susceptible patient.

Lymphoma

Lymphoma, rarely confined to the thorax, is well described in AIDS patients. Lymphoma occurs with increased frequency in AIDS patients probably as a consequence of B-lymphocyte proliferation due to long-term stimulation by the HIV virus, and Epstein–Barr virus infection. When the presentation is with thoracic disease, there may be atypical mediastinal nodal enlargement, pleural or pericardial effusions, areas of pulmonary infiltrate or single or multiple pulmonary masses (Figs 5.71, 5.72).

Lung cancer

There are several reported series of lung carcinoma occurring in patients with AIDS. It is not clear from these studies whether AIDS

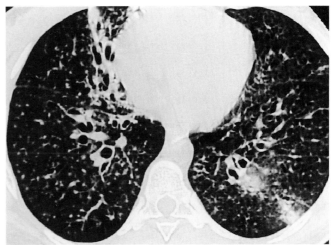

Fig. 5.70 Non-specific interstitial pneumonitis. A nodular infiltrate with patches of confluence is present in addition to widespread bronchiectasis, most marked in the middle lobe. The appearances have been slowly evolving over 3 years.

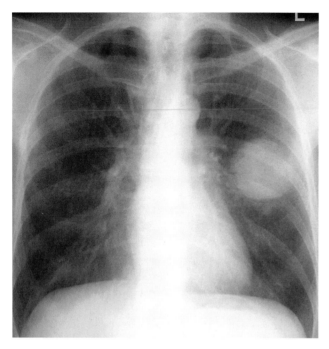

Fig. 5.71 AIDS-related lymphoma. There is a well-defined mass in the left mid zone. Percutaneous needle biopsy was undertaken to confirm the diagnosis.

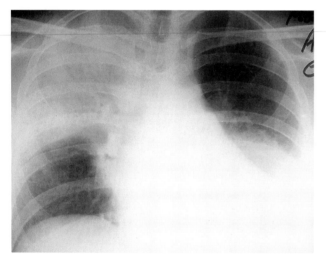

Fig. 5.72 AIDS-related lymphoma causing extensive consolidation in the right upper lobe. Infiltration of the left lower lobe in association with a pleural effusion is also evident.

patients have an increased risk of developing primary malignant lung tumours. Unlike KS and lymphoma, no associated mutagenic viral agent has been identified in relation to the development of lung cancer in AIDS patients and if there is a true increase in the prevalence of lung carcinoma it may be secondary to deficiencies in immunoregulation although the CD4+ count does not appear to correlate with the development of lung carcinoma.

REFERENCES AND SUGGESTIONS FOR FURTHER READING

Armstrong, P., Wilson, A. G., Dee, P., Hansell, D. M. (2000) AIDS and other forms of immunocompromise. In: *Imaging of Diseases of the Chest*, 3rd end, pp. 255–304. St Louis: Mosby–Year Book.

Armstrong, P., Wilson, A. G., Dee, P., Hansell, D. M. (2000) Infections of the lung and pleural. In: *Imaging of Diseases of the Chest*, 3rd edn, pp. 163–254. St Louis: Mosby–Year Book.

Berkmen, Y. M. (1980) Aspiration and inhalalation pneumonias. *Seminars in Roentgenology*, **15**, 73–84.

Berkmen, Y. M. (1980) Uncommon acute bacterial pneumonias. *Seminars in Roentgenology*, **15**, 17–24.

Boiselle, P. M., Crans, Jr, C. A., Kaplan, M. A. (1999) The changing face of *Pneumocystis carinii* pneumonia in AIDS patients. *American Journal of Roentgenology*, **172**, 1301–1309.

Conces, Jr, D. J., (1998) Pulmonary infections in immunocompromised patients who do not have acquired immunodeficiency syndrome: a systematic approach. *Journal of Thoracic Imaging*, **13**, 234–246.

Goodman, P. C. (1995) Tuberculosis and AIDS. *Radiologic Clinics of North America*, **33**, 707–717.

Goodman, L. R., Putman, C. E. (1984) Diagnostic imaging in acute cardiopulmonary disease. *Clinics in Chest Medicine*, **5**, 247–264.

Haramati, L. B., Jenny-Avital, E. R. (1998) Approach to the diagnosis of pulmonary disease in patients infected with the human immunodeficiency virus. *Journal of Thoracic Imaging*, **13**, 247–260.

Kuhlman, J. E. (1999) Imaging pulmonary disease in AIDS: state of the art. *European Radiology*, **9**, 395–408.

McGuinness, G. (1997) Changing trends in the pulmonary manifestations of AIDS. *Radiology Clinics of North America*, **35**, 1029–1082.

Maki, D. D. (2000) Pulmonary infections in HIV/AIDS. *Seminars in Roentgenology*, **35**, 124–139.

Marik, P. E. (2001) Aspiration pneumonitis and aspiration pneumonia. *New England Journal of Medicine*, **344**, 665–667.

Miller, W. T. (ed.) (1996) Fungus diseases of the chest. *Seminars in Roentgenology*, **31**, 1.

Palmer, P. E. S. (1979) Pulmonary tuberculosis—usual and unusual radiographic presentations. *Seminars in Roentgenology*, **141**, 204–243.

Reeder, M. M., Palmer, P. E. S. (1980) Acute tropical pneumonias. *Seminars in Roentgenology*, **15**, 35–49.

Staples, C. A., Kang, E. Y., Wright, J. L., Phillips, P., Muller, N. L. (1995) Invasive pulmonary aspergillosis in AIDS: radiographic, CT, and pathologic findings. *Radiology*, **196**, 409–414.

Shah, R.M., Salazar, A. M. (1998) CT manifestations of human immunodeficiency virus (HIV)-related pulmonary infections. *Seminars in Ultrasound CT and MR*, **19**, 167–174.

6

DISEASES OF THE AIRWAYS: COLLAPSE AND CONSOLIDATION

Michael B. Rubens and Simon P. G. Padley

THE TRACHEA

Congenital abnormalities

Tracheo-oesophageal fistula usually occurs in association with oesophageal atresia, but it may also occur as an isolated anomaly. On the plain film, air may be visible in the oesophagus (Fig. 6.1), but the diagnosis is usually made by a contrast study of the oesophagus. Barium or low osmolarity contrast medium must be used. If a simple swallow does not show the fistula, contrast medium should be injected into a nasogastric tube with the patient prone. As the

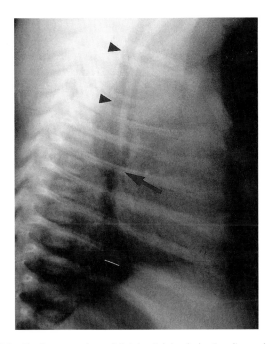

Fig. 6.1 Tracheo-oesophageal fistula. A lateral chest radiograph shows the fistula between the trachea and the oesophagus (arrow). The oesophagus is air filled (arrowheads).

tube is withdrawn the fistula is usually seen. Tracheo-oesophageal fistula may also be associated with other congenital anomalies such as the VATER complex (i.e. vertebral, anal, tracheo-oesophageal and renal anomalies). Other congenital causes of tracheal narrowing are hypoplasia of the tracheal cartilage, and compression by a distended oesophageal pouch.

Tracheal narrowing

Tracheal narrowing may be due to an extrinsic mass or mediastinal fibrosis or an intrinsic abnormality of the tracheal wall. *Laryngotracheobronchitis* or *croup* is the commonest cause of tracheal narrowing. It is usually viral and affects the upper trachea, most often in young children. Pyogenic bacteria and tuberculosis may cause a more generalized acute tracheitis. Tuberculosis may cause fibrosis and chronic tracheal stenosis.

Fibrosing mediastinitis, which may be due to tuberculosis or histoplasmosis, can cause both tracheal and bronchial stenosis. Rarer chronic inflammatory causes of tracheal narrowing include *sarcoidosis, chronic relapsing polychondritis* (Fig. 6.2), *Wegener's granulomatosis, rhinoscleroma* and *tracheopathia osteoplastica*.

Saber-sheath trachea is a condition which usually occurs in elderly men and is almost invariably associated with chronic obstructive airways disease. The abnormality affects only the intrathoracic part of the trachea which is narrowed from side to side, probably as a result of abnormal intrathoracic pressures. This theory is supported by the calibre of the extrathoracic part of the trachea being normal.

Primary tumours of the trachea are rare. Benign tumours present as small, well-defined intraluminal nodules. They are mostly papillomas, fibromas, chondromas or haemangiomas. Malignant tumours of the trachea tend to occur close to the carina. They are mostly squamous, adenoid cystic or adeno-carcinomas (Fig. 6.3). They may cause a localised mass or a long stricture. Their extraluminal extent is best assessed by CT (Fig. 6.4).

Tracheal stenosis may be the result of previous injury. This includes incomplete laceration of the trachea as well as iatrogenic causes such as previous tracheostomy or prolonged tracheal intubation (Fig. 6.5). Stricture development following prolonged

161

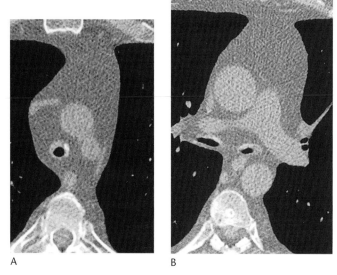

A B

Fig. 6.2 Relapsing polychondritis. (A) CT scan just above level of aortic arch shows diffuse thickening of tracheal wall with abnormal calcification and narrowing of the tracheal lumen. (B) CT scan just below level of carina shows identical abnormalities extending into both main bronchi.

intubation is thought to be secondary to ischaemia of the tracheal mucosa due to overinflation of the cuff of the endotracheal tube. Low pressure cuffs have now become widespread to prevent this complication. Other rare causes of tracheal wall thickening and stenosis are *amyloidosis, tracheopathia osteoplastica* and *tracheomalacia*.

Tumours of the thyroid, oesophagus or lung may displace or compress the trachea, and if malignant may invade the trachea. Rarely the trachea is the site of metastases from a distant primary tumour such as melanoma.

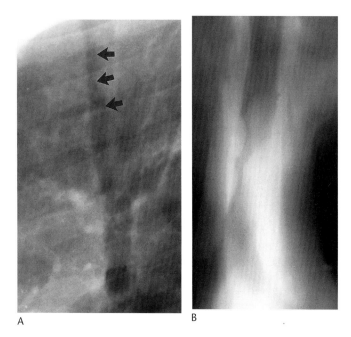

A B

Fig. 6.3 Squamous carcinoma of the trachea. (A) Close-up of the lateral chest X-ray demonstrates narrowing of the trachea with irregularity of the posterior wall (arrows). (B) AP tomogram demonstrating lobulated filling defects within the tracheal air column.

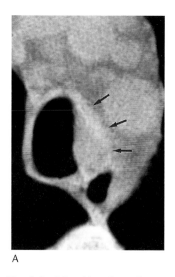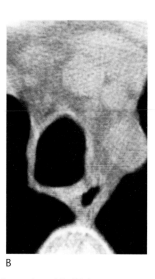

A B

Fig. 6.4 Adenoid cystic carcinoma of the trachea. (A) CT demonstrates a mass within the left lateral tracheal wall causing only slight distortion of the lumen. The extraluminal component extends into the adjacent mediastinal fat (arrows). (B) CT image 2 cm cranial to the lesion demonstrates normal tracheal wall thickness.

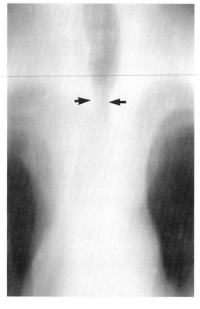

Fig. 6.5 There is a stricture (arrows) of the trachea following tracheostomy 10 years earlier.

Tracheal widening

The normal dimensions of the trachea have been assessed using a variety of techniques, most recently computed tomography. The trachea becomes slightly larger with increasing age. On CT scanning the maximum coronal diameter of the trachea is 23 mm in a male and 20 mm in a female. Dilatation of the trachea is rare, and it may result from a defect of connective tissue. This may be an isolated abnormality as in *tracheobronchomegaly* (Mounier–Kuhn syndrome—Fig. 6.6) or associated with Ehlers–Danlos syndrome or cutis laxa. In *Mounier–Kuhn syndrome* the trachea may be as wide as the vertebral bodies and of uneven contour, with bulging of the mucosa between the cartilage rings. The dilatation may proceed

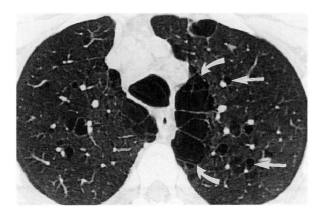

Fig. 6.6 Mounier–Kuhn syndrome. There is dilatation of the trachea in association with bronchiectasis (arrows). There are also multiple paraseptal bullae (curved arrow).

no further than the main bronchi, or it may be associated with a generalized bronchiectasis. The hypothesis that it results from a defect of connective tissue receives some support from its occasional association with Ehlers–Danlos syndrome, a generalized connective tissue disorder.

THE BRONCHI

Bronchiectasis

Bronchiectasis is the irreversible dilatation of one or more bronchi, and is usually the result of severe, recurrent or chronic infection. Childhood pneumonias, especially *pertussis* and *measles*, and *tuberculosis* are important causes. Other predisposing factors include *chronic sinusitis, bronchial obstruction* and *abnormalities of the cilia, mucus and immune system* (e.g. *Kartagener syndrome*— Fig. 6.7), *cystic fibrosis and agammaglobulinaemia*). Non-infective causes include bronchopulmonary aspergillosis and inhalation of noxious fluids or gases. In addition bronchiectasis is seen in association with intrinsic connective tissue abnormalities such as Ehlers–Danlos syndrome, Marfan syndrome and tracheobronchomegaly, and rarely in association with more common conditions such as rheumatoid disease and Sjögren syndrome. In patients with interstitial pulmonary fibrosis distortion and dilatation of segmental and subsegmental bronchi is a frequent occurrence producing so-called 'traction bronchiectasis'.

Bronchiectasis may be localised or generalised. It is frequently basal but, in tuberculosis and cystic fibrosis, it usually involves the upper zones. Dilated bronchi may produce tramline shadows (Fig. 6.8) or ring shadows (Fig. 6.9), and dilated, fluid-filled bronchi may cause 'gloved finger' shadows. Accumulation of pus or secretions in ectatic bronchi may produce fluid levels (Figs 6.7, 6.9). Chest infections frequently complicate bronchiectasis so that areas of consolidation may obscure the above signs. *Bronchography* was until relatively recently the definitive method of diagnosing bronchiectasis but has now been completely superseded by HRCT. Traditionally bronchiectasis has been described as cylindrical, varicose or saccular.

Cylindrical (or tubular) bronchiectasis (Fig. 6.10) produces a dilated bronchus with parallel walls, in *varicose bronchiectasis* the walls are irregular, and in *saccular (or cystic) bronchiectasis* (Fig. 6.11) the airways terminate as round cysts. In an individual

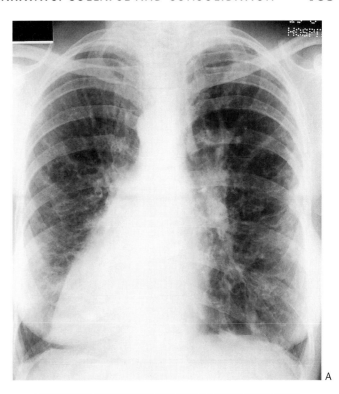

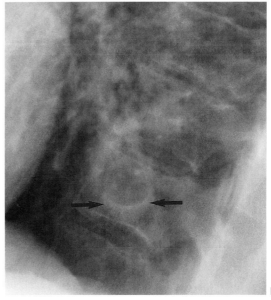

Fig. 6.7 Kartagener's syndrome. (A) There is dextrocardia and widespread bronchiectasis, most obvious at the left base. (B) A lateral view demonstrates an air–fluid level (arrows) within a dilated bronchus.

patient it is common to see more than one pattern. Bronchiectasis usually involves the peripheral bronchi more severely than the central bronchi. Although it has long been held that in bronchopulmonary aspergillosis this pattern may be reversed, overall the distribution and morphology of bronchiectatic change demonstrated by CT gives no more than a clue to the underlying aetiology.

The CT signs of bronchiectasis are those due to dilated bronchi, which often have thickened walls and may or may not contain secretions (Fig. 6.12). The common appearances of bronchiectasis on CT include non-tapering bronchi extending into the peripheral

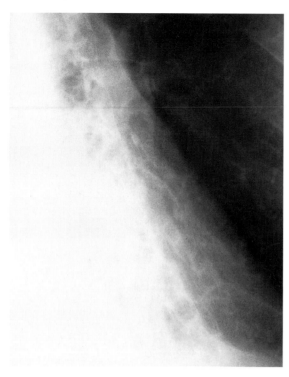

Fig. 6.8 Bronchiectasis. Tramline shadows are visible through the heart shadow.

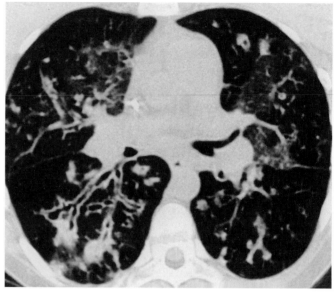

Fig. 6.10 Cylindrical or tubular bronchiectasis. CT image at the level of the hila demonstrates widespread bronchiectasis, particularly well seen in the apical segment of the right lower lobe. The bronchi fail to taper and have irregular thickened walls.

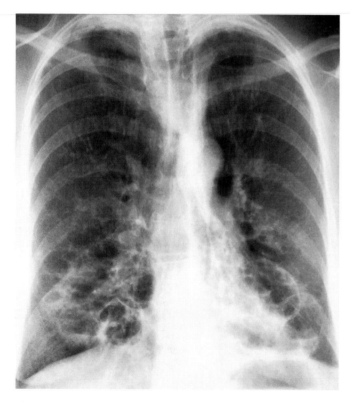

Fig. 6.9 Bronchiectasis. Multiple ring shadows, many containing air–fluid levels, are present throughout the lower zones of this patient with cystic bronchiectasis.

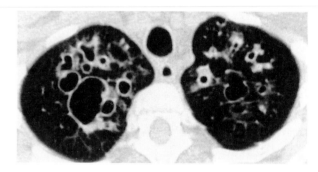

Fig. 6.11 Cystic bronchiectasis. A CT image through the upper lobes demonstrates multiple ring shadows. More caudal images reveal these to be due to irregularly dilated bronchi.

third of the lung. This is best appreciated when the bronchus lies in the plane of the CT section (Fig. 6.10). Normally a bronchus is the same size as or fractionally larger than the adjacent artery, although attention to the arterial bifurcation should be made to avoid overdiagnosis. When the bronchus is more markedly dilated and passes through the axis of the scan a typical signet ring appearance may be seen (Fig. 6.13). The wall of the bronchus may or may not be thickened. On expiratory scans there is frequently evidence of air trapping (Fig. 6.14). Peripheral airways may become plugged producing small subpleural branching opacities (Fig. 6.13).

Bronchial arteriography is sometimes useful in the management of haemoptysis secondary to bronchiectasis. Severe haemoptysis may be secondary to bronchial artery hypertrophy. If the site of bleeding can be identified, it may be treated by therapeutic embolisation.

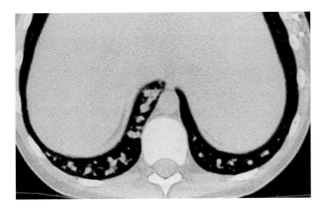

Fig. 6.12 Bronchiectasis with mucus plugging. A CT scan through the posterior costophrenic recesses showing multiple fluid-filled dilated bronchi causing a string of rounded opacities in the posterior costophrenic angle. (Same patient as illustrated in Fig. 6.13.)

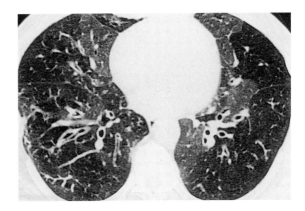

Fig. 6.14 Bronchiectasis with air trapping. CT image at end expiration demonstrates areas of relatively higher and lower attenuation. The lower attenuation areas indicate air trapping.

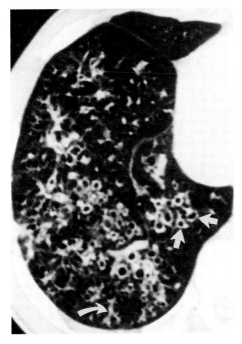

Fig. 6.13 Bronchiectasis. CT image through the right lower lobe reveals dilated subsegmental bronchi. Note how the bronchi are larger than the accompanying vessels. Several bronchi demonstrate the signet ring sign (arrows). Plugging of peripheral smaller bronchi is evident (curved arrow).

CYSTIC FIBROSIS

Cystic fibrosis was formerly a condition seen only in children. However, with improved management many patients now reach adulthood (see Ch. 19).

The increased viscosity of the bronchial secretions in cystic fibrosis causes bronchial obstruction. This leads to air trapping and also predisposes to bronchiectasis. The *chest radiograph* may, therefore, show signs of air trapping with flattening of the diaphragm, bowing of the sternum and increased dorsal kyphosis, and also signs of bronchiectasis (Fig. 6.15). Peribronchial thickening, peripheral nodular opacities and ring shadows may be visible. Areas of emphysema may develop. Chest infections are common,

staphylococci and *Pseudomonas* being important pathogens, so that areas of consolidation may be seen (Fig. 6.15). In response to chronic pulmonary infection the hilar lymph nodes may enlarge. The central pulmonary arteries may also enlarge due to pulmonary arterial hypertension. In later stages of the disease spontaneous pneumothorax may occur (Fig. 6.16).

OBSTRUCTIVE AIRWAYS DISEASE

Chronic obstruction to bronchial airflow is an abnormality that unites the group of conditions termed *chronic obstructive pulmonary disease* (COPD) or *chronic obstructive airways disease (COAD)*. This group is the most common form of chronic lung disease and includes chronic bronchitis, pulmonary emphysema and asthma, which are discussed in this section.

Definitions
Chronic bronchitis
This is defined in clinical terms as 'a chronic cough without demonstrable cause, with expectoration on most days during at least three consecutive months for more than two consecutive years'.

Asthma
Asthma is a clinical term referring to 'widespread narrowing of the bronchi, which is paroxysmal and reversible'.

Emphysema
This is defined in morphological terms as 'an increase beyond the normal in the size of the air spaces distal to the terminal bronchioles, with dilatation and destruction of their walls'.

Clinically and radiologically a patient may have manifestations of more than one kind of chronic obstructive airways disease.

ASTHMA

The clinical syndrome of asthma results from hyper-reactivity of the larger airways to a variety of stimuli, causing narrowing of the bronchi, wheezing and often dyspnoea.

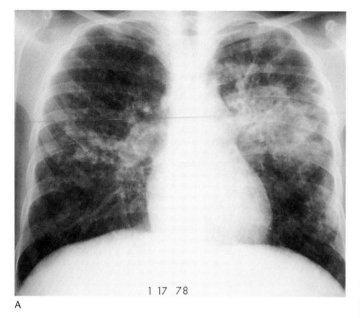

A

1 17 78

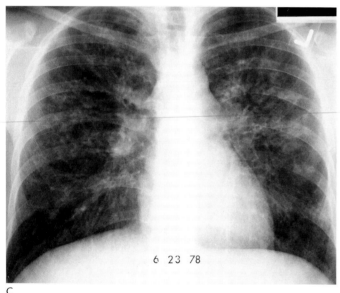

C

6 23 78

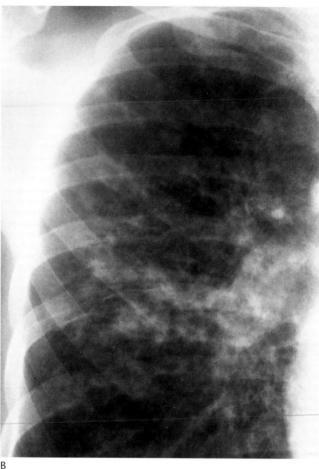

B

Fig. 6.15 Cystic fibrosis. (A) Chest X-ray during an acute chest infection showing left perihilar and right midzone consolidation. (B) Close-up of the right midzone demonstrating multiple ring shadows and tramlines due to extensive bronchiectasis. (C) Six months later the acute changes have resolved leaving a background of bronchiectasis.

Extrinsic or atopic asthma is usually associated with a history of allergy and raised plasma IgE. An important cause of extrinsic asthma is aspergillosis; this is discussed in detail in Chapter 5. *Intrinsic* or non-atopic asthma may be precipitated by a variety of factors such as exercise, emotion and infection. In acute exacerbation of chronic bronchitis due to a chest infection, wheezing is a common feature.

The role of radiology in asthma is limited. Most asthmatics show a normal chest X-ray during remissions. During an asthmatic attack the chest X-ray may show signs of hyperinflation (Fig. 6.17), with depression of the diaphragm and expansion of the retrosternal air space. Mediastinal emphysema may occur secondary to a rupture at terminal bronchiolar level or beyond, and occasionally this may lead to a pneumothorax. The peripheral pulmonary vessels appear normal, but if the central pulmonary arteries are enlarged, irreversible pulmonary arterial hypertension is probably present. The importance of radiology is to exclude complications such as a pulmonary infection, atelectasis due to mucus plugging or pneumothorax. High-resolution CT (HRCT) scanning of asthmatic patients may show one or more of the following: bronchial wall thickening, tubular bronchiectasis, mucoid impaction and areas of decreased attenuation in the lung parenchyma.

CHRONIC BRONCHITIS

The most consistent pathological finding in chronic bronchitis is hypertrophy of the mucus-secreting glands of the bronchi. Their secretions are more viscous than usual, leading to interference with

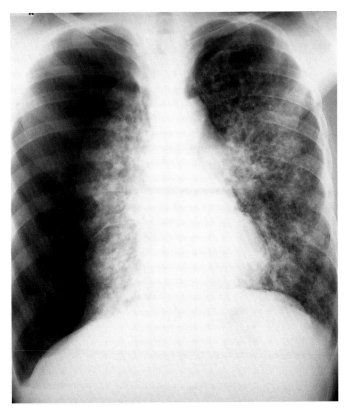

Fig. 6.16 Cystic fibrosis. There are widespread bronchiectatic changes and a large right pneumothorax; a small left apical pneumothorax is also present.

the mucociliary transport mechanisms and plugging of the small airways.

Chronic bronchitics are almost always smokers, and are usually male. Other important aetiological factors are urban atmospheric pollution, a dusty work environment and low socio-economic group.

The role of radiology in chronic bronchitis is to detect and assess complications of the condition and also to detect coincidental diseases. Pulmonary emphysema is a common complication which can be assessed radiographically, as can the development of cor pulmonale. The presenting symptoms of pulmonary tuberculosis and lung cancer can be masked by chronic bronchitis, and again the chest X-ray may help.

Radiological appearances

Approximately 50% of patients with chronic bronchitis have a normal chest X-ray. In patients with a plain film abnormality, the signs are due to emphysema, superimposed infection or possibly bronchiectasis.

An appearance which suggests chronic bronchitis is the so-called '*dirty chest*' (Fig. 6.18). There is generalized accentuation of the bronchovascular markings. Small, poorly defined opacities may be seen anywhere in the lungs, but their perception can be extremely subjective. There is some correlation between the 'dirty chest' and the presence of perivascular and peribronchial oedema, chronic inflammation and fibrosis. If this pattern is particularly obvious, with fine linear shadows and hazy nodular opacities, the appearance may resemble interstitial fibrosis, lymphangitis carcinomatosis or bronchiectasis.

Thin tramline or tubular shadows may also be seen, suggesting bronchiectasis, but the precise nature of these shadows is uncertain. These opacities are usually related to the hila, and may be clearly demonstrated by tomography, but again are only suggestive and not diagnostic of chronic bronchitis.

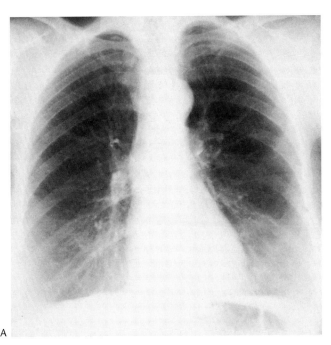

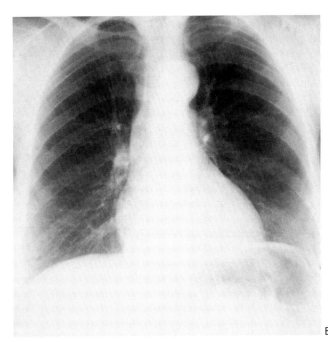

A   B

Fig. 6.17 Asthma in a woman of 64. (A) During an asthmatic attack the lungs are hyperinflated, the diaphragms being depressed and flattened. (B) During remission the chest radiograph is normal.

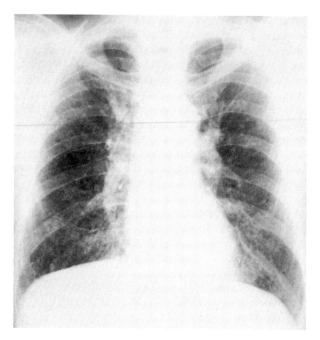

Fig. 6.18 Chronic bronchitis in a man of 62. Small poorly defined opacities are present throughout both lungs, producing the 'dirty chest'. This contrasts with the clear lungs in Fig. 6.17B.

If emphysema with air trapping is present the lung volumes increase, the diaphragm becomes flattened and the retrosternal air space increases. The number and size of the peripheral vessels decrease, and the central pulmonary arteries may enlarge. If cor pulmonale supervenes the heart enlarges.

EMPHYSEMA

As stated above, emphysema is defined in morphological terms as enlargement of the airways beyond the terminal bronchi, with dilatation and destruction of their walls. Classification of emphysema is also based, in part, on morphology, and a basic knowledge of lung structure is therefore pertinent. The trachea, bronchi and terminal bronchioles are strictly conducting airways. Beyond the terminal bronchioles, gas exchange takes place, so that respiratory bronchioles, alveolar ducts and alveolar sacs are both conducting and respiratory structures. The alveoli are purely respiratory in function. The secondary pulmonary lobule is a unit of lung structure supplied by between three and five terminal bronchioles; lung distal to a terminal bronchiole is called an acinus, and a secondary pulmonary lobule, therefore, comprises 3–5 acini.

Types of emphysema and associated conditions
Involvement of the secondary pulmonary lobule by emphysema may be non-selective or selective.

1. *Panacinar emphysema* This is a non-selective process characterized by destruction of all of the lung distal to the terminal bronchiole. It is sometimes termed panlobular emphysema. The lung may be involved locally or generally, but distribution throughout the lung is rarely uniform, although there tends to be a basal predominance. It may be associated with centriacinar emphysema, especially in chronic bronchitis, and is also seen in α_1-antitrypsin deficiency.

2. *Centriacinar or centrilobular emphysema* This is a selective process characterized by destruction and dilatation of the respiratory bronchioles. The alveolar ducts, sacs and alveoli are spared until a late stage. The upper zones tend to be more severely involved than the lung bases. It is usually found in smokers, frequently in association with chronic bronchitis.

3. *Paraseptal emphysema* This type of emphysema involves the periphery of the secondary lobules, usually in the lung periphery, sometimes combined with pan- or centriacinar emphysema, and occasionally causes bulla formation.

4. *Paracicatricial emphysema* This term refers to distension and destruction of terminal air spaces adjacent to fibrotic lesions, and is most frequently seen as a result of tuberculosis.

5. *Obstructive emphysema* This is strictly a misnomer, and the condition is better termed 'obstructive hyperinflation', since the distal airways are dilated but not necessarily destroyed. It is discussed here for the sake of completeness. It occurs when a larger bronchus is obstructed in such a way that air enters the lung on inspiration but is trapped on expiration. Such one-way valve obstruction may be due to an inhaled foreign body (e.g. peanuts or teeth) or due to an endobronchial or peribronchial tumour. The lung beyond the obstruction becomes hyperinflated.

6. *Compensatory emphysema* Another process that is better regarded as hyperinflation. If part or all of a lung collapses, shrinks or is removed, the resulting space is occupied by displacement of the mediastinum or diaphragm, or usually, more significantly, by hyperinflation of the unaffected or remaining lung. This is discussed in the section on lobar collapse later in this chapter.

7. *Bulla* A bulla is an emphysematous space with a diameter of more than 1 cm in the distended state, and its walls are made up of compressed surrounding lung or pleura, depending on its location.

Emphysema may be classified according to the presence or absence of air trapping at respiratory bronchiolar level. Panacinar, obstructive and congenital lobar emphysema are associated with air trapping and usually cause symptoms. Centriacinar, paraseptal and compensatory emphysema are not associated with air trapping and are usually asymptomatic.

Radiological appearances
1. *Panacinar emphysema* The radiographic features of panacinar emphysema are the results of destruction of lung tissue altering the vascular pattern, interference of ventilation decreasing lung perfusion, and air trapping. The effects of panacinar emphysema are almost always apparent clinically by the time the radiographic manifestations occur, but a normal chest X-ray virtually excludes severe generalised emphysema.

The main radiographic signs are (Fig. 6.19):

a. Reduction of pulmonary vascularity peripherally
b. Hyperinflation of the lungs
c. Alteration of the cardiac shadow and central pulmonary arteries.

The vascular pattern in affected areas of lung is attenuated. Involvement of the lung may be localised or generalised, but if

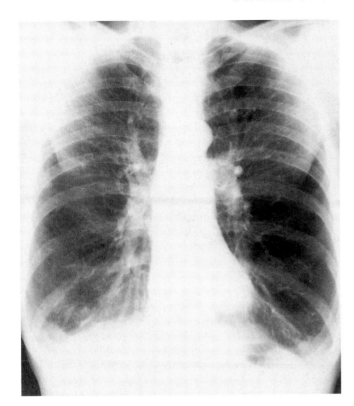

Fig. 6.19 Emphysema in a man of 54. The lungs are hyperinflated, the diaphragm being low and flat. The peripheral vascular pattern is attenuated in the right mid and left mid and lower zones. The central pulmonary arteries are enlarged, indicating pulmonary arterial hypertension. The heart is elongated.

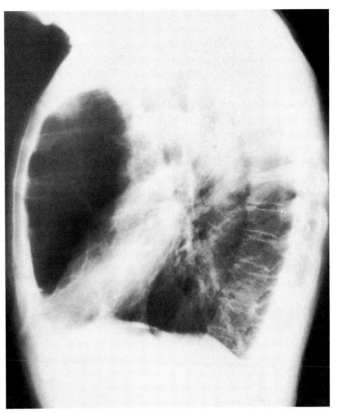

Fig. 6.20 Emphysema in a man of 52. Lateral film shows increased lung volume, which is producing a barrel chest. The retrosternal space is deeper than normal and extends more inferiorly than normal.

generalised is usually patchy. Involved areas have fewer vessels than normal, and those vessels that remain are small. Mild degrees of vascular attenuation are difficult to perceive, so it is worth comparing the size of vessels in different zones. If vessels are diminished in calibre and number in a particular zone, compared to another, that zone is likely to be emphysematous.

Peripheral vascular attenuation is due to a number of factors. Perfusion of emphysematous lung is less than normal, and pulmonary blood flow is diverted to less affected areas of lung. Pulmonary vessels are displaced around emphysematous areas and bullae. Small arteries are obliterated by the primary emphysematous process, but these vessels are too small to be visualised radiographically, and this process, therefore, probably does not contribute to the oligaemic appearances, but may be a factor in increased radiolucency of affected areas.

Panacinar emphysema has a tendency to affect the lung bases and may cause diversion of blood flow to the upper zones, which should not be mistaken for pulmonary venous hypertension. In α_1-antitrypsin deficiency the changes of emphysema tend to be basal. Air trapping causes hyperinflation of the lungs, and may lead to flattening of the diaphragm and increased anteroposterior diameter of the thorax. Flattening of the diaphragm is often best seen on the lateral projection, the level of the diaphragm often being as low as the eleventh rib posteriorly. Some normal individuals can push their diaphragm as low on full inspiration, but on expiration the diaphragm will rise 5–10 cm, whereas in emphysema excursion of the diaphragm is usually less than 3 cm. In severe emphysema the diaphragm may actually be inverted.

The 'barrel chest' is caused by bowing of the sternum and increased thoracic kyphosis. The retrosternal air space may increase in depth, and extend inferiorly between the anterior surface of the heart and the sternum (Fig. 6.20).

The heart often appears long and narrow. This is probably due primarily to the low position of the diaphragm altering the projection of the heart. Enlargement of the central pulmonary arteries usually signifies pulmonary arterial hypertension (Fig. 6.19). If cor pulmonale develops, the heart may enlarge due to right ventricular dilatation. In patients with emphysema who develop left heart failure, the signs of hyperinflation may decrease, and the level of the diaphragm will rise. This is due to pulmonary oedema decreasing the compliance of the lung and thus reducing the lung volume. In these patients the distribution of oedema fluid within emphysematous lung may be bizarre.

CT is more sensitive than the plain chest X-ray in detecting the presence and distribution of emphysema (Fig. 6.21). Vascular attenuation may be detected earlier, and bullae may be identified by CT when not visible on the chest X-ray. In addition expiratory scans may identify areas of air trapping.

2. Bullous disease of the lungs Bullae are usually present in the lung in association with some form of emphysema, but occasionally bullae occur locally in otherwise normal lung (Fig. 6.22). They commonly occur in paraseptal emphysema, and in emphysema associated with scarring, but clinically the most important bullae are those due to panacinar emphysema, with or without chronic bronchitis.

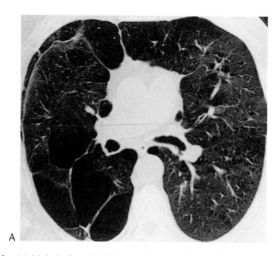
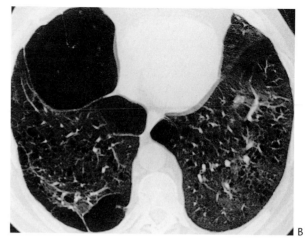

A   B

Fig. 6.21 Multiple bullae. (A) CT scan through the level of the right main pulmonary artery reveals multiple bullae predominantly in the right lung. (B) CT scan further toward the lung bases revealing several further bullae. Some of these have well-defined walls.

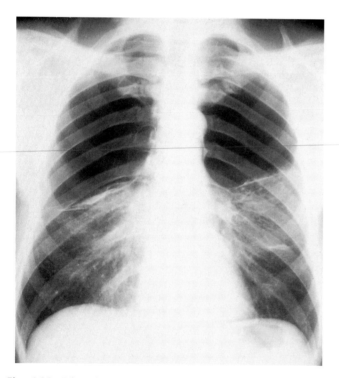

Fig. 6.22 Bilateral upper zone bullae in a man of 35. 'Routine' chest X-ray—no history or symptoms of respiratory disease. Both upper zones are occupied by large bullae which are compressing the upper lobes. There is no evidence of generalised emphysema or air trapping. The level and shape of the diaphragm are normal.

Bullae appear as round or oval translucencies varying in size from 1 cm in diameter to occupation of almost an entire hemithorax (Fig. 6.23). They may be single or multiple, and are usually peripheral. In asymptomatic patients and in those with pulmonary scarring, bullae tend to be apical, but in chronic obstructive airways disease bullae are found throughout the lungs (Fig. 6.21). Their walls may be visible as a smooth, curved, hairline shadow. If the walls are not visible, displacement of vessels around a radiolucent area may indicate a bullous area.

Bullae are usually air-filled but may become infected and filled with fluid. Associated inflammatory change may be present in the surrounding lung. A bulla will show a fluid level if it is partially fluid-filled, or will appear solid if completely fluid-filled (Fig. 6.24).

A giant bulla may be difficult to differentiate from a loculated pneumothorax, and CT may be necessary to demonstrate the wall of the bulla or thin strands of lung tissue crossing it.

3. *Emphysema with chronic bronchitis* Many patients with chronic obstructive airways disease have emphysema *and* chronic

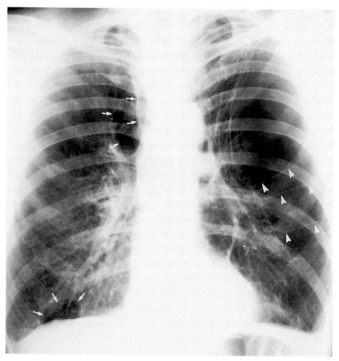

Fig. 6.23 Emphysema with bullae in a man of 61. The lungs are hyperinflated. A giant bulla occupies most of the left hemithorax, compressing the left lung. Strands of lung tissue (arrowheads) are seen crossing this bulla. Small bullae (arrows) are also present in the right lung.

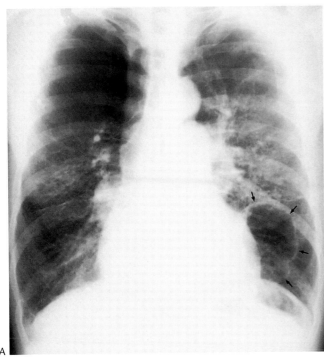
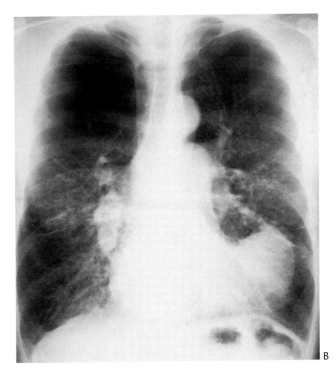

Fig. 6.24 Emphysema with infected bulla in a man of 48. (A) The lungs are hyperinflated. The right upper zone is occupied by a large bulla, and another bulla is seen adjacent to the left heart border (arrows). The central pulmonary arteries are enlarged. (B) Following a chest infection the left-sided bulla has filled with fluid and appears completely opaque.

bronchitis. The chest X-ray may then show a combination of changes of hyperinflation, pulmonary arterial hypertension and increased bronchovascular markings of the so-called 'dirty chest'.

At one end of the clinical spectrum is the 'pink puffer' who, by major effort, ventilates sufficient alveoli to maintain normal blood gases; since there is no hypoxaemia, normal pulmonary artery pressure is preserved. Pink puffers tend to have predominantly panacinar emphysema, and the chest X-ray shows peripheral vascular attenuation and hyperinflation. This appearance may be termed the 'arterial deficiency' pattern.

At the other end of the clinical spectrum is the 'blue bloater', who chronically retains carbon dioxide due to poor alveolar ventilation. The respiratory centre becomes insensitive to the persistently raised concentration of arterial carbon dioxide, and chronic cyanosis occurs. Chronic hypoxaemia causes pulmonary arteriolar constriction, and in due course pulmonary arterial hypertension and cor pulmonale occur. Blue bloaters tend to have centriacinar emphysema and less extensive panacinar emphysema. The chest X-ray shows increased bronchovascular markings, enlarged central pulmonary arteries and possibly cardiac enlargement. This appearance may be termed the 'increased markings' pattern of emphysema, and signs of hyperinflation are rarely severe. Most patients with chronic bronchitis and emphysema exhibit features between these extremes.

4. *Swyer–James or MacLeod's syndrome* Classically this syndrome is based on the chest X-ray appearance of a hypertransradiant hemithorax. It is probably the result of a childhood viral infection causing bronchiolitis and obliteration of the small airways; the involved distal airways are ventilated by collateral air drift, and air trapping may lead to panacinar emphysema.

However, CT of patients shows that although one lung tends to be more affected than the other, there are usually bilateral abnormalities characterised by bronchiectasis and areas of hypertransradiancy. The basic pathology is a constrictive obliterative bronchiolitis (see below), although it has previously, inappropriately been called 'unilateral or lobar emphysema'.

The affected lung is hypertransradiant, due to decreased perfusion, and may be smaller than normal. The ipsilateral pulmonary artery is visible, but small, and the peripheral vascular pattern is attenuated. Air trapping occurs in the affected lung, which tends to maintain its volume on expiration, resulting in displacement of the mediastinum to the more normal side, and restriction of the ipsilateral hemidiaphragm (Fig. 6.25).

The syndrome may also be illustrated by radionuclide scanning, when a perfusion scan will show reduced flow to the affected lung, and a ventilation scan, using xenon, will demonstrate air trapping.

The differential diagnosis of the chest X-ray appearance includes proximal interruption of the pulmonary artery, the hypogenetic lung syndrome and pulmonary artery obstruction due to embolism. However, none of these entities exhibits air trapping.

5. *Centriacinar emphysema* This occurs principally in chronic bronchitis and uncomplicated coal miner's pneumoconiosis. The radiological appearance is that of the primary condition. In later stages panacinar and bullous emphysema may become apparent.

6. *Obstructive 'emphysema'* Obstructive hyperinflation may affect an entire lung, a lobe or a segment. The cause—such as an inhaled foreign body or tooth, or a central tumour—may be apparent on the chest X-ray. The vascular pattern of the affected part of the lung is attenuated, and this area may appear hypertransradiant.

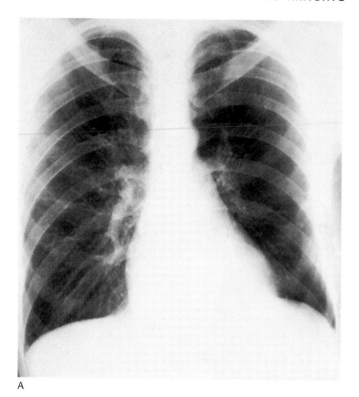

A

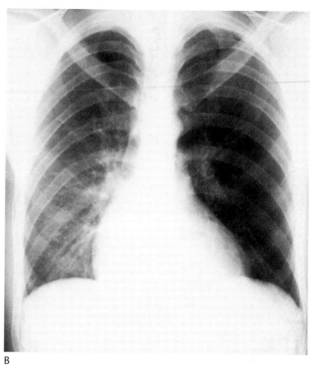

B

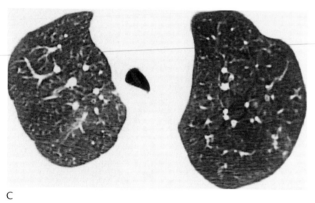

C

Fig. 6.25 Unilateral emphysema in a man of 30 with a history of repeated chest infections as a child, but no current respiratory symptoms. (A) Inspiratory film shows normal right lung and hypertransradiant left lung with small left pulmonary artery. (B) Expiratory film demonstrates displacement of mediastinum to the right and restricted movement of the left hemidiaphragm, indicating air trapping in the left lung. (C) CT scan through the upper lobes of a different patient with unilateral emphysema. At end expiration there is air trapping within the left lung where the vessels are relatively attenuated.

Fluoroscopy or an expiratory film will demonstrate air trapping in the affected area with deviation of the mediastinum to the normal side, and restriction of the ipsilateral hemidiaphragm on expiration.

7. Compensatory 'emphysema' The radiological signs resulting from collapse or removal of all or part of a lung are discussed in the section on lobar collapse (see pp. 176–179).

8. Congenital lobar emphysema This is discussed in Chapter 9.

BRONCHIOLITIS

The term bronchiolitis encompasses a range of conditions.

1. Acute bronchiolitis This occurs in children, usually in the first year of life, and is most commonly the result of respiratory syncytial virus infection. The condition is usually self limiting;

nevertheless, in the UK, it is the main cause of paediatric hospital admission during the winter months. Radiologically the appearances are most frequently hyperinflation of the lungs and perihilar prominence and indistinctness. When it is due to respiratory syncitial or adenovirus infection there is an increased risk of subsequent development of constrictive obliterative bronchiolitis.

2. Obliterative bronchiolitis (OB) Bronchiolar obliteration may result from peribronchiolar inflammation and scarring which causes constrictive obliterative bronchiolitis, or from development of intraluminal granulation tissue, which causes a proliferative bronchiolitis and may be found in association with chronic organising pneumonia (see below). *Constrictive OB* may result from a viral bronchiolitis (often in childhood), from inhalation of toxic fumes, drug therapy (classically penicillamine) or rheumatoid disease. It may also complicate lung or heart-lung transplantation and bone marrow transplantation. Obliterative bronchiolitis resulting from childhood viral infection may present in adult life as Swyer-James syndrome. The chest radiograph may show evidence of pulmonary hyperinflation, and decreased vascularity in the mid and lower zones. Changes on HRCT include bronchial dilatation with or without patchy (mosaic) areas of hypertransradiancy, probably due to air trapping (Fig. 6.26).

3. *Respiratory bronchiolitis — associated interstitial lung disease (RB-ILD)* This condition is seen in heavy smokers and is due to an inflammatory process involving the respiratory bronchioles, alveolar ducts and alveoli. It may be responsible for some of the abnormal ill-defined opacities often seen on the chest X-rays of smokers (Fig. 6.18). HRCT may show patchy, ground-glass shadowing and thickening of interlobular septa.

4. *Panbronchiolitis* Diffuse panbronchiolitis, often referred to as Japanese panbronchiolitis because of its relative frequency in Japan and the Far East, is a disorder characterised by bronchial

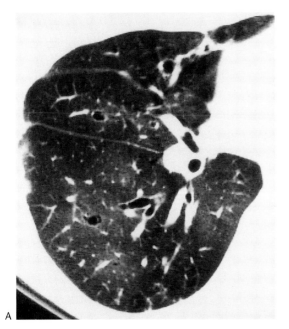

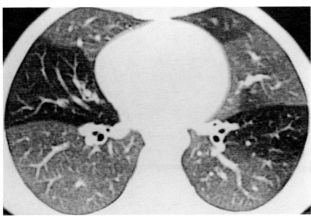

Fig. 6.26 Obliterative bronchiolitis due to graft-versus-host disease. (A) Close-up view of the right lower zone reveals patchy areas of higher and lower attenuation and thin-walled dilated bronchi. (B) Obliterative bronchiolitis in a different patient. A CT scan obtained at end expiration shows marked variation in the CT attenuation within the lungs. The relatively hypodense areas have failed to deflate due to small airways disease.

inflammation and chronic sinus infection. Eventually pulmonary function tests become obstructive, and bronchiectasis and respiratory failure may develop. Although the chest radiograph may demonstrate mid and lower zone nodules, becoming more profuse and widespread as the disease progresses, the bronchiolitis is best demonstrated by HRCT. This demonstrates small branching opacities which pathologically correspond to respiratory bronchioles surrounded by and containing an inflammatory infiltrate (Fig. 6.27). Treatment involves low-dose long-term erythromycin and supportive measures.

CRYPTOGENIC ORGANIZING PNEUMONITIS AND BRONCHIOLITIS OBLITERANS ORGANIZING PNEUMONIA

COP and *BOOP*, two recently recognised entities, are effectively the same condition, described independently in the UK and the USA at approximately the same time. To avoid confusion with the largely separate condition of obliterative bronchiolitis, COP is suggested as the preferred term. It probably represents one possible response of the lung to an inflammatory stimulus. Numerous drugs have been implicated as causing COP, as well as various infections (viral, bacterial and fungal), most connective tissue diseases and many immune disorders.

Patients are typically middle aged, and there is no preponderance of either sex. Frequently the patient has had a systemic illness lasting a few weeks or months with a non-productive cough, dyspnoea, malaise and a low-grade fever. Often antibiotics have been administered without response, and no organism has been identified. The chest radiograph usually demonstrates consolidation which is patchy, non-segmental and chronic (Fig. 6.28). On HRCT there is air-space consolidation, usually in the lower half of the lungs: in 50% of cases with a predominantly subpleural distribution, and in 30–50% of cases in a peribronchovascular distribution (Fig. 6.29). Lung biopsy, which characteristically demonstrates small airways and adjacent air spaces plugged with granulation tissue, may be required to make the diagnosis, and there is often a dramatic clinical and radiological response to corticosteroid therapy.

Bronchocele and mucoid impaction

Obstruction of a segmental bronchus may lead to accumulation of secretions and pus in the lung distally. If collateral air drift allows

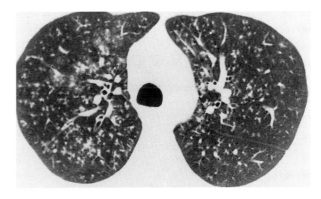

Fig. 6.27 Panbronchiolitis. There are multiple branching opacities representing distended and occluded small airways.

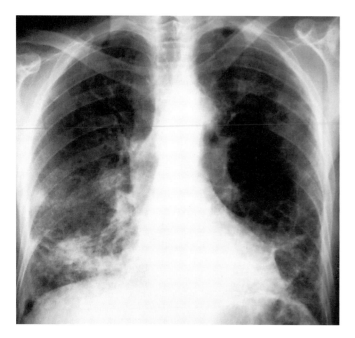

Fig. 6.28 Cryptogenic organising pneumonia in a 70-year-old man with chronic consolidation. The appearances had been unchanged for several weeks despite multiple courses of antibiotics.

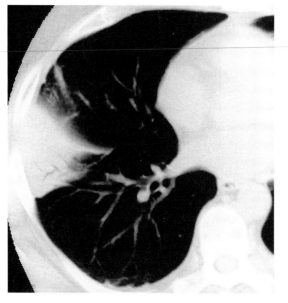

Fig. 6.29 Cryptogenic organising pneumonia. There is a wedge-shaped pleurally based patch of consolidation containing an air bronchogram. The diagnosis was confirmed following a percutaneous needle biopsy.

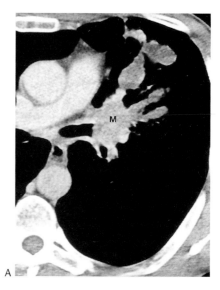

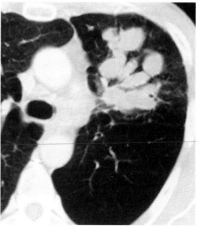

Fig. 6.30 Bronchocele secondary to a left hilar tumour. (A) On mediastinal windows there are fluid density opacities radiating out from the left hilar mass (M). (B) A scan at a slightly more cranial level on lung window settings shows multiple rounded opacities in the left upper lobe due to mucoid impaction within obstructed bronchi.

the affected lung to remain aerated, a bronchocele or bronchial mucocele may develop. The obstruction may be congenital or due to endobronchial tumour or inhaled foreign body, or to inflammatory stricture or extrinsic compression. Mucoid impaction in asthma, allergic bronchopulmonary aspergillosis and cystic fibrosis may produce a similar obstruction. The typical appearance on the chest radiograph is a group of oval or cigar-shaped shadows, which may appear to branch (Fig. 6.30): they lie along the axis of the bronchial tree and point toward the hilum.

Bronchial atresia

Bronchial atresia is an uncommon condition that usually presents as an incidental well-defined pulmonary opacity, most frequently in the left upper lobe. The surrounding lung is emphysematous, a feature best demonstrated on CT (Fig. 6.31). Pathologically there is mucus impaction and dilatation distal to a short atresia in a segmental bronchus. Although the diagnosis can be suggested confidently from the typical HRCT appearances, resection of the affected segment is often undertaken due to the remote possibility of a small occluding neoplasm. The majority of cases occur in the left upper lobe, with the right upper lobe and lower lobes being involved with reducing frequency.

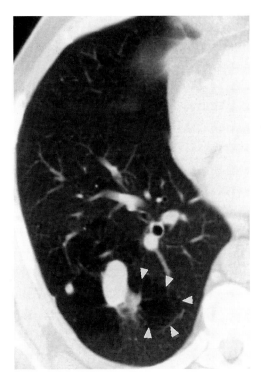

Fig. 6.31 Bronchial atresia. There is a well-defined opacity in the right lower lobe surrounded by a patch of emphysematous lung (arrowheads).

THE LUNGS—COLLAPSE AND CONSOLIDATION

COLLAPSE

Partial or complete loss of volume of a lung is referred to as collapse or atelectasis. Current usage has made these terms synonymous, and they imply a diminished volume of air in the lung with associated reduction of lung volume. This contrasts with consolidation, in which a diminished volume of air in the lung is associated with normal lung volume. There are several different mechanisms which may cause pulmonary collapse.

Mechanisms of collapse

Relaxation or passive collapse

This is the mechanism whereby the lung tends to retract toward its hilum when air or increased fluid collects in the pleural space. It is discussed above under diseases of the pleura.

Cicatrisation collapse

As discussed in the section on the pleura, normal lung expansion depends upon a balance between outward forces in the chest wall and opposite elastic forces in the lung. When the lung is abnormally stiff, this balance is disturbed, lung compliance is decreased and the volume of the affected lung is reduced. This occurs with pulmonary fibrosis.

Adhesive collapse

The surface tension of the alveoli is decreased by surfactant. If this mechanism is disturbed, as in the respiratory distress syndrome, collapse of alveoli occurs, although the central airways remain patent.

Resorption collapse

In acute bronchial obstruction the gases in the alveoli are steadily taken up by the blood in the pulmonary capillaries and are not replenished, causing alveolar collapse. The degree of collapse may be modified by collateral air drift if the obstruction is distal to the main bronchus, and also by infection and accumulation of secretions. If the obstruction becomes chronic, subsequent resorption of intra-alveolar secretions and exudate may result in complete collapse. This is the usual mechanism of collapse seen in carcinoma of the bronchus.

Radiological signs of collapse

The radiographic appearance in pulmonary collapse depends upon the mechanism of collapse, the degree of collapse, the presence or absence of consolidation, and the pre-existing state of the pleura. Signs of collapse may be considered as direct or indirect. Indirect signs are the results of compensatory changes which occur in response to the volume loss.

Direct signs of collapse

Displacement of interlobar fissures
This is the most reliable sign, and the degree of displacement will depend on the extent of the collapse.

Loss of aeration
Increased density of a collapsed area of lung may not become apparent until collapse is almost complete. However, if the collapsed lung is adjacent to the mediastinum or diaphragm, obscuration of the adjacent structures may indicate loss of aeration.

Vascular and bronchial signs
If a lobe is partially collapsed, crowding of its vessels may be visible; if an air bronchogram is visible, the bronchi may appear crowded.

Indirect signs of collapse

Elevation of the hemidiaphragm
This sign may be seen in lower lobe collapse, but is rare in collapse of the other lobes.

Mediastinal displacement
In upper lobe collapse the trachea is often displaced toward the affected side, and in lower lobe collapse the heart may be displaced.

Hilar displacement
The hilum may be elevated in upper lobe collapse, and depressed in lower lobe collapse.

Compensatory hyperinflation

The normal part of the lung may become hyperinflated, and it may appear hypertransradiant, with its vessels more widely spaced than in the corresponding area of the contralateral lung. If there is considerable collapse of a lung, compensatory hyperinflation of the contralateral lung may occur, with herniation across the midline.

Patterns of collapse

An air bronchogram is almost never seen in resorption collapse, but is usual in passive and adhesive collapse, and may be seen in cicatrisation collapse if fibrosis is particularly dense.

Pre-existing lung disease such as fibrosis and pleural adhesions may alter the expected displacement of anatomic landmarks in lung collapse. There also tends to be a reciprocal relationship between the compensatory signs: e.g. in lower lobe collapse, if diaphragmatic elevation is marked, hilar depression will be diminished.

Complete collapse of a lung

Complete collapse of a lung, in the absence of pneumothorax or large pleural effusion or extensive consolidation, causes opacification of the hemithorax, displacement of the mediastinum to the affected side and elevation of the diaphragm. Compensatory hyperinflation of the contralateral lung occurs, often with herniation across the midline (Fig. 6.32). Herniation most often occurs in the retrosternal space, anterior to the ascending aorta, but may occur posterior to the heart or under the aortic arch (Fig. 6.33).

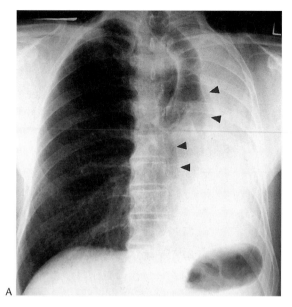

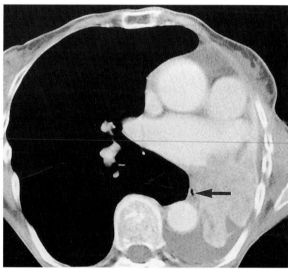

Fig. 6.33 Complete collapse of the left lung due to a left hilar tumour. (A) The chest radiograph demonstrates deviation of the trachea and shift of the mediastinum to the left. Air–soft-tissue interfaces are seen due to herniation of the right lung across the midline (arrowheads). (B) CT scan demonstrates herniation of both the retrosternal lung and the azygo-oesophageal reflection. The oesophagus contains a small amount of air (arrow).

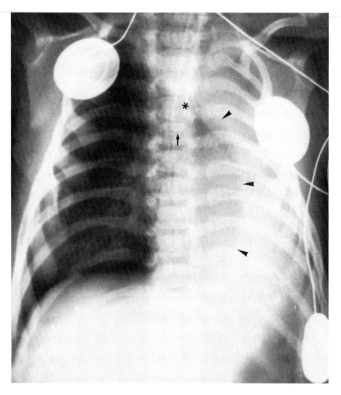

Fig. 6.32 Complete collapse of the left lung. A newborn child with complex cyanotic heart disease. The tip of the endotracheal tube (arrow) is beyond the carina (asterisk) and down the right bronchus, causing collapse of the left lung and compensatory hyperinflation of the right lung which has herniated across the midline (arrowheads).

Lobar collapse

The following descriptions apply to collapse of individual lobes, uncomplicated by pre-existing pulmonary or pleural disease. The line drawings (Figs 6.34, 6.36, 6.38, 6.40, 6.43) represent the alteration in position of the fissures, as seen in the frontal and lateral projections, resulting from increasing degrees of collapse. Only the fissures are represented. The indirect signs of collapse are not indicated.

Right upper lobe collapse *(Figs 6.34, 6.35)* The normal horizontal fissure is usually at the level of the right fourth rib anteriorly. As the right upper lobe collapses, the horizontal fissure pivots about the hilum, its lateral end moving upward and medially toward the superior mediastinum, and its anterior end moving

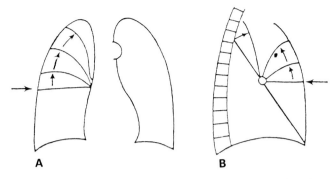

Fig. 6.34 Right upper lobe collapse. (A) PA projection. Note how lesser fissure is drawn upward, and often curved, toward the apex and mediastinum. (B) Right lateral view. Lesser fissure also displaced upward. Note some forward displacement of greater fissure above the hilum.

upward toward the apex. The upper half of the oblique fissure moves anteriorly. The two fissures become concave superiorly. In severe collapse the lobe may be flattened against the superior mediastinum, and may obscure the upper pole of the hilum. The hilum is elevated, and its lower pole may be prominent. Deviation of the trachea to the right is usual, and compensatory hyperinflation of the right middle and lower lobes may be apparent.

Right middle lobe collapse *(Figs 6.36, 6.37)* In right middle lobe collapse the horizontal fissure and lower half of the oblique fissure move toward one another. This can best be seen in the lateral projection. The horizontal fissure tends to be more mobile, and therefore usually shows greater displacement. Signs of right middle lobe collapse are often subtle on the frontal projection, since the horizontal fissure may not be visible, and increased opacity does not become apparent until collapse is almost complete. However, obscuration of the right heart border is often

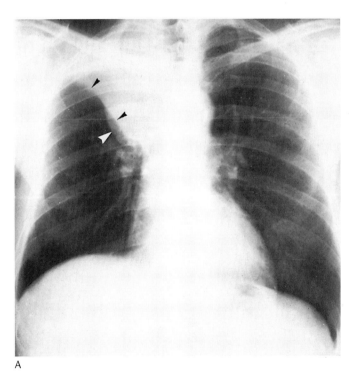

A

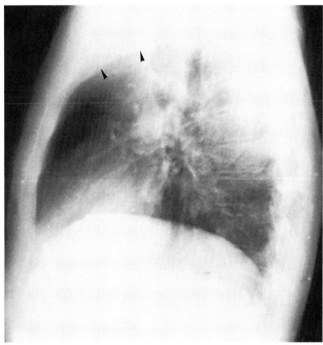

B

Fig. 6.35 (A) PA film shows a mass (white arrowhead) above the right hilum, and elevation of the horizontal fissure (black arrowheads). There is compensatory hyperinflation of the right lower lobe. (B) Lateral film shows anterior displacement of part of oblique fissure (arrowheads). (C) CT scan of right upper lobe collapse in a different patient (images on mediastinal window settings.)

C

present, and may be the only clue in this projection. The *lordotic AP projection* brings the displaced fissure into the line of the X-ray beam, and may elegantly demonstrate right middle lobe collapse. Since the volume of this lobe is relatively small, indirect signs of volume loss are rarely present.

Lower lobe collapse *(Figs 16.38–16.41)* The normal oblique fissures extend from the level of the fourth thoracic vertebra posteriorly to the diaphragm, close to the sternum, anteriorly. The position of these fissures on the lateral projection is the best index of lower lobe volumes. When a lower lobe collapses its oblique

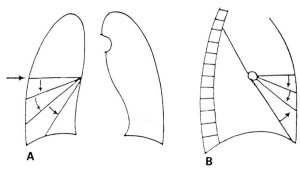
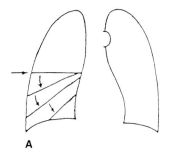
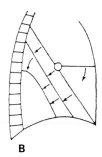

Fig. 6.36   Right middle lobe collapse. In both projections the lesser fissure is drawn downward. In the PA view (A) the fissure finally merges with the mediastinum and disappears. Note in the lateral view (B) that the lower part of the greater fissure may be displaced forward.

Fig. 6.38   Right lower lobe collapse. In the PA projection (A) the greater fissure is not visible until the collapse is fairly complete. The lesser fissure is displaced downward as in collapse of the middle lobe. The degree of displacement seen may be greater in collapse of the lower lobe than of the middle lobe, as the middle lobe tends to retract toward the hilum and the fissure may disappear. In the lateral view (B), the oblique fissure moves backward, tending to retain its obliquity. The upper part of the oblique fissure may curve backward and downward, so becoming visible in the PA projection.

fissure moves posteriorly but maintains its normal slope. In addition to posterior movement, the collapsing lower lobe causes medial displacement of the oblique fissure, which may then become visible in places on the frontal projection.

Right lower lobe collapse   This causes depression of the horizontal fissure, which may be apparent on the frontal projection. Increased opacity of a collapsed lower lobe is usually visible on the frontal projection. A completely collapsed lower lobe may be so small that it flattens and merges with the mediastinum, producing a thin, wedge-shaped shadow. On the left this shadow may be obscured by the heart, and a penetrated view with a grid may be required for its visualisation. If complete *left lower lobe collapse* is still in doubt, a right oblique film may demonstrate the wedge of tissue between spine and diaphragm. Mediastinal struc-

tures and parts of the diaphragm adjacent to the non-aerated lobe are obscured.

The hilum is usually depressed and rotated medially, and upper lobe hyperinflation is evident, but diaphragmatic elevation is not usual.

Lingula collapse *(Fig. 6.42)*   The lingula is often involved in collapse of the left upper lobe, but it may collapse individually, when the radiological features are similar to right middle lobe collapse. However, the absence of a horizontal fissure on the left makes anterior displacement of the lower half of the oblique

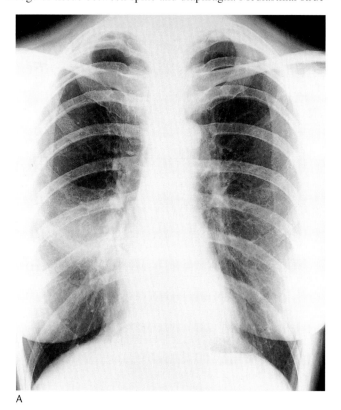

A

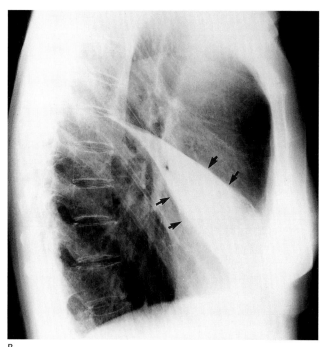

B

Fig. 6.37   Right middle lobe collapse. (A) PA film shows loss of definition of the right heart border indicating loss of aeration of the middle lobe. (B) A lateral film shows partial collapse of the middle lobe evident as a wedge-shaped opacity (arrows).

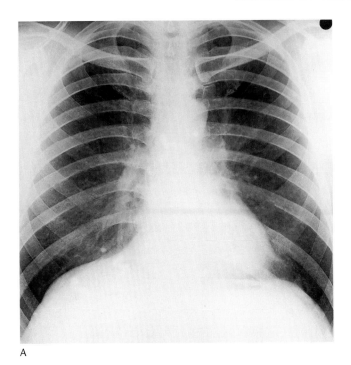

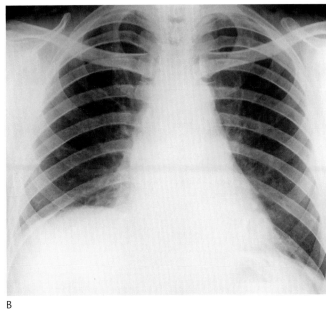

A

B

Fig. 6.39 Right lower lobe collapse. (A) Normal preoperative film. (B) Following coronary artery bypass surgery there is right lower lobe collapse with depression and medial rotation of the hilum, elevation of the right hemidiaphragm and hyperinflation of the right upper lobe.

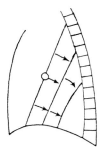

Fig. 6.40 Left lower lobe collapse. No fissure is visible in the PA projection. The lateral view shows that the greater fissure is displaced posteriorly as in collapse of the right lower lobe. The upper part of the fissure may also be drawn downward as well as backward.

fissure and increased opacity anterior to it important signs. On the frontal projection the left heart border becomes obscured.

Left upper lobe collapse *(Figs 6.42–6.44)* The pattern of upper lobe collapse is different in the two lungs. Left upper lobe collapse is apparent on the lateral projection as anterior displacement of the entire oblique fissure, which becomes oriented almost parallel to the anterior chest wall. With increasing collapse the upper lobe retracts posteriorly and loses contact with the anterior chest wall. The space between the collapsed lobe and the sternum becomes occupied by either hyperinflated left lower lobe or herniated right upper lobe. With complete collapse, the left upper lobe may lose contact with the chest wall and diaphragm and retract medially against the mediastinum. On a lateral film, therefore, left upper lobe collapse appears as an elongated opacity extending from the apex and reaching, or almost reaching, the diaphragm; it is anterior to the hilum and is bounded by displaced oblique fissure posteriorly, and by hyperinflated lower lobe anteriorly.

A collapsed left upper lobe does not produce a sharp outline on the frontal view. An ill-defined hazy opacity is present in the upper, mid and sometimes lower zones, the opacity being densest near the hilum. Pulmonary vessels in the hyperinflated lower lobe are usually visible through the haze. The aortic knuckle is usually obscured, unless the upper lobe has collapsed anterior to it, allowing it to be outlined by lower lobe. If the lingula is involved, the left heart border is obscured. The hilum is often elevated, and the trachea is often deviated to the left.

Rounded atelectasis *(Fig. 6.45)* This is an unusual form of pulmonary collapse which may be misdiagnosed as a pulmonary mass. It appears on the plain film as a homogenous mass, up to 5 cm in diameter, with ill-defined edges. It is always pleural-based and associated with pleural thickening. Vascular shadows may be seen to radiate from part of the opacity, resembling a comet's tail. The appearance is caused by peripheral lung tissue folding in on itself. It is often related to asbestos exposure, but may occur secondary to any exudative pleural effusion. It is not of any other pathological significance. The CT appearance is usually diagnostic, and enables differentiation from other pulmonary masses.

CONSOLIDATION

Functionally the pulmonary airways can be divided into two groups. The proximal airways function purely as a conducting network; the airways distal to the terminal bronchioles are also conducting structures, but, more importantly, are the site of gaseous exchange. These terminal airways are termed acini, an acinus comprising respiratory bronchioles, alveolar ducts, alveolar

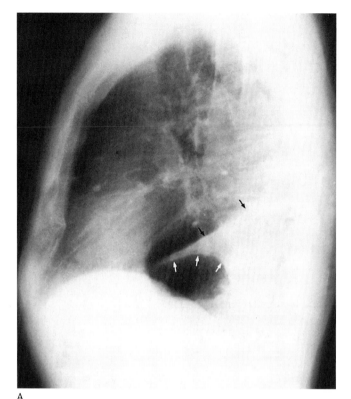

A

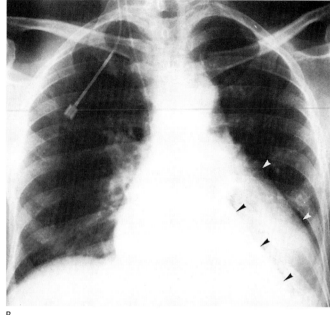

B

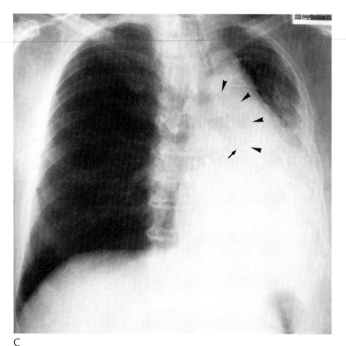

C

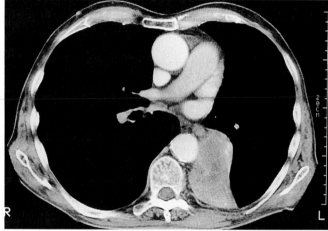

D

Fig. 6.41 (A) Sixty-six-year-old man with squamous cell carcinoma of the left lower lobe. The oblique fissure is displaced posteriorly (black arrows). The left hemidiaphragm is obscured by the collapsed lobe, but the position of the stomach bubble (white arrows) indicates that the left hemidiaphragm is elevated. (B) Postoperative film of patient with aortic valve replacement. The shadow of the collapsed left lower lobe (black arrowheads) is seen through the shadow of the heart (white arrowheads). (C) Fifty-seven-year-old man with oat cell carcinoma occluding the left bronchus (arrow). The left lower lobe is collapsed, obscuring the left hemidiaphragm. The mediastinum is shifted to the left, and part of the hyperinflated right lung has herniated across the midline (arrowheads). (D) Left lower lobe collapse demonstrated on CT. There is mixed density within the collapsed lung, probably due to fluid-filled bronchi.

sacs and alveoli arising from a terminal bronchiole. Consolidation implies replacement of air in one or more acini by fluid or solid material, but does not imply a particular pathology or aetiology. The smallest unit of consolidated lung is a single acinus, which casts a shadow approximately 7 mm in diameter. Communications between the terminal airways allow fluid to spread between adjacent acini, so that larger confluent areas of consolidation are generally visible and are frequently not confined to a single segment.

The commonest cause of consolidation is acute inflammatory exudate associated with pneumonia. Other causes include *cardiogenic pulmonary oedema, non-cardiogenic pulmonary oedema, haemorrhage* and *aspiration. Neoplasms* such as alveolar-cell carcinoma and lymphoma can produce consolidation, and *alveolar proteinosis* is a rare cause. In an individual patient, consolidation may be due to more than one basic aetiology. For example, a patient with major head trauma may be particularly susceptible to infection, aspiration and non-cardiogenic pulmonary oedema.

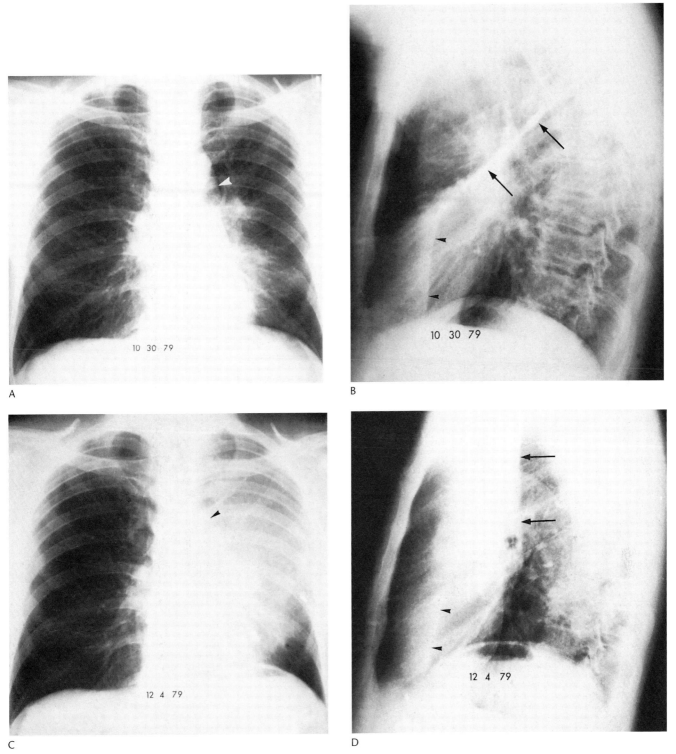

Fig. 6.42 Lingula and left upper lobe collapse in a man with carcinoma at the left hilum. (A) PA film shows hazy left heart border, indicating loss of aeration of the lingula. A mass is present in the aortopulmonary window (arrowhead). (B) Lateral film shows collapse-consolidation of the lingula, with anterior displacement of the lower part of the oblique fissure (arrowheads). The upper part of the oblique fissure (arrows) is thickened, but in normal position. (C) Five weeks later the left upper lobe has collapsed. A hazy opacity covers most of the left hemithorax. Vessels in the hyperinflated left lower lobe can just be seen through the haze, and the aortic knuckle is obscured (arrowhead). (D) Lateral film shows that the oblique fissure is now displaced anteriorly (arrows).

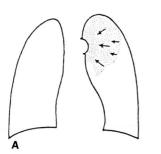
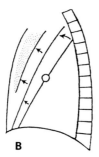

Fig. 6.43 Left upper lobe collapse. (A) The greater fissure does not become visible in the PA projection. When the degree of collapse is fairly complete the lobe shows a uniform loss of translucency (this may be due to accompanying consolidation), which increases in density as the degree of collapse increases. Vessel markings seen through this opacity are those in the overexpanded lower lobe. (B) In the lateral view, initially the fissure moves bodily forward, the lingula remaining in contact with the diaphragm. With increasing collapse the lingula retracts upward, and the bulk of the upper lobe moves posteriorly, and becomes separated from the sternum by aerated lung. This is usually overexpanded lower lobe, though occasionally a portion of the right lung may herniate across the midline.

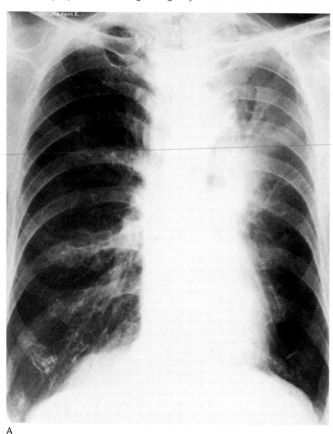

A

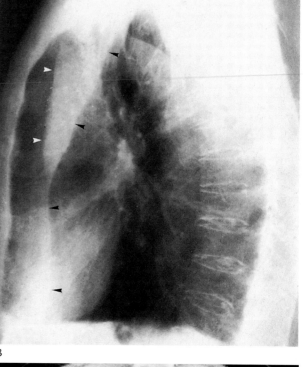

B

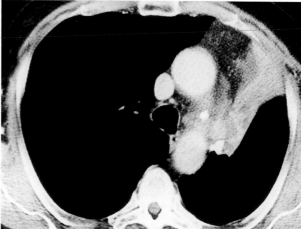

C

Fig. 6.44 Left upper lobe collapse due to squamous cell carcinoma. (A) PA film shows typical upper zone haze, through which is seen the elevated and enlarged left hilum, and vessels of the hyperinflated lower lobe. The contour of the aortic knuckle is indistinct, but the descending aorta is sharply outlined. (B) Lateral film shows the collapsed left upper lobe between the anteriorly displaced oblique fissure (arrow heads) and part of the hyperinflated lower lobe. (C) CT demonstration of left upper lobe collapse. Calcified lymph nodes due to previous tuberculosis are visible.

When consolidation is associated with a patent conducting airway an *air bronchogram* (Fig. 6.46) is often visible. This sign is produced by the radiographic contrast between the column of air in the airway and the surrounding opaque acini. If consolidation is secondary to bronchial obstruction, however, the air in the conducting airway is resorbed and replaced by fluid, and the affected area is of uniform density.

The volume of purely consolidated lung is similar to that of the normal lung since air is replaced by a similar volume of fluid or solid. However, collapse and consolidation are often associated with one another. When consolidation is due to fluid, its distribution is influenced by gravity, so that in acute pneumonitis consolidation is often denser and more clearly demarcated inferiorly by a pleural surface, and is less dense and more indistinct superiorly.

Ultrasound may demonstrate consolidation in adjacent lung (Fig. 6.47). When air bronchograms are evident on the chest radiograph these may be manifest as echogenic linear structures. When

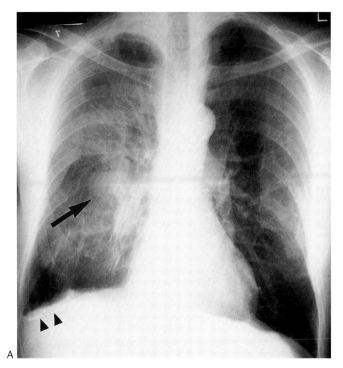

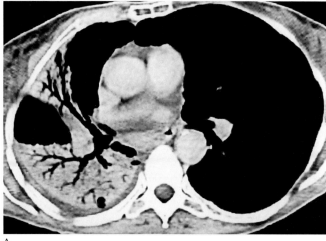

A

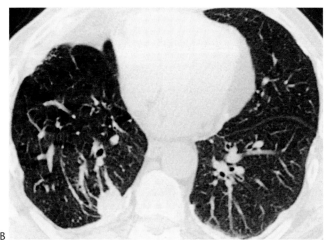

B

Fig. 6.45 Rounded atelectasis in a patient with a history of asbestos exposure. (A) Chest radiograph shows en face pleural plaque on the right with calcified pleural plaques over the dome of the right diaphragm (arrowheads). There is the suggestion of a right infrahilar mass. (B) High-resolution CT demonstrates indrawing of the bronchovascular structures into a pleurally based mass. The appearances are typical of rounded atelectasis. There is widespread calcified pleural plaque.

the bronchi become fluid filled they are more clearly demonstrated as echo-free branching structures.

Lobar consolidation

Consolidation of a complete lobe produces a homogenous opacity, possibly containing an air bronchogram, delineated by the chest wall, mediastinum or diaphragm and the appropriate interlobar fissure or fissures. Parts of the diaphragm and mediastinum adjacent to the non-aerated lung are obscured.

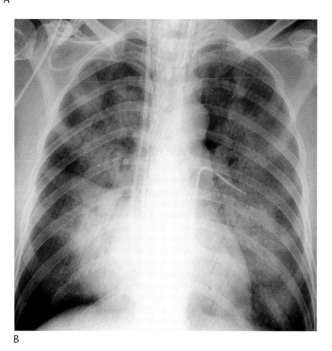

A

B

Fig. 6.46 Air bronchogram. (A) CT shows patent air-filled bronchi surrounded by widespread pulmonary consolidation due to an acute bacterial chest infection. (B) Chest radiograph of a different patient following aspiration of gastric contents demonstrating widespread air-space shadowing containing air bronchograms.

Right upper lobe consolidation *(Fig. 6.48)* This is confined by the horizontal fissure inferiorly and the upper half of the oblique fissure posteriorly, and may obscure the right upper mediastinum.

Right middle lobe consolidation *(Fig. 6.49)* This is limited by the horizontal fissure above, and the lower half of the oblique fissure posteriorly, and may obscure the right heart border.

Lower lobe consolidation *(Fig. 6.50)* This is limited by the oblique fissure anteriorly, and may obscure the diaphragm.

Left upper lobe and lingula consolidation *(Fig. 6.51)* These are limited by the oblique fissure posteriorly. Lingula consolidation may obscure the left heart border, and consolidation of the upper lobe may obscure the aortic knuckle.

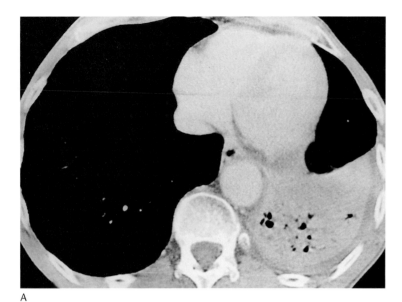

A

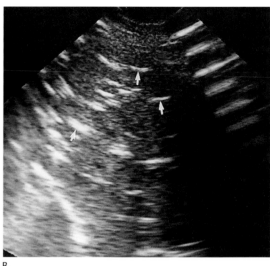

B

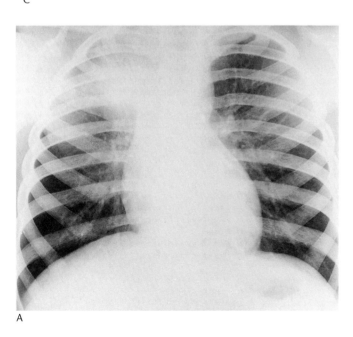

C

Fig. 6.47 (A) Right lower lobe consolidation associated with volume loss demonstrated on CT. Note the air-filled bronchi. (B) Ultrasound scan. The air bronchograms are evident as echogenic linear structures (arrows). (C) Fluid bronchograms in a different patient (arrows); arrowheads indicate the position of the diaphragm.

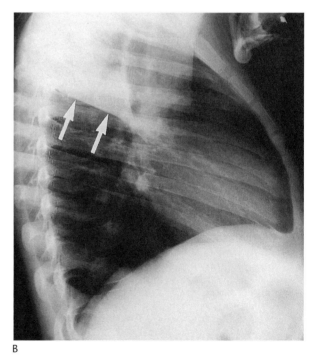

B

A

Fig. 6.48 Right upper lobe consolidation in a 6-year-old boy with aortic valve disease. (A) Opacity in the right upper zone obscures the upper mediastinum. (B) The lateral film shows consolidation anterior to the upper part of the oblique fissure (arrows), mostly in the posterior segment of the right upper lobe.

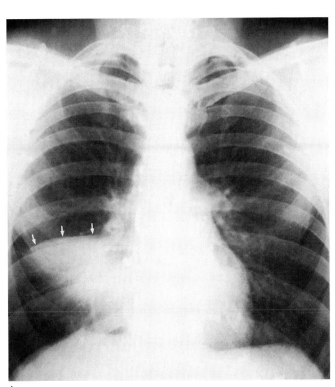
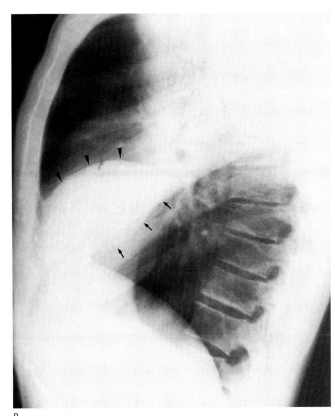

A
B

Fig. 6.49 Right middle lobe consolidation in a 37-year-old man with squamous cell carcinoma of the right middle lobe. (A) PA film shows homogeneous opacity limited by horizontal fissure (arrows) and obscuring the right heart border. (B) Lateral film shows consolidation bounded by horizontal fissure (arrowheads) and lower half of oblique fissure (arrows).

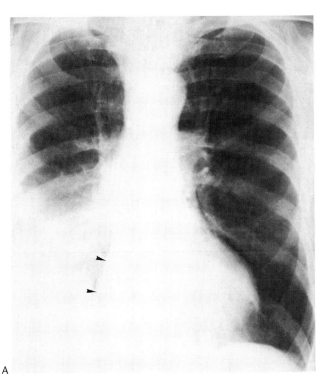
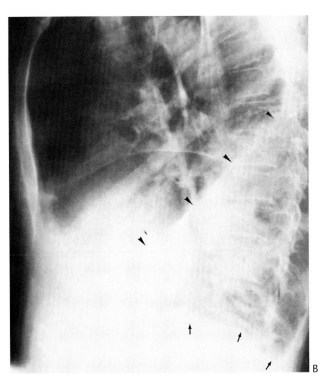

A
B

Fig. 6.50 Right lower lobe consolidation. Pneumonia complicating chronic bronchitis. (A) PA film shows right lower zone shadowing obscuring the diaphragm but not the right heart border (arrowheads). (B) Lateral film shows shadowing with air bronchogram, limited by oblique fissure anteriorly (arrowheads). The left hemidiaphragm is visible (arrows) but the right is obscured.

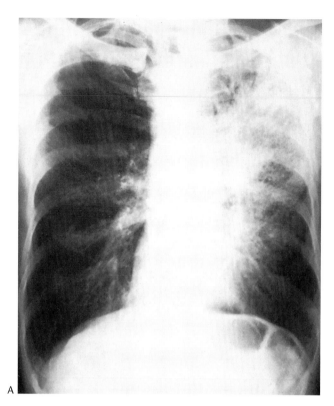
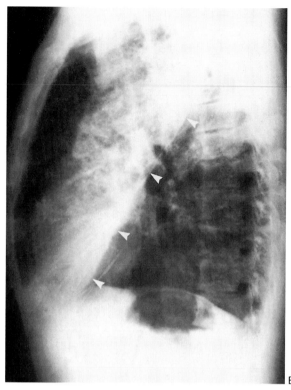

Fig. 6.51 Left upper lobe and lingula consolidation. A 70-year-old man with left upper lobe carcinoma. (A) Patchy consolidation obscures the left heart border and aortic knuckle. (B) The consolidation is bounded posteriorly by the oblique fissure (arrowheads).

REFERENCES AND SUGGESTIONS FOSR FURTHER READING

Atelectasis Part I (1996) *Journal of Thoracic Imaging*, **11**, 91–149.

Bergin, C. J., Müller, N. L., Miller, R. R. (1986) CT in the qualitative assessment of emphysema. *Journal of Thoracic Imaging*, **1**, 94–103.

Breatnach, E., Kerr, I. H. (1982) The radiology of cryptogenic obliterative bronchiolitis. *Clinical Radiology*, **33**, 657–661.

Carr, D. H., Pride, N. B. (1984) Computed tomography in preoperative assessment of bullous emphysema. *Clinical Radiology*, **35**, 43–45.

Fletcher, C. M., Pride, N. B. (1984) Editorial. Definitions of emphysema, chronic bronchitis, asthma and air flow obstruction: 25 years on from the CIBA Symposium. *Thorax*, **39**, 81–85.

Foster, W. L., Giminez, E. I., Roubidoux, M. A., et al (1993) The emphysemas: radiologic–pathologic correlations. *RadioGraphics*, **13**, 311–328.

Garg, K., Lynch, D. A., Newell, J. D., et al (1994) Proliferative and constrictive bronchiolitis: classification and radiologic features. *American Journal of Roentgenology*, **162**, 803–808.

Grenier, P., Cordeau, M. P., Beigelman, C. (1993) High-resolution computed tomography of the airways. *Journal of Thoracic Imaging*, **8**, 213–229.

Gückell, C., Hansell, D. M. (1998) Imaging the dirty lung—has high resolution computed tomography cleared the smoke? *Clinical Radiology*, **53**, 717–720.

Kwong, J. S., Müller, N. L., Miller, R. R. (1992) Diseases of the trachea and main-stem bronchi: correlation of CT with pathological findings. *RadioGraphics*, **12**, 645–657.

Macleod, W. M. (1954) Abnormal transradiancy of one lung. *Thorax*, **9**, 147–153.

Nishimura, K., Kitaichi, M., Izumi, T., et al (1992) Diffuse panbronchiolitis: correlations of high-resolution CT and pathologic findings. *Radiology*, **184**, 779–785.

Padley, S. P. G., Adler, B. D., Hansell, D. M., et al (1993) Bronchiolitis obliterans: high resolution CT findings and correlation with pulmonary function tests. *Clinical Radiology*, **47**, 236–240.

Patheram, I. S., Kerr, T. H., Collins, J. V. (1981) Value of chest radiographs in severe acute asthma. *Clinical Radiology*, **32**, 281–282.

Proto, A. V., Tocino, I. (1980) Radiographic manifestations of lobar collapse. *Seminars in Roentgenology*, **15**, 117–173.

Robbins, L. L., Hale, C. H. (1945) The roentgen appearance of lobar and segmental collapse of the lung; preliminary report. *Radiology*, **44**, 107–114.

Schneider, H. J., Felson, B., Gonzalez, L. L. (1980) Rounded atelectasis. *American Journal of Roentgenology*, **134**, 225–232.

Simon, G. (1964) Radiology and emphysema. *Clinical Radiology*, **15**, 293–306.

Swyer, P. R., James, G. C. W. (1953) A case of unilateral emphysema. *Thorax*, **8**, 133–136.

Thurlbeck, W. M., Churg, A. M. (eds) (1995) *Pathology of the Lung*, 2nd edn, pp. 739–826. New York: Thieme Medical.

Thurlbeck, W. M., Simon, G. (1978) Radiographic appearance of the chest in emphysema. *American Journal of Roentgenology*, **130**, 429–440.

Tomashefski, J. F. (1977) Definition, differentiation and classification of COPD. *Postgraduate Medicine*, **162**, 88–97.

Vock, P., Spiegel, T., Fram, E. K., et al (1984) CT assessment of the adult intrathoracic cross section of the trachea. *Journal of Computer Assisted Tomography*, **8**, 1076–1082.

Webb, W. R. (1997) Radiology of obstructive pulmonary disease. *American Journal of Roentgenology*, **169**, 637–647.

Webb, W. R., Müller, N. L., Naidich, D. P. (1996) *High Resolution CT of the Lung*, pp. 227–270. Philadelphia: Lippincott–Raven.

Weber, A. L. (1996) Radiologic evaluation of the trachea. *Chest Surgical Clinics of North America*, **6**, 637–673.

7

DIFFUSE LUNG DISEASE

Simon P. G. Padley and Michael B. Rubens

There are many causes of diffuse lung disease in addition to infection, neoplasia or a primary abnormality of the airways. The chest radiograph remains the basic radiological tool in the investigation of these patients. However plain radiography is a relatively insensitive test, and is normal in 10–20% of patients with histologically proven interstitial lung disease.

Computed tomography

There is no doubt that CT and, particularly, high-resolution CT (HRCT) can play a major role in the assessment of patients with chronic diffuse lung disease (CDLD) (Box 7.1). HRCT has been shown to have a high sensitivity and specificity, and as a result there has been much recent interest in the role of this imaging technique in the diagnosis and management of many diffuse lung diseases. Because there is no superimposition of structures HRCT allows better assessment of parenchymal abnormalities compared with plain radiography. Conventional CT uses contiguous 10-mm-thick sections and is ideal for many clinical situations, but due to volume averaging there is some loss of fine detail. To avoid volume averaging HRCT uses thin-section CT images 1–2 mm thick and 10–15 mm apart. Resolution is further improved by using a high-spatial-frequency algorithm. This combination produces images with striking anatomical detail. All current CT scanners have the ability to generate HRCT images of high quality.

HRCT is particularly useful in the patient with suspected CDLD but with a normal radiograph or with only questionable abnormalities evident. In many cases HRCT allows the radiologist to make a confident diagnosis, and in some cases biopsy can be avoided. In others the site and type of biopsy (open lung biopsy, biopsy at video-assisted thoracoscopic surgery or transbronchial biopsy) most likely to provide the diagnosis can be suggested.

HRCT has repeatedly been demonstrated to be accurate in the diagnosis of many common causes of CDLD including fibrosing alveolitis, sarcoidosis, lymphangitis carcinomatosa, silicosis and asbestosis. HRCT is also remarkably accurate in the diagnosis of some of the rarer causes of CDLD such as lymphangioleiomyomatosis and Langerhan's cell histiocytosis. HRCT has a further role in the assessment of disease activity in some types of CDLD, particularly in fibrosing alveolitis and sarcoidosis.

SARCOIDOSIS

Sarcoidosis is a multisystem disease of unknown aetiology. Pathologically it is characterised by the development of non-caseating granulomas which either resolve completely or leave a legacy of fibrotic scarring. It may occur at any age but usually presents in young adults. Although worldwide in distribution there are racial differences in incidence, natural history and radiographic patterns. There is evidence of a genetic predisposition from clustering of familial cases and a higher frequency in monozygotic than dizygotic twins. Blacks are 12 times more likely to develop sarcoidosis than whites, and black females are twice as susceptible as black males. By contrast, the disease is almost unknown amongst the Chinese and South East Asian populations. Patients most commonly present with one or more of erythema nodosum, arthralgia, an abnormal chest radiograph and respiratory symptoms. The diagnosis is usually made by the combination of symptoms, clinical signs and histology. When the chest radiograph is abnormal transbronchial biopsy is usually diagnostic and demonstrates non-caseating epithelioid granulomas. Within the lungs these are distributed along the bronchovascular bundles and often lie adjacent to pleural surfaces and interlobular septa. Healing frequently involves fibrosis which may progress whilst the disease remains active. The final radiographic appearances range from a return to normal to severe fibrosis. A Kveim test is still occasionally performed to confirm the diagnosis. A Kveim test requires an intradermal inoculation of an extract of sarcoid tissue. The resulting skin reaction is biopsied and is deemed positive if it displays typical sarcoid histology.

Box 7.1   **Indications for the use of HRCT in diffuse lung disease**

- Confirmation of abnormality in patients with symptoms suggestive of diffuse lung disease with a normal or near normal chest radiograph
- Specific diagnosis or further assessment in patients with an abnormal but non-diagnostic chest radiograph
- As a guide to the site and method of biopsy
- As a guide to the assessment of disease activity especially in fibrosing alveolitis
- To diagnose superimposed complications such as infection or tumour when they are clinically suspected but not visible on the chest radiograph
- To determine the relative importance of each condition in patients with more than one chronic diffuse lung disease

---

Radiological appearances

Sarcoidosis commonly causes *thoracic lymphadenopathy* and *parenchymal lung opacities*. Adenopathy almost always precedes pulmonary shadowing, but they are often present simultaneously. The chest radiograph is abnormal at some time in 90% of patients with sarcoidosis.

Typically there is bilateral, symmetrical hilar enlargement involving both tracheobronchial and bronchopulmonary nodes (Fig. 7.1). Bilateral hilar lymph node enlargement, in the correct clinical setting, is often regarded as sufficient evidence of sarcoidosis to negate the need for biopsy. Right paratracheal lymphadenopathy is also common, and left paratracheal adenopathy is occasionally seen. Enlargement of other mediastinal nodes is rarely appreciated on the chest radiograph but may be seen on CT (Fig. 7.2). If the hilar adenopathy is very asymmetrical or anterior mediastinal adenopathy is a feature, other diagnoses should be considered. Rarely the involved lymph nodes may calcify, sometimes peripherally, causing 'egg-shell' calcification (Fig. 7.3).

Nodal enlargement usually resolves, and recurrence following resolution is unusual. In some patients nodal enlargement may persist for many years, and despite a long period of non-progression the development of parenchymal disease may still occur. Overall approximately 50% of cases will progress from radiographically evident bilateral hilar lymph node enlargement to nodal and pulmonary disease. Virtually all patients with intrathoracic adenopathy due to sarcoid develop pulmonary granulomas histologically. It is therefore not surprising that the incidence of parenchymal abnormality is significantly higher on HRCT scanning than on chest radiography. Typically HRCT reveals multiple small irregular nodular opacities which, although widespread, tend to have a predominantly peribronchovascular and subpleural distribution (Fig. 7.4). The midzones are most profusely involved and nodules may be so numerous as to create fine ground-glass opacification or appear as miliary shadows (Fig. 7.5). Larger nodules of the order of 1 cm in diameter may be present. They may be well or poorly marginated and may coalesce to form larger opacities (Fig. 7.6). Air bronchograms are occasionally visible, and rarely nodules may cav-

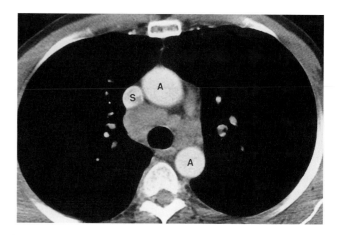

Fig. 7.2 Sarcoidosis. There are multiple mediastinal lymph nodes. S = superior vena cava; A = aorta.

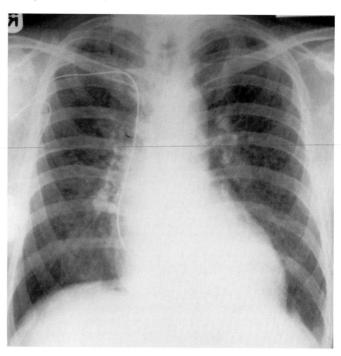

Fig. 7.3 Sarcoidosis. There is bilateral hilar lymph node calcification. Some of the nodes are calcified peripherally ('egg-shell' calcification). A pacing electrode is present. Heart block is an occasional complication of sarcoidosis.

itate. Parenchymal nodules evident on chest radiography often appear most profuse in the lung bases where the anteroposterior dimension of the lungs is maximised. A reticular pattern may be evident, usually radiating from the hila. Septal lines are uncommon. When present they do not indicate lymphatic obstruction from nodal disease but rather reflect micronodular disease related to intralobular septa. Nodules up to 2–3 cm in size are rarely seen in the UK but are recognised in the USA, most commonly in Afro-Caribbean patients.

Most cases of parenchymal involvement resolve completely, but approximately one-third develop *pulmonary fibrosis*. This tends to involve the mid and upper zones more than the bases (Fig. 7.6). The commonest pattern is of a few inconspicuous linear midzone scars. Coarse linear shadows, ring shadows and bullae may be seen in

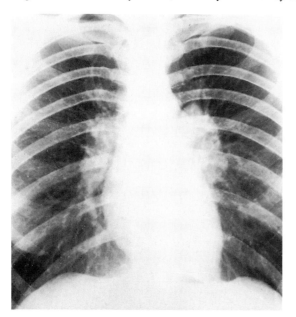

Fig. 7.1 Sarcoidosis. Bilateral hilar node enlargement.

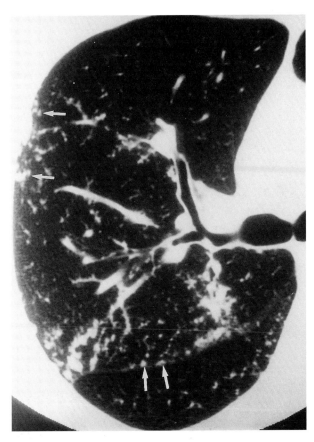

Fig. 7.4 Sarcoidosis. HRCT scan through the right lung shows nodularity of the bronchovascular bundles due to multiple sarcoid granulomas. Nodules are also evident in the subpleural regions adjacent to the chest wall and major fissure (arrows).

more severe cases. Occasionally, confluent fibrotic areas develop and on HRCT a typical perihilar and posterior midzone pattern is evident (Fig. 7.7).

Unusual manifestations of sarcoidosis include basal septal lines, pleural effusions, spontaneous pneumothorax and bronchostenosis. Rarely endobronchial disease may result in fibrotic strictures causing segmental or even lobar collapse. Evidence of air trapping is well recognised on expiratory HRCT scanning (Fig. 7.8).

The isotope gallium-67 is taken up by involved lymph nodes and lung, and has been used to assess the activity and extent of the disease. However there is no clear role in the initial assessment of patients with possible sarcoidosis, except in the occasional patient with disease that is entirely extrathoracic, or in the differentiation between inactive fibrotic tissue and active sarcoidosis.

THE PNEUMOCONIOSES

The pneumoconioses are diseases caused by inhalation of *inorganic dusts*. The diagnosis depends on a history of exposure to the dust, and an abnormal chest radiograph and respiratory function tests. Only occasionally is a lung biopsy required to confirm the diagnosis. The history of exposure may include living near a mine or a factory or living with an exposed worker, as well as working directly with dust. Dusts may be termed active or inactive. Active dusts are fibrogenic in the lung, and inactive dusts are relatively

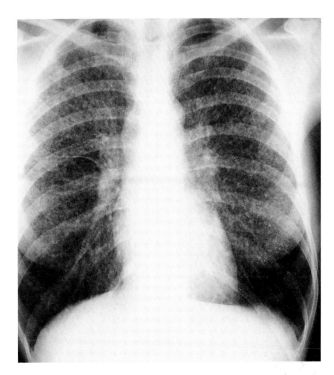

Fig. 7.5 Sarcoidosis. Miliary, nodular opacities are present throughout both lungs. One year later the appearances were entirely normal.

inert. Inhaled dusts—such as coal dust—are often a combination of active and inactive materials. The important active dusts are asbestos and silica. The reaction of an individual to dust exposure depends on several factors in addition to the nature of the dust, including the duration of exposure, concentration of particles and individual susceptibility.

Dust particles larger than 5 μm in diameter are usually deposited onto the bronchial and bronchiolar walls and are coughed up. Smaller particles may reach the alveoli. Asbestos fibres are the exception, fibres longer than 30 μm sometimes penetrating the lung parenchyma.

SILICOSIS

In addition to exposure related to coal mining, exposure to silica may occur in granite, slate and sandstone quarrying, gold mining, sandblasting and in foundry, ceramic and pottery works. Exposure of several years may lead to pulmonary fibrosis. Fibrosis may continue after exposure has ceased.

Radiology

Simple silicosis causes multiple, nodular shadows, 2–5 mm in diameter (Fig. 7.9). These initially appear in the mid and upper zones, eventually involving all lung zones but relatively sparing the bases. HRCT confirms that they are most profuse in the mid and upper zones but also demonstrates a predilection for the posterior aspect of the lungs not evident on the chest radiograph (Fig. 7.10). The nodules are well defined, uniform in density and size (2–5 mm) and rarely calcify. Linear shadows and septal lines may also appear. In *complicated silicosis* the nodules become confluent and form homogeneous, non-segmental areas of shadowing. This tends to occur in the upper lobes, and the areas of fibrosis may migrate

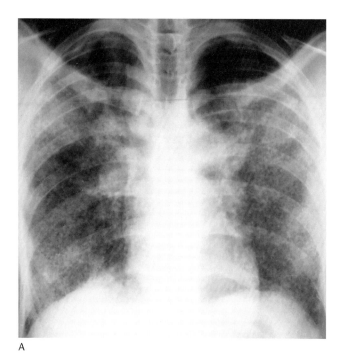

A

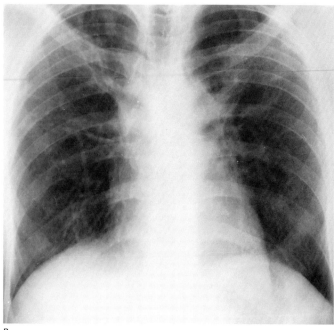

B

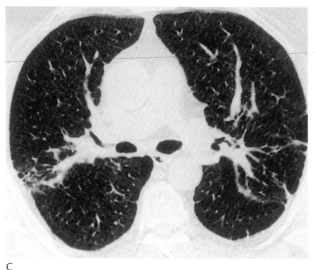

C

Fig. 7.6 Sarcoidosis. (A) Miliary nodules with areas of coalescence peripherally. (B) After resolution of the nodular shadowing there is mild mid and upper zone linear scarring. (C) CT image through the midzones in a different patient demonstrating mild residual fibrotic change causing minor traction bronchiectasis on the right.

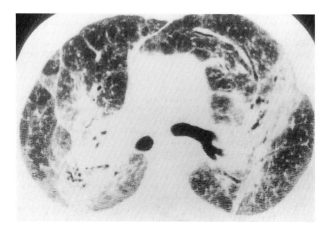

Fig. 7.7   HRCT scan at the level of the hila showing conglomerate fibrotic masses with radiation into the surrounding lung.

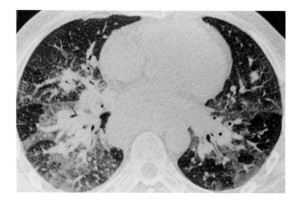

Fig. 7.8   Sarcoidosis. Expiratory HRCT scan through the lower zones. There is air trapping as evidenced by areas of parenchyma that remain as lower attenuation on expiration. Some of these correspond to individual secondary pulmonary nodules.

toward the hila, creating areas of emphysema in the lung periphery. These changes may be seen on plain radiography (Fig. 7.11), but are detected at an earlier stage by conventional or HRCT (Fig. 7.12).

When complicated silicosis develops the possibility of tuberculosis should be considered, although cavitation of 'massive shadows' may also be due to ischaemic necrosis (Fig. 7.11). HRCT also has a role in patients with silicosis in whom the pulmonary function tests and radiological appearances do not correlate. The impairment in pulmonary function correlates with the severity of emphysematous changes, often best assessed with HRCT, rather than the profusion of pulmonary nodules.

Extensive fibrosis may be complicated by pulmonary arterial hypertension and cor pulmonale. Hilar lymphadenopathy is common in silicosis, and the nodes may calcify diffusely or with a peripheral 'egg-shell' pattern (Fig. 7.13). Patients with silicosis and rheumatoid disease may develop *Caplan's syndrome*, but like massive fibrosis this is commoner in coal worker's pneumoconiosis.

COAL WORKER'S PNEUMOCONIOSIS

Coal dust is mostly carbon, but it may contain silica. Coal workers are prone to coal worker's pneumoconiosis, silicosis, chronic bronchitis and emphysema. Coal dust is not fibrogenic and deposits in the lung are surrounded by emphysema. The corresponding radiographic appearance is simple pneumoconiosis. As in silicosis, simple pneumoconiosis may progress to a complicated variety with the development of *progressive massive fibrosis (PMF)* (Fig. 7.14). This is usually associated with prolonged exposure and sometimes a complicating factor such as infection or an autoimmune process.

In *simple pneumoconiosis*, small, faint, indistinct nodules, 1–5 mm in diameter, appear in the midzones. Eventually nodules may be seen throughout the lungs, but remain most numerous in the midzones. The development of PMF is marked by coalescence of the small nodules or the appearance of larger opacities of 1 cm

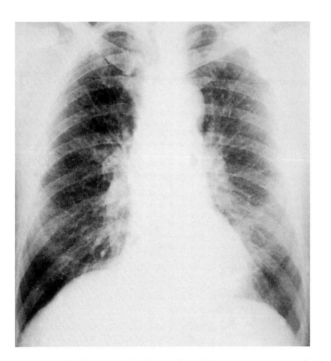

Fig. 7.9 Simple silicosis. Multiple, small nodules are present throughout both lungs.

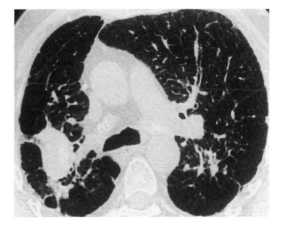

Fig. 7.11 Progressive massive fibrosis (PMF). Large confluent masses have formed. Cavitation is evident on the left (arrow).

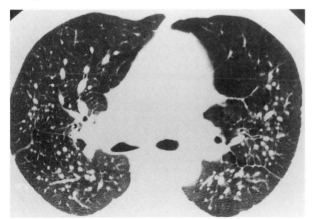

Fig. 7.10 Simple silicosis. CT scan demonstrates multiple well-defined pulmonary nodules, most numerous in the posterior lung parenchyma.

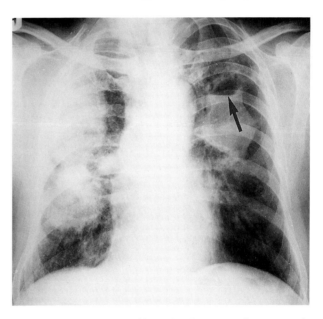

Fig. 7.12 Early complicated silicosis. CT scan demonstrates coalescence of nodules into pulmonary masses.

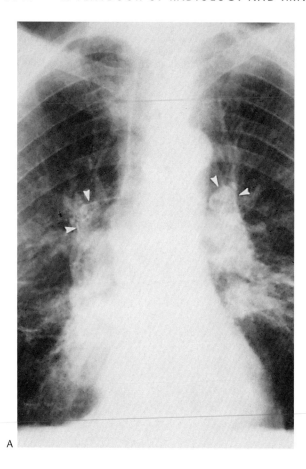

A

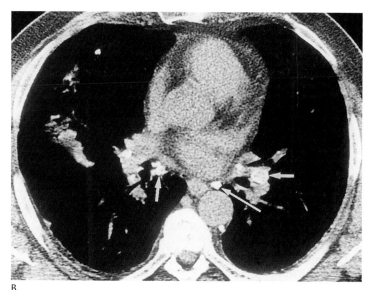

B

Fig. 7.13 Silicosis. (A) There is bilateral hilar lymphadenopathy. Many of the nodes are calcified, some of them peripherally. (B) Similar changes on CT.

diameter or more. As in silicosis, areas of massive fibrosis associated with coal worker's pneumoconiosis are usually mid or upper zone and bilateral; they are round or oval and tend to migrate toward the hila creating peripheral areas of emphysema and bullae. The fibrotic masses may calcify or cavitate (Fig. 7.14). Simple coal worker's pneumoconiosis does not usually develop further if exposure ceases, but PMF often does progress.

Patients with rheumatoid disease and coal worker's pneumoconiosis may develop *Caplan's syndrome*. Multiple, round, well-defined opacities, 1–5 cm in diameter, may appear in the lungs (Fig. 7.15). These usually appear in crops, and are often accompanied by cutaneous rheumatoid nodules. These represent necrobiotic nodules, but if the underlying pneumoconiosis is not appreciated they may be misdiagnosed as metastases. Nodules may regress, remain static, calcify or cavitate (Fig. 7.16).

ASBESTOSIS

Asbestos exposure may occur in asbestos mining and processing, in construction and demolition work, in shipbuilding and in the manufacture of some textiles. Living near such workplaces, or with exposed workers, also carries some risk of exposure. Manifestations of exposure may not become apparent for many years.

Asbestos is a group of crystalline silicates that form fibres. There is a confusing nomenclature surrounding asbestos. The virtue of distinguishing between the different subtypes of fibre lies in their relative importance in the pathogenesis of asbestos-associated conditions. In brief there are two geometric forms, serpentine (twisted and flexible) and amphibole (stiff and brittle). The serpentine group includes chrysotile asbestos, the commonest form used industrially and of relatively low pathogenicity. The amphibole group includes crocidolite, amosite and anthophyllite, which have much greater pathogenicity, especially for the induction of mesothelioma. Indeed there is some evidence that the few cases of mesothelioma that arise in patients exposed to serpentine forms of asbestos are probably induced by contamination of the serpentine fibres by amphibole asbestos. Both groups of fibres are fibrogenic, and there is a dose–response relationship for all the asbestos-related diseases except for mesothelioma.

Fibrosis is probably the result of physical and chemical irritation in addition to an autoimmune mechanism. Inhaled fibres, sometimes longer than 30 μm, may reach the alveoli and penetrate the pleura and occasionally the diaphragm. The fibres gravitate to the lower lobes, so that changes are more severe in the lower zones than in the mid and upper zones.

Symptoms of asbestosis are often not apparent until 20 or 30 years after exposure. Malignant disease is an important complication. Lung cancer is relatively common, especially when asbestos exposure is combined with cigarette smoking. Compared to the non-smoker without exposure to asbestos, asbestos alone increases the likelihood of lung cancer by a factor of 5, cigarette smoking alone by a factor of 10, and the combination of asbestos and cigarettes by a factor of 50. The combination of asbestos and cigarettes also predisposes to carcinomas of the oesophagus, larynx and oropharynx. Mesothelioma of the pleura is the other malignancy closely associated with asbestos exposure, and may develop after a latent period of 20 years. Other neoplasms associated with asbestos exposure are carcinomas of the large bowel and renal tract and peritoneal mesothelioma.

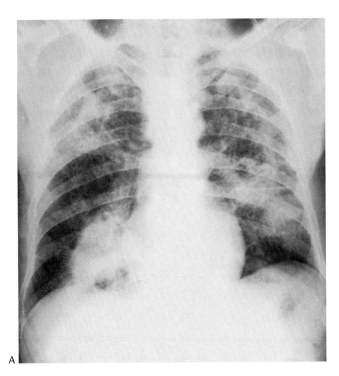
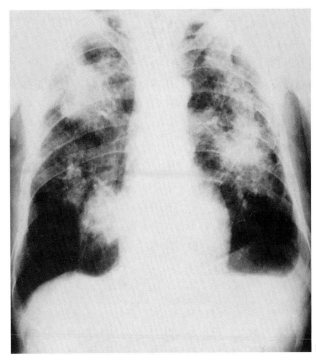

A
B

Fig. 7.14 Progressive massive fibrosis in a coal miner of 52. (A) Nodular opacities are present throughout both lungs, and several areas of more confluent shadowing are present. (B) Four years later, lower zone masses have migrated centrally, leaving peripheral areas of emphysema. The upper lobe opacities have enlarged.

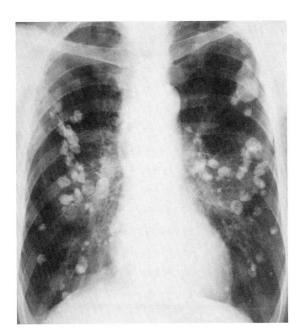

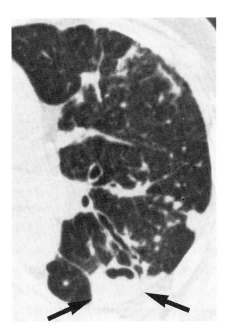

Fig. 7.15 Male aged 54 with Caplan's syndrome. Coal worker with rheumatoid arthritis. Multiple rounded opacities are present (some partly calcified).

Fig. 7.16 Caplan's syndrome. There is a left-sided cavitating pulmonary nodule (arrows) on a background of pneumoconiosis.

Radiological appearance

Asbestos exposure may produce changes in the lung parenchyma and in the pleura. Pleural changes, which include plaques, calcification, diffuse thickening and effusions, are seen on the chest X-ray more often than parenchymal changes.

Pleural plaques and fibrosis Plaques develop bilaterally. They tend to occur in the midzones and over the diaphragm (Figs 3.20 and 3.29) and are the most frequent manifestation of previous exposure. Small plaques may be difficult to see on the standard chest radiograph, but may be demonstrated with oblique views or by *ultrasound* or *HRCT* (Fig. 7.17). The plaques often calcify and may produce bizarre opacities that have been described as resembling holly leaves (Fig. 3.27). Unlike pleural plaques, diffuse pleural thickening is not specific to asbestos exposure. Diffuse pleural thickening rarely calcifies and may be associated with short parenchymal lines extending into the adjacent lung. It is unclear if this appearance heralds asbestosis. A CT definition of diffuse pleural thickening, as suggested by Lynch and coworkers (1989), is a continuous sheet of pleural thickening greater than 5 cm by 8 cm and at least 3 mm thick. The importance in distinction between diffuse pleural thickening and pleural plaques lies in the fusion of parietal and visceral pleural layers in the former condition, with subsequent impairment in lung function. By contrast, pleural plaques are usually isolated discrete lesions that involve the parietal pleura.

Benign pleural effusions Small pleural effusions may occasionally occur. These usually arise within a decade of exposure, and may be bilateral or unilateral. They may recur, and although frequently asymptomatic, may give rise to pleuritic symptoms. The effusions are usually small (less than 500 ml), and may be blood stained. Resolution may be complete or associated with infolded lung or diffuse pleural thickening. Large effusions should raise the possibility of an underlying carcinoma or mesothelioma.

Pulmonary fibrosis This may be seen with or without pleural changes. While the chest radiograph remains the first investigation in patients with suspected asbestosis, HRCT is indicated in those patients with clinical or functional abnormalities compatible with asbestosis in which the chest radiograph is normal or shows questionable abnormalities. Between 5% and 25% of asbestos-exposed patients with a normal chest radiograph have HRCT abnormalities suggestive of asbestosis. On plain radiography the earliest signs are a fine reticular or nodular pattern in the lower zones (Fig. 7.18). With progression this becomes coarser and causes loss of clarity of the diaphragm and cardiac shadow—the so-called 'shaggy heart' (Fig. 7.19). Eventually the whole lung may become involved, but the basal preponderance persists and areas of emphysema may develop. HRCT demonstrates fibrosis initially in the periphery of the lung (Fig. 7.19). Parenchymal bands that extend inward from the pleural surface may develop with resultant distortion in the lung architecture (7.20). Subpleural linear opacities may also be present (Fig. 7.21). A pattern of interstitial fibrosis indistinguishable from

idiopathic pulmonary fibrosis may develop, and the presence of asbestos-related pleural disease can be helpful in differentiating between the two conditions.

BERYLLIOSIS

Acute berylliosis causes a chemical pneumonitis, which radiographically has the appearance of non-cardiogenic pulmonary oedema. *Chronic berylliosis* is a systemic disease characterised by widespread non-cavitating granulomas. The thoracic radiological manifestations are identical to sarcoidosis (Fig. 7.22). Both diseases have become increasingly rare since the toxic effects of beryllium have become widely appreciated with subsequent improvements in industrial practice.

OTHER PNEUMOCONIOSES DUE TO INACTIVE DUSTS

Inactive dusts do not cause fibrosis in the lungs, but may produce changes on the chest X-ray simply by accumulating in the lungs. Symptoms are usually absent.

Siderosis

This is a result of prolonged exposure to iron oxide dust. Widespread reticulonodular shadowing occurs. When exposure ceases the shadowing may regress. In *silicosiderosis* fibrosis may occur, with a picture resembling that of silicosis.

Stannosis

This condition is caused by inhalation of tin oxide. Multiple, very small, very dense, discrete opacities of 0.5–1 mm diameter are distributed throughout the lungs. Particles may collect in the inter-

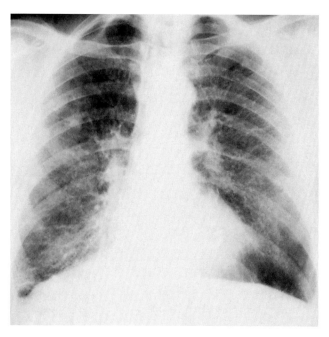

Fig. 7.18 Asbestos exposure of 25 years. Fine reticulonodular shadowing in the mid and lower zones is best seen on the right. Bullous disease is present at the left base.

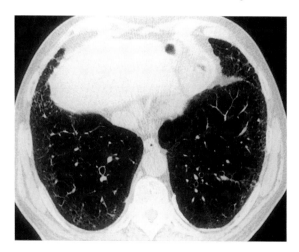

Fig. 7.17 Asbestosis. There is a fine subpleural reticular infiltrate associated with low-volume calcified pleural plaques (best seen in a left paravertebral position).

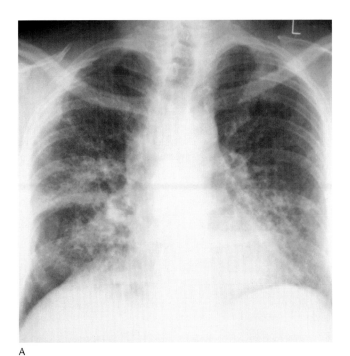

A

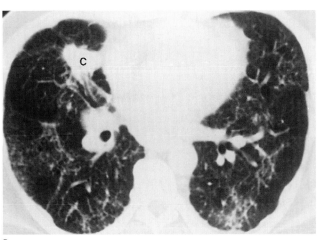

B

Fig. 7.19 Asbestosis. (A) Chest radiograph demonstrating loss of clarity of the cardiac silhouette (shaggy heart). (B) HRCT reveals linear opacities and also a carcinoma (on part B) adjacent to the right heart border.

lobular lymphatics and produce dense septal lines. The opacities are denser than calcium because of the high atomic number of tin.

Barytosis

This results from inhalation of particulate barium sulphate, causing very dense nodulation throughout the lungs. Following cessation of exposure the changes regress.

ASPIRATION AND INHALATION

Aspiration of liquid or solid material into the airways may cause mechanical obstruction, and depending on the nature of the aspirate, a variable amount of inflammation.

Mendelson's syndrome

Mendelson described aspiration of gastric contents in women during parturition. However Mendelson's syndrome is often taken to include massive aspiration of gastric contents for whatever reason. Intense bronchospasm is followed by a chemical pneumonitis. The chest radiograph shows widespread pulmonary oedema. Similar changes are seen in patients after near drowning.

Lipoid pneumonia

This results from aspiration of mineral oil, which is usually being taken for chronic constipation. Aspirated oil tends to collect in the dependent parts of the lungs where it causes a chronic inflammatory response. The chest radiograph usually shows large, dense, tumour-like opacities.

Petrol or paraffin aspiration

This may cause a pneumonitis, which is usually basal. It may be followed by the development of pneumatoceles.

Inhalation of irritant gases

Chlorine, ammonia and oxides of nitrogen may produce pulmonary oedema followed by obliterative bronchiolitis and emphysema.

Oxygen toxicity

This may occur following prolonged administration of oxygen in concentrations above 50%. Damage to the alveolar epithelium causes pulmonary oedema followed by interstitial fibrosis.

EXTRINSIC ALLERGIC ALVEOLITIS

Extrinsic allergic alveolitis, also known as *hypersensitivity pneumonitis*, is an allergic inflammatory granulomatous reaction of the lungs caused by the inhalation of dusts containing certain organisms or proteins. Inhaled particles less than 10 μm in diameter are capable of reaching the alveoli, where their potential for causing damage to the gas-exchanging parts of the lungs is considerable. If the particles are antigenic and the lung previously sensitised, a hypersensitivity reaction ensues. Antibodies are meant to neutralise potentially harmful foreign material, but sometimes the combination of antigen and antibody is itself damaging and constitutes a disease process. In *farmer's lung* the offending organism is usually *Micropolyspora faeni* from damp mouldy hay. *Pigeon breeders* inhale dust from feathers or desiccated droppings containing bird serum protein. *Fungal spores from the compost used affects mushroom growers. Sugar cane workers* exposed to mouldy sugar cane residue may develop bagassosis. *Air-conditioning systems* may circulate fungal spores and amoebae. A similar reaction in the lungs may be induced by drugs, in this case blood borne, the most common examples being *nitrofurantoin* and *salazopyrine*, although the number of drugs known to result in a hypersensitivity-type reaction in the lungs is ever increasing.

Precipitating antibodies directed specifically against the antigen are found in the serum of patients but their presence only implies exposure, not necessarily disease. Some 40% of pigeon breeders

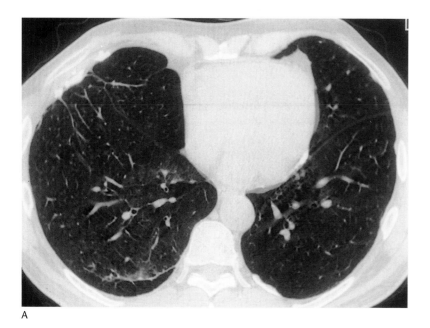

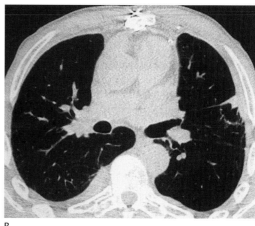

A   B

Fig. 7.20 (A) Asbestos exposure has resulted in pleural plaques. There are coarse parenchymal bands extending arising from these plaques that are causing some distortion of the lung architecture. (B) In a different patient the result of asbestos exposure is the development of diffuse pleural thickening. This predated the sternotomy.

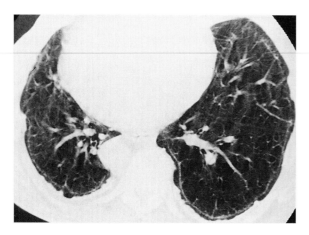

Fig. 7.21 HRCT demonstrating an extensive subpleural linear stripe due to asbestosis.

have precipitins but few suffer from the disease; however, the presence of precipitins to extracts of budgerigar excreta in those exposed is stronger evidence in favour of disease. The immunological reactions are predominantly Type III, that is free-circulating antigen and antibody combine in the presence of complement to form complexes, which are deposited in the alveolar walls. Activation of complement sets in train a sequence of reactions liberating a variety of damaging substances. The time-scale of the reaction is intermediate, which corresponds well with the clinical presentation. Type IV reactions also play a part, and here the antibody is produced and transported by lymphocytes, which then aggregate at the site where the reaction takes place. The granulomas, a characteristic feature of Type IV reactions, are the fundamental histological lesion of extrinsic allergic alveolitis.

Typically the patient develops headache, fever, chills, a cough and dyspnoea 5 or 6 hours after exposure. Smaller and more frequent exposure to the antigen may result in progressive dyspnoea,

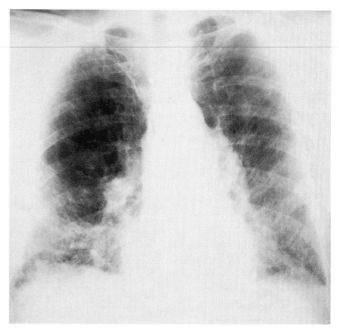

Fig. 7.22 Berylliosis. The patient had spent 35 years in the glass-blowing industry making neon lights. The chest radiograph shows diffuse reticular shadowing. The appearance is indistinguishable from end-stage sarcoidosis.

and is typical of disease due to budgerigars. On auscultation there are usually inspiratory crepitations. Lung function tests show restricted ventilation and impaired gas transfer but little airways obstruction. The best test is a bronchial challenge by the inhalation of the allergen to reproduce the symptoms and functional abnormalities. It is now rarely used, but it was instrumental initially in establishing the pathogenesis of the disease.

Treatment is by removal from exposure or, if that is not possible, reduction of contact to a minimum. Steroids are of doubtful value.

In only 50–60% of patients does the lung function return to normal and some continue to deteriorate after elimination of exposure.

Radiological appearances

The radiographic appearances are dependent on the length of allergen exposure and the balance between continuing inflammatory change and the development of fibrosis. A mixture of inflammatory and fibrotic changes is the most common pattern. In the early stages the chest radiograph may be normal, but may show diffuse fine nodular opacities or a generalised, 'ground-glass' haze (Fig. 7.23). HRCT frequently reveals a combination of small (1–3 mm) pulmonary nodules and areas of ground-glass change even in those patients with a normal chest radiograph (Fig. 7.24). Patchy consolidation and septal lines, similar to pulmonary oedema, may also be seen in acute attacks (Fig. 7.25). With the development of fibrosis reticulonodular shadows may progress to coarse linear opacities, typically in the mid and upper zones. Finally, severe contraction of the upper and midzones with 'honeycombing', cyst formation and bronchiectasis may occur.

Lung fibrosis is a common end-stage of a number of disparate diseases, including extrinsic allergic alveolitis, cryptogenic fibrosing alveolitis, tuberculosis, bronchopulmonary aspergillosis, ankylosing spondylitis and many others. At this stage it is often impossible to differentiate between them on the basis of the chest radiograph alone, although HRCT frequently still allows the underlying aetiology to be identified.

CONNECTIVE TISSUE DISEASES

This group of conditions, also known as the collagen vascular diseases, comprises a number of chronic inflammatory, autoimmune disorders. They may involve any tissue in any part of the body; joints, serous membranes and blood vessels are frequently involved, and all connective tissue diseases involve the lungs and pleura to some extent. The acute inflammatory episodes characteristically lead to fibrosis and collagen production. While many patients show

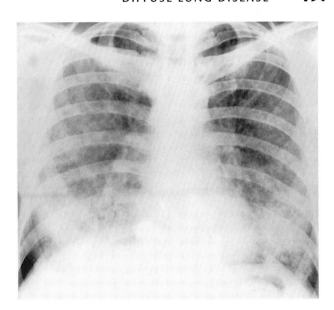

Fig. 7.23 Farmer's lung. Patchy alveolar opacification superimposed on a miliary nodulation. The costophrenic angles are clear.

clinical or radiological features that allow the diagnosis of a specific connective tissue disorder, some patients exhibit signs of more than one of the conditions. Consequently it is not always possible to make a precise diagnosis.

Conventionally, the connective tissue diseases comprise rheumatoid arthritis, systemic lupus erythematosus (SLE), systemic sclerosis (SS), mixed connective tissue disease (MCTD), polyarteritis nodosa (PAN) and dermatomyositis/polymyositis (PMS). CREST syndrome is a subset of SS characterised by cutaneous calcinosis, Raynaud's phenomenon, oesophageal abnormalities, sclerodactyly and telangiectasis. Mixed connective tissue disease consists of combined features of SLE, SS and PMS. The term 'overlap syndrome' has been extended to include almost any combination so that it now lacks a precise definition.

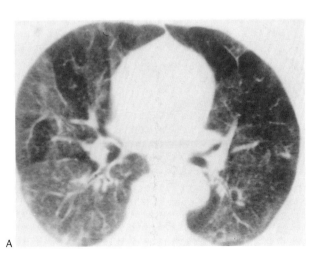
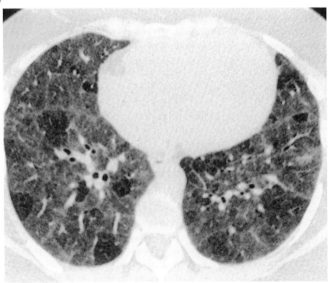

Fig. 7.24 Extrinsic allergic alveolitis. (A) CT demonstrates widespread patchy areas of increased attenuation (ground-glass shadowing) representative of areas of inflammatory infiltrate. (B) Similar appearances in a different patient. Note the characteristic sparing of single, or small clusters of, secondary pulmonary nodules.

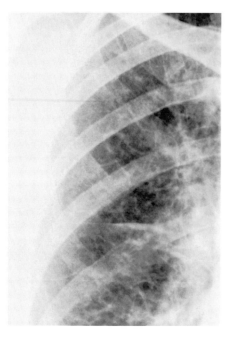

Fig. 7.25 Allergic alveolitis due to monoamine oxidase inhibitor drug. The interstitial shadowing was generalised throughout both lungs. Complete resolution within 7 days.

SYSTEMIC LUPUS ERYTHEMATOSUS

SLE is typically a disease of young women (F : M = 9 : 1), and blacks are affected more frequently than whites. Features usually include some or all of a butterfly facial rash, arthralgias, Raynaud's phenomenon, renal involvement and CNS disease. The lungs or pleura are involved in approximately 50% of cases. Interstitial fibrosis is relatively rare, occurring in less than 5% of cases.

Pleuritic pain with a small *pleural effusion* is a common manifestation, and may occur bilaterally (Fig. 7.26). Movement of the diaph-

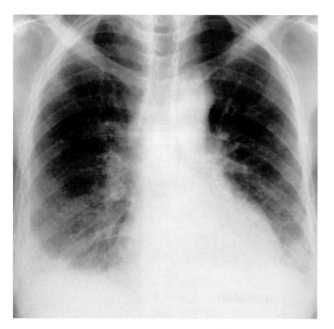

Fig. 7.26 Systemic lupus erythematosus. Bilateral pleural effusions are present.

ragm is decreased secondary to the pleurisy and may cause areas of *atelectasis* in the lower lobes. This may produce bilateral, horizontal basal band shadows and elevation of the diaphragm on the chest radiograph. The reduction in lung volume is not usually accompanied by pleural or parenchymal disease, even on HRCT. It is probably a reflection of SLE-related chest wall or diaphragmatic myopathy.

Patchy consolidation

This may be seen, sometimes with cavitation, and is most often due to infection, pulmonary oedema or pulmonary infarction. Lupus pneumonitis and diffuse pulmonary haemorrhage occasionally occur. Vascular thrombosis, either in the lungs or elsewhere, is related to the lupus anticoagulant that paradoxically increases coagulability in vivo.

Enlargement of the cardiac shadow

This may be due to pericardial effusion, myocarditis or endocarditis, and should be investigated by cardiac ultrasound in the first instance.

RHEUMATOID DISEASE

Rheumatoid disease may cause pleural effusions, pulmonary nodules, fibrosing alveolitis and bronchiolitis obliterans. These occur more often in males than females, occasionally being apparent before joint disease. Overall, only a few per cent of patients with rheumatoid arthritis develop fibrosing alveolitis, although conversely rheumatoid arthritis is a relatively common aetiology in a mixed population of patients with fibrosing alveolitis.

Pleural effusion

Effusions are the commonest thoracic manifestation. These may be unilateral or bilateral, are usually larger than in SLE and are often asymptomatic. Rheumatoid pleural effusions often become chronic but may resolve with pleural fibrosis. Rarely a cholesterol effusion may develop and remain unchanged over several years.

Rheumatoid pulmonary nodules

These are uncommon but are characteristic of this condition (Fig. 7.27). The necrobiotic nodules are usually associated with subcutaneous nodules, and are similar histologically. They produce well-defined, round opacities up to 7 cm in diameter and may be single or multiple and may cavitate. In Caplan's syndrome rheumatoid nodules develop against a background of simple pneumoconiosis. The two diseases modify each other in a distinctive fashion and numerous round opacities up to 5 cm in diameter, resembling metastases, may appear (Fig. 7.15). The solid fibrotic lesions eventually become hyalinised and may calcify. The syndrome was first described in coal miners but it is also found in asbestosis, silicosis and other industrial pneumoconioses.

Fibrosing alveolitis

This is apparent on the chest radiograph in approximately 5% of patients. However evidence of interstitial fibrosis is more common on HRCT, pulmonary function testing and histological examination.

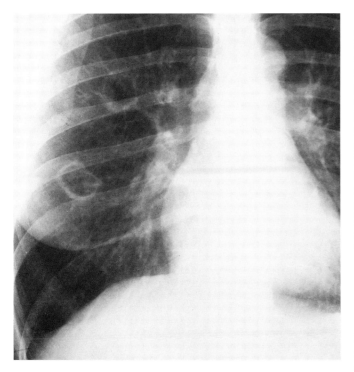

Fig. 7.27 Rheumatoid disease. Two cavitating necrobiotic nodules are visible in the right lung.

The pattern of disease is indistinguishable from cryptogenic fibrosing alveolitis, and opinion is divided as to whether the prognosis is any better than cryptogenic fibrosing alveolitis. Radiologically there is usually basal reticulonodular shadowing that may progress to honeycombing and severe volume loss (Fig. 7.28).

Obliterative bronchiolitis is a potential cause of respiratory failure and the chest radiograph may be normal, although evidence of small airways disease may be evident on HRCT.

Progressive upper lobe fibrosis with bullous cystic changes indistinguishable from those found in ankylosing spondylitis has also been reported.

SYSTEMIC SCLEROSIS

Systemic sclerosis has the highest incidence of pulmonary fibrosis amongst the connective tissue diseases, with almost all patients eventually developing lung disease that is indistinguishable from idiopathic pulmonary fibrosis. However progression is slower and the outlook slightly better than in cryptogenic fibrosis. Oesophageal involvement resulting in abnormal motility may cause reflux and aspiration. Occasionally a dilated oesophagus, sometimes demonstrating an air–fluid level, is visible on the chest radiograph (Fig. 7.29). Pulmonary artery hypertension may be seen with or without pulmonary fibrosis. As in other conditions with fibrosing alveolitis, the usual appearance on the chest radiograph is of basal reticulonodular shadowing, with progressive pulmonary volume loss (Fig. 7.29). Eventually honeycomb change may develop. Eggshell lymph node calcification is a recognised feature. Associated pleural disease is rare. There is an increased prevalence of *lung cancer*.

OTHER CONNECTIVE TISSUE DISORDERS

Dermatomyositis and polymyositis

Primary lung involvement is unusual. A basal fibrosing alveolitis may occur and involvement of the pharyngeal muscles may predispose to aspiration pneumonitis (Fig. 7.30).

Ankylosing spondylitis

In 1–2% of cases of longstanding ankylosing spondylitis, upper lobe fibrosis develops. It is usually bilateral and associated with apical pleural thickening. The radiological appearances are indistinguishable from other causes of upper lobe fibrosis. With severe fibrosis bullae develop and may become colonised by *Aspergillus* (Fig. 7.31).

Sjögren's syndrome

Sjögren's syndrome comprises dry eyes, dry mouth and one of the other connective tissue disorders. If the latter is missing it is called the sicca syndrome or primary Sjögren's syndrome. Women are

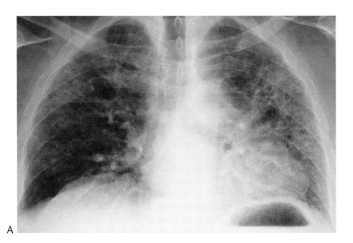

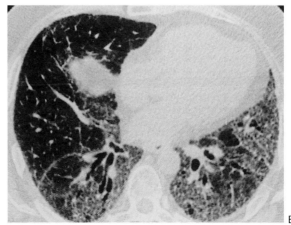

A   B

Fig. 7.28 Rheumatoid disease. Chest radiograph (A) and HRCT (B) demonstrating typical subpleural honeycomb changes of pulmonary fibrosis. There is considerable volume loss.

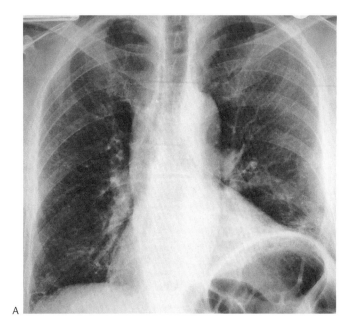

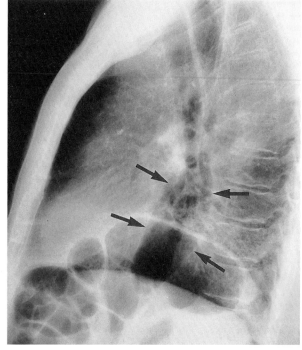

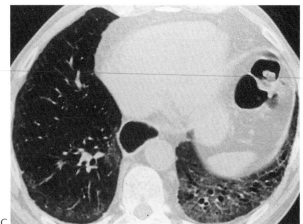

Fig. 7.29 Systemic sclerosis. (A,B) The chest radiograph demonstrates early fibrosis and dilatation of the oesophagus, best appreciated on the lateral film (arrows). (C) HRCT demonstrating fine basal fibrosis with some honeycomb changes. The left diaphragm is elevated.

more often affected than men. The salivary, lacrimal and mucous glands of the mouth, nose, eyelids, pharynx, bronchial tree and stomach may all be the site of the pathological changes, which consist of a massive lymphoid infiltration with eventual atrophy of the gland acini. There are minor salivary glands in the lip and this is the easiest site for diagnostic biopsy. Although sarcoidosis may involve the salivary glands, with the same functional effects, it is by convention excluded from the definition of Sjögren's and sicca syndromes. In addition to the features of an associated connective tissue disease there may also be pleural effusion, fibrosing alveolitis, recurrent chest infections and lymphocytic interstitial pneumonitis. As a result there is no characteristic pattern.

SYSTEMIC VASCULITIDES

This section also includes diseases that have traditionally been classified together as *pulmonary angiitis* and *granulomatosis*. This subgroup comprises Wegener's granulomatosis, allergic angiitis and granulomatosis (Churg–Strauss syndrome), necrotising sarcoid granulomatosis, lymphoid granulomatosis and bronchocentric granulomatosis.

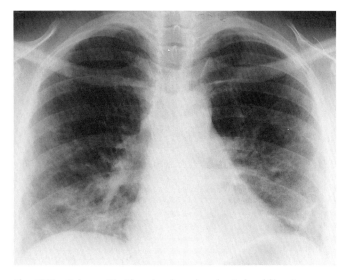

Fig. 7.30 Polymyositis. There is volume loss due to basal fibrosis.

Wegener's granulomatosis

Classic Wegener's granulomatosis is a necrotising vasculitis, which involves the upper respiratory tract, the lungs and the kidneys. There is a limited variant, which is more or less confined to the thorax.

Symptoms referable to the upper air passages are almost always present at some time in the course of the disease: nasal obstruction, purulent discharge, sinusitis, chronic ulceration—even, in some cases, necrosis of nasal cartilage and bone. Cough, haemoptysis and pleurisy are usually accompanied by constitutional symptoms of malaise, weakness and fever. Rheumatoid and antinuclear factors are commonly found in the blood. Untreated, the disease has a poor prognosis with an average survival of 5 months, but steroids and cyclophosphamide have transformed the outlook.

Lesions occur in any part of the respiratory tract and take the form of inflammatory necrosis in the walls of small arteries and veins leading to occlusion of the lumen. Granulation tissue containing lymphocytes, polymorphs and giant cells represents a reparative process, but this also undergoes necrosis. The necrotic granulation tissue forms rubbery pulmonary masses, which may be single or multiple. Granulomatous masses up to several centimetres in diameter may be apparent on the chest radiograph (Fig. 7.32). These are fairly well defined and often cavitate; they may resolve spontaneously, while new masses appear. Cavitating lesions may have thick or thin walls, depending on how much of the necrotic material is expectorated. Multiple cavities can closely mimic tuberculosis.

A diffuse pattern of disease, where the area of involved lung is still aerated but contains vaguely reticular or irregular nodular opacities, is also recognised. Relapse may occur in previously affected areas.

Other frequent radiographic signs are small pleural effusions and paranasal sinus opacification. Occasional complications are pneumothorax and subglottic stenosis, and granulomas may also develop in the trachea or bronchi and cause pulmonary collapse. Reactive hilar or mediastinal lymphadenopathy may be seen.

Polyarteritis nodosa (PAN)

Classic PAN is a vasculitis of medium sized arteries which involves the kidneys and liver more often than the lungs. There is inflammation in and around the vessel, followed by necrosis of the wall, which is thereby weakened and gives way, forming small aneurysms, the 'nodosa' of the title. The process also occludes vessels. It is predominantly a male disease, in the ratio 3 : 1. The protean symptomatology reflects the widespread distribution of the lesions, affecting gut, skin, kidney, heart, central nervous system, joints and muscle. Visceral angiography shows aneurysms or other arterial abnormalities in over 60% of cases.

PAN may be associated with eosinophilia, and may present as asthma with transient pulmonary opacities. Pulmonary oedema may occur secondary to cardiac or renal failure, and areas of consolidation may be due to pulmonary haemorrhage.

Radiological appearances

Abnormalities in the lungs are unusual but nodules, segmental opacities, atelectasis, small pleural effusions and diffuse interstitial fibrosis may be found. Opacities are usually transient, except for those caused by diffuse fibrosis.

The rare disease of *relapsing polychondritis* has similarities to polyarteritis nodosa and the two conditions are sometimes found together. There is inflammation, necrosis and fibrosis of cartilage and other tissues with a high glycosaminoglycan content. The destruction of the cartilage of the bronchial tree produces collapsible airways and ultimately fibrotic strictures. The lungs are exposed to the risk of infection because of defective clearance of secretions.

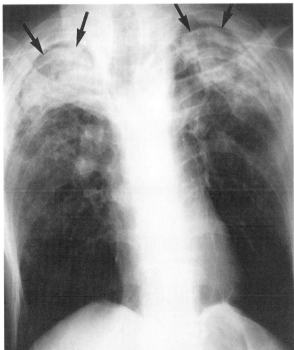

A

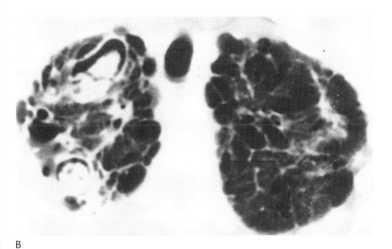

B

Fig. 7.31 Ankylosing spondylitis. (A) Chest radiograph demonstrating bilateral apical mycetoma (arrows). (B) Ankylosing spondylitis in a different patient with mycetoma formation confirmed on CT.

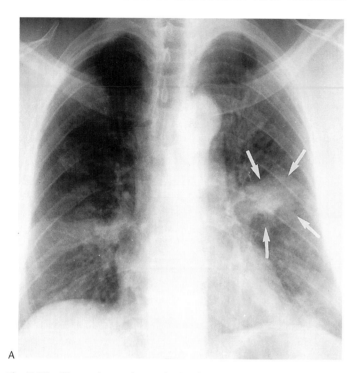
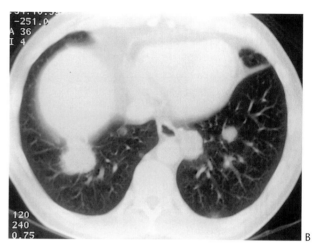

Fig. 7.32 Wegener's granulomatosis. (A) There are several poorly defined pulmonary masses, the largest in the left midzone (arrows). (B) CT through the lung bases of a man with biopsy-proven Wegener's. There are multiple mass-like lesions up to several centimetres in size.

Allergic granulomatosis and angiitis (*Churg–Strauss disease*)

This lies at one end of a scale with classic polyarteritis nodosa at the other (see below), the middle ground being occupied by the overlap syndrome with features common to both. Like classic PAN, allergic granulomatosis and angiitis is a generalised necrotising vasculitis but with certain differences. The lungs are always involved; it occurs in patients with asthma; there is a blood eosinophilia; the pathology is granulomatous; and eosinophils figure more prominently in the infiltrations. The differences are therefore mostly of degree rather than of kind. It is to be suspected in asthmatics with a multisystem disorder and affects the same organs as classic PAN.

Lung opacities are alveolar consolidations, sometimes massive, or a diffuse coarse reticulation, and typically they wax and wane. Infarcts following pulmonary arteritis account for some of the opacities. Sometimes the presentation is acute, suggesting a precipitating insult, and drugs, serum sickness or infection can induce this hypersensitivity vasculitis. Henoch–Schönlein purpura is a vasculitis of this type. These transient lung opacities are nodular, diffuse or patchy.

Necrotising sarcoid angiitis

It is still unclear if this condition represents a form of sarcoidosis in which there is necrosis in the granulomas and vessels, or a necrotising angiitis with a sarcoid-like reaction. Unlike other angiocentric granulomatous diseases this condition spares the upper airways, glomeruli and systemic circulation, and shares histological and clinical features of sarcoidosis. It has been suggested that a more appropriate name would be nodular sarcoidosis. Within the lungs there are sarcoid-like granulomas and a granulomatous vasculitis.

Multiple or solitary pulmonary nodules, with or without infiltrates, and hilar lymph node enlargement are the radiological features.

Lymphomatoid granulomatosis

This is similar to Wegener's granulomatosis but involves the lymphoreticular tissues. Indeed many of the features of this condition also occur in various lymphomas and it is probable that it may be a form of lymphoma itself. Indeed approximately 10% of cases will develop more classic features of lymphoma. Radiology is non-specific and biopsy is required for diagnosis.

Bronchocentric granulomatosis

This condition resembles allergic bronchopulmonary aspergillosis. Vasculitis is probably only a secondary phenomenon to airways disease and only occurs adjacent to necrotising granulomatous lesions. The disease may occur in asthmatics, in which case there may be pulmonary and peripheral eosinophilia and precipitins to aspergillus. When the disease is encountered in non-asthmatics, the patients are older and have milder symptoms. Radiologically the appearances are non-specific. There may be a single or multiple opacities, consolidation, atelectasis, cavitation or a reticulonodular infiltrate (Fig. 7.33). Changes are usually unilateral. Diagnosis requires biopsy.

PULMONARY EOSINOPHILIA

A number of conditions cause transient opacities on the chest radiograph in association with an excess of eosinophils in the blood. The pulmonary opacities are due to an eosinophilic exudate. These con-

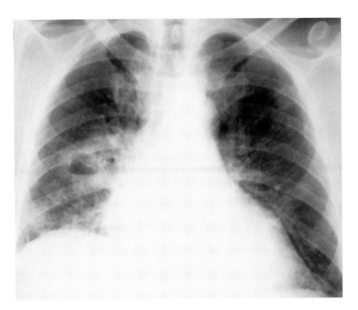

Fig. 7.33 Bronchocentric granulomatosis. There is a cavitating pulmonary mass. Diagnosis was made following resection.

ditions are sometimes referred to as the PIE syndrome (pulmonary infiltrates with eosinophilia).

Simple pulmonary eosinophilia (*Löffler's syndrome*)

This is usually a mild, transient condition. A large number of allergens have been found to be responsible, but often the cause is not identified. Box 7.2 lists some of the causes. The chest radiograph shows areas of ill-defined, non-segmental consolidation, which may change position over a few days, but usually resolve within a month. HRCT may reveal areas of ground-glass attenuation (Fig. 7.34).

Chronic pulmonary eosinophilia

This rare condition is associated with fever, malaise, cough and prolonged eosinophilia. One-third of patients give a history of asthma or atopy. Pathological examination demonstrates alveolar exudate containing eosinophilia and macrophages and mild alveolar wall infiltration. A few patients will have eosinophilic infiltration in other organs, including the myocardium. The radiological features

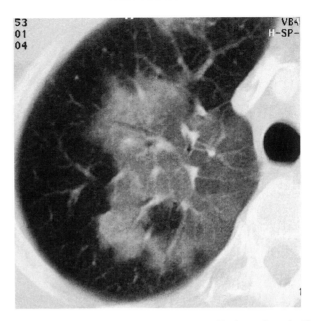

Fig. 7.34 Simple pulmonary eosinophilia (Loffler's syndrome). This patient had a marked transient blood and pulmonary eosinophilia, with non-specific chest symptoms. CT revealed patchy areas of ground-glass density in both lung apices that cleared rapidly on prednisolone therapy.

are similar to Löffler's syndrome, but persist for a month or more, and the areas of consolidation tend to be peripheral in distribution (Fig. 7.35). A particularly distinctive pattern that is virtually diagnostic in the appropriate clinical setting is a vertical band of consolidation paralleling the chest wall but separated from it, not being restricted by the pulmonary fissures. This distribution is even more apparent on CT (Fig. 7.36). The differential diagnosis of this radiological appearance should include cryptogenic organising pneumonia, particularly when the changes are peripheral and basal. Treatment with steroids usually produces a dramatic radiological and symptomatic improvement, although initial doses

---

Box 7.2 Pulmonary eosinophilia: types and causes

Simple pulmonary eosinophilia	Chronic pulmonary eosinophilia
Parasites	Aetiology uncertain
Ascaris lumbricoides	Tropical pulmonary eosinophilia
Ankylostoma	Filariasis
Strongyloides	Asthmatic pulmonary eosinophilia
Taenia	*Aspergillus fumigatus*
Toxocara	Connective tissue disorders
Drugs	Wegener's granulomatosis
PAS	Other systemic vasculitides
Aspirin	
Penicillin	
Nitrofurantoin	
Sulfonamides	

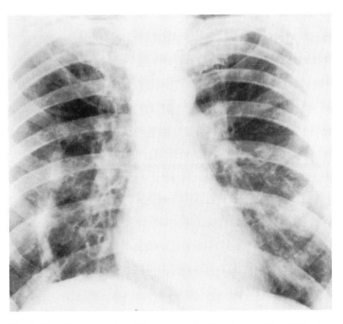

Fig. 7.35 Chronic eosinophilic pneumonia. Alveolar opacities distributed peripherally. The vertical band in the right lung is characteristic.

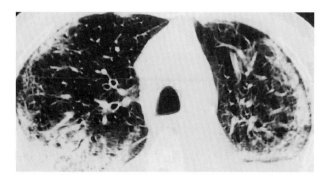

Fig. 7.36 Chronic eosinophilic pneumonia in a retired farmer. There is consolidation paralleling the chest wall bilaterally.

need to be high and therapy at a reduced dose may need to be prolonged.

Tropical pulmonary eosinophilia

This is caused by *filariasis* and presents with a cough, wheeze and sometimes fever. The chest radiograph shows fine, bilateral, diffuse nodular shadowing, with occasional confluent areas.

Asthmatic pulmonary eosinophilia

This is most commonly caused by *Aspergillus fumigatus* but often no allergen is identified. In uncomplicated asthma the chest radiograph is usually normal between attacks or may show hyperinflation during an episode of wheezing. In chronic severe asthma hyperinflation may persist. Lobar or segmental collapse due to bronchial mucosal swelling and mucus plugging may occur and often resolves completely and rapidly. When asthmatic pulmonary eosinophilia develops bronchial casts may be coughed up during attacks, and there may be fever. The chest radiograph may then show transient infiltrates, but after repeated attacks there may also be irreversible changes due to fibrosis and bronchiectasis.

Pulmonary eosinophilia associated with the systemic vasculitides

The radiographic features are those of the underlying connective tissue disorder.

DIFFUSE PULMONARY FIBROSIS

Pulmonary fibrosis may be a localised or generalised occurrence. Localised pulmonary fibrosis is commonly the result of pneumonia or radiotherapy. Diffuse pulmonary fibrosis is usually the result of a systemic condition or is due to inhalation of dusts or fumes (Box 7.3).

Fibrosing alveolitis

Fibrosing alveolitis describes a number of conditions in which there is pulmonary fibrosis associated with a chronic inflammatory reaction in the alveolar walls. It includes such conditions as diffuse idiopathic pulmonary fibrosis, diffuse interstitial fibrosis and

Box 7.3 Diffuse pulmonary fibrosis: causes	
Cryptogenic fibrosing alveolitis	Infection
Radiation	Tuberculosis
Drugs and poisons	Fungi
Connective tissue diseases	Viral
Systemic sclerosis	Sarcoidosis
SLE	Histiocytosis
Rheumatoid disease	Neurofibromatosis
Organic and inorganic dusts	Tuberose sclerosis
Pneumoconioses	Lymphangiomyomatosis
Silicosis	
Extrinsic allergic alveolitis	
Noxious gases	
Chronic pulmonary venous hypertension	
Adult respiratory distress syndrome	

Hamman–Rich disease. The aetiology is frequently uncertain, but many cases are associated with a known cause (Box 7.3).

Cryptogenic fibrosing alveolitis

This condition is also known as *usual interstitial pneumonitis* (UIP) and may be regarded as an interstitial pneumonitis. Histologically most cases show fibrosis and cellular infiltrate confined to the alveolar walls. Rarely the predominant finding is a mononuclear cell infiltrate in the alveoli and may be termed *desquamative interstitial pneumonitis* (DIP) (Fig. 7.37). Other variants are associated with bronchiolitis obliterans and diffuse alveolar damage, lymphocytic interstitial pneumonitis or a giant cell interstitial pneumonitis.

Patients present with increasing dyspnoea, a dry cough, finger clubbing, widespread basal crackles, and impaired ventilation and gas exchange. The disease may be rapidly progressive with death from respiratory or cardiac failure within a few weeks, or it may continue for many years.

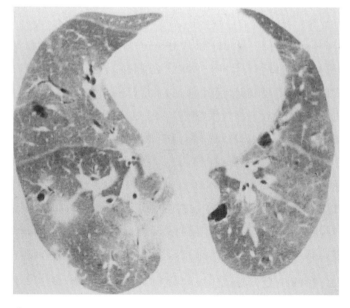

Fig. 7.37 Desquamative interstitial pneumonitis (DIP). There is diffuse ground-glass change throughout the lungs due to inflammatory infiltrate. Note the relatively low density of the larger bronchi and small bullae compared with the remainder of the lungs.

Desquamative histology has a better prognosis, but it can hardly be called benign, with a reported mortality of 27% and a mean survival time of 12 years. Carcinoma of the lung of all histological types, including bronchioloalveolar cell, complicates the disease process in about 10% of cases.

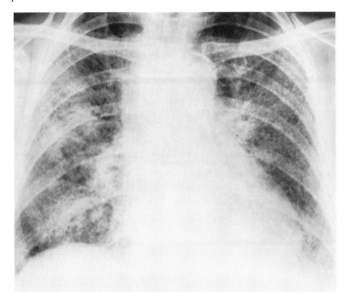

Fig. 7.38 Cryptogenic fibrosing alveolitis. Miliary opacities and a little reticulation. The apices are spared.

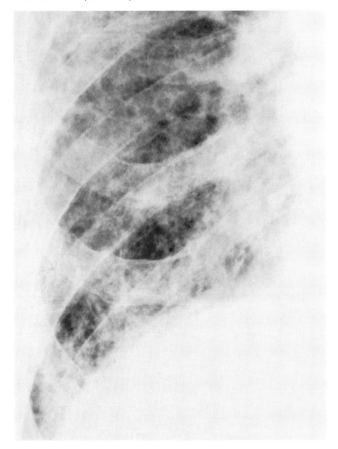

Fig. 7.39 Cryptogenic fibrosing alveolitis. Ring shadows are well seen in the right lower zone due to coarse fibrosis and honeycomb formation.

The earliest *radiographic change* is bilateral, basal, ground-glass shadowing. This is followed by a fine nodular pattern, and then coarser, linear shadows develop, predominantly basally but spreading throughout the lungs (Fig. 7.38). There is progressive pulmonary volume loss. Ring shadows appear and may produce a honeycomb pattern (Fig. 7.39), and basal septal lines may be visible. Pleural effusion is rare.

HRCT is of particular value in idiopathic pulmonary fibrosis, in which the appearances may be sufficiently diagnostic to avoid the necessity of an open lung biopsy (Fig. 7.40). In addition, HRCT allows some assessment of the relative degrees of inflammation and fibrosis, and so is able to predict the likelihood of success of steroid therapy (Fig. 7.41). Hilar and mediastinal lymph node enlargement is well recognised, but only usually apparent on CT. Pleural effusions are rare. Cor pulmonale, pulmonary embolism and infection

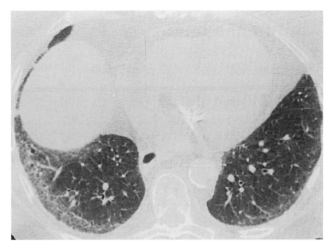

Fig. 7.40 Cryptogenic fibrosing alveolitis. HRCT through the lung bases shows subpleural fibrosis. Lung biopsy is likely to reveal established fibrosis.

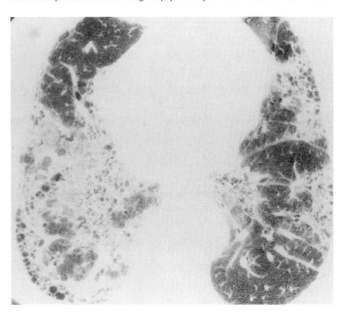

Fig. 7.41 Cryptogenic fibrosing alveolitis. HRCT shows a mixture of fibrosis and areas of ground-glass change. Histological assessment of lung biopsy will reveal a mixture of inflammation and fibrosis. This patient may benefit from steroids although the established fibrous component may remain.

are all complications that may further contribute to radiographic changes.

Langerhans cell histiocytoses

In the past this disorder was known as histiocytosis X and divided into three subtypes: Letterer–Siwe disease, Hand–Schüller–Christian disease and eosinophilic granuloma. They are now felt to be manifestations of the same disorder, and are collectively known as Langerhans cell histiocytosis. The three patterns of clinical presentation overall involve the lung in about 20% of cases. Letterer–Siwe is the disseminated form of disease that usually presents before 2 years of age. Eosinophilic granuloma, which may be multifocal or unifocal, usually involves the skeleton, but may be confined to the lungs.

Pulmonary Langerhans cell histiocytosis may present without symptoms, or with a dry cough, dyspnoea, fever, chest pain or spontaneous pneumothorax. Patients are often young, sex incidence is probably equal, and 95% of patients are smokers. Histologically there is infiltration of alveolar walls by histiocytes and eosinophils, followed by fibrosis. The presence of Langerhans cells is regarded as specific. There is no association with atopy or allergy and there is no blood eosinophilia.

Radiology

The earliest reported manifestation is ill-defined transient patchy consolidation, but this is rarely seen. A fine reticulonodular pattern throughout both lungs, but predominantly in the mid and upper zones, is more usual (Fig. 7.42). The diagnosis usually requires confirmation with lung biopsy, although the HRCT changes are characteristic and show a mixture of discrete nodules and cystic spaces, sometimes with sparing of the lung bases. The range of severity of lung involvement and associated pulmonary impairment is wide. As fibrosis progresses, a coarser linear pattern appears, with development of ring shadows, honeycombing and bullae. The lung volumes are usually normal. There is a 20% incidence of spontaneous pneumothorax. In severe cases transplantation has been undertaken, although even then the disease may recur in the donor lungs (Fig. 7.43).

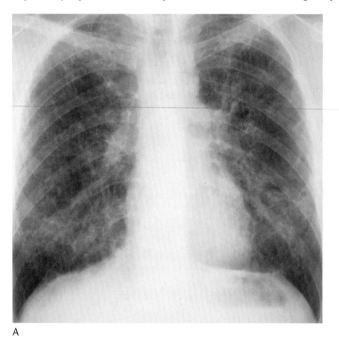

A

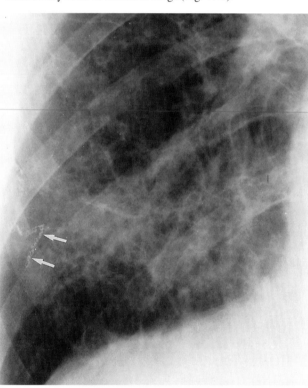

B

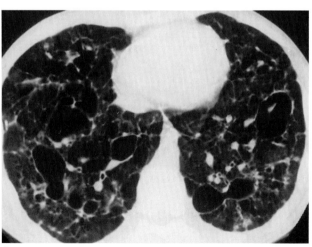

C

Fig. 7.42 Histiocytosis. (A,B) Fine reticulonodular shadowing is present throughout both lungs, producing a honeycomb pattern. Note the line of biopsy staples (arrows). (C) CT demonstrates cystic spaces and discrete nodules characteristic of histiocytosis.

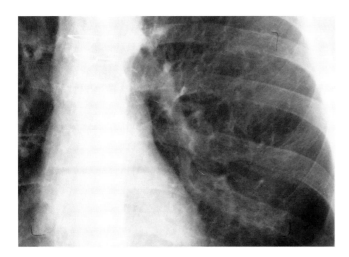

Fig. 7.43 Histiocytosis recurring following transplantation. Note the sternotomy suture wires.

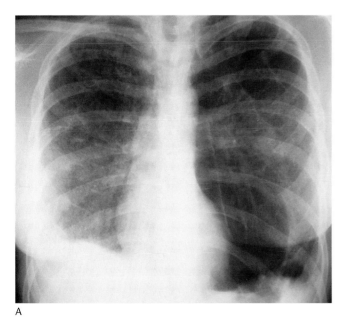

A

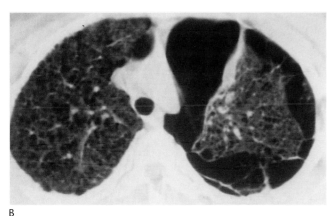

B

Fig. 7.44 Tuberous sclerosis. (A) There is a fine reticular infiltrate. The right costophrenic angle is blunted following pleurodesis. There is a loculated left pneumothorax. (B) HRCT demonstrates multiple thin-walled cystic spaces, and loculated pneumothorax.

Tuberous sclerosis

This is an autosomal dominant neurocutaneous disorder that classically consists of the triad of mental retardation, epilepsy and adenoma sebaceum. Only about 1% of patients with tuberous sclerosis will develop lung involvement. The majority of patients developing lung involvement are older and with a lower incidence of mental retardation than the population of tuberous sclerosis patients as a whole. If pulmonary disease does develop it is often the most important clinical consequence of the disease. Recurrent pneumothoraces are frequent (Fig. 7.44), and respiratory failure or cor pulmonale is often progressive and fatal. Diffuse hyperplasia of smooth muscle in the small airways, alveolar walls and peripheral vessels produces reticulonodular shadowing and eventually *honeycombing* on the chest radiograph.

As with histiocytosis X the diagnosis can be suggested with HRCT, which demonstrates multiple thin-walled cysts, with normal areas of intervening lung, usually affecting all lung zones equally (Fig. 7.45). Chylous pleural effusions are rare but may be large, bilateral and persistent.

Lymphangioleiomyomatosis (LAM)

The condition is radiologically and pathologically very similar to tuberous sclerosis. There is proliferation of smooth muscle and lymphatics in the alveolar walls, interlobular septa and pleura. However in LAM the distribution of muscle proliferation is initially perilymphatic, and the disease may also involve the mediastinal and retroperitoneal lymph nodes. Hence chylothorax and chyloperitoneum are commoner than in tuberous sclerosis. LAM is confined to females, and almost all are premenopausal. Clinical features of pneumothorax, dyspnoea and haemoptysis are the same as those encountered in tuberous sclerosis. Anti-oestrogen therapy has resulted in some improvement in prognosis.

The chest radiographic and HRCT features (Fig. 7.46) are identical to tuberous sclerosis apart from occasional associated changes in the ribs.

Neurofibromatosis

Pulmonary fibrosis occurs in approximately 10% of patients with neurofibromatosis Type I. Disease progression is slow, in contrast to

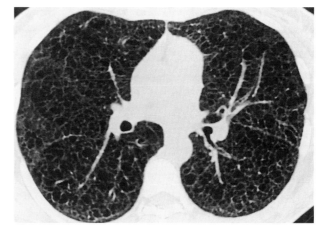

Fig. 7.45 Tuberous sclerosis. The lungs are almost completely replaced by multiple thin-walled cysts.

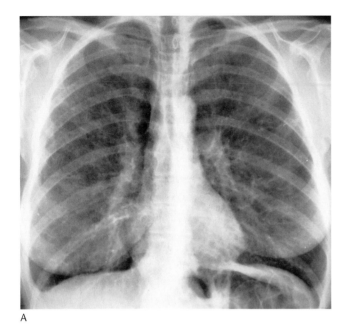

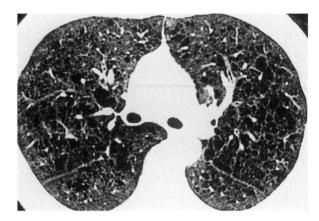

Fig. 7.47 Neurofibromatosis. There are multiple thin-walled cysts replacing the normal lung parenchyma.

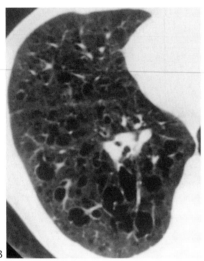

Fig. 7.46 Lymphangioleiomyomatosis. (A) Chest radiograph demonstrating normal lung volumes and multiple thin-walled cysts. (B) HRCT shows normal lung between the discrete cystic spaces.

tuberous sclerosis. Radiographically neurofibromatosis may produce reticular shadowing and honeycombing on the chest radiograph. Bullae may develop in the mid and upper zones (Fig. 7.47).

PULMONARY HAEMORRHAGE AND HAEMOSIDEROSIS

Haemorrhage into the lungs and airways may complicate lung cancer, pneumonia, bronchiectasis, pulmonary venous hypertension, blood dyscrasias, anticoagulant therapy, disseminated intravascular coagulation and trauma. Multifocal bleeding into the alveoli not associated with any of these conditions may be referred to as pulmonary haemosiderosis.

Pulmonary haemosiderosis

This may be either idiopathic or associated with renal disease. In *Goodpasture's syndrome* pulmonary haemosiderosis occurs with a glomerulonephritis associated with circulating antiglomerular basement membrane antibodies. Immunofluorescence microscopy shows a linear deposit of the immunoglobulin on the glomerular capillaries, sometimes with similar deposits on the alveolar capillaries. In other cases the nephritis may be due to Wegener's granulomatosis, systemic lupus erythematosus, polyarteritis nodosa or penicillamine hypersensitivity.

Infection, fluid overload, smoking and inhalation of toxic fumes are factors which are known to precipitate episodes of bleeding. Pulmonary function tests often indicate airways obstruction and there may be an increased uptake of inhaled radioactive carbon monoxide by the leaked blood. The latter test is useful in differentiating haemorrhage from oedema and infection. Treatment regimens include steroids, immunosuppression and plasmapheresis, and these are more effective in Goodpasture's syndrome than in the other types.

Haemoptysis is a common symptom but its severity does not match the large volumes of blood lost into the lungs, as most of it is beyond the mucociliary clearing processes. Bleeding is severe enough to cause anaemia, even at times requiring blood transfusion. Macrophages with engulfed red cells and haemosiderin fill the alveolar spaces and infiltrate the walls. These macrophages in the sputum or bronchoalveolar lavage fluid are a diagnostic feature. After repeated attacks of bleeding, interstitial fibrosis is initiated but this is not sufficiently extensive to cause gross scarring or destruction of lung architecture.

Radiology

During an acute episode of pulmonary haemorrhage patchy, ill-defined areas of consolidation appear on the chest radiograph (Fig. 7.48). They may become confluent and demonstrate an air bronchogram. The appearance may be indistinguishable from pulmonary oedema. HRCT is more sensitive than the chest radiograph in detecting abnormalities in patients with suspected pulmonary haemorrhage (Fig. 7.49). When bleeding stops, the opacities resolve within a few days. Following repeated episodes of bleeding, pulmonary fibrosis may develop and produce a diffuse hazy nodular or reticular pattern (Fig. 7.50).

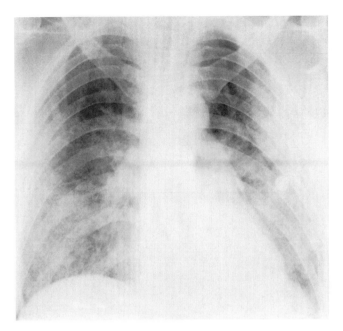

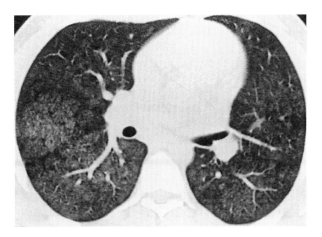

Fig. 7.50 Pulmonary haemosiderosis, chronic phase. There is diffuse ill-defined nodular change, mainly in the posterior aspect of the lungs.

Fig. 7.48 Pulmonary haemorrhage. Goodpasture's syndrome. Large alveolar opacities.

Patients with nephritis are prone to pulmonary oedema and pneumonia, and the differentiation from pulmonary haemorrhage may be difficult. Pneumonic consolidation tends to resolve more slowly than oedema or haemorrhage. Cardiomegaly, septal lines and pleural effusion suggest cardiogenic pulmonary oedema.

Pulmonary haemosiderosis is also well recognised in some patients with heart disease which chronically elevates left atrial pressure, such as occurs secondary to mitral stenosis. The radio-

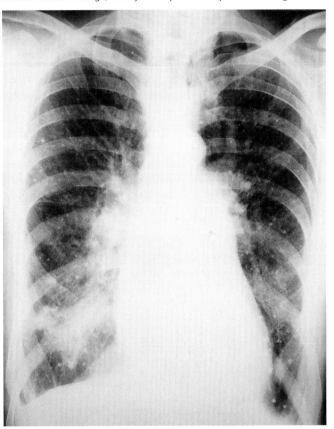

Fig. 7.51 Mitral stenosis with pulmonary ossification due to haemosiderosis.

graphic features in the lungs are distinctive, consisting of a permanent miliary stippling due to the focal nature of the bleeding (Fig. 7.51).

DRUG-INDUCED PULMONARY DISEASE

Many drugs in common use are toxic to the lungs and may produce diffuse pulmonary abnormalities. Although in some patients there is

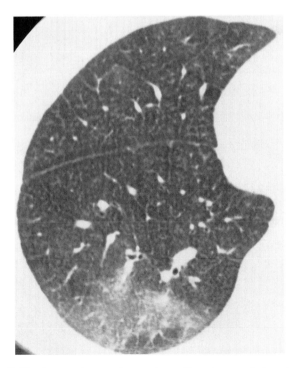

Fig. 7.49 Acute pulmonary haemorrhage. There is ground-glass change in the posterior aspect of the right lung, due to alveolar haemorrhage. Note the generalised nodularity due to the effects of recent haemorrhage.

a clear temporal relationship between the onset of symptoms and the introduction of drug therapy, in others there may be a lag time of several years before lung disease becomes clinically apparent. As a result the development of toxicity may go undetected.

When interpreting a chest radiograph with diffuse shadowing it is important to be aware of what therapy the patient has received or is undergoing. Some drugs are intrinsically toxic to the lungs (e.g. many cancer chemotherapeutic agents) and their effect on the lung may be dose related or cumulative. Other drugs seem to cause pulmonary abnormalities in a minority of recipients who show a hypersensitivity or idiosyncratic response. There are a variety of lung responses to drug toxicity. HRCT has been shown to be more sensitive than chest radiography in the detection of parenchymal changes in those patients suspected of having drug-induced lung disease.

Pulmonary fibrosis

Many cytotoxic drugs (e.g. azathioprine, bleomycin, busulfan, cyclophosphamide, chlorambucil) and non-cytotoxic drugs (amiodarone, nitrofurantoin) cause alveolitis which may progress to pulmonary fibrosis. The fibrogenic effect of cytotoxic drugs is enhanced by radiotherapy and high levels of inspired oxygen. The chest radiograph may show reticulonodular shadowing, often with a basal predominance (Fig. 7.51).

Pulmonary eosinophilia

Para-aminosalicylic acid (PAS), aspirin, penicillin, nitrofurantoin, sulfonamides and methotrexate are some of the substances that may produce an eosinophilia and pulmonary infiltrates. This hypersensitivity may, after prolonged drug administration, lead to pulmonary fibrosis.

Adult respiratory distress syndrome (ARDS)

This may result from the administration of a variety of agents, particularly cytotoxic agents such as cyclophosphamide, bleomycin and busulfan (Fig. 7.52).

Bronchiolitis obliterans

This condition may be drug induced, most commonly as a result of penicillamine therapy.

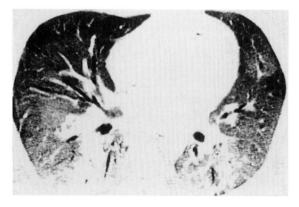

Fig. 7.52 ARDS reaction to methotrexate administration. Note the anterior posterior gradient of increase in lung density.

SLE reaction

Some drugs—such as penicillin, procainamide, isoniazid and methyldopa—may cause pleural effusions, pneumonitis and pulmonary fibrosis.

Pulmonary oedema

Pulmonary oedema may be a complication of narcotic overdose. It may also be caused by overinfusion of intravenous fluids and by hypersensitivity to transfused blood or blood products.

Pulmonary thromboembolism

This may arise from the use of oral contraceptives.

Opportunistic infection

Drugs that suppress the immune system (e.g. cancer chemotherapeutic agents and steroids) predispose to infection. Pneumonias that are likely to be seen in this context may be due to tuberculosis, Gram-negative bacteria, viruses, *Pneumocystis* and *Aspergillus*.

Mediastinal adenopathy

Phenytoin and amiodarone may cause lymph node enlargement (Fig. 7.53).

Pulmonary talcosis

Chronic intravenous drug abuse may lead to pulmonary talcosis as a result of chronic deposition of magnesium silicate (talc) within the lungs. The most common source of intravenous talc is as a binding agent used in most tablets, which may then be ground up and injected. The pulmonary inflammatory reaction produced by talc deposition may initially appear as a fine nodular or ground-glass appearance on the chest radiograph and HRCT scan (Fig. 7.54). Eventually the pulmonary fibrosis results in severe emphysema, with a radiological pattern that may resemble progressive massive fibrosis or end-stage sarcoidosis (Fig. 7.55).

AMYLOIDOSIS

Amyloid is a proteinaceous substance with specific chemical and staining properties. Amyloidosis is a group of conditions in which amyloid in unusually large amounts is deposited in connective tissue, around parenchymal tissue cells and in the walls of blood vessels. The conditions are grouped into primary and secondary categories according to whether there is a prior precipitating cause. Secondary amyloidosis may arise as a complication of chronic infection such as tuberculosis, osteomyelitis, bronchiectasis or leprosy, but in western countries infection now assumes less importance and the most common causes are rheumatoid disease and neoplasia.

Both primary and secondary amyloidosis can occur in localised and generalised forms. Once generalised amyloidosis is established, it tends to be progressive and has a poor prognosis when vital organs become involved. In 75% of cases of the generalised disease

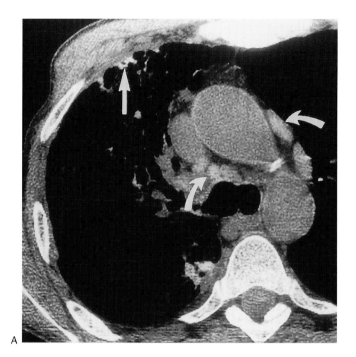

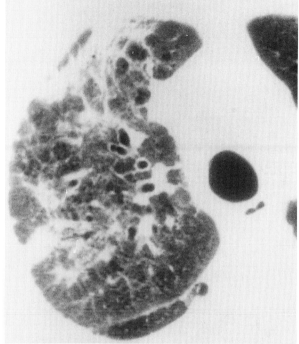

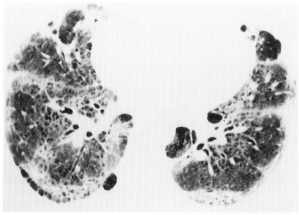

Fig. 7.53 (A) Amiodarone toxicity. There are enlarged mediastinal lymph nodes (curved arrows). Note the area of dense peripheral consolidation due to amiodarone deposition (arrow). (B) Same patient on lung windows demonstrating coarse fibrosis. (C) Lung fibrosis in a different patient on long-term pizotifen therapy.

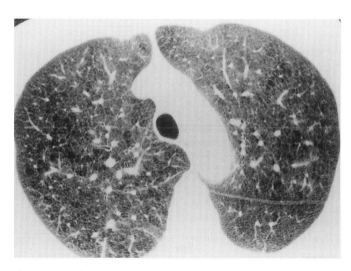

Fig. 7.54 Pulmonary talcosis due to repeated injection of ground-up tablets. There is diffuse increase in attenuation of the lung compared with the trachea.

there are amyloid deposits in the mucosa of rectal biopsy specimens. Secondary amyloid does not invoke an inflammatory response in the lungs, whereas primary amyloid does. For this reason secondary amyloidosis in the lungs seldom causes symptoms, and the chest radiograph is normal unless the initiating cause is intrapulmonary.

Primary amyloidosis may produce a variety of abnormalities in the airways and lungs. There may be multiple nodular angular opacities which can cavitate or calcify (Fig. 7.56). These nodules may be up to several centimetres in size and grow slowly. Calcification is usually in the form of fine stippling. Alternatively there may be diffuse reticulonodular shadowing or honeycombing due to diffuse deposition of amyloid within alveolar walls, lobular septa and pulmonary arterioles. Occasionally amyloid deposition is confined to hilar and mediastinal lymph nodes. Alternatively lymph node involvement may accompany tracheobronchial or parenchymal amyloid. Enlarged lymph nodes may contain calcification, and nodal size is occasionally massive.

Tracheobronchial amyloid may take the form of a solitary endobronchial tumour mass or polyp, or it may grow down the trachea

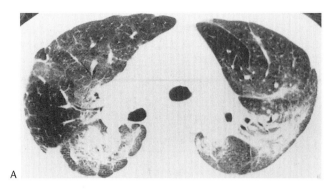

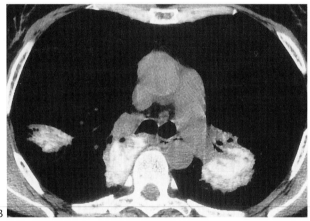

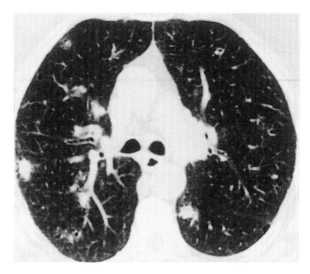

Fig. 7.56 Amyloidosis. CT scan reveals multiple small pulmonary nodules scattered through the lungs. In this patient these were non-calcified.

and into the bronchi in the form of nodular submucosal plaques. Radiologically, the effects are those of obstruction, namely atelectasis, distal bronchiectasis and infection. There is a nodularity of the wall of the air passages and multiple strictures. Surgical resection may be required. Amyloid material is sometimes found in relation to bronchial neoplasms, and caution is required in the interpretation of biopsy appearances as they may not be typical of the whole lesion.

Tracheobronchopathia osteochondroplastica is a very rare condition in which cartilaginous masses occur within the walls of the trachea and major bronchi. The masses contain amyloid deposits, calcific bodies and ossifications, and the condition may represent an end-stage of tracheobronchial amyloidosis.

Fig. 7.55 Pulmonary talcosis. (A) There are perihilar masses with radiating strands of fibrosis distorting the surrounding pulmonary architecture. Compare with Fig. 7.7. (B) CT scan on mediastinal window setting in a different patient demonstrating high attenuation in the perihilar masses.

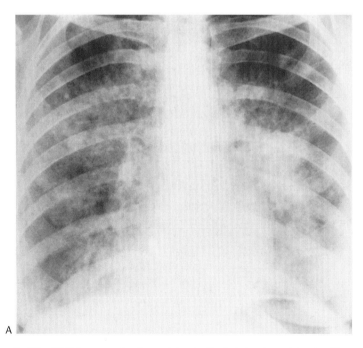

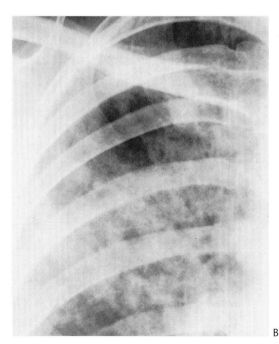

Fig. 7. 57 (A) Pulmonary alveolar proteinosis. Central alveolar patchy densities and vague nodulation. (B) Close-up. Ill-defined alveolar opacities; air bronchogram visible.

PULMONARY ALVEOLAR PROTEINOSIS

This is a rare disease of unknown aetiology in which Type II pneumocytes overproduce a proteinaceous lipid-rich material to a degree that overwhelms the capacity of the lung to remove it. This is probably the result of a response by the lungs to an irritant. Histologically there is a striking lack of reaction within the alveolar walls. The disease is three times more common in men than in women and can occur at any age.

The radiographic appearance resembles pulmonary oedema, with small, acinar, perihilar opacities present in both lungs (Fig. 7.57). These opacities may become confluent. There may be thickening of the interlobular septa in addition to ground-glass shadowing and consolidation on HRCT, producing the 'crazy-paving' appearance that is typical of this condition (Fig. 7.58). The disease predisposes to pulmonary infection from both common respiratory pathogens and opportunistic organisms. It may also be associated with lymphoma, leukaemia and immunoglobulin deficiency. Diagnosis is made by lung biopsy or bronchoalveolar lavage. Approximately 25% of cases are fatal within 5 years.

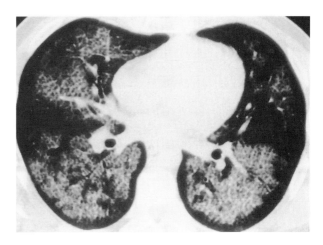

Fig. 7.58 Alveolar proteinosis. Typical crazy-paving appearances with alveolar filling and septal wall thickening.

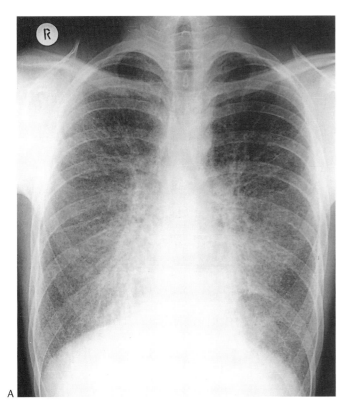

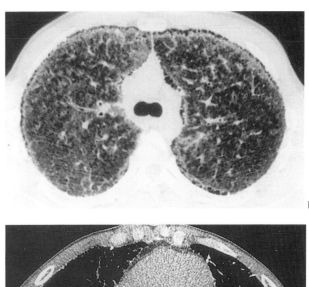

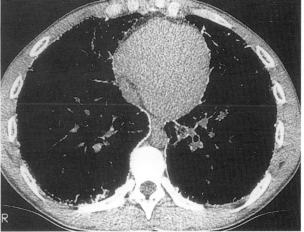

Fig. 7.59 (A) Pulmonary alveolar microlithiasis. Multiple, fine, dense opacities are visible throughout the lungs. HRCT on lung (B) and mediastinal (C) window settings. Innumerable tiny nodules are present, and there is a marked subpleural lucent line that may be apparent on scrutiny of the chest radiograph. The high-density nature of the lesions is apparent adjacent to the mediastinum.

PULMONARY ALVEOLAR MICROLITHIASIS

This is a disease of unknown aetiology which may be familial. It is characterised by the presence of multiple, fine sand-like calculi in the alveoli. The calculi are calcified and produce widespread, minute, but very dense opacities on the chest radiograph (Fig. 7.59). The strikingly abnormal radiograph contrasts with a relative lack of symptoms, although later in the disease there may be pulmonary fibrosis.

IDIOPATHIC PULMONARY OSSIFICATION

This rare condition has also been described under a variety of other names, including ossifying pneumonitis, bony metaplasia of lung and arboriform pulmonary ossification. In its usual form the delicate branching or lace-like pattern of dystrophic bone formation in the lower parts of the lungs is sufficiently distinctive to suggest the diagnosis. The cause is unknown and there are no symptoms attributable to the condition.

REFERENCES AND SUGGESTIONS FOR FURTHER READING

Aberle, D. R., Gamsu, G., Ray, C. S., et al (1988) Asbestos-related pleural and parenchymal fibrosis: detection with high-resolution CT. *Radiology*, **166**, 729–734.

Adler, B. D., Padley, S. P. G., Müller, N. L., et al (1992) Chronic hypersensitivity pneumonitis: high-resolution CT and radiographic features in 16 patients. *Radiology*, **185**, 91–95.

Akira, M., Yokoyama, K., Yamamoto, S., et al (1991) Early asbestosis: evaluation with high-resolution CT. *Radiology*, **178**, 409–416.

Begin, R., Ostiguy, G., Fillion, R., et al (1991) Computed tomography scan in the early detection of silicosis. *American Review of Respiratory Disease*, **144**, 697–705.

Bergin, C. J., Muller, N. L., Vedal, S., et al (1986) CT in silicosis: correlation with plain films and pulmonary function tests. *American Journal of Roentgenology*, **146**, 477–483.

Blesovsky, A. (1966) The folded lung. *British Journal of Diseases of the Chest*, **60**, 19–22.

Breatnach, E., Kerr, I. H. (1982) The radiology of cryptogenic obliterative bronchiolitis. *Clinical Radiology*, **33**, 657–661.

Brennan, S. R., Daly, J. J. (1979) Large pleural effusions in rheumatoid arthritis. *British Journal of Diseases of the Chest*, **73**, 133–140.

Buschman, D. L., Waldron, J. A., King, T. E. (1990) Churg–Strauss pulmonary vasculitis: high-resolution computed tomography scanning and pathologic findings. *American Review of Respiratory Disease*, **142**, 458–461.

Caplan, A. (1953) Certain unusual radiological appearances in the chest of coal-miners suffering from rheumatoid arthritis. *Thorax*, **8**, 29–37.

Caplan, A. (1962) Correlation of radiological category with lung pathology in coal-workers' pneumoconiosis. *British Journal of Industrial Medicine*, **19**, 171–179.

Cotes, E., Gibson, J. C., McKerrow, C. B., et al (1983) A long term follow-up of workers exposed to beryllium. *British Journal of Industrial Medicine*, **40**, 13–21.

Demling, R. H. (1987) Smoke inhalation injury. *Postgraduate Medicine*, **82**, 63–68.

Doig, A. T. (1976) Barytosis: a benign pneumoconiosis. *Thorax*, **31**, 30–39.

Epler, G. R., McLoud, T. C., Gaensler, E. A., et al (1978) Normal chest roentgenograms in chronic diffuse infiltrative lung disease. *North American Journal of Medicine*, **298**, 934–939.

Epler, G. R., McLoud, T .C., Gaensler, E. A. (1982) Prevalence and incidence of benign asbestos pleural effusion in a working population. *Journal of the American Medical Association*, **247**, 617.

Farrelly, C. A. (1982) Wegener's granulomatosis: a radiological review of the pulmonary manifestations at initial presentation and during relapse. *Clinical Radiology*, **33**, 545–551.

Feigin, D. S. (1986) Talc: understanding its manifestations in the chest. *American Journal of Roentgenology*, **146**, 295–301.

Frazier, A. R., Miller, R. D. (1974) Interstitial pneumonitis in association with polymyositis and dermatomyositis. *Chest*, **65**, 403–407.

Gaensler, E. A., Carrington, C. B. (1977) Peripheral opacities in chronic eosinophilic pneumonia: the photographic negative of pulmonary edema. *American Journal of Roentgenology*, **128**, 1–13.

Gaensler, E. A., Carrington, C. B. (1980) Open biopsy for chronic diffuse infiltrative lung disease: clinical, roentgenographic and physiological correlation in 502 patients. *Annals of Thoracic Surgery*, **30**, 411–426.

Gaensler, E. A., Carrington, C. B., Coutre, R. E., et al (1972) Pathological, physiological and radiological correlations in the pneumoconioses. *Annals of the New York Academy of Sciences*, **200**, 574–607.

Hansell, D. M., Moskovic, E. (1991) High-resolution computed tomography in extrinsic allergic alveolitis. *Clinical Radiology*, **43**, 8–12.

Hartman, T. E., Primack, S. L., Swensen, S. J., et al (1993) Desquamative interstitial pneumonia: thin section CT findings in 22 patients. *Radiology*, **187**, 787–790.

Hunninghake, G. W., Fauci, A. S. (1979) Pulmonary involvement in the collagen vascular diseases. *American Review of Respiratory Disease*, **119**, 471–503.

Julsrud, P. R., Brown, I. R., Li, C-Y., Rosenow, E. C., Crowe, J. K. (1978) Pulmonary processes of mature-appearing lymphocytes: pseudolymphoma, well-differentiated lymphocytic lymphoma and lymphocytic interstitial pneumonitis. *Radiology*, **127**, 289–296.

Kuhlman, J. E. (1991) The role of chest computed tomography in the diagnosis of drug-related reactions. *Journal of Thoracic Imaging*, **6**, 52–61.

Kuhlman, J. E., Hruban, R. H., Fishman, E. K. (1991) Wegener's granulomatosis: CT features of parenchymal lung disease. *Journal of Computer Assisted Tomography*, **15**, 948–952.

Landay, M. J., Christensen, E. E., Bynum, L. J. (1978) Pulmonary manifestations of acute aspiration of gastric contents. *American Journal of Roentgenology*, **131**, 587–592.

Levin, D. C. (1971) Proper interpretation of pulmonary roentgen changes in systemic lupus erythematosus. *American Journal of Roentgenology*, **111**, 510–517.

Locke, G. B. (1963) Rheumatoid lung. *Clinical Radiology*, **14**, 43–53.

Lynch, D. A., Gamsu, G., Aberle, D. R. (1989) Conventional and high resolution tomography in the diagnosis of asbestos-related diseases. *Radiographics*, **9**, 523–551.

Lynch, D. A., Rose, C. S., Way, D., et al (1992) Hypersensitivity pneumonitis: sensitivity of high-resolution CT in a population-based study. *American Journal of Roentgenology*, **159**, 469–472.

McDonald, T. J., Neel, H. B., DeRemee, R. A. (1982) Wegener's granulomatosis of the subglottis and the upper portion of the trachea. *Annals of Otology, Rhinology and Larnyngology*, **91**, 588–592.

MacFarlane, J. D., Diepe, P .A., Rigden, B. G., Clark, T. J. H. (1978) Pulmonary and pleural lesions in rheumatoid disease. *British Journal of Diseases of the Chest*, **72**, 288–300.

McLoud, T. C., Epler, G. R., Colby, T. V., Gaensler, E. A., Carrington, C. B. (1986) Bronchiolitis obliterans. *Radiology*, **159**, 1–8.

Mana, J. (1997) Nuclear imaging. 67-Gallium, 201-thallium, 18F-labeled fluoro-2-deoxy-D-glucose positron emission tomography. *Clinics in Chest Medicine*, **18**, 799–811.

Mayo, J. R., Müller, N. L., Road, J., et al (1989) Chronic eosinophilic pneumonia: CT findings in six cases. *American Journal of Roentgenology*, **153**, 727–730.

Mendelson, C. L. (1946) The aspiration of stomach contents into the lungs during obstetric anesthesia. *American Journal of Obstetrics and Gynecology*, **52**, 191–205.

Müller, N. L., Miller, R. R., Webb, W. R., et al (1986) Fibrosing alveolitis: CT–pathologic correlation. *Radiology*, **160**, 585–588.

Müller, N. L., Staples, C. A., Miller, R. R., et al (1987) Disease activity in idiopathic pulmonary fibrosis: CT and pathologic correlation. *Radiology*, **165**, 731–734.

Neeld, E. M., Limacher, M. C. (1978) Chemical pneumonitis after the intravenous injection of hydrocarbon. *Radiology*, **129**(1), 36.

Padley, S. P. G., Hansell, D. M., Flower, C. D. R., et al (1991) Comparative accuracy of high resolution, computed tomography in the diagnosis of chronic diffuse infiltrative lung disease. *Clinical Radiology*, **44**, 222–226.

Padley, S. P. G., Adler, B., Hansell, D. M., et al (1992) High-resolution computed tomography of drug-induced lung disease. *Clinical Radiology*, **46**, 232–236.

Peacock, C., Copley, S. J., Hansell, D. M. (2000) Asbestos-related benign pleural disease. *Clinical Radiology*, **55**, 422–432.

Primack, S. L., Hartman, T. E., Hansell, D. M., et al (1993) End-stage lung disease: CT findings in 61 patients. *Radiology*, **189**, 681–686.

Remy-Jardin, M., Degreef, J. M., Beuscart, R., et al (1990) Coal workers pneumoconiosis: CT assessment in exposed workers and correlation with radiographic findings. *Radiology*, **177**, 363–371.

Remy-Jardin, M., Remy, J., Deffontaines, C., et al (1991) Assessment of diffuse infiltrative lung disease: comparison of conventional CT and high-resolution CT. *Radiology*, **181**, 157–162.

Remy-Jardin, M., Remy, J., Wallaert, B., et al (1993) Pulmonary involvement in progressive systemic sclerosis: sequential evaluation with CT, pulmonary function tests, and bronchoalveolar lavage. *Radiology*, **188**, 499–506.

Sargent, E. N., Gordonson, J. S., Jacobson, G. (1977) Pleural plaques: a signpost of asbestos dust inhalation. *Seminars in Roentgenology*, **12**, 287–297.

Schurawitzki, H., Stiglbauer, R., Graninger, W., et al (1990) Interstitial lung disease in progressive systemic sclerosis: high-resolution CT versus radiography. *Radiology*, **176**, 755–759.

Staples, C. A., Gamsu, G., Ray, C. S., et al (1989) High resolution computed tomography and lung function in asbestos-exposed workers with normal chest radiographs. *American Review of Respiratory Diseases*, **139**, 1502–1508.

Talner, L. B., Gmelich, J. T., Liebow, A. A., Greenspan, R. H. (1970) The syndrome of bronchial mucocele and regional hyperinflation of the lung. *American Journal of Roentgenology*, **110**, 675–686.

Turner-Warwick, M. (1974) A perspective view on widespread pulmonary fibrosis. *British Medical Journal*, **ii**, 371–376.

Turner-Warwick, M., Dewar, A. (1982) Pulmonary haemorrhage and pulmonary haemosiderosis. *Clinical Radiology*, **33**, 361–370.

Wells, A. U., Hansell, D. M., Corrin, B., et al (1992) High resolution computed tomography as a predictor of lung histology in systemic sclerosis. *Thorax*, **47**, 738–742.

Yoshimura, H., Hatakeyama, M., Otsuji, H., et al (1986) Pulmonary asbestosis: CT study of subpleural curvilinear shadow. *Radiology*, **158**, 653–658.

8

MISCELLANEOUS CHEST CONDITIONS

Simon P. G. Padley and Michael B. Rubens

TRAUMA

The thorax may be affected by direct trauma, or by effects of trauma elsewhere in the body. Direct trauma may be the result of penetrating or non-penetrating injury. The usual causes of penetrating injury are shooting, stabbing and shrapnel wounds.

Thoracic surgery is a special category of penetrating trauma. Falls, blows, blasts or automobile accidents may cause non-penetrating injuries. Trauma to other areas of the body may have thoracic complications. For example, bone fractures may cause fat emboli, and pulmonary complications following abdominal surgery are common.

Radiological techniques

The severely injured patient, the postoperative patient and the patient in the intensive care ward are true tests of the radiographer's skill. In no areas of radiography are good-quality films more necessary or more difficult to produce.

The injured patient is usually brought to the X-ray department, where, if possible, an erect PA film should be taken. A high-kV technique is desirable in order to see mediastinal detail. A lateral film may be useful. If the patient is severely injured it is necessary to make do with supine films. Acutely multiple views for rib fractures are not indicated, as it is complications of the fractures that really matter, whether or not fractures are seen.

The use of *computed radiography* is becoming more common-place in the intensive care setting. Whilst the X-ray source is a standard portable generator, the image is captured on a phosphor plate detector which is then laser scanned to produce a digital chest radiograph. This technique has advantages over conventional radiography, because the latitude of the detector system is wide, reducing the need for repeat examinations for technical reasons, and maintaining a consistent quality of image between examinations. Although the radiograph can be laser printed onto film, in common with all digital information, the radiograph may be sent to a remote location for reporting or viewing, and the current radiograph can be compared with previous films retrieved from a digital archive.

Ultrasound is an excellent method for examining the pleura, diaphragm and subphrenic areas.

Aortography, *CT* and *trans-oesophageal ultrasound* may be indicated when vascular injuries are suspected.

The postoperative patient and the patient in the intensive care ward will usually be examined with mobile X-ray equipment. An erect PA film, with the patient sitting up, is preferable, but a supine film at end inspiration is better than a film taken with the patient slouched and at end expiration. The highest kV and mA possible and high-speed screens will minimise motion blurring. Horizontal-beam lateral decubitus films are occasionally useful to assess pleural fluid, pneumothoraces and fluid levels.

The films of intensive care ward patients need to be examined in the light of full clinical information, because many of the pathological processes to which these patients are susceptible produce similar radiographic manifestations. Serial films need to be evaluated for general trends, as day-to-day changes may not be apparent, and special attention needs to be given to monitoring and life-support devices.

INJURIES TO THE THORACIC CAGE

Rib fractures are common, and may be single, multiple, unilateral or bilateral. Healed rib fractures are a fairly frequent incidental finding on the chest X-ray. Acute rib fractures are often difficult to detect if there is no displacement, and their presence may only be inferred by surrounding haematoma producing an extrapleural opacity. In cases of chest trauma, the chest X-ray is more important in detecting a complication of rib fracture than the fracture itself. However, fracture of the first three ribs is often associated with major intrathoracic injury, and fracture of the lower three ribs may be associated with important hepatic, splenic or renal injury.

Complications of rib fracture include a flail segment, pneumothorax, haemothorax and subcutaneous emphysema. A *flail segment* is usually apparent clinically, the affected part of the chest wall being sucked in during inspiration, possibly compromising the underlying lung. The chest X-ray will show several adjacent ribs to be fractured in two places, or bilateral rib fractures.

The fractured ends of ribs may penetrate underlying pleura and lung and cause a *pneumothorax, haemothorax, haemopneumothorax* (Fig. 8.1) or *intrapulmonary haemorrhage*. Air may also escape into the chest wall and cause *subcutaneous emphysema* (Fig. 8.2).

Stress fractures of the first and second ribs are sometimes an incidental finding on the chest X-ray. *Cough fractures* usually affect

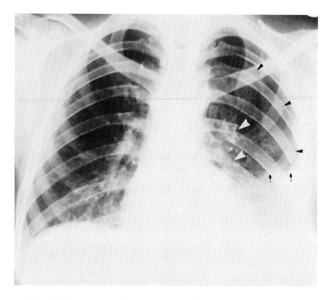

Fig. 8.1 Rib fractures and haemopneumothorax in a woman injured in an automobile accident. The left seventh and eighth ribs are fractured (white arrowheads). A pneumothorax (black arrowheads) is present, and a fluid level (arrows) is seen in the pleural space.

the sixth to ninth ribs in the posterior axillary line, but may not be visible until callus has formed.

Fractures of the *sternum* usually require a lateral film or CT for visualisation.

Fractures of the *thoracic spine* may be associated with a paraspinal shadow which represents haematoma.

Fractures of the *clavicle* may be associated with injury to the sub-clavian vessels or brachial plexus, and posterior dislocation of the clavicle at the sternoclavicular joint may cause injury to the trachea, oesophagus, great vessels or nerves of the superior mediastinum.

Herniation of lung tissue is usually associated with obvious rib fractures, but may only be apparent on tangential views in full inspiration.

INJURIES TO THE DIAPHRAGM

Laceration of the diaphragm may result from penetrating or non-penetrating trauma to the chest or abdomen. Ruptures of the left hemidiaphragm are encountered more frequently in clinical practice than ruptures on the right. The typical plain film appearance is of obscuration of the affected hemidiaphragm and increased shadowing in the ipsilateral hemithorax due to herniation of stomach, omentum, bowel or solid viscera (Fig. 8.3), although such herniation may be delayed. Ultrasound may demonstrate diaphragmatic laceration and free fluid in both the pleura and peritoneum. Barium studies may be useful to confirm herniation of stomach or bowel into the chest.

INJURIES TO THE PLEURA

Pneumothorax, as mentioned above, may be a complication of rib fracture, and is then usually associated with a haemothorax (Fig. 8.1). If no ribs are fractured, pneumothorax is secondary to a pneumomediastinum, pulmonary laceration or penetrating chest

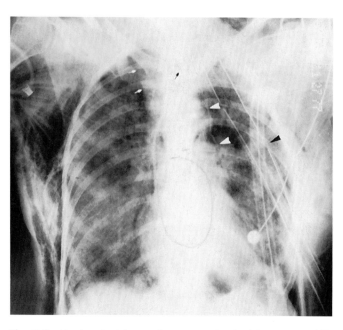

Fig. 8.2 Massive chest trauma in a woman involved in an automobile accident. Gross subcutaneous emphysema extends over the chest wall, outlining muscle planes. The right clavicle is fractured. Several ribs were fractured, but this is not seen on this film. Mediastinal emphysema separates pleura from the descending aorta (white arrowheads). A mediastinal haematoma is present (white arrows). Widespread lung contusion is obscured by the subcutaneous emphysema. Note tracheostomy tube (black arrow), left pleural tubes, with side hole indicated (black arrowhead), Swan–Ganz catheter and ECG lead.

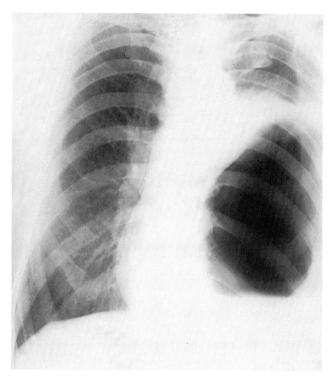

Fig. 8.3 Rupture of diaphragm in a man of 58 who fell from a building 13 years before, breaking ankles and injuring chest, and now presenting with persistent vomiting. The chest radiograph demonstrates distended stomach in the left hemithorax, confirmed by barium swallow. Thoracotomy revealed stomach herniating into left pleural cavity through a 5-cm rent in the left hemidiaphragm.

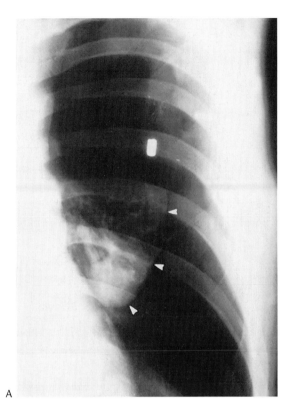
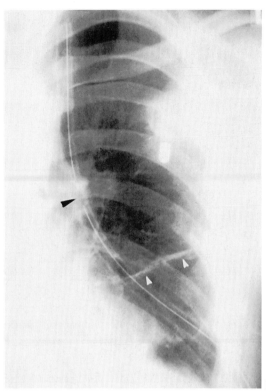

A   B

Fig. 8.4 Penetrating chest injury—man with bullet wound. (A) Large pneumothorax (arrowheads), and bullet in chest wall. (B) Following insertion of pleural tube (black arrowhead), the lung re-expands, revealing haematoma in bullet track. Band shadow in lower zone (white arrowheads) represents subsegmental atelectasis.

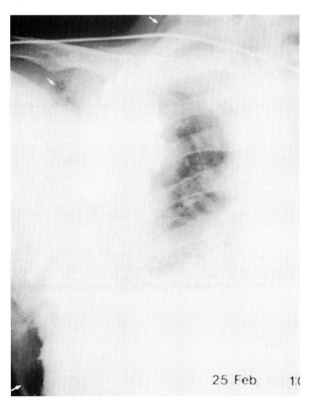

Fig. 8.5 Pulmonary contusion and haemothorax in a man with a gunshot injury. Subcutaneous emphysema is present over the chest wall (arrows), and dense shadowing extends over most of the hemithorax.

injury (Fig. 8.4). Pneumothorax due to a penetrating injury is liable to develop increased pressure, resulting in a tension pneumothorax which may require emergency decompression.

Haemothorax may also occur with or without rib fractures (Fig. 8.5), and is a result of laceration of intercostal or pleural vessels. If a pneumothorax is also present a fluid level will be seen on a horizontal-beam film (Fig. 8.1).

Pleural effusion may also result from trauma. Open injuries to the pleura are prone to infection and development of an empyema.

INJURIES TO THE LUNG

Pulmonary contusion is a result of haemorrhagic exudation into the alveoli and interstitial spaces and appears as patchy, non-segmental consolidation (Figs 8.5, 8.6). Shadowing appears within the first few hours of penetrating or non-penetrating trauma, usually shows improvement within 2 days, and clears within 3–4 days (Fig. 8.7). When contusion due to a bullet wound clears, a longitudinal haematoma in the bullet track may become visible (Fig. 8.4).

Pulmonary lacerations as a result of non-penetrating trauma may appear as round thin-walled cystic spaces. When the injury is acute, the laceration may be obscured by pulmonary contusion, but as the surrounding consolidation resolves, laceration will become evident. If the laceration is filled with blood it appears as a homogeneous round opacity, and if partly filled with blood it may show a fluid level (Fig. 8.8). Such pulmonary haematomas or blood cysts gradually decrease in size, but may take a few months to resolve completely (Fig. 8.9). Pulmonary haematomas are often multiple (Fig. 8.6).

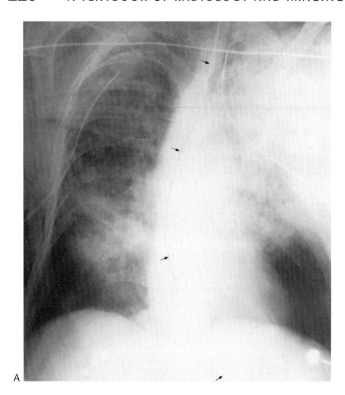

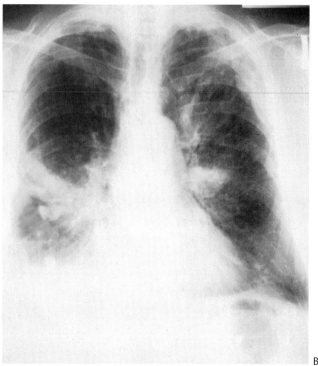

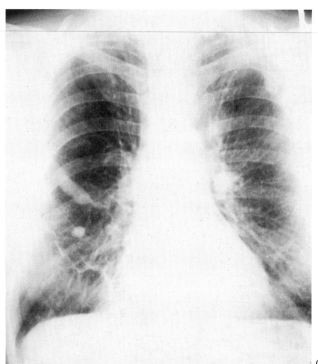

Fig. 8.6 Pulmonary contusion and haematoma in a youth of 18 trampled on by a bull. (A) Extensive consolidation is present throughout both lungs, particularly in the left upper zone. Subcutaneous emphysema is seen over the right hemithorax. Bilateral pleural tubes and a nasogastric tube (arrows) are present. (B) Six days later the contusion has resolved and multiple pulmonary haematomas and some extrapleural haematomas have become visible. (C) One month later the haematomas are smaller.

Torsion of a lung is a rare result of severe thoracic trauma, usually to a child. The lung twists about the hilum through 180°. If unrelieved the lung may become gangrenous and appear opaque on the chest X-ray.

Atelectasis and compensatory *hyperinflation* after a chest injury may be due to aspiration of blood or mucus into the bronchi. Atelectasis may also occur secondary to decreased respiratory movement.

Pulmonary oedema as a manifestation of the adult respiratory distress syndrome may occur after major trauma.

Fat embolism is a rare complication of multiple fractures, due to fat globules from the bone marrow entering the systemic veins and embolising to the lungs. Poorly defined nodular opacities appear throughout both lungs; the opacities resolve within a few days. The diagnosis is confirmed if fat globules are present in the sputum or urine.

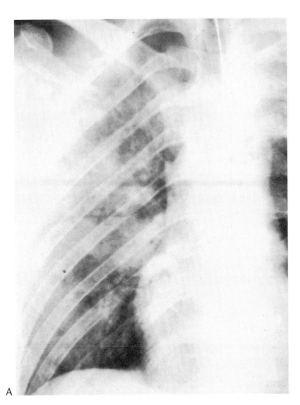
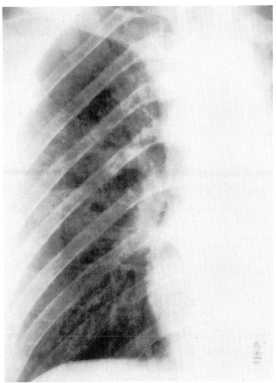

Fig. 8.7 Pulmonary contusion in a man following an automobile accident. (A) Extensive consolidation throughout right lung. Left lung was clear. No rib fractures. (B) Four days later the shadowing has resolved.

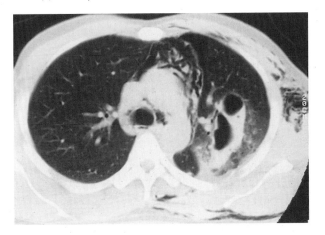

Fig. 8.8 Pulmonary contusion and pulmonary laceration. CT through the chest demonstrates mediastinal and chest wall emphysema following trauma. There is also a thin-walled loculated air/fluid collection within the lung due to a pulmonary laceration surrounded by ground-glass change indicative of contusion.

INJURIES TO THE TRACHEA AND BRONCHI

Laceration or rupture of a major airway is an uncommon result of severe chest trauma, usually in an automobile accident. Fracture of the first three ribs is often present, and mediastinal emphysema and pneumothorax are common (Fig. 8.10). The injury is usually in the *trachea* just above the carina, or in a *main bronchus* just distal to the carina. If the bronchial sheath is preserved there may be no immediate signs or symptoms, but tracheostenosis or bronchiectasis may occur later. CT may be helpful in diagnosis, but bronchoscopy is the best diagnostic method in the acute stage.

INJURIES TO THE MEDIASTINUM

Pneumomediastinum and *mediastinal emphysema* describe the presence of air between the tissue planes of the mediastinum. Air may reach here as a result of pulmonary interstitial emphysema, perforation of the oesophagus, trachea or bronchus, or from a penetrating chest injury. Pulmonary interstitial emphysema is a result of alveolar wall rupture due to high intra-alveolar pressure, and may occur during violent coughing, asthmatic attacks or severe crush injuries, or be due to positive-pressure ventilation. Air dissects centrally along the perivascular sheath to reach the mediastinum. Rarely, air may dissect into the mediastinum from a pneumoperitoneum. A pneumomediastinum may extend beyond the thoracic inlet into the neck, and over the chest wall. Pneumothorax is a common complication of pneumomediastinum, but the converse rarely occurs.

Pneumomediastinum usually produces vertical translucent streaks in the mediastinum. This represents gas separating and outlining the soft-tissue planes and structures of the mediastinum. Gas shadows may extend up into the neck (Fig. 8.11), or dissect extrapleurally over the diaphragm, or extend into the soft-tissue planes of the chest wall, causing subcutaneous emphysema (Figs 8.11, 8.12). The mediastinal pleura may be displaced laterally, and become visible as a linear soft-tissue shadow parallel to the mediastinum (Figs 8.2, 8.10–8.12). If mediastinal air collects beneath the pericardium the central part of the diaphragm may be visible, producing the 'continuous diaphragm' sign (Fig. 8.12).

Sometimes it may be difficult to differentiate between *pneumopericardium* and pneumomediastinum. In pneumopericardium gas does not extend beyond the aortic root or much beyond the main pulmonary artery (Fig. 8.21). In pneumomediastinum, gas often outlines the aortic knuckle and extends into the neck. In pneumopericardium a

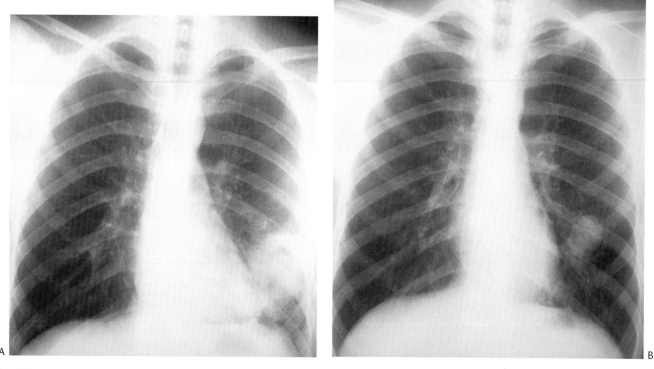

Fig. 8.9 (A) Chest radiograph obtained immediately following a stab wound to the chest. There is a pulmonary haematoma evident on the left. (B) Radiograph 3 months later demonstrates only partial resolution.

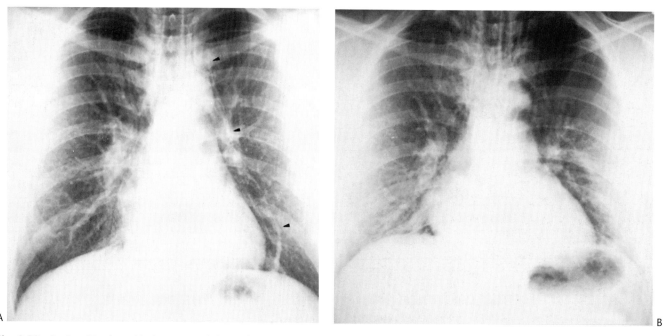

Fig. 8.10 Ruptured trachea with dyspnoea and chest pain in a man suffering a deceleration injury. (A) Pneumomediastinum with linear lucencies in the mediastinum and displacement of mediastinal pleura (arrowheads). (B) One hour later, following a bout of coughing, a left pneumothorax has developed. Bronchoscopy revealed a ruptured trachea.

fluid level is often seen on horizontal-beam films, and the distribution of air may alter with changes in the patient's position. The patient's position has little or no effect on a pneumomediastinum. Pneumomediastinum is relatively more common in neonates and infants, and may displace the thymus or resemble a lung cyst.

Mediastinal haemorrhage may result from penetrating or non-penetrating trauma, and be due to venous or arterial bleeding. Many cases are probably unrecognised, as clinical and radiographic signs are absent. Important causes include automobile accidents, aortic rupture and dissection, and introduction of central venous catheters.

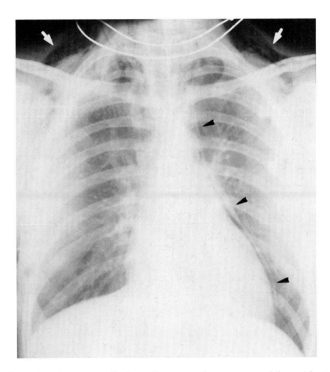

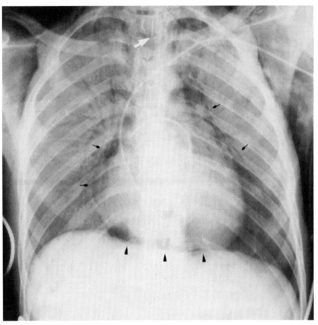

Fig. 8.11 Pneumomediastinum in a man after an automobile accident. Note linear lucencies in the mediastinum extending into the neck, and subcutaneous emphysema over the supraclavicular fossae (arrows). The mediastinal pleura is outlined by air and displaced laterally (arrowheads).

Fig. 8.12 Complications of positive-pressure ventilation. Diffuse consolidation in a boy aged 15 following presumed viral pneumonia. Note endotracheal tube (white arrow) and Swan–Ganz catheter, both well positioned. Pneumomediastinum is indicated by linear lucencies in the mediastinum, lateral displacement of the mediastinal pleura (black arrows) and infrapericardial air, producing the 'continuous diaphragm' sign (arrowheads). There is extensive bilateral subcutaneous emphysema.

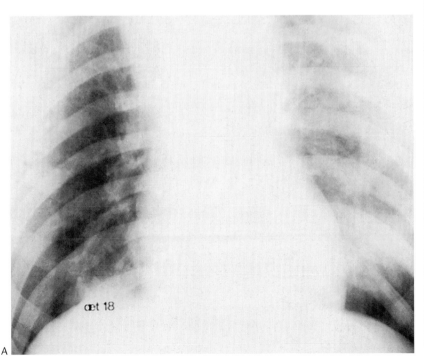

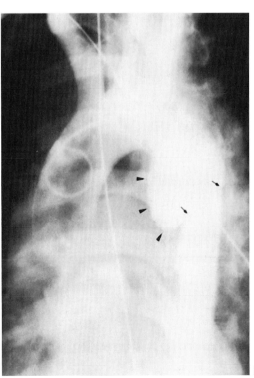

Fig. 8.13 Mediastinal haemorrhage in a youth of 18 after an automobile accident. (A) Chest radiograph shows bilateral widening of the superior mediastinum. The aorta is obscured. (B) Arch aortogram demonstrates an aneurysm of the aortic isthmus (arrowheads) with intimal tear (arrows).

There is usually bilateral mediastinal widening (Fig. 8.13), but a localised haematoma may occur (Figs 8.2, 8.30).

Aortic rupture is usually the result of an automobile accident. Most non-fatal aortic tears occur at the aortic isthmus, the site of the ligamentum arteriosum. Only 10–20% of patients survive the acute episode, but a small number may develop a chronic aneurysm at the site of the tear. The commonest acute radiographic signs are widening of the superior mediastinum, and obscuration of the aortic knuckle (Fig. 8.13). Other radiographic signs include deviation of the left main bronchus anteriorly, inferiorly and to the right, and rightward displacement of the trachea, a nasogastric tube or the right parasternal line. A left apical extrapleural cap or a left haemothorax may be visible. Whilst aortography is the definitive investigation, CT, transoesophageal echocardiography or MRI may be diagnostic. In everyday practice many departments will have emergency access to a CT scanner but will not be centres of cardiothoracic surgery. A properly conducted CT scan demonstrating a normal mediastinum has a very high negative predictive value for aortic rupture. However, if CT is equivocal or shows a mediastinal haematoma, then generally angiography will be required prior to surgery (Fig. 8.14).

Cardiac injury may result from penetrating or blunt trauma. Penetrating injuries are usually rapidly fatal but may cause tamponade, ventricular aneurysm or septal defects. Blunt trauma may cause myocardial contusion and infarction and may be associated with transient or more permanent rhythm disturbance.

Oesophageal rupture is usually the result of instrumentation or surgery (Fig. 8.15), but occasionally occurs in penetrating trauma, and is rarely spontaneous and due to sudden increase of intra-oesophageal pressure (Boerhaave's syndrome). Clinically there is acute mediastinitis; radiographically there are signs of pneumo-mediastinum, with or without a pneumothorax or hydropneumo-thorax, which is usually left-sided. The diagnosis should be confirmed by a swallow. This should initially be with water-soluble contrast medium in order to avoid the small risk of granuloma formation in the mediastinum that has been described following barium leakage.

Chylothorax due to damage to the thoracic duct may become apparent hours or days after trauma. Thoracic surgery is the commonest cause.

THE POSTOPERATIVE CHEST

Intrathoracic surgery is performed most frequently for resection of all or part of a lung, or for cardiac disease. This section will discuss the usual acute and long-term changes apparent radiographically following such surgery, followed by a description of complications.

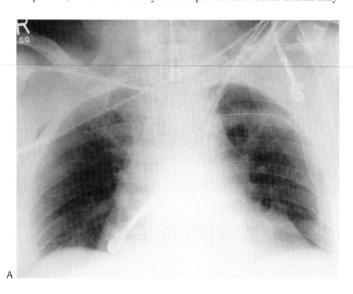

A

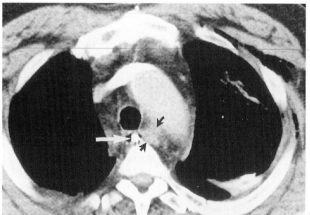

B

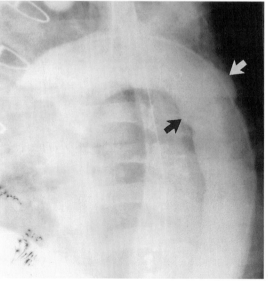

C

Fig. 8.14 Aortic rupture. Fifty-six-year-old male patient with a severe deceleration injury and a remote history of sternotomy for coronary artery bypass grafting. (A) Supine chest radiograph demonstrates questionable mediastinal widening, surgical emphysema and a left chest tube. (B) Contrast-enhanced CT scan at the level of the aortic arch reveals a small mediastinal haematoma (black arrows) adjacent to the oesophagus, which contains a nasogastric tube. The mediastinum is of normal width. (C) Arch aortogram demonstrating an intimal tear at the usual site (arrows).

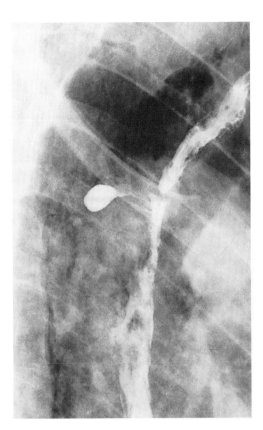

Fig. 8.15 Oesophageal rupture following difficult endoscopy. Following the procedure a check radiograph demonstrated pneumomediastinum (not shown) and a localised perforation was detected on contrast swallow.

THORACOTOMY

Lung resections are usually performed posterolaterally through the fourth or fifth intercostal space. Part of a rib may be resected, the periosteum may be stripped or the ribs may simply be spread apart following a muscle incision (Fig. 8.16). Rib fractures sometimes occur, but often the surgical route is not obvious on the chest X-ray, or is marked only by some narrowing of the intercostal space, or some overlying soft-tissue swelling and subcutaneous emphysema.

Following *pneumonectomy* it is important for the remaining lung to be fully expanded, and for the mediastinum to remain close to the midline. Excessive mediastinal shift may compromise respiration and venous return to the heart. On the initial postoperative film the trachea should be close to the midline, the remaining lung should appear normal or slightly plethoric. The pneumonectomy space also usually contains a small amount of fluid. A drainage tube may or may not be present in the space. Over the next several days the pneumonectomy space begins to obliterate by gradual shift of the mediastinum to that side, and accumulation of fluid. The space is usually half-filled within about a week, and completely opacifies over the next 2–3 months (Fig. 8.17). If the mediastinum moves toward the opposite side, this may indicate too rapid accumulation of fluid in the pneumonectomy space, or atelectasis in the remaining lung. A sudden shift may indicate a bronchopleural fistula (Fig. 8.18).

Following *lobectomy* the remaining lung should expand to fill the space of the resected lobe. Immediately postoperatively, pleural drains are present, preventing accumulation of pleural fluid, and the mediastinum may be shifted to the side of the operation. With hyperinflation of the remaining lung the mediastinum returns to its

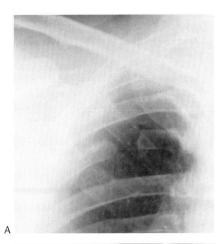

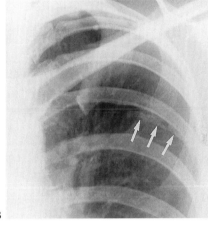

Fig. 8.16 (A) Typical sharply truncated rib defect following right thoracotomy (right upper lobectomy for carcinoma). (B) Late postsurgical changes following periosteal stripping at time of left fifth interspace thoracotomy for mitral valvotomy. There is a wavy line of calcification below the affected rib (arrows).

normal position. When the drains are removed a small pleural effusion commonly occurs but usually resolves within a few days, perhaps leaving residual pleural thickening.

With *segmental* or *subsegmental lung resections* a cut surface of the lung is oversewn, and air leaks are fairly common, sometimes causing persistent pneumothorax which may require prolonged drainage. Wire sutures or staples may be visible at the site of a bronchial stump or lesser lung resection.

Complications of thoracotomy

Postoperative spaces

These may persist following lobectomy and segmental or subsegmental resections. They are air spaces that correspond to the excised lung. Fluid may collect in them, but they usually resolve after a few weeks or months. If they persist and are associated with constitutional symptoms, increasing fluid and pleural thickening, an empyema or bronchopleural fistula should be suspected.

Empyema

Empyema complicating pneumonectomy, or rarely lobectomy, usually occurs a few weeks after surgery, although it may occur

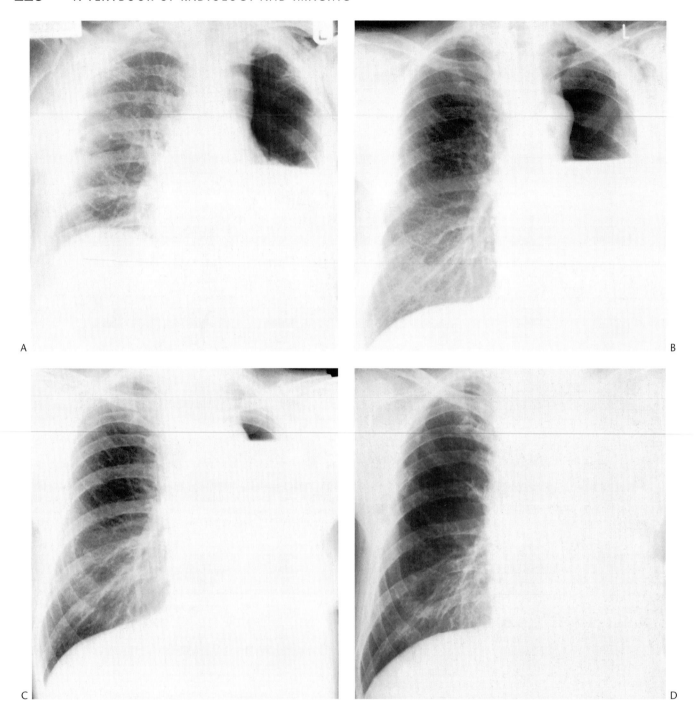

Fig. 8.17 Normal postpneumonectomy appearance: 1 day (A), 6 days (B), 5 weeks (C) and 8 weeks (D) postoperatively. The pneumonectomy space is gradually obliterated by the rising fluid level and mediastinal shift.

months or years later. Rapid accumulation of fluid may push the mediastinum to the normal side. If a fistula develops between the pneumonectomy space and a bronchus or the skin, the air–fluid level in the space will suddenly drop (Fig. 8.18). Increasing gas in the pneumonectomy space may also indicate infection by a gas-forming organism.

Bronchopleural fistula

This is a communication between the bronchial tree (or lung tissue) and the pleural space. The commonest cause is a complication of

lung surgery, but it may be the result of rupture of a *lung abscess*, erosion by a *lung cancer* or *penetrating trauma*. Bronchopleural fistula complicating complete or partial lung resection may occur early, when it is due to faulty closure of the bronchus, but it more commonly occurs late due to infection or recurrent tumour of the bronchial stump. The usual radiographic appearance is the sudden appearance of, or increase in the amount of, air in the pleural space, with a corresponding decrease in the amount of fluid in the space. A fluid level is almost always present (Fig. 8.18). If fluid enters the airways and is aspirated into the remaining lung,

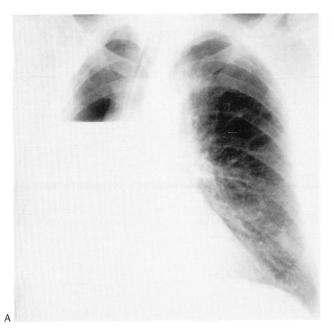
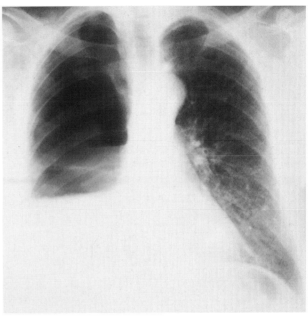

A   B

Fig. 8.18 Bronchopleural fistula. (A) Thirteen days after right pneumonectomy the space is filling with fluid and the mediastinum is deviated to the right. (B) Two days later, after the patient coughed up a large amount of fluid, the fluid level has dropped and the mediastinum has returned to the midline. Bronchoscopy confirmed a right bronchopleural fistula.

widespread consolidation may be seen on the chest X-ray. Sinography of the pleural space or bronchography may demonstrate the fistula.

Pleural fluid

This is usually seen on the chest X-ray following thoracic surgery. If the amount is excessive it may be due to bleeding or chylothorax.

Diaphragmatic elevation

Elevation may indicate phrenic nerve damage and is best assessed by fluoroscopy or ultrasound.

Other pulmonary complications of thoracic surgery include *atelectasis*, *aspiration pneumonia*, *pulmonary embolism* and *pulmonary oedema*, both cardiogenic and non-cardiogenic. These may also complicate non-thoracic surgery and are discussed below.

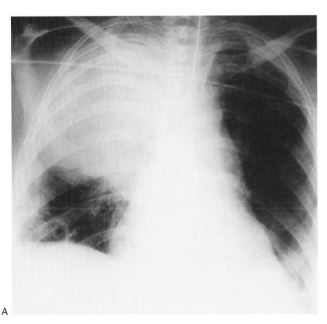
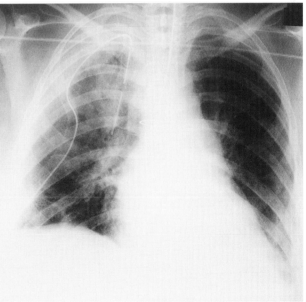

A   B

Fig. 8.19 Haemorrhage following cardiac transplantation. (A) Four hours following return from surgery the chest radiograph reveals opacification of the right upper zone. Ultrasound at the patient's bedside confirmed a large fluid collection. (B) After insertion of a chest drain there has been partial resolution of the appearances.

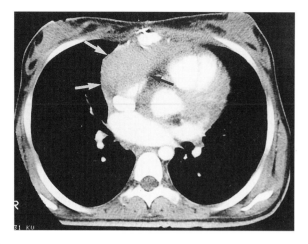

Fig. 8.20 Mediastinal haematoma. Enhanced CT scan demonstrates a soft-tissue density non-enhancing mass in the anterior mediastinum 3 days following cardiac surgery (arrows).

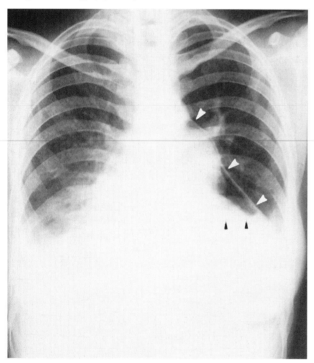

Fig. 8.21 Haemopneumopericardium in a woman 2 days after closure of atrial septal defect. The pericardium is outlined by air (white arrowheads), which does not extend as high as the aortic arch. A fluid level (black arrowheads) is present in the pericardium, and there are bilateral pleural effusions.

CARDIAC SURGERY

Most cardiac operations are performed through a *sternotomy* incision, and wire sternal sutures are often seen on the postoperative films (Figs 8.35, 8.36). Mitral valvotomy is now rarely performed via a *thoracotomy* incision (Fig. 8.16), but this route is still used for surgery of coarctation of the aorta, patent ductus arteriosus, Blalock–Taussig shunts and pulmonary artery banding.

Following cardiac surgery, some widening of the cardiovascular silhouette is usual, and represents bleeding and oedema. Marked widening of the mediastinum suggests significant *haemorrhage*, but

the necessity for re-exploration is based upon the overall clinical situation (Figs 8.19, 8.20). Some air commonly remains in the pericardium following cardiac surgery, so that the signs of *pneumopericardium* may be present (Fig. 8.21).

Pulmonary opacities are very common following open heart surgery, and left basal shadowing is almost invariable, representing *atelectasis*. This shadowing usually resolves over a week or two. Small *pleural effusions* are also common in the immediate postoperative period.

Pneumoperitoneum is sometimes seen, due to involvement of the peritoneum by the sternotomy incision. It is of no pathological significance.

Violation of left or right pleural space may lead to a *pneumothorax*. Damage to a major lymphatic vessel may lead to a *chylothorax* or a more localised collection—a *chyloma*. Phrenic nerve damage may cause paresis or paralysis of a hemidiaphragm.

Surgical clips or other metallic markers have sometimes been used to mark the ends of coronary artery bypass grafts. *Prosthetic heart valves* are usually visible radiographically, but they may be difficult to see on an underpenetrated film. Their assessment—fluoroscopically, angiographically or ultrasonographically—is outside the scope of this chapter.

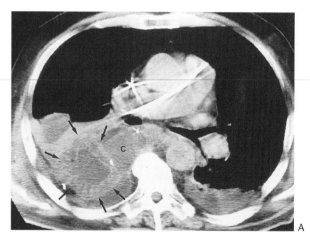

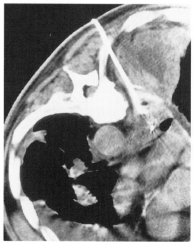

Fig. 8.22 Infected mediastinal collection following oesophagectomy. (A) The gastric conduit (arrows) is discernible separately from the collection (C) and small bilateral effusions. (B) Drainage accomplished by CT-guided pigtail catheter insertion with the patient in a semiprone position.

Sternal dehiscence may be apparent radiographically by a linear lucency appearing in the sternum and alteration in position of the sternal sutures on consecutive films. The diagnosis is usually made clinically and may be associated with osteomyelitis. A first or second rib may be fractured when the sternum is spread apart. The importance of this observation is that it may explain chest pain in the postoperative period.

Acute mediastinitis may complicate mediastinal surgery although it is more commonly associated with oesophageal perforation or surgery. Radiographically there may be mediastinal widening or pneumomediastinum, and these features are best assessed by CT scan (Figs 8.22, 8.23).

Chronic mediastinal infection including sternal osteomyelitis may follow median sternotomy, and may be difficult to differentiate from postsurgical granulation tissue and haematoma. Mediastinal gas may persist for some weeks or months after surgery, and only increasing amounts of gas on subsequent examination is a reliable indication of the presence of a gas-forming organism.

The *postpericardotomy syndrome* is probably an autoimmune phenomenon, usually occurring in the month after surgery. It presents with fever, pleurisy and pericarditis. Pleural effusions may be visible and the cardiac silhouette may enlarge. Ultrasound will demonstrate pericardial fluid. Patchy consolidation may occur in the lung bases.

LATE APPEARANCES AFTER CHEST SURGERY

Following thoracotomy, the appearance of the chest X-ray may return to normal, or evidence of surgery may persist. Resected ribs or healed rib fractures are usually obvious (Figs 8.13, 8.24). There may be irregular regeneration of a rib related to disturbed periosteum. A rib space may be narrowed where a thoracotomy wound has been closed (Fig. 8.24). Rib notching may result from a Blalock–Taussig shunt between subclavian and pulmonary arteries. Pleural thickening often remains after a thoracotomy.

Rearrangement of the remaining lung occurs after lobectomy, so that the anatomy of the fissures may be altered. Following oesophageal surgery, stomach or loops of bowel may produce unusual soft-tissue opacities or fluid levels if they have been brought up into the chest (Fig. 8.25). A contrast swallow frequently clarifies the appearances.

Surgery is now rarely performed for pulmonary tuberculosis, but many patients who have had such surgery are still alive. The object of surgery was to reduce aeration of the infected lung, usually an upper lobe. *Thoracoplasty* involved removal of the posterior parts of usually three or more ribs so that the underlying lung collapsed (Fig. 8.26). Occasionally, thoracoplasty was combined with pneumonectomy for the treatment of chronic tuberculous empyema. An alternative approach was *plombage*, which was the extrapleural insertion of some inert material to collapse the underlying lung. Solid or hollow *lucite balls* (Fig. 8.27) were commonly used. Other substances included crumpled *cellophane packs* and *kerosene (paraffin)* (Fig. 8.28).

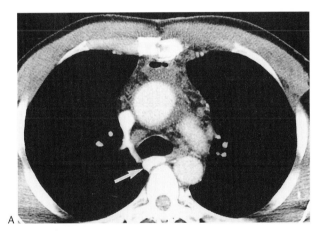
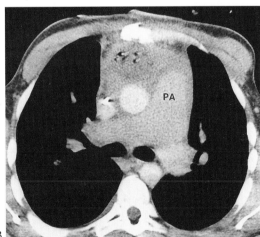

Fig. 8.23 Postsurgical mediastinitis. Two cases. (A) CT 3 weeks following aortic valve replacement in a patient with signs of infection. There is a small retrosternal air and fluid collection, subsequently drained. Note the enlarged azygos vein (arrow) due to previous thrombosis of the superior vena cava. (B) Infected mediastinal collection in a different patient several weeks following atrial septal defect closure. Note the large pulmonary trunk (PA).

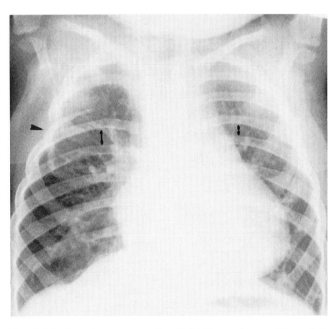

Fig. 8.24 Post-thoracotomy ribs. Right thoracotomy with partially excised regenerating right fourth rib (arrowhead) after repair of tracheo-oesophageal fistula. Left thoracotomy, indicated by narrowed fifth intercostal space, for pulmonary artery banding for multiple ventricular septal defects.

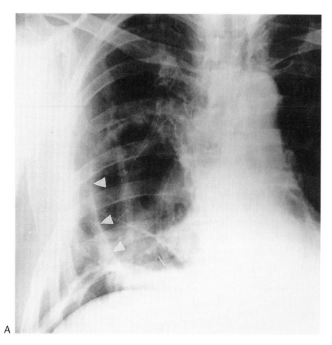

A

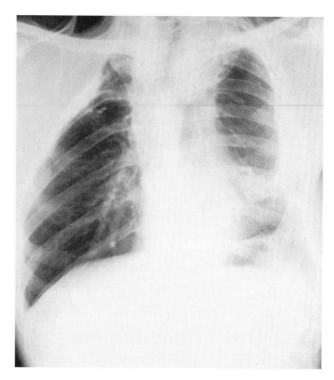

Fig. 8.26 Thoracoplasty. The first five right ribs have been removed. Left upper lobe fibrosis, bilateral apical calcification and extensive left pleural calcification are due to tuberculosis.

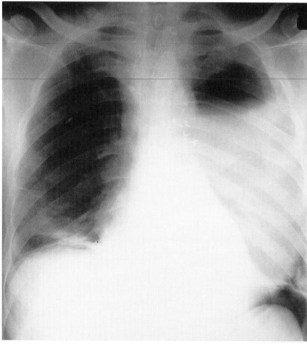

B

Fig. 8.25 (A) Ivor Lewis oesophagectomy. There is a rib defect, air under the diaphragm and a gas-filled gastric conduit in the right chest. This is outlined by a rim of pleural fluid (arrowheads). (B) Dilated gastric pull-up in a different patient. An air–fluid level is seen in the distended conduit in the left chest due to outflow obstruction at the site of the mobilised pylorus. Right basal atelectasis is present.

THORACIC COMPLICATIONS OF GENERAL SURGERY

Atelectasis

This is the commonest pulmonary complication of thoracic or abdominal surgery (Fig. 8.25B). Predisposing factors are a long anaesthetic, obesity, chronic lung disease and smoking. It is a result of retained secretions and poor ventilation. Postoperatively it is painful to breathe deeply or cough. The chest X-ray usually shows elevation of the diaphragm, due to a poor inspiration. Linear, sometimes curved, opacities are frequently present in the lower zones, and probably represent a combination of subsegmental volume loss and consolidation (Fig. 8.4B). These shadows usually appear about 24 hours postoperatively and resolve within 2 or 3 days.

Pleural effusions

These are common immediately following abdominal surgery and usually resolve within 2 weeks. They may be associated with pulmonary infarction. Effusions due to subphrenic infection usually occur later.

Pneumothorax

When it complicates extrathoracic surgery pneumothorax is usually a complication of positive pressure ventilation or central venous line insertion. It may complicate nephrectomy.

Aspiration pneumonitis

This is common during anaesthesia but fortunately is usually insignificant. When significant, patchy consolidation appears within a few hours, usually basally or around the hila (Fig. 8.29). Clearing occurs within a few days, unless there is super-infection.

Pulmonary oedema

In the postoperative period oedema may be cardiogenic or non-cardiogenic. The latter includes fluid overload and the adult respiratory distress syndrome.

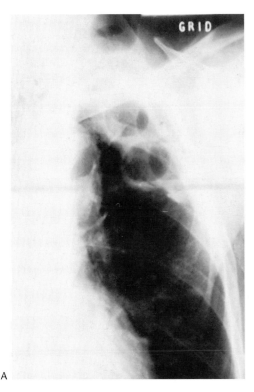

A

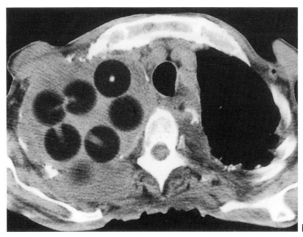

B

Fig. 8.27 Plombage. (A) Several hollow balls have been inserted extrapleurally at the left apex. The balls are slightly permeable, and the shallow fluid levels do not indicate a complication. (B) CT through right apical Lucite balls in a different patient demonstrating characteristic appearance.

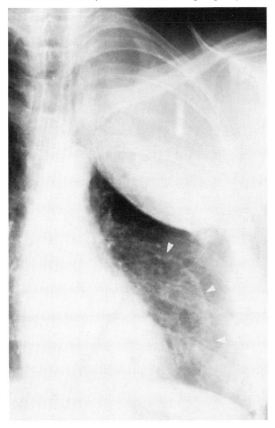

Fig. 8.28 Oleothorax. Plombage has been performed by instilling kerosene (paraffin) extrapleurally through a thoracotomy with excision of the fifth rib. A thin rim of calcification has developed in the extrapleural collection. Some keresone has tracked inferiorly behind the lung and produced a calcified pleural plaque which is seen en face (arrowheads).

Pneumonia

Postoperative atelectasis and aspiration pneumonitis may be complicated by pneumonia. Postoperative pneumonias, therefore, tend to be associated with bilateral basal shadowing.

Subphrenic abscess

This usually produces elevation of the hemidiaphragm, pleural effusion and basal atelectasis. Loculated gas may be seen below the diaphragm, and fluoroscopy may show splinting of the diaphragm. Subphrenic abscess can be demonstrated by CT or ultrasound.

Pulmonary embolism

This may produce pulmonary shadowing, pleural effusion or elevation of the diaphragm. However, a normal chest X-ray does not exclude pulmonary embolism, and the initial investigation of choice is a perfusion lung scan. There is also an emerging role for spiral CT scanning in the investigation of acute pulmonary embolism (see below).

THE PATIENT IN INTENSIVE CARE

Patients are admitted to an intensive care ward postoperatively, following major trauma or following circulatory or respiratory failure. A number of monitoring and life-support devices may be used in their care. Radiology plays an important part in the management of these devices.

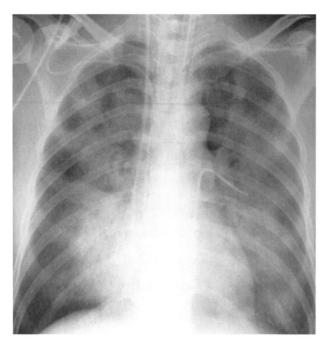

Fig. 8.29 The admission chest radiograph (not shown) of a patient with acute viral encephalitis was clear. Six hours later a film following emergency intubation reveals extensive bilateral basal and perihilar air space shadowing due to massive aspiration of gastric contents. A Swan–Ganz catheter is in situ with the tip projected more peripherally than ideal in the left lung.

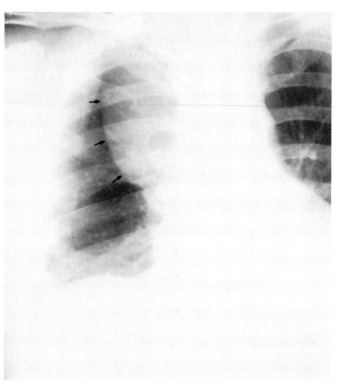

Fig. 8.30 Mediastinal haematoma. Following unsuccessfully attempted placement of a central venous line via the right subclavian vein, a large extrapleural haematoma (arrows) is present.

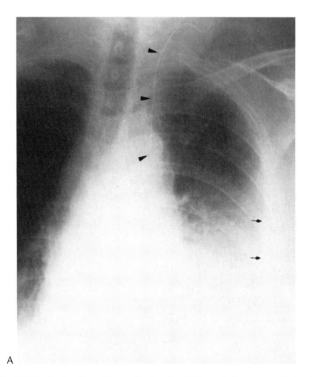

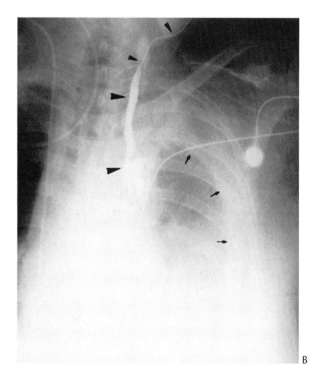

A

B

Fig. 8.31 Perforation of innominate vein. (A) A central venous catheter (arrowheads) has been introduced via the left jugular vein. Its tip points inferiorly, rather than to the right along the axis of the innominate vein. A pleural effusion (arrows) is present. (B) Next day the effusion is larger. Injection of contrast medium into the catheter (larger arrowheads) demonstrates extravasation and communication with the pleural effusion.

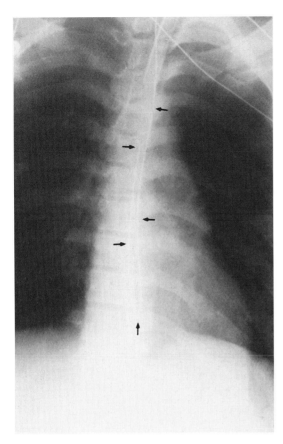

Fig. 8.32 Nasogastric tube coiled in oesophagus. The tube does not reach the stomach, but has folded back on itself (arrows).

Central venous pressure (CVP) catheters

These are used to monitor right atrial pressure. The end of a CVP line needs to be intrathoracic, and is ideally in the superior vena cava (Fig. 8.33B). CVP lines may be introduced via an antecubital, subclavian or jugular vein. Subclavian venous puncture carries a risk of pneumothorax and mediastinal haematoma (Fig. 8.30). Rarely, perforation of the subclavian vein leads to fluid collecting in the mediastinum or pleura (Fig. 8.31). All catheters have a potential risk of coiling and knotting, or fracture leading to embolism.

Swan–Ganz catheters (pulmonary artery flotation catheters)

These are used to measure pulmonary artery and pulmonary wedge pressures. The latter is an index of left atrial pressure. These catheters are usually introduced via an antecubital or jugular vein. An inflatable balloon at the catheter tip guides it through the right heart. Ideally the end of the catheter should be maintained 5–8 cm (2–3 in) beyond the bifurcation of the main pulmonary artery in either the right or left pulmonary artery (Figs 8.12, 8.34). When the pulmonary wedge pressure is measured the balloon is inflated, and the flow of blood carries the catheter tip peripherally, to a wedged position. After the measurement has been made the balloon is deflated and the catheter returns to a central position, otherwise there is a risk of pulmonary infarction. The inflation balloon is radiolucent. The balloon should normally be kept deflated to minimise the risk of thrombus formation.

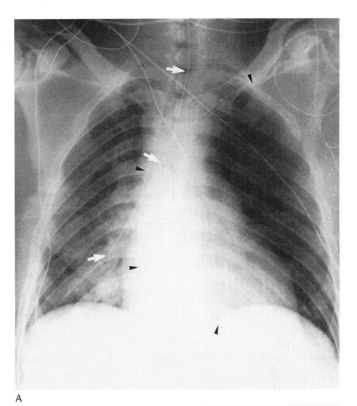

A

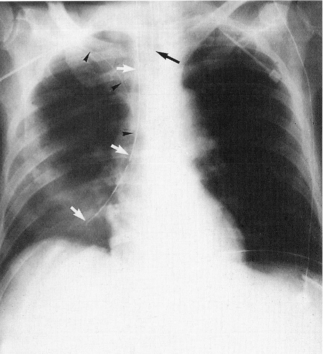

B

Fig. 8.33 Nasogastric tubes in right bronchus. (A) The nasogastric tube (arrows) passes down the trachea and into the right bronchus. The patient had been 'fed' via the tube, causing patchy consolidation in the right lung. A temporary pacing electrode (arrowheads) is present. (B) This patient, with chronic renal failure, developed peritonitis following peritoneal dialysis. Drains are present in the abdomen. A nasogastric tube (white arrows) has been passed beyond an endotracheal tube (black arrow) and into the right bronchus. Two venous lines are present; the right-sided catheter (arrowheads) is well placed for central venous pressure measurements.

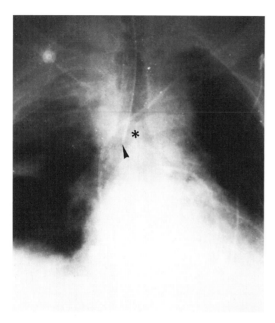

Fig. 8.34   Endotracheal tube too low. The tip of the endotracheal tube (arrowhead) is beyond the carina (asterisk) and in the right bronchus. A well-positioned Swan–Ganz catheter is present.

Nasogastric tubes

These may not reach the stomach or may coil in the oesophagus (Fig. 8.32) or occasionally are inserted into the trachea and into the right bronchus (Fig. 8.33).

Endotracheal tubes

These are used for access to the airways for ventilation and management of secretions, and also to protect the airway. The chest X-ray is important in assessing the position of the tip of the endotracheal tube relative to the carina. Extension and flexion of the neck may make the tip of an endotracheal tube move by as much as 5 cm. With the neck in neutral position the tip of the tube should ideally be about 5–6 cm above the carina. A tube that is inserted too far usually passes into the right bronchus (Fig. 8.34), with the

risk of collapse of the left lung. If the inflated cuff of the tube dilates the trachea, there is a risk of ischaemic damage to the tracheal mucosa. A late complication of an overinflated cuff is tracheostenosis.

Tracheostomy tubes

These are usually inserted for long-term ventilatory support, either percutaneously using a Seldinger type technique, or by formal surgical tracheostomy. The tube tip should be situated centrally in the airway at the level of T3 (Fig. 8.2). Acute complications of tracheostomy include pneumothorax, pneumomediastinum and subcutaneous emphysema. Long-term complications include tracheal ulceration, stenosis and perforation.

Positive-pressure ventilation

Complications may include interstitial emphysema, pneumomediastinum, pneumothorax and subcutaneous emphysema (Fig. 8.12).

Pleural tubes

These are used to treat pleural effusions and pneumothoraces. If the patient is being nursed supine, the tip of the tube should be placed anteriorly and superiorly for a pneumothorax, and posteriorly and inferiorly for an effusion. A radiopaque line usually runs along pleural tubes, and is interrupted where there are side holes. It is important to check that all the side holes are within the thorax (Figs 8.2, 8.4). Tracks may remain on the chest X-ray following removal of chest tubes, causing tubular or ring shadows. When doubt remains about tube position then CT scanning should be considered (Fig. 8.35).

Mediastinal drains

These are usually present following sternotomy. Apart from their position, they look like pleural tubes.

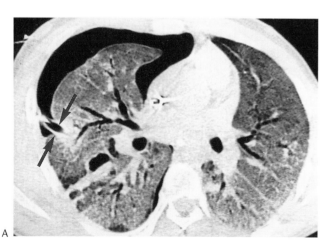
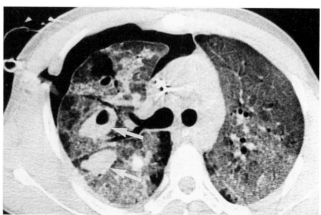

Fig. 8.35   (A,B) Multiple injuries in a patient following an automobile accident. CT obtained due to a persistent pneumothorax despite apparently satisfactory tube position. The chest tube can be seen entering the lung parenchyma (black arrows). Note also the extensive parenchymal changes due to ARDS, and the right-sided pulmonary haematomas (white arrows).

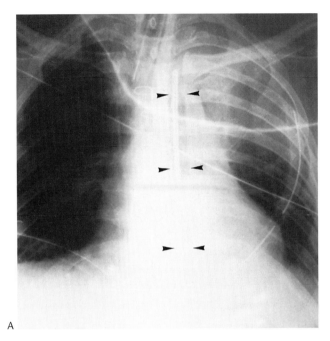 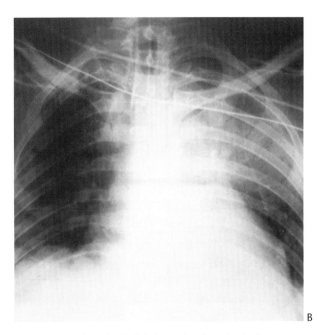

A   B

Fig. 8.36   Intra-aortic balloon pump. Postcoronary artery bypass surgery. (A) Bilateral pleural and mediastinal drains and endotracheal tube are present. The pump is well sited, and its balloon is seen to be inflated (arrowheads). (B) The drains have been removed. When this radiograph was exposed the balloon was deflated.

Intra-aortic balloon pumps

These are used in patients with cardiogenic shock, often following cardiac surgery. The pump comprises a catheter, the end of which is surrounded by an elongated, inflatable balloon. It is inserted via a femoral artery and is positioned in the descending thoracic aorta. The pattern of inflation and deflation of the balloon is designed to increase coronary perfusion during diastole, and to reduce the left ventricular afterload. The ideal position of the catheter tip is just distal to the origin of the left subclavian artery (Fig. 8.36). If the catheter tip is advanced too far it may occlude the left subclavian artery, and if it is too distal the balloon may occlude branches of the abdominal aorta.

Pacemakers

These may be permanent or temporary. Temporary epicardial wires are sometimes inserted during cardiac surgery, and may be seen as thin, almost hair-like metallic opacities overlying the heart. Temporary pacing electrodes are usually inserted transvenously via a subclavian or jugular vein (Fig. 8.33A). If a patient is not pacing properly, a chest X-ray may reveal that the position of the electrode tip is unstable, or a fracture in the wire may be seen (Fig. 8.37). A full discussion of the radiology of pacemakers is outside the scope of this chapter.

RADIATION INJURY OF THE LUNG

Radiation injury of the lung usually results from treatment of a pulmonary or mediastinal neoplasm by radiotherapy. It may also be a complication of the treatment of breast cancer. The changes seen on the chest X-ray are often remarkably geometrical, and correspond to the shape of the treatment portal.

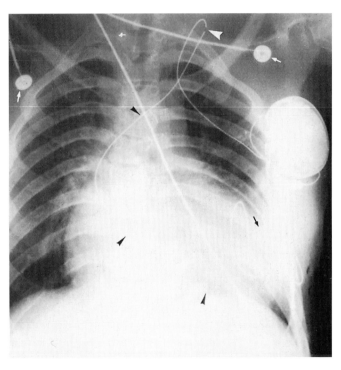

Fig. 8.37   Fractured pacing wire. Patient with surgically repaired complete atrioventricular canal. A permanent transvenous pacing system is present; the power unit is in the left axilla; the electrode (arrowheads) reaches the right ventricle by traversing the innominate vein, superior vena cava and right atrium. The electrode is fractured (white arrowhead). Note disconnected epicardial electrodes (black arrow) and ECG electrodes (white arrows).

The earliest pathological changes in the lung are alveolar and bronchiolar desquamation and accumulation of exudate in the alveoli. This is followed by organisation and fibrosis.

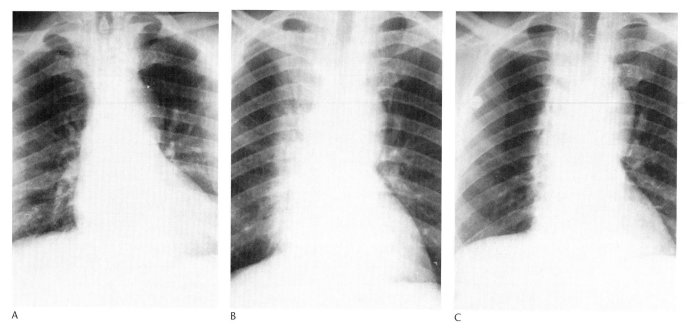

A   B   C

Fig. 8.38 Radiation pneumonitis in a man of 45 with diffuse histiocytic lymphoma who developed upper thoracic spinal cord compression. (A) After surgical decompression the lungs are clear and the patient commenced radiotherapy to the spine. (B) Ten weeks later there is paraspinal consolidation with air bronchograms. (C) Fourteen weeks after treatment paraspinal pulmonary fibrosis has developed. The changes correspond to the shape of the treatment portal.

The effect of radiation on the lung depends upon several factors. Healthy lung tissue is more resistant to damage than diseased lung. Previous radiotherapy and associated chemotherapy increase the likelihood of fibrosis. The total dose, the time over which it is given and the volume of lung irradiated are other factors. Radiographic changes are rare at a dose rate of 20 Gy (2000 rad) over 2–3 weeks, but are usual with doses of 60 Gy (6000 rad) or more over 5–6 weeks.

The radiological changes correspond to the pathology. The acute or exudative phase is not usually evident until a month or more after treatment, and may take up to 6 months to appear.

Consolidation, usually with some volume loss, occurs. It is not segmental or lobar, but corresponds to the shape of the radiation portal. An air bronchogram may be visible. The patient is usually asymptomatic, but may have a pyrexia or cough. Fibrosis then occurs, and is usually complete by 9–12 months (Figs 8.38, 8.39). Fibrosis, if extensive and severe enough, may cause displacement of fissures, the hila or mediastinum, and compensatory hyperinflation of the less affected lung (Fig. 8.40). Very dense fibrosis may produce an air bronchogram (Fig. 8.41).

A *pleural effusion* as a result of irradiation is rare, and is more likely to be due to the malignant disease being treated. Pericardial effusion may occur as a late complication of irradiation. Necrosis of ribs or a clavicle may be seen on the chest X-ray following radiotherapy (Fig. 8.42) and radiation-induced sarcomas are well recognised although rare.

The diagnosis of *radiation pneumonitis* and *fibrosis* is usually easy, based on the history and characteristic shape, but occasionally apical fibrosis following treatment of breast cancer may resemble tuberculosis.

Late complications of radiation treatment are various and include arteriosclerosis and occlusion of large and medium sized arteries,

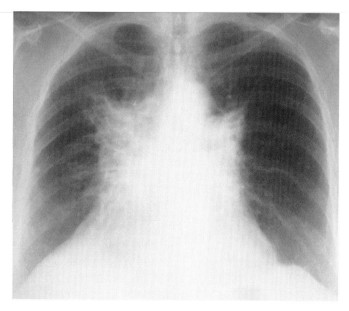

Fig. 8.39 Mediastinal fibrosis following radiotherapy several years previously. The sharp margins of the fibrosis correspond to the edges of the radiation field.

myocardial fibrosis and tracheal or bronchial strictures. Late bone changes include demineralisation and osteonecrosis, with associated patchy changes in bone density. Spontaneous fractures may occur with subsequent non-union being common. The aortic and subclavian *radiation-induced sarcomas* are a rare but well-recognised complication, the latent period ranging from 5 to 28 years (mean 13 years) in one study (Fig. 8.43).

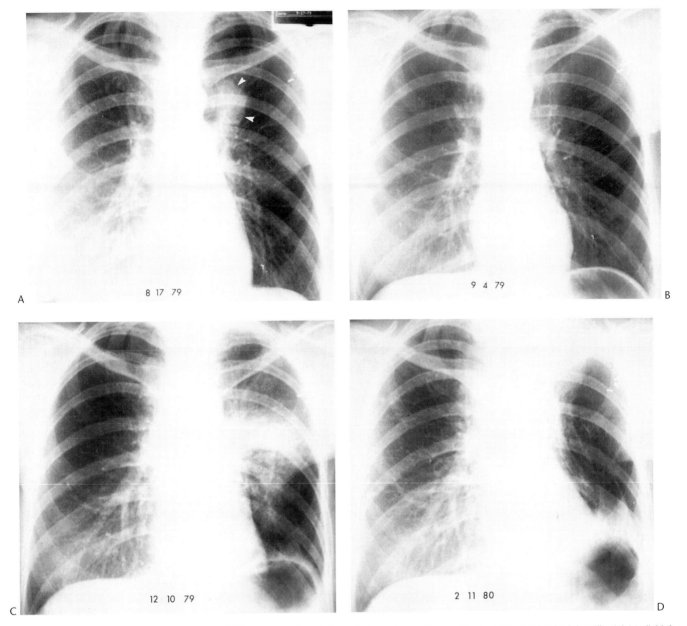

Fig. 8.40 Radiation pneumonitis in a woman of 32, one year after a left mastectomy for carcinoma. Surgical clips overlie the left axilla. (A) Medial left upper zone opacity (arrowheads) is caused by metastasis to left internal mammary lymph nodes. (B) Eighteen days later, following radiotherapy, the left upper mass has gone. (C) Sixteen weeks after treatment there is extensive consolidation in the left mid and upper zones. (D) Five months after treatment there is gross left upper lobe fibrosis, the mediastinum has shifted to the left and the left hemidiaphragm is elevated. The patient remained asymptomatic throughout this time.

PULMONARY EMBOLISM

Most pulmonary emboli arise in the pelvic or lower limb vessels and when acute above knee deep vein thrombosis (DVT) is left untreated clinical pulmonary embolism (PE) will occur in up to half of patients. A significant number of asymptomatic patients will undergo subclinical PE. The mortality rate from untreated PE is usually quoted as 30%, and the institution of anticoagulation, nowadays with low molecular weight heparin, has been shown to greatly reduce subsequent morbidity and mortality.

Radiological investigation of PE usually commences with a *chest radiograph*. Whilst this is rarely able to confirm the diagnosis of an embolism it is rarely normal and will frequently serve as an important guide for planning subsequent investigations.

The next most commonly undertaken investigation is a *perfusion scintigram*. This investigation can only provide indirect evidence of the presence of an embolus, and there have been a number of attempts to clarify and improve reporting methods. Many of these refinements have been instituted since the PIOPED study, but even the most widely accepted of them, such as those proposed by the PISA–PED study, leave a large cohort of patients without a defini-

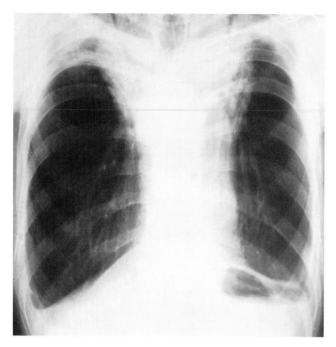

Fig. 8.41 Massive radiation fibrosis. Patient with Hodgkin's disease treated with mediastinal irradiation and chemotherapy (MOPP–bleomycin). Note gross bilateral upper lobe fibrosis with extensive air bronchogram.

tive diagnosis. Nevertheless in a sizeable group of patients scintigraphy remains of great utility, namely those patients in whom the clinical assessment and ventilation perfusion scan results are concordant and either give a normal or high probability result. The proportion of patients falling into this category varies from study to study but is almost certainly less than 50%.

An ideal test for PE would provide non-invasive direct visualisation of thrombus within pulmonary arteries; *CT pulmonary angiography* (CTPA) comes close to fulfilling this description (Fig. 8.44).

The sensitivities and specificities for pulmonary emboli detection by CTPA at main, lobar and segmental levels are almost always reported as greater than 90%. Many of these studies of CTPA have also emphasised the improved interobserver agreement of CTPA (83–95%) compared with V/Q scintigraphy for intermediate or low probability studies (70%), the ability to make alternative diagnoses in those patients without a PE, and the relatively low incidence of non-diagnostic studies. The technique of CTPA may be extended to include assessment of the pelvic and lower limb veins.

The optimal technique required for CTPA is being constantly refined, most recently following more widespread availability of multislice systems, with a tendency towards narrower collimation, and so more reliable depiction of segmental and subsegmental arteries (Fig. 8.45). Workstation-based image analysis rather than traditional hard copy images is also increasing, an approach that has been shown to result in greater detection rates. The CT signs of pulmonary embolism are now well defined, and the cardinal sign of an intraluminal filling defect remains the central diagnostic criterion for an embolus (Figs 8.44, 8.45).

The prevalence and significance of *subsegmental emboli* remains open to question. A number of studies suggest that the prevalence rates in patients investigated for suspected PE varies from as low as 5% to as high as 36%. A reasonable estimate would suggest that about 10% of patients in an unselected population of patients with PE will have isolated subsegmental emboli. These small emboli may herald the arrival of a subsequent significant embolus; however, follow up studies of patients with negative CT studies, some of whom are presumed to have undetected small emboli but are left untreated, suggest a representation rate following a normal CT of less than 1%, similar to that found after a normal V/Q scan or angiography. Whilst subsegmental emboli may be difficult to detect on CTPA, it should be borne in mind that interobserver agreement for two observers for these emboli on angiography has been demonstrated to be only 66%, falling to only 13% for agreement between three observers. More recent work assessing the relative

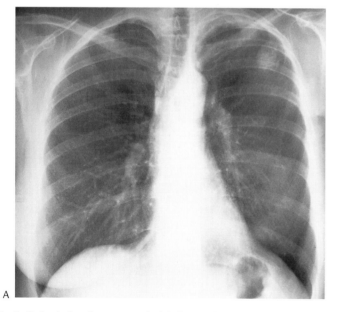

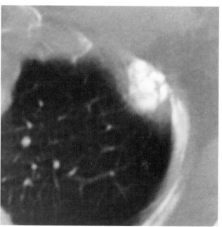

Fig. 8.42 Radiation-induced osteonecrosis. (A) Chest radiograph obtained 15 years after left mastectomy and radiation therapy demonstrates a dense opacity projected over the left second rib. (B) On CT there is a calcified mass arising from the second rib. Long-term follow-up showed no evidence of progression.

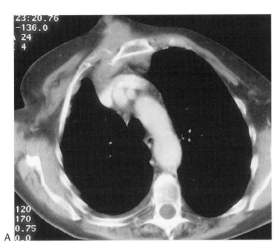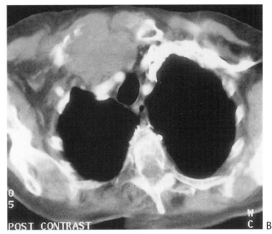

Fig. 8.43 Radiation-induced sarcoma. (A, B) There is a soft-tissue mass arising within the anterior chest wall in a patient treated 14 years previously for a right breast carcinoma. Note direct extension from subcutaneous tissues through the chest wall musculature into mediastinal fat.

accuracies of CTPA and conventional angiography for the detection of subsegmental-size thrombi found no significant differences in the abilities of the two tests.

Lung scintigraphy continues to play an important role in a significant proportion of patients presenting with possible PE, with approximately 25% of patients with suspected PE having the diagnosis refuted by normal scintigraphy, and another 25% with suspected PE having a high probability study. Either result could be taken as an investigational end-point. However when other acute or chronic chest disease is present and scintigraphy is unable to allow definitive diagnosis, further investigation is required. The evidence available increasingly suggests that CT is capable of replacing angiography as the definitive test for suspected PE.

TRANSPLANTATION

Cardiopulmonary transplantation is an uncommon procedure, with only a few thousand cases undertaken worldwide each year. Heart transplantation remains the most frequent procedure, with conges-

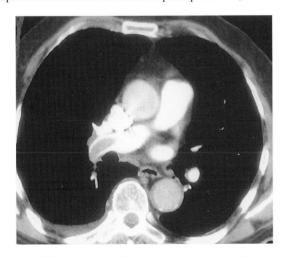

Fig. 8.44 CT image from a CT pulmonary angiogram at the level of the right main pulmonary artery. There is a large filling defect due to thrombus. Note the minor streak artefact arising from the dense contrast in the superior vena cava, and the small right pleural effusion.

tive cardiomyopathy or coronary artery disease being the usual indications. The combined frequencies of single or double lung transplantation and combined heart and lung transplantation remain significantly less than heart transplantation alone. Patients undergoing these procedures will suffer from complications common to many types of thoracic surgery, in addition to conditions that are more specific to transplantation.

HEART TRANSPLANTATION

Following surgery there is frequently evidence of basal atelectasis, especially in the left lower lobe. This may in part be due to the effects of cardioplegia upon the diaphragm and the left phrenic nerve. There are often small effusions present. Following surgery there is the possibility of haematoma collection within the pleura or mediastinum. Chest drains are usually placed during surgery, and pneumothoraces and mediastinal air are frequent findings. Intraperitoneal air may also be observed in the immediate postoperative period. Increasing amounts of gas in any of these spaces is not expected on serial postoperative radiographs and may herald one of a number of complications. If cardiac function is depressed in the postoperative period then ionotropic or mechanical assistance may be required and there may be evidence of pulmonary oedema. Appearances may return to normal within a few weeks, with little evidence of previous surgery (Fig. 8.46).

Complications related to rejection are usually manifest by cardiac failure. Rejection may be due to acute, usually within 3 months of surgery, or more chronic, in the subsequent months or years.

In keeping with other patients on long-term immunosuppression to prevent rejection, there is also an increased risk of lymphoproliferative disorders including lymphoma (Figs 8.47, 8.48). Complications specific to heart transplantation also include accelerated coronary artery atherosclerosis.

LUNG TRANSPLANTATION

Lung transplantation success was harder to achieve than heart transplantation for two main reasons. In the normal individual the lung is exposed to many pathogens each day without succumbing to infection. Following lung transplantation, the high levels of steroid

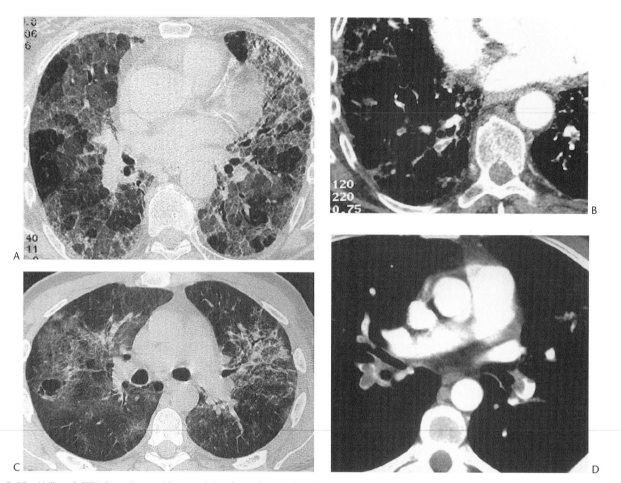

Fig. 8.45 Utility of CTPA in patients with pre-existing lung disease. (A) The initial HRCT through the lungs of this patient with sudden worsening of breathlessness demonstrates changes consistent with the known extrinsic allergic alveolitis. (B) The CTPA images demonstrate thrombus in the segmental and subsegmental vessels in the right lower lobe. (C) HRCT in a different patient at the time of CTPA. There are diffuse lung changes consistent with the known diagnosis of *Pneumocystis carinii* pneumonia. (D) The CTPA study demonstrates that there are also multiple pulmonary emboli.

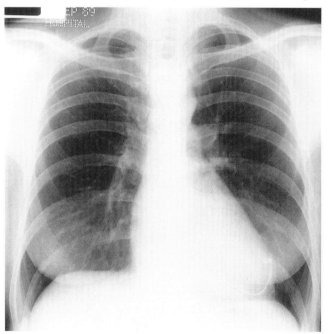

Fig. 8.46 Chest radiograph of patient 2 weeks after heart and lung transplantation. Apart from the epicardial pacing wire there is little evidence of the recent surgery.

immunosuppression required to prevent rejection result in a lowering of resistance to infection and a reduction in tissue-healing properties. Thus historically many lung transplants failed due to a combination of rejection and/or infection, or due to breakdown of the bronchial anastomoses. The introduction of cyclosporine, with its steroid-sparing effects, together with refinements in surgical technique, has now greatly reduced these problems.

The technique of single lung transplantation has become favoured over double lung transplantation, which is now reserved for pulmonary hypertension and suppurative lung disease. Single lung transplantation is suitable for conditions resulting in destruction of lung parenchyma such as fibrosing alveolitis, sarcoidosis, silicosis, chronic obstructive pulmonary disease, alpha-1 antitrypsin deficiency, etc. (Fig. 8.49). Both lungs may be transplanted as a single organ, with the left being technically easier to perform.

Selection of the donor organ and proper selection and preparation of the recipient are complex tasks that require a multidisciplinary approach and are beyond the scope of this text. However radiology plays an important part in this process, particularly in excluding occult contraindications such as incidental lung tumours or infection in the opposite lung, and for assessing the degree and extent of pleural abnormality.

As with cardiac transplantation, complications can be usefully divided into acute and chronic phases. In the initial postoperative

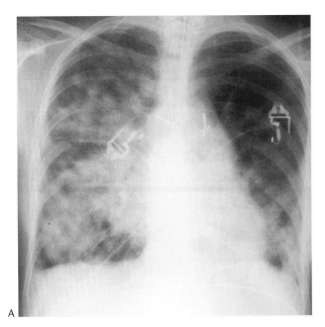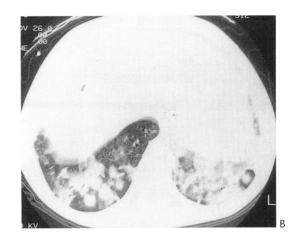

Fig. 8.47 Post-transplantation lymphoma following heart and lung transplantation. The chest radiograph (A) and CT (B) demonstrate widespread pulmonary nodules 2–3 cm in size which developed within 2 months of surgery. There was also mediastinal and hilar lymph node enlargement. Needle biopsy confirmed B-cell lymphoma which proved rapidly fatal.

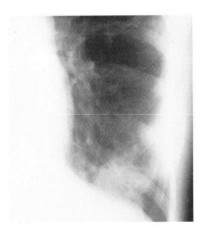

Fig. 8.48 Two years following heart and lung transplantation there is a large pulmonary nodule at the left lung base. This was one of several coexistent nodules that cleared rapidly following antiviral treatment administered after biopsy confirmed benign polyclonal lymphoproliferation.

phase *reperfusion oedema* is very common and varies greatly in severity and duration. It is usually apparent by day 3 and clears by day 10, assuming further complications have not supervened. Possible explanations for reimplantation oedema include prolonged ischaemic time resulting in increased capillary permeability, or lymphatic or autonomic nerve supply interruption as a result of the surgery. The duration and severity of the reimplantation response can be reduced by minimising ischaemic time and by careful restriction of postoperative fluid replacement.

Acute rejection tends to occur after the fifth postoperative day and may overlap with the reimplantation response. These processes may prove difficult to distinguish and may also coexist. The chest radiograph may remain normal in acute rejection, or may demonstrate diffuse interstitial oedema with pleural fluid, usually without increase in the heart size. Distinction between causes of pulmonary

infiltrate in the early postoperative period therefore usually requires bronchoscopy and transbronchial biopsy.

Infection may complicate the postoperative period. A number of factors increase susceptibility to infection, including colonisation of the upper airway by virulent hospital flora, impaired clearance of aspirated nasopharyngeal secretions in the perioperative period, and reduced immunity as a result of antirejection immunosuppression. There is also impairment of the normal mucociliary escalator as a result of the bronchial surgery. In the first month following transplantation bacterial infections are the most common organisms, and the radiological appearances are similar to those encountered in the general population. In addition opportunistic infections may occur, and these include fungal pathogens, most importantly *Aspergillus* species (Fig. 8.50).

The transplanted lung may fail in the postoperative period for a number of reasons other than rejection or infection, the commonest being *ischaemic damage* sustained during the transplantation process. In addition *anastomotic failures*, occasionally vascular but more frequently bronchial, may result in dehiscence or stenosis. Modern radiological and surgical techniques, previously with omental wrapping of the anastomosis, but more recently with telescoping of the recipient and donor bronchi, have reduced but not eliminated these problems. Bronchial anastomosis dehiscence may result in the development of mediastinal emphysema and the diagnosis can usually be confirmed by CT demonstration of mediastinal air collections around the point of anastomosis. On occasion CT is able to identify the bronchial wall defect itself.

A number of *late complications* are also recognised including chronic rejection, opportunistic and other infections and complications with anastomoses.

Most episodes of acute rejection occur in the first month following surgery. Occasionally similar episodes of illness occur at longer intervals after the surgery, usually with fever and breathlessness. Radiographic changes may be absent, or may be akin to pulmonary

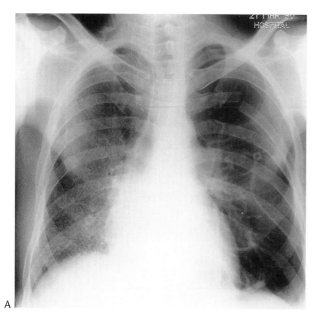

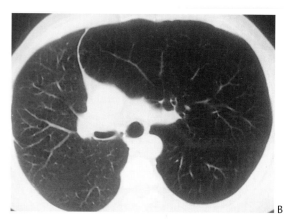

Fig. 8.49   (A) Chest radiograph in a patient 2 weeks following left lung transplantation for fibrosing alveolitis. Note the surgical defect in the posterior part of the left fifth rib. (B) HRCT through the lungs of a patient who has recently undergone right lung transplantation for emphysema related to alpha-1-antitrypsin deficiency. Note the displacement of the midline structure due to the relatively large emphysematous left lung.

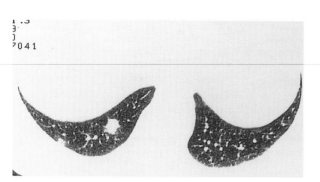

Fig. 8.50   Invasive *Aspergillus* infection following heart and lung transplantation. HRCT reveals the presence of small foci of infection in the posterior costophrenic recesses. Despite the development of new symptoms the chest radiograph had been normal.

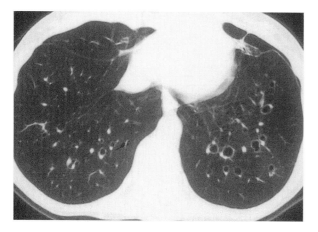

Fig. 8.51   Bronchiolitis obliterans following transplantation. There is marked bronchial dilatation in the lower lobes bilaterally, although the lung parenchyma appears unremarkable.

oedema. Diagnosis usually depends on exclusion of infection and appropriate response to high-dose pulsed steroids. The more common form of *chronic rejection* is manifest radiographically and physiologically as *bronchiolitis obliterans*. Thus there is progressive reduction in FEV_1, with increasing respiratory impairment. Although the chest radiograph is frequently normal, there may be hyperexpansion. By contrast, HRCT is more sensitive and usually demonstrates variation in attenuation of pulmonary parenchyma, a finding accentuated on expiratory images and reflecting regional air trapping. There may also be evidence of bronchial dilatation, usually with minimal bronchial wall thickening (Fig. 8.51). Chronic rejection is more common after repeated episodes of acute rejection. Pathologically there is scarring and obliteration of the terminal and respiratory bronchioles.

Lymphoproliferative diseases may occur at any time following transplantation, and vary in severity from a benign polyclonal lymphoproliferation, historically related to Epstein–Barr virus infection (Fig. 8.48), to highly malignant forms of non-Hodgkin's lymphoma (Fig. 8.47). The benign forms of lymphoproliferation respond rapidly to antiviral agents and reduction in immunosuppression, but the malignant forms of disease are extremely difficult to treat and are frequently lethal. There are usually multiple pulmonary nodules or masses, and there may be mediastinal or hilar nodes evident on CT, a combination highly suggestive of post-transplantation lymphoproliferation.

ADULT RESPIRATORY DISTRESS SYNDROME

Adult respiratory distress syndrome (ARDS) may be due to a large number of causes (Box 8.1), and presents as acute respiratory failure in patients without previous lung disease, usually following major trauma or shock. Clinically the patient becomes hypoxaemic 12–24 hours after the precipitating event. There is then progressive

Box 8.1   Common causes of ARDS

Major trauma	Burns
Septicaemia	Viral pneumonia
Hypovolaemic shock	Pancreatitis
Fat embolism	Oxygen toxicity
Near-drowning	Disseminated intravascular coagulation
Mendelson's syndrome	

respiratory failure over several days requiring ventilator support. During this time there may be superimposed infection, or various complications of positive-pressure ventilation may develop. In excess of 50% of cases are fatal, and survivors may be left with chronic lung disease.

There are three broad pathological stages in the evolution and resolution of ARDS with roughly corresponding radiographic features. *Stage 1* (0–24 hours) (Fig. 8.52) represents the acute phase where there is widespread shedding of the alveolar epithelium and endothelial lining of the alveolar capillaries. Despite these marked pathological changes there is little increase in extracellular fluid content in the lungs and so the radiograph is often normal. *Stage II* (24–36 hours) (Fig. 8.53) corresponds to the leak of fluid into the lungs from the damaged capillary bed, together with the development of hyaline membranes. Radiographically there is increased general opacification in the lungs which progresses rapidly to widespread air-space infiltrate. This may initially appear patchy before becoming diffuse, and is characterised by air bronchograms and usually the absence of pleural fluid. Appearances often remain static for 2–3 days until the start of *Stage III* (3–14 days). During this last stage there is slow pathological and radiological resolution, with interstitial fibrosis and proliferation of Type II pneumocytes. The chest radiograph may never return completely to normal as a result of scarring.

One of the more common and difficult radiological assessments required for patient management in the intensive care setting is distinguishing between *cardiogenic* and *non-cardiogenic* oedema.

Although accurate diagnosis is frequently not possible from the chest radiograph alone, radiographic signs found to be suggestive of cardiogenic oedema include pulmonary vascular upper lobe redistribution, widening of the vascular pedicle, and perihilar distribution of alveolar oedema.

Complications frequently occur during the evolution of ARDS, and many of these result from the need for aggressive ventilatory support. These include pneumomediastinum, pneumothorax and subcutaneous emphysema, in addition to pulmonary interstitial emphysema (Fig. 8.54). Air may also track into the peritoneum and retroperitoneum. Complications of ARDS may supervene at any

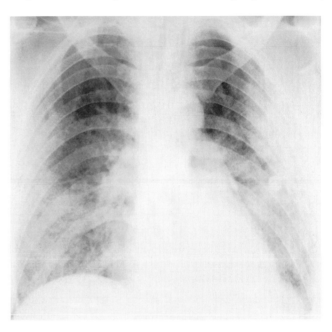

Fig. 8.52 ARDS. Fat embolism from multiple skeletal trauma. Diffuse alveolar opacities.

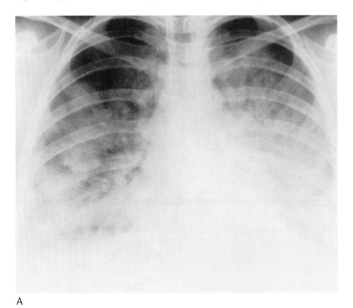

A

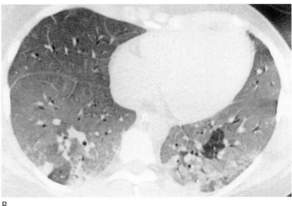

B

Fig. 8.53 (A) Staphylococcal toxic shock. Extensive alveolar opacification. *Staphylococcus aureus* was isolated from a vaginal tampon. (B) HRCT in a different patient with ARDS demonstrates the anterior–posterior gravitational gradient of lung density, with occasional spared secondary pulmonary lobules.

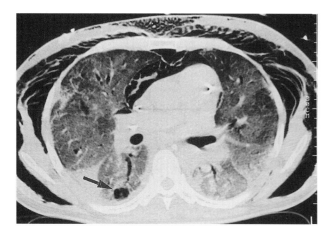

Fig. 8.54   ARDS. CT demonstrates extensive mediastinal and subcutaneous emphysema as well as a parenchymal bulla (arrow) possibly related to high-pressure ventilation. Note the typical anterior–posterior density gradient in lung attenuation due to the effects of gravity.

time and one of the primary roles of radiography and CT examination at this time is in detection and management. The development of barotrauma is usually related to large tidal volumes, high inflationary pressures and the presence of pre-existing lung disease. Usually air leak is initially into the lung interstitium, and although this is frequently difficult to detect, if present is almost always the precursor of pneumothorax and pneumo-mediastinum.

Superadded infection is a further common problem during ARDS. Due to the widespread lung changes already present diagnosis is usually far from easy, with departure from the expected evolution of pulmonary changes often providing the first radiological clue.

CT has a small but vital role in the management of the critically ill patient with ARDS. A number of important insights into the pathophysiology of ARDS have been provided by HRCT. In the context of day-to-day management CT is valuable for the detection of complications not clearly delineated by the chest radiograph, particularly loculated pneumothoraces, abscesses, empyema and mediastinal collections (Fig. 8.55). In addition, CT may aid deci-

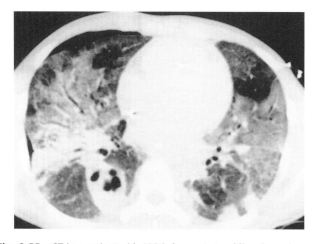

Fig. 8.55   CT in a patient with ARDS demonstrates diffuse lung changes and a shallow pneumothorax on the right. In addition there is a loculated rounded abscess in the right lower lobe that was not apparent on the chest radiograph.

sions regarding mode of ventilation support, including recruitment of dependent non-aerated lung by turning the patient prone.

REFERENCES AND SUGGESTIONS FOR FURTHER READING

Trauma

Ball, T., McCrory, R., Smith, J. O., Clements, Jr J. L., (1982) Traumatic diaphragmatic hernia: errors in diagnosis. *American Journal of Roentgenology*, **138**, 633–637.

Batra, P. (1987) The fat embolism syndrome. *Journal of Thoracic Imaging*, **2**(3), 12–17.

Cochlin, D. L., Shaw, M. R. P. (1978) Traumatic lung cysts following minor blunt chest trauma. *Clinical Radiology*, **29**, 151–154.

Crass, J. R., Cohen, A. M., Motta, A. O., et al (1990) A proposed new mechanism of traumatic aortic rupture: the osseous pinch. *Radiology*, **176**, 645–649.

Feliciano, D. V., Rozycki, G. S. (1999) Advances in the diagnosis and treatment of thoracic trauma. *Surgical Clinics of North America*, **79**, 1417–1429.

Fishman, J. E. (2000) Imaging of blunt aortic and great vessel trauma. *Journal of Thoracic Imaging*, **15**, 97–103.

George, P. Y., Goodman, P. (1992) Radiographic appearance of bullet tracks in the lung. *American Journal of Roentgenology*, **159**, 967–970.

Goarin, J. P., LeBret, F., Riou, B., et al (1993) Early diagnosis of traumatic thoracic rupture by transesophageal echocardiography. *Chest*, **103**, 618–619.

Hartley, C., Morritt, G. N. (1993) Bronchial rupture secondary to blunt chest trauma. *Thorax*, **48**, 183–184.

Mirvis, S. E., Shanmuganathan, K. (2000) MR imaging of thoracic trauma. *Magnetic Resonance Imaging Clinics of North America*, **8**, 91–104.

Parkin, G. J. S. (1973) The radiology of perforated oesophagus. *Clinical Radiology*, **24**, 324–332.

Raptopoulos, V., Sherman, R. G., Phillips, D. A., et al (1992) Traumatic aortic tear: screening with chest CT. *Radiology*, **182**, 667–673.

Richardson, P., Mirvis, S. E., Scorpio, R., et al (1991) Value of CT in determining the need for angiography when the findings of mediastinal hemorrhage on chest radiographs are equivocal. *American Journal of Roentgenology*, **156**, 273–279.

Rollins, R. J., Tocino, I. (1987) Early radiographic signs of tracheal rupture. *American Journal of Roentgenology*, **148**, 695–698.

Scaglione, M., Pinto, A., Pinto, F., Romano, L., et al (2001) Role of contrast-enhanced helical CT in the evaluation of acute thoracic aortic injuries after blunt chest trauma. *European Radiology*, **11**, 2444–2448.

Schild, H. H., Strunk, H., Weber, W., et al (1989) Pulmonary contusion: CT vs plain radiograms. *Journal of Computer Assisted Tomography*, **13**, 417–420.

Sefczek, D. M., Sefczek, R. J., Deeb, S. L. (1983) Radiographic signs of acute traumatic rupture of the thoracic aorta. *American Journal of Roentgenology*, **141**, 1259–1262.

Shanmuganathan, K., Killeen, K., Mirvis, S. E., White, C.S. (2000) Imaging of diaphragmatic injuries. *Journal of Thoracic Imaging*, 15, 104–111.

Somers, J. M., Gleeson, F. V., Flower, C. D. R. (1990) Rupture of the right hemidiaphragm following blunt trauma: the use of ultrasound in diagnosis. *Clinical Radiology*, **42**, 97–101.

Valliers, E., Shamji, F. M., Todd, T. R. (1993) Post pneumonectomy chylothorax. *Annals of Thoracic Surgery*, **55**, 1006–1008.

Wiot, J. F. (1975) The radiologic manifestations of blunt chest trauma. *Journal of the American Medical Association*, **231**, 500.

The postoperative chest and intensive care

Carter, A. R., Sostman, H. D., Curtis, A. M., Swett, H. A. (1983) Thoracic alterations after cardiac surgery. *American Journal of Roentgenology*, **140**, 475–481.

Goodman, L.R. (1980) Postoperative chest radiograph: I. Alterations after abdominal surgery. *American Journal of Roentgenology*, **134**, 533–541.

Goodman, L. R. (1980) Postoperative chest radiograph: II. Alterations after major intrathoracic surgery. *American Journal of Roentgenology*, **134**, 803–813.

Goodman, L. R., Kuzo, M. D. (eds) (1996) Intensive care radiology. *Radiologic Clinics of North America*, **34**, 1.

Spirn, P. W., Gross, G. W., Wechsler, R. J., Steiner, R. M. (1988) Radiology of the chest after thoracic surgery. *Seminars in Roentgenology*, **23**, 9–31.

Thorsen, M. K., Goodman, L. R. (1988) Extracardiac complications of cardiac surgery. *Seminars in Roentgenology*, **23**, 32–48.

Radiation injury of the lung

Boushy, S. F., Belgason, A. H., Borth, L. B. (1970) The effect of radiation on the lung and bronchial tree. *American Journal of Roentgenology*, **108**, 284–292.

Davis, S. D., Yankelevitz, D. F., Henschke, C. I. (1992) Radiation effects on the lung: clinical features, pathology and imaging findings. *American Journal of Roentgenology*, **159**, 1157–1164.

Huvos, A. G., Woodward, H. Q., Cahan, W. B., et al (1985) Post irradiation osteogenic sarcoma of bone and soft tissue: a clinico-pathologic study in 66 patients. *Cancer*, **55**, 1244–1255.

Ikezoe, J., Takashima, S., Morimoto, S., et al (1988) CT appearance of acute radiation-induced injury in the lung. *American Journal of Roentgenology*, **150**, 765–770.

Libshitz, H. I., Shuman, L. S. (1984) Radiation-induced pulmonary change: CT findings. *Journal of Computer Assisted Tomography*, **8**, 15–19.

Polansky, S. M., Ravin, C. E., Prosnitz, I. R. (1980) Lung changes after breast irradiation. *American Journal of Roentgenology*, **139**, 101–105.

Rowinsky, E. K., Abeloff, M. D., Wharam, M. D. (1985) Spontaneous pneumothorax following thoracic irradiation. *Chest*, **88**, 703–708.

Wencel, M. L., Sitrin, R. G. (1988) Unilateral lung hyperlucency after mediastinal irradiation. *American Research into Respiratory Disease*, **137**, 955–957.

Pulmonary embolism

Baile, E. M., King, G. G., Muller, N. L., et al (2000) Spiral computed tomography is comparable to angiography for the diagnosis of pulmonary embolism. *America Journal of Respiratory and Critical Care Medicine*, **161**, 1010–1015.

Burkill, G. J., Bell, J. R., Padley, S. P. (1999) Survey on the use of pulmonary scintigraphy, spiral CT and conventional pulmonary angiography for suspected pulmonary embolism in the British Isles. *Clinical Radiology*, **54**, 807–810.

Garg, K., Welsh, C. H., Feyerabend, A. J., et al (1998) Pulmonary embolism: diagnosis with spiral CT and ventilation-perfusion scanning—correlation with pulmonary angiographic results or clinical outcome. *Radiology*, **208**, 201–208.

Goodman, L. R., Lipchik, R. J. (1996) Diagnosis of acute pulmonary embolism: time for a new approach. *Radiology*, **199**, 25–27.

Huisman, M. V., Buller, H. R., ten Cate, J. W., et al (1989) Unexpected high prevalence of silent pulmonary embolism in patients with deep venous thrombosis. *Chest*, **95**, 498–502.

Invasive and noninvasive diagnosis of pulmonary embolism. Preliminary results of the Prospective Investigative Study of Acute Pulmonary Embolism Diagnosis (PISA–PED). (1995) *Chest*, **107** (1 Suppl), 33S–38S.

Remy-Jardin, M., Remy, J., Deschildre, F., et al (1996) Diagnosis of pulmonary embolism with spiral CT: comparison with pulmonary angiography and scintigraphy. *Radiology*, **200**, 699–706.

Robinson, P. J. (1996) Ventilation-perfusion lung scanning and spiral computed tomography of the lungs: competing or complementary modalities? *European Journal of Nuclear Medicine*, **23**, 1547–1553.

Task force report (2000) Guidelines on the diagnosis and management of acute pulmonary embolism. *European Heart Journal*, **21**, 1301–1336.

Value of the ventilation/perfusion scan in acute pulmonary embolism. Results of the prospective investigation of pulmonary embolism diagnosis (PIOPED). The PIOPED Investigators. (1999) *JAMA*, **263**, 2753–2759.

van Erkel, A. R., van Rossum, A. B., Bloem, J. L., Kievit, J., Pattynama, P. M. (1996) Spiral CT angiography for suspected pulmonary embolism: a cost-effectiveness analysis. *Radiology*, **201**, 29–36.

Wells, P. S., Anderson, D. R., Ginsberg, J. (2000) Assessment of deep vein thrombosis or pulmonary embolism by the combined use of clinical model and noninvasive diagnostic tests. *Seminars in Thrombosis and Hemostasis*, **26**, 643–656.

Transplantation

Anderson, D. C., Glazer, H. S., Semenkovich, J. W., et al (1995) Lung transplant edema: chest radiography after lung transplantation—the first 10 days. *Radiology*, **195**, 275–281.

Collins, J., Kuhlman, J. E., Love, R. B. (1998) Acute, life-threatening complications of lung transplantation. *RadioGraphics*, **18**, 21–43.

Collins, J., Muller, N. L., Leung, A. N., et al (1998) Epstein–Barr virus-associated lymphoproliferative disease of the lung: CT and histologic findings. *Radiology*, **208**, 749–759.

Dauber, J. H., Paradis, I. L., Dummer, J. S. (1990) Infectious complications in pulmonary allograft recipients. *Clinics in Chest Medicine*, **11**, 291–308.

Herman, S. J. (1994) Radiologic assessment after lung transplantation. *Radiologic Clinics of North America*, **32**, 663–678.

Kesten, S., Chaparro, C. (1999) Mycobacterial infections in lung transplant recipients. *Chest*, **115**, 741–745.

Levine, S. M., Angel, L., Anzueto, A., et al (1999) A low incidence of posttransplant lymphoproliferative disorder in 109 lung transplant recipients. *Chest*, **116**, 1273–1277.

Leung, A. N., Fisher, K., Valentine, V., et al (1998) Bronchiolitis obliterans after lung transplantation: detection using expiratory HRCT. *Chest*, **113**, 365–370.

Loubeyre, P., Revel, D., Delignette, A., Loire, R., Mornex, J. F. (1995) High-resolution computed tomographic findings associated with histologically diagnosed acute lung rejection in heart-lung transplant recipients. *Chest*, **107**, 132–138.

Mihalov, M. L., Gattuso, P., Abraham, K., Holmes, E. W., Reddy, V. (1996) Incidence of post-transplant malignancy among 674 solid-organ-transplant recipients at a single center. *Clinical Transplantation*, **10**, 248–255.

Murray, J., McAdams, H., Erasmus, J., Patz Jr, E., Tapson, V. (1996) Complications of lung transplantation: radiologic findings. *American Journal of Roentgenology*, **166**, 1405–1411.

Schulman, L. L., Scully, B., McGregor, C. C., Austin, J. H. (1997) Pulmonary tuberculosis after lung transplantation. *Chest*, **111**, 1459–1462.

Shepard, J. A. (1999) Imaging of lung transplantation. *Clinics in Chest Medicine*, **20**, 827–844.

Shreeniwas, R., Schulman, L. L., Berkmen, Y. M., McGregor, C. C., Austin, J. H. (1996) Opportunistic bronchopulmonary infections after lung transplantation: clinical and radiographic findings. *Radiology*, **200**, 349–356.

Spiekerkoetter, E., Krug, N., Hoeper, M., et al (1998) Prevalence of malignancies after lung transplantation. *Transplantation Proceedungs*, **30**, 1523–1524.

Rappaport, D. C., Chamberlain, D. W., Shepherd, F. A., Hutcheon, M. A. (1998) Lymphoproliferative disorders after lung transplantation: imaging features. *Radiology*, **206**, 519–524.

Venuta, F., Boehler, A., Rendina, E. A., et al (1999) Complications in the native lung after single lung transplantation. *European Journal of Cardiothoracic Surgery*, **16**, 54–58.

ARDS

Andrews, C. P., Coalson, J. J., Smith, J. D., Johanson Jr., W. G. (1981) Diagnosis of nosocomial bacterial pneumonia in acute, diffuse lung injury. *Chest*, **80**, 254–258.

Bernard, G. R., Artigas, A., Brigham, K. L., et al (1994) The American–European Consensus Conference on ARDS: definitions, mechanisms, relevant outcomes, and clinical trial coordination. *American Journal of Respiratory and Critical Care Medicine*, **149**, 818–824.

Chastre, J., Trouillet, J. L., Vuagnat, A., et al (1998) Nosocomial pneumonia in patients with acute respiratory distress syndrome. *American Journal of Respiratory and Critical Care Medicine*, **157**, 1165–1172.

Desai, S. R., Wells, A. U., Rubens, M. B., Evans, T. W., Hansell, D. M. (1999) Acute respiratory distress syndrome: computed tomographic abnormalities at long-term follow-up. *Radiology*, **210**, 29–35.

Gattinoni, L., Pelosi, P., Vitale, G., Pesenti, A., D'Andrea, L., Mascheroni, D. (1991) Body position changes redistribute lung computed-tomographic density in patients with acute respiratory failure. *Anesthesiology*, **74**, 15–23.

Gattinoni, L., Bombino, M., Pelosi, P., et al (1994) Lung structure and function in different stages of severe adult respiratory distress syndrome. *Journal of the American Medical Association*, **271**, 1772–1779.

Gattinoni, L., Pelosi, P., Suter, P. M., Pedoto, A., Vercesi, P., Lissoni, A. (1998) Acute respiratory distress syndrome caused by pulmonary and extrapulmonary disease: different syndromes? *American Journal of Respiratory and Critical Care Medicine*, **158**, 3–11.

Goodman, L. R., Fumagalli, R., Tagliabue, P., et al (1999) Adult respiratory distress syndrome due to pulmonary and extrapulmonary causes: CT, clinical, and functional correlations. *Radiology*, **213**, 545–552.

Hansell, D. M. (1996) Imaging the injured lung. In: Evans, T.W., Haslett, C. (eds) *ARDS: Acute Respiratory Distress in Adults*, pp. 361–379. London. Chapman & Hall.

Snow, N., Bergin, K. T., Horrigan, T. P. (1990) Thoracic CT scanning in critically ill patients: information obtained frequently alters management. *Chest*, **97**, 1467–1470.

Winer-Muram, H. T., Rubin, S. A., Ellis, J. V., et al (1993) Pneumonia and ARDS in patients receiving mechanical ventilation: diagnostic accuracy of chest radiography. *Radiology*, **188**, 479–485.

Wright, J. L. (1995) Adult respiratory distress syndrome. In: Thurlbeck, W. M., Churg, A. M. (eds) *Pathology of the Lung*, 2nd edn, pp. 385–399. New York: Thieme.

9

THE PAEDIATRIC CHEST

Catherine M. Owens and Karen E. Thomas

Paediatric chest radiology is a complex subject and hence a full understanding of all the relevant pathologies is beyond the scope of this text. The aim of this chapter is to give a brief overview of the more important pathologies within the paediatric chest with an emphasis on congenital respiratory problems. There are however numerous excellent texts which focus on the imaging of the respiratory system and other review articles monographs and textbooks which deal more specifically with the newborn chest, respiratory tract emergencies and intensive care imaging.

TECHNIQUES

Plain radiographs

These remain the basis for the evaluation of the chest in childhood. In the neonate, satisfactory films can be obtained in incubators using modern mobile X-ray apparatus. The baby lies on the cassette and the film is exposed. Although automatic triggering of the exposure can be made using variations of temperature at the nostril and of electrical impedance across the chest in the differing phases of respiration, an experienced radiographer will usually be able to judge the end of inspiration. An adequate inspiration will be with the right hemidiaphragm at the level of the eighth rib posteriorly. Films in expiration frequently show a sharp kink in the trachea to the right and varying degrees of opacification of the lung fields, with apparent enlargement of the heart. Films should be well collimated, the baby positioned as straight as possible and lordotic films avoided, especially if the heart size is of particular interest. As much monitoring equipment as possible should be removed.

Computed radiography is particularly useful in intensive care, and the facility of data manipulation (edge enhancement) improves visualisation of supportive apparatus such as tubes and lines.

Children over 5 years can usually cooperate sufficiently to stand for a PA film like adults. Below this age some form of chest stand is needed in which an assistant, preferably the mother, can hold the child in front of a cassette with a suspended protective lead apron behind which she stands. With proper collimation, the dose to the mother is small and her position allows the child to be held straighter than from a position to the side. The difference between a PA and an AP projection in the small child is usually negligible.

High kilovoltage techniques with added filtration and the use of a grid allow evaluation of the trachea and major bronchi, which is important in stridor.

Fluoroscopy

Limitation of radiation exposure is vital in childhood, but quick fluoroscopic examination (using pulsed rather than continuous fluoroscopy) of the chest can frequently prove extremely useful, in particular in the evaluation of differing lung radiolucencies in suspected foreign body aspiration. With obstructive emphysema, the affected lung will show little volume change with respiration and the mediastinum will swing contralaterally in expiration.

Lateral fluoroscopy is also valuable for dynamic evaluation of tracheomalacia.

Barium swallow

Vascular rings, extrinsic masses, laryngeal clefts and tracheo-oesophageal fistula can be ruled out with good quality single contrast barium or water soluble contrast studies.

Computed tomography

CT is an invaluable technique in many paediatric chest diseases, however it is vital to assess the diagnostic benefit versus radiation risk to the patient. In the younger child (less than 5 years of age) sedation or general anaesthesia is often required, and this, again, has risk management issues.

CT demonstrates anatomy in a transaxial manner and has an increased sensitivity over the conventional chest radiograph. CT is ideal for chest/pleural lesions and can detect extension of mediastinal masses through the chest wall. The trachea and major bronchi are well visualised and extrinsic and intrinsic airway masses are easily diagnosed. The pulmonary parenchyma is visualised in great detail with both spiral, volumetric and high-resolution lung CT. The increased sensitivity of chest CT versus the chest X-ray for the detection of pulmonary nodules has been extensively studied.

High-resolution CT (HRCT) allows early detection of diffuse pulmonary parenchymal disease to the level of the secondary pulmonary lobule. HRCT is also useful in the characterisation of opportunistic infection in the immunocompromised patient and can act as a road map for minimally invasive thoracoscopic procedures. The recommended technique in children with diffuse pulmonary disease includes HRCT slices of approximately 1–2-mm thickness at 1–2-cm intervals from lung apices to lung bases (depending on the size of the thorax). A high-resolution (bone algorithm) is mandatory. If possible, CT slices should be obtained at total lung capacity (TLC), i.e. at end inspiration to diminish vascular crowding, particularly in the dependent areas of the lung, where oedema is more obvious in children than in adults.

There are many advantages of conventional CT over the plain chest X-ray, however the added problems of cardiac and respiratory motion artefacts may significantly degrade images and the paucity of mediastinal fat in children compared to adults make tissue contrast less good. Spiral CT, ultrafast electron beam CT (EBCT) and volumetric CT are particularly useful to investigate the major intrathoracic airways, cardiovascular and mediastinal abnormalities, and the advantage of quick scan times in children is particularly useful, reducing the need for sedation and giving excellent vascular opacification with relatively lower contrast volumes.

In uncooperative children acquisition of expiratory scans can be problematical where there is a suspicion of small airways disease. The decubitus position is then useful, as when the child is placed decubitus the dependent hemithorax is splinted, and its motion restricted, causing underaeration of the dependent lung plus hyperaeration of the upper lung, i.e. providing effectively an expiration view of the dependent lung and an inspiration view of the upper lung. This is useful for the detection of air trapping in the dependent lung.

Magnetic resonance imaging

The multiplanar imaging capabilities of cardiac gated MR and magnetic resonance angiography (MRA) make these important methods for investigating cardiac lesions, anomalies of the great vessels and mediastinal vessels, masses such as bronchopulmonary foregut malformations, chest wall masses, bone marrow infiltrations, tracheobronchial abnormalities and neurogenic masses. The capability of MRI to characterise tissue allows more specific diagnoses of some mediastinal masses. Ongoing refinements with improved gating techniques and shorter scan times are under continuous redevelopment and continue to further enhance the role of MRI in evaluating the pulmonary hila, lung parenchyma, heart and diaphragm.

The importance of non-ionising radiation techniques in paediatrics cannot be overemphasised, and MRI is a highly desirable tool for investigating children, although the setbacks include the enhanced use of sedation or general anaesthesia due to the prolonged scan times.

Ultrasonography

Ultrasound is particularly important in paediatric practice as it obviates the need for ionising radiation. The real-time and portable application of ultrasound make it even more useful, especially in intensive care units. As air is highly reflective, the applications of chest ultrasound are limited, however in evaluation of pleural fluid, pleural masses, peridiaphragmatic masses and neck masses, pericardial disease, diaphragmatic eventeration, diaphragmatic motion and the evaluation of the thymus, ultrasound is invaluable.

Doppler ultrasound with colour flow and power Doppler aid in the evaluation of vascular status and patency, and abnormal vascular anatomy.

Radionuclide imaging

Nuclear medicine techniques help delineate cardiac function, right to left shunts, pulmonary embolism, inflammatory lung disease, neoplasia and lung ventilation/perfusion.

Bronchography

High-resolution thin-section CT has almost eliminated the need for bronchography in children, however the technique is still used for functional bronchography, plus assessing the dynamics of tracheobronchomalacia.

Angiography

In extracardiac chest pathology, angiography is used relatively infrequently. MRI is a useful non-invasive technique with no radiation burden.

Interventional techniques such as embolisation of bronchial arteries is performed in cases of severe haemorrhage/haemoptysis in cystic fibrosis.

SPECIFIC FEATURES OF THE CHEST RADIOGRAPH IN CHILDREN

The thymus

The normal thymus is a frequent cause of widening of the superior mediastinum during the first years of life. The lateral margin often shows an undulation—the thymic wave—which corresponds to the indentations of the ribs on the inner surface of the thoracic cage. Particularly on the right, the thymus may have a triangular 'sail-like' configuration. The thymus may involute in times of stress, and a decrease in size can be induced by steroids.

At times, the differentiation of physiological thymus from pathology in the anterior mediastinum can be difficult. Ultrasound examination will usually differentiate cystic lesions from the homogeneous normal thymic tissue. Occasionally the normal thymus can act as a significant space-occupying lesion in the superior mediastinum and in such cases differentiation may be helped by

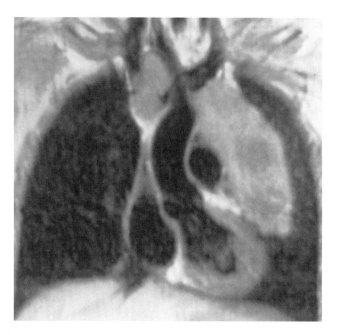

Fig. 9.1 Coronal MRI scan (T₁-weighted) in a child with a mediastinal mass. Note how the heart and great vessels are readily differentiated by signal void due to blood flow from the glandular masses due to Hodgkin's disease.

MRI, which shows homogeneous signal with a normal thymus, and heterogenous signal with pathology (Fig. 9.1).

The cardiothoracic ratio

In toddlers, the cardiothoracic ratio can at times exceed 50% and care should be exercised in overdiagnosis of cardiomegaly.

Kink of trachea to the right

This is a frequent feature of a chest film taken in less than full inspiration. This is a physiological buckling and does not represent a mass lesion.

The soft tissues

These may be prominent in children, and the anterior axillary fold crossing the chest wall can at times mimic a pneumothorax. Similarly, skin folds can at times cast confusing shadows. Plaits of hair over the upper chest can mimic pulmonary infiltrations.

Pleural effusions

Whereas in adults an early sign of pleural effusion is blunting of the costophrenic angles, in childhood it is more common to see separation of the lung from the chest wall with reasonable preservation of the clarity of the costophrenic angles, and accentuation of the lung fissures.

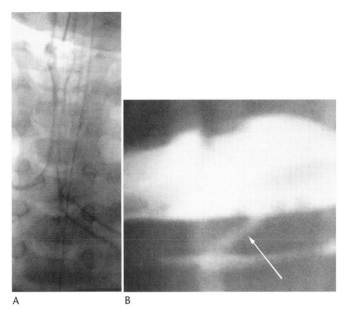

A   B

Fig. 9.2 (A) Bronchogram. Water-soluble contrast has been introduced into the trachea and bronchi showing long segment tracheal stenosis. Right apical (pig) bronchus also present. (B) Prone oesophagogram showing good bolus distension of the oesophagus with a hairline communication between the oesophagus and trachea (which contains contrast along its posterior wall) representing the 'N' or 'H' type tracheo-oesophageal fistula (arrow).

CONGENITAL LUNG ABNORMALITIES

TRACHEOBRONCHIAL ABNORMALITIES

Tracheal agenesis

This is exceedingly rare and commonly associated with maternal polyhydramnios. The presentation is immediate and acute with severe respiratory distress, absent cry and inability to intubate the airway. There are three main forms of tracheal agenesis:

- **Type 1.** Absent upper trachea, lower trachea connecting to the oesophagus.
- **Type 2.** Common bronchus connecting right and left main bronchi to the oesophagus with absent trachea.
- **Type 3.** Right and left main bronchi arising independently from the oesophagus. There are associated congenital heart, radial ray and duodenal (atresia) anomalies. Diagnosis can be confirmed via the cautious injection of water-soluble contrast into the oesophagus.

Tracheal stenosis

Acquired tracheal stenosis occurs as a consequence of long-term intubation or traumatic suctioning, but congenital stenosis due to complete cartinogenous rings is rare. Fifty per cent of congenital tracheal stenoses are focal, 30% generalised (Fig. 9.2A) and 20% funnel shaped; the latter is commonly seen with pulmonary artery sling.

The diagnosis of congenital tracheal stenosis should prompt a detailed search for associated abnormalities (tracheo-oesophageal fistula (TOF), lung agenesis or hypoplasia, pulmonary artery sling and bronchial stenosis). Ninety per cent of affected children present in the first year of life with biphasic stridor. The determination of the cause of a fixed tracheal narrowing in a symptomatic child is crucial, and bronchoscopy may not be adequate alone. CT is useful in showing the presence and extent of tracheal narrowing, MRI is also useful in assessing the anatomy and has the added advantage of angiographic capabilities.

Tracheomalacia

This is due to softening of the tracheal wall, supposedly due to cartilaginous abnormalities. The commonest type is secondary to tracheostomy, oesophageal atresia/TOF, chronic inflammation (associated with cystic fibrosis, recurrent aspiration, immunodeficiency), extrinsic compression (vascular rings, slings or aberrancy) and neoplasia. Tracheomalacia causes expiratory wheeze, which is exacerbated with crying, and may disappear at rest. Lateral fluoroscopy shows an exaggerated decrease in the sagittal width of the trachea during expiration. Dynamic CT can be useful to assess the cross-sectional anatomy and compliance of the trachea.

Tracheo-oesophageal fistula (TOF)

TOF may present with choking, cyanosis, coughing at the time of feeding or, in a more insidious way, with chronic respiratory infection. In cases associated with oesophageal atresia the diagnosis is more obvious.

The majority of cases are associated with the presence of oesophageal atresia. However, when in isolation, tracheo-oesophageal fistula can be difficult to diagnose, and the contrast oesophagram is used to demonstrate the presence of a fine hair-like structure connecting the oesophagus and trachea with linear opacification of the posterior tracheal wall (Fig. 9.2B).

Bronchial atresia

The upper lobe bronchi are more frequently affected by congenital atresia of lobar or segmental bronchi. In the newborn period this presents as a mass, occupying part or all of an upper lobe due to retention of fetal lung fluid trapped behind the atresia. In later childhood, the fetal lung fluid escapes (via pores or Kohn and canals of Lambert), revealing a round opacity at the site of the atresia central to the air trapping. There may be associated abnormalities such as bronchogenic cyst, intralobar sequestration or cystic adenomatoid malformation.

Tracheal bronchus (PIG bronchus)

The incidence of tracheal bronchus is 1% of the normal population, where the right upper lobe bronchus arises directly from the trachea (Fig. 9.1).

Other bronchial tree abnormalities

Isomerism syndromes are associated with unique bronchial branching patterns. Asplenia or Ivermark's syndrome includes bilateral right lung (trilobed bronchial pattern), absent spleen and complex cyanotic congenital heart disease.

Polysplenia is left lung isomerism including bilateral left lung bronchial patterns, intestinal malrotation, multiple small spleens, interruption of the IVC and atrial or ventricular septal defects.

PULMONARY UNDERDEVELOPMENT

Pulmonary underdevelopment including absent lung is fairly common. The three types of pulmonary underdevelopment are agenesis, aplasia and hypoplasia.

Agenesis is complete absence of a lung or lobe with absent bronchi (Fig. 9.3), aplasia is absence of lung tissue but the presence of a rudimentary bronchus, and hypoplasia is the presence of both bronchi and alveoli in an underdeveloped lobe (Fig. 9.4).

Lung agenesis

Complete agenesis is easily recognisable with a small opaque hemithorax and displacement of mediastinal structures towards that side (Fig. 9.3). Right lung agenesis has a higher mortality rate, possibly because of the higher incidence of cardiovascular abnormalities. Bronchography or bronchoscopy confirms the absent main stem bronchus, and angiography shows no pulmonary or bronchial arterial circulation on the same side as the absent lung. Associated abnormalities include the Vater syndrome (vertebral segmentation anomalies, anorectal atresia, tracheo-oesophageal fistula, oesophageal atresia, radial ray and renal anomalies).

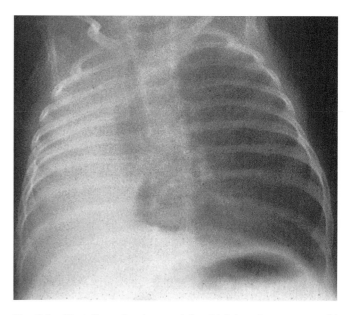

Fig. 9.3 Chest X-ray showing overinflated left lung in a neonate with crowding of the ribs and opacification of the right hemithorax due to agenesis of the right lung.

Lobar underdevelopment

Pulmonary hypoplasia is caused by factors directly or indirectly compromising the thoracic space available for lung growth. These

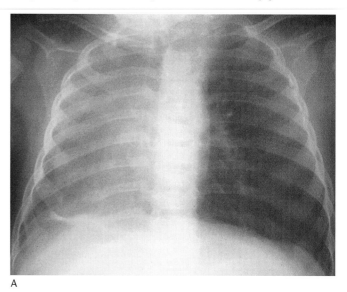

A

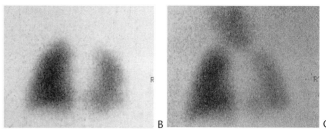

B C

Fig. 9.4 (A) Chest X-ray showing hypoplasia of the right lung with mediastinal shift to the right. (B, C) VQ scans show reduced ventilation and perfusion to the abnormal hypoplastic right lung (posterior view).

may be intrathoracic (diaphragmatic hernia, extralobar sequestration) or extrathoracic (oligohydramnios/arthrogryphosis). Lobar underdevelopment (agenesis, aplasia, hypoplasia) classically involves the right lung and may be associated with right-sided or obstructive congenital heart defects, and this suggests that pulmonary blood flow is an important factor in normal development of the tracheobronchial tree. With lung hypoplasia there is a decrease in volume of the right hemithorax, with an increased density of tissues and displacement of the heart and mediastinum towards the abnormal side (Fig. 9.4). There is obscuration of the heart border due to extrapleural areolar tissue. Associated abnormalities are diaphragmatic hernia and renal dysgenesis/agenesis.

Scimitar syndrome (congenital pulmonary venolobar syndrome)

This is a unique form of lobar agenesis or aplasia, associated with other abnormalities of pulmonary vessels and the thorax. The common feature in all cases of pulmonary venolobar syndrome is hypoplasia or aplasia of one or more lobes of the right lung. The variable components including partial anomalous pulmonary venous return from the abnormal lung (often seen as a scimitar-shaped vein; absent or small pulmonary artery perfusing the abnormal lung; arterial supply to the abnormal segment of lung partly or wholly from the thoracic aorta, abdominal aorta or coeliac axis; ipsilateral hemidiaphragm anomalies; absent IVC and anomalies of the bony thorax with excessive extrapleural areolar tissue). This syndrome may be inherited with an autosomal dominant inheritance with variable expression. The hemithorax is small, with obscuration of the heart border and a retrosternal soft-tissue density, and on the AP film the anomalous vein has the appearance of a Turkish scimitar, which normally drains to the IVC but may drain to the portal vein, hepatic veins or the right atrium. The right pulmonary artery may be absent with a systemic vessel arising from the lower thoracic or upper abdominal aorta supplying the right lower lobe. This may be associated with a mass of abnormal lung tissue in the right lower lobe (pulmonary sequestration).

OTHER PULMONARY DEVELOPMENTAL ANOMALIES

The sequestration spectrum, the commonest clinically significant pulmonary developmental anomalies, span a continuum of maldevelopment, and include bronchopulmonary foregut malformations. At one end of the spectrum normal pulmonary vessels attach to abnormal parenchyma, for example congenital lobar emphysema/overinflation, at the other end of the spectrum abnormal pulmonary vessels course through normal pulmonary tissue (pulmonary arterior venous malformation). In between these two extremes are anomalies with varied combinations of pulmonary and vascular maldevelopment, with the continuum known as the sequestration spectrum.

Congenital lobar overinflation/ emphysema

Congenital lobar overinflation/emphysema (CLO/CLE) is characterised by progressive overdistension of a lobe or occasionally two lobes, with emphysema being a misnomer, as there is no alveolar

wall destruction. The aetiology is unknown in 50% of cases, but is probably related to obstruction of the bronchus by a ball valve mechanism. Postulated reasons for this include abnormal bronchial cartilage deficiency/dysplasia, inflammatory changes, inspissated mucus, mucosal folds or webs, bronchial stenosis and extrinsic vascular or mass compression. Histological examination of the 'emphysematous' lobes reveals distended alveoli with thin septa, which may sometimes be associated with an increase in the alveolar number (polyalveolar type). The male to female ratio is 3:1 and other associated anomalies occur in up to 50% of children. These frequently involve the cardiovascular system, with patent ductus arteriosus, ventricular septal defect and tetralogy of Fallot being the most common abnormalities. The upper lobes, or right middle lobe, are more commonly involved. (Distribution left upper = 43%, right middle = 32%, right upper = 20% and lower lobes = 5%.)

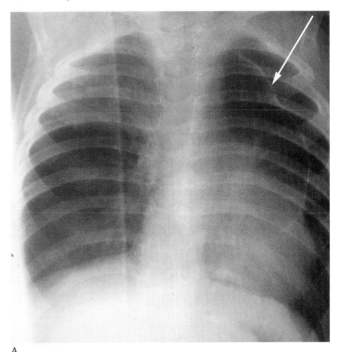

A

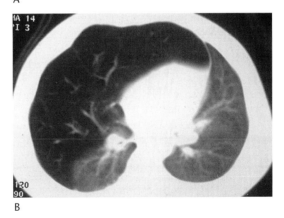

B

Fig. 9.5 (A) Congenital lobar emphysema/overinflation. Chest X-ray shows gross overinflation of the right lung which is hypovascular with marked shift of the mediastinum to the left and herniation of the lung into the left hemithorax (arrow). (B) CT of right middle lobe congenital lobar overinflation/emphysema causing shift of the mediastinum to the left with marked distortion of the pleural reflections to the left of the midline.

During the first few days of life, lung fluid may become trapped in the involved lobe, giving an opaque enlarged hemithorax, but this gradually clears via vascular and lymphatic re-absorption, resulting in the classical radiographic appearance of a grossly overinflated lobe with generalised hypertransradiency (Fig. 9.5). Marked attenuation of the pulmonary vessels through the hyper-transradient lobe occurs and compression of adjacent lobes is marked.

Definitive treatment for congenital lobar emphysema (which is compromising the patient) is surgical resection of the involved lobe with an excellent prognosis.

Bronchopulmonary foregut malformations

This refers to a number of developmental abnormalities resulting from abnormal budding of the embryonic foregut and tracheo-bronchial tree. Bronchopulmonary foregut malformations include foregut cysts, bronchogenic cysts, enteric and neurenteric cysts. Cystic hamartomatous (adenomatous) malformation and pulmonary sequestration are also included in this spectrum.

Bronchogenic cysts account for approximately half of all congenital thoracic cysts and may be intrapulmonary or mediastinal. The latter are more common and represent an earlier budding abnormality; intrapulmonary bronchogenic cysts result from later budding defects and the cysts are all lined by ciliated epithelium. They may contain smooth muscle and cartilage. Mediastinal bronchogenic cysts can be paratracheal (usually right sided, carinal or hilar) and the carinal location is most common. Bronchogenic cysts do not usually communicate with the tracheobronchial tree but instrumentation of the cyst or infection may lead to an air-filled cyst or an air–fluid level. The differential diagnosis includes an acquired cyst, or one of the extremely rare but potentially malignant cystic mesenchymal hamartomas.

Enteric cysts

Enteric cysts form earlier in embryogenesis and are generally located in the posterior mediastinum. If present in the oesophageal wall these are referred to as oesophageal cysts or duplication cysts and present early with acid secretion which may rupture into the tracheobronchial tree and cause haemoptysis. There is usually a large posterior mediastinal (right-sided) mass. Mediastinal uptake of ^{99}Tc-MDP (pertechnetate) is strong evidence that the enteric cysts contain gastric mucosa.

Neuroenteric cysts

Neuroenteric cysts present as posterior mediastinal masses with associated vertebral abnormalities. MRI is the most useful tool for evaluating the thoracic and spinal components of neuroenteric cysts (Fig. 9.6).

Most bronchogenic, enteric and neuroenteric cysts are filled with serous or mucoid fluid and are typically solitary and unilocular. Cross-sectional imaging has an important role in the evaluation of intrathoracic foregut cysts, with the capabilities for localising and defining the extent in relation to other structures and characterising the intrinsic density. Cysts may be watery or viscous and attenuation values are therefore variable. Regardless of the CT density,

lack of enhancement is expected but complex cysts (following infection) may however show wall enhancement. T_1-weighted spin-echo MR images show intrinsic signal intensity ranging from low to high depending on cyst content (serous, mucinous, proteinaceous, milk of calcium). On T_2-weighted spin-echo images the cysts are typically of high signal intensity. Both MR and contrast-enhanced CT confidently exclude vascular lesions such as pulmonary artery slings.

Congenital cystic adenomatoid (hamartomatous) malformation

This malformation (acronym: CCAM) of the lung consists of hamartomatous proliferation of terminal bronchioles at the expense of alveolar development, and the lesions are often composed of both cystic and solid tissue. The cysts are lined by respiratory epithelium

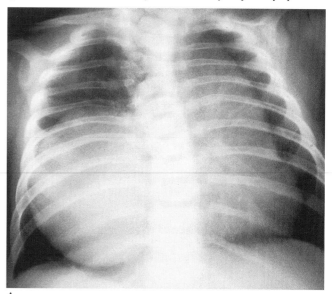

A

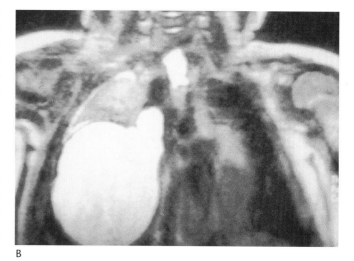

B

Fig. 9.6 (A) Neurenteric cyst. Chest X-ray showing multiple segmentation anomalies affecting the cervicothoracic spine with a large soft-tissue mass occupying the right hemithorax. (B) Coronal T_2-weighted spin-echo image showing the high-signal cystic mass originating from the cervicothoracic spine causing compressive atelectasis of the right upper lobe.

and usually communicate with the tracheobronchial tree with a slight predilection for the upper lobes. Malformations are classified on the basis of clinical, radiographic and histological features:

- **Type 1.** This is the most common type (50%) and is composed of variable cysts with at least one dominant cyst (greater than 2 cm in diameter). Prognosis is excellent and there is an infrequent association with other congenital abnormalities (5%).
- **Type 2.** This type (41%) is composed of smaller, more uniform cysts up to 2 cm in diameter. Congenital malformations (renal, intestinal, cardiac, skeletal) are common in up to 50% of children.
- **Type 3.** This is the least common type (9%). These cysts are composed of microcysts and appear solid upon visual inspection. Fetal hydrops and maternal polyhydramnios are common in type 3 CCAM, and because of associated congenital

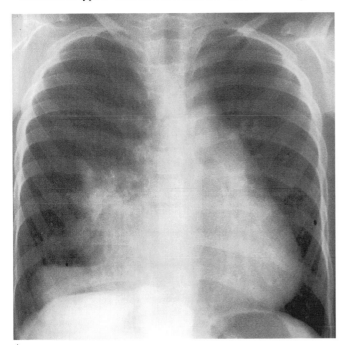

A

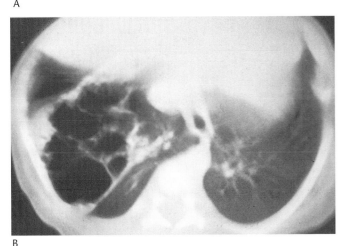

B

Fig. 9.7 (A) Chest X-ray: right cystic hamartomatous/adenomatous malformation type 1 with multiple cystic lesions in the right lower lobe showing air-fluid levels consistent with infection. (B) Axial CT scan through the lung bases show the thick-walled cysts in the right lower lobe.

abnormalities and severe respiratory compromise prognosis is poor. All types of CCAM have normal vascular supply and drainage.

Radiographically Type 1 lesions have one or more dominant cysts with adjacent smaller cysts (Fig. 9.7). Type 2 lesions display more heterogeneous and smaller cysts. Type 3 CCAMs appear as a solid mass with mass effect and a ground-glass appearance on CT (Fig. 9.8). Air–fluid levels may be seen with or without superadded infection.

Pulmonary sequestration

Sequestrated lung is defined as 'a congenital mass of aberrant pulmonary tissue that has no normal connection with the bronchial tree or with the pulmonary arteries'. The sequestration is usually supplied by an anomalous artery arising from the aorta and its venous drainage is via the azygos system, the pulmonary veins or the inferior vena cava. Although frequently asymptomatic, children with sequestrations usually present because of superadded infection and the sequestration is usually located in one of the basal segments of the lower lobe. Bronchograms show normal bronchi draping around the sequestration and aortography demonstrates one or more systemic vessels entering the mass, usually arising from the aorta at or below the diaphragm (Fig. 9.9). Intralobar sequestration (ILS) is contained within the lung with no separate pleural covering and is intimately connected to adjacent lung. Venous drainage is usually via the pulmonary veins.

ILS is confined to a lower lobe in 98% of cases and the medial part of the left lower lobe is most often involved. Anomalies elsewhere are present in only 12% of patients with ILS. Anomalies are common in extralobar sequestration (ELS) (65%), congenital lobar emphysema (42%) and Type 2 CCAM (26%). Extralobar sequestration (ELS) is located between the lower lobe and the diaphragm and has its own pleural covering. Ninety-eight per cent of ELSs are left sided and usually drain via the azygos system. The venous drainage is not always clear cut (Fig. 9.10).

Modes of presentation of the two types are very different as most cases of intralobar sequestration are diagnosed after adolescence with symptoms of pneumonia which is either recurrent or refractory to therapy. It is uncommon to see symptomatic ILS in neonates and infants, however extralobar sequestrations usually present within the first 6 months of life with dyspnoea, cyanosis and feeding difficulties. The incidence of other associated abnormalities is common (65%), including pulmonary hypoplasia, horseshoe lung, CCAM, bronchogenic cysts, diaphragmatic hernia and cardiovascular anomalies such as truncus arteriosus and total anomalous pulmonary venous return (TAPVR).

Imaging is directed to identification of sequestrated or dysplastic lung tissue, identification of aberrant arterial and venous connections and evaluation of possible bronchial or gastrointestinal connections, and exclusion of other associated lung anomalies such as horseshoe lung or hypoplasia, and assessment of diaphragmatic integrity. The imaging modality of choice for sequestration is ultrasound, especially in the newborn period presenting with a mass adjacent to the liver or diaphragm. Antenatal sonography often depicts a fetal chest mass and strongly suggests the diagnosis of extralobar sequestration. Doppler ultrasound readily demonstrates the vascular connections to the sequestration (Fig. 9.9). CT of the lung in the intralobar sequestration localises and shows the extent

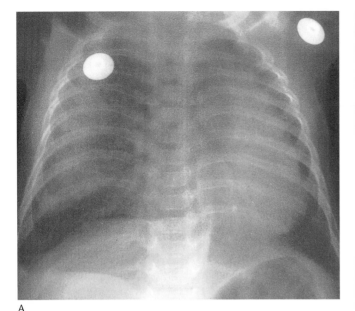

A

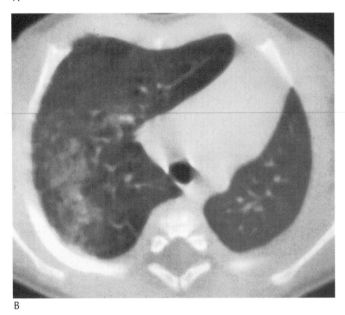

B

Fig. 9.8 (A) Chest X-ray: cystic hamartomatous/adenomatous malformation type 3. Extensive ground-glass shadowing with gross overinflation of the right lung and herniation across the midline due to the presence of a CCAM type 3. (B) CT scan of the same patient with extensive overexpansion of the right lung and ground-glass shadowing due to microcysts beyond the resolution of the CT.

of the abnormality, showing a multicystic mass at the lung base. The extralobar sequestration is a solid soft-tissue mass with avid contrast enhancement adjacent to the diaphragm (Fig. 9.10). MRI can be useful for identifying the pulmonary abnormality and vascular connections in a multiplanar fashion.

Pulmonary arteriovenous malformations

Abnormal communication between the blood vessels are either congenital or acquired. The acquired connections are called pulmonary

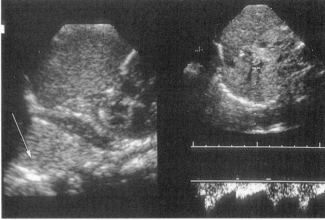

A

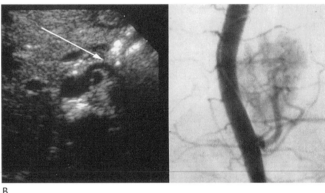

B

Fig. 9.9 (A) Coronal ultrasound examination of a pulmonary sequestration (arrow) in left lower lobe. The Doppler scan shows a large systemic vessel arising from the aorta to supply the sequestration. (B) Axial ultrasound shows the origin of systemic vessel (arrow) from aorta, confirmed at aortography.

fistulas associated with either liver disease, cyanotic heart disease, chronic pulmonary infection or emphysema. Congenital arteriovenous malformations are abnormal communications between pulmonary arteries and veins without an intervening capillary bed and are often clinically silent, however cyanosis, polycythaemia, dyspnoea and digital clubbing sometimes develop. Multiple lesions are common (33–50%), as are bilateral lesions (8–20%). Sixty per cent are in the lower lobes and 6% occur in patients with the autosomal dominant disorder hereditary haemorrhagic telangiectasia. Typical appearances are of a well-defined pulmonary mass which is often lobulated.

DIAPHRAGMATIC ABNORMALITIES

Anomalies of the diaphragm such as hernia, eventeration and agenesis may be associated with lung malformations and cause severe respiratory symptoms.

Congenital diaphragmatic hernia

Bochdalek's hernia (through the posteropleuroperitoneal foramen) usually causes severe respiratory distress in the neonate and is one of the commonest congenital anomalies of the thorax. The diagno-

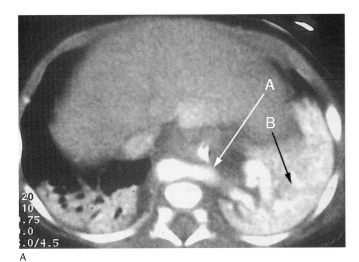

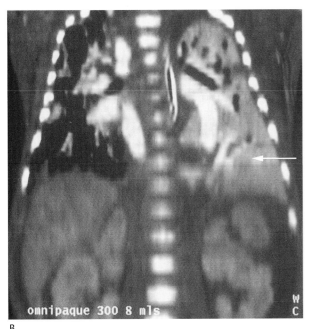

Fig. 9.10 (A) Axial contrast-enhanced CT scan through the lung bases with a large systemic vessel arising from the left side of the aorta (arrow A) supplying a very vascular left-sided extralobar sequestration (ELS) (arrow B). (B) Coronal CT multiplanar reconstruction (MPR) showing the normal lung and beneath this (arrow) the left-sided basal ELS with a draining vein entering the azygous system below the diaphragm.

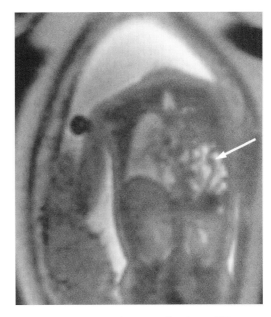

Fig. 9.11 Left congenital diaphragmatic hernia. HASTE sequence from coronal MRI of a 32-week fetus showing presence of a left-sided congenital diaphragmatic hernia. The normal right lung is of intermediate to high signal intensity and meconium within the bowel in the left chest is hyper-intense (arrow) (similar signal to the amniotic fluid surrounding the fetus).

Congenital eventeration of the diaphragm

Eventeration is either partial or complete and often right sided, due to hypoplasia of the diaphragmatic muscle. Symptomatic patients require surgical plication. The differential diagnosis of diaphragmatic herniation is sometimes difficult but most eventerations are

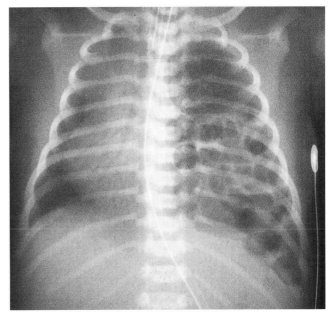

Fig. 9.12 A chest X-ray taken at 2 days of age showing a left-sided congenital diaphragmatic hernia with loops of bowel in the left hemithorax and shift of the heart and mediastinum to the right. The stomach is delineated by the presence of the nasogastric tube below the level of the diaphragm.

sis is now frequently made prenatally at antenatal ultrasound or MRI (Fig. 9.11) and involves the left pleuroperitoneal foramen in 75% of cases. The neonatal radiograph shows a left-sided large intrathoracic mass of soft-tissue density, and the more characteristic pattern of intrathoracic air-filled loops develops after several hours (Fig. 9.12). There is absence of the normal gas-containing bowel in the abdomen which is usually scaphoid on examination. The prognosis correlates with the degree of underlying lung hypoplasia. The differential diagnoses are of other cystic-appearing intrathoracic masses in the newborn, such as lobar emphysema, cystic adenomatoid malformations, sequestration, bronchogenic cysts and other developmental abnormalities of the lung.

minor, transitory, local diaphragmatic elevations found incidentally within the first few years of life and disappear with age.

NEWBORN CHEST RADIOLOGY

Immature lung disease

This is a condition of small, premature infants with clinical, radiological and prognostic features differing from respiratory distress syndrome (RDS). These infants have birth weights of less than 1500 g (average 1000 g). Unlike RDS the cardinal signs of respiratory distress are absent until days 4–7 of life. Surfactant phospholipid components are present because of accelerated production of surfactant from intrauterine stress, but insufficient surfactant is present to maintain alveolar ventilation. Chest radiography shows diffuse granularity of the lungs which can be confused with RDS but there is a relative absence of air bronchograms and little or no underaeration of the lungs. The granular appearance of the lungs is due to summation of densities within thickened interstitium. Complications of immature lung disease include apnoea and bradycardia with persistent patent ductus arteriosus. These complications require ventilation and the incidence of barotrauma-induced lung disease is much lower than with RDS because very low ventilatory pressures and rates are required for ventilatory support. However other factors such as intraventricular cerebral haemorrhage, bronchopulmonary dysplasia, necrotising enterocolitis and death are fairly common in infants born at less than 1000 g. The entity should be distinguished from RDS as the overall survival (82%) with immature lung diseases is considerably better than RDS.

Respiratory distress syndrome

Respiratory distress syndrome (RDS), also known as hyaline membrane disease (HMD), is a manifestation of pulmonary immaturity and seen predominantly in newborns under 36 weeks' gestation, weighing less than 2.5 kg. Despite recent advances in ventilatory therapy RDS remains a leading cause of death in liveborn infants with symptoms beginning shortly after birth characterised by chest wall retraction, cyanosis and grunting. Postmortem changes show non-compliant atelectatic lung with thickening of the interstitium and dilatation of the terminal airways which are usually lined with hyaline membranes. RDS is due to a deficiency in pulmonary surfactant, a phospholipid complex synthesised by Type 2 pneumocytes which coats alveolar lining cells and prevents atelectasis by lowering alveolar surface tension, which increases pulmonary compliance and decreases breathing effort. However hyaline membranes are not specific to this disease and paradoxically are frequently absent in patients with RDS who die at less than 4 hours of age. Hence the more correct term 'respiratory distress syndrome' rather than the emphatic term of hyaline membrane disease should be used to describe this condition. The spectrum of abnormalities in RDS ranges from mild to severe, correlating with the clinical severity, and the hallmark features are reticular granularity of the lungs due to superimposition of multiple acinar nodules, related to atelectatic alveoli and diffuse pulmonary underaeration (Fig. 9.13). Aeration may appear normal when the child is ventilated. The development of air bronchograms is dependent on the coalescence of areas of atelectasis around dilated terminal bronchioles. Rupture of alveolar air sacs can lead to pulmonary interstitial emphysema (Fig. 9.14). The same factors, prematurity, perinatal asphyxia, caesarean section, etc., also predispose to wet lung disease with extensive alveolar and

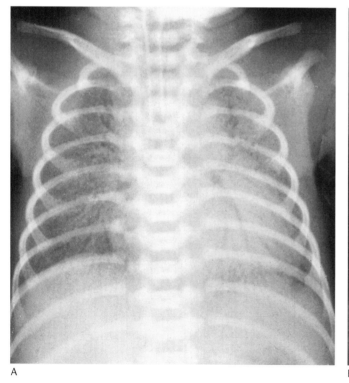

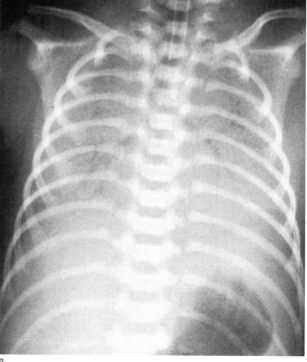

A　　　　　　　　　　　　　　　　　B

Fig. 9.13 Hyaline membrane disease. (A) Mild changes aged 1 day—fine reticulonodular shadowing with prominent air bronchograms. (B) More advanced changes aged 3 days—marked pulmonary opacification with loss of diaphragmatic and cardiac contours.

interstitial opacities in both processes. As fluid clears from the lungs through the bronchial lymphatic and capillaries, the associated wet lung syndrome disappears and one is left with a more classic appearance of RDS. A normal chest X-ray at 6 hours of age excludes RDS. The granular densities and hypoaeration persists for 3–5 days in mild to moderate RDS, and clearing extends from peripheral to central and upper to lower lobes. In more severe RDS the progressive underaeration of the lungs and diffuse bilateral opacities become complicated by interstitial and alveolar oedema with or without superimposed parenchymal haemorrhage, and this type of severe RDS often leads to death within the first 72 hours of life. Other entities producing similar reticular granular densities include immature lung, wet lung disease, neonatal pneumonia (particularly group B *Streprococcus pneumoniae*), idiopathic hypoglycaemia, congestive heart failure, maternal diabetes and early pulmonary haemorrhage.

Air block phenomena/pulmonary interstitial emphysema (PIE)

pneumomediastinum/pneumothorax

As the premature infant's lungs are immature and vulnerable to damage, alveolar rupture leads to various air block complications including parenchymal pseudocysts, pulmonary interstitial emphysema (PIE), pnuemomediastinum, pneumothorax, pneumopericardium, intravascular air and air in the extrathoracic soft tissues. The pathophysiology involves increase in the transalveolar pressure leading to alveolar rupture, dissection of air along peribronchial and perivascular spaces of the interstitium to reach the mediastinum with subsequent decompression of this pneumomediastinum into the pleural spaces and pneumothorax. In addition, interstitial air (primarily within lymphatics) may rupture directly through the visceral pleura to produce a pneumothorax. PIE is

almost always preceded by positive-pressure-assisted ventilation and is manifest as tortuous linear lucencies of uniform size radiating from the hila through the lungs (Fig. 9.14). Another manifestation is with small rounded lucencies in the lungs which if peripheral can produce subpleural blebs that ultimately rupture into the pleural space to produce a pneumothorax (Fig. 9.15) or extend medially to produce pneumomediastinum or pneumopericardium.

It is sometimes difficult to distinguish pneumomediastinum from pneumopericardium or medially located pneumothorax. In cases of pneumopericardium air completely outlines the heart on both AP and lateral projections and air is (by definition) limited to the pericardium so cannot extend beyond the origins of the aorta and pulmonary artery. Pneumopericardium and medial pneumothorax do not elevate or outline the thymus on either AP or lateral shoot-through radiographs.

If the child is moved to the decubitus position (rarely necessary) a medial pneumothorax will shift to the less dependent part of the pleural space whereas a pneumomediastinum remains fixed and central.

The Mikity–Wilson syndrome

This is a radiological appearance describing diffuse interstitial infiltrations giving rise to a multicystic appearance. The onset is usually accompanied with apnoea and cyanosis in premature babies later in the first week of life. There is no preceding history of RDS, and episodes of gastro-oesophageal reflux and aspiration may account for at least part of this syndrome, which may progress to full-blown bronchopulmonary dysplasia/chronic lung disease.

Bronchopulmonary dysplasia/chronic lung disease of prematurity

Bronchopulmonary dysplasia (BPD) or chronic lung disease of prematurity (CLD) is an important and significant complication of ven-

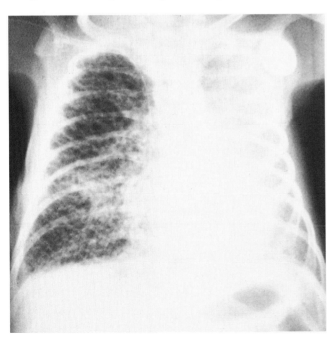

Fig. 19.14 Pulmonary interstitial emphysema. Fine reticular shadowing in the right lung with deviation of the mediastinum contralaterally. RDS affecting the left lung.

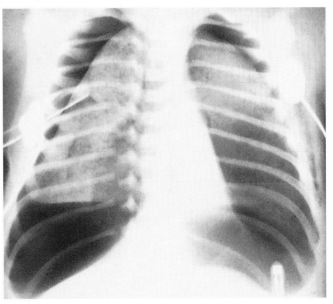

Fig. 9.15 Bilateral pneumothoraces in hyaline membrane disease. Right intercostal drain.

tilation in the newborn. The pathological, radiological and clinical features were originally described by Northway and Rosin in 1967. There have been numerous publications since its recognition. This distinct pulmonary disease affects all developing lung tissue following prolonged oxygen or ventilator therapy for RDS, and was initially thought to represent pure oxygen toxicity. Four clear stages were defined by Northway and Rosin.

- *Stage 1.* Identical to RDS. Pathology of mucosal necrosis is present.
- *Stage 2 (4–10 days).* Bilateral 'white out' occurs due pathologically to necrosis and alveolar epithelial repair with hyaline membranes and bronchiolar necrosis accompanied by interstitial oedema.
- *Stage 3 (10–20 days).* Bubbly appearance of lungs due to alveolar overdistension and scarred acini. Pathologically this represents persistent epithelial injury with superimposed bronchial and bronchiolar mucosal metaplasia, +/– hyperplasia with exudation of alveolar macrophages.
- *Stage 4 (after 1 month of age).* This is the classic appearance of BPD with bubbly appearances to the lungs with alternating cyst-like lucencies surrounded by curvilinear stranding of soft-tissue density (Fig. 9.16). The long-term prognosis, although improved, still has a mortality of 40% for Stage 4 disease. Sequential chest radiographs show persistent overinflation during infancy, which gradually clears to some degree, although the majority of patients show pulmonary function abnormalities and an increased predisposition to lower respiratory tract infections.

Transient tachypnoea of the newborn or wet lung disease

Wet lung disease is due to delayed resorption and clearance of fetal lung fluid, and one of the commoner causes of respiratory distress in a newborn with characteristic radiological and clinical features. The radiological appearances represent delayed clearance of normal

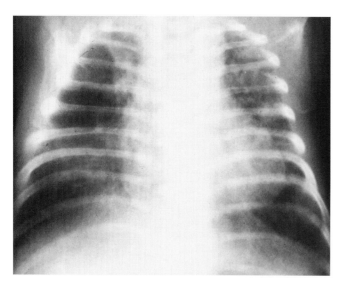

Fig. 9.16 Bronchopulmonary dysplasia. Patchy shadowing from areas of loss of volume and fibrosis, with areas of compensatory emphysema, especially in the right upper lobe.

lung fluid which is usually cleared through the bronchi via thoracic squeeze during vaginal delivery (30%), lymphatic clearance (30%) and capillary clearance (40%). Predisposing conditions include prematurity, maternal diabetes, precipitous delivery/ caesarean section.

Chest radiographs within the first 6 hours show fluid within the lungs with prominent vascular markings and hazy margins. There may be small pleural effusions and in more severe cases alveolar oedema occurs. Lung clearance begins within 10–12 hours and during this phase the reticular granular densities may mimic RDS however with transient tachypnoea/wet lung syndrome there is normal or hyperinflation of the lungs (not underinflation as in RDS). Gradually clearance occurs from peripheral to central and the chest film becomes normal at 48–72 hours of age.

As the condition is benign treatment is conservative and supportive with an excellent prognosis.

Persistent fetal circulation syndrome—persistent pulmonary hypertension of the newborn

In normal circumstances the high pulmonary vascular resistance in the fetus drops in the newborn period in response to pulmonary expansion and oxygenation. If this physiological transition fails and the high pulmonary vascular resistance persists it may result in right to left shunting at the level of the foramen ovale or ductus arteriosus. If pulmonary artery pressures exceed systemic arterial pressures, PFC (persistent fetal circulation) may occur as a primary form of pulmonary hypertension with a sinister and unknown aetiology.

Secondary PFC is related to hypoxia due to other causes of pulmonary hypoplasia (e.g. meconium aspiration syndrome, diaphragmatic hernia, etc.). The chest radiograph may appear normal or show slight olegaemia with diminished pulmonary vascularity and mild cardiomegaly in primary PFC. Neonates with secondary PFC have radiographic pictures reflecting the primary cause.

Meconium aspiration syndrome

Meconium aspiration syndrome (MAS) is caused by intrauterine or intrapartum aspiration of meconium-stained amniotic fluid. Approximately 1% of newborns develop MAS defined as 'meconium in the airway below the level of the vocal cords'. The mechanism involves intrauterine hypoxaemia causing fetal defaecation and gasping leading to aspiration of meconium-containing amniotic fluid directly into the tracheobronchial tree. This causes bronchial obstruction and chemical pneumonitis.

The radiological features vary according to the severity of aspiration but involve bilateral patchy asymmetrical areas of opacification associated with marked overinflation, complicated by pneumothorax and pneumomediastinum in approximately 25% of cases. Meconium causes a chemical pneumonitis and therefore clearing of the radiological opacification may take several weeks, often despite clinical improvement, with radiological clearance lagging behind the clinical status.

In the past treatment was supportive with antibiotics and ventilation, however due to a mortality rate of up to 25% in babies with meconium aspiration, extracorporeal membrane oxygenation (ECMO) is being increasingly used to treat this condition, as well as other causes of intractable respiratory failure. ECMO provides circulatory bypass for the lungs with minimal pulmonary inflation but maintains oxygen tension and oxygen saturation at physiological levels. On ECMO therapy the lungs are almost airless. The two main types of ECMO include arteriovenous and venovenous ECMO (Fig. 9.17).

Neonatal pneumonia

This may be acquired in utero as ascending or transplacental infection, during delivery or after birth. An abnormal chest X-ray may be the first sign of infection.

Group B streptococcal infection is the commonest form of newborn pneumonia (at least 25% of women in labour are colonised with this organism) and the radiology is identical to RDS but pleural effusions are common (up to 67% of cases). The latter are rare in uncomplicated RDS. Other viruses, bacteria, protozoa and fungi do occur but are rare.

THE CHEST RADIOGRAPH IN THE OLDER CHILD

This subject is dealt with briefly and readers are advised to consult other texts for more details. Only a brief summary of some relevant diseases will be entertained.

Pulmonary infection

Respiratory tract infection is the most common human illness with viruses the major cause in children, especially below 5 years of age. Bacteria become increasingly important in older children and in the hospitalised child. As children's peripheral airways are smaller and more collapsible than those in adults, and there is a higher concentration of mucus glands lining the airway, partial or complete occlusion of bronchi or bronchioles and consequent air trapping or atelectasis is commoner. At about 8 years of age pulmonary architecture is similar to the adult, however. The role of imaging in pneumonia is to confirm the presence, extent, anatomical location and evaluate progress or complications. Radiology is not specific for the various organisms involved and radiographs must always be interpreted with clinical information.

In the neonate, streptococcus, staphylococcus, *Escherichia coli* and *Haemophilus influenzae* are the commonest bacterial organisms. Viral pneumonia tends to affect ambulatory children under the age of 5 years of age with respiratory syncytial virus (RSV) occurring in epidemics but parainfluenza, adenovirus and influenza also causing pneumonia in preschool children.

Mycoplasma pneumoniae plays an increasingly important role in school-aged children (causing 30% of all childhood pneumonias).

Tuberculosis

There has been an alarming increase in the frequency of TB in the western world, especially in areas inhabited by immigrants and refugees. Other factors include poverty, homelessness and the epidemic of human immunodeficiency virus (HIV).

Primary tuberculosis

Primary tuberculosis produces a localised air-space disease in a pulmonary segment or lobe with regional lymph node enlargement and pleural effusions in some cases. Infection spreads from a peripheral air-space focus to central lymph nodes by lymphatic channels.

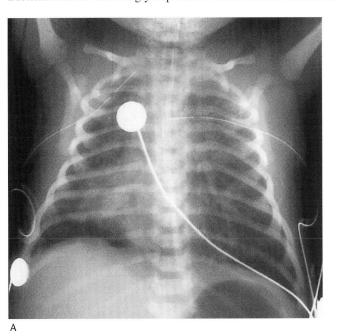

A

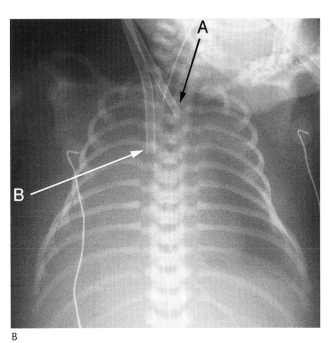

B

Fig. 9.17 (A) Meconium aspiration. There is marked overinflation of the lungs with coarse nodular shadowing secondary to meconium aspiration. Bilateral chest drains drain pneumothoraces (persistent in right subpulmonic distribution). (B) Arteriovenous ECMO catheters are present/in situ. Diffuse ground-glass shadowing is present within the collapsed lungs. The arterial cannula (arrow A) has been inserted into the right common carotid artery with its tip in the aortic arch. The venous cannula (arrow B) has been inserted into the right internal jugular vein, and its tip should lie in the right atrium.

Several weeks later hypersensitivity develops with regional lymph node enlargement +/– caesation and necrosis in the inflammatory foci. As resistance develops the inflammatory reaction in the lung parenchyma and lymph nodes involute and sometimes calcify resulting in a peripheral Gohn focus or a Ranke complex (calcification in the parenchyma and central lymph nodes). If host resistance is poor or overwhelming infection occurs, the primary parenchymal focus extends involving larger volumes of lung, and this is often associated with pleural effusions. Spread of organisms from the lymphatic system into the venous system through the thoracic duct may result in seeding of mycobacteria into the lungs resulting in miliary (Fig. 9.18) or secondary TB. Incidentally, infants with miliary tuberculosis may have few symptoms despite showing the characteristic radiological appearance of multiple small nodular opacities of relatively uniform size (2–3mm) scattered throughout the lungs. HRCT confirms the interstitial thickening and nodularity of miliary TB.

The immune compromised child

This can be primary or secondary. Primary immune deficiency is usually related to a congenital abnormality of the B and/or T cells resulting in an increased incidence of infection or lymphoproliperative disease and other malignancies. Immunologically compromised children often develop pneumonia caused by less common pathogens. Pneumocystis is important as is cytomegalovirus, fungus and nocardial infection. Pulmonary opacification in children with AIDS may be due to infection or lymphoid hyperplasia in association with lymphocytic interstitial pneumonitis. AIDS in childhood is usually transmitted vertically (from mother to child) and children are prone to bacterial infections as well as an increased incidence of viral and opportunistic infection such as *Pneumocystis carinii* pneumonia (Fig. 9.19).

Disseminated infiltrative lymphocytic syndrome (DILS) is caused by widespread polyclonal lymphocytic and plasma cell proliferation which results in lymphocytic interstitial pneumonitis in the lungs manifest as diffuse nodular opacification throughout the lungs. This is a relatively benign disease thought to be related to Epstein–Barr infection in immunocompromised patients.

Inhaled foreign body

Children manage to inhale all forms of foreign body, radiopaque and non-radiopaque. The overall tendency is for the foreign bodies to enter the more vertically orientated right main bronchus. Complete obstruction leads to peripheral collapse but partial obstruction leads to obstructive emphysema. Films taken in expiration (or in the decubitus position) as well as inspiration, supplemented if necessary by fluoroscopy, will show mediastinal shift away from the obstructive emphysema on expiration/decubitus position (abnormal lung dependent) (Fig. 9.20).

Bronchoscopy should be performed if there is any clinical doubt, even when radiographs are normal.

ASTHMA

Longstanding reactive airways disease usually results in a radiograph showing overinflation of the lungs with a low, flat diaphragm, sternal bowing and peribronchial thickening seen as rings end-on or tram lines longitudinally, with occasional patchy shadowing. Pneumomediastinum may occur with extension into the subcutaneous tissues of the neck. Pneumothorax may, uncommonly, complicate asthma.

CYSTIC FIBROSIS

With the exception of asthma, cystic fibrosis is the most important chronic respiratory illness amongst children, adolescents and young adults. The cystic fibrosis gene is located on chromosome 7 and is inherited as an autosomal recessive trait. Gene carriage rate is

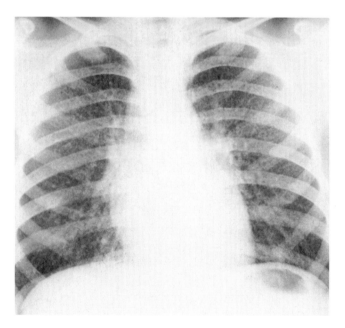

Fig. 9.18 Miliary tuberculosis. Fine nodularity throughout both lungs.

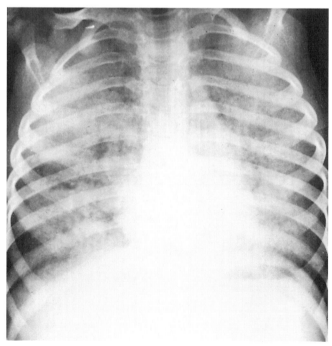

Fig. 9.19 *Pneumocystis* pneumonia. Widespread alveolar shadowing.

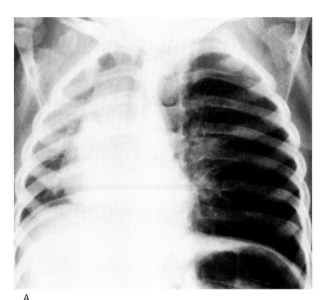

A

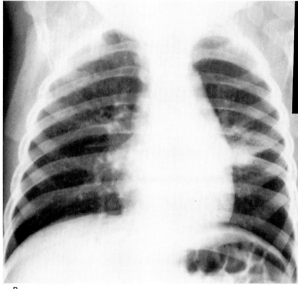

B

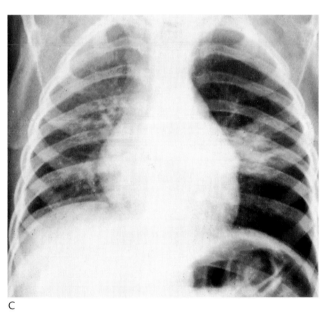

C

Fig. 9.20 Foreign body inhalation. (A) Obstructive emphysema from a foreign body in the left main bronchus. (B, C) Another child showing loss of volume in the left lung with patchy collapse in the apex of the left lower lobe; in inspiration (B) the mediastinum is slightly to the left; in expiration (C) the volume of the left lung changes little with the mediastinum swinging to the right.

approximately 1 in 25 individuals of Northern European extraction, with a disease prevalence of approximately 1 in 2500. Infants with cystic fibrosis are prone to develop atelectasis, focal or generalised overinflation with mucus plugging partially obstructing the airway producing secondary hyperinflation. This is often initially thought to be related to viral pneumonitis and early radiological appearances are identical.

In older children chest radiographs show overinflation with bronchial wall thickening, dilatation and bronchial mucus plugging with frank bronchiectasis. The established bronchiectatic cavities may contain air–fluid levels, and eventually hilar adenopathy or pulmonary hypertension resulting in large central pulmonary arteries develops.

HRCT demonstrates the early changes in a more sensitive fashion with extensive central bronchiectasis the hallmark feature. Complications such as pneumothorax (Fig. 9.21) are not uncommon. Haemoptysis, although uncommon, can be a devastating com-

plication, and bleeding sites may be demonstrated by selective bronchial arteriography and embolisation in the intractable cases. Corpulmonale and pulmonary hypertension eventually develop, and the definitive treatment at the present time is lung/heart–lung transplantation. Patients also have sinus, pancreatic and gut disease simultaneously.

Langerhans cell histiocytosis or histiocytosis X

In childhood bone and central nervous system manifestations are frequently more prominent than lung involvement, but fine widespread nodularity can at times resemble miliary tuberculosis (Fig. 9.22).

The chest X-ray shows diffuse reticulonodular change which may progress to honeycomb lung and the patients develop complicating pneumothoraces.

Bronchiectasis

Bronchiectasis is much less commonly seen outside the setting of the immunocompromised patient, but may follow local damage to the airways from a retained foreign body or following severe infection such as measles, etc.

Intrathoracic masses

Detailed discussion of the various tumours involving the thoracic cavity is beyond the scope of this chapter. However neurogenic tumours such as neuroblastoma (Fig. 9.23) and ganglioneuroma typically occur in the posterior mediastinum, frequently deforming

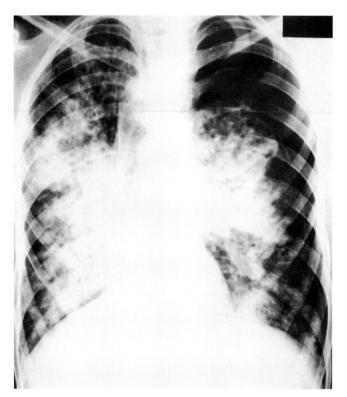

Fig. 9.21 Advanced cystic fibrosis (mucoviscidosis). Gross peribronchial shadowing with confluent pneumonic shadowing. There is a left pneumothorax with slight displacement of the mediastinum to the right.

and distorting the thoracic rib cage. Calcification may occur within the tumour and pleural effusions are often seen. Congenital neuro-enteric cysts may show connections with the spinal canal (Fig. 9.6).

Cystic hygromas usually have a component in the neck as well as extension into the upper thoracic cavity, and ultrasound helps to demonstrate their characteristic mainly cystic appearance.

Idiopathic pulmonary haemosiderosis

This disease is of unknown aetiology caused by intra-alveolar haemorrhage and is thought to be autoimmune with some cases related to sensitivity due to protein in cows' milk. Symptoms include cough, fever and respiratory distress with failure to thrive, fatigue and pallor. Severe bleeding leads to haemoptysis and haematemesis with development of anaemia due to chronic blood loss. Following an acute haemorrhage there are bilateral hazy opacifications in the lungs identical to pulmonary oedema, but as blood is cleared from the alveoli, haemosiderin is deposited into the lung septa, and the pattern evolves into a reticulonodular interstitial pattern (Fig. 9.24). The definitive diagnosis is made by identifying haemosiderin-laden macrophages in the sputum or gastric washings.

Pulmonary alveolar proteinosis

Pulmonary alveolar proteinosis (PAP) is an uncommon disease of unknown aetiology characterised by deposition of lipoproteinacious deposits within the alveolar spaces. The male to female ratio is 2 : 1 and most patients present around the age of 20 years, although an

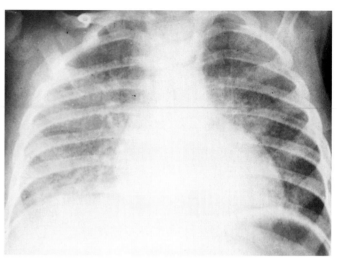

Fig. 9.22 Histiocytosis X. Fine nodularity in both lung fields.

infantile form (which is more aggressive) has been described which is possibly related to immune compromise. The pathological and radiological abnormalities are identical to surfactant protein B deficiency.

Clinically the patients have diarrhoea and vomiting, failure to thrive, exertional dyspnoea and cyanosis.

Chest radiographs show multiple acinar nodules assuming a miliary pattern, which may coalesce to form larger densities and conglomorate areas of consolidation (Fig. 9.25A). CT of the chest shows scattered alveolar densities more marked in the dependent areas of the lungs which correspond to the histological appearances (Fig. 9.25B,C). These appearances are reflected in the histological PAS-positive staining of material within the alveoli. Bronchial lavage is the therapy of choice for childhood PAP with a decreased mortality rate in this previously uniformly fatal condition.

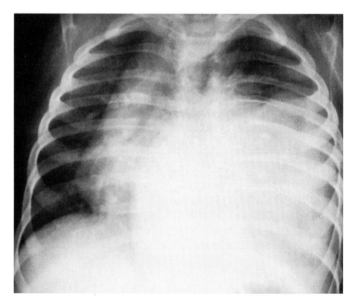

Fig. 9.23 Neuroblastoma. A large left posterior mass deviates the mediastinum to the right, with thinning and separation of the adjacent posterior ends of the ribs.

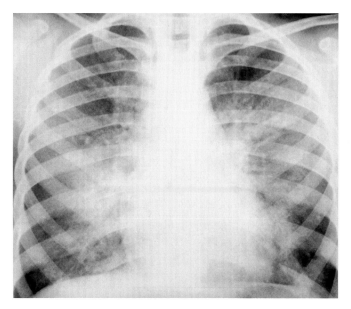

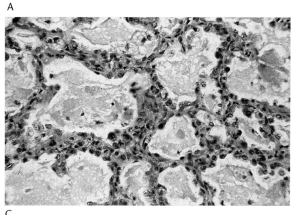

A

Fig. 9.24 Idiopathic pulmonary haemosiderosis. Perihilar shadowing with a reticulonodular pattern in the peripheral lung fields.

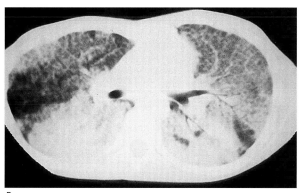

B

C

Fig. 9.25 (A) Pulmonary alveolar proteinosis. Chest X-ray showing diffuse alveolar shadowing in a perihilar distribution with some fine linear change in the upper zones. (B) High-resolution CT scan confirming these appearances showing diffuse alveolar exudate with interstitial thickening most marked in the non-dependent areas of the lung. (C) Histological specimen from video-assisted thoracoscopic biopsy of the lung showing diffuse glycoproteinaceous exudate within the alveolar spaces with thickening of the interstitium of the lung which shows marked increase in cellularity.

REFERENCES AND SUGGESTIONS FOR FURTHER READING

Alford, B.A. (1995) Neonatal chest: conditions requiring intervention or surgery. In: Kirks, D.R. (ed.) *Emergency Pediatric Radiology. A Problem-oriented Approach,* pp. 205–209. Reston, VA: American Roentgen Ray Society.

Chernick, V. (ed.)(1990) *Kendig's Disorders of the Respiratory Tract in Children,* 5th edn. Philadelphia: W.B. Saunders.

Cleveland, R.H. (1995) Imaging of the newborn chest: medical disease. In: Kirks, D.R. (ed.) *Emergency Pediatric Radiology. A Problem-oriented Approach,* pp. 197–203. Reston, VA: American Roentgen Ray Society.

Cleveland, R.H. (1995) A radiologic update on medical diseases of the newborn chest. *Pediatric Radiology,* **25,** 631–637.

Felman, A.H. (1987) *Radiology of the Pediatric Chest: Clinical and Pathological Correlations.* New York: McGraw-Hill.

Fowler, C.L., Pokorny, W.J., Wagner, M.L., Kessler, M.S. (1988) Review of bronchopulmonary foregut malformations. *Journal of Pediatric Surgery,* **23,** 793–797.

Griscom, N. T. (1993) Diseases of the trachea, bronchi, and smaller airways. *Radiologic Clinics of North America,* **31,** 605–615.

Hedlung, G. L., Kirks, D. R. (1990) Emergency radiology of the pediatric chest. *Current Problems in Diagnostic Radiology;* **19,** 133–164.

Kirks, D. (1998) *Practical Paediatric Imaging,* 3rd edn. chap. 7. Philadelphia: Lippincott-Raven.

Lefebvre, J. (1979) *Clinical Practice in Pediatric Radiology,* vol. 2. *The Respiratory System.* New York: Masson.

Lynch, D. A., Brasch, R. C., Hardy, K. A., Webb, W. R. (1990) Pediatric pulmonary disease: assessment with high-resolution ultrafast CT. *Radiology,* **176,** 243–248.

Markowitz, R. I. (1995) Chest radiology in the pediatric intensive care unit. In: Kirks, D. R. (ed.), pp. 217–223. *Emergency Pediatric Radiology. A Problem-oriented Approach.* Reston, VA: American Roentgen Ray Society.

Putman, C. E. (ed.) (1981) *Pulmonary Diagnosis: Imaging and Other Techniques.* New York: Appleton-Century-Crofts.

Silverman, F. N. (1977) Chronic lung disorders in children. In: Eklof, O. (ed.) *Current Concepts in Pediatric Radiology,* vol. 1, pp.13–27. New York: Springer.

Simoneaux, S. F., Bank, E. R., Webber, J. B., Parks, W. J. (1995) MR imaging of the pediatric airway. *RadioGraphics,* **15,** 287–298.

Singleton, E. B., Wagner, M. L., Dutton, R. V. (1988) *Radiologic Atlas of Pulmonary Abnormalities in Children,* 2nd edn. Philadelphia: W.B. Saunders.

Stocker, J. T. (1986) Sequestrations of the lung. *Seminars in Diagnostic Pathology,* **3,** 106–121.

Stocker, J. T., Drake, R. M., Madewell, J. E. (1978) Cystic and congenital lung disease in the newborn. *Perspectives in Pediatric Pathology*, **4**, 93–154.

Sty, J. R., Wells, R. G., Starshak, R. J., Gregg, D. C. (1992) *Diagnostic Imaging of Infants and Children*, vol. 3. Gaithersburg, MD: Aspen.

Swischuk, L. E. (1989) *Imaging of the Newborn, Infant, and Young Child.* 3rd edn. Baltimore: Williams & Wilkins.

Swischuk, L. E. (1994) *Emergency Imaging of the Acutely Ill or Injured Child.* 3rd edn. Baltimore: Williams & Wilkins.

Swischuk, L. E., John, S. D. (1995) *Differential Diagnosis in Pediatric Radiology,* 2nd edn. Baltimore: Williams & Wilkins.

Wagner, R. B., Crawford Jr, W. O., Schimpf, P. P. (1988) Classification of parenchymal injuries of the lung. *Radiology,* **167**, 77–82.

Wesenberg, R. L. (1973) *The Newborn Chest.* Hagerstown, MD: Harper & Row.

Wood, B. P., Davitt, M. A., Metlay, L. A. (1989) Lung disease in the very immature neonate: radiographic and microscopic correlation. *Pediatric Radiology,* **20**, 33–40.

10

THE NORMAL HEART: ANATOMY AND TECHNIQUES OF EXAMINATION

Peter Wilde and Mark Callaway

NORMAL ANATOMY

The description of cardiac anatomy in this chapter is accompanied by a variety of images which are taken by different imaging techniques which show specific anatomical features. An overview of the anatomy of the heart and associated structures will most easily be appreciated by reference to the accompanying series of normal MRI scans taken in the transverse, coronal and sagittal planes (Figs 10.1–10.3).

The heart lies in the anterior mediastinum immediately posterior to the sternum and closely related to the central portion of the diaphragm. The heart lies within a fibrous pericardial sac which is continuous with the central tendon of the diaphragm and which extends to the root of the aorta and the pulmonary artery. The pericardium is lined by two serous layers, the parietal pericardium which is a thin layer lining the fibrous pericardial sac and the visceral pericardium which is a thin layer over the surface of the heart itself. Between these two layers is a very small amount of fluid, which allows free movement of the heart within the pericardial sac. The heart is freely mobile within this sac apart from the attachments at the site of entry of the great vessels. The great veins, the superior and inferior vena cava and the pulmonary veins are all enclosed within a single fold of pericardium, which contains a recess known as the oblique sinus (Fig. 10.4). The outflow from the heart through the aorta and pulmonary artery is enveloped separately and between the major inflow and outflow vessels there is a transverse pericardial sinus. The left and right lungs, contained within their plural cavities, extend around the lateral aspects of the heart and most of the anterior portion of the heart with only a small portion of the right ventricle being directly related to the posterior aspect of the sternum. This small area extends just to the left of the midline where the heart is in direct contact with the costal cartilages and intercostal spaces (Fig. 10.5).

The apex of the heart is normally orientated downwards and leftwards but there is considerable variation in the orientation according to the build of an individual patient. In tall slim individuals, particularly those with hyperinflated lungs, there is a very vertical orientation to the heart whereas in patients with a short, wide build and poor air entry there will be a much more horizontal orientation of the ventricular mass. The orientation of the heart is governed very much by surrounding structures as well as the intrinsic anatomy and differential chamber enlargement will often change the alignment of the heart.

The left ventricle is the most muscular chamber in the heart as its function is to pump systemic flow into the aorta at high pressure. In a normal adult the left ventricle will have a wall thickness measuring 1 cm in diastole and the cross-section of the left ventricular chamber is circular, reflecting the high-pressure function of the chamber. The right ventricle has a thinner free wall, measuring up to 4 or 5 mm in thickness (Fig. 10.6). The left ventricle fills through the mitral valve, which has two leaflets, an anterior leaflet and a posterior leaflet (Fig. 10.7). The anterior leaflet is deeper than the posterior leaflet but has a slightly smaller circumference. The mitral leaflets are attached to chordae tendinae, which arise from two large papillary muscles that are both attached to the free wall of the left ventricle. Each papillary muscle (the anterolateral and posteromedial) gives rise to chordae to both mitral leaflets (Fig. 10.8). The endocardium of the left ventricle is lined with fine lattice-like trabeculation, apart from the basal half of the interventricular septum which is smooth. The outflow of the left ventricle is through the aortic valve. The posterior part of the aortic valve annulus is in fibrous continuity with the base of the anterior leaflet of the mitral valve (Fig. 10.9). The anterior portion of the aortic valve annulus is in continuity with the interventricular septum.

The right ventricle has a much thinner free wall and of course shares the septum with the left ventricle. The interventricular septum curves convex towards the right ventricle due to the higher pressure in the left ventricle. The right ventricle is rhomboid in shape compared to the elliptical shape of the left ventricle. The inner surface of the right ventricle has heavier trabeculation than the left ventricle and several small papillary muscle groups that arise from both the free wall and the septal surface support the tricuspid valve. The tricuspid valve has three leaflets, an anterior leaflet, a septal leaflet and an inferior leaflet. The outflow portion of the right ventricle forms a muscular tube that curves around the septal and anterior surface of the left ventricle to reach the pulmonary valve (Fig. 10.10). The pulmonary valve and tricuspid valve are separated by this muscular infundibulum. The pulmonary valve

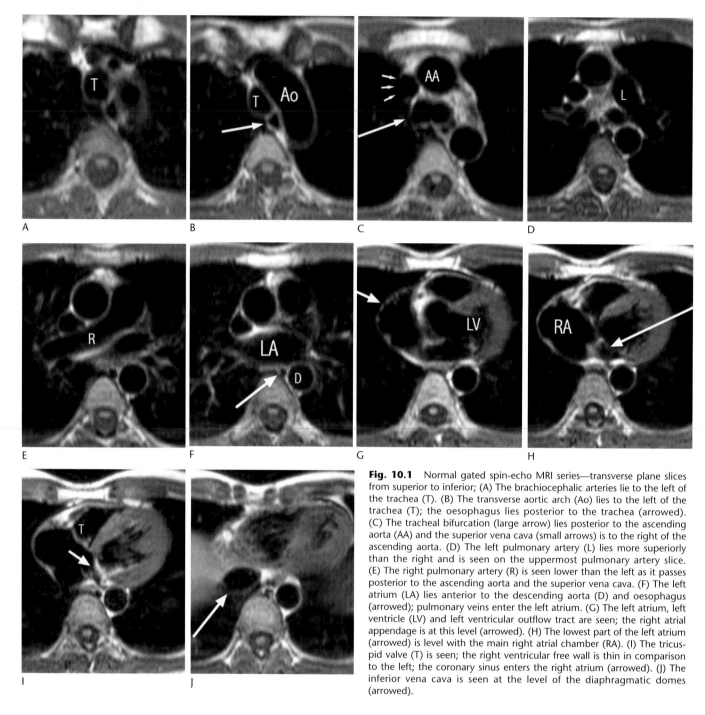

Fig. 10.1 Normal gated spin-echo MRI series—transverse plane slices from superior to inferior; (A) The brachiocephalic arteries lie to the left of the trachea (T). (B) The transverse aortic arch (Ao) lies to the left of the trachea (T); the oesophagus lies posterior to the trachea (arrowed). (C) The tracheal bifurcation (large arrow) lies posterior to the ascending aorta (AA) and the superior vena cava (small arrows) is to the right of the ascending aorta. (D) The left pulmonary artery (L) lies more superiorly than the right and is seen on the uppermost pulmonary artery slice. (E) The right pulmonary artery (R) is seen lower than the left as it passes posterior to the ascending aorta and the superior vena cava. (F) The left atrium (LA) lies anterior to the descending aorta (D) and oesophagus (arrowed); pulmonary veins enter the left atrium. (G) The left atrium, left ventricle (LV) and left ventricular outflow tract are seen; the right atrial appendage is at this level (arrowed). (H) The lowest part of the left atrium (arrowed) is level with the main right atrial chamber (RA). (I) The tricuspid valve (T) is seen; the right ventricular free wall is thin in comparison to the left; the coronary sinus enters the right atrium (arrowed). (J) The inferior vena cava is seen at the level of the diaphragmatic domes (arrowed).

lies close to the aortic valve but the flow is directed posteriorly, whereas the aortic valve has flow directed superiorly, anteriorly and slightly rightwards.

The interventricular septum is a complex curved shape running from the base to the apex of the heart and from the inferior (diaphragmatic) surface of the heart to the outflow portion near the pulmonary valve. The anatomy of the septum shows considerable curvature, which must be borne in mind in any examination that evaluates the interventricular septum.

The relationship of the inlet valves, the tricuspid and mitral valves is of considerable importance. The annulus of the tricuspid valve lies slightly more apically than the annulus of the mitral valve and this

creates a small segment of septum lying between the left ventricle and the right atrium. This is termed the 'ventriculoatrial septum' and is an important identifier of normal atrioventricular valve anatomy. The most superior part of the ventriculoatrial septum becomes very thin (the membranous septum) before it reaches its insertion in the aortic valve annulus. The muscular portion of the interventricular septum lying between the mitral and tricuspid valves is normally termed the inlet or basal septum and further down the ventricle the septal areas are described as mid and apical muscular septal regions. As the septum curves towards the infundibulum passing over the anterior wall of the right ventricle the septum is known as the outflow or conal septum.

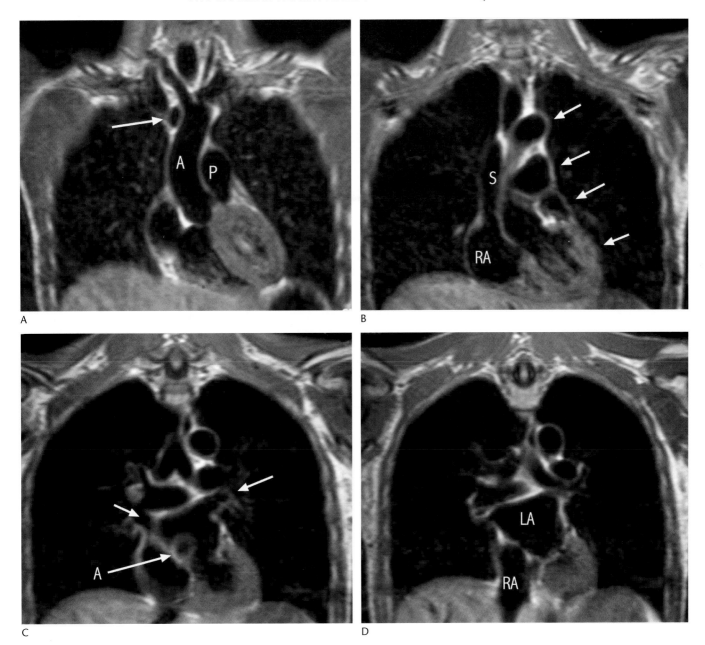

Fig. 10.2 Normal gated spin-echo MRI series—coronal plane slices from anterior to posterior. (A) The most anterior coronal section shows the ascending aorta (A) curving to the right of the main pulmonary trunk (P); the brachiocephalic venous confluence lies to the right of the first brachiocephalic branch (arrowed). (B) The next slice shows how the superior vena cava (S) and the right atrium (RA) form the right heart border; the aortic knuckle, the pulmonary trunk, the left atrial appendage and the left ventricle form the left heart border (arrowed). (C) Pulmonary veins (arrowed) are seen entering the left atrium in the plane of the tracheal bifurcation; the most posterior part of the aortic root is just visible in the slice (A). (D) The left atrium (LA) lies below the tracheal bifurcation and the right pulmonary artery; the interatrial septum lies obliquely above the right atrium (RA); the IVC is to the right of the descending aorta.

The right atrium is characteristically identified by its triangular and broad-based right atrial appendage with trabeculation extending into the free wall of the atrial chamber. The superior vena cava drains into the right atrium immediately posterior to the right atrial appendage and the inferior vena cava drains into the floor of the right atrium, passing for a short distance through the pericardium before entering the atrium. The interatrial septum has a central indentation, the fossa ovalis, marked by a superior limbus. This area represents the region of the patent foramen ovale of fetal life. Just below the interatrial septum

and close to the tricuspid valve lies the opening of the coronary sinus that drains into the right atrium. There is frequently a fibrous fold lying between the inflow of the inferior vena cava and the tricuspid valve; this is known as the Eustachian valve. Frequently this valve extends into the right atrial chamber as a collection of mobile fronds known as the Chiari malformation (Fig. 10.11). This is a normal variant of no clinical significance.

The left atrium is a smooth-walled chamber which gives rise to a narrow-based and anteriorly pointing finger-like left atrial

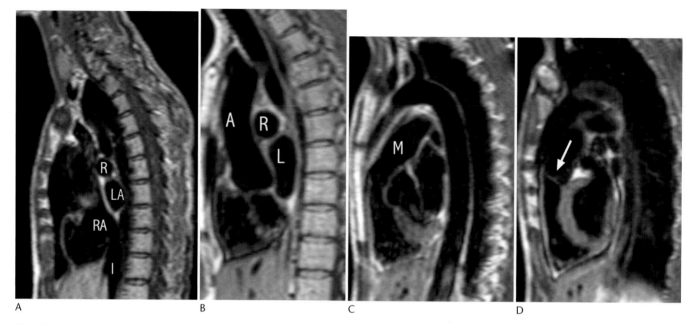

A   B   C   D

Fig. 10.3 Normal gated spin-echo MRI series—sagittal plane slices from right to left. (A) The inferior vena cava (I) enters the right atrium (RA) near the Eustachian valve; the left atrium lies above and posterior to the right atrium and below the right pulmonary artery (R). (B) The ascending aorta (A) lies anterior to the left atrium (L) and right pulmonary artery (R). (C) The transverse and posterior aortic arch lie at the same level as the main pulmonary artery (M). (D) The relationship between the right and left ventricles is clearly seen; the pulmonary valve lies above the right ventricular outflow tract (arrowed).

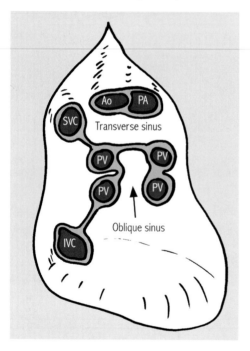

Fig. 10.4 The posterior aspect of the pericardial space. The transverse sinus lies between the aorta/pulmonary artery and the great veins. The oblique sinus lies between the pulmonary venous confluence. Ao = aorta; PA = pulmonary artery; PV = pulmonary vein; SVC = superior vena cava; IVC = inferior vena cava.

appendage that contains trabeculation (Fig. 10.12). The pulmonary veins drain into the posterior part of the left atrium, usually in four separate openings from the left and right upper and lower pulmonary veins (Fig. 10.13). The left atrium usually lies slightly higher than the right atrium and in transverse sectional imaging techniques this can be clearly demonstrated.

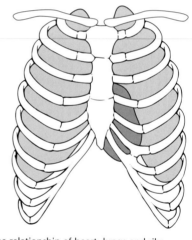

Fig. 10.5 The relationship of heart, lungs and ribs.

The aorta commences with the three leaflet aortic valve. This semilunar valve has leaflets related to the three slightly bulging sinuses of Valsalva (Fig. 10.14). The normal orientation of the ascending aorta as it leaves the heart is directed superiorly with slight anterior and rightward angulation. The ascending aorta passes upwards close to the sternum and slightly right of the midline before turning posteriorly into the aortic arch and crossing back to the left side as it passes down the descending aorta. The aortic arch normally gives rise to three branches, the first being the right brachiocephalic branch which divides into the right subclavian artery and the right common carotid artery. The second branch is the left common carotid artery and the third is the left subclavian artery. The subclavian arteries both give rise to vertebral arteries, but in a small proportion of cases the left vertebral artery arises separately from the aorta. Another common variant is a common origin of the right brachiocephalic artery with the left common

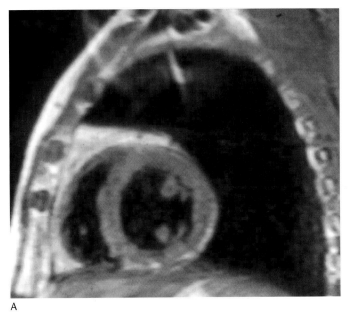

A

Fig. 10.6 (A) Gated spin-echo MRI short-axis section of the left and right ventricles. The papillary muscles are clearly seen in the left ventricle comparative TOE image (B) showing a short-axis section of both ventricles—the gastric position of the transducer is at the bottom of the image.

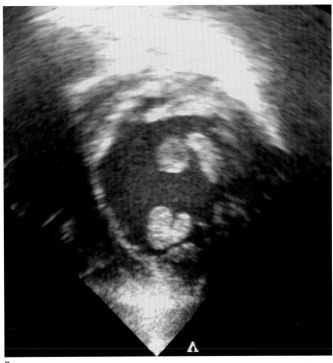

B

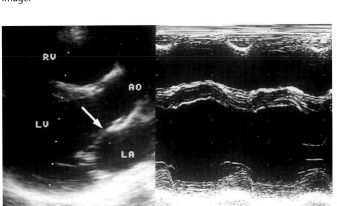

A   B

Fig. 10.7 Transthoracic echocardiogram showing a long-axis view of the left ventricle (A) with a corresponding M-mode trace. (B) The anterior leaflet of the mitral valve arises from the posterior aortic annulus (arrowed).

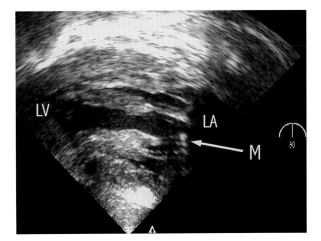

Fig. 10.8 Transoesophageal long-axis view from the transgastric window showing the chordae running from the papillary muscles to the mitral valve (M). LA = left atrium; LV = left ventricle.

carotid artery. A less common variant is the anomalous right subclavian artery; the right brachiocephalic artery only giving rise to the right common carotid artery, with the anomalous right subclavian artery being the last branch from the aorta which passes posteriorly behind the oesophagus to reach its normal position (Fig. 10.15). In a small proportion of cases patients may have a right-sided aortic arch, the arch passing to the right of the trachea rather than to the usual left side. In the case of a right aortic arch the branching may be mirror image (an exact reverse of the normal pattern) or it may be of a type that give branches as left common carotid, right common carotid, right subclavian, anomalous left subclavian artery. The latter type is the most common branching pattern in isolated right-sided aortic branch, whereas the former (mirror image) type is more often associated with cyanotic congenital heart disease.

The main pulmonary artery passes almost directly posteriorly past the ascending aorta and bifurcates, giving a right pulmonary artery

that traverses the middle mediastinum immediately posterior to the ascending aorta before reaching its termination at the right hilum (Fig. 10.16). The left pulmonary artery passes directly posteriorly to reach the left hilum. The left pulmonary artery arches over the left main bronchus where as the right pulmonary artery lies anterior to the right main bronchus. The left pulmonary artery is slightly higher in position than the right pulmonary artery and is often demonstrated on higher slices of sectional imaging techniques.

The aortic root gives rise to left and right coronary arteries. The three sinuses of Valsalva lie anatomically in anterior, leftward posterior and rightward posterior positions. The anterior sinus is also known as the right coronary sinus that gives rise to the right coronary artery and the leftward posterior sinus is also known as the left

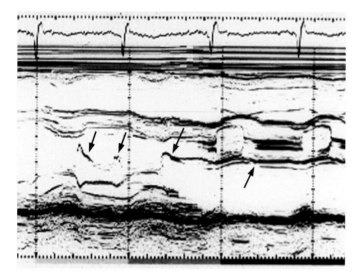

Fig. 10.9 M-mode sweep from mitral to aortic valve. The anterior leaflet of the mitral valve (arrowed) is in continuity with the posterior wall of the aortic root. The anterior wall of the aorta is in continuity with the interventricular septum.

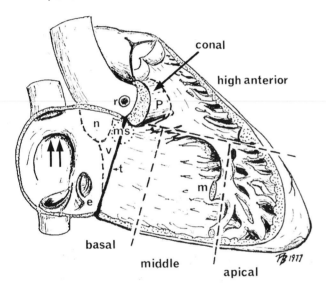

Fig. 10.10 The anterior view of the septal surface of the right ventricle. The basal, middle, apical, conal and high anterior portions of the septum are marked. The Eustachian valve (e) lies between the opening of the inferior vena cava and the tricuspid valve annulus (t). The limbus of the fossa ovalis is arrowed. The membranous septum (ms) lies on the upper aspect of the tricuspid valve annulus and forms part of the ventriculoatrial septum (v). The transected moderator band of the right ventricle (m) lies in the mid septum. The parietal band of muscle (P) forms the conal or outflow septum. The right (r) and non-coronary (n) aortic sinuses are marked.

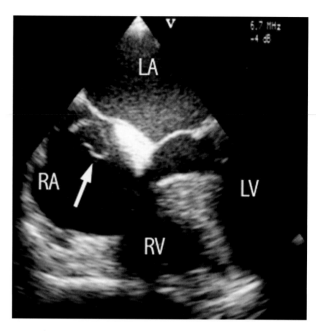

Fig. 10.11 Four-chamber transoesophageal echocardiogram showing the mobile sinuous appearance of a Chiari malformation in the right atrium. RA = right atrium; LA = left atrium; RV = right ventricle; LV = left ventricle.

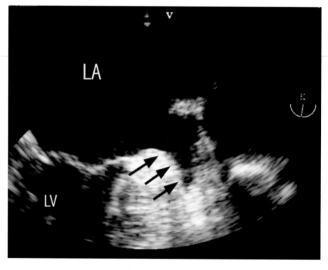

Fig. 10.12 Longitudinal transoesophageal echocardiogram showing the left atrial appendage (arrowed). LA = left atrium; LV = left ventricle.

sinus of Valsalva that gives rise to the left coronary artery. The rightward posterior sinus is also known as the non-coronary sinus. The angulated orientation of the ascending aorta means that all sinuses are not at the same level, the non-coronary sinus usually being the lowest and the left coronary sinus being the highest (Fig. 10.17).

The coronary anatomy in the accompanying description can be identified in the series of accompanying figures (Fig. 10.18). The left coronary artery arises as a left main stem which initially is directed leftwards and posteriorly but which curves immediately

around to an anterior orientation where it bifurcates to the left anterior descending artery and the circumflex artery. In some cases the left main coronary artery can be very short and occasionally the left anterior descending and circumflex coronary arteries can have separate origins from the left sinus of Valsalva. The left anterior descending artery runs along the superior aspect of the interventricular septum emerging into the anterior interventricular groove as a superficial vessel which runs right down to the apex of the heart. The left anterior descending artery gives rise to penetrating septal branches and surface diagonal branches. The circumflex artery passes around the left atrioventricular groove giving off free wall branches to supply the left ventricular myocardium. These branches are commonly known as marginal or obtuse marginal branches. The circumflex artery will also frequently supply important left atrial

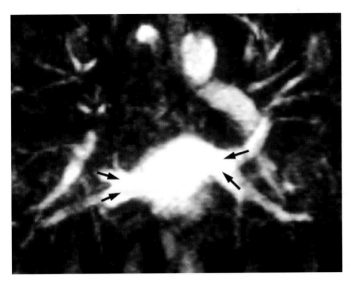

Fig. 10.13 Gadolinium contrast MRI angiography in the coronal plane showing the four pulmonary veins entering the left atrium.

branches. In some cases the left main stem will divide into three branches rather than two, the third branch lying between the left anterior descending artery and the circumflex artery and being termed the intermediate branch. This supplies free wall muscle between the diagonal and obtuse marginal territories.

The right coronary artery arises from the right sinus of Valsalva and immediately turns rightward and inferiorly to follow the right atrioventricular groove. One of the earliest branches from the right coronary artery passes over the surface of the right ventricular outflow tract and is known as the conus branch. This branch can sometimes have a separate origin immediately adjacent to the right coronary stem. During this course the vessel gives off several right ventricular free wall branches which are generally smaller than the corresponding obtuse marginal branches. As the right coronary artery reaches the posterior ventricular groove it gives rise to the posterior descending artery and frequently continues in the atrioventricular groove to terminate in branches supplying the inferior myocardium of the left ventricle. The posterior descending artery supplies penetrating branches into the septum, corresponding to those from the anterior descending artery. The point of division of the right coronary artery into the posterior descending and left ventricular branches is commonly termed the crux and at this point there is often a vertical penetrating branch to the atrioventricular node.

The asymmetrical orientation of the heart within the thorax has led to confusion over nomenclature of orientation of the heart. The conventional terms of anterior, posterior, superior and inferior are not used in exactly the same way with anatomical descriptions of the heart. The oblique orientation of the heart has led to some slightly adjusted terms, which are now in common descriptive use. The left ventricular free wall conventionally divided into three main areas which are termed the anterior, the lateral and the posterior (or inferior) segments. Strictly the anterior wall of the left ventricle is more anterosuperior, and the lateral wall of the left ventricle is leftward posterior in orientation. The posterior wall of the left ventricle would more conventionally be called inferior. These terms must be appreciated when dealing with cardiological descriptions.

TECHNIQUES

There are numerous imaging techniques available for examination of the heart and it is essential that the most appropriate technique is applied according to any given situation. The main techniques for examining the heart are plain chest radiography, echocardiography (cardiac ultrasound), CT scanning, MRI scanning, radionuclide imaging and angiography. Each of these techniques has particular applications and each technique must be considered in the context of its diagnostic appropriateness, cost, availability, associated hazards and accuracy. In straightforward situations well-established protocols will allow selection of the most appropriate examination without difficulty. In more complex clinical situations however it is important to discuss the appropriate examination with an experienced radiologist in order to evaluate the condition most appropriately.

CHEST X-RAY

The chest X-ray is the commonest type of imaging examination of the heart, although frequently the examination is used for other aspects of examination of the thorax and the heart is examined as part of this overall investigation.

The chest X-ray can be extremely valuable in cardiac assessment in three ways. First cardiac size and contour can be clearly demonstrated and the silhouette of the heart produced in this way will give many important clues as to chamber enlargement. The second and most crucial aspect of the chest X-ray is the evaluation of the lung fields. Careful analysis of the pulmonary appearances will give vital clues to the cardiac function. Third the chest X-ray will demonstrate additional features related to cardiac disease which may

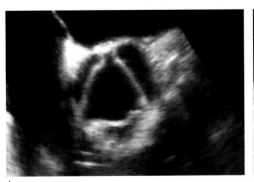

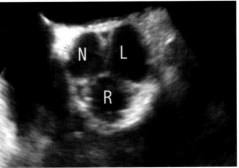

Fig. 10.14 Short-axis transoesophageal echocardiogram of the aortic valve in systole (A) and diastole (B). The right (R), left (L) and non-coronary (N) sinuses are shown. The lower part of the images lie anteriorly.

A   B

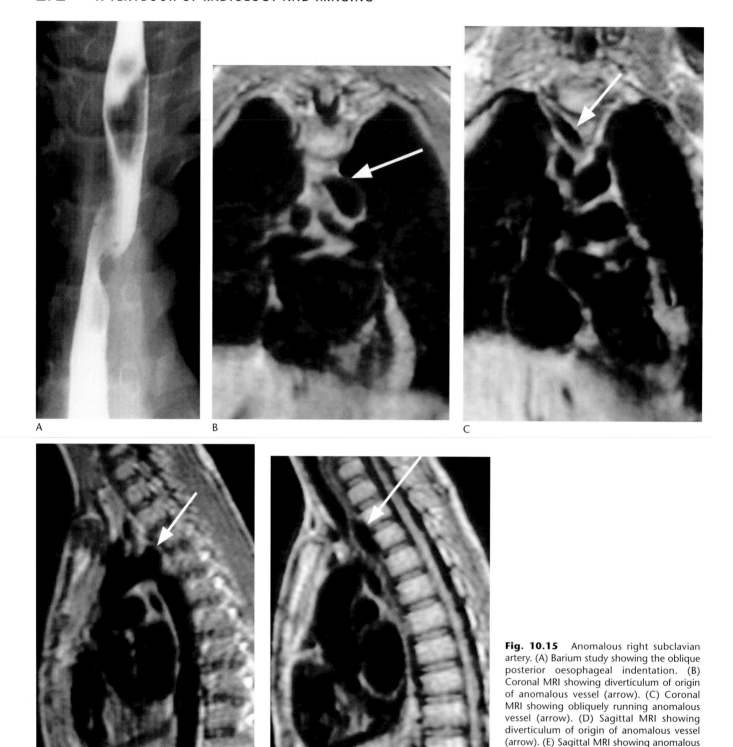

Fig. 10.15 Anomalous right subclavian artery. (A) Barium study showing the oblique posterior oesophageal indentation. (B) Coronal MRI showing diverticulum of origin of anomalous vessel (arrow). (C) Coronal MRI showing obliquely running anomalous vessel (arrow). (D) Sagittal MRI showing diverticulum of origin of anomalous vessel (arrow). (E) Sagittal MRI showing anomalous vessel posterior to oesophagus (arrow).

include metallic or other implants, calcifications or bony anomalies which are related to the underlying heart abnormality.

The normal chest X-ray should show clear definition of the cardiac contour and it should be possible in an adult chest film to identify the aortic knuckle, the main pulmonary artery and the left ventricle (Fig. 10.19). The area between the main pulmonary artery and the left ventricle may be occupied by additional structures if they are slightly enlarged, namely the left atrial appendage and the right ventricular outflow tract. The superior vena cava and the right atrium usually form the right heart border but in some cases where there is enlargement or unfolding of the ascending aorta this structure may comprise part of the upper right heart border. On a conventional PA chest film the cardiothoracic ratio can be measured. This expresses the proportion of heart size to internal thoracic

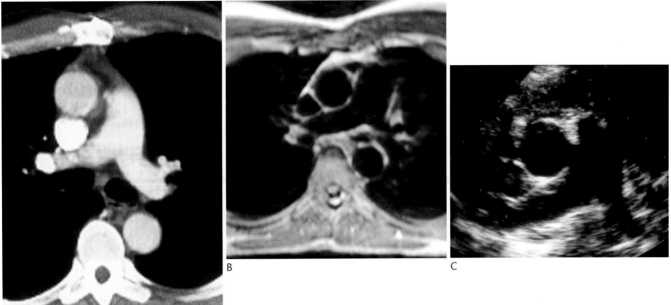

Fig. 10.16 Main pulmonary artery bifurcation. (A) Contrast-enhanced CT. (B) Gated spin-echo MRI. (C) Transthoracic echocardiogram.

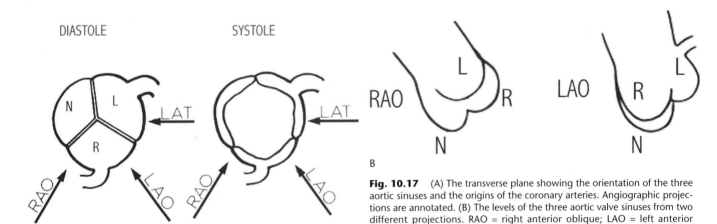

Fig. 10.17 (A) The transverse plane showing the orientation of the three aortic sinuses and the origins of the coronary arteries. Angiographic projections are annotated. (B) The levels of the three aortic valve sinuses from two different projections. RAO = right anterior oblique; LAO = left anterior oblique; LAT = lateral; L = left sinus; R = right sinus; N = non-coronary sinus.

diameter. Cardiothoracic ratio is normally well below 50% but in AP films (usually mobile or portable films) normal value can be accepted as 55%. In infants the normal value can also be 55%.

In the assessment of the pulmonary vascularity on an erect PA film in an adult, it should be quite easy to identify segmental branching vessels passing from the hilum regions into both lung fields. If it is not possible to identify branching vessels in the lungs then there may be either a technical or a pathological explanation. In an erect film normal pulmonary vasculature should always show substantially larger vessels in the lower zones compared to the upper zones. This feature should always be sought in routine examination of the chest film. There should also be progressive tapering in size from the left and right pulmonary arteries at the hilum to the peripheral vessels, which are normally seen extending about two-thirds of the distance across the lung fields. In general it is difficult to distinguish pulmonary arteries from pulmonary veins on a chest radiograph but in the right lower zone the anatomical features make this task easier. In this area horizontal vessels are likely to be pulmonary veins passing into the left atrium, whilst in the same region

pulmonary arteries are more vertically orientated towards the more superiorly positioned hilum.

ECHOCARDIOGRAPHY

Echocardiography is a highly versatile technique that had become central in cardiological diagnosis but it is also a very operator dependent technique and requires considerable experience before reliable diagnostic results can be achieved. Echocardiography is generally performed from the transthoracic route using a small 'footprint' sector scanner. Careful positioning of the patient is essential to maximise access to the heart through the intercostal spaces whilst avoiding interposition of pulmonary air. Usually the patient rests in a 45° semi-erect position rotated towards their left side to enhance the cardiac contact with the chest wall.

Echocardiography employs a number of different modalities for cardiac diagnosis. Two-dimensional imaging or real-time sector scanning gives direct imaging information about the anatomy and

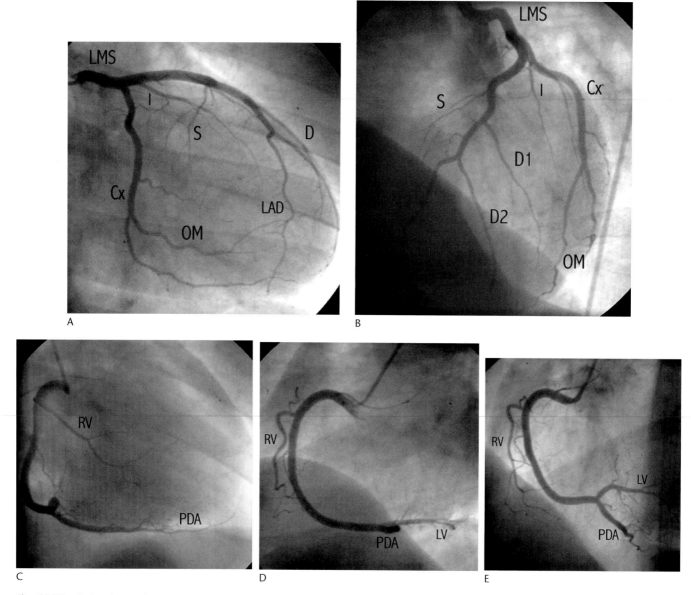

Fig. 10.18 Series of normal coronary artery angiograms. LMS = left main stem; LAD = left anterior descending artery; D = diagonal branch; S = septal branch; I = intermediate branch; Cx = circumflex artery; OM = obtuse marginal branch; PDA = posterior descending artery; RV = right ventricular branch; LV = inferior left ventricular branch. (A) Right anterior oblique view of the left coronary artery. (B) Cranially angulated view of the left coronary artery. (C) Right anterior oblique view of the right coronary artery. (D) Left anterior oblique view of the right coronary artery. The posterior descending artery is foreshortened. (E) Cranially angulated left anterior oblique view of the right coronary artery. The posterior descending artery is now well profiled.

physiology of the heart. M-mode imaging is a one-dimensional evaluation using a single line of ultrasound interrogation down a specific orientation through cardiac structures. This technique is particularly useful for precise measurement and timing of cardiac events. Doppler echocardiography allows evaluation of blood flow through the heart and is carried out using continuous-wave, pulsed-wave and colour flow Doppler techniques. Each of these techniques has particular advantages and in current cardiac ultrasound equipment all the above modalities are normally available interchangeably from the control panel.

Two-dimensional echocardiography techniques rely on the operator identifying particular anatomical planes within the heart. These planes are orthogonal in orientation and are termed the long-axis plane, the short-axis plane and the four-chamber plane. Each of

these planes can be achieved by scanning from at least two different positions or 'windows' on the chest wall. The most commonly used windows are the left parasternal (second or third left interspace), the apical and the subcostal (or xiphisternal). Table 10.1 shows the imaging planes that can be obtained from each window.

Two-dimensional imaging has the great advantage of demonstrating overall cardiac anatomy and movement and this allows excellent evaluation of many cardiac abnormalities. There are however limitations in the technique and precision measurement and timing can be limited due to the rapid movement of the heart and the need for a high frame rate. The two-dimensional image however allows measurement of area to be calculated and allows relative motion of different structures to be studied.

Table 10.1   Imaging planes obtainable in each window

Window	Planes obtainable
Left parasternal	Long axis
Left parasternal	Short axis
Apical	Long axis
Apical	Four chamber
Subcostal (subxiphoid)	Four chamber
Subcostal (subxiphoid)	Short axis

In its early days M-mode echocardiography was a technique that required great skill, as there was no two-dimensional image to guide the M-mode beam. Modern systems however allow the two-dimensional image to guide M-mode placement and for this reason very accurate positioning of the M-mode beam can be achieved, which means much more reliable measurements can be made.

Doppler examination

Continuous-wave Doppler examination. This technique employs a continuously emitting transducer adjacent to a continuously receiving transducer. This allows a continuous interrogation down the length of the ultrasound beam but the technique does not allow differentiation of structures at any particular depth along the beam. The advantage of continuous-wave Doppler examination is that high-velocity flows can easily be recorded and in pathological conditions within the heart this is extremely important. Pulsed-Doppler examination uses time delays to interrogate at specific depths along the beam. This means that measurements can be made at precise sites within the heart (Fig. 10.20) but the time limitations of the

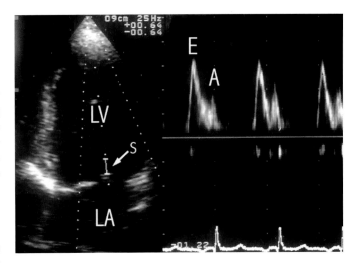

Fig. 10.20   Pulsed-Doppler study showing normal mitral inflow. The left panel shows an apical image with the sample volume (S) placed in the mitral orifice between left atrium (LA) and left ventricle (LV). The right panel shows the normal inflow pattern with an initial large passive flow (E) followed by a later smaller active flow (A) produced by atrial systole.

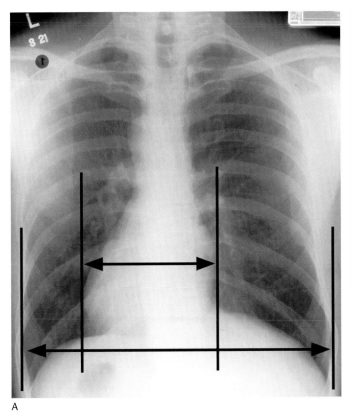

A

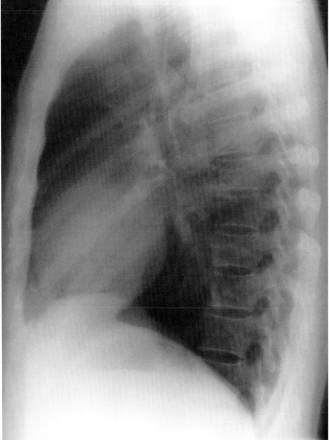

B

Fig. 10.19   Normal chest X-ray. (A) PA view annotated to show measurements for cardiothoracic ratio. (B) Lateral view.

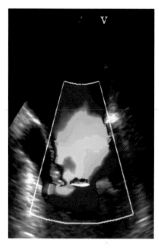

Fig. 10.21 Transoesophageal echocardiogram showing colour flow through a normal mitral valve. There is aliasing (yellow and red) in the central part of the flow where the velocity is highest.

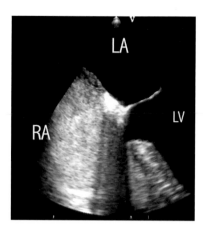

Fig. 10.22 Transoesophageal echocardiogram showing agitated saline contrast in the right atrium (RA). There is no evidence of bubble contrast in the left atrium (LA), indicating an intact atrial septum. LV = left ventricle.

pulsed-Doppler technique mean that the highest velocities cannot easily be measured. Pulsed-Doppler evaluation is often used for flow measurement and calculations but cannot be used for the highest velocity pathological jets. Continuous-wave studies are frequently used in techniques to derive pressure differences within the heart from the velocities of flow through stenotic or regurgitant valves.

Colour flow Doppler examination is based on the principle of pulsed-Doppler technique and as such it is limited by high-velocity flows. For this reason aliasing (or misregistration of colour) is a common phenomenon in colour-flow imaging (Fig. 10.21). Nevertheless this technique is highly valuable in demonstrating normal and abnormal flows quickly and easily and in many cases, once the flow has been identified, a more precise evaluation can be achieved using specific continuous-wave or pulsed-Doppler interrogation.

Transoesophageal echocardiography

This has become an extremely important adjunct to the overall echo repertoire. Examination of the heart from within the oesophagus or stomach allows high-frequency transducers to be used from very close range and this leads to excellent quality images, particularly of the more deep posterior structures such as the left atrium or mitral valve. Modern instruments now employ multiplane transducers, which can rotate to produce a wide range of image planes through the cardiac anatomy. Transoesophageal echocardiography can be performed on an outpatient basis usually with mild sedation, and is indicated in a wide range of abnormalities including pros-

thetic heart valve malfunction, endocarditis, evaluation of thrombus in the left atrium and congenital heart defects. All the imaging and Doppler modalities are generally available on current transoesophageal echo systems. The transoesophageal endoscopes themselves are purely ultrasound imaging devices and do not have any direct viewing capacity. For this reason intubation must be carefully performed but in experienced hands and in patients without contraindications the complication rate is extremely low.

Contrast echocardiography

This technique has some useful applications. In its simplest form, a very effective contrast echo study can be achieved with the intravenous injection of an agitated blood and saline mixture containing microbubbles. This technique is easily performed but great care must be taken to avoid the injection of visible bubbles. This technique will provide dense opacification of right-sided structures and is most commonly used for the identification of right to left shunting or other mixing at atrial or ventricular level (Fig. 10.22). These bubbles will be absorbed during transit through the lungs and the technique is therefore not of use in studying left-sided structures.

Box 10.1

Continuous-wave Doppler examination
  Adjacent transducer elements act as simultaneous transmitter and receiver
  High-velocity flow recordable
  No depth resolution possible

Pulsed-wave Doppler examination
  The same transducer used to transmit and receive
  Pulse repetition frequency limits high-velocity recording—aliasing will result
  Sample volume can be placed at a specific depth

Colour flow Doppler examination
  Multiple pulsing down each line allows colour encoding for flow
  Image frame rate reduced due to multiple sampling
  Aliasing easily induced

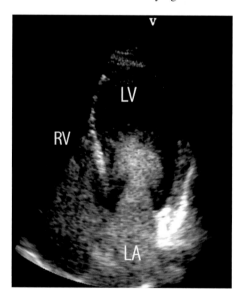

Fig. 10.23 Transthoracic apical four-chamber view showing a bolus of transpulmonary contrast agent entering the left ventricle through the mitral valve after peripheral intravenous injection. LV = left ventricle; RV = right ventricle; LA = left atrium.

Transpulmonary echo contrast agents are now commercially available for the study of left-sided structures. These agents, some of which are based on albumen-encapsulated microbubbles, can be used to enhance visibility of left-sided structures (Fig. 10.23). They can also be used for myocardial perfusion studies. The latter are still in limited use due to some of the associated technical difficulties.

Stress echocardiography

These studies in some selected situations have been very sensitive in the detection of myocardial ischaemia. Important coronary artery stenoses may allow adequate flow at rest but may become flow limiting under conditions of exercise or pharmacological stress. In such circumstances normally contracting myocardium may become abnormal in function and this will reveal the presence of important

underlying coronary artery disease. The same principle underlies electrocardiographic stress tests (exercise ECG) and radionuclide perfusion scans. All three techniques have relative advantages and disadvantages and their utility depends on specialist experience.

Radionuclide imaging

Radionuclide imaging of the heart has traditionally been of two types, blood pool imaging and myocardial imaging. The former technique involves the labelling of red cells with a technetium tracer, usually in vivo, followed by image acquisition using electrocardiographic gating. The technique allows counts to be detected in the cardiac chambers during a series of frames acquired through the cardiac cycle. The technique has some technical limitations including the difficulties of chamber superimposition and the need for

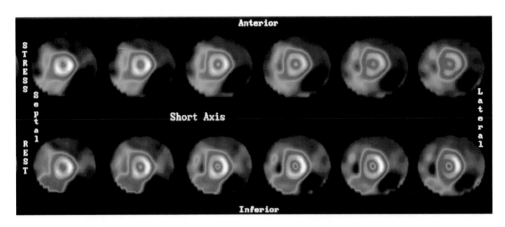

Fig. 10.24 Technetium SPECT study showing a normal series of short-axis slices along the left ventricle after exercise stress (top) and at rest (bottom).

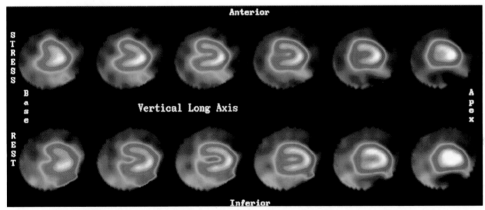

Fig. 10.25 Technetium SPECT study showing a normal series of vertical long-axis slices of the left ventricle after exercise stress (top) and at rest (bottom).

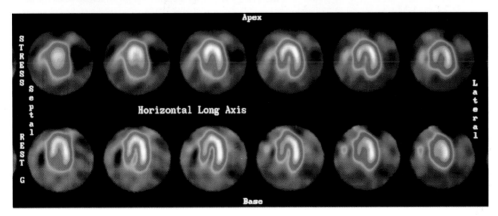

Fig. 10.26 Technetium SPECT study showing a normal series of horizontal long-axis slices of the left ventricle after exercise stress (top) and at rest (bottom).

background count subtraction. In recent years the rapid development of other non-invasive techniques such as echocardiography and MRI has meant that blood pool imaging has decreased in application and is now a relatively rare technique.

By contrast, however, perfusion imaging is still of considerable importance and this can be carried out using a wide range of techniques. The principle is based on myocardial tissue labelling, usually comparing stress and rest situations. Until recently thallium was the preferred radionuclide agent for these studies but the suboptimal radiation imaging characteristics of thallium meant higher radiation doses and anatomically poor images. The advantage of the thallium scan is that a single study, injected at stress, can be scanned immediately for stress abnormalities and after 4–6 hours a resting (redistribution) scan can be performed. The more recently introduced technetium agents (e.g. sestamibi) allow higher image quality studies to be achieved but separate stress and rest studies must be performed on different days.

The imaging technology for myocardial scanning usually involves tomographic acquisition of data using a rotating gamma camera and electrocardiographic gating. This allows relatively high-resolution images to be acquired in selected anatomical planes. The short-axis plane corresponds to echocardiographic short-axis views, the vertical long-axis view is close in orientation to the echocardiographic long-axis view and the horizontal long-axis view corresponds to the four-chamber view (Figs 10.24–10.26). The slices produced in these views can be displayed in a number of ways for ease of interpretation and quantitation, the 'bull's eye' view being a common way of demonstrating the full extent of the left ventricular myocardium (Fig. 10.27). An additional benefit of this technique is its use in outlining the left ventricular chamber to produce a functional ventriculogram at stress and rest (Fig. 10.28).

Positron emission tomography is a sensitive technique that is very valuable in the detailed assessment of functional myocardial physiology. The requirement for sophisticated equipment and an adjacent cyclotron make it limited in availability and application.

Computed tomography

CT can give excellent quality images of intrathoracic anatomy. Unfortunately the temporal resolution of even the fastest multislice CT scanners does not freeze cardiac motion completely and therefore the technique is more useful for assessing major cardiac structures and great vessels than detailed internal cardiac anatomy. The technique has proved highly effective in the diagnosis of abnormalities of the great arteries and masses adjacent to the heart. In combination with high-dose contrast injection this is often the first-line technique for diagnosing acute aortic disease, including aortic dissection. Recent advances in high-speed multislice CT have allowed much higher precision to be achieved in the detection of calcification in the coronary arteries, which is of great prognostic value. Early work in some advanced systems now allows proximal coronary anatomy to be evaluated with high-resolution contrast studies (Fig. 10.29).

Contrast-enhanced multislice CT scanning is currently an alternative to some types of cardiac MRI scanning. The advantage of multislice CT is in its temporal resolution and practical utility but it offers high radiation doses and cannot image directly in complex oblique planes. Electron-beam CT systems are based on the same principle as conventional CT but the rotating electron beam eliminates the need for rotation of heavy equipment in the gantry around the patient and therefore faster scan times can be achieved, good quality images being obtained in as little as 50 ms. The equipment is, however, limited in availability due to its expense.

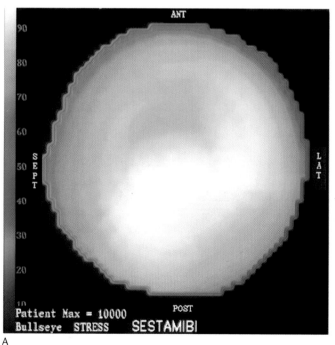

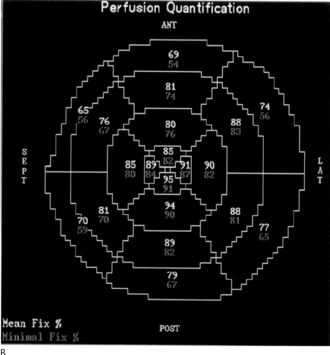

A   B

Fig. 10.27 Technetium SPECT study showing a normal 'bull's eye view' display (A). The apex of the left ventricle is represented at the centre of the image and the regions around the ventricle are annotated. (B) Quantitation of the same display showing only minor variation in counts across the left ventricular myocardium.

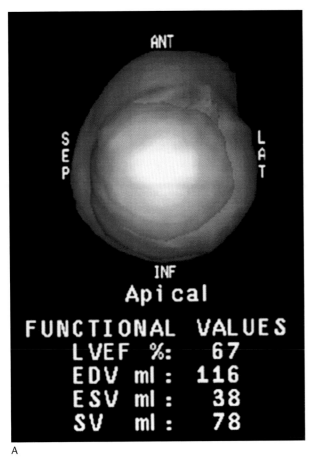

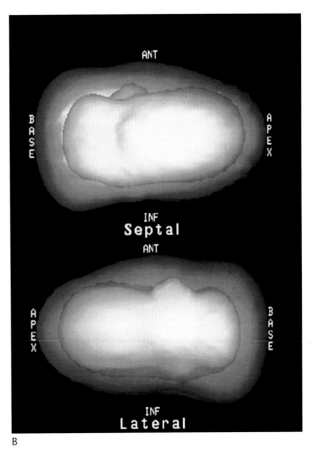

Fig. 10.28 Technetium SPECT study showing surface-rendered images of a normally contracting left ventricle. The systolic contour is represented within the diastolic contour short-axis view (A) and vertical (top) and horizontal (bottom) long-axis views (B).

Magnetic resonance imaging

This area of cardiac examination is progressing rapidly and there is a very considerable amount of potential for future development. MRI can produce highly detailed examination of both the external and internal cardiac structures without the use of contrast medium. The technique can distinguish blood from adjacent tissues and appropriate sequences will demonstrate flow. MRI can demonstrate anatomy in a full range of imaging planes including transverse, coronal, sagittal and complex obliques (Fig. 10.30). The combination of the above features makes MRI a particularly powerful tool for evaluating cardiac disease. Unfortunately the limitations are that image acquisition is still prolonged such that in the majority of anatomical imaging cases (spin-echo technique) it is necessary to gate to the electrocardiogram and collect imaging across many cardiac cycles. This type of techniques gives the typical 'black blood' image. Flow sequences (white blood imaging) are performed using a gradient-echo technique and ciné sequences can be achieved through the cardiac cycle in a selected examination plane (Fig. 10.31). Once again, however, it is necessary to obtain data over several cardiac cycles with the aid of cardiac gating. Newer techniques and equipment are now beginning to introduce 'real-time' acquisition of cardiac images.

Coronary anatomy can be evaluated to a certain extent using MRI techniques but, as with CT scanning, the technique is not sufficiently advanced to give comprehensive evaluation of all the coronary artery anatomy and at present only proximal or large vessels can be reliably identified.

The main strength of cardiac MRI techniques lies in their flexibility and the combination of anatomical and functional studies. Pharmacological stress studies on the myocardium are now routinely achievable and, together with anatomical imaging of coronary arteries, offers the potential of full assessment of coronary heart disease by one technique. MRI flow studies are also possible and this will lead to the more complete assessment of haemodynamic lesions such as valve abnormalities and congenital heart defects.

Angiography

In spite of the wide range of imaging techniques available, many of which are non-invasive, angiography still remains an important technique for the evaluation of cardiac and great vessel anatomy.

Perhaps the commonest form of cardiac angiography at the present time is coronary angiography. This examination is by far the commonest angiographic technique performed in advanced countries and this is due to the widespread availability of revascularisation techniques such as coronary artery bypass grafting and coronary angioplasty. Coronary angiographic equipment has very high X-ray specifications because diagnostic demands are extremely high. Image resolution must be capable of demonstrating coronary anatomical detail down to structures of 0.3 mm or less and exposure

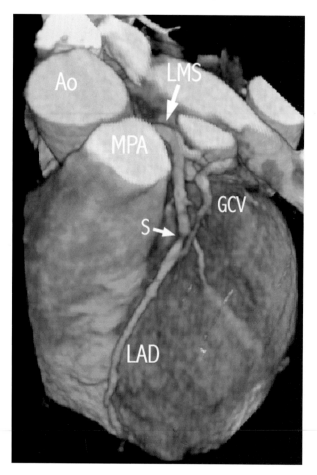

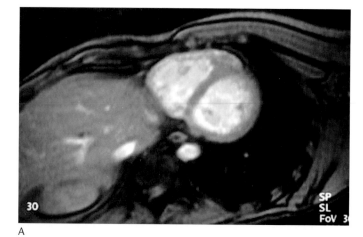

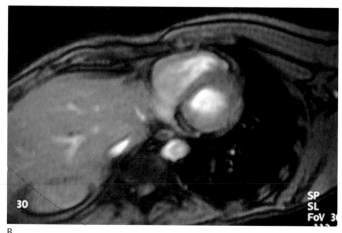

Fig. 10.29 High-resolution multislice contrast CT demonstrating the left coronary artery with a stenosis (S) in the mid left anterior descending branch. Ao = aorta; MPA = main pulmonary artery; LMS = left mainstem; LAD = left anterior descending artery; GCV = great cardiac vein. (Courtesy of Dr A. Baumbach and Dr S. Schroeder.)

Fig. 10.30 Double oblique MRI gradient-echo ciné sequence of the left ventricular short axis in diastole (A) and systole (B).

times must be no more than 5 ms. This must be achievable with frame rates of 12.5 frames/s (digital) or 25 frames/s (ciné). The equipment must be capable of performing multiple runs without excessive heat load of the X-ray tube and the X-ray gantry must be capable of a wide range of angulations to evaluate the three-dimensional cardiac anatomy.

Coronary angiography is usually performed via the percutaneous Seldinger approach from the femoral route. Commonly used catheter shapes such as Judkins or Amplatz allow selective cannulation of the left and right coronary ostia. In the case of each coronary artery a series of angiograms is taken in a variety of angulations to ensure full exposure of all branches and bifurcations. Iodine as the contrast medium at 320–370 mg/ml is generally employed, but currently it is increasingly common to use non-ionic media that offer a lower contrast load to the circulation. At the time of coronary angiography, it is also frequently useful to carry out left ventricular angiography (Fig. 10.32). This is generally done as a matter of practicality but in theory it would be possible to omit this step and carry out non-invasive evaluation of the left ventricle.

Aortography (of the ascending aorta) is normally carried out for anatomical assessment or functional assessment of the aortic valve. In both cases high-density contrast in the aorta must be achieved, but this can only be accomplished with a large volume of contrast

injected at a higher rate through an injection pump. Typically an adult male would require 40–50 ml of contrast medium injected at 20 ml/s to give good quality opacification of the ascending aorta.

Pulmonary angiography can be performed for the assessment of possible pulmonary embolism. The technique is relatively straightforward but it does require sufficient experience to pass a venous catheter through the right atrium, right ventricle and main pulmonary artery. In performing such an examination the patient should be fully monitored for pressure and ECG evaluation in order to be aware of any cardiac irregularity caused by passage of the catheter. Dense opacification of the pulmonary artery should be achieved to assess peripheral vascular detail and in the case of possible high pulmonary vascular resistance it is important to use low osmolarity contrast medium. This type of angiogram still offers extremely high resolution imaging of the heart and great vessels. Appropriate timing of the imaging sequence will allow the pulmonary arterial, capillary and venous phases to be imaged as well as the later laevophase, which will show the left ventricle and aorta (Fig. 10.33).

In the case of paediatric angiography a wide variety of sites and angiographic projections are used to evaluate paediatric cardiac anatomy.

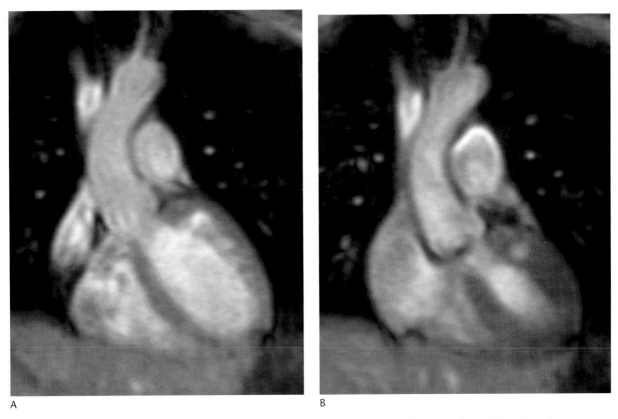

Fig. 10.31 Coronal MRI gradient-echo ciné sequence of the left ventricular outflow tract and aortic valve in diastole (A) and systole (B).

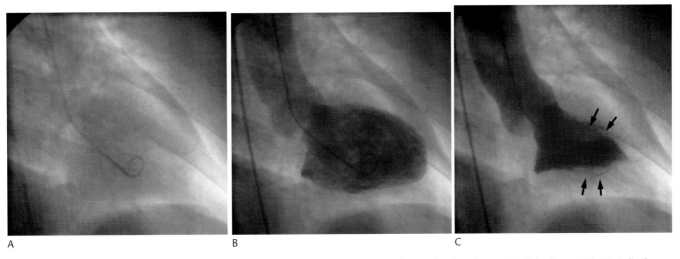

Fig. 10.32 Left ventricular angiogram in the right anterior oblique projection using a pigtail catheter. (A) Plain frame. (B) Diastolic frame. (C) Systolic frame. The papillary muscles are arrowed.

Angiography and associated angiographic techniques are an essential part of interventional cardiology. There is now a wide range of interventional procedures for treating cardiac disease, perhaps the commonest of which is percutaneous transluminal coronary angioplasty (PTCA). There are numerous additional techniques that can be performed in the heart, including balloon valvuloplasty, stenting of stenosed vessels and closure of abnormal communications. In each case high-resolution angiography together with X-ray screening and sometimes ultrasound evaluation are important for the conduct of these procedures.

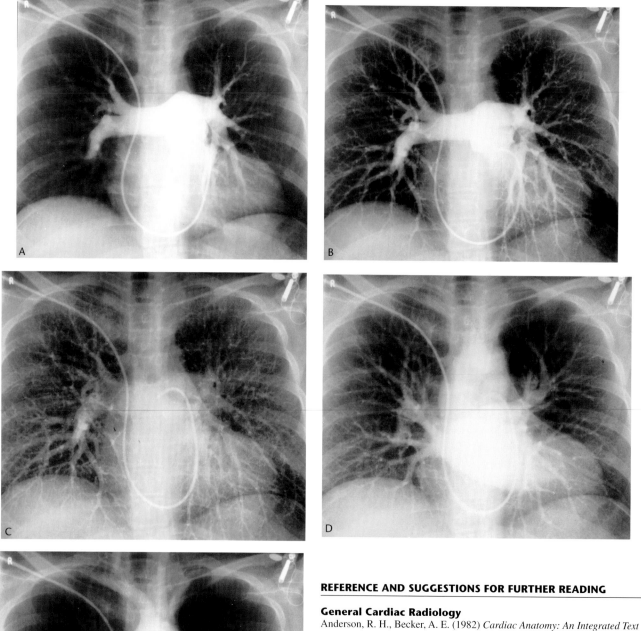

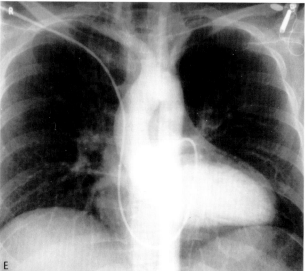

Fig. 10.33 Cut film pulmonary angiogram series. (A) Early arterial phase. (B) Late arterial phase. (C) Capillary phase. (D) Pulmonary venous phase. (E) Laevophase.

REFERENCE AND SUGGESTIONS FOR FURTHER READING

General Cardiac Radiology

Anderson, R. H., Becker, A. E. (1982) *Cardiac Anatomy: An Integrated Text and Colour Atlas*. Edinburgh, Churchill Livingstone.

Chiles, C., Putman, C. E. (1997) Pulmonary and Cardiac Imaging. Marcel Dekker Inc.

Higgins, C. B. (1992) Essentials of Cardiac Radiology and Imaging. J. B. Lippincott Company.

Pohost, G. M., O'Rourke, R. A. (1991) *Principles and Practice of Caardiovascular Imaging*. Little Brown and Company USA.

Skorton, D. J., Schelbert, H. R., Wolf, G. L., Brundage, B. H. (1996) Marcus Cardiac Imaging: A Companion to Braunwald's Heart Disease. W. B. Saunders, USA.

11

ACQUIRED HEART DISEASE I: THE CHEST RADIOGRAPH

Mark Callaway and Peter Wilde

INTRODUCTION

In spite of the rapid development of imaging technologies in recent years, the chest radiograph still remains the most frequently performed radiographic examination. This examination is often one of the most difficult to interpret, requiring a logical and methodical approach to examining each aspect of the chest and cardiovascular system to ensure no detail is missed. This is however a rewarding exercise with a great deal of clinical information being available. Often a great deal of emphasis is placed on the respiratory diseases that can be diagnosed from the chest radiograph, but a large amount of clinical information about the cardiovascular system can also be obtained.

To obtain all the available information a systematic approach is required. Evaluation of the heart and its individual chambers, the pulmonary vasculature, the aortic arch and the non-cardiac review areas can all provide important diagnostic information. This basic examination can provide a good diagnostic basis to progress to the next appropriate form of imaging and this opportunity is often overlooked in the rush to more complex investigations.

The chest radiograph with its low radiation dose and relatively low expense is an easily repeatable examination. This, together with its ability to show the heart size and pulmonary vascularity, very clearly makes it an ideal monitoring examination to follow the progress of a disease or its treatment. It is thus not only a primarily diagnostic technique but also a management tool, allowing the radiologist and physician together to evaluate the progress of a patient's condition.

APPROACH TO CARDIAC DISEASE ON THE CHEST X-RAY

Heart size and shape

A good quality PA chest radiograph is an important indicator of cardiac size. Not only can global cardiac enlargement be detected but individual chamber enlargement can also be identified.

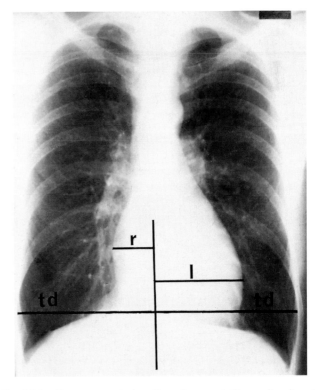

Fig. 11.1 The assessment of cardiac enlargement. The cardiac diameter should be the maximum cardiac diameter (r + l). The transverse thoracic diameter is measured in various ways; here it is measured as the maximum internal diameter of the thorax.

The most common method of describing the heart size is by use of the cardiothoracic ratio (Fig. 11.1). This is derived by measuring: (i) the internal diameter of the thoracic cavity from the medial border of the ribs at the level of the right hemidiaphragm and (ii) the transverse cardiac measurement as the horizontal distance the most lateral aspects of the left and right margins of the heart. The cardiothoracic ratio is expressed as a percentage of the heart size with respect to internal thoracic diameter. It is sometimes useful to record the actual measurements from the radiograph.

283

While the most common figure used as a normal cardiothoracic ratio is a maximum of 50%, some important caveats need to be observed. This ratio refers to measurement in the adult Caucasian chest. In non-Caucasian adults the normal ratio can be slightly higher than this. The cardiothoracic ratio is often increased in the neonate and can also be increased in the elderly, often being associated with an unfolding of the aorta or a thoracic scoliosis.

Enlargement of the heart is often associated with specific chamber enlargement and by assessing from the plain film which chambers are enlarged the observer can begin to assess what dynamic changes are present, for example stenosis or regurgitation of a valve. Isolated enlargement of individual cardiac chambers is less common than multichamber enlargement, the latter often being the consequence of sequential effects of one lesion upon several parts of the cardiovascular circulation. A dilated and failing left ventricle can lead to left atrial enlargement and this in turn can produce raised pulmonary pressures and increased size of the right-sided chambers. Single chamber enlargement will, however, be discussed in detail, as this will provide clues to the assessment of multichamber enlargement as well as highlighting several important conditions.

Left atrial enlargement

There are several well-documented features of left atrial enlargement. A 'double' right heart border, elevation of the left main bronchus, splaying of the carina and enlargement of the left atrial appendage (Fig. 11.2) (prominence of the portion of the left heart border at the level of the left main bronchus) all suggest left atrial enlargement. The left atrium is a roughly spherical chamber lying in the posterior part of the cardiac mass and if it is enlarged, the increased density of the enlarged chamber itself is often evident, particularly on a penetrated (PA) or a lateral film (Fig. 11.3). The extra shadow along the right heart border on the PA film is formed

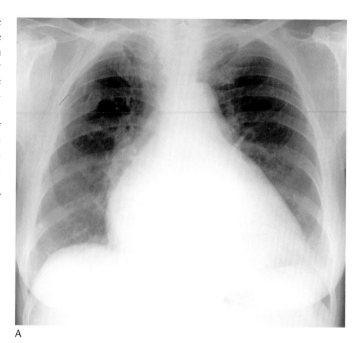

A

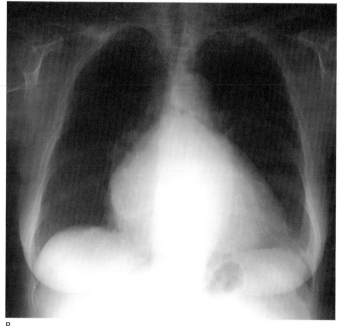

B

Fig. 11.3 Left atrial enlargement. A PA (A) and penetrated chest film (B) in the same patient. The double right heart border and splaying of the carina, due to enlargement of this posterior chamber, is easily visualised on the penetrated film.

by the projection of the distended rightward margin of the left atrial mass lying close to the usual right atrial margin. While these features are usually well recognised, exact measurements have been suggested. A distance between the middle of the double density and the left main bronchus of greater than 7 cm has been shown to indicate left atrial enlargement in over 90% of cases.

Right atrial enlargement

The features of right atrial enlargement can be subtle and difficult to determine in mild and moderate cases. The most common is a

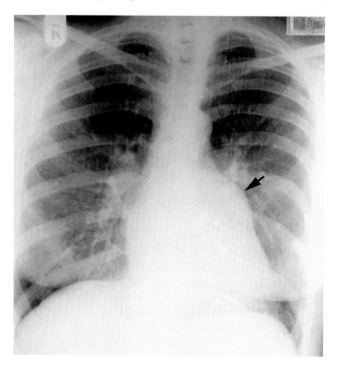

Fig. 11.2 Rheumatic mitral stenosis. This frontal film shows marked enlargement of the left atrial appendage (arrow).

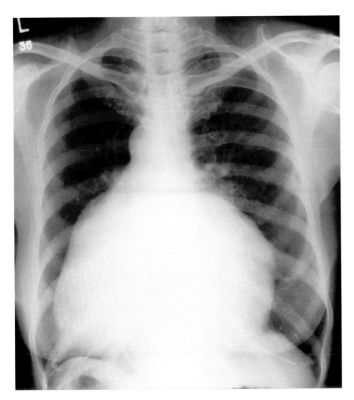

Fig. 11.4 Right atrial enlargement. Right atrial enlargement is often difficult to detect with only subtle enlargement of the right heart border present on the PA view.

lateral prominence of the right heart border, often associated with an increase convexity. In severe chronic cases the right heart border can become massively distended towards the right side (Fig. 11.4).

Left ventricular enlargement

As the left ventricle enlarges there is usually an increase in the cardiothoracic ratio and the curvature of the lower left heart border takes on a larger radius. The ventricle enlarges towards the lateral wall of the thorax in a downward direction, displacing the apex laterally and inferiorly. A measurement to assess left ventricular enlargement on a lateral film has been defined (Fig. 11.5). This is the Hoffman–Rigler sign, and is the distance from the posterior aspect of the IVC to the posterior border of the heart horizontally at the level 2 cm above the intersection of the diaphragm and the IVC. A distance of greater than 1.8 cm indicates left ventricular enlargement. Such measurements can be helpful but great reliance cannot be placed on them as individual anatomical variation can cause discrepancies.

Right ventricular enlargement

While right ventricular enlargement may also cause lateral displacement of the left heart border, it is the position of the apex and the different curvature of the heart border that suggests right ventricular enlargement. The apex is often displaced laterally but not inferiorly and the curvature at the apex remains small (if the left ventricle remains small). The right ventricle enlargement occurs somewhat higher on the left heart border, between the left ventricular contour and the pulmonary outflow tract (Fig. 11.6). The lateral view will

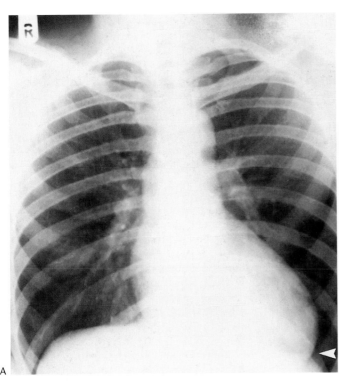

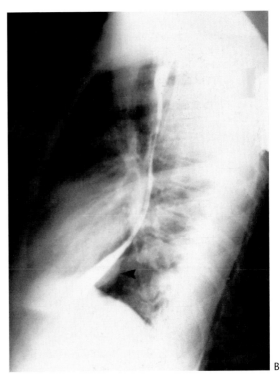

Fig. 11.5 Selective left ventricular enlargement in aortic incompetence. (A) Frontal view shows that the left ventricle has enlarged along its long axis, taking the apex of the heart to the left and downward (white arrow). (B) Lateral view shows the left ventricle extending behind the line of the barium-filled oesophagus (arrow).

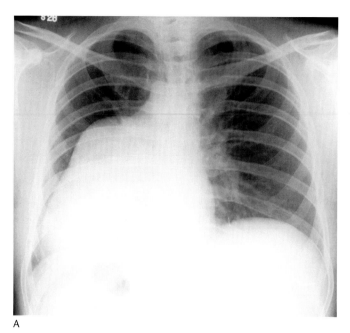

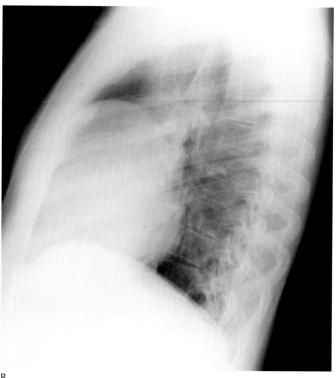

Fig. 11.6 Gross right ventricular enlargement due to isolated right ventricular cardiomyopathy. The right ventricular enlargement occurs on the left heart border between the left ventricular contour and the pulmonary outflow tract (A) and is well seen on the lateral film (B).

frequently show an enlarged right ventricle, the increased size of the chamber being more prominent in the retrosternal area.

Pulmonary vascular patterns

The pulmonary vascular pattern composed of a combination of arteries and veins can provide a great deal of information, apparent on the plain film, about the cardiovascular system. There is often difficulty in recognising and interpreting the pathological changes in this vasculature and some important points should be made. Visualisation of the pulmonary vessels and their abnormalities can only be achieved reliably with a technically good erect PA chest film. Supine films or AP films will often be misleading. The visualisation of any vessels in the lungs will depend on the silhouette sign, namely the outlining of the vascular structures by intrapulmonary air. If for any reason such as infiltration, pulmonary oedema or consolidation there is no air adjacent to the vessels then they will not be visible in their own right and conclusions about vascularity will be hard to draw. The degree of exposure of the film must not detract the radiologist from examination of the vessels and their size. A light (underexposed) film may make vessels appear more prominent but this will not alter their size, and it is the size and distribution of the vessels that is of major importance.

Normal pulmonary vascular pattern

The pulmonary circulation begins with the main pulmonary artery, which can be identified on the standard plain PA film. This artery forms the convexity on the left mediastinal border between the arch of the aorta and the straight left heart border. Subtle prominence of this convexity can be difficult to identify but can suggest significant enlargement of the main pulmonary artery. However, in children and young women mild prominence may be normal.

The main pulmonary artery divides after a variable distance into the left and right pulmonary arteries. The left pulmonary artery continues as a branch of the main pulmonary artery before branching. The left upper lobe artery arises as the left pulmonary artery passes over the left main bronchus. This portion of the circulation can be identified on the plain PA film as the upper part of the left hilum.

The right pulmonary artery arises sharply from the main pulmonary artery, passing rightwards into the mediastinum as an immediate posterior relation of the ascending aorta. The right pulmonary artery divides in the mediastinum. The descending branch of the right pulmonary artery is the first vessel to be identified and forms, on the PA film, the lower border of the right hilum. Within the lung the arteries can be identified as they divide in a constant manner, these branches tapering smoothly, and can usually be identified as far as the outer third of the lung.

The pulmonary veins can be distinguished from the pulmonary arteries under some circumstances but their identification is not always easy. Pulmonary veins can be differentiated on the plain film by position and course in some areas only. Pulmonary veins in the right lower zone tend to run in a horizontal direction entering the left atrium, compared with the more vertical course taken by the arteries. The difficulty in clearly distinguishing pulmonary arteries and veins in most circumstances means that the term 'pulmonary vessels' or 'pulmonary vascularity' are more practical than potentially inaccurate attempts to distinguish the two types of vessel.

On a normal erect PA film the upper lobe vessels tend to be small or not visible because left atrial pressure is inadequate to distend these vessels and there is little arterial blood flow directed to the upper lobes. The pulmonary vascular bed is very compliant, the pulmonary vascular resistance being very low compared to the systemic circulation. In the normal adult in the erect position there is adequate pulmonary perfusion through the lower parts of the lungs

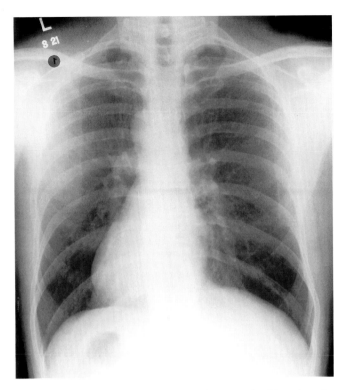

Fig. 11.7 Normal chest radiograph. In the normal subject there is a marked difference between the size of the upper and lower zone vasculature, the lower zone vessels being much more prominent.

with only a minimal flow in the apices. This means that normal pulmonary vascularity shows a marked differential between upper and lower zones (Fig. 11.7). The normal diameter of the upper lobe vessels in the first interspace is rarely more than 3 mm. Normal values have been calculated for the descending branch of the right pulmonary artery, which usually does not exceed 16 mm in men and 15 mm in women.

Changes in the pulmonary circulation can occur within the arterial or venous system due to an increase or reduction in flow. In addition there can be a change in the pulmonary vascular resistance as a result of intrinsic lung disease. Maintaining this low-pressure system is a complex balance, the pulmonary vascular resistance being about 20% that of the systemic circulation, hence the pulmonary artery pressure is approximately 20% of normal systemic arterial pressure (25/10 mmHg).

Abnormal pulmonary vascular patterns

Pulmonary vascular patterns can alter for a number of different reasons, occurring either together or in combination. The pressure in the pulmonary arteries may be increased (pulmonary arterial hypertension) or the pressure in the pulmonary veins may be increased (pulmonary venous hypertension), or both of these may be present. Overall pulmonary flow may increase above normal (pulmonary plethora) or it may fall below normal (pulmonary oligaemia). There may also be patchy changes in the pulmonary vascular pattern due to inhomogeneous pulmonary disease or localised perfusion variations due to acquired or congenital differences in regional blood supply.

Pulmonary arterial hypertension

This is defined as a systolic pressure of greater than 30 mmHg in the presence of a normal systemic pressure. An increase in pulmonary artery pressure most commonly occurs as a result of intrinsic lung disease, which results in an increase in pulmonary vascular resistance and a subsequent increase in pulmonary artery pressure. Other causes of increased pulmonary vascular resistance include chronic pulmonary embolic disease and reactive pulmonary vascular disease. The latter may occur as a result of increase flow as in left to right shunt. Pulmonary artery pressure can also increase as a result of an increase in pulmonary venous pressure. This secondary increase in pulmonary venous pressure arises from an obstruction to left-sided cardiac flow, the classic example being mitral stenosis. Impaired left ventricular function is probably the commonest cause of raised pulmonary venous pressure. This increase is then transmitted back through the pulmonary capillary bed to the pulmonary artery.

Eisenmenger's syndrome develops in patients with large untreated left to right shunts, usually at ventricular or arterial level. The pulmonary vascular bed is thus subjected to both high flow and high pressure. In this situation secondary changes occur at an arteriolar level, which lead to an increase in pulmonary vascular resistance. Eventually, the pulmonary vascular resistance increases to a pressure greater than that of the main pulmonary artery and the shunt is reversed. The plain chest film demonstrates a large, triangular heart with large main and central pulmonary arteries. The enlargement can often be extremely large with complete infilling of the pulmonary artery/ventricular concavity on the left heart border. The pulmonary arteries within the lungs are enlarged but there is

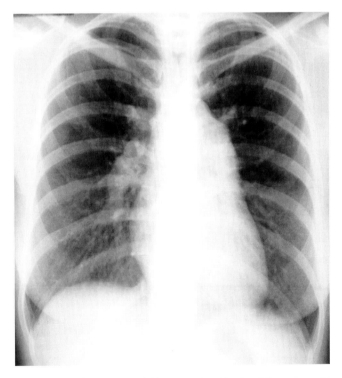

Fig. 11.8 Pulmonary arterial hypertension. The heart has a large triangular shape with large main and central pulmonary arteries. There is complete infilling of the pulmonary artery/ventricular concavity on the left heart border. The pulmonary arteries within the lungs are enlarged but there is rapid tapering of the vessels as they run towards the periphery.

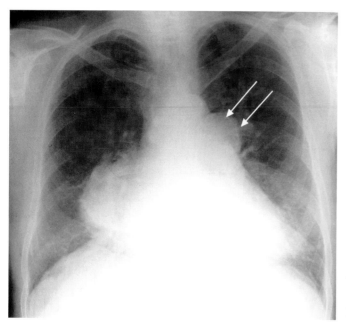

Fig. 11.9 Pulmonary arterial hypertension. If the pulmonary artery hypertension is severe and chronic, the pulmonary arteries may become very large and calcified (arrows).

rapid tapering of the vessels as they run towards the periphery (Fig. 11.8). The key observation is the discrepancy between central and peripheral vessel size, large central pulmonary arteries being associated with inappropriately small peripheral vessels. In some cases the central vessels are near normal in size but peripherally the arteries are still disproportionately small.

The features of Eisenmenger's syndrome on the plain film are initially pronounced tapering of the pulmonary arteries, usually associated with cardiomegaly caused by the volume overload of the shunt. As the syndrome progresses less blood flows through the pulmonary vascular bed and the pulmonary vessels become less prominent. This change is associated with the reduction in left to right shunt and the cardiomegaly may diminish. A late film in Eisenmenger's syndrome may be difficult to distinguish from normal until the old film is reviewed. Calcification of the main and proximal pulmonary arteries, although uncommon, can develop and can be identified on a plain film (Fig. 11.9). Pulmonary artery calcification is often curvilinear in appearance and can be easily mistaken for egg-shape calcification of enlarged hilar lymph nodes, although in the latter condition there is an absence of peripheral pruning.

Pulmonary venous hypertension

If impairment to the forward flow of blood through the left side of the heart develops, then left atrial pressure rises. This can be a result of impaired left ventricular function, the development of mitral stenosis or other left-sided pathology. This increase in atrial pressure is directly transmitted to the pulmonary veins, producing pulmonary venous hypertension. The changes in pulmonary venous hypertension are well defined on the plain film and increase as the left atrial pressure increases, the first radiological feature being enlargement of the upper zone vessels. The physiological reasons surrounding upper lobe blood diversion are not always well understood.

There is always a balance between the intrinsic pressure in the pulmonary vascular bed that tends to lead to extravasation of fluid into the extracellular space, and the plasma osmotic pressure that will tend to retain fluid in the vascular compartment. In the normal person the plasma osmotic pressure is sufficient to retain fluid and keep the extracellular space 'dry'. If the pulmonary venous pressure rises to exceed this level (around 25 mmHg), there will be extravasation of fluid into the small but important extracellular space. This makes the lung 'stiff' and decreases the compliance in the affected part of the lung, in turn raising the vascular resistance and reducing flow. As there is always higher pressure in the lower zones than in the upper zones due to the hydrostatic pressure across the lungs, this leakage will first occur at the lung bases. The consequence of this is redistribution of flow to the mid and upper zones of the lungs. (These changes are related to lung zones, not anatomical lobes.) This redistribution does not just lead to increased upper zone flow, but it also causes reduction of flow in the lower zones and attenuation of the size of the lower zone pulmonary arteries. This phenomenon is actually the earliest manifestation of pulmonary oedema, even though the fluid has not extended to pulmonary lymphatics or air spaces.

Other factors affecting vascular redistribution include factors that address the normal ventilation perfusion mismatch and enhance oxygenation of the blood. Normal perfusion is predominantly to the lower zones while ventilation is directed to the upper lobes.

If the intravascular pressure remains consistently elevated there will be continuous leakage of fluid into the interstitium. This must be constantly drained back to the central circulation and this occurs

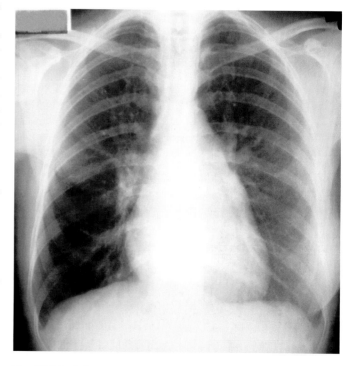

Fig. 11.10 Pulmonary venous hypertension. There is a mild haziness in the lower zones with attenuation of the lower zone vessels and prominence of the upper zone vessels. There is loss of definition of the heart and mediastinal contours. This is most notable when viewing the branches of the right pulmonary artery. The difference in density at the lung bases is due to a right mastectomy.

via the intrapulmonary lymphatics. These intrapulmonary lymphatic channels become visible, producing the development of Kerley B lines. As pulmonary pressure rises alveolar pulmonary oedema may develop. Alveolar oedema appears when the pulmonary pressure increases to above 25 mmHg in the acute phase or 30–35 mmHg or more in the chronic phase. Alveolar oedema occurs when the leakage of fluid into the interstitium exceeds the capacity of pulmonary lymphatics to drain it away. This can occur at relatively low pressures in the acute situation but at higher pressures in patients with chronic pulmonary hypertension and well-developed lymphatic channels.

The chest X-ray appearances of pulmonary venous hypertension are characterised by a mild haziness in the lower zones with attenuation of the lower zone vessels and prominence of the upper zone vessels (Fig. 11.10). There may be slight loss of definition of the heart and mediastinal contours. This is most notable when viewing the branches of the right pulmonary artery. These changes result as the normally sharp interfaces between the interstitum and air become obscured because of the presence of extravascular fluid. Chronic changes are associated with Kerley B lines—horizontal subpleural lines, 1–3 mm in thickness and up to 1 cm in length most frequently identified at the costophrenic angles (Fig. 11.11). Interstitial oedema may cause thickening of the interlobar fissures, seen in the horizontal fissure in the PA film and in both horizontal and oblique fissures in the lateral film. Pulmonary effusions may also develop. The effusions are usually bilateral and can be large.

Longstanding pulmonary venous hypertension can occasionally be associated with the development of two other features. The first is haemosiderosis, which appears on the plain film as a series of fine punctate calcifications that are scattered throughout both lungs.

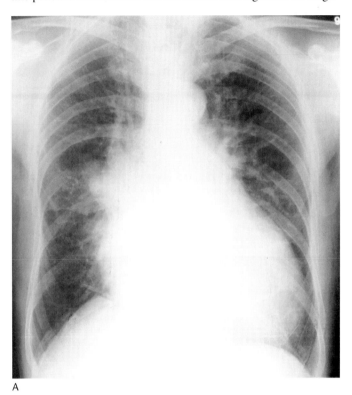

A

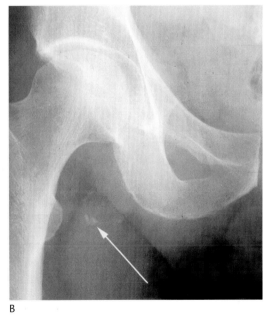

B

Fig. 11.12 Pulmonary plethora due to high-output cardiac failure. This PA chest radiograph demonstrates pulmonary plethora (A). The pulmonary vessels are considerably enlarged and also more tortuous than usual. The central pulmonary arteries are also large. This patient had a large femoral arteriovenous fistula (arrow) due to venous surgery 20 years previously. The calcified fistula is evident on a plain film (B).

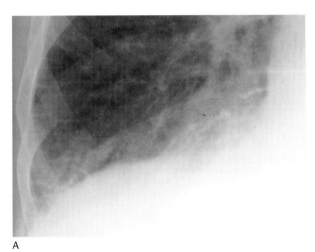

A

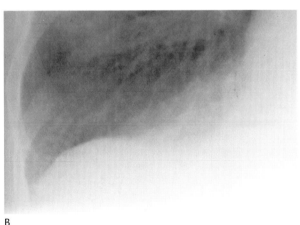

B

Fig. 11.11 Kerley B lines are caused by interstitial fluid and are defined as subpleural perpendicular lines 1–3 cm in length (A). These lines often resolve following treatment (B).

If pulmonary hypertension remains severe for a long period of time pulmonary ossific nodules can develop. These are small areas of bone formation in the lungs. These nodules are never larger then 1cm in diameter and can appear to have a trabecular structure.

Pulmonary plethora

This appearance is most commonly due to above-normal flow through the pulmonary vascular circuit. It is usually associated with intracardiac shunting from left to right. It is most easily appreciated in longstanding low-pressure shunts such as atrial septal defect, but will be evident in any large shunt including ventricular septal defect, patent ductus arteriosus, anomalous pulmonary venous drainage and common arterial trunk. The increased flow may be associated with heart failure and pulmonary oedema, particularly in large high-pressure shunts in infancy, but is commonly seen without evidence of interstitial oedema. Left to right shunting must be at least 2 to 1 to produce plethora on the PA chest film and a pulmonary to systemic flow ratio of 3 to 1 is necessary before the plethora is easily seen. In large shunts of longstanding the pulmonary vessels will be considerably enlarged and also more tortuous than usual. The central pulmonary arteries will also be large.

Other less common causes of increased pulmonary flow can also cause plethora. Hyperdynamic circulation due to increased metabolic states can produce plethora. Systemic arteriovenous shunts can give rise to a high output cardiac state, which will lead to high pulmonary flow and consequent plethora (Fig. 11.12).

An early sign in mild cases of pulmonary plethora is the equalisation in size of upper and lower zone vessels. This contrasts with the appearances of pulmonary venous hypertension because there will not be any attenuation of lower zone vessels and there will usually be no haziness of interstitial oedema.

Prolonged pulmonary plethora may lead to pulmonary arterial hypertension, particularly if the shunt is large and between ventricles or great arteries.

Pulmonary oligaemia

Pulmonary oligaemia is a state of below-normal flow through the pulmonary circuit. It is usually due to congenital heart disease in which there is right to left shunting, taking flow away from the lungs. It is generally associated with some degree of cyanosis. In some cases of reduced overall cardiac output there may be pulmonary oligaemia but this is not a common finding as all normal compensation mechanisms in the circulation act to preserve normal cardiac output wherever possible.

The appearances on the chest film are of generalised decrease in size of the pulmonary vessels in all zones. The differential between upper and lower zones is usually maintained although it is less obvious. The underperfusion of the lung fields is often associated with hyperlucent lung fields but it is important to avoid interpreting any overpenetrated film as being due to oligaemia. The size of the pulmonary vessels themselves must always be assessed.

Regional abnormalities in pulmonary vascularity

Regional variations in pulmonary vascularity can be due to many causes. Patchy areas of pulmonary disease will be associated with variations in perfusion. Chronic obstructive airways disease, bullous disease, pulmonary fibrosis, pulmonary embolism, pulmonary infection and pulmonary collapse will all affect regional pulmonary blood flow. In cases of congenital cyanotic heart disease the presence of collateral vessels and surgical shunts will affect the distribution of flow in different parts of the lungs. These variations must be assessed in the context of the known history, the recognised overall pattern of pulmonary vascularity and the features of regional lung disease.

Other chest radiographic features associated with cardiovascular disease

It is very important to assess all the extra information that is available on the chest radiograph so that the presence of underlying cardiac disease can be detected. One area that is easily overlooked is the thoracic cage. The shape of the bony structures is important; pectus excavatum (Fig. 11.13) is important to identify, as this appearance is associated with both Marfan's disease and prolapse of the mitral valve. The definition of pectus excavatum is a narrowed AP thoracic diameter, less than 8 cm, between the anterior border of the vertebral bodies and the sternum.

Another subtle abnormality is the presence of rib notching in the presence of a coarctation of the thoracic aorta, this usually occurs in ribs 3–8. It can rarely be unilateral on the left side only in the presence of an anomalous right subclavian artery. It is unusual to identify this appearance in the asymptomatic adult as most cases are now identified in childhood, but it is important to assess the ribs in the young hypertensive patient.

POSTINTERVENTION CHEST RADIOGRAPHS

The general postoperative chest radiograph

The chest radiograph obtained from the intensive care unit is often obtained in suboptimal conditions; the patient is supine or semierect and often ventilated and the radiograph is portable. The daily chest radiograph is, however, an important integral part of the management of the seriously ill patient. The image is used to assess the position of the lines and tubes and to identify any potential complications, to assess any change in the cardiopulmonary status of the patients and to assess the lungs.

As the portable film is taken in an AP projection, this will lead to an increase in the magnification of the cardiac shadow, which can be increased in size by up to 20%. The upper limit of a cardiothoracic ratio in the AP film has been reported at 57%. Often the patients are supine, making examination of the lungs difficult. In this position there is poor air entry (Fig. 11.14), without ventilation the lungs appearing to be of small volume, and because of the loss of gravitational forces there is redistribution through both lungs. This appearance can mimic upper lobe blood diversion. In addition, the supine position makes the diagnosis of both a pneumothorax and pleural fluid extremely difficult. Due to the redistribution of fluid the only clue can be the small veil-like opacity in the apex. Air in the pleural cavity also rises to the non-dependent portion of the chest; this can be either medial or lateral producing an area of radiolucency.

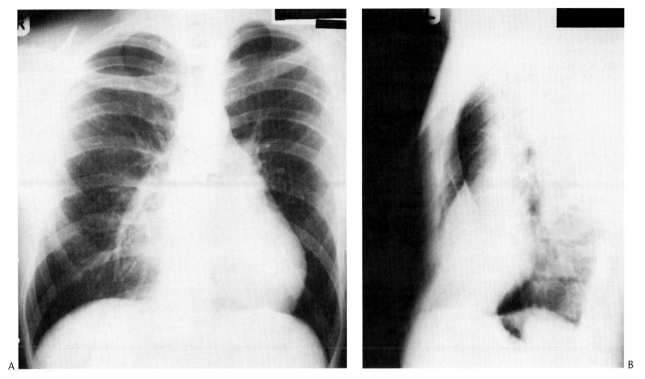

Fig. 11.13 Depressed sternum. (A) Frontal view. The heart is displaced to the left. Its left border is straight and there is a prominence in the position of the main pulmonary artery. There is an ill-defined shadow to the right of the vertebral column. The clue to those appearances is given by the visualisation of the intervertebral discs at the level of the lower thoracic spine where normally they would disappear. (B) Lateral view. This demonstrates the enormous sternal depression. This patient was thought to have a normal heart.

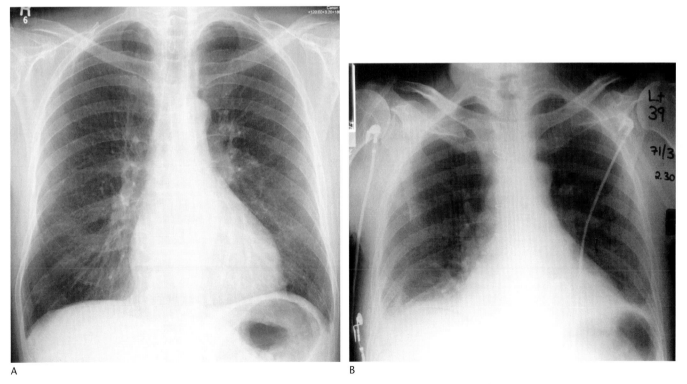

Fig. 11.14 Pre- and post-mitral valve replacement. The preoperative film shows mild cardiac enlargement and pulmonary venous hypertension with good aeration of both lungs (A). On the mobile AP film (B) on the second postoperative day there is poor air entry to the chest leading to basal atelectasis. Small bilateral pleural effusions are also present and the mitral prosthesis can be identified.

Postcardiac surgery

Most adult cardiac operations are performed through a central midline sternotomy with wire midline sutures being used to close the wound. Following cardiac surgery some widening of the mediastinum occurs, due to a combination of bleeding and oedematous change. Marked mediastinal widening can represent major mediastinal haemorrhage, and the necessity to re-explore the chest. The demonstration of a pneumopericardium post procedure is also common. The increased use of the right and left internal mammary arteries for coronary grafting has led to an increase in damage to the underlining pleura during dissection of the vessels, with an increase in the pneumothorax rate.

The distribution of metal clips can indicate which vessels have been used when performing the surgery and should be used in the overall assessment of the surgery (Fig. 11.15). When assessing the immediate postoperative radiograph all the hardware present on the film needs to be assessed to ensure that the tube or catheter has been correctly positioned with no evidence of radiographic complications.

When the patient is ventilated, the position of the endotracheal tube should routinely be assessed. Several important variables need to be considered. The standard endotracheal tube should be two-thirds the width of the normal tracheal and the tip should be between 5 and 7 cm above the carina. This position allows up to 4 cm of movement that can occur when the head is moved from flexion to extension. Any deviation from this position should be interpreted in the context of the patient's head position at the time of the radiograph. The carina is often easily visualised but can be estimated at the level of T5–T7. Complications of ventilation should also be considered and the lungs inspected for the presence of pneumothorax or air within the mediastinum.

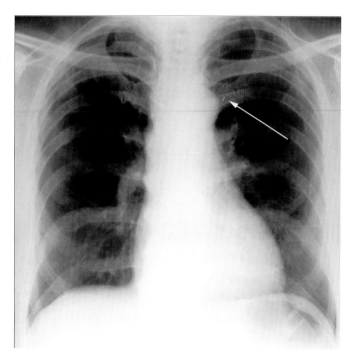

Fig. 11.15 Post cardiac surgery. The midline sternotomy sutures are difficult to visualise on the PA film. There are surgical clips in the anterior mediastinum which have been used to occlude small side branches of the left internal mammary artery (arrow), which has being used as a graft.

Following most cardiac surgery, mediastinal and chest drains are placed prior to the closure of the sternotomy wound. Often there is a straight tube into the anterior mediastinum and an angled tube over the left diaphragm, which tends to lie in a more posterior posi-

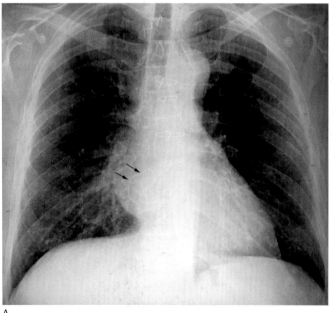

A

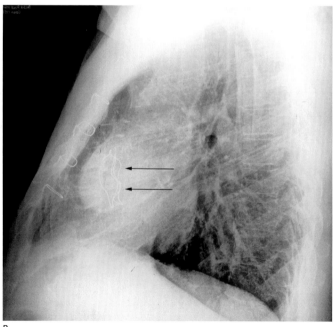

B

Fig. 11.16 Cardiac surgery complication. On the PA chest radiograph (A) the right heart border has an unusual configuration and on closer inspection a metallic strip can be visualised (arrows). This soft-tissue opacity is anterior to the heart and clearly visualised (arrows) on the lateral film (B). This was a retained swab.

tion. These tubes allow both air and fluid to escape in the immediate postoperative period.

Virtually all patients being intensively monitored will have a central line in position to administer drugs and monitor the central venous pressure. Most of these lines are placed via the subclavian or the jugular vein and the tip should be within the distal subclavian vein where possible, avoiding placing the catheter directly into the right atrium. Following percutaneous placement a check radiograph should be obtained in order to assess the position of the catheter tip and to identify any complications (Fig. 11.16).

It is important to be familiar with all the 'hardware' used in the perioperative period (Box 11.1).

It is also important to be aware of the common appearances on the early postoperative chest radiograph, which may include basal collapse, lobar collapse (left > right), linear atelectasis, consolidation, pleural effusion, pericardial effusion, pneumothorax, pneumomediastinum. Box 11.2 outlines typical features that may be seen on postoperative films after coronary artery bypass grafting.

Heart transplantation

Cardiac transplantation is now widely accepted as a form of treatment for end-stage heart disease. The most common complications of heart transplantation are rejection of the donor heart and infections of the lungs and other organs. Lymphoma and other cancers sometimes occur following transplantation. Two methods of transplantation exist; the first is where the donor heart is 'piggy-backed' into the recipient's heart with the native right atrium being preserved. The second method is for the native heart to be completely removed.

The chest radiograph will demonstrate many of the changes previously described associated with a midline sternotomy and cardiac surgery. In addition the chest radiograph can demonstrate an altered configuration of the cardiac contour, this is often a double heart border where there is a double right atrial shadow produced by the lateral position of the native right atrium. If there has been a discrepancy in the size of the donor and native aorta there can be an abrupt change in diameter at the site of anastomosis. In the immediate postoperative period an increase in the cardiothoracic ration can indicate a pericardial effusion, however beyond this period this increase in size can suggest cardiac rejection.

Box 11.1   Devices that may be seen on the postcardiac surgical chest radiograph

Endotracheal tube, tracheostomy
Nasogastric tube, oesophageal temperature line
Central venous line, pulmonary artery catheter, left atrial line
Sternal wires, surgical clips
Epicardial pacing electrodes, temporary pacing wire
Mediastinal/pericardial drain, left or right chest drain
Valve prostheses, annuloplasty rings, conduits
Intra-aortic balloon pump
External devices (ECG, oxygen lines, etc.)

Box 11.2   Features that may be seen on postoperative films after coronary artery bypass grafting

Immediate postoperative film
Patient usually artificially ventilated. Lungs well inflated. Often no focal lesion seen. Check for pneumothorax, position of endotracheal tube, central venous line, site of drains, nature of sternal wires and surgical clips. Note any other 'hardware'

24 hours postoperative film
Lungs often less well aerated than during ventilation. Endotracheal tube removed. Usually no focal lung lesion

48 hours postoperative film
Chest drains removed. Some loss of volume at both bases, usually more on the left side. Possible areas of atelectasis in the midzones. Possible small pleural effusion on the left

4 days postoperative film
Central venous line removed. Probable persisting left lower lobe loss of volume, some improvement in air entry

6 days postoperative film
Continued improvement in air entry. Partial re-expansion of basal collapse

6 weeks postoperative film
Full re-expansion of lungs. Minor residual basal changes

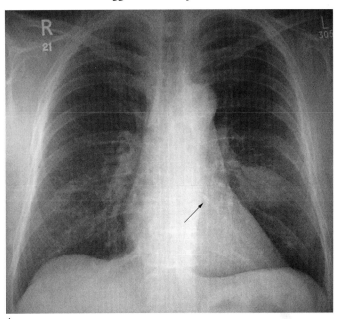

A

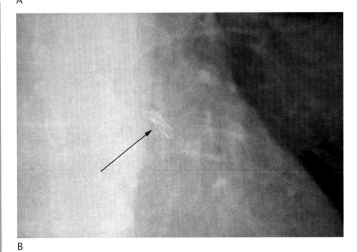

B

Fig. 11.17 Coronary artery stent. This patient presented with a cough. On the PA chest radiograph (A), a 3-cm soft-tissue mass is present due to an adenocarcinoma of the left bronchus. A stent is seen in the left anterior descending coronary artery (arrow). The detailed configuration of the stent is clearly seen (arrow) on the magnified view (B).

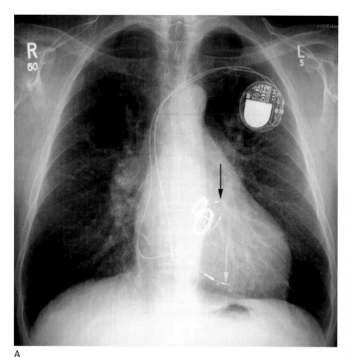

A

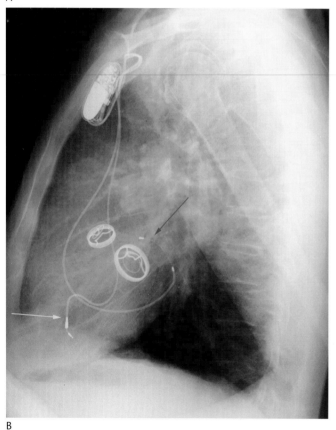

B

Fig. 11.18 Prosthetic mitral and aortic valves with biventricular pacemaker insertion. This treatment for heart failure allows synchronous contraction of both ventricles. There is one lead with its tip in the coronary sinus (black arrow) to pace the left ventricle (A). This position is best visualised on the lateral view (B). The other lead has its tip in the apex of the right ventricle (white arrow).

Occasionally single or multiple nodules can develop after transplantation, in one series this occurred in 10% of recipients, usually between 2 and 6 months post transplantation. In this series the commonest cause was infection usually from *Aspergillus* or *Nocardia*, although in a small percentage of patients the nodule was due to a B-cell lymphoma. In half of the nodules cause by *Aspergillus* cavitation was present. Both *Aspergillus* and *Nocardia* are inhaled which was thought to be the route of infection in these immune-compromised patients.

Implants

Nowadays an increasing number of patients have had previous operative intervention to the heart and it is important to identify any sternal wires, surgical clips, valve prostheses, pacemakers, coronary artery stents (Fig. 11.17) or other signs of previous medical or surgical treatment. There is a great variety of such devices and it is important to identify such implants even if it is not entirely clear as to their nature. Referral to the clinical history will usually resolve the problem. Some of these devices will be seen more clearly on the lateral film. In the case of permanent pacemaker implants it is important to check the lung fields on the immediate postimplantation film in order to exclude pneumothorax. It is also important to check the course of the electrode on successive films in case of possible lead displacement. Current pacing technology is developing rapidly and a variety of lead patterns will be seen including single lead pacing, dual lead pacing (one atrial and one ventricular lead) and biventricular pacing (one lead in the right ventricle and one to the left ventricle via the coronary sinus (Fig. 11.18). Automatic implantable cardiac defibrillators are in increasing use and these resemble permanent pacing systems but they have a larger generator box and a more bulky intracardiac electrode (Fig. 11.19).

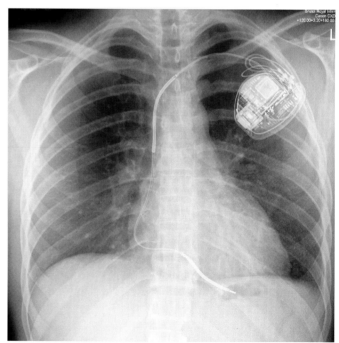

Fig. 11.19 Automatic implantable defibrillator. The electrode is heavier than a normal pacing electrode with additional discharge electrodes in the SVC and the right ventricle. The generator is larger than the current generation pacemaker generators.

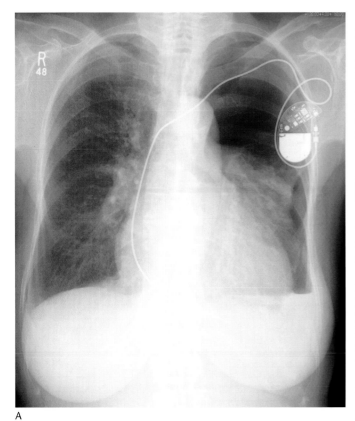

A

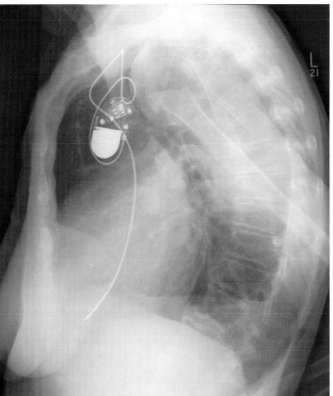

B

Fig. 11.20 Pneumothorax post pacemaker placement. A single-chamber pacemaker has been inserted. The tip is in a good position on both the PA film (A) and lateral film (B) in the apex of the right ventricle. The lateral film taken within 24 hours of pacemaker insertion is obtained using a non-standard method with the arms by the side. There is a large left pneumothorax.

A chest radiograph should routinely be taken in PA and lateral projections after pacemaker implantation to exclude lead displacement, pneumothorax or other complication (Fig. 11.20). In all patients with implanted pacemakers or defibrillators the radiologist must be aware that MRI is absolutely contraindicated as it can cause malfunction of these devices. The remainder of implanted devices are safe in the MRI scanner apart from some of the oldest implanted metallic cardiac valves. In any case of doubt it is important to check on the MRI compatibility of any device.

CORONARY HEART DISEASE

Coronary heart disease is the commonest cause of premature death in the developed world and is the commonest cause of acute medical admission to hospital in developed countries. In the UK alone 1.4 million people suffer from angina and 300 000 people have myocardial infarction each year (Department of Health, National Service Framework in Coronary Heart Disease 2000). This has raised the subject of coronary heart disease to the top of most health priorities and the diagnosis and management of the many forms of this disease are heavily dependent on cardiac imaging techniques.

The process of development of coronary atheroma is complex and multifactorial and depends on a number of risk factors including smoking history, lipid profile, family history, obesity, diet and exercise, hypertension, diabetes and a number of others. Much is still not fully understood about the disease process. The development of atheromatous plaques in the coronary arteries (as with other important arteries elsewhere in the body) can lead to a variety of clinical syndromes according to the nature, site and progress of these plaques. Chronic increase in the size and occlusive nature of the plaques will lead to conditions such as stable angina or ischaemic cardiomyopathy. Acute changes, especially plaque rupture, will lead to a variety of 'acute coronary syndromes', the most important of which will be unstable angina and myocardial infarction.

Stable angina

The investigation of stable angina is predominantly clinical and will depend heavily on clinical symptoms and the ECG. A stress study, in most cases an exercise ECG study, is usually needed for the diagnosis. The chest radiograph of a patient with stable angina is usually normal unless there have been previous events such as myocardial infarction or other coexisting heart disease which have altered the heart size and pulmonary vascularity. Careful examination of the penetrated film may reveal some abnormalities.

Coronary artery calcification is best seen in the proximal left coronary artery and may be identified near the aortic root on both PA and lateral views (Fig. 11.21). The significance of this finding is dependent on the patient's age. In the elderly, over 70, the finding is common and may not relate directly to plaque calcification but may simply be due to degenerative calcification in the vessel walls. In patients under 50 years of age, however, the finding is highly significant and will usually indicate calcified atheromatous plaques. There is intermediate significance between 50 and 70 years of age. In some cases of hyperlipidaemia there may be prominent calcified plaques in the aortic root just above the sinuses of Valsalva. This is

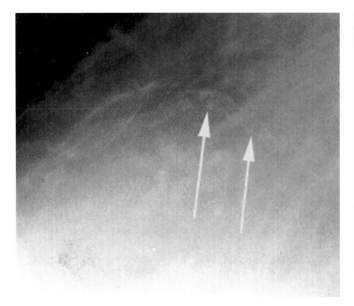

Fig. 11.21   Coronary calcification. Calcification of the coronary arteries is often best seen on the lateral view. The calcification of the vessels is shown well on this magnified view (arrows).

normally an uncommon site for aortic calcification and if this finding is present it should raise the probability of coronary heart disease.

In patients who have had stable angina for many years but who have never had a documented myocardial infarction, there may still be left ventricular damage, presumably due to chronic ischaemia and fibrosis, which may be manifest as a dilated and impaired left ventricle. The diagnostic findings in this condition are very similar to those in other forms of dilated cardiomyopathy.

The definitive diagnosis of stable angina will be made by a combination of functional studies and coronary arteriography.

Acute myocardial infarction

The plain chest radiograph is usually obtained in all patients presenting with acute myocardial infarction. It will be normal in the acute phase (less than 24 hours after onset of symptoms) in the majority of patients if they have had a normal preceding film. The chest radiograph remains an important piece of the diagnostic jigsaw, providing some insight into the severity of the myocardial infarction. In addition, over the course of the acute illness serial films can provide important diagnostic and prognostic information. The larger the infarct and the more acute its onset, the more likely early changes are seen.

The most common feature identified is the development of pulmonary oedema. The features of this can vary, with haziness of the pulmonary arteries at the lung bases and prominence of upper lobe vessels indicating pulmonary venous hypertension. This may progress to perihilar and peripheral parenchymal clouding, leading to the formation of septal lines and alveolar pulmonary oedema. Pleural effusions can develop if the left heart failure is prolonged.

Mortality has been estimated from radiographic features. The presence of pulmonary oedema indicates a one-year mortality of 44%. If there is no evidence of heart failure, this indicates a good prognosis with an 8% one-year mortality.

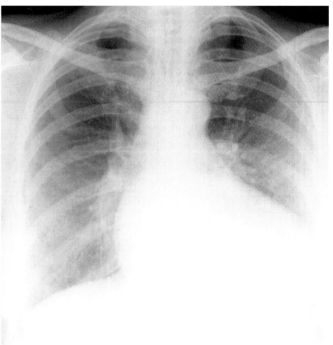

Fig. 11.22   Cardiac failure post myocardial infarction. A previous PA film obtained before the infarction is normal. Marked cardiomegaly is seen 2 weeks after a large anterior myocardial infarction, indicating left ventricular damage. Pulmonary venous hypertension has also developed.

The chest radiographic features of acute myocardial infarction include progressive enlargement of the heart, more often identified in anterior myocardial infarction (Fig. 11.22). If the serial films taken over the first few days or weeks following myocardial infarction show progressive cardiac enlargement, this is an important adverse prognostic sign that should be further evaluated. Comparison of films may be difficult if there is poor or inconsistent technical film quality.

Several of the important complications of an acute myocardial infarction can be suggested from the plain chest radiograph. Although the chest radiograph is not the primary method of diagnosing these conditions, it is a useful adjunct.

Acute mitral regurgitation

The acute left ventricular damage caused by myocardial infarction may precipitate mitral regurgitation by a number of mechanisms. Acute dilatation of the left ventricle will cause annular dilatation and consequent 'functional' mitral regurgitation. An infarct affecting the papillary muscle(s) can lead to malfunction of the mitral closure mechanism and consequent mitral regurgitation. Depending on the severity and the speed of onset, the mitral regurgitation may lead to cardiomegaly or pulmonary venous hypertension but this is not always seen. The chest radiographic features of chronic mitral regurgitation are similar to those produced by other causes of mitral regurgitation.

Rupture of the papillary muscle is rare but devastating, occurring in about 1% of acute myocardial infarction. Rupture of either papillary muscle can occur but it is more common to involve the posterior muscle as a result of an inferior myocardial infarction. The condition carries a grave prognosis with a mortality of near 70% in

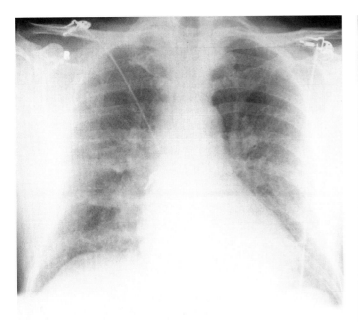

Fig. 11.23 Post myocardial infarction ventricular septal defect. This patient developed breathlessness on day 4 after an acute myocardial infarction. The interventricular septum has ruptured producing left to right shunting and heart failure. There is engorgement of the pulmonary vasculature (pulmonary plethora).

the first 24 hours. The muscular rupture leads to acute mitral valve insufficiency; on the chest radiograph, pulmonary oedema develops with little increase in the cardiac size or more particularly the left atrium. The definitive diagnosis may be hard to make from the chest film and the final diagnosis is clinical and echocardiographic.

Rupture of the interventricular septum

This is also a rare complication of an acute myocardial infarction but is the major differential diagnosis of papillary muscular rupture. This condition occurs in up to 2% of all acute cases. The interventricular septum is most likely to rupture between 4 and 21 days postinfarction, leading to rapid-onset left to right shunting and heart failure. There is engorgement of the pulmonary vasculature (pulmonary plethora) and pulmonary oedema is frequently seen (Fig. 11.23). The definitive diagnosis is clinical and echocardiographic.

Left ventricular rupture

If the profoundly damaged segment of the left ventricle affected by an acute infarct lies in the free wall, then acute rupture into the pericardium can occur. This is normally an acute fatal complication but in rare instances the rupture may be contained in the pericardium and this can lead to the late development of a false aneurysm with cardiomegaly and possible heart failure. The diagnosis of this condition is rarely made acutely.

Left ventricular aneurysm

If an infarcted segment is large and sustains full-thickness ischaemia, then it may develop over a few weeks into a left ventricular aneurysm. This is most commonly seen at the cardiac apex in association with an anterior infarct (Fig. 11.24), but it can also

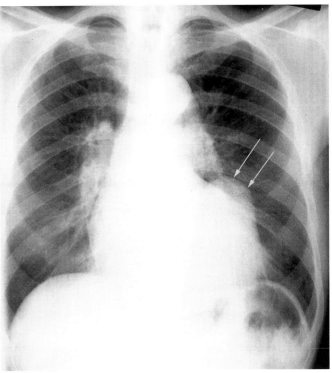

A

B

Fig. 11.24 Anterior left ventricular aneurysm. There is a bulge of the anterior border of the left ventricle shown on both the PA (A) and lateral (B) films (arrows). This patient suffered a large infarct and has developed an anterior aneurysm of the left ventricle.

occur in the posterior position (Fig. 11.25). This may lead to several complications including the development of heart failure or the development of intracardiac thrombus and possible systemic

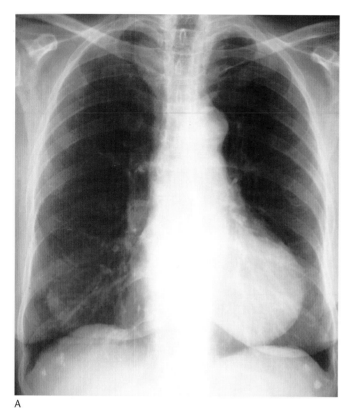

A

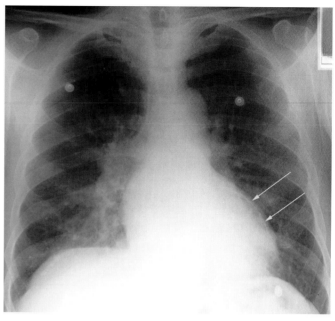

Fig. 11.26 Calcification of a left ventricular aneurysm. In a small number of cases a fine line of calcification within the aneurysm can be identified (arrows).

embolism. The chest radiograph will frequently develop a localised bulge on the left heart border but if the aneurysm is not well demarcated or if it lies in a less prominent position it may not be identified on the plain film. The wall of a longstanding aneurysm (or a non-aneurysmal infarct) may show calcification (Fig. 11.26) .

Pericardial effusion

Acute pericardial effusion is a bad prognostic feature, being most commonly associated with partial ventricular rupture. Later in the course of the condition a pericardial or pleural effusion can occur

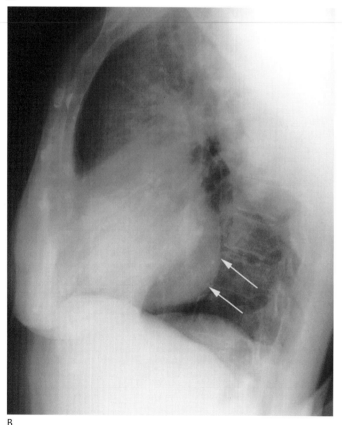

B

Fig. 11.25 Posterior left ventricular aneurysm. The PA chest radiograph shows a sharply defined and rounded left heart border due to the profiling of the margin of the aneurysm (A). The bulge of the posterior border of the left ventricle due to the aneurysm is clearly seen on the lateral film (B) (arrows).

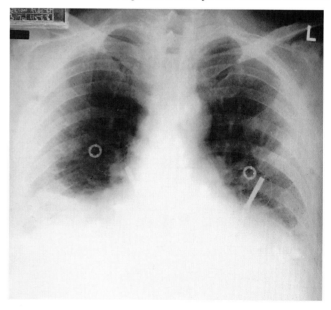

Fig. 11.27 Postmyocardial infarction (Dressler's) syndrome. Small effusions are seen in both costophrenic angles, together with ill-defined basal shadows resembling pulmonary infarcts.

with Dressler's syndrome, which is an inflammatory reaction to the infarct (Fig. 11.27). There may be mild cardiomegaly with this condition.

HEART MUSCLE DISEASE

The development of heart failure without a recognisable cause suggests an underlying abnormality of the heart muscle. The most common cause is dilatation of the left ventricle as a result of coronary heart disease. However, the development of heart failure may be a result of disease of the cardiac muscle, cardiomyopathies. Three distinct types of cardiomyopathies are recognised—dilated, hypertrophic and restrictive—but there can be elements of more than one type in any individual case.

Dilated cardiomyopathy

The classic features of a dilated cardiomyopathy are the dilatation of the left ventricle with impairment of ventricular emptying, leading to a reduction in the ejection fraction. The condition is often postviral but the cause is often not found.

The plain film is often abnormal, demonstrating cardiac enlargement of all four chambers or of just the left ventricle. Rarely the dilatation of the left ventricle is demonstrated on the lateral film only. In the untreated patient there is often volume overload of the left atrium leading to engorgement of the pulmonary vasculature. The dilatation of the ventricle is a compensatory mechanism, and it is by this compensation that some patients may have very poor left

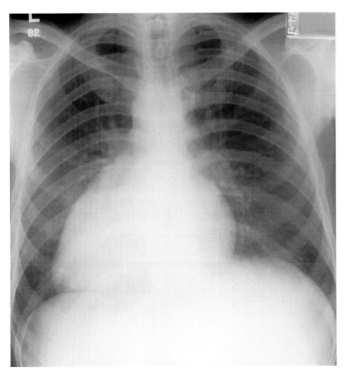

Fig. 11.28 Ischaemic cardiomyopathy. There is biventricular dilatation of the ventricles producing a globular large heart in this patient with ischaemic cardiac failure.

ventricular function but the pulmonary vascularity remains within normal limits. These individuals, however, have very poor reserves and can easily run into heart failure with any minor adverse circulatory event. The right ventricle may also be prominent in ischaemic cardiomyopathy (Fig. 11.28).

The differential diagnosis of dilated cardiomyopathy is wide and includes ischaemic changes, left ventricular aneurysm or valvular disease. The diagnosis cannot be made on the chest radiograph alone.

Hypertrophic cardiomyopathy

More than half the patients with hypertrophic cardiomyopathy (HCM) have a normal chest radiograph. In those who do show changes, these are often non-specific. The most common abnormality is pulmonary venous hypertension as a result of the reduction in left ventricular compliance. There may be evidence of left atrial enlargement, but the overall heart size remains normal. In a very small number of patients a degree of focal enlargement of the heart does occur. This is a result of extreme enlargement of the outflow portion of the left ventricle producing a prominent convexity on the upper left heart border. In general this diagnosis is not made on the chest radiograph.

Restrictive cardiomyopathy

This is the least common of all cardiomyopathies, occurring as either an idiopathic primary disease or as a result of various forms of infiltration into the left ventricle wall. The functional abnormality is essentially an impairment of diastolic function of the left ventricle. This means that the compliance of the ventricle is poor and it requires a higher pressure to fill the chamber. Systolic function (as measured by ejection fraction) is usually maintained. Types of disease processes that infiltrate the wall include sarcoidosis, haemochromatosis and amyloid, all producing a reduction in the left ventricular compliance without an increase in muscle wall volume.

The heart size is normal with left atrial enlargement and pulmonary venous hypertension, features mimicking mitral valve disease, which is the major differential diagnosis. In some cases there is coexisting right ventricular restrictive change which produces right atrial dilatation in addition. As the disease process progresses there is often late ventricular dilatation, producing mild to moderate cardiomegaly on the plain film. Unlike other cardiomyopathies the chest radiograph does produce an assessment of the severity of the disease in this condition. The radiographic development and progression of pulmonary venous hypertension reflects the overall reduction in left ventricular compliance.

ACQUIRED VALVE DISEASE

There is a wide variety of structural change that can affect the heart valves, but in terms of their function valvular disease can either be pure stenosis or pure regurgitation, or more likely a combination of both. The appreciation of the dynamics of flow through the cardiac chambers is important and allows the interpreter to assess from the features on the radiograph exactly what changes are occurring at the valvular level.

Aortic valve disease

Aortic stenosis

Rheumatic heart fever leading to the inflammatory fusion of the commissures is a less likely cause of aortic stenosis in the current era, with the most common reason for the development of aortic stenosis in adult life being changes secondary to a congenital bicuspid valve.

Significant aortic stenosis may be present with a virtually normal heart shadow although it is rare not to detect some evidence of ventricular enlargement in either the frontal or lateral view. The chest radiograph often shows rounding of the left ventricular apex indicative of left ventricular hypertrophy. There is also dilatation of the ascending aortic arch, a result of the impact of the stenotic jet on the vessel wall (Fig. 11.29). The poststenotic dilatation caused by this jet is variable as the jet itself will vary in direction from patient to patient. The degree of dilatation does not correlate with the severity of stenosis. These appearances can be difficult to detect in the older patient in whom the aorta often becomes unfolded and slightly dilated.

On the lateral film the presence of calcification in the position of the aortic valve is an important sign, usually indicating important valve stenosis. Some authors suggest this calcification represents severe aortic stenosis with a gradient of at least 50 mmHg.

In most cases of aortic stenosis the pulmonary vascularity is normal but in advanced cases there will be left ventricular impairment and associated changes of heart failure. In patients with aortic stenosis, normal pulmonary vascularity should not be taken as an indication that the stenosis is mild.

Aortic regurgitation

There are many causes of aortic regurgitation including damage to the valvular cusps as a result of either endocarditis or rheumatic fever, dilatation of the aortic root due to Marfan's syndrome or degenerative ectasia of the root, and also as a solitary consequence of bicuspid aortic valve. The condition can occur in combination with aortic stenosis. Occasionally aortic regurgitation can develop as a complication of a primary disease of the aortic wall, such as aortitis. A dissection of the aorta can produce valvular regurgitation if the false lumen dissects towards the aortic valve ring.

The appearances described are those that develop in association with chronic aortic regurgitation. The plain radiograph demonstrates a large heart with a predominantly left ventricular configuration. The heart size reflects the severity of the disease. Calcification of the aortic valve is not a feature of pure aortic regurgitation but can be visualised if there is a combination of regurgitation and stenosis. The ascending aorta and often the aortic arch are large, and can sometimes be visualised as a bulge on the right of the mediastinum. In many patients with pure aortic regurgitation there is excellent compensation for the increased flow in the left ventricle and there is normal pulmonary vasculature. The combination of a large left ventricle, no other chamber enlargement and normal pulmonary vessels is very suggestive of severe chronic aortic regurgitation (Fig. 11.30).

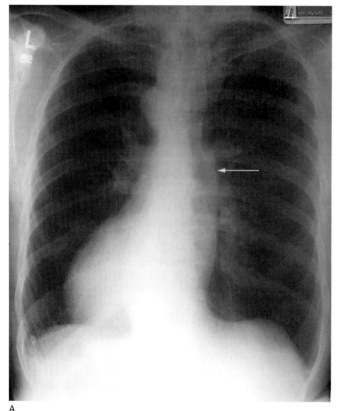
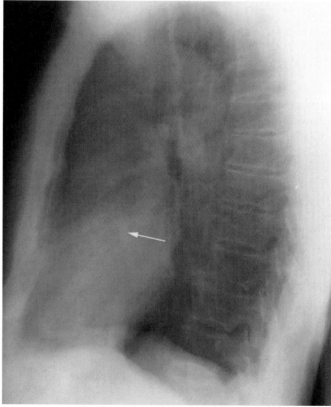

A   B

Fig. 11.29   Calcified aortic stenosis. The heart has a slightly prominent left ventricular contour on the PA chest radiograph and there is dilatation of the ascending aortic arch (arrow) caused by the poststenotic dilatation (A). Calcification of the aortic valve (arrow) is more apparent on the lateral film (B).

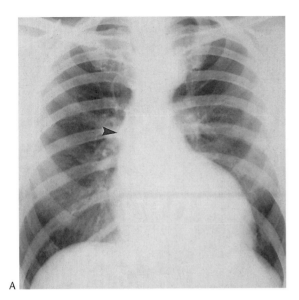

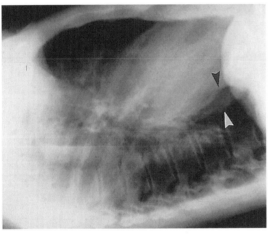

Fig. 11.30 Gross left ventricular dilatation from chronic aortic incompetence. (A) The axis of the heart is elongated to the left with rounding of the apex. There is slight prominence of the ascending aorta (black arrow). (B) The body of the left ventricle (white arrow) can be seen bulging behind the line of the right atrium (black arrow).

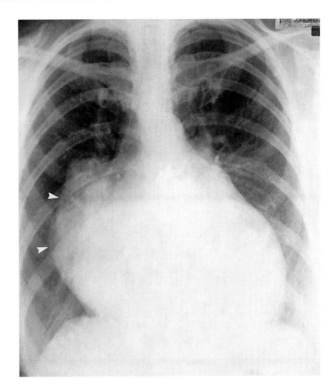

Fig. 11.31 Left atrial dilatation in mitral stenosis. The grossly enlarged left atrium (arrows) extends beyond the right heart border. Note that the border of the right atrium can be identified where it is joined by the IVC coming up through the diaphragm.

Mitral valve disease

Mitral stenosis

The most common cause of mitral stenosis is rheumatic fever. The reduction of flow occurs as a result of fusion of the leaflet commissures. In addition, thickening of the valve leaflets occurs with shortening and thickening of the chordae tendinae which further restricts valve movement. The symptoms of flow restriction (dyspnoea and heart failure) may be few until the valve becomes critically narrowed. The condition does however predispose to thrombus formation in the left atrium and consequent systemic embolus. The condition may present with a systemic embolism.

The chest radiograph demonstrates selective left atrial enlargement, which can vary from trivial to gross (Fig. 11.31). If the mitral stenosis is a result of rheumatic fever there is often marked enlargement of the left atrial appendage, which forms a bulge on the left

heart border just below the main pulmonary artery. This enlargement can again range from the trivial to the marked with a large protrusion. In the early years of this chronic disease there is often a normal heart size with only subtle signs of left atrial enlargement being evident (Fig. 11.32). In causes of unexplained heart failure with a normal heart size it is important not to overlook mitral stenosis. Even in late stages of the condition, the atria may be large but the left ventricular contour is still of small radius, indicating the small size of the ventricular chamber.

If the mitral stenosis is both severe and longstanding then calcification of the valve can develop. This feature is best visualised in the lateral position (Fig. 11.33) but can sometimes be visualised in the PA projection if the film is penetrated. This calcification needs to be differentiated from the far more common C- or J-shaped calcification that occurs in the valve annulus (Fig. 11.34). In severe mitral valve disease with associated atrial fibrillation, calcification of the left atrium, or thrombus within the left atrium, can occur.

The development of mitral stenosis can lead to marked changes in the pulmonary circulation that can be identified on the plain film. These changes result from a chronically raised left atrial pressure. Often there is upper lobe blood diversion, with enlargement of the main and central pulmonary arteries indicating pulmonary arterial hypertension. The right-sided cardiac chambers will often be considerably enlarged and the presence of a 'double right heart border' is often due to considerable enlargement of both atria. A very large left atrium, aneurysmal if it reaches to within 2.5 cm of the thoracic wall, may be associated with segmental or even lobar collapse. This is more common on the right side.

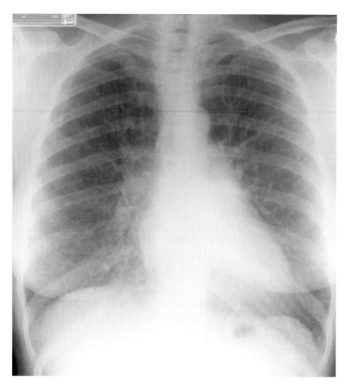

Fig. 11.32 Mitral stenosis with a normal size heart. In the early years of this chronic disease there is often a normal heart size with only subtle signs of left atrial enlargement being evident. The left atrial appendage is prominent and there is pulmonary venous hypertension.

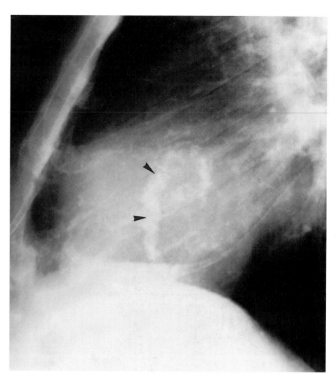

Fig. 11.34 Calcification in the mitral ring. In this lateral view the calcified mitral valve ring (arrows) appears as a characteristic C-shape; it may take a J-shape.

Mitral stenosis is one of the causes of longstanding pulmonary venous hypertension and thus chronic features may be visible which are not seen in conditions with a shorter natural history. Haemosiderosis and pulmonary ossific nodules may occasionally be seen (Fig. 11.35).

Mitral regurgitation

The commonest cause of mitral regurgitation in western countries is degeneration of the valve. There are several variants of this degeneration, including myxomatous degeneration of the valve tissue with prolapse of part or all of the valve. Degeneration of the chordae can lead to rupture and a consequent flail portion of leaflet,

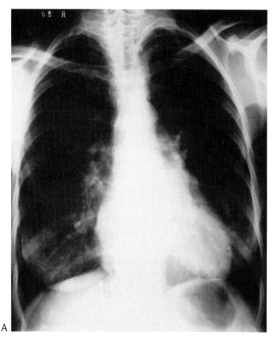

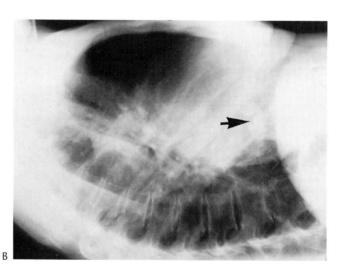

Fig. 11.33 (A, B) Calcified mitral valve in rheumatic mitral stenosis. The calcification is best seen in the lateral view (arrow).

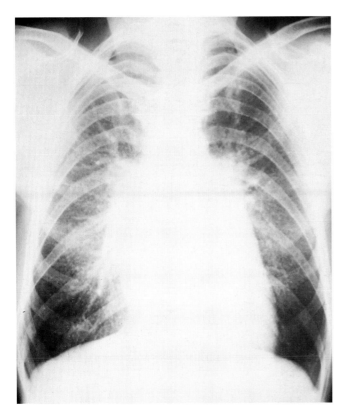

Fig. 11.35 Pulmonary haemosiderosis secondary to longstanding mitral valve disease. The fine granular background pattern to the lung is typical of haemosiderosis. In addition, note changes suggestive of mitral valve disease: straightening of the left heart border and some upper-lobe blood diversion.

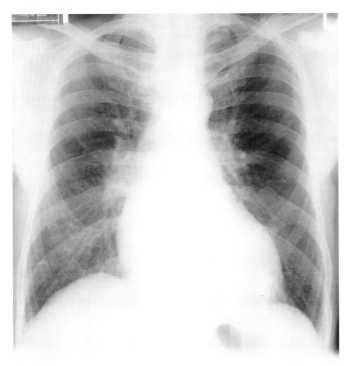

Fig. 11.36 Longstanding severe mitral regurgitation due to mitral valve prolapse. There is prominence of the left ventricular contour and subtle evidence of left atrial enlargement. There is also pulmonary venous hypertension.

this condition often occurring with abrupt onset of symptoms as the chordae rupture. Infective endocarditis will also cause damage of the valve with consequent regurgitation but this will usually be on an already abnormal valve. In the case of an impaired left ventricle, mitral regurgitation can occur due to annular dilatation or papillary muscle dysfunction.

In most of these cases the plain film appearances are very different from those of mitral regurgitation associated with rheumatic disease. In the chronic phase the heart tends to enlarge with a left ventricular configuration, left atrial enlargement being proportionately less prominent with enlargement of the left atrial appendage occurring rarely (Fig. 11.36). In longstanding cases, however, there can still be very marked left atrial enlargement. Calcification does not occur. If the mitral valve prolapse is associated with Marfan's disease there may also be enlargement of the aortic root. In the acute phase the heart size is likely to remain normal even in the presence of a high left atrial pressure. This high pressure in the acute phase often leads to the formation of acute pulmonary oedema (Fig. 11.37).

The regurgitation associated with rheumatic fever results from the destruction of the actual cusps, usually at the free edges leading to leakage. The commonest result of rheumatic valve disease is a combination of both stenosis and regurgitation. The valve fails to open fully in diastole, but the thickened and rolled edges of the cusps do not fully coapt (seal).

The pulmonary vascular appearances are very similar to those of mitral stenosis but the heart is often larger. There is often greater enlargement of the left atrium, which can be massive or even aneurysmal. The presence of left ventricular dilatation in mitral regurgitation (seen as enlargement of the left ventricular contour with a larger radius curve) will indicate left ventricular volume overload or end-stage left ventricular dilatation.

Tricuspid valve disease

The tricuspid valve is very commonly regurgitant as a consequence of left-sided heart disease but it is unusual for the secondary effects to cause diagnostic changes on the chest radiograph. It is relatively rare to see primary tricuspid valve disease, which can occur as a complication of bacterial endocarditis or as a late feature of rheumatic heart disease. Often the endocarditis in tricuspid valve disease is a complication of intravenous drug abuse and the most common pathogen is staphylococcal. As well as cardiac manifestations there is often consolidation within the lungs, this often progressing to cavitation. A number of congenital conditions will affect tricuspid valve function.

Metastatic carcinoid disease will also affect the right-sided heart valves, producing deformity and some regurgitation of both tricuspid and pulmonary valves.

Important tricuspid valve disease will cause enlargement of the right atrium, producing a prominent, bulging or elongated right heart border (Fig. 11.38). This appearance has a single margin and is distinct from the 'double heart border' produced by left atrial enlargement. The difference can be distinguished by the position of entry of the IVC, this structure limiting the expansion of the right atrium. Significant cardiomegaly can be caused by right atrial enlargement.

Pulmonary valve disease

It is very rare to see acquired disease of the pulmonary valve. Carcinoid disease and endocarditis can occasionally affect the valve.

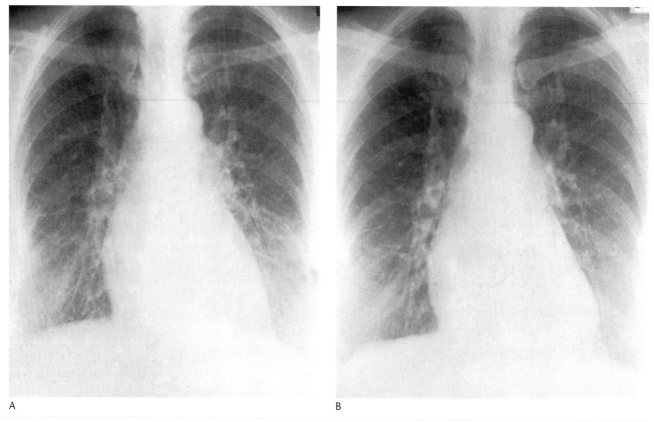

Fig. 11.37 Acute non-rheumatic mitral regurgitation. (A) Frontal view in the acute phase. The heart size is virtually normal, even in the presence of high left atrial pressure as evidenced by the preferential dilatation of the upper-lobe vessels and interstitial oedema. (B) Frontal film 2 weeks later. This shows clearing of the oedema though upper-lobe blood diversion can still be seen.

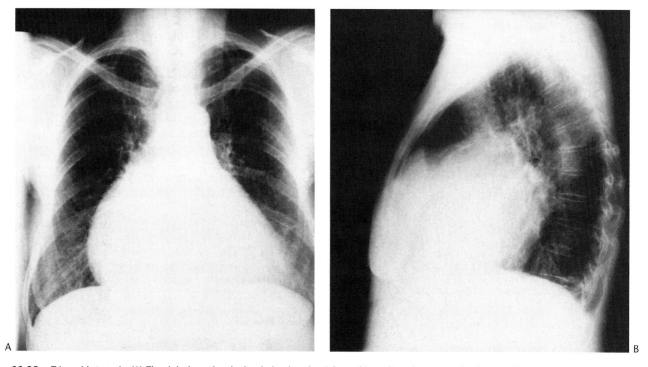

Fig. 11.38 Tricuspid stenosis. (A) The right heart border has bulged to the right and its radius of curvature has increased. (B) In the lateral view, the gap between the front of the heart and the sternum is filled in.

PERICARDIAL DISEASE

The normal pericardial sac is composed of two layers separated by a space containing a few millilitres of fluid. The outer layer of parietal pericardium is a tough fibrous sac enclosing the heart and attached to the central tendon of the diaphragm. The inner or visceral pericardium is closely associated with the surface of the heart. Both layers are fused to the heart at the entry of the pulmonary veins to the left atrium and at the entry of the inferior vena cava. The pericardial reflection extends up the ascending aorta, fusing with the structure about half way between the aortic valve and the innominate artery. The pericardium also extends along the main pulmonary artery, fusing with it before the artery bifurcates.

On a chest radiograph the pericardium has the same radiographic density as the heart. However, sometimes a substantial amount of epicardial fat is present and this leads to identification of the pericardium, the radiolucent fat line lying within the cardiac shadow (Fig. 11.39). Pericardial fat pads, which develop in the cardiophrenic angles, are often visualised as low-density triangles and can occasionally be quite large and can alter the cardiac silhouette. In the assessment of cardiac size on the chest radiograph the fat pads should be ignored.

Pericardial effusion

The main causes of pericardial effusion are listed in Box 11.3.

A pericardial effusion is the commonest abnormality of the pericardium that is encountered in clinical practice. Symptoms of a

---

Box 11.3   Main causes of pericardial effusion

Transudates
  Heart failure
  Hypoalbuminaemia
  Uraemia
Exudates
  Viral infection (pericarditis or myocarditis)
  Acute or chronic bacterial infection (including tuberculosis)
  Inflammation (e.g. Dressler's syndrome)
  Tumour (malignant infiltration or invasion) (Fig. 11.40)
Haemopericardium
  Postcardiac surgery
  Perforation of the heart by catheter (angiogram, pacemaker or angioplasty)
  Bleeding disorders (including anticoagulation)

---

pericardial effusion depend on the rapidity with which the fluid collects. Three hundred millilitres of rapidly accumulating fluid can cause more symptoms than a chronic effusion of more than a litre.

The appearances that can be identified on the plain film depend on the amount of fluid present. A very large collection of fluid can cause massive enlargement of the cardiac shadow. This shadow has a rounded, globular appearance with no particular chamber enlargement being identified. It is often noted that the cardiac contour is very clearly demarcated, this being due to the static outer margin of the distended pericardial sac. If large enough the effusion will lead to an obstruction of the venous return to the right heart, which leads to a reduction of flow and pressure through the lungs. This produces the characteristic appearance of a large effusion on the plain film of

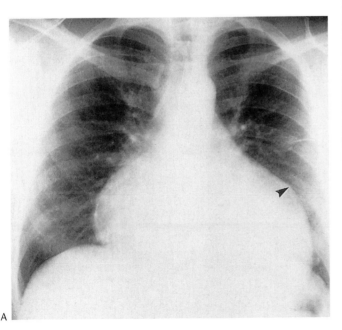

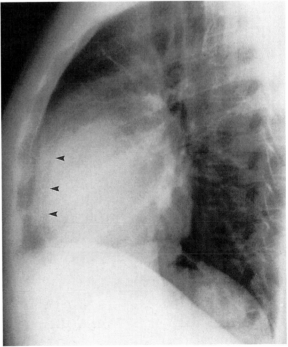

A   B

Fig. 11.39   Pericardial effusion. A chest film taken 6 months previously was normal. (A) Frontal chest film. The heart silhouette has dramatically increased in size. There is an ill-defined bulge (arrow) above the cardiac apex. The lungs show no features of cardiac failure, which might be expected if this were a dilated heart. (B) Lateral chest film. Epicardial fat is clearly identified (arrows), displaced away from the edge of the cardiac silhouette and indicating the presence of a pericardial effusion.

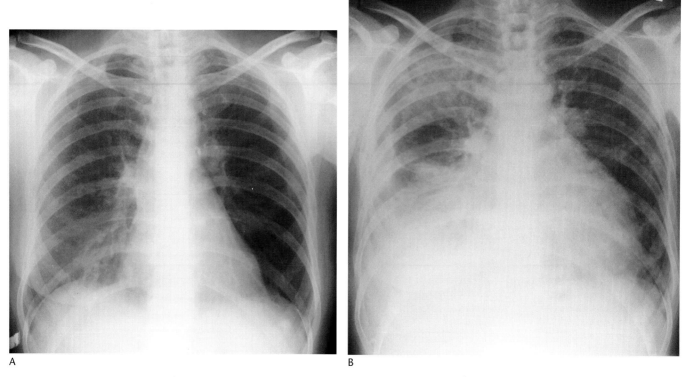

A   B

Fig. 11.40 Pericardial effusion. The first film in a patient who has had a left mastectomy for a carcinoma of the breast demonstrates a normal heart (A). However, during the course of treatment the patient became breathless and a follow-up film (B) shows marked enlargement of the cardiac silhouette as a result of a malignant pericardial effusion. A right-sided pleural effusion has also developed.

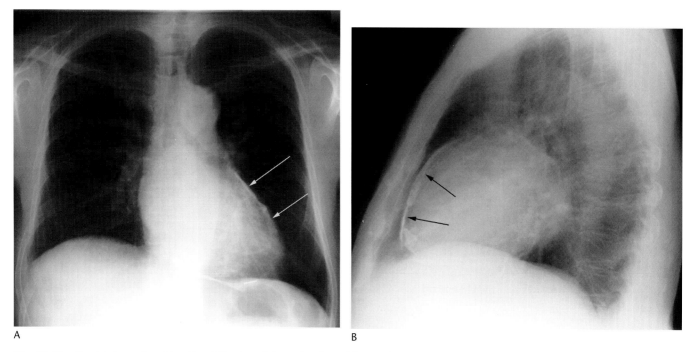

A   B

Fig. 11.41 Constrictive pericarditis with calcification of the pericardium. Often with constrictive pericarditis there is straightening of the right heart border and roughening of the cardiac outline as a result of pleuropericardial thickening. Calcification often has a characteristic distribution involving the anterior and lateral aspects of the heart as shown on the PA (A) and lateral films (B) (arrows).

a large globular heart with clear rather than congested lungs. The other feature often demonstrated is a rapidly increasing heart size on several serial films as the effusion accumulates. Drainage of a large effusion will lead to an abrupt decrease in cardiac size.

Constrictive pericarditis

This condition is a result of inflammation of the pericardial sac leading to thickening and a reduction in compliance; this leads to a reduction in left ventricular filling. The commonest causes are viral and tuberculous but a haemopericardium or infiltrative process can lead to the development of this condition.

On the plain film the heart is often normal but can be non-specifically enlarged. Straightening of the right heart border and roughening of the cardiac outline as a result of pleuro-pericardial adhesions have been described. Calcification has been described in approximately half of the cases; it often has a characteristic distribution involving the front and lateral aspects of the heart (Fig. 11.41). Calcification does not occur at the back of the heart as fluid cannot collect around the insertion of the pulmonary veins. The presence of calcification in the atrioventricular groove can obstruct left atrial emptying and pulmonary oedema can develop but calcification may not necessarily be associated with constriction. The lungs are usually clear due to constriction over the right heart, although a pleural effusion is not uncommon.

MASSES AND TUMOURS

The most common 'masses' associated with the heart are the pericardial fat pads, these arise from the cardiophrenic angle but can

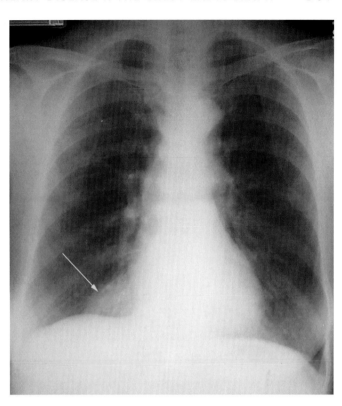

Fig. 11.42 Cardiac fat pad. There is a low-density soft-tissue opacity adjacent to the right heart border (arrow). The triangular nature of the lesion with the characteristic position suggests the diagnosis of a pericardial fat pad.

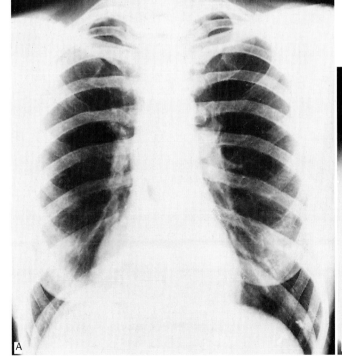

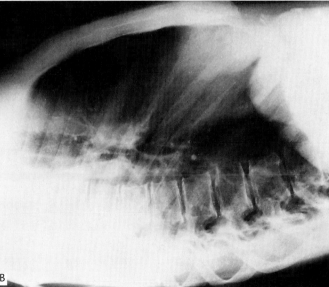

Fig. 11.43 Pericardial cyst. (A) Frontal chest radiograph, there is a sharply defined abnormal shadow in the right pericardiophrenic angle. (B) Lateral view. This is seen to lie anteriorly, and is one of the characteristic sites for a pericardial cyst.

mimic disease. The triangular nature of the lesion with the characteristic position suggests the diagnosis (Fig. 11.42). A benign pericardial or springwater cyst is usually unilocular and is intimately related to the pericardium. The cyst is thin walled, occurring in the lower half of the mediastinum, and is more common on the right (Fig. 11.43). It does communicate with the pericardial cavity and the diagnosis is usually straightforward on the plain radiograph. The cyst is rounded, sharply defined and is usually situated in the anterior cardiophrenic angle. The differential diagnosis includes a Morgagni hernia in the elderly that can be filled with omentum; an echocardiogram will differentiate the two conditions. An isolated pericardial defect is usually left sided and will allow prolapse of the left atrium beyond the normal left heart contour (Fig. 11.44). Other uncommon masses adjacent to or in continuity with the heart border include aneurysmal coronary fistulas and multiple infective pericardial cysts, tuberculous or hydatid (Figs 11.45, 11.46).

Tumours of the heart

Primary tumours

A primary tumour of the heart is rare, and the majority are benign. The most common is the myxoma, accounting for up to 50% of cardiac tumours, but other less common examples include a rhabdomyoma or fibroma. The clinical manifestation and radiological changes depend on the site of the tumour, most intracavity tumours are pedunculated and mobile causing obstruction and embolic symptoms whereas an infiltrating tumour is much more likely to produce an arrhythmia or cardiac failure.

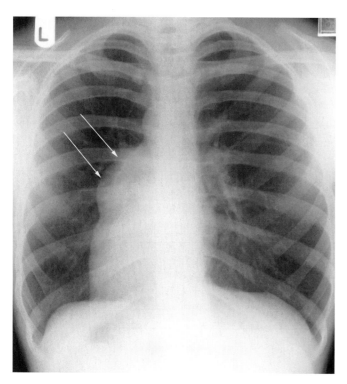

Fig. 11.44 A congenital pericardial defect. An isolated pericardial defect is usually left sided (arrows) and can allow prolapse of the left atrium beyond the normal left heart contour.

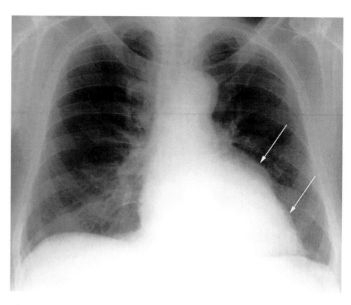

Fig. 11.45 Pericardial cysts. The outline of the left ventricle has an undulating appearance (arrows); this was due to the presence of multiple pericardial cysts, which were tuberculous in origin.

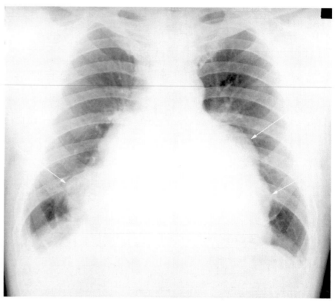

Fig. 11.46 Hydatid pericardial disease. Multiple large cysts (arrows) distort the cardiac outline.

Myxoma

The atrial myxoma is the most common benign tumour of the heart. It occurs most frequently in middle age, 30–60 years, and has an association with pituitary adenoma, testicular tumours and Cushing's disease.

The symptoms are often non-specific with a relatively short history and often rapid progression. Malaise, fever, arthralgia and weight loss have all been described. On examination there is often a tachyarrhythmia and a murmur that is positional. The patient may rarely develop finger clubbing. Embolic complications can also develop. A raised ESR and anaemia can often be detected.

The most common location for an atrial myxoma is within the left atrium attached to the left side of the interatrial septum.

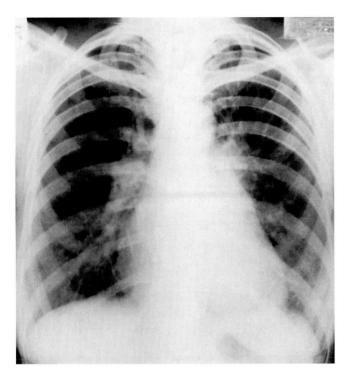

Fig. 11.47 Left atrial myxoma. The chest X-ray shows selective enlargement of the left atrium; the left atrial appendage is also enlarged.

The plain film appearances can vary from a normal examination to an enlarged heart with selective left atrial and left atrial appendage enlargement (Fig. 11.47). Rarely if obstruction develops upper lobe blood diversion can occur leading to the development of pulmonary oedema. Calcification of a mxyoma has been reported with associated movement detected on fluoroscopy.

Secondary tumours

The most common secondary tumour involvement of the heart originates from either carcinoma of the breast or bronchus. This, according to postmortem studies, occurs frequently, but rarely manifests clinically. The most frequent abnormality is the development of a large pericardial effusion from direct pericardial involvement.

THORACIC AORTA

The thoracic aorta is the main vessel of the systemic circulation, carrying 5 litres of blood per minute to the brain and all other parts of the body. The anatomy of the thoracic aorta is often poorly understood, as the vessel is composed of four anatomical regions, the aortic root, the ascending aorta, the aortic arch and the isthmus and descending aorta.

The aortic root is the region from the aortic valve annulus to the superior margin of the sinuses of Valsalva. This area is composed of three sinuses, and gives rise to the first aortic branches, the coronary arteries. Above the sinuses of Valsalva is the ascending aorta, a 4–8-cm segment that arches superiorly, rightwards and then posteriorly to the origin of the right brachiocephalic artery. This is usually situated at the level of the fourth/fifth thoracic vertebrae. The diam-

eter of the ascending aorta is variable and will be discussed more in Chapter 12 on cross-sectional imaging.

The arch of the aorta gives rise to the brachiocephalic branches and then extends to the aortic isthmus, a region of slight narrowing, especially in the child. This is an important anatomical region. It is the point at which the thoracic aorta becomes fixed, by both the left subclavian artery and thoracic arteries, and is therefore the region that is most prone to transection in an injury where rapid acceleration and deceleration occur. The aorta then passes inferiorly to the level of the twelfth thoracic vertebra where it passes through the diaphragm to enter the abdomen. The aorta is fixed by the aortic valve, the vessels of the head and neck, the ligamentum arteriosum and the diaphragm. Despite this there is a great deal of movement of the ascending aorta throughout the normal cardiac cycle, in contrast to the posterior segment that remains relatively fixed. The wall of the aorta is extremely durable, allowing changes in both pressure and flow rates; it is composed of three layers, the intima, the media and the adventitia. The intima is a thin inner lining that is easily damaged, the media provides the vessel's strength with spiralling elastic layers of elastic tissue and the adventitia is the layer that contains the supportive tissue and the aorta's blood supply, the vasa vasorum.

Aortic dissection

Aortic dissection is a devastating disease that occurs as a result of degeneration of the thoracic aorta. Despite modern treatment the mortality from this condition remains high, with death in 25% of patients with a dissection of the ascending aorta within the first 24 hours and a mortality of over 75% within the first month. The major contributing factor is hypertension and the incidence is between 5 and 10 cases per million population. Middle-aged men are the most often affected with only 5% of dissections occurring in the under 40 age group. Aortic dissection in younger patients usually occurs in high-risk groups such as patients with Marfan's syndrome, Ehlers–Danlos disease or in pregnancy. There is also an association with aortic valve disease. In many cases there is associated aneurysmal dilatation of the aorta.

The primary event still remains unclear and there is debate to whether the dissection is caused by rupture of the intima with secondary extension into the media or a haemorrhagic event within the diseased media followed by disruption of the adjacent intima and propagation through the intimal tear. However caused, the most common pattern of dissection involves the right anterior aspect of the ascending aorta and the posterior left lateral aspect of the descending aorta. Dissection in the descending aorta can extend down to the abdominal aorta and may lead then to dissection of the left renal artery with associated ischaemic change.

The classic clinical presentation is a sudden onset of a razor-sharp pain between the shoulder blades but many cases are atypical, making diagnosis difficult. Accurate and prompt diagnosis is important, as early surgical treatment of a dissection of the ascending aorta can dramatically reduce mortality. There are two major types of classification, the De Bakey and the Stanford.

De Bakey introduced a classification of three divisions:

• *De Bakey Type I.* A dissection commences in the ascending aorta and extends through the arch into the descending portion, sometimes as far as the iliac arteries. Occurs in 45% of cases.

- *De Bakey Type II.* A dissection commences in the ascending aorta but does not extend further than the aortic arch. This is an uncommon pattern of dissection occurring in only 10% of cases, but is the most common type in patients with Marfan's disease.
- *De Bakey Type III.* A dissection that commences in the descending arch, beyond the origin of the brachiocephalic arteries, and extends into the abdominal aorta. This type of dissection is often treated by a reduction of blood pressure. Occurs in 45% of patients.

The Stanford classification is simpler with two types of dissection described, Type A and Type B. Type A is equivalent to a De Bakey Type I or Type II dissection, involving the ascending arch, whereas Type B just involves the descending aorta. Type A is generally treated with urgent surgery with Type B generally being treated conservatively.

It is essential to understand the descriptive terms used in aortic disease. These are commonly used incorrectly and it is essential to be aware that dissection, aneurysm and rupture can all occur separately or together in any combination. Correct interpretation of any imaging technique should evaluate the possibility of each of these entities (Box 11.4).

The signs apparent on the chest radiograph are often subtle and comparison with any previous films is particularly useful. The most common abnormality is widening of the mediastinum, which occurs in 50–80% of cases. This is often associated with an indistinct

outline of the aorta or an irregular wavy contour. Loss of clarity of the anatomy implies mediastinal haematoma due to aortic rupture or associated vascular damage. A more characteristic but a less frequent radiological finding is localised dilatation of the aortic knuckle and upper descending aorta, giving rise to a prominent hump sign which will indicate aneurysmal dilatation or unfolding of the arch. Lateral displacement of either the trachea or oesophagus (sometimes identified by the course of a nasogastric tube) has also been described (Fig. 11.48). In addition the descending aorta may bulge to the left.

The medial displacement of a calcified plaque of intima at the aortic knuckle has been described but this is a rare finding and can be difficult to visualise. A pleural effusion caused by blood in the chest occurs in about 20% of cases.

Traumatic aortic transection

This is a devastating condition caused by the forces exerted on the thoracic aorta by a rapid declaration. The most common cause of such a force is a road traffic accident. This condition can be extremely difficult to diagnose on both clinical and radiological evidence, particularly as two-thirds of patients will have multiple other injuries. Prompt diagnosis is required however, as this condition has a time-related mortality. The longer the diagnosis and subsequent treatment takes, the higher the mortality is likely to be. The mortality overall is extremely high, 80% of patients dying within the first hour, 85% of patients within the first 24 hours

---

Box 11.4   Aortic lesions
Dissection—Separation of the layers of the intima of the vessel Aneurysm—Abnormal dilatation of the vessel beyond its normal size Rupture—Leakage of blood outside the adventitia of the vessel

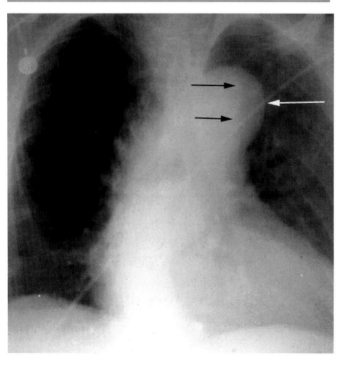

Fig. 11.48   Aortic dissection. There is unfolding of the aorta on this PA film in a patient who presented with severe back pain. There is a double density within the aortic arch that is unusual but suggests the possibility of a false lumen. A type A dissection was diagnosed on CT (black/white arrows).

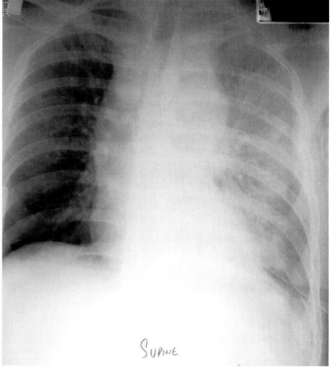

Fig. 11.49   Traumatic aortic rupture. This patient was involved in a high-speed road traffic accident. The film demonstrates several important features of a transected aorta. There is a widened mediastinum. This is non-specific finding, but a mediastinal width of greater than 8 cm or a mediastinum to chest ratio of greater than 0.25 are highly suggestive of a large mediastinal haematoma associated with this diagnosis. There is a left pleural effusion producing hazy opacification in this supine patient. There is also poor definition of the lateral border of the descending aorta.

and only 2% of all cases survive at 10 weeks. Surgical intervention improves outcome with 15% of patients surviving at 10 weeks.

Most transection takes place at the point where the aortic arch becomes fixed to the descending aorta at the isthmus. Transection should be considered in all patients who have suffered a rapid deceleration injury, particularly as the clinical features can be extremely non-specific. The initial radiological chest examination is usually of low quality performed in the supine patient who is often fixed to a spinal board. However, there are several important radiological features that can be identified on this film (Fig. 11.49). The most common finding is a widened mediastinum. This is non-specific finding, but a mediastinal width of greater than 8 cm or a mediastinum to chest ratio of greater than 0.25 are highly suggestive of a large mediastinal haematoma associated with this diagnosis. Although the descending aorta may have a poorly defined outline, this is an extremely non-specific sign. The relationship of the aorta to the surrounding mediastinal structures is also important. The oesophagus, which can be identified if it contains a nasogastric tube, is deviated to the right of the transverse process of the fourth thoracic vertebra in 60% of cases. In addition, there can be compression or deviation of the trachea to the right; again this being detected in 60% of cases. The left main stem bronchus is depressed anteroinferiorly towards the right side in about one half of cases.

Although it has been reported that fractures of the first two ribs should suggest the possibility of transection, any fracture of the vertebra from sixth cervical to the eighth thoracic indicates a high degree of force and transection should actively be excluded. Late presentation may occur with a well-defined saccular aneurysm of the aortic arch that follows previously undetected but contained traumatic rupture (Fig. 11.50).

Recently, several studies using spiral CT have demonstrated a high proportion of normal chest radiographs in the context of CT-demonstrated transection. In one recent study this proportion was as high as 44% of patients in whom this subsequent diagnosis was made.

The aorta can of course suffer trauma from other forms of injury including penetration injury; the acute appearances are similar (Fig. 11.51).

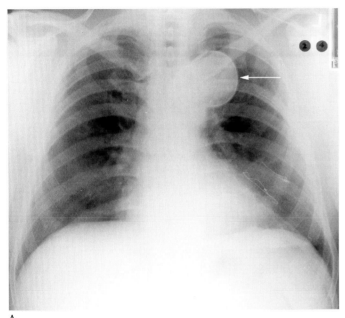

A

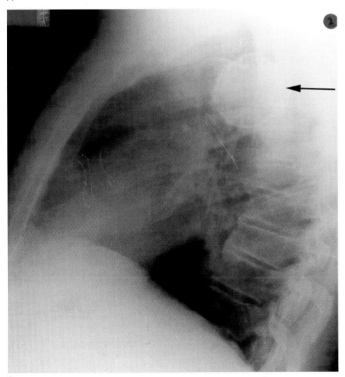

B

Fig. 11.50 Calcified saccular aneurysm of the aortic arch. Both the PA (A) and lateral films (B) demonstrate the large saccular aneurysm of the aortic arch (arrow). The aneurysm has calcified.

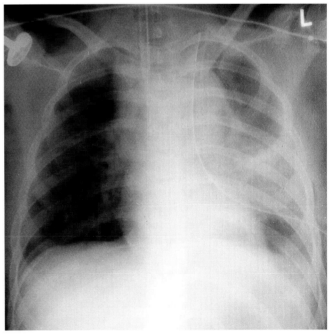

Fig. 11.51 Aortic stab wound. The supine view shows marked widening of the mediastinum indicating haemorrhage. There is also an increase in density in the left hemithorax, due to the presence of a left-sided pleural effusion.

Thoracic aortitis and aortic aneurysms

Atheromatous disease of the thoracic aorta

Atheromatous diseases are now the leading cause of aneurysmal dilatation of the thoracic aorta. Aneurysmal dilatation is defined as a diameter of greater than 4 cm, with the dilatation involving all three layers of the aorta. While this definition is based on size, the prognosis of this condition is also size related. Although less data is available regarding the follow-up of this type of aneurysm as compared to information about the abdominal aorta, most studies suggest rupture is unusual in an aorta of less than 5 cm and most ruptures occur when the vessel diameter exceeds 6 cm. Additionally, the presence of clinical symptoms from the aneurysm is a bad prognostic feature. The aneurysm may be localised or extensive and it may involve the ascending aorta (Fig. 11.52), the descending aorta (Fig. 11.53) or both.

Marfan's syndrome

Marfan's syndrome gives rise to a weakening of the aortic wall leading to ectasia and eventually aneurysm formation, often involving the sinuses of Valsalva and the ascending aorta (Fig. 11.54). Marfan's syndrome can also affect the aortic ring, resulting in aortic regurgitation. Characteristically the aortic root aneurysm associated with Marfan's syndrome is 'flask shaped' with loss of the usual indentation at the sino-tubular junction. Widening of the mediastinum, and in particular the aortic arch, are the most common radiological features noted on the chest radiograph. Large aneurysms of the upper ascending aorta or transverse arch displace the oesophagus and trachea to the left.

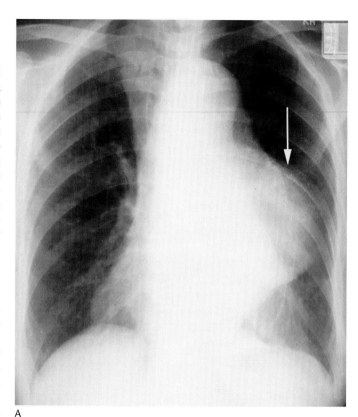

A

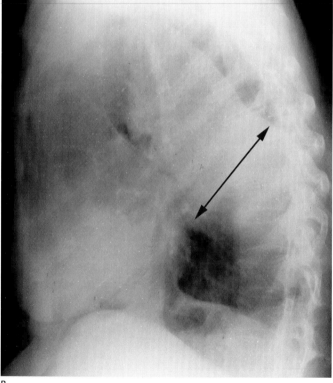

B

Fig. 11.53 Aneurysm of the descending aorta. The descending aorta has become dilated and tortuous with a marked increase in size (arrows). These changes are often well visualised on both PA (A) and lateral (B) films.

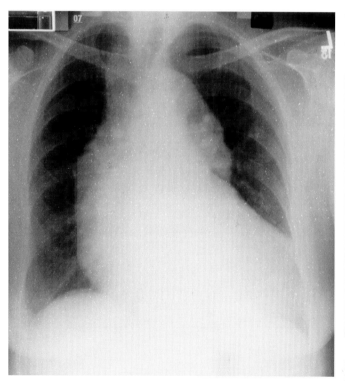

Fig. 11.52 Aneurysm of the ascending and descending aorta. This PA film demonstrates marked dilatation of the ascending aorta consistent with a large aneurysm, in a patient with atheromatous disease.

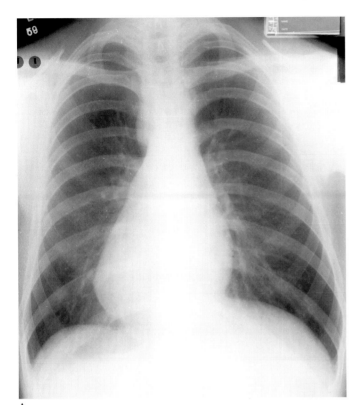

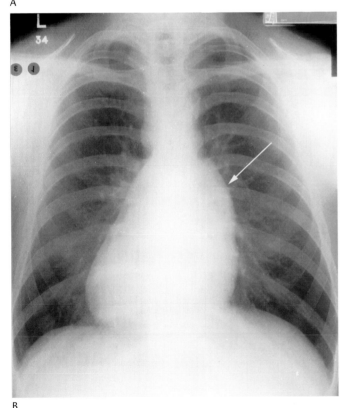

Fig. 11.54 Expanding aortic aneurysm. These serial PA films of a patient with Marfan's disease demonstrate expansion of the ascending aorta as an aneurysm develops. The initial film shows mild prominence of the ascending aorta, unusual in a young adult male (A). The second film taken 2 years later shows obvious increase in prominence of the ascending aorta (arrow) as the aortic root has expanded (B).

Syphilitic aortitis

Although this condition used to be the most common cause of an aneurysm of the ascending aorta it is now much less common. Syphilitic aortitis developed in 12% of untreated patients, usually between 10 and 30 years after the initial infection, the dilatation usually being asymmetrical, most commonly in the ascending aorta commencing near the aortic root. Syphilitic aortitis can in some cases also involve the descending aorta. This condition also leads to the development of aortic regurgitation. The aneurysm is most often saccular in nature with classic pencil-thin dystrophic calcification (Fig. 11.55), this sometimes being obscured by the secondary coarse calcification of atherosclerosis. Once developed, treatment will not stop further degeneration, and only surgical repair is offered in symptomatic or larger aneurysms.

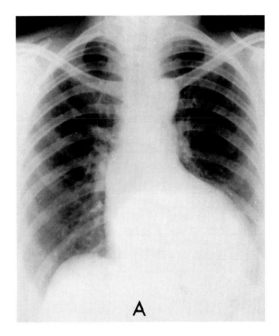

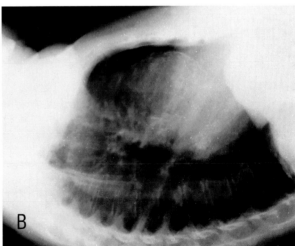

Fig. 11.55 Aortic incompetence due to syphilitic aortic root aneurysm. (A) Frontal view, showing left ventricular dilatation extending to the left and only a slight prominence in the position of the ascending aorta, with a barely visible rim of calcium. (B) Lateral view, showing a large saccular aortic root aneurysm clearly outlined by calcification.

Takayasu's aortitis

Takayasu's aortitis is a chronic inflammatory panarteritis of unknown pathogenesis, which affects segments of aorta, including the main aortic branches. This condition can also affect the pulmonary arteries. The disease process affects young adolescents or adults, predominantly females, especially of oriental ethnic background. The condition often presents in a non-specific manner with a fever in adolescence. The patient then loses the pulse from major vessels in the arms. The chest radiograph findings are non-specific with a subtle widening of the supracardiac shadow, particularly if this shadow increases in size to greater than 3 cm in diameter. In a small proportion of patients aortic calcification is present, and occasionally rib notching can develop.

Mycotic aneurysm

This is a rare cause of an aneurysm of the thoracic aorta, induced by bacteria invading the arterial wall. This type of aneurysm accounts for 2.5% of all thoracic aneurysms and is important to diagnose because of the extremely poor prognosis. The cause can often be difficult to determine but there may be direct bacterial infection of an atheromatous plaque or secondary spread from a thoracic infection such as tuberculosis. Other predisposing causes such as infected prosthetic valves or sternal wires are also important. The prognosis is poor because the aneurysm often expands quickly, leading to rupture.

Sinus of Valsalva aneurysm

The sinus of Valsalva aneurysm is a congenital abnormality resulting in a deficiency between the aortic media and the annulus fibrosus of the aortic valve. The blood flow distends this region, leading to eventual aneurysm formation. This usually occurs in the non-coronary sinus but it can involve the right coronary sinus. The weakness may lead to rupture, leading to a tract between the aortic root and the right ventricle if the abnormality involves the right coronary sinus, or to the right atrium if the non-coronary sinus is the site.

There is an association of this condition with Marfan's syndrome, Turner's syndrome and abnormality of the aortic valve. An association has also been reported in patients with a ventricular septal defect.

PULMONARY VASCULATURE

Pulmonary embolism

Pulmonary embolic disease remains one of the true causes of a sudden death. This condition represents a spectrum of clinical outcomes, from the devastating acute massive central pulmonary embolism to pulmonary arterial hypertension as a result of multiple or chronic pulmonary embolic disease.

Acute massive pulmonary embolism

Acute massive pulmonary embolism occurs when an organised thrombus, usually from the lower limbs, embolises to the central pulmonary arteries. If the embolism is large enough, this leads to acute right heart failure and possible circulatory collapse and death. The clinical diagnosis of pulmonary embolism remains difficult, with several studies suggesting no clear pattern of signs and symptoms.

The best quality radiograph of the chest should be obtained, allowing for the clinical situation. The most likely scenario is a portable chest radiograph obtained on an ill patient in the accident and emergency department and this examination can be of limited

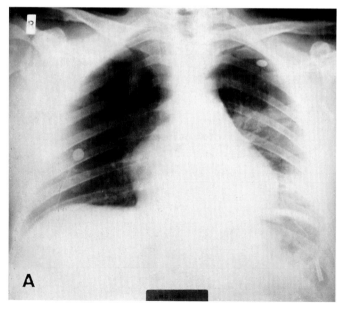 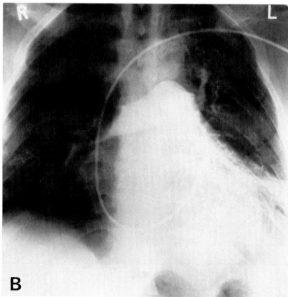

Fig. 11.56   Acute massive pulmonary embolism. (A) Frontal chest film (portable). The right lung and the left upper zone are hypertransradiant due to oligaemia, and there is overperfusion of the left mid and lower zones. (B) Pulmonary arteriogram, same patient. The leading edge of an embolus is seen impacted in the right pulmonary artery, producing virtually complete obstruction. Another embolus is seen in the supply to the left upper lobe which is also impaired. Only the left lower lobe fills adequately with contrast medium.

quality. It is frequently stated that the presenting film is normal but often the plain film is not normal, with signs that can be difficult to visualise and interpret. There is often slight enlargement of the heart. There is often an area of pulmonary underperfusion (the Westermark sign), although this can be extremely difficult to detect, particularly if large portions of the lung are affected (Fig. 11.56). An extremely rare appearance is an increased density of the lungs with peripheral cut-off. Any previous films are of considerable use as they allow direct comparison, highlighting changes.

Non-acute pulmonary embolic disease

If the thrombus breaks up as it travels through the IVC, smaller emboli are produced and these lodge in smaller more peripheral vessels. Pulmonary infarction can occur due to these smaller emboli but this is relatively uncommon as the bronchial circulation usually protects the lungs. Once the smaller pulmonary arteries become blocked, there is certainly underperfusion of the lung, leading to a reduction in the aeration of the lung and often a loss of volume. Continued hypoventilation will lead to atelectasis and eventually collapse. The classic triangular or wedge-shaped area of infarct can sometimes be detected but remains rare, this being termed 'Hampton's hump'. Often small areas of abnormality develop as linear shadows that are non-specific but often reversible. The pleurae are invariably involved and often a small amount of pleural fluid will develop. This is sometimes large enough to be detected in the costophrenic angle.

Chronic pulmonary embolic disease

If the patients have continued small emboli over a long period of time, irreversible pulmonary hypertension will eventually become established, leading to right heart failure. The chest radiograph will show the changes of pulmonary arterial hypertension.

Pulmonary artery thrombosis

Thrombosis of the main pulmonary artery and its branches is a rare complication of a variety of conditions of the lung, heart and blood. The condition has been reported in association with rheumatic heart disease, congenital abnormality and sickle cell anaemia. The plain film appearances mimic pulmonary artery hypertension.

Pulmonary artery aneurysm

Generalised dilatation of the pulmonary artery occurs in many situations where there are altered pulmonary haemodynamics. This can result from the presence of a shunt, an increase in pulmonary artery pressures or even longstanding mitral valve disease. These dilatations do not constitute aneurysms. Localised aneurysm of the pulmonary artery is very rare.

Scimitar syndrome

One relatively common form of partial vascular anomalous drainage that can often present in adult life is the Scimitar syndrome. The syndrome describes an abnormal pulmonary vein draining the right lower lobe, inserting below the diaphragm,

usually into the IVC. This condition often presents with a non-specific respiratory infection and can be an incidental finding on a plain chest radiograph. It can be associated with an atrial septal defect.

The plain film has characteristic appearance giving rise to the name of the syndrome. There is a soft-tissue opacity shaped like an inverted Scimitar sword within the right lower zone, terminating at or below the diaphragm. The condition can be associated with a hypoplastic right lower lobe, with associated shift of the mediastinum towards the right side.

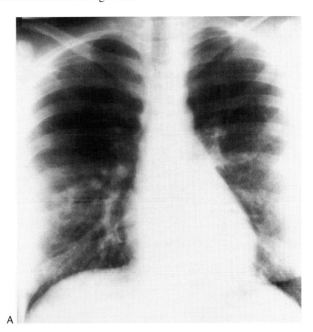

A

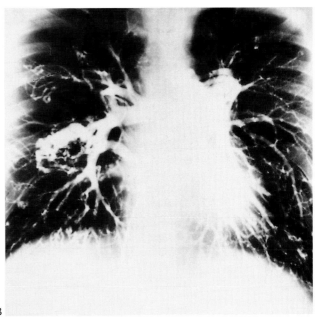

B

Fig. 11.57 Pulmonary arteriovenous malformations. (A) Frontal chest film. Abnormal pulmonary shadows, typically elongated, can be identified in the right mid zone. (B) Pulmonary arteriogram. The pulmonary arteriovenous malformations in the right mid zone, associated with premature venous filling, can be identified. Additional abnormal pulmonary vessels are clearly visible in the right upper zone and throughout the left lung.

Pulmonary arteriovenous malformation

This is a rare congenital condition where a direct arterial–venous connection has developed. This occurs between small pulmonary arteries and veins in the vast majority of cases (95%), but can occur between the systemic artery and the pulmonary vein. The condition is usually manifest in adulthood. There is dilatation of the terminal portions of the vessel due to the increased flow that produces soft-tissue opacification in the periphery of the lungs. In one-third of cases these lesions are multiple and in one-third of cases they form part of a spectrum, the Osler–Weber–Rendu syndrome or hereditary haemorrhagic telectangiectasia (Fig. 11.57).

On the plain film there are often multiple small soft-tissue lesions that can enlarge rapidly, the differential diagnosis being multiple metastasis. In a small proportion of cases the vasculature leading to the abnormality can be identified, and very rarely it may calcify, phleboliths being identified.

Pulmonary varix

A pulmonary varix is a rare localised dilatation of the pulmonary vein with no direct arterial input. These lesions are associated with both congenital and acquired heart disease and can develop in isolation. They are usually recognised by the presence of rounded or even lobulated shadows near the hilum.

REFERENCE AND SUGGESTIONS FOR FURTHER READING

General cardiac radiology

Chiles, C., Putman, C. E. (1997). *Pulmonary and Cardiac Imaging* New York: Marcel Dekker.
Shapiro (2001) *Heart*, **85**, 218–222.
Higgins, C. B. (1992) *Essentials of Cardiac Radiology and Imaging*. New York J. B. Lippincott.
Skorton, D. J., Schelbert, H. R., Wolf, G. L., Brundage, B. H. (1996) *Marcus Cardiac Imaging*, 2nd edn. *A Companion to Braunwald's Heart Disease*. Philadelphia W. B. Saunders.

Non-invasive cardiac imaging

Blackwell, G. G., Cranney, G. B., Pohost, G. M. (1992) *MRI: Cardiovascular System*. London: Gower.
DePuey, E. G., Berman, D. S., Garcia, E. V. (1995) *Cardiac SPECT Imaging*. New York: Raven Press.
Globits, S., Higgins, C. B., Edelman, R. E., et al (eds) (1996) *Clinical Magnetic Resonance Imaging; Adult Heart Disease*. Philadelphia: W. B. Saunders.
Manning, W. J., Pennell, D. J. (2001) *Cardiac Magnetic Resonance Imaging*. Edinburgh: Churchill Livingstone.
Meire, H. Cosgrove. D., Dewbury, K., Wilde, P. (1993) *Clinical Ultrasound: Cardiac Ultrasound*. Edinburgh: Churchill Livingstone.
Otto, C. M. (1999) *Textbook of Clinical Echocardiography*, 2nd edn. Philadelphia: W. B. Saunders.
Roelandt, J. R. T. C., Sutherland, G. R., Iliceto, S., Linker, D. T. (1993) *Cardiac Ultrasound*. Edinburgh: Churchill Livingstone.
Walsh, C. Wilde, P. (1999) *Practical Echocardiography*. London: Greenwich Medical Media.
Zaret, B. L., Beller, G. A. (1999) *Nuclear Cardiology. State of the Art and Future Directions*. St Louis: Mosby.

Angiography and intervention

Kern, M. J. (1998) *The Cardiac Catheterization Handbook,* 3rd edn. St Louis: Mosby.
Nienaber, C. A., Sechtem, U. (1996) *Imaging and Intervention in Cardiology.* London Kluwer Academic Publishers.
Norell, M. S., Perrins, J. (2001) *Essential Interventional Cardiology.* Philadelphia: W. B. Saunders.
Topol, E. J. (1998) *Textbook of Interventional Cardiology.* Philadelphia: W. B. Saunders.

Congenital heart disease

Elliott, L. P. (1991) *Cardiac Imaging in Infants, Children and Adults.* Philadelphia: J. B. Lippincott.
Freedom, R. M., Mawson, J. B., Yoo, S. J., Benson, L. N. (1997) *Congenital Heart Disease; Textbook of Angiocardiography*. London: Futura.
Higgins, C. B., Silverman, N. H., Kersting, S., Sommerhoff, B. A., Schmidt, K. (1990) *Congenital Heart Disease; Echocardiography and Magnetic Resonance Imaging*. New York: Raven Press.
Linker, D. T. (2000) *Practical Pediatric Echocardiography of Congenital Heart Disease*. Edinburgh: Churchill Livingstone.

12

ACQUIRED HEART DISEASE II: NON-INVASIVE IMAGING

Mark Callaway and Peter Wilde

INTRODUCTION

'Non-invasive' is a term that is used imprecisely and can mean different things to different people. If 'invasive' is taken to mean hazardous or potentially hazardous, then even a chest X-ray presents potential danger from ionising radiation. If 'invasive' means introducing medical equipment into the body, then an intravenous injection of contrast medium or endoscopic ultrasound examination is 'invasive'. This chapter will use a broad definition of 'non-invasive imaging' which will include echocardiography (including transoesophageal echocardiography), nuclear medicine, CT and MRI. Chest X-rays and other plain film X-rays have been covered in a previous chapter. Conventionally, angiography and interventional endovascular treatments have been considered 'invasive' and these techniques are covered in a subsequent chapter. An alternative but equally valued interpretation of 'non-invasive' and 'radiation free' will be found in Ch. 15 p. 000.

In the last two decades there has been a huge development in non-invasive imaging techniques in cardiac disease. This has followed the development of these techniques in other organ systems of the body but has been more difficult to achieve for several reasons.

The first of several additional challenges encountered in cardiac imaging concerns cardiac movement. No other organ system has such fast moving structures and in a number of pathological circulations the velocity of blood flow itself can be very high. Parts of the cardiac anatomy such as heart valve leaflets and even major structures such as atrial walls or coronary arteries can move at several hundred centimetres per second.

In addition to this the cardiac anatomy itself poses a variety of challenges. The asymmetrical anatomy of the heart and cardiac structures within the chest means that the conventional planes of examination which relate to external body reference points may be of less use than specialised cardiac planes of examination. Many organs can be examined without difficulty using conventional transverse, coronal and sagittal planes of examination, but in addition to these the cardiac examination may need to employ specialised planes such as the short-axis or long-axis planes. These planes may vary from patient according to individual cardiac chamber orientation or anatomy.

The oblique nature of the heart has also led historically to the development of terminology that does not correspond exactly with conventional descriptive terms. The anterior and posterior walls of the left ventricle, for example, are not situated in conventional anterior or posterior positions, rather the anterior wall is antero-supero-leftward in orientation and the posterior wall is postero-infero-rightward in orientation. Clearly these precise but cumbersome terms have been dropped for practical utility. There are several other examples of specialised terminology used in cardiac descriptions.

Finally the nature of cardiac structure and function is such that physically small structures or variations in structure can be of crucial importance in the health of a patient. The difference in calibre of a coronary artery of 1 mm can be of profound significance. A tiny vegetation on a cardiac valve may have vital prognostic implications.

The development of non-invasive cardiac imaging has thus been driven by these exacting demands and as yet not all the challenges have been overcome. It is for this reason that the experienced cardiac radiologist or imager will have to understand fully the potential of a wide range of techniques. The choice of technique will depend on factors such as diagnostic potential, available equipment, available expertise and cost and, of course, any potential hazards for the patient.

TECHNIQUES

In selecting a technique to examine the heart, many factors must be considered. No final recommendations can usually be made for an individual situation but Table 12.1 indicates the diagnostic utility of most major cardiac imaging techniques together with their advantages and disadvantages.

CHEST X-RAY

The chest X-ray is used as an overview technique for assessment of the heart size and shape, individual chamber enlargement and the state of the lungs and pulmonary circulation. It is also very useful for identifying the presence of calcification and implants in the heart

Table 12.1 Diagnostic utility, advantages and disadvantages of most major cardiac imaging techniques

Diagnostic utility	Chest X-ray	Transthoracic echocardiogram	Transoesophageal echocardiogram	Nuclear medicine techniques	Multislice CT	MRI	Angiography
Anatomy							
Myocardium	+	++	+++	+	++	+++	++
Valves	+	++	+++	0	+	++	++
Coronaries	0	0	+	0	++	++	+++
Pericardium	+	+	+	0	++	+++	+
Pulmonary vessels	+++	0	0	0	+++	++	++
Calcification	+++	+	+	0	+++	+	+++
Function							
Myocardium	++	++	+++	++	+	+++	++
Valves	+	++	+++	0	+	+	++
Coronaries	0	0	+	++	++	+	+++
Limitations							
Radiation hazard	–	0	0	– –	– – –	0	– – –
Risk/discomfort	0	0	– –	–	–	–	– – –
Spatial resolution	– –	– –	–	– – –	–	–	0
Temporal resolution	– –	–	–	– – –	– –	– –	0
Operator skills	–	– – –	– – –	– –	–	– – –	– – –
Cost	–	–	– –	– –	– –	– – –	– – –

+++ = Major utility; ++ = moderate utility; + = minor utility; 0 = no utility/no limitation; – = minor limitation; – – = moderate limitation; – – – = major limitation.

and thorax. It will be essential for identifying bony anomalies associated with cardiac conditions as well as incidental pathologies. Perhaps the most common use of the chest X-ray is as a clinical management tool, useful for following the progress of a disease or treatment. In taking advantage of the relative simplicity and low cost of the examination, it must still be remembered that the investigation carries a potential, although small, radiation hazard. The chest X-ray should therefore never be requested or performed 'routinely' but only where there is a clear justification for the procedure.

TRANSTHORACIC ECHOCARDIOGRAPHY

Transthoracic echocardiography is the most commonly used cardiac imaging examination after the chest X-ray and probably approaches the electrocardiogram in its clinical utility. It is harmless and relatively comfortable for the patient and is the first-line technique for evaluating most abnormalities of the cardiac chambers, valves and great vessels. The multi-modality nature of the technique offers two-dimensional and M-mode imaging as well as pulsed-wave (PW), continuous-wave (CW) and colour flow Doppler studies. This means that echocardiography is not only very important in assessing structural cardiac abnormalities but will also be valuable in the detection and quantitation of many functional abnormalities. Colour flow Doppler techniques will identify normal and abnormal flow patterns, and together with PW and CW Doppler interrogation will allow the quantitation of valve stenosis, regurgitation, intracardiac shunts and in some cases will facilitate intracardiac pressure estimation.

Further applications of echocardiography include stress studies, usually with pharmacological stress, that can be used to reveal functional abnormalities of ventricular function which are not apparent on a conventional resting study. This technique has been reported as more sensitive than stress ECG in the detection of occult coronary disease.

Contrast echocardiography using the new agents that will cross the lungs after intravenous injection are now being used to assess myocardial perfusion, although these techniques are still in a relatively early stage of development.

Common indications for echocardiography include:

- Assessment of left ventricular function
- Determination of the cause of cardiac failure
- Evaluation of a patient with a cardiac murmur
- Evaluation of a patient with an abnormal chest X-ray
- Assessment of known or suspected cardiac valve disease
- Assessment or exclusion of congenital heart lesion(s)
- Follow-up of any of the above.

The major adverse feature of echocardiography is its dependence on operator skill in both carrying out and interpreting the examination. It takes many hundreds of supervised examinations before complete expertise is achieved and misinterpretation of the study is common with inexperienced operators. Many national and international societies specify precise training requirements for echocardiography.

TRANSOESOPHAGEAL ECHOCARDIOGRAPHY

Transoesophageal echocardiography (TOE) is a more complex examination which requires more skill than transthoracic echocardiography and the transducer is considerably more expensive than a conventional transducer. The examination is uncomfortable and requires topical anaesthesia of the throat and mild sedation is usually employed. The patient should be carefully monitored during the procedure and, again, there are precise standards set out for the safe conduct of the examination. Having said this, the procedure is easily performed on outpatients and most do not regard it as excessively unpleasant. The technique also has applications in the operating theatre and intensive care unit. The benefits of the examination are the high-quality studies that can be obtained, particularly in deeper structures and in 'hard to image' patients.

The risks associated with TOE are few, provided normal precautions are taken and the incidence of complications is very low. Perforation of the pharynx or oesophagus is potentially the most dangerous complications but in experienced hands these complications are rare. Cardiac arrhythmias, hypoxia and hypotension have also been reported. The reported mortality of the technique is hard to establish but only a few cases of mortality related to the procedure have been reported in the literature with tens of thousands of procedures being performed in the UK alone each year. In about 2–3% of cases the examination is not possible due to intolerance of the probe.

Common indications for transoesophageal echocardiography include:

- Detailed assessment of the left atrium for thrombus
- Detailed assessment of native or prosthetic mitral valve
- Assessment of the interatrial septum
- Assessment of heart valves in known or suspected endocarditis
- Assessment of abnormalities of the aortic valve
- Diagnosis of dissection of the thoracic aorta
- General echocardiography indications in 'hard to image' patients
- Assessment of some forms of congenital heart disease
- Assessment of some right-sided cardiac lesions
- Assessment of left ventricular function perioperatively
- Assessment of cardiac surgical repairs perioperatively.

Limitations related to the technique include the poorer imaging of distant structures (such as the cardiac apex) by the high-frequency probe and the confinement of the probe to the oesophagus or gastric fundus. In spite of the multiplane technology of modern transducers, the investigation will not be capable of answering all questions and as such it must be used appropriately in conjunction with other techniques including transthoracic echocardiography.

CARDIAC NUCLEAR MEDICINE STUDIES

This group of techniques is very much more functional than structural and requires considerable specialist knowledge of radionuclide techniques, cardiac pathophysiology, cardiac pharmacology and detailed understanding of myocardial perfusion and contractility. A detailed account of these techniques is beyond the scope of this chapter but it is important for the cardiac radiologist to understand the principles of the commoner technique.

Radionuclide cardiac studies have long been grouped into two main categories, blood pool imaging and myocardial imaging. Blood pool imaging was most commonly performed as an electrocardiographically (ECG) gated blood pool scan, performed at rest or under stress conditions. This technique produced valuable data on overall and regional left ventricular function. The technique is becoming much less commonly used as such information is becoming more easily available from echocardiography and MRI techniques.

Myocardial perfusion scanning is, however, still a technique of major practical importance and this includes conventional radionuclide scanning as well as positron emission tomography (PET). Routine myocardial perfusion scanning now employs technetium agents more than thallium agents due to the improved imaging characteristics and improved radiopharmaceuticals available with the former. The standard stress thallium scan followed by resting images after 4 hours is now superseded by a 2-day protocol for rest and stress. The stress technique follows a variety of protocols, depending on the information required and the ability of the patient to exercise. Adenosine and dobutamine are employed in a variety of pharmaceutical stress protocols. PET scanning is not widely available as it depends on the close proximity of a cyclotron but this sophisticated technique will give more detailed insight into complex phenomena such as hibernating (recoverable), infarcted or stunned (temporarily impaired) myocardium.

Current scanners can use ECG gating to achieve functional studies of the left ventricle as an addition to the myocardial perfusion study.

The most common indication for radionuclide scanning is the assessment of myocardial perfusion and viability. This can be as a first-line technique for the diagnosis of coronary artery disease, as an adjunct to coronary arteriography or as a specific decision-making tool in the planning of coronary interventions.

COMPUTED TOMOGRAPHY

CT has for many years had limited application in the study of the heart due to its poor temporal resolution and the need for contrast injection. Current generations of CT scanners now use spiral and multislice technology and the acquisition times can be considerably reduced. Contrast resolution of CT scans is good and the technique has been proposed as a good screening tool for the detection of coronary calcification. This screening approach has not yet gained wide acceptance. High-resolution multislice CT studies with contrast injection can now be used to demonstrate the major coronary vessels in impressive detail, but not yet with as much detail as can be achieved with angiography. Even more advanced are electron beam CT systems that are not widely available but can acquire slices in 50–100 ms, allowing functional ventricular studies to be carried out for the first time using CT technology.

In most cases, however, CT examination of the heart is confined to examination of masses in or near the heart and studies of the aorta and pulmonary artery.

Common indications for CT examination of the heart include:

- Assessment of masses in or near the heart
- Assessment of the thoracic aorta
- Assessment of the pulmonary artery and its major branches.

The use of CT is associated with relatively high doses of radiation and so care must be taken to ensure that the technique is used only when appropriate benefit to the patient is likely.

MAGNETIC RESONANCE IMAGING

This technique is potentially the most comprehensive cardiac imaging modality available. High-resolution intracardiac imaging is possible without the use of ionising radiation or contrast media. The technique allows imaging in any spatial orientation, which makes it particularly suited to the complex, variable and asymmetrical cardiac anatomy. In addition to this, MRI can be used to perform a variety of flow studies within the heart and great vessels.

The assessment of ventricular function is an important application for MRI. The technique can be used to define the cardiac chambers very accurately and technically good gated studies now offer the 'gold standard' in assessing systolic function of the ventricles, having less interobserver variability than echocardiography. Perfusion studies are now becoming possible and the current generation of scanners can be used to perform pharmacological stress and perfusion examination of the myocardium. Flow studies are beginning to match the potential of echocardiography and again tend to have less observer variability. It is likely that most valve pathology will be diagnosed and quantitated by MRI in the near future.

In spite of these benefits, MRI is still limited in both spatial and temporal resolution. Although detail of major coronary arteries can be resolved, the luminal detail required for planning coronary interventions is not yet achievable. The acquisition times are becoming less but the majority of cardiac MRI scans still require ECG gating to resolve intracardiac motion. There is, however, rapid development of these techniques and real-time intracardiac imaging with fine spatial resolution is only a few years away.

Typical current indications for cardiac MRI studies include:

- Assessment of complex structural cardiac abnormalities
- Assessment of left and right ventricular function
- Assessment of the aorta and pulmonary artery
- Assessment of congenital heart disease.

The main disadvantage of the technique is currently its limited availability and the considerable time and expertise required to achieve high-quality results.

In the next decade it is likely that MRI will supplant echocardiography as the 'first-line' cardiac imaging technique.

ANGIOGRAPHY

In spite of all the potential of the non-invasive imaging techniques, angiography still offers the highest temporal and spatial resolution of all cardiac imaging techniques. It is currently the primary tool for the detailed study of the coronary arteries and is integral to the conduct of most interventional cardiac techniques such as angioplasty or valve dilatation.

CORONARY HEART DISEASE

SCREENING FOR CORONARY HEART DISEASE

The high incidence of coronary heart disease has introduced the concept of screening for the condition before symptoms become apparent in order to modify the progress of the condition.

Isotope stress perfusion studies are potentially capable of detecting occult coronary disease and positron emission tomography is perhaps the most sensitive of the tests available. In spite of this, the sensitivity is not sufficiently high to recommend the technique as a routine screening tool even if finances permitted it. Stress echocardiography is another tool that offers the potential for screening, but again insufficient sensitivity of the technique and the associated costs are prohibitively limiting factors.

The association of coronary artery calcification and underlying atheromatous disease has been known for several decades, early authors suggesting a poor prognosis if coronary artery calcification was detected on fluoroscopic screening.

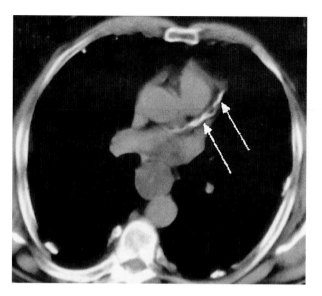

Fig. 12.1 Non-contrast-enhanced CT scan of the thorax. There is heavy calcification of the left anterior descending coronary artery (arrows). In addition there is a hiatus hernia and calcification of the pleurae indicating previous asbestos exposure.

Recently, with the development of fast CT scanning techniques, there has been a resurgence of interest in the detection of calcification in the coronary arteries (Fig. 12.1). This method has several advantages in that it can be performed quickly and is non-invasive. Motion artefact has been a problem in the assessment of coronary calcification and recent investigators have utilised ultrafast, multislice technology and electron beam CT. The latter uses an extremely fast method of beam generation, allowing a marked reduction in motion artefact and potentially 'freezing' cardiac movement.

Several groups have shown that the presence of calcification is easily detected in the coronary arteries but that just the presence or absence of a calcified artery offers little prognostic information. An increase in both the sensitivity and specificity of this method is achieved if a calcium score is calculated as a product of the attenuation value of the calcification and the area of coverage. This value is said to correlate with the degree of stenosis.

As yet the presence of coronary artery calcification indicates that there is likely to be underlying atheromatous disease but a direct correlation with the degree of stenosis cannot be assumed. This test has not been accepted as suitable for screening either low- or high-risk individuals by the American Heart Association. However, the presence of this abnormality can be easily detected even on standard thoracic CT scans and has been associated with adverse events in individuals undergoing thoracic surgery, so the presence of calcification should always be reported.

MRI is less suited to the detection of calcification and the potential for using MRI as a screening tool for coronary artery disease must wait until high-resolution studies of coronary arteries are achieved on a routine basis.

The whole principle of screening for coronary artery disease is, however, dependent on the principle that detection of asymptomatic disease will be a benefit for patients. As yet this is not proven and in an era of 'evidence-based medicine' we must await further data on this subject.

STABLE ANGINA

This condition is generally diagnosed clinically and non-invasive imaging techniques are usually confined to stress studies that can detect areas of abnormal myocardial function which are not apparent at rest. Stress echocardiography, usually using a dobutamine infusion protocol, has been shown to be more sensitive than isotope perfusion scanning in the identification of reversible areas of ischaemia in the left ventricular myocardium.

The majority of patients presenting for the first time with angina will have a normal chest X-ray and normal resting ventricular function. Angiography will be needed to identify the site and exact extent of coronary artery disease.

In the management of patients with angina, it may be necessary to use non-invasive stress techniques after angiography in order to identify areas that would most benefit from revascularisation. Isotope scanning, stress-echo and stress MRI studies have all been used for this purpose (Fig. 12.2).

ACUTE MYOCARDIAL INFARCTION

The clinical management of acute myocardial infarction is a complex matter, depending on the precise mode of presentation and the site and size of the infarct. The chest X-ray is used as a guide to cardiac function and heart failure but other imaging techniques are not routinely used in the first few days after myocardial infarction unless there are haemodynamic complications. Sudden deterioration of the patient, the onset of a new murmur or clinical signs of specific complications will indicate the need for echocardiography, sometimes at the bedside in the coronary care unit.

The echocardiogram will usually demonstrate the site, size and severity of the infarct and will allow an assessment of overall left ventricular function. Large infarcts, particularly at the apex, may contain fresh thrombus, indicating the need for anticoagulation. The mitral valve will be assessed in detail, both by imaging and Doppler flow studies and regurgitation due to acute annular dilatation, papillary muscle dysfunction and papillary muscle rupture should be

differentiated. In severe haemodynamic upset, rupture of the interventricular septum should be sought and the presence of significant pericardial fluid in the early postinfarct phase is a bad prognostic sign, indicating possible myocardial rupture. The right ventricle should also be assessed, as major infarction involving this chamber has a poor prognosis.

TOE is occasionally helpful in the acute phase but the potential imaging benefits must be seen in the context of the patient's clinical condition, and therefore this procedure should only be performed when there is a clear clinical management decision to be made.

There is little role for cross-sectional imaging in assessing the early complications of myocardial infarction.

LATE COMPLICATIONS OF MYOCARDIAL INFARCTION

Several complications of myocardial infarction may develop in the weeks following the acute event. A large full-thickness infarction, particularly involving the anterior wall and apex of the left ventricle, may evolve into a left ventricular aneurysm over a period of weeks. This may be seen clearly on echocardiography as a thin-walled, non-contractile and echogenic portion of the left ventricular wall. The aneurysm is often associated with dyskinetic movement, namely an outward bulging at a time when the remainder of the myocardium is contracting inwards. There may be thrombus contained in the aneurysm which has the potential for systemic embolisation (Fig. 12.3). Both CT and MRI have an important complementary role in identifying and quantifying the effect on ventricular function of a left ventricular aneurysm.

In the first few weeks following myocardial infarction there can be an inflammatory pericarditis, Dressler's syndrome, which may be associated with a small or moderate size pericardial effusion. This will easily be detected by transthoracic echocardiography.

The management of patients following myocardial infarction requires ongoing assessment of ventricular and valvular function. It is now commonplace for patients to have a baseline echocardiogram after initial recovery so the appropriate therapy can be

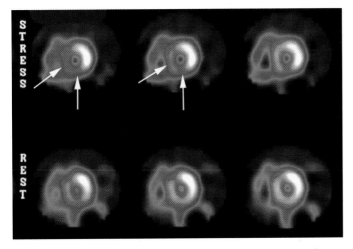

Fig. 12.2 A ^{99m}technetium myocardial perfusion scan showing SPECT images. This study is performed after exercise stress of the myocardium (top images) and a later study was performed at rest (bottom images). The images are through the short axis of both the left and right ventricle and demonstrate a partially reversible perfusion defect in the interventricular septum and posterior wall of the left ventricle (arrows).

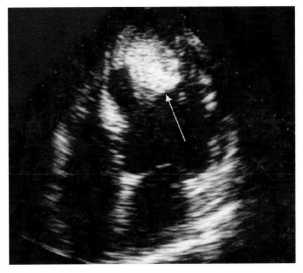

Fig. 12.3 A transthoracic echocardiogram demonstrating an apical four-chamber view. There is an aneurysm of the apex of the left ventricle that has developed as a complication of a previous myocardial infarction. Within the aneurysm is a hyperechoic thrombus (arrow).

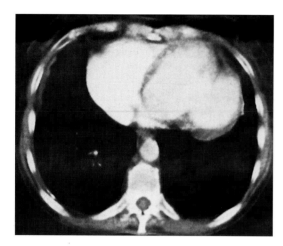

Fig. 12.4 Left ventricular aneurysm. Contrast enhancement demonstrates neck of apical and posterior aneurysm communicating with left ventricular cavity. This has the typical appearance of a false aneurysm of the left ventricle.

used to reduce the chances of later heart failure or other complications.

Left ventricular aneurysms may be associated with persistent angina, life-threatening arrhythmias and congestive cardiac failure. The aneurysm occasionally calcifies after several months or years and this is well seen on CT as well as the chest X-ray. Several studies have used both CT and MRI to identify the presence of an aneurysm, accurately delineating the transitional zone from fibrous band to myocardium. In a minority of cases surgical resection of the aneurysm is appropriate and both types of scan have been used to quantify left ventricular function and to follow-up patients pre and post resection. In rare cases the left ventricular aneurysm may be a false aneurysm (Fig. 12.4). This is a cavity formed after a contained rupture of the left ventricular free wall. In longstanding cases it can be hard to distinguish from a true aneurysm but the key differentiating feature is the discontinuity of the myocardium of the left ventricular myocardium. The clinical history may reveal a particularly difficult postinfarct recovery period.

In some cases a patient may sustain multiple small infarcts which may not be clinically detected and these can lead to diffuse left ventricular impairment or 'ischaemic cardiomyopathy'.

HEART MUSCLE DISEASE

Most of the non-invasive imaging techniques are capable of diagnosing cardiomyopathy, but for some years the dominant technique has been echocardiography. The utility of MRI scanning in functional evaluation of ventricular function has increased considerably in recent years and this technique may take over as the 'gold standard'.

DILATED CARDIOMYOPATHY

This is a heart muscle disorder defined by the presence of a dilated and poorly functioning left ventricle in the absence of abnormal loading conditions such as aortic stenosis or hypertension. There is a large number of causes of the condition but all produce similar effects of increased diastolic volume of the ventricle and decreased ejection fraction. The patient may present with heart failure characterised by dyspnoea, exertional symptoms and fatigue. The condition may be detected on routine screening or chest radiography.

Causes of dilated cardiomyopathy include:

- Postviral myocarditis
- Induced by chronic alcohol overuse
- Drug related (e.g. anthracyclines, cocaine)
- Peripartum
- Endocrine
- Inherited (e.g. muscular dystrophy)
- Nutritional (e.g. thiamine deficiency)
- Inborn errors of metabolism (e.g. haemochromatosis)
- Endocrine
- Arrhythmogenic right ventricular dysplasia
- Ischaemic cardiomyopathy (not always included as a true cardiomyopathy but the appearances are similar)
- Idiopathic dilated cardiomyopathy—the commonest type.

Echocardiographic diagnosis of dilated cardiomyopathy

The diagnosis based on echocardiography is taken as a short-axis diastolic ventricular dimension more than two standard deviations above the normal upper limit. Typically the upper limit of this dimension in an adult male is 6.0 cm (depending on height and weight), with an ejection fraction below 50% (Fig. 12.5).

The ventricular volumes can be derived from the short-axis dimension of the ventricle providing that the measurement is taken appropriately between papillary muscles and mitral valve and there is no regional wall motion variation. In the case of unusually shaped ventricles or those with obvious regional differences, a more detailed area length calculation is required.

$$\text{Ejection fraction (\%)} = \frac{(\text{Diastolic volume} - \text{systolic volume})}{\text{Diastolic volume}} \times 100$$

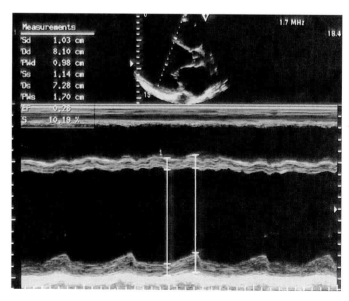

Fig. 12.5 Transthoracic echocardiogram showing a dilated cardiomyopthy. The top 2D reference image shows the left parasternal long-axis view and the lower panel shows the corresponding M-mode trace. The left ventricle is markedly dilated with a diastolic diameter of 8.1 cm and a systolic diameter of 7.3 cm. There is poor contractility overall but the posterior wall contracts slightly better than the septum.

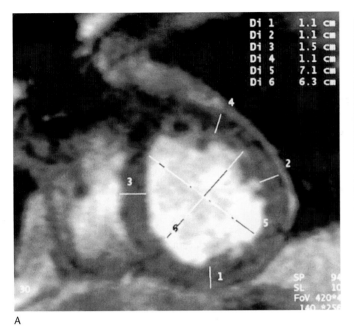
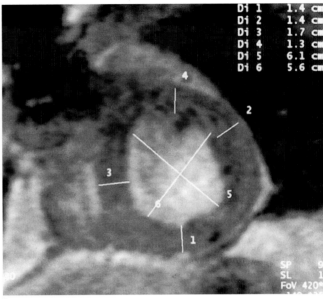

Fig. 12.6 Short-axis ECG-gated white blood MRI of the left ventricle in diastole (A) and systole (B) in a patient with a dilated cardiomyopathy performed at the level of the papillary muscles. The left ventricular diameter in both phases of the cardiac cycle has been measured, allowing calculation of the ejection fraction. The mean diastolic diameter was 6.7 cm and the mean systolic diameter was 5.9 cm. In addition the ventricular wall thickness has been measured, increasing from a mean of 1.2 cm in diastole to 1.45 cm in systole.

MRI assessment of ventricular function

The estimation of cardiac function using MRI depends on the ability to gate the image such that a single cardiac cycle can be divided into 15–20 phases. The smallest and largest volumes of the left ventricle can be obtained from this data, representing end-diastolic and end-systolic volumes and a range of functional measurements produced. The accuracy of this method can be improved further if multiple sections through the left ventricle are obtained along the short axis, and a true three-dimensional estimation of the ventricle produced. This technique is probably more accurate than echocardiography in patients with dilated cardiomyopathy. If the wall thickness values are taken in addition to the cavity measurements, a measure of the myocardial mass can be produced (Fig. 12.6).

If the images are viewed in short axis a visual demonstration of the contraction of the ventricle can be produced. Several cardiac packages allow the interpreter to assess regional wall motion, a measurement of the wall thickness being made at end-diastolic and end-systolic portions of the cycle and wall thickening calculated. In normal subjects normal wall thickening is greater than 2 mm.

Myocardial tagging is another method to assess both thickening and motion of individual sections of the ventricular wall. This method utilises an automated grid, which is superimposed onto the ventricle at the beginning of a cycle. If the ventricle is uncoordinated or has areas of regional wall motion abnormality the grid becomes distorted.

Haemochromatosis is an interesting cardiomyopathy from the point of view of MRI with deposition of iron in the heart muscle occurring in both primary and secondary haemochromatosis. One recent study has suggested that ciné gradient echo magnetic resonance scanning can detect this iron deposition. This produces an image where the ration of signal intensity of the myocardial signal to skeletal muscle is abnormally low.

ARRHYTHMOGENIC RIGHT VENTRICULAR DYSPLASIA

Arrhythmogenic right ventricular dysplasia (ARVD) is a heart muscle disorder of unknown aetiology. This condition is characterised by fibrofatty replacement of the right ventricular myocardium. This condition is probably underdiagnosed but presents with a spectrum of clinical manifestations ranging from a subtle cause of congestive cardiac failure to an important cause of sudden death in an otherwise fit, young healthy person. The disease demonstrates familial tendencies with an autosomal inheritance. There is a spectrum of electrographic abnormalities including ventricular tachycardia or left bundle branch block. Morphological changes are confined to the right ventricle where there is often dilatation. In addition, right ventricular aneurysms are common and are often distributed within the regions referred to as the 'triangle of dysplasia', the right ventricular outflow tract, the apex and the infundibulum. Indeed aneurysm at any of these sites is considered pathognomonic of ARVD.

Radionuclide studies in this condition demonstrate moderately depressed right ventricular ejection fraction while the left ventricular ejection fraction remains normal. The gold standard method of imaging this condition remains contrast angiography, but the versatility of MRI is providing a very good non-invasive alternative. MRI can provide excellent morphological images of the right ventricle in both a static and ciné mode. The technique has a specific advantage in demonstrating fatty infiltration in the right ventricular wall as a bright signal against the normal low signal of the myocardium (Fig. 12.7).

HYPERTROPHIC CARDIOMYOPATHY

Hypertrophic cardiomyopathy (HCM) is a rare condition that is important to diagnose, as it remains an important cause of sudden

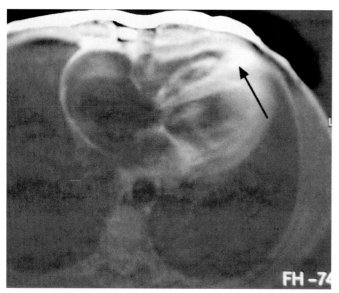

Fig. 12.7 A gradient-echo T$_1$-weighted axial MRI scan of the right ventricle. The right ventricular wall contains fat, high signal on both T$_1$- and T$_2$-weighting (arrow). This fatty replacement is diagnostic of arrhythmogenic right ventricular dysplasia.

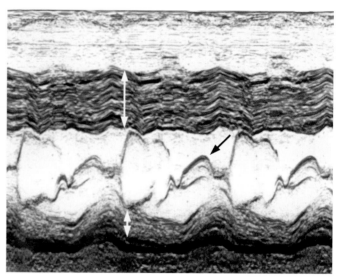

Fig. 12.8 An M-mode echocardiogram, showing systolic anterior motion of the mitral valve apparatus (black arrow). This abnormal motion of the valve apparatus is a feature of hypertrophic obstructive cardiomyopathy caused by the altered haemodynamics of the small ventricular cavity and the prominent septum. The marked septal hypertrophy contrasts with the almost normal thickness posterior left ventricular wall (white arrows).

death in the young adult. This is caused by the arrhythmia caused by the abnormal thickness of the ventricular wall, which leads to electrical instability or acute outflow obstruction. The condition is characterised by excessive thickening of the myocardial muscle with disarray of the myofibrils. There is a hereditary tendency to the condition but sporadic cases are common. This thickening invariably involves the left ventricle, and can be symmetrical or asymmetrical in nature. The mainstay of diagnosis remains echocardiography.

Echocardiographic diagnosis of hypertrophic cardiomyopathy

The classical finding is of asymmetrical hypertrophy (ASH) with a ratio of at least 1.5 to 1 in thickness of the septum and left ventricu-

lar free wall (Fig. 12.8). The echo texture of the myocardium may be 'brighter' than normal. It is important to obtain accurate measurements from both two-dimensional and M-mode imaging, as misinterpretation of septal measurements is common. In elderly patients there is often localised thickening and angulation of the basal septum and this should not be considered as HCM.

In many cases there is systolic anterior motion (SAM) of the mitral anterior leaflet towards the septum, caused by the altered haemodynamics of the small ventricular cavity and the prominent septum. This may in part be responsible for the left ventricular

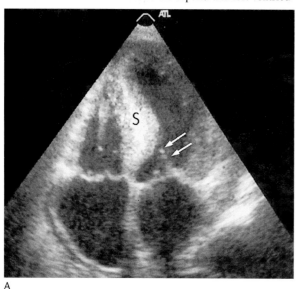

A

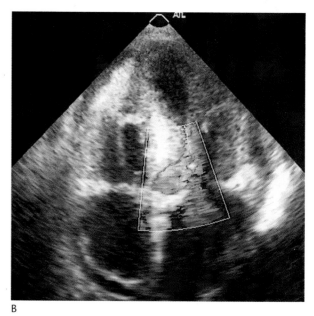

B

Fig. 12.9 Apical four-chamber transthoracic echocardiogram in a patient with hypertrophic cardiomyopathy. (A) Septal hypertrophy (S) and systolic anterior motion of the mitral valve (arrows). Image (B) is taken from the same site in systole and shows the generation of a high-velocity turbulent colour flow Doppler signal by the outflow tract obstruction. There is also associated mitral regurgitation.

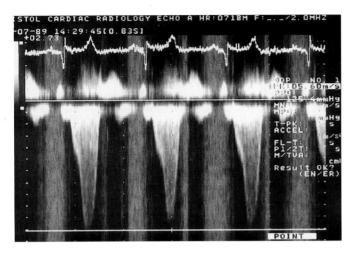

Fig. 12.10 Apical continuous-wave Doppler trace in a patient with dynamic left ventricular outflow tract obstruction due to hypertrophic cardiomyopathy. The curve has a characteristic late systolic peak with a peak velocity of 5.6 m/s. This indicates a peak instantaneous pressure drop at this site of 125 mmHg.

outflow tract obstruction that occurs in some (but not all) patients with this condition (Figs 12.9, 12.10). The outflow tract obstruction may also be due to the obstructive effect of the hypertrophied septum itself. In some cases there is premature or mid-systolic closure of the aortic valve due to the restriction of flow in the left ventricular outflow tract.

The condition is most commonly confined to the septum but there is a spectrum of appearances that can be detected in the condition. The most common abnormality involves the entire septum but there can be localised hypertrophy involving the outflow septum causing obstruction. There are in addition rare forms of this disease that involve the midventricular region or the apex. In a minority of cases there is concentric involvement of the left ventricle. Often there is associated increase in the right ventricular mass.

In view of the risks of sudden death in this condition, particularly in association with athletic pursuits, it is common to screen other family members of patients with the condition. It is also becoming common to screen professional athletes for this condition as part of their medical examination.

MRI diagnosis of hypertrophic cardiomyopathy
The major role for MRI is in the characterisation of the atypical forms of the disease, particularly the rare apical form of the condition. The role of MRI in HCM is to identify the morphological changes in addition to providing data about the ventricular mass and the degree of outflow obstruction. Due to the variability of the distribution of the disease, information about abnormalities in regional wall motion can be difficult to acquire, but ECG-gated myocardial tagging has led to an improvement in detection of these regional abnormalities. Tagging the myocardium has demonstrated that in the thickened regions there is a reduction in the fractional and circumferential thickening compared with healthy volunteers.

Several studies have shown a close correlation between echocardiography and MRI in diagnosing conventional septal HCM, but MRI is more sensitive in the diagnosis of the rare apical form of the disease. Several studies have described a 'spade-like' deformity of the apex demonstrated on angiography and this can be reproduced using MRI directed through the long axis of the left ventricle. This appearance has been renamed as the 'ace of

spades' deformity and is thought to be pathognomonic of this rare condition.

Recently, there has been interest in developing the non-surgical management of this condition, particularly using selective embolisation of the septal branches. MRI has been used to assess the pre- and post-intervention appearances.

RESTRICTIVE CARDIOMYOPATHY

This group of conditions is characterised by diastolic dysfunction of one or both ventricles. Typically the chamber size is normal and the ejection fraction is normal, indicating normal systolic function. The myocardium in many cases does not show any characteristic changes. The restrictive aspect of the condition, however, impairs the diastolic filling of the ventricle and causes raised atrial pressures and atrial dilatation, the latter sometimes being quite marked. An abnormal diastolic filling pattern may be identified on Doppler examination of the mitral valve. There are a number of causes of restrictive cardiomyopathy but many cases are of unknown cause. The majority of the identified causes involve infiltration of the myocardium by a pathological process.

AMYLOIDOSIS

In this condition the amyloid infiltration causes a brighter than normal echo pattern from the myocardium. The left ventricular wall thickness is increased but this is not associated with increased contractility as would be seen with hypertrophy.

ENDOMYOCARDIAL FIBROSIS

This is a rare condition most frequently identified in areas of equatorial Africa, Southern India and Brazil but a very similar clinical condition can be found in Caucasians in Northern Europe and North America. In Europe the condition is associated with hypereosinophilia (Loeffler's endomyocarditis).

A restrictive cardiomyopathy develops as a layer of fibrosis becomes deposited in the endocardium. The fibrosis usually begins at the apex and extends to the atrioventricular grove. Both ventricles can be affected. In the non-Caucasian population the right side of the heart is often involved, leading to marked tricuspid regurgitation. In the later phases of the disease the contractility of the ventricle is also affected. A similar disease process has been described in patients with Behçet's disease.

The diagnosis on echocardiography is characterised by the dilated atria and in some cases the endomyocardial fibrosis can be identified. In advanced cases there is obliteration of the apical portion of the ventricular cavity.

The infiltrative process can have a variable signal on MRI, but initial work with animal models suggests that enhancement of the areas of infiltration occurs using ECG-gated T_1-weighted postgadolinium-DTPA imaging.

SARCOIDOSIS

Cardiac sarcoidosis occurs in about 20% of patients who develop the chronic form of the disease and the condition is probably underdiagnosed. Infiltration can produce arrhythmia or even congestive cardiac failure. MRI has been shown to be an accurate method of identifying the larger non-caseating granulomas, which produce a high signal on T_2-weighting.

ACQUIRED VALVE DISEASE

At the present time the assessment of heart valve disease is heavily dominated by echocardiography which is extremely well suited to this purpose, being able to image valve morphology as well as assess function using Doppler studies and other functional techniques.

AORTIC VALVE STENOSIS

The commonest cause of aortic stenosis in the adult is a degenerative bicuspid aortic valve. Strictly this is a congenital condition, occurring in about 2% of the population, but it most commonly becomes manifest in middle or later life and so will be considered in this section. A bicuspid valve will easily be recognised on a two-dimensional echocardiogram in childhood or early adult life, showing two leaflets in the short-axis view and some doming in the long-axis view, related to the fact that even a non-degenerate bicuspid valve will have mild restriction of opening. There may be concomitant aortic regurgitation of a variable degree in a minority of cases. As the valve degenerates, it will become harder to detect the underlying bicuspid morphology. The characteristic feature of aortic valve stenosis on echocardiography is the thickening, increased echogenicity and reduced mobility of the valve leaflets. Fibrotic thickening will increase the echo pattern but calcified leaflets will be extremely echogenic and there will be acoustic shadowing behind the calcification. MRI will show the calcification as a signal void (Fig. 12.11). Rheumatic aortic stenosis is much less common and is usually associated with rheumatic mitral valve disease. The valve usually has normal tricuspid morphology but in advanced stages it will be difficult to distinguish this from a bicuspid valve.

Many elderly people develop aortic valve sclerosis which is a simple degenerative process affecting a normal tricuspid valve. The leaflets will be somewhat thickened and the valve annulus will also be thickened and echogenic, encroaching slightly onto the valve orifice. This condition will often be associated with a systolic murmur but it rarely leads to significant obstruction.

Longstanding aortic stenosis with significant obstruction will be associated with the development of concentric left ventricular hypertrophy that may be severe. In most patients the left ventricular cavity is normal or small in size with preserved contractility and only in the later stages of untreated disease will the left ventricle dilate and fail.

Quantitation of aortic stenosis is achievable with continuous-wave Doppler interrogation of the jet passing through the narrow orifice (Fig. 12.12). Use of the simplified Bernoulli equation will permit estimation of the peak and mean pressure drop ('gradient') across the valve. The jet direction can be variable from patient to patient and it is important to interrogate from a variety of angles to ensure that the best alignment is achieved. It is also possible to estimate valve orifice area by means of the continuity equation. Both these techniques are very operator dependent and experience is required to achieve an accurate result.

The simplified Bernoulli equation gives

$$P = 4V^2$$

where P is the pressure drop across the valve in mmHg and V is the recorded velocity in m/s.

The continuity equation gives

$$A_2 = \frac{A_1 \times V_1}{V_2}$$

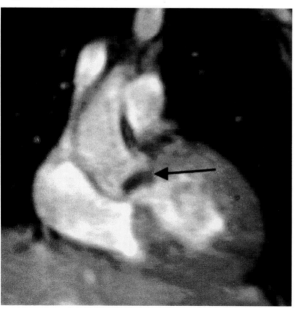

Fig. 12.11 Coronal gradient-echo MRI image (ECG gated) through the left ventricular outflow tract and aortic valve in a patient with calcific aortic stenosis. There is calcification of the aortic valve which produces a signal void (arrow).

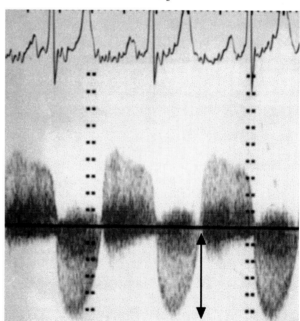

Fig. 12.12 Continuous-wave apical spectral Doppler recording through the aortic valve in a patient with both aortic stenosis and regurgitation. The peak velocity across the valve in systole is 5.5 m/s (arrow), suggesting a peak gradient of 120 mmHg as calculated by the simplified Bernoulli equation.

Where A_2 is aortic valve orifice area, A_1 is left ventricular outflow area (measured by two-dimensional imaging), V_1 is left ventricular outflow tract velocity (measured by pulsed-wave Doppler sampling in the outflow tract) and V_2 is aortic orifice velocity (measured by continuous-wave Doppler interrogation of the orifice jet).

Measurement of the orifice area by planimetry of two-dimensional images is inaccurate and should only be used with great care. The overall evaluation of a stenotic aortic valve depends on assessment of both valve and left ventricular characteristics.

AORTIC VALVE REGURGITATION

A congenital bicuspid aortic valve is the commonest cause of this condition but there is a variety of other causes including:

* Aortic annular ectasia
* Marfan's syndrome
* Infective endocarditis
* Dissection of the aorta
* Rheumatic heart disease
* Connective tissue diseases.

The most obvious feature on echocardiography is a jet of regurgitation seen on colour flow Doppler imaging (Fig. 12.13). The size, shape, distribution and intensity of the jet appearance give valuable clues about the severity of the lesion. The regurgitation can also be detected and quantified by continuous-wave Doppler interrogation of the regurgitant jet in the left ventricle and pulsed-wave Doppler sampling of flow in the aortic arch to detect any abnormal reversal of flow (Fig. 12.14). The left ventricular function is an important guide to severity, a dilated and hypercontractile ventricle indicating the volume overload that is associated with the condition.

The classical M-mode appearance of the condition is the high-frequency fluttering of the anterior leaflet of the mitral valve, as the regurgitant jet strikes it. This elegant sign, analogous to the Austin Flint murmur, is unfortunately not useful in assessing the severity of the lesion.

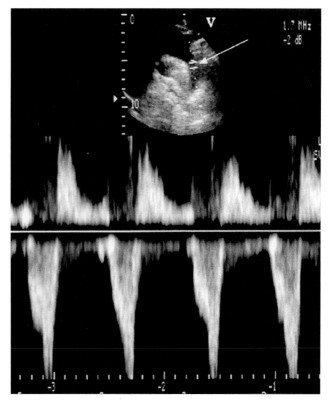

Fig. 12.14 An echocardiogram performed with the transducer positioned in the suprasternal notch with extension of the patient's neck to demonstrate the aortic arch. The sample volume for pulsed-wave Doppler interrogation has been positioned in the descending portion of the arch (arrow) (top) and the Doppler spectral trace illustrates normal forward flow into the descending aorta in systole and prominent reversal of flow in diastole, due to the presence of severe aortic regurgitation.

Many patients can tolerate significant isolated aortic regurgitation for many years but regular echocardiographic review is necessary to ensure that the left ventricle does not dilate excessively before surgery is undertaken.

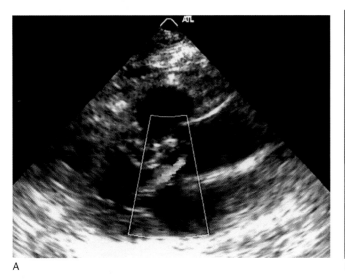 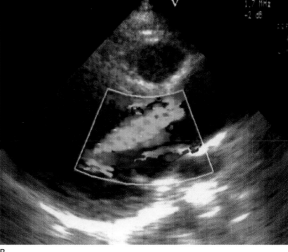

A   B

Fig. 12.13 Both images show colour flow Doppler images taken in the parasternal long-axis view. (A) A very small central regurgitant jet indicating mild aortic regurgitation. (B) A much broader based jet in a patient with severe aortic regurgitation.

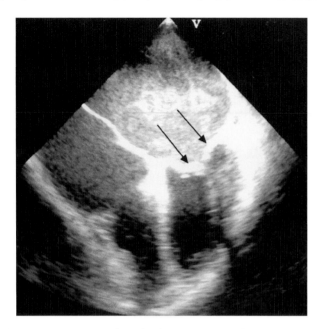

Fig. 12.15 A transoesophageal echocardiogram, at the level of the left atrium, showing a four-chamber view of the heart in a patient with mitral stenosis. The left atrium is at the top of the image and contains spontaneous echo formation due to the stagnation of flow in the distended chamber. The thickened and restricted mitral leaflets are indicated by arrows.

MITRAL VALVE STENOSIS

This condition is almost exclusively caused in adults by rheumatic heart disease. Congenital mitral stenosis is rare and virtually never presents in adult life. Annular thickening of the mitral valve in the elderly can reduce the orifice size slightly but it hardly ever causes significant obstruction.

Echocardiography of rheumatic mitral stenosis shows thickening of both mitral leaflets with restricted mobility and a characteristic

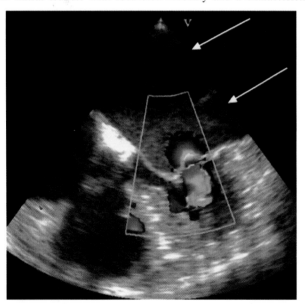

Fig. 12.16 A transoesophageal echocardiogram, at the level of the left atrium (arrows), showing a four-chamber view of the heart. A colour Doppler flow examination through the mitral valve shows a small mitral orifice size with acceleration of flow and turbulence at the site of narrowing.

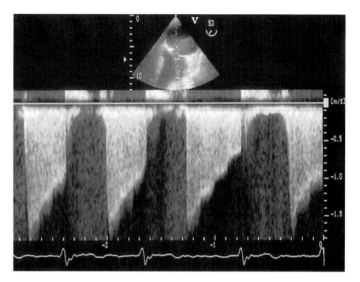

Fig. 12.17 Continuous-wave Doppler examination of the mitral valve from a transoesophageal echo examination. The patient is in atrial flutter. The diastolic flow into the left ventricle has a high peak velocity of 1.8 m/s. The characteristic shape of the curve shows only a slow diminution of flow velocity during diastole. This trace can be used to calculate pressure half-time and estimate the mitral orifice area.

doming appearance to the valve in diastole (Fig. 12.15). There may be prominent fibrosis and possible calcification of the valve, its commissures, the chordae and papillary muscles. The restricted flow through the valve (Fig. 12.16) can be measured with Doppler interrogation and the peak and mean pressure gradients can be derived from the simplified Bernoulli equation (Fig. 12.17). A useful guide to severity is provided by the pressure half-time calculation. This can be measured from a good quality Doppler trace of the flow through the valve; the pressure half-time being the time taken for the pressure drop at the commencement of flow to fall to half its original level. This has been shown to correlate well with valve orifice area:

$$\text{Orifice area (cm}^2) = \frac{220}{\text{Half-time (ms)}}$$

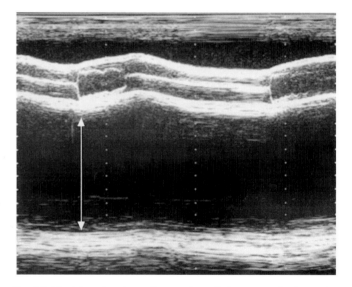

Fig. 12.18 M-mode echocardiogram through the aortic valve from a left parasternal position. There is a massively enlarged left atrium (arrow) with a diameter of 9 cm.

Measurement of orifice size by planimetry from two-dimensional imaging is unreliable.

Mitral stenosis is associated with dilatation of the left atrium, which may become severe and may be associated with thrombus in the atrium or left atrial appendage. Evaluation of the valve and left atrium can be elegantly carried out using transoesophageal echocardiography, which is necessary prior to percutaneous mitral balloon commissurotomy.

The left ventricle remains small and well contracting in pure mitral stenosis whilst the left atrium may become massively dilated in longstanding cases (Fig. 12.18). Right-sided chambers will be affected by chronic elevation of the pulmonary pressures and dilatation of both right ventricle and right atrium are seen. Measurement of the tricuspid regurgitant jet velocity will give an estimate of pulmonary artery pressure that is often elevated.

MITRAL VALVE REGURGITATION

There are several causes of mitral regurgitation, which include:

- Degenerative valve or chordal tissue
  Prolapsed leaflet
  Ruptured chordae
  Myxomatous degeneration
- Secondary to ischaemic heart disease or cardiomyopathy
  Dilated mitral annulus
  Papillary muscle dysfunction
  Papillary muscle rupture
- Rheumatic mitral disease
- Infective endocarditis
- Hypertrophic cardiomyopathy.

The diagnosis of mitral regurgitation will include identification of the morphological abnormality of the valve by two-dimensional echocardiography together with the assessment of the regurgitation by Doppler studies (Fig. 12.19). Degenerative leaflets are often thickened and echogenic but this is not always the case. Careful study of the coaptation (valve closure line) of the mitral leaflets together with the jet direction in the left atrium is necessary to understand the cause of the regurgitation. In the case of a prolapse of part of or the entire posterior leaflet, the regurgitant jet will be directed superiorly to the roof of the left atrium near the aortic root and with anterior leaflet prolapse, the jet will be directed inferiorly (Fig. 12.20).

The left atrium will usually be enlarged, although this feature depends more on the duration of the regurgitation than its severity. In moderate or severe cases of mitral regurgitation the left ventricle shows signs of volume overload with a dilated and hyperkinetic chamber. The right-sided chambers will often be dilated and there may be signs of pulmonary hypertension. Grading of the severity of mitral regurgitation still remains challenging in many cases.

Transoesophageal echocardiography can be a very valuable technique for assessing the exact nature and severity of the lesion (Fig. 12.21), often vital in making decisions about surgery. The technique is often used peroperatively to assess valve repair.

TRICUSPID VALVE DISEASE

This valve frequently shows evidence of regurgitation secondary to lesions of the right heart or pulmonary hypertension. This is rarely a severe leak but it can be used advantageously to assess right heart pressures (Fig. 12.22). Primary acquired disease of the tricuspid valve is rare but rheumatic tricuspid stenosis is sometimes seen in advanced rheumatic heart disease which usually has accompanying involvement of mitral and aortic valves. Infective endocarditis of the tricuspid valve can be due to a venous portal of entry of infection, sometimes being caused by intravenous drug abuse. Metastatic carcinoid syndrome can produce toxic metabolites that can damage the tricuspid valve.

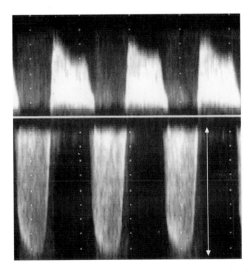

Fig. 12.19 Transthoracic continuous-wave Doppler examination of the mitral valve from the apex. The flow pattern of mixed mitral valve disease is shown. The restricted forward ventricular filling pattern of mitral stenosis is demonstrated, together with the large regurgitant jet (arrow) which has a peak velocity of 5 m/s.

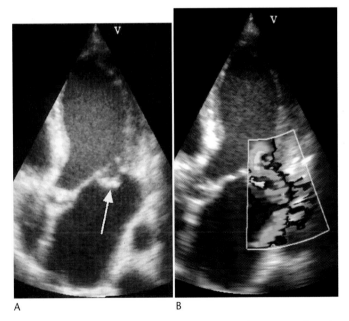

Fig. 12.20 An apical long-axis view of the heart from a transthoracic examination. (A) Prolapse of the anterior mitral valve leaflet (arrow). Colour flow Doppler examination (B) taken from the same position shows prominent eccentric regurgitant flow directed towards the inferior wall of the dilated left atrium.

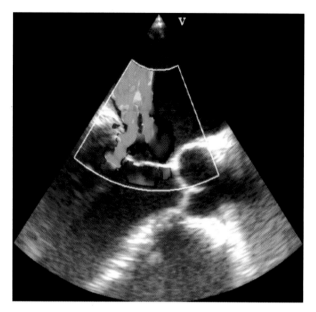

Fig. 12.21 A transoesophageal long-axis echocardiogram with colour flow Doppler examination that demonstrates clearly a prominent jet of severe mitral regurgitation. The green colours indicate 'variance' due to high-velocity turbulence in the jet.

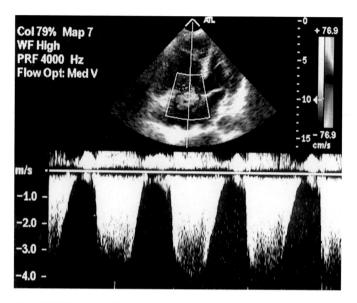

Fig. 12.22 An apical four-chamber view from a transthoracic examination in a patient with pulmonary hypertension. A colour flow (top) and continuous-wave Doppler examination of the tricuspid valve is shown. The spectral trace demonstrates regurgitation through the valve into the right atrium and measurement of the flow velocity of the jet allows an assessment of the right heart pressure. In this case the peak jet velocity of 4 m/s suggests an estimated right ventricular pressure of at least 70 mmHg.

PROSTHETIC HEART VALVES

Prosthetic heart valves may be mechanical or biological and may be seen in any position, most commonly the aortic and mitral valves. Mechanical valves are of the ball and cage type (Starr–Edwards—now rarely used) or the tilting disc type. The single tilting disc (Bjork–Shiley) has now given way to the commonly employed bileaflet types (St Jude or CarboMedic). These valves are clearly identified by echocardiography as they give rise to strong reverberant echo patterns. Nevertheless it is usually possible to evaluate their function and see the leaflets moving. In the case of mitral regurgitation the valves may shield the left atrium from the ultrasound beam and assessment of the regurgitant jet may require transoesophageal echocardiography. Biological valves can be stent-mounted porcine xenografts (pig valve tissue mounted on a frame) or homograft valves (human tissue, usually without additional

mechanical support). The mobile leaflets of these valves are usually visible with good quality echocardiography (Fig. 12.23).

All prosthetic valves offer a smaller orifice size than the original native valve and Doppler flow patterns in these valves always show a slightly restrictive pattern. Valve regurgitation with either type of valve can be paraprosthetic (outside the valve sewing ring) but degenerative change in biological valves can produce regurgitation directly through the valve ring. Study of prosthetic valve function requires considerable experience in echocardiography. Transoesophageal echocardiography is often important in the assessment of these valves if malfunction is suspected.

INFECTIVE ENDOCARDITIS

This condition can affect any valve but abnormal valves and prosthetic valves are much more commonly affected. The condition is

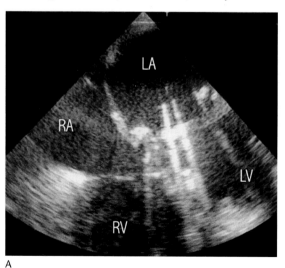

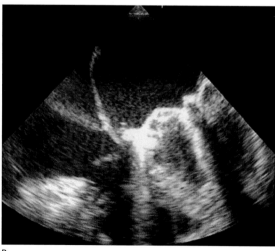

Fig. 12.23 Transoesophageal echocardiogram of a patient with a bileaflet prosthetic mitral valve. The two leaflets are shown open in diastole (A) and closed in systole (B). Prominent ultrasonic artefacts are generated from the prosthetic material. LA = left atrium; LV = left ventricle; RA = right atrium; RV = right ventricle.

A

B

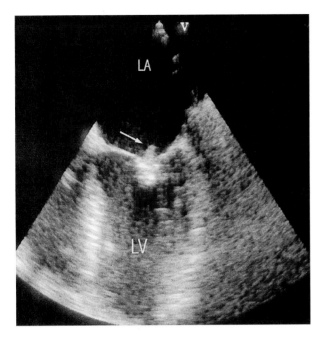

Fig. 12.24 Transoesophageal echocardiogram of a patient with mitral stenosis and infective endocarditis of the mitral valve. A small vegetation is seen prolapsing into the left atrium in systole (arrow). LA = left atrium; LV = left ventricle.

The condition is dangerous and can be rapidly progressive, so a high level of suspicion is required and early echocardiography is an important part of clinical management of the condition.

Sectional imaging in acquired valve disease

The role of CT is limited in assessing degrees of valvular dysfunction but this imaging modality has a role in identifying postoperative complications from valve replacements.

There is an established role for MRI in the diagnosis and quantification of valvular heart diseases, particular in confirming changes that are often difficult to determine by echocardiographic methods. Most clinical studies have used cardiac gated ciné MRI which produces a set of images at different stages of the cardiac cycle that can be viewed dynamically (usually with white blood). Any marked turbulence of flow of blood is demonstrated as black signal void (Fig. 12.26), hence both regurgitation and stenotic

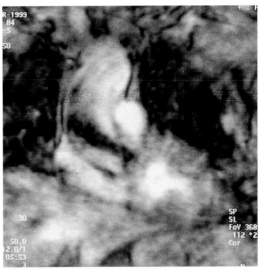

Fig. 12.26 Coronal gradient-echo MRI scan at the level of the aortic valve in a patient with aortic valve stenosis. The high-velocity turbulent jet entering the aortic root is seen as a signal void.

diagnosed clinically but strong diagnostic support can be obtained from echocardiography. In many cases, transoesophageal echocardiography is essential to make a detailed examination of the valves. The characteristic feature of infective endocarditis is the vegetation, an infected echogenic mass usually adherent to the free edge of a valve cusp. Vegetations can be small (1–5 mm) or they can be very large (2–3 cm) (Figs 12.24, 12.25). There is a high risk of embolisation with large vegetations. The infective process can lead to valve regurgitation by damaging the free edge of the leaflets or by leaflet perforation. Abscess formation can form in the valve annulus, particularly in the aortic root.

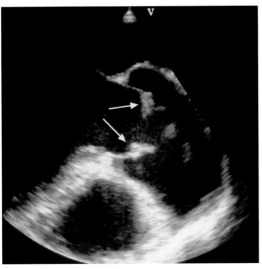

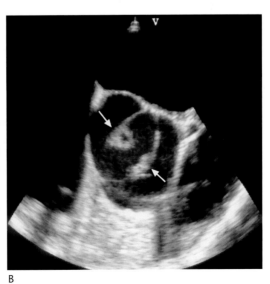

Fig. 12.25 Transoesophageal echocardiogram in the long-axis plane. The bicuspid aortic valve shows large vegetations on opposing leaflets (A) (arrow). The short-axis view confirms the bicuspid anatomy and shows the 'kissing' vegetations on opposing leaflets (B) (arrow).

A   B

valves can be highlighted. This method is particularly important in attempting quantification of the degree of incompetence of a valve, and has been used in both aortic and mitral regurgitation. Other early methods have directly measured the volume of the signal void. This method has shown promising correlation between both echocardiographic and angiographic findings in differentiating between mild, moderate and severe regurgitation.

Most recent research has centred on the use of velocity-encoded ciné MRI to try to quantify the degree of regurgitation present. This method utilises the principles of flow measurement incorporated in echocardiographic practice. If the combination of a flow velocity and area of a vessel are known then an estimation of the stroke volume can be produced.

Most of these methods are still research tools, because the time taken to estimate the degree of valvular dysfunction in each patient makes it an impractical method in the context of a busy scanner. However, as the availability of scanners increases and the methods of measurements become more automated MRI will be of increasing use in solving these difficult clinical problems.

PERICARDIAL DISEASE

Echocardiography of pericarditis and pericardial effusion

The diagnosis of pericardial effusion was one of the earliest applications of echocardiography and it remains today an important application of the technique. The characteristic echo-free space around the heart characterises a fluid collection and it is well demonstrated using both two-dimensional and M-mode imaging (Fig. 12.27). Several types of fluid that may collect in the pericardial space, including transudates, exudates, purulent fluid and

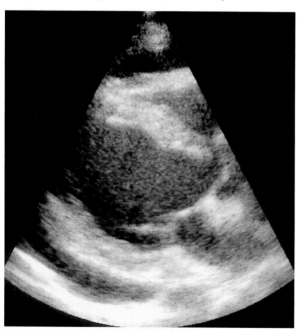

Fig. 12.27 Transthoracic echocardiogram in the parasternal long-axis view showing a moderate size pericardial effusion both anteriorly and posteriorly. LV = left ventricle; LA = left atrium; RV = right ventricle; Eff = pericardial effusion.

blood. It is not always possible to distinguish one from another but the clinical history will of course help. Exudates tend to contain fibrous strands and the pericardial surfaces may be shaggy. Purulent fluid will often have a fluid nature with echogenic material within it; it may also be loculated. Haemopericardium may be seen as a simple fluid collection or as a mixture of thrombotic and fluid material.

Inflammation of the pericardium alone will not be obvious on most types of imaging unless there is additional pathological change such as pericardial effusion, thickening or calcification.

The examination of the effusion must carefully distinguish between a pericardial effusion and an adjacent pleural effusion. In a good quality scan the separate layers can be identified but in case of doubt the collapsed lung tissue in the pleural effusion will be a clear identification sign.

Simple pericarditis can occur after a simple viral infection. The presence of fluid is detected up to 6 weeks after the onset of illness and is often associated with fever and pain. Occasionally this condition leads to constriction.

The presence of pus in the pericardium is unusual, but is often a result of direct local spread. This can occur from such sources as infective endocarditis, a subphrenic collection, or if the patient is immunosuppressed when fungal and atypical infections can develop. One important cause for a purulent pericarditis is tuberculosis. Although this condition is thought to result from direct spread from infected mediastinal lymph nodes, less than half of the cases have pulmonary involvement. Features that suggest tuberculosis as a diagnostic possibility include progressive thickening of the pericardium associated with a large, often loculated, effusion.

Constrictive pericarditis is a rare complication of pericardial inflammation but is increasing in frequency. The classically described cause of the condition is post-tuberculous constrictive pericarditis with calcification. Viral pericarditis complicated by development of fibrous adhesions is not uncommon, but there are an increasing number of iatrogenic cases. The most common is following the development of a haemopericardium post cardiac surgery. Another iatrogenic cause of the recent past is mediastinal irradiation, although great care is now used to avoid irradiating the heart. Radiation therapy often affects the parietal pericardium, leading to the development of a large effusion. This has been reported as a late complication of this therapy.

Examination of a pericardial effusion must include full evaluation of the extent of the collection, particularly if it is loculated. Retrosternal and posterior loculations can be particularly difficult to diagnose. Size and movement of the cardiac chambers must be assessed. If the right atrium and ventricle are small, this may indicate pericardial tamponade (restricted filling of the heart due to compression by the fluid). If diastolic collapse of either chamber is seen, this is an even stronger indication of tamponade (Fig. 12.28). Doppler evaluation of the tricuspid and mitral valve inflow can also assist in the diagnosis of tamponade. The normal inspiratory increase in tricuspid inflow is exaggerated. The normal mitral flow velocity tends to decrease in inspiration and this finding is also exaggerated in cardiac tamponade.

If the effusion is large and there are clinical or echocardiographic signs of tamponade, then ultrasound-guided pericardiocentesis is often indicated. This is based on the clear identification of the site of the maximal collection of fluid and the most direct access site. The drainage may be carried out from a parasternal or apical position and does not have to be from the traditional subcostal route,

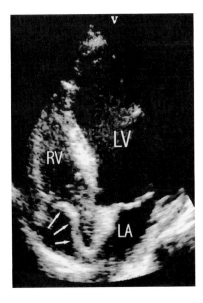

Fig. 12.28 Transthoracic echocardiogram from the apex showing diastolic collapse of the right atrial free wall (arrows). LV = left ventricle; LA = left atrium; RV = right ventricle.

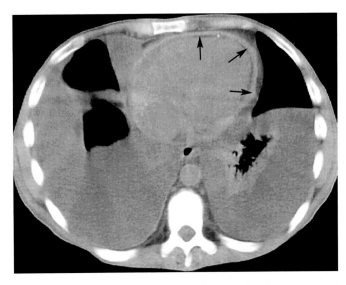

Fig. 12.30 Pericardial thickening (arrows) in a patient in chronic renal failure.

indeed the latter often involves a transhepatic route for the needle. A multihole drainage catheter may be left in situ. This technique requires special training, as there are risks of cardiac trauma (Fig. 12.29).

CT of pericarditis and pericardial effusion

Diseases of the pericardium can be clearly visualised using CT. The normal appearance of the pericardium is of a linear opacity up to 3 mm thick anterior to the right ventricle. The pericardium is clearly visualised because it is bordered by epicardial and mediastinal fat. Most imaging of the thorax using CT is with the patient in the supine position and any small amount of excess fluid tends to collect in a dependent portion of pericardium; this is usually posterior to the left atrium. If an effusion becomes large it tends to surround the heart and motion artefact from within the fluid may be detected. Sometimes there are fibrous components to the pericardial collection resulting in loculations. Chronic pericardial effusions can also result in thickening of the pericardium (Fig. 12.30).

If the pericardial collection is large enough often it can be characterised by assessing the attentuation value. A transudate will have

a value of Hounsfield units similar to 0. An exudate has slightly higher values of attenuation, very close to the value of the parietal pleura, or higher if the effusion is blood stained. Hounsfield values of 50–60 suggest a haemopericardium. CT also detects thickening of the pericardium and calcification with a high degree of sensitivity and specificity. This method of imaging also provides information about the adjacent structures in the thorax including the pleura and the lungs.

CT can be used to demonstrate not only thickening of the pericardium by direct visualisation, but also bilateral disproportionate dilatation of the atria, generated by the increase in atria pressure. In addition to atrial deformity, reflux of contrast media into the coronary sinus has also been reported. CT is the most accurate method of demonstrating the extent and distribution of pericardial calcification. Pericardial calcification occurs in approximately one-third of cases of constrictive pericarditis, usually characterised as a fine irregular line of calcification (Fig. 12.31).

CT will also demonstrate the presence of additional pleural effusions or ascites associated with the increase in both right and left

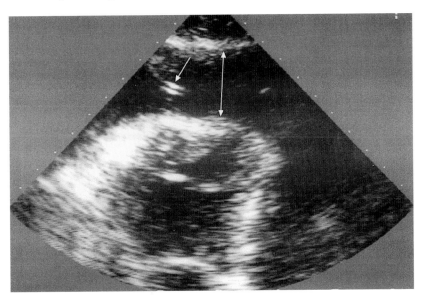

Fig. 12.29 Transthoracic echocardiogram demonstrating a large pericardial effusion (double-headed arrow). This effusion is large enough to compromise the cardiac output and a 6Fr pigtail catheter (arrow) has been placed under ultrasound guidance into the effusion to allow drainage.

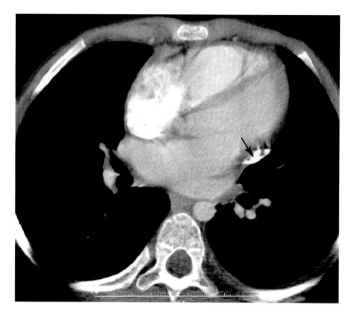

Fig. 12.31 Chronic constrictive pericarditis with focal pericardial calcification (arrow).

atrial pressures. An increase in the size of the SVC and IVC, and azygos system can be detected.

MRI of pericarditis and pericardial effusion

Diseases of the pericardium are clearly visualised using MRI (Fig. 12.32) and this method should be considered in cases where the diagnosis using echocardiography is unclear. MRI has many advantages; haemopericardium can be distinguished from conventional fluid and it is the best imaging modality for differentiating the diagnosis of constrictive pericarditis from a restrictive cardio-

myopathy. MRI is the method of choice in identifying the rare congenital absence of the pericardium, as MRI allows direct visualisation of the pericardium. Although a thickness of 3 mm or greater on MRI is consistent with the diagnosis of pericarditis, this finding has to be interpreted in the clinical context. Several studies have demonstrated thickening of the pericardium in the postoperative period, lasting for several months.

MRI is very sensitive at detecting even small amounts of fluid within the pericardium; a small amount of fluid is detected in the normal subject particularly in the superior pericardial recess. Both T_1- and T_2-weighted axial images should be acquired as a haemorrhagic effusion will have a high signal on both images.

If cardiac-gated ciné MRI is performed in the axial plane, vital information about the haemodynamics of the chambers is produced. Often in constrictive pericarditis there is disproportionate dilatation of the atrium compared to the ventricles. If assessment of the valves excludes the diagnosis of regurgitation and imaging of the pericardium shows pathological thickening, then the diagnosis of constrictive pericarditis is likely. Occasionally, constriction of the pericardium is localised to the right side of the heart and sometimes the pericardial thickening is localised to the atrioventricular groove with consequent narrowing of the tricuspid valve orifice.

CONGENITAL ABSENCE OF THE PERICARDIUM

A complete or partial absence of the pericardium can occur and can be detected by both CT and MRI. A partial absence of the pericardium is almost always left sided. Associated congenital anomalies are more common when a partial absence occurs and are present in about one-third of cases. The partial absence of the left pericardium was found in 1 in 13 000 postmortems. This condition is more common in men. The common associations include tetralogy of Fallot, patent ductus ateriosus, atrial septal defects and lung

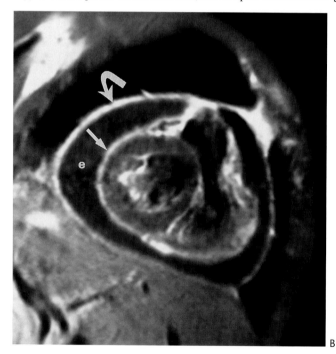

Fig. 12.32 Inflammatory pericarditis on transverse (A) and parasagittal (B) ECG-gated T_1-weighted spin-echo (SE 750/15) images following intravenous administration of gadolinium chelate. There is a large low-signal pericardial effusion (e) with marked enhancement of the parietal (curved arrow) and visceral (straight arrow) pericardia.

defects such as interlobular sequestration and a bronchogenic cyst. The defect occurs in front of and below the left hilum and measures up to 5 cm. Rarely, herniation of the left atrial appendage or pulmonary artery through this structure has been reported and the outcome can be fatal.

PERICARDIAL MASSES

Both CT and MRI are excellent imaging modalities for characterising pericardial masses. The commonest pericardial 'mass' is the pericardial cyst. A pericardial cyst is an asymptomatic cyst that is more common in men and on the right side of the pericardium. The cyst can be large, measuring up to 8 cm in diameter and containing clear fluid, referred to as 'spring water'. The pericardial cyst represents about 10% of all mediastinal masses. Occasionally the pericardial cyst contains calcification and differentiation from other mediastinal masses

can be difficult. This can be compounded in the cyst in an unusual location. CT allows demonstration of the attenuation of the fluid in the cyst; simple pericardial cysts have an attenuation of between 20 and 40 HU, if the attenuation is higher than this figure then diagnostic aspiration should be performed (Fig. 12.33). Cysts of the pericardium can also be due to infective conditions such as tuberculosis and hydatid disease (Fig. 12.34). These cysts may also be identified by echocardiography if they are in a suitable position.

Secondary invasion of the pericardium can complicate disease processes such as bronchogenic carcinoma or carcinoma of the breast (Fig. 12.35). MRI is very sensitive at detecting invasion, particularly when a STIR sequence is used. This sequence, whilst lacking the resolution of other sequences, will demonstrate high signal associated with infiltration. Often infiltration through the pericardium produces a haemorrhagic pericardial effusion and this can be detected, with high signal on T_1-weighting, on MRI.

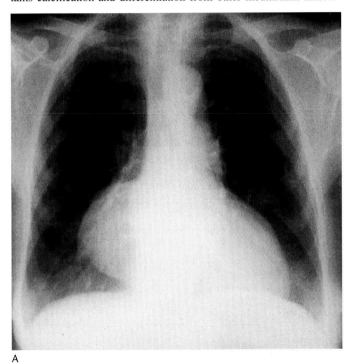

A

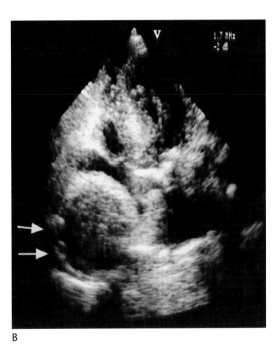

B

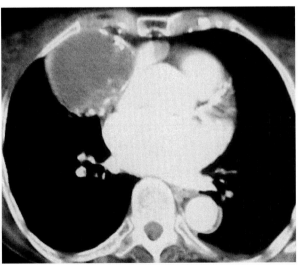

C

Fig. 12.33 In the frontal chest radiograph (A) there is a convex abnormality of the right heart border which is the classic appearance of a simple pericardial cyst. The transthoracic echocardiogram (B) confirms the presence of a cyst adjacent to the right atrium (arrows). A contrast-enhanced CT scan (C) confirms the presence of a simple cyst, containing fluid of a low attenuation. This CT scan also demonstrates fine calcification in the cyst wall, an uncommon feature of simple pericardial cysts.

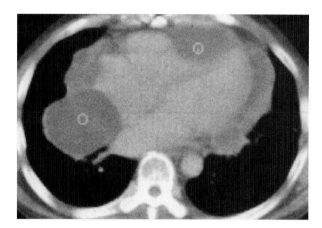

Fig. 12.34 A non-contrast-enhanced CT of the heart. There are multiple pericardial cysts of varying size surrounding the heart in a patient with hydatid disease. The attenuation value has been measured in two of the cysts (O). The attenuation was less than 30 Hounsfield units, consistent with a simple cyst. Hydatid disease is a rare cause of pericardial cysts.

CARDIAC MASSES AND TUMOURS

The development of non-invasive cardiac imaging has been central to the diagnosis and management of cardiac tumours. Identification of the site, size and nature of cardiac tumours is usually made by echocardiographic techniques. MRI may add specific information as an additional technique.

Primary cardiac tumours are rare, with a necropsy incidence of only 0.05%; secondary tumours are more common, occurring in 1% of postmortem examinations, especially in the context of widespread malignancy. Clinical presentation of cardiac tumours is very variable but embolisation, obstruction, systemic illness and arrhythmia are common presenting features.

PRIMARY BENIGN CARDIAC TUMOURS

The incidence of these tumours is shown in Table 12.2.

Atrial myxoma is the commonest cardiac tumour. These tumours can occasionally be familial and may be associated with facial freckling and endocrine adenomas. Ninety per cent are in the left atrium and 90% are solitary. Echocardiographic diagnosis is key

Table 12.2 Incidence of cardiac tumours. (Reproduced from Shapiro 2001)

	Adults (%)	Children (%)
Myxoma	45	15
Lipoma	20	–
Papillary fibroelastoma	15	–
Angioma	5	5
Fibroma	3	15
Haemangioma	5	5
Rhabdomyoma	1	45
Teratoma	<1	15

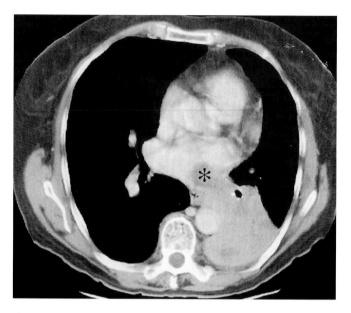

Fig. 12.35 Carcinoma of the bronchus invading the left atrium (*), transgressing the pericardium.

and both transthoracic and transoesophageal echocardiography will elegantly demonstrate the site and size of the tumour. The commonest appearance is a polypoid and mobile tumour with a heterogeneous echogenic appearance that arises from the interatrial septum, most commonly on the left side, and occasionally it may be difficult to distinguish the lesion from thrombus. The lesion may prolapse through the mitral valve in diastole and cause obstruction, mimicking mitral stenosis (Fig. 12.36). Urgent surgery is usually indicated for the condition, and regular echocardiographic follow-up is essential, as local recurrence is common.

The lesion is often diagnosed on transthoracic echocardiography but transoesophageal studies are frequently needed for establishing more diagnostic detail (Fig. 12.37).

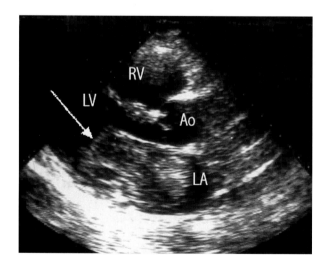

Fig. 12.36 A transthoracic echocardiogram in the parasternal long-axis view. An echogenic mass can be identified prolapsing through the mitral valve (arrow). This was an atrial myxoma. LA = left atrium; LV = left ventricle; RV = right ventricle; Ao = aortic root.

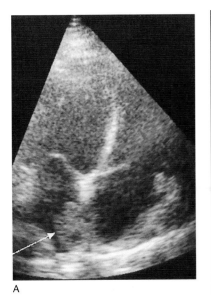

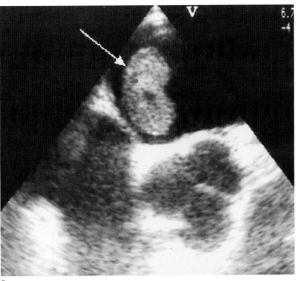

A   B

Fig. 12.37 Two different echo-cardiograms in a patient with an atrial myxoma. (A) A transthoracic apical four-chamber view. The soft-tissue mass (arrow) is difficult to identify. However, a trans-oesophageal examination (B) clearly shows the tumour (arrow). Trans-oesophageal echocardiography is the method of choice for visualising the posterior structures of the heart.

Papillary fibroelastoma

These small tumours occur on valves and valve apparatus and there is a risk of embolisation. Surgical excision may be appropriate in some cases. The differential is that of vegetation.

Rhabdomyoma

This is the commonest cardiac tumour of childhood and it is associated with tuberous sclerosis. The mass may lie within the myocardium or it may be pedunculated and obstructive. Spontaneous tumour resolution is common.

Lipoma

They usually occur in a subepicardial position and rarely cause symptoms. Large lipomas will predispose towards obstruction and arrhythmias. These tumours must be distinguished from lipomatous hypertrophy of the atrial septum, a non-neoplastic condition that may be found in elderly obese patients.

Fibroma

These tumours are usually intraventricular and can become quite large, causing obstruction or arrhythmia.

Angioma

These are rare and occur in the interventricular septum.

PRIMARY MALIGNANT CARDIAC TUMOURS

Approximately 25% of primary cardiac tumours have features of malignancy, 95% of these being sarcomas and 5% lymphomas. Sarcomas are commonest and are more common in middle-aged males (Fig. 12.38).

Angiosarcomas are most common and occur most often in the right atrium and may spread locally to the pericardium, pleura or mediastinum. Angiosarcomas may give rise to pulmonary metastases.

Rhabdomyosarcomas can occur in any chamber and are slightly less aggressive in terms of local invasion and distant metastasis.

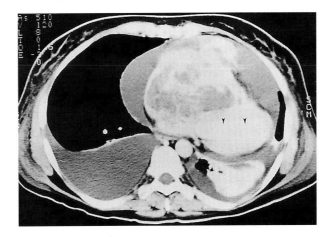

Fig. 12.38 Malignant angiosarcoma—CT scan with contrast. The tumour mass appears as an irregular filling defect in the right atrium and ventricle. The left ventricle is displaced posteriorly (arrows). A large pericardial effusion surrounds the heart.

Fibrosarcoma, histiocytoma and lymphoma are all rare although lymphoma is increasing in frequency in association with the acquired immunodeficiency syndrome (AIDS).

SECONDARY MALIGNANT CARDIAC TUMOURS

The majority of these tumours are epicardial but they may occur at any site. Pericardial effusion is common. They are 20 times more common than primary cardiac tumours and usually form part of a disseminated malignant process. They are clinically silent in 90% of cases.

Secondary malignancy may spread by direct invasion, usually from the mediastinum or lung, or by extension of the tumour from the upper abdomen through the inferior vena cava, usually from a liver, kidney or adrenal primary. The most common tumour to cause direct invasion is bronchogenic in origin but mediastinal lymphoma can often extend into the heart (Fig. 12.39).

Melanoma, lymphoma and leukaemia have a particular predisposition for blood-borne metastasis to the heart.

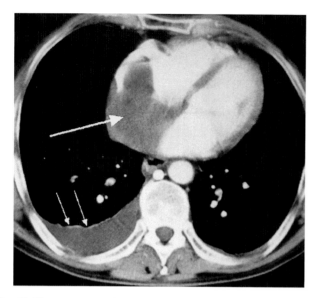

Fig. 12.39 A contrast-enhanced CT scan in a patient with non-Hodgkin's lymphoma. There is a large soft-tissue defect filling the right atrium (large arrow). This mass was biopsied and was shown to be a lymphoma. In addition, a right-sided pleural effusion has also developed (small arrows).

MRI of cardiac tumours

MRI has several advantages over CT when imaging and diagnosing intracardiac masses (Fig. 12.40). The gated method for performing most cardiac MRI means there is a reduction in cardiac motion, improving the resolution of the image. The signal characteristic of the lesion demonstrated on both T_1- and T_2-weighting can also suggest the composition of the mass. Differentiating a clot from an intracardiac mass can be difficult. If spin-echo MR is used the signal intensity of the clot will vary with the age of the clot. A relatively fresh thrombus will have high signal intensity on T_2-weighting, producing lower signal intensity as the clot matures. Most tumours have a high signal on T_2-weighted imaging.

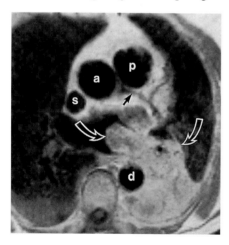

Fig. 12.40 Enhancing bronchial carcinoma (curved arrows) invading the left lower lobe bronchus, left atrium and descending aorta on a transverse gated T1-weighted post-gadolinium–DTPA spin-echo image (TE 26 ms). Note the associated lower-lobe collapse, which is difficult to differentiate from the tumour. The left coronary artery (straight arrow), with its anterior descending and circumflex branche, is shown. a = ascending aorta; d = descending aorta; la = left atrium; p = pulmonary artery; s = superior vena cava.

Gradient-echo sequencing is particularly useful, a tumour usually having medium signal intensity on T_2-weighting, while a thrombus will have a lower intensity than the surrounding tissue.

An atrial myxoma can be well demonstrated on MRI but there are limitations to the technique and small tumours less then 1.5 cm have been missed on MRI but detected by transoesophageal imaging. Atrial myxomas are often indistinguishable from thrombus because of the presence of calcification, fibrosis or even iron, all leading to a low signal. These tumours are best demonstrated by using white blood gradient-echo techniques where the mass is demonstrated as a low signal lesion surrounded by high signal blood.

A lipoma will have a characteristic high signal on T_1-weighting because of the high fat composition. If the diagnosis remains in doubt then a fat-saturation or STIR sequence will suppress the signal from the lesion.

Angiosarcoma can have a low signal when compared to the surrounding cardiac muscle on T_2-weighted imaging. The tumour does not enhance following intravenous gadolinium.

DISEASES OF THE THORACIC AORTA

A wide variety of pathological conditions can affect the aorta. These include atherosclerosis, degenerative change, connective tissue disorder, hypertensive disease, trauma and inflammation. The aortic structure may also be changed by pathology of the aortic valve and the reverse may also occur. It is not always possible to distinguish the aetiology of aortic pathology by imaging techniques alone, but it should be possible to assess the size and shape of the aorta, the abnormalities of its wall and the function of the aortic valve.

The major non-invasive imaging techniques of echocardiography (including transoesophageal echocardiography), CT and MRI should be capable of assessing the structural pathology of the aorta in almost all cases. The application of the different techniques will depend on the underlying condition, the clinical setting and the availability of equipment and expertise in each imaging modality. In rare cases it may still be necessary to use angiography for the assessment of aortic disease.

Three main structural abnormalities may affect the aorta:

1. Aneurysm—enlargement of the aorta beyond accepted normal limits.
2. Dissection—separation of the layers of the aortic intima with a communicating tear to the lumen to produce a 'false lumen'.
3. Rupture—leakage of blood outside the normal confines of the aortic adventitia.

These three conditions may all occur independently or they may also occur together in any combination. The three abnormalities may occur to different degrees at different sites.

The task of the radiologist is to use the most appropriate imaging techniques to determine the nature of these structural abnormalities as accurately as necessary for the correct management of the patient. In some cases, such as potential dissection or rupture, there will be a need to achieve accurate diagnosis as quickly as possible to hasten treatment and improve prognosis.

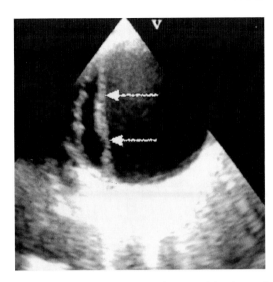

Fig. 12.41 A transoesophageal echocardiogram of the descending aorta clearly identifies a dissection flap present (arrows). This region is poorly visualised by transthoracic echocardiography because of its posterior location.

Echocardiography

Transthoracic echocardiography is an excellent technique for assessing the heart, the aortic valve and the pericardium but it is more limited in the assessment of the aorta. In some cases reasonable quality images of the aortic root and the aortic arch can be obtained but generally the technique is insufficient to make accurate and complete diagnoses of aortic disease. Transoesophageal echocardiography, however, can give excellent detail of much of the aorta. The aortic valve, aortic root, lower portion of the ascending aorta and the descending aorta are all seen with great clarity by the technique (Fig. 12.41). The upper half of the ascending aorta and the arch as far posteriorly as the isthmus are very hard to image well by the technique due to the interposition of the major airways. Doppler studies will enhance diagnostic accuracy by showing flow in the true and false lumens as well as demonstrating the site of the tear in many cases.

The technique has the advantage of convenience, as it is suitable for use at the bedside in the ward or in the operating theatre, but it remains a somewhat uncomfortable procedure and there are risks of causing increased hypertension if the examination is not conducted atraumatically.

In some settings, for example specialist cardiac surgical units, this technique is frequently employed as the first-line investigation for dissection and rupture. In other settings these specialised skills and equipment will not be available. The study will allow assessment of the aortic root from the level of the aortic valve, it will demonstrate flow in any true or false lumens, and it will usually identify the initiating tear of the dissection. Care must be taken to avoid misinterpretation of reverberant artefacts as intimal flaps.

In the case of aortic aneurysm without the concern of acute pathology, echocardiography is less likely to be the first-line investigation due to its lack of complete coverage.

AORTIC DISSECTION

Contrast-enhanced CT

This is now the mainstay of diagnosis in aortic dissection in most departments without transoesophageal echocardiography. There is

also a role for MRI in aortic dissection, particularly because of its multiplanar capability, but most MRI scanners do not have anaesthetic- or resuscitation-compatible equipment and therefore safe conduct of the examination in compromised acute patients is not possible.

Every effort should be made to maximise the quality of the CT scan, which is often performed as an emergency in a patient with an unstable cardiovascular system. Care should be taken to remove all possible potential external artefacts from the plane of imaging. Spiral and multislice CT scanners can now cover a large volume of tissue in a short acquisition time, and the patient should be imaged from above the origins of the great vessels in the thorax to the aortic bifurcation. Further scanning should be performed if the dissection flap is visualised at the bifurcation to determine the extent of the dissection in the lower limb vessels.

Typically 100–150 ml of contrast medium at a concentration of 300 mg of iodine per ml is injected using a pump at a rate of 3–5 ml per second. The imaging sequence is started after 75% of the injection or by automatic trigger on detection of arrival of the contrast bolus in the systemic vessels.

Often the intimal flap can be identified by demonstration of two lumens within the aorta originating from the point of the dissection tear dissection (Fig. 12.42). In 95% of all Type A dissections the origin will be within 2–3 cm of the aortic root and in Type B dissections the tear will usually be just distal to the origin of the left subclavian artery. Two-thirds of all dissections involve the ascending aorta. Often a differential bloodflow within the true and false lumens can be detected by the variable enhancement patterns following the intravenous contrast. This is an important consideration when an extensive dissection has occurred, because sometimes absence of perfusion of the abdominal organs such as the kidneys can be identified (Fig. 12.43). This is important information for the clinicians in the postoperative period. Another important consideration is the need to determine if the dissection extends into any of the great vessels arising from the aortic arch—very important information for the surgeon.

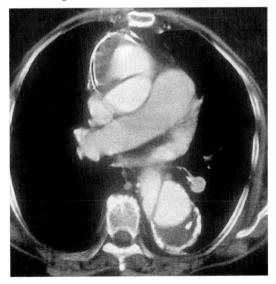

Fig. 12.42 A contrast-enhanced CT scan of the mediastinum at the level of the right pulmonary artery. The ascending and descending aorta are both heavily calcified and dilated. A dissection flap is clearly visualised in both components of the aorta, with equal contrast opacification in both the false and true lumen. This is a Stanford type A dissection.

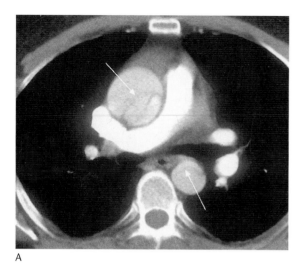

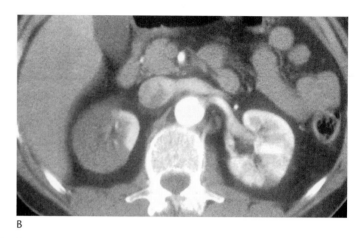

Fig. 12.43 A contrast-enhanced CT scan of the mediastinum (A) at the level of the right pulmonary artery. The timing of the scan shows the maximum contrast opacification in the pulmonary arteries but a dissection flap can be identified in both the ascending and descending components of the aorta. In this patient with a Stanford type A dissection the dissection extended into the abdomen and involved the main right renal artery leading to renal ischaemia (B). A small part of the kidney enhances supplied by an accessory renal artery.

Often in aortic dissection the CT will demonstrate periaortic haematoma caused by venous bleeding within the aortic wall. The technique may also demonstrate a pericardial effusion (haemopericardium), related to a tear extension into the aortic root. One of the major disadvantages of CT in the detection of aortic dissection is that this imaging modality produces little information about the function of the aortic valve. Often a dissection extends into the aortic root leading to the development of aortic regurgitation. This extension can also involve the origins of either coronary artery and can lead to myocardial infarction.

There are some pitfalls to be avoided in CT diagnosis of dissection. Linear artefacts across the aortic lumen can mimic an intimal flap. Leads or metallic lines on the patient's chest, or more commonly opacification of an adjacent venous structure such as the superior vena cava, can generate these artefacts. Use of a less concentrated contrast, which reduces the streaking artefact, can reduce this effect, but if doubt remains a repeat scan or alternative technique may be necessary. The overall volume of contrast medium administered should be monitored to avoid circulatory overload. Occasionally periaortic structures can be interpreted as periaortic haematoma; a classic area that can give rise to confusion is the presence of fluid in the superior pericardial recess. Perhaps the most common misinterpretation is caused by tortuosity of the aorta, which can give rise to an apparent inward projection of the aortic wall.

CHRONIC DISSECTION IN THE THORACIC AORTA

The major role for imaging aortic dissection is in assessing the medically treated Type B dissection and in assessing the ascending

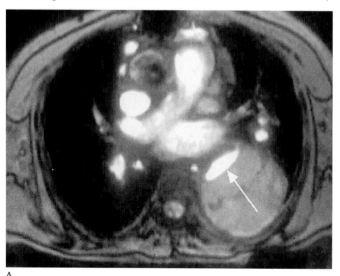

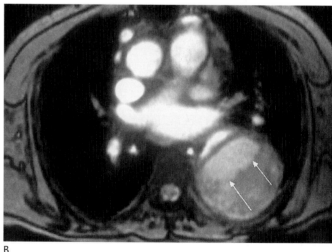

Fig. 12.44 A gradient-echo axial MRI through a dilated descending aorta using a white blood ciné sequence. Several images are obtained at this level over a period of time. Initially blood flowing in the true lumen is white (arrow), indicating a previous dissection (A). However, when the full sequence is assessed there is an increase in the signal of a second false lumen on (B) (arrows). A further lumen fails to opacify. This suggests there are three components to this chronic dissection.

aorta and aortic root in the postoperative patient. In both these conditions the patient is haemodynamically stable and can therefore be imaged easily. The multiplanar nature of MRI allows a tortuous aorta to be imaged more easily. In addition, the use of ciné sequences in both the oblique and axial planes allows important information about the aortic valve and flow within the false lumen to be obtained. It is not unusual for further dissection to occur in the treated group. Ciné MRI will often demonstrate variable flow patterns in the true lumen and one or more false lumens. At the time of follow-up MRI examination, the heart can also be imaged to assess the degree of aortic regurgitation and to assess left ventricular function. Sometimes haematoma can be visualised in the aortic wall, this finding has been reported in isolation, and is often referred to in this context as a penetrating ulcer of the aortic wall or as a precursor to a full dissection (Fig. 12.44).

ANEURYSM OF THE THORACIC AORTA

This can occur at any site in the aorta depending on the aetiology. In atherosclerotic and degenerative disease, the arch and descending aorta are commonly involved but in Marfan's syndrome it is the aortic root that is most commonly affected. Marfan's syndrome is an autosomal disease with a variable penetrance, 15% of cases being in new mutations. The disease leads to the development dilatation of the aortic root, which extends into the aortic arch, although this dilatation rarely extends further than the innominate artery. It is important to diagnose the presence of dilatation of the aorta in members of a family of a patient with known Marfan's syndrome. The dilatation starts in the sinuses of Valsalva with all three sinuses dilating and causing loss of the normal angle between the sinuses and the ascending aorta itself (the sino-tubular junction). The aneurysm usually extends to involve the proximal ascending aorta.

Assessment of any aneurysm must include determination of the site, shape and size of the lesion as well as its relationship to aortic branches. The wall must be evaluated to see if there is any associated thrombus formation or dissection. All these features are well demonstrated by sectional imaging MRI, has the most flexible options to demonstrate both form and function. It is usually stated that risk of spontaneous rupture of an aortic aneurysm rises significantly once the diameter increases beyond 5 cm.

A rare cause of aortic aneurysm is a post-traumatic aneurysm, commonly saccular and seen at the isthmus or arch. It is debatable whether this type of aneurysm is a true or false aneurysm.

Syphilitic aortic aneurysm is uncommon but can involve the ascending or descending aorta.

AORTIC RUPTURE

The commonest cause of isolated aortic rupture is high-velocity trauma but rupture is also commonly associated with dissection, aneurysm or atherosclerotic disease (Fig. 12.45). The diagnosis of rupture depends on the identification of haematoma outside the aortic lumen but in close association with the course of the vessel. This must be seen in addition to the features of any underlying pathology. The haematoma will not usually show contrast enhancement on CT examination unless there is severe bleeding. In some cases where the haematoma cannot be correlated with a bleeding

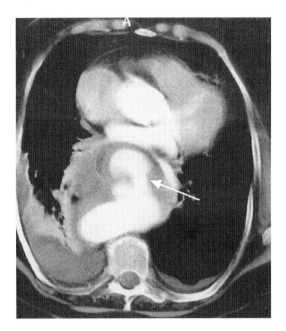

Fig. 12.45 Contrast-enhanced CT scan of the lower descending aorta demonstrating a penetrating ulcer (arrow), which has ruptured into the para-aortic space. This ulcer has developed as a result of atherosclerotic disease.

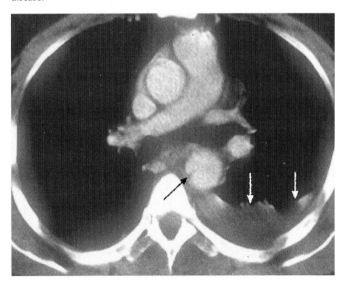

Fig. 12.46 Contrast-enhanced CT scan of a young man who was involved in a high-speed road traffic accident. There is a small mediastinal collection and a left-sided pleural effusion (white arrows). In addition a small defect can be identified in the lumen of the descending aorta (black arrow). This small defect represents a transection of this vessel, which was confirmed on angiography.

site, the source of the haemorrhage may be periaortic veins or small arteries (Fig. 12.46). There will often be an associated pleural effusion and of course the presence of a haemopericardium is most likely due to rupture of the aortic root.

In any assessment of possible traumatic aortic rupture, the great vessels arising from the arch must be fully examined as rupture or avulsion of these vessels is not an uncommon association. In some cases of traumatic or atherosclerotic rupture, the definitive diagnosis can be hard to make and this is one of the clinical situations where angiography may still be necessary (Fig. 12.47).

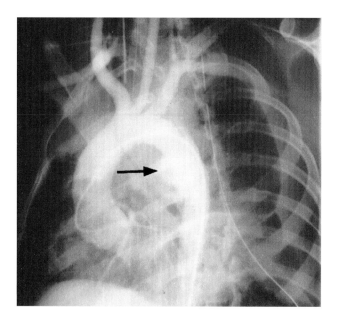

Fig. 12.47 Aortic angiogram in the left anterior oblique view. This shows aortic transection with localised extravasation and a left pleural effusion.

PULMONARY VESSELS

There can be few areas of imaging that have produced such controversy over the last 10 years than the correct method to image pulmonary embolic disease and the role of cross-sectional imaging modalities in establishing this diagnosis. The situation is compounded by the wide availability of radionuclide imaging at a time when CT scanners are becoming increasingly busy with a wide variety of applications. It has been established that properly performed spiral CT allows uniform opacification of the central pulmonary arteries, which allows clear visualisation of central vessels; the identification of the more peripheral emboli remains difficult. Maximal visualisation of the more peripheral vessel requires careful technique with exact timings. Often the data needs to be reviewed on a workstation where the images of the pulmonary arteries can be scrolled through to try and identify an abrupt cut-off that indicates an embolus.

Echocardiography has little role in establishing the diagnosis of pulmonary embolus. The right heart may show signs of acute dilatation and rarely large emboli may be visualised in the central pulmonary arteries. The peripheral lung fields are not accessible to echocardiography.

CT scanning in pulmonary embolism

There is no current accepted technique for maximising the identification of pulmonary emboli, every aspect of imaging being assessed with varying degrees of controversy; these include the collimation, the pitch, the rate and concentration of contrast and the algorithm of reconstruction. Several of these factors have also recently changed with the advent of multislice technology.

There is controversy as to whether a plain scan of the entire thorax should initially be performed. This scan will identify any other pathological processes that may have mimicked a PE, which is important as the entire thorax will not be imaged post-contrast and in the absence of a plain scan certain areas of the chest will be omitted. It also allows accurate localisation of the area to be imaged in the single breathhold post-contrast angiography phase.

There is a trade-off between the needs for thin-slice acquisition and short (single breath-hold) acquisition time. The distance that needs to be covered in this breath-hold is from the aortic arch to the inferior pulmonary vein, a distance of 12 cm. Although there is now an increased availability of sub-second scanners, most researchers have used a pitch of between 1.7 and 2. This combination produces images of acceptable quality but maintaining overall coverage in an acceptable breath-hold.

There are currently two methods of administering the contrast media used to opacify the pulmonary arteries. The difference in methods arises from work suggesting that the higher concentration contrast leads to streak artefacts that can be misinterpreted. To reduce this problem low iodine contrast has been injected at a high rate of flow, between 3 and 5 ml per second. This compares with a slow rate of flow used when injecting the high concentration contrast at 2–3 ml per second. Some researchers also minimise the effect of streak artefacts by scanning in a caudal–cranial direction.

Once a rate of injection has been decided, the timing of the bolus becomes crucial. Again there is little consensus about what is best delay but many researchers use a 20-second delay between commencement of injection and start of the imaging sequence. Some CT scanners have an automated scan-acquisition package which scans at low dose repeatedly through a particular level with a defined region of interest, and as soon as the attenuation level reaches a trigger value the scan is performed. If these automated systems are not available, the correct timing of the scan can be estimated from using a timing bolus. This is a simple technique in which a small amount of contrast (10–20 ml) is injected at the predetermined rate, and images are obtained at the level of the pulmonary outflow tract every 5 seconds over a 30-second period, the time to maximum opacification then being estimated.

The role of MRI in identifying pulmonary embolic disease is less well defined but it does have a great deal of potential, particularly with the recent interest in hyperpolarised gases. MRI does have the potential of producing a 3D ventilation perfusion study. Most of the early work was limited by the speed of scanning, but with the advent of faster gradients and magnetic systems it is now possible to produce a pulmonary angiogram in a single breath-hold using a 3D volume of acquisition. Most centres would use a gadolinium-enhanced technique to produce the 3D angiogram, as this shortens the T_1 relaxation times of the blood. The 3D dataset has the benefit of reducing the respiratory and cardiac motion artefacts. In combination with the phased array body coils, which provide a higher signal-to-noise ratio, segmental branches of the pulmonary circulation can be identified.

Some centres have tried other sequences where there is limited enhancement of the blood pool, emphasis being placed on imaging the clot, with techniques designed to maximise the properties of a resolving thrombus, but these still remain research tools.

THE DIAGNOSIS OF ACUTE PULMONARY EMBOLISM

The diagnosis of pulmonary emboli can be made by CT scanning if a filling defect outlined by a thin rim of contrast is visualised within the lumen of the vessel (Fig. 12.48). If this occurs in a vertically situated artery a central filling defect can be produced, the 'Polo

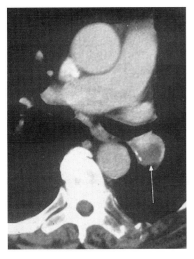

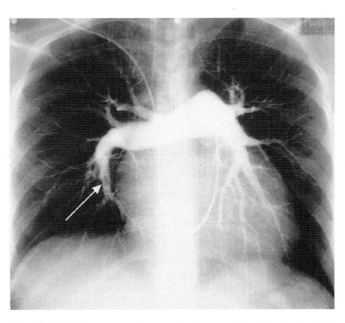

Fig. 12.48 Contrast-enhanced CT pulmonary angiogram demonstrating a large filling defect in an enlarged left lower lobe pulmonary artery (arrow). This is a large proximal pulmonary embolism.

mint sign'. If the embolus is in a horizontally orientated artery a 'tram-track' filling defect may be produced. Another common finding in the more peripheral arteries is 'the complete cut-off sign': this is produced when the thrombus completely occludes the lumen. This sign is easy to miss unless the interpreter scrolls through the images on a workstation where the abrupt cessation of a vessel becomes easier to visualise.

CT has the benefit of providing extra diagnostic information from the lungs, pleura and heart to indicate the presence of a pulmonary embolism. These findings are similar to the changes that have been described in this disease on the plain chest X-ray. Within the lungs wedge-shaped areas of consolidation can be identified abutting the pleurae; linear atelectasis and consolidation have also been reported. The presence of small unilateral or bilateral pleural effusions can be detected. Acute right heat dilatation with a marked increase in the diameter of the right ventricle has been described in association with a large embolus. The diameter of the right ventricle on the standard axial plain should be less than the diameter of the left ventricle; a reversal of this ratio suggests acute right ventricular strain (Fig. 12.49).

Major controversies surround the production of an imaging algorithm for clear assessment of the pulmonary arteries in establishing the diagnosis of pulmonary embolus. This debate is compounded if factors such as a positive D-dimer are also utilised. As yet no clear guidelines exist as the best method to image. Another controversial

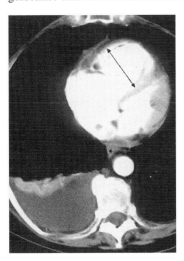

Fig. 12.49 This contrast-enhanced CT pulmonary angiogram identifies additional features that can be detected on CT and supports the diagnosis of pulmonary embolism. There is a right-sided pleural effusion and dilatation of the right ventricle (arrow).

Fig. 12.50 Pulmonary angiogram showing a small embolus in the right lower lobe artery (arrow). Angiography remains the most sensitive method of identifying small subsegmental pulmonary emboli.

area includes establishing what test can now be assumed to be the gold standard examination, many authorities believing that pulmonary angiography is an underperformed examination (Fig. 12.50).

CT has several important advantages over ventilation/perfusion scanning. The CT pulmonary angiogram is designed to directly visualise the thrombus, as opposed to a flow defect on a perfusion image. Currently, the speed of acquisition limits the amount of tissue that can be imaged in a single breath-hold. This problem is compounded because the patients with an indeterminate scan on radionuclide imaging are the patients least likely to be able to suspend respiration for a prolonged period of time due to their coexisting pulmonary disease.

A ventilation perfusion scan is a difficult image to interpret with a high degree of interobserver variation, with particular areas of disagreement including indeterminate scans and the identification of subsegmental emboli. There are, however, advantages in using ventilation perfusion scanning in combination with the chest X-ray as a first-line imaging investigation. Ventilation perfusion imaging is very accurate if the scan is interpreted as normal or high probability of pulmonary embolism. However, these two groups represent only 40% of all patients (Prospective Investigation of Pulmonary Embolism (PIOPED) study). In other studies, no patient reported as having a normal VQ scan suffered a further pulmonary embolic event in the next 6 months, and all patients in the high probability group had emboli demonstrated on subsequent angiography.

In this indeterminate group, 66% of patients were shown to have subsequent pulmonary emboli. The likelihood of any one patient having an indeterminate scan is increased in the presence of coexisting lung disease, usually evident on the initial chest X-ray.

Emphasis should be placed on the initial examination in deciding the most appropriate form of investigation. If the patient has a normal chest X-ray, a VQ scan should be performed because there is a low chance of an indeterminate scan. If there is a background of lung disease then a CT pulmonary angiogram should be performed, but the clinicians should be aware of the limitations of this form of imaging.

The relevance of subsegmental emboli is an additional area of controversy. There is a great deal of debate about the clinical importance of the subsegmental emboli. In the PIOPED study only 6% of patients had subsegmental emboli with only 1% of patients developing further emboli episodes. However, several angiographic studies have suggested that emboli can occur in isolation in up to 30% of patients. The relevance of isolated emboli in clinical practice has also been questioned—in a separate arm of the PIOPED study researchers found no difference in mortality or morbidity in two groups of patients, one treated and one untreated, with very mild ventilation perfusion abnormalities. There is little doubt that in patients with established cardiovascular disease a small embolus can make a significant clinical impact and if the diagnosis is of this importance then pulmonary angiography should be performed.

RADIONUCLIDE STUDIES OF LUNG PERFUSION AND VENTILATION

Radionuclide studies remain the most common method of trying to diagnose pulmonary embolic disease because of the high specificity of the positive test and the availability of the imaging technique. However, multiple studies have demonstrated that VQ scanning will produce an indeterminate result in up to 70% of cases, particularly if there is background lung disease producing an abnormal chest radiograph. A recent chest radiograph and ventilation images are both required to interpret perfusion scanning fully. While a normal perfusion scan excludes a pulmonary embolus, the certainty of the diagnosis in the context of the abnormal perfusion scan is dependent on the associated changes on both radiograph and ventilation study (Fig. 12.51).

The perfusion study is produced by injection intravenously of ^{99m}Tc-labelled human albumin microspheres (HAM) or macroaggregates. These albumin particles, which have a diameter of between 20 and 40 μm, occlude small terminal branches of the pulmonary artery. The perfusion scan will therefore demonstrate areas of the lung that are perfused by the pulmonary circulation. This examination is contraindicated in patients with known left to right shunts where the emboli may lodge in either the brain or the kidney.

The ventilation part of the examination is often performed using a technetium generator, which produces an aerosol that is inhaled. Although particles are physiologically different from gases, they can give an accurate assessment of ventilation if the particle size is small enough to ensure alveolar deposition. Care must be taken to ensure that the particle sizes do not become too

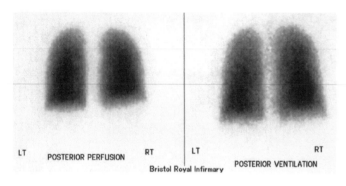

Fig. 12.51 Normal perfusion (A) and ventilation (B) scans in the posterior projection. There are no significant differences in appearances and there is no evidence of pulmonary embolus.

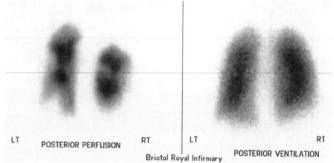

Fig. 12.52 Abnormal perfusion (A) scan and normal ventilation (B) scan in the posterior projection. There are multiple perfusion defects in both lungs that are not matched by ventilation defects.

Table 12.3   PIOPED criteria for the diagnosis of pulmonary embolism (Reproduced from PIOPED 1990)

Probability of pulmonary embolism	Normal chest radiograph	Abnormal chest radiograph	Interpretation not dependent on chest radiograph
Normal			Normal perfusion
Very low probability	1–3 small perfusion defects		
Low probability	1. Single moderate perfusion defect 2. VQ match in <50% of 1 lung including <75% of 1 lung zone	1. Perfusion defect substantially smaller than chest X-ray abnormality, ventilation findings irrelevant 2. 3 or fewer small perfusion/chest film matches	More than 3 small perfusion defects
Indeterminate probability			Abnormality that is not defined clearly by any other criteria
High probability	1. 2 or more large perfusion defects 2. 2 or more moderate perfusion defects and one large perfusion defect 3. 4 or more moderate perfusion defects	2 or more perfusion defects in which perfusion is substantially larger than either matching ventilation or chest film defect	

large too ensure alveolar deposition and hot spots may be seen in patients with chronic airways disease. Krypton-81m was used in the past but has several disadvantages including a short half-life.

For both the ventilation and perfusion components of the examination between four and six views of the lungs are obtained, and by convention the comparable views of ventilation and perfusion are demonstrated together (Fig. 12.52).

Most centres have adopted the PIOPED study findings to predict the probability of a pulmonary embolism. These criteria are listed in Table 12.3.

REFERENCES AND SUGGESTIONS FOR FURTHER READING

Blackwell, G. G., Cranney, G. B., Pohost, G. M. (1992) *MRI: Cardiovascular System.* London: Gower.

DePuey, E. G., Berman, D. S., Garcia, E. V. (1995) *Cardiac SPECT Imaging.* New York: Raven Press.

Globits, S., Higgins, C. B. (1996) Adult heart disease. In: Edelman, R. E. et al (eds) *Clinical Magnetic Resonance Imaging,* 2nd edn. Philadelphia: W. B. Saunders.

Manning, W. J., Pennell, D. J. (2001) *Cardiac Magnetic Resonance Imaging.* Edinburgh: Churchill Livingstone.

Meire, H., Cosgrove, D., Dewbury, K., Wilde, P. (1993) *Clinical Ultrasound: Cardiac Ultrasound.* Edinburgh: Churchill Livingstone.

Otto, C. M. (1999) *Textbook of Clinical Echocardiography,* 2nd edn. Philadelphia: W. B. Saunders.

Pioped Investigators (1990) JAMA **263(20)**: 2753–9.

Roelandt, J. R. T. C., Sutherland, G. R., Iliceto, S., Linker, D. T. (1993) *Cardiac Ultrasound.* Edinburgh: Churchill Livingstone.

Shapiro, L. M. (2001) Incidence of Cardiac Tumours *Heart* **85(2)**: 218–22.

Walsh, C., Wilde, P. (1999) *Practical Echocardiography.* London: Greenwich Medical Media.

Zaret, B. L., Beller, G. A. (1999) *Nuclear Cardiology State of the Art and Future Directions.* St Louis, MO: Mosby.

Non-invasive Cardiac Imaging

Blackwell, G. G., Cranney, G. B., Pohost, G. M. (1992) MRI: *Cardiovascular System.* London. Gower.

DePuey, E. G., Berman, D. S., Garcia, E. V. (1995) *Cardiac SPECT Imaging.* London. Raven Press.

Globits, S., Higgins, C. G. (1996) *Clinical Magnetic Resonance Imaging; Adult Heart Disease,* 2nd edn., Philadelphia, W. B. Saunders.

Meire, H., Cosgrove, D., Dewbury, K., Wilde P. (1993) *Clinical Ultrasound: Cardiac Ultrasound.* Edinburgh. Churchill Livingstone.

Roelandt, J. R. T. C., Sutherland, G. R., Iliceto, S., Linker, D. T. (1993) *Cardiac Ultrasound.* Edinburgh. Churchill Livingstone.

13

INVASIVE IMAGING AND INTERVENTIONAL TECHNIQUES

Peter Wilde and Mark Callaway

INTRODUCTION

In spite of the rapid development of non-invasive imaging in the past two decades there has been an ever-increasing expansion in the number of invasive cardiac examinations performed. The main reason for this is the very high incidence of coronary heart disease in developed countries coupled with the increasing therapeutic opportunities for treatment once precise anatomy and pathology of the coronary arteries has been determined. High-quality image resolution is required as typical major coronary artery branches have an internal diameter of 2.5–3.5 mm, with the left main stem being only 4 or 5 mm in internal diameter. Subdivisions of the major vessels can cause important clinical abnormalities, including those 1 mm or less in diameter. Lesion morphology is increasingly important in determining optimal selection of treatments and submillimetre resolution is now essential in coronary diagnosis (Figs 13.1, 13.2).

The coronary anatomy generally follows a recognised pattern, but in each individual there are variations and in many cases the variable branching and tortuosity of the surface vessels can be quite

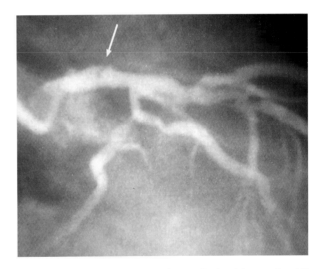

Fig. 13.2 Selective left coronary angiogram in the right anterior oblique projection. The arrow indicates a membranous plaque obstructing the left mainstem.

complex. Movement of the heart can be rapid, particularly in the right atrioventricular groove, and in order to 'freeze' motion imaging, exposure times of 5 ms or less must be achieved. Any other form of imaging technique, including the most advanced sectional techniques, cannot currently meet these demands and therefore coronary angiography remains the mainstay of advanced diagnosis in coronary heart disease.

Besides the study of coronary arteries there is only a limited number of other indications for cardiac catheterisation and angiography. In some cases where there is diagnostic doubt following non-invasive examination, it may be necessary to perform angiography together with detailed intracardiac pressure measurement or oximetry to resolve any diagnostic uncertainties. It is, however, unusual to have to rely on cardiac catheterisation and angiography to make routine evaluations of valvular lesions that are generally well evaluated with echocardiography or possibly MRI. There may be other cases where fine detail can only be resolved by angiography, for example in the evaluation of peripheral pulmonary branching patterns by pulmonary angiography. Left ventriculography, while conveniently performed in

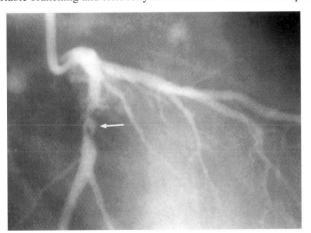

Fig. 13.1 Selective left coronary angiogram in the right anterior oblique projection. The arrow indicates a well-demarcated ulceration of an atheromatous plaque in the circumflex artery.

conjunction with coronary arteriography, is rarely needed as a primary tool to evaluate left ventricular function. Diseases of the aorta, particularly in emergency situations, have traditionally been diagnosed with aortography. CT or MRI have almost completely superseded this function and it is now rare to use angiography in this situation. Occasionally critically ill patients may be difficult to investigate in the MRI scanner due to difficulties with monitoring and intensive care support and angiography may be an appropriate alternative.

The investigation of congenital heart disease still makes frequent demands on angiography because fine detail of anatomy cannot always be identified by echocardiography, particularly as important structures may be close to pulmonary air spaces and may be difficult to image. In particular the pulmonary vascular structures may be hard to image by any other means. The fine resolution required for imaging paediatric cardiac anatomy may be impossible to achieve with sectional imaging techniques. The assessment of sophisticated haemodynamic measurements such as pulmonary vascular resistance or intracardiac shunt ratios may require intracardiac measurements and therefore the combined use of angiography may well be appropriate.

There is an increasing number of interventional or therapeutic techniques for the treatment of heart disease. These techniques include the dilatation of narrowings or obstructions, closure of abnormal communications, retrieval of foreign bodies, electrical stimulation or ablation and cardiac biopsy. All these techniques require X-ray imaging and may be combined with angiography to achieve a satisfactory outcome. It is for this reason that cardiac catheterisation and angiography remain major tools in the investigation and treatment of cardiac disease. Angiography facilities will be found in all major cardiology units and cardiac surgical centres.

In developed countries with a high incidence of coronary artery disease it will be usual to see between two thousand and five thousand cardiac angiography procedures performed annually for every million population. In some countries the figures will be even higher.

using a pigtail catheter which has multiple side-holes and an end-hole, the pigtail curve being designed to be atraumatic within the ventricular chamber. The left ventricle should be outlined with a contrast injection of sufficient duration to demonstrate three or four cardiac cycles but the pump injection should not be delivered so fast as to precipitate multiple ventricular ectopic beats or ventricular tachycardia which can impair the interpretation of the angiogram. A right anterior oblique projection is usually used to demonstrate the long axis of the left ventricle and care must be taken to analyse the contractility of all regions. Not only must the overall movement of the endocardium be assessed but the trabecular contraction must also be evaluated. In cases of extensive full-thickness previous myocardial infarction the abnormalities may be obvious (Fig. 13.4), but in some cases the abnormalities may be subtle and significant experience is needed to recognise them. In the case of any major abnormality a second projection in the left anterior oblique view is frequently employed. Valvular function is also assessed on the left ventricular angiogram and in particular, mitral regurgitation is well seen (Fig. 13.3). Care must be taken to avoid creating artefactual appearances by ectopic ventricular contractions or by malpositioning the catheter (Fig. 13.5). It is essential to position the pigtail catheter freely in the centre of the left ventricular cavity, between the papillary muscles; if the end-hole or side-holes are impacted against the endocardium an intramyocardial extravasation can result (Fig. 13.6). Modern digital equipment will usually allow an estimated calculation of left ventricular volume study and the ejection fraction, all of which will be derived from known magnification factors and recognised volume algorithms. The left ventricular angiogram will also be useful to delineate functioning of the aortic valves and in addition may add information about the overall pattern of coronary artery anatomy, bypass graft anatomy or unusual aortic anatomy. Aortic regurgitation will not be detectable by left ventricular angiography, this assessment requiring an aortic root injection.

DIAGNOSTIC CARDIAC ANGIOGRAPHY

The commonest diagnostic technique involves examination of the left ventricle and both coronary arteries in cases of known or suspected coronary artery disease—commonly referred to as a 'left heart catheter'. The approach is usually a percutaneous trans-femoral one using the Seldinger technique and it should be carried out with high-specification cardiac angiography equipment supported by continuous monitoring of the ECG and blood pressure through the catheter. All normal safety and resuscitation equipment should be immediately available including cardiac drugs, oxygen and a defibrillator. There must be trained support staff present, including a nurse, cardiac technician and radiographer all with cardiac experience and training.

LEFT VENTRICULAR ANGIOGRAPHY

The usual left heart examination is carried out using 6Fr or 5Fr catheters and most commonly begins with left ventriculography

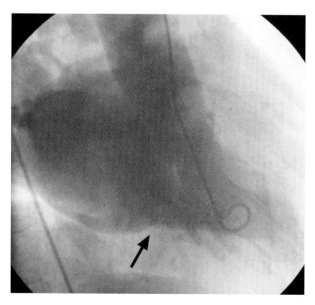

Fig. 13.3   Left ventricular angiogram in the right anterior oblique projection showing severe mitral regurgitation. The large left atrium is densely opacified and the mitral valve is arrowed.

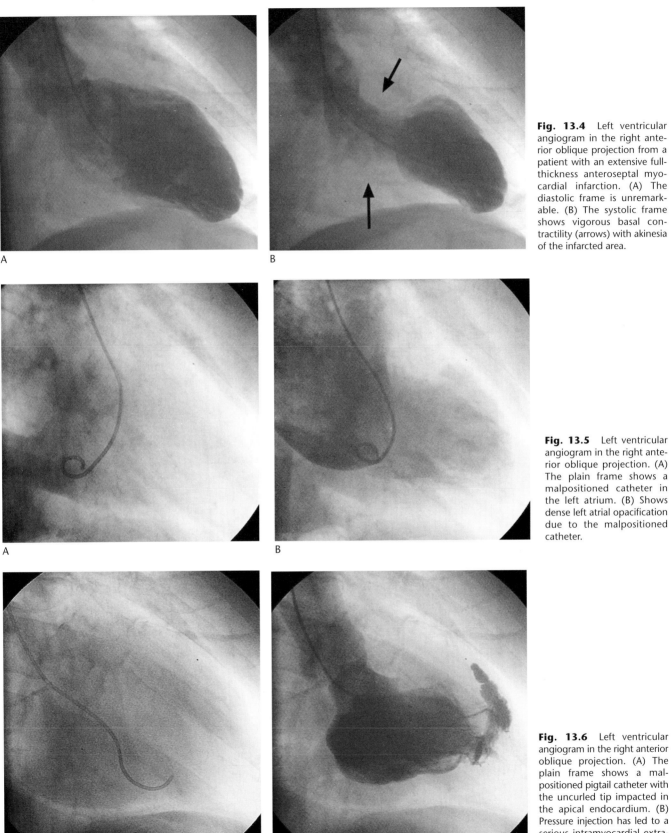

Fig. 13.4 Left ventricular angiogram in the right anterior oblique projection from a patient with an extensive full-thickness anteroseptal myocardial infarction. (A) The diastolic frame is unremarkable. (B) The systolic frame shows vigorous basal contractility (arrows) with akinesia of the infarcted area.

Fig. 13.5 Left ventricular angiogram in the right anterior oblique projection. (A) The plain frame shows a malpositioned catheter in the left atrium. (B) Shows dense left atrial opacification due to the malpositioned catheter.

Fig. 13.6 Left ventricular angiogram in the right anterior oblique projection. (A) The plain frame shows a malpositioned pigtail catheter with the uncurled tip impacted in the apical endocardium. (B) Pressure injection has led to a serious intramyocardial extravasation of contrast medium.

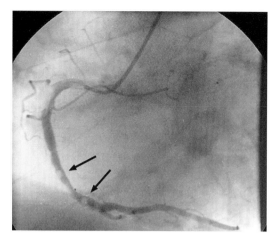

Fig. 13.7 Selective right coronary angiogram in the left anterior oblique projection. There has been inadvertent injection of a small amount of air. Arrows show small bubbles.

CORONARY ANGIOGRAPHY

Coronary angiography is normally carried out selectively using pre-formed end-hole catheters. The Judkins pattern is most usually employed with different shapes being utilised for left and right coronary arteries and indeed different curves are available for different configurations of aortic root and coronary anatomy. A

Box 13.1 Safety requirements for coronary angiography

Equipment
  High-resolution dedicated imaging equipment
  Multiangular projections available
  High-quality physiological monitoring
  Full resuscitation equipment immediately available
  Full range of catheter shapes available
  Low osmolar contrast medium preferable

Staff
  Operator fully trained in imaging and cardiological aspects
  Experienced support staff—radiographer, technician and nurse

Technique
  Care with catheter passage to aortic root
  Full awareness of catheter tip positioning
  Full awareness of any physiological changes
  Understanding of aortic and coronary anatomy
  Continuous angiographic interpretation during procedure

Box 13.2 Possible complications of coronary angiography

Femoral
  Dissection of femoral/iliac artery or aorta
  Haematoma

Aorta
  Damage to aortic intima
  Embolus to head and neck vessels
  Aortic root dissection

Coronary
  Ostial dissection
  Coronary embolus
  Arrhythmia due to catheter wedging or contrast medium
  Spasm due to catheter or contrast medium

General
  Hypotension
  Left heart failure—contrast overload
  Contrast allergy

---

wide range of alternative shapes of catheter is available, the most common being the Amplatz shape. Coronary injections are carried out using contrast medium containing 320–370 mg of iodine per ml and it is increasingly usual to see non-ionic media employed. Injection is normally made by hand from a closed manifold system, which has direct access to pressure monitoring, and the volume injected will depend on the size of the coronary distribution. It is essential that meticulous technique is employed to avoid introduction of air into the coronary circulation. Even small amounts of air can cause severe symptoms (Fig. 13.7). Typically the left coronary artery is well filled with 6–8 ml of contrast medium, with a typical smaller right coronary distribution requiring 3–5 ml. The injection should be made sufficiently fast to cause reflux of contrast medium to the ostium in order to demonstrate the artery completely.

During the conduct of coronary angiography it is vital to be aware of many important safety aspects (Boxes 13.1, 13.2). It is essential that the catheter tip does not wedge into a narrow coronary ostium and cause occlusion of flow. It is also essential that the tip of the catheter must be axially orientated in the proximal vessel rather than being angulated against the side-wall which can cause intimal damage (Fig. 13.8). Contrast injection with a catheter tip impacted on the side-wall of a proximal coronary artery can cause ostial dissection, one of the most serious and potentially fatal complications of the technique. Wedging of the catheter tip in an ostial stenosis will also be hazardous as there will be obstruction to flow

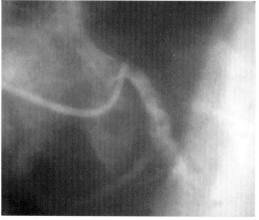

A

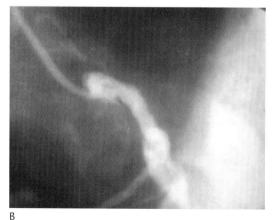

B

Fig. 13.8 Selective left coronary angiogram in the left anterior oblique projection. (A) The left Judkins catheter tip is upwardly angled against the wall of the left mainstem. (B) An improved position with the catheter tip axially aligned.

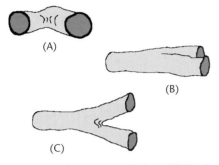

Fig. 13.9 Bifurcation in three orthogonal views. (A) Foreshortening of the branches. (B) Overlapping of the branches. (C) The only projection that fully demonstrates the bifurcation.

and ischaemia and arrhythmia will soon follow. It is for these reasons that constant visualisation of the catheter tip and continuous monitoring of catheter tip pressure is essential.

Coronary anatomy is very variable from patient to patient and it is essential to take a series of views in a range of obliques, some of which will include significant cranial or caudal angulation. A coronary arterial study cannot be considered complete until all major branches and bifurcations have been adequately profiled. All major bifurcations must be fully assessed if important lesions are not to be missed. The examination beam must be tangential to the opened bifurcation. This is only possible in one main orientation, the other

Table 13.1 Typical contrast injection doses and angulations in cardiac angiography

	Contrast volume (ml)	Injection rate (ml/s)	Typical projections (variable depending on anatomy)
Coronary angiography			
Left coronary	6–10	Hand (4–6)	RAO 50, RAO 20, LAO 40 + cranial 20, LAO 60, left lateral. (also optional PA + cranial 40 for additional LAD visualisation and PA + caudal 20 for left mainstem visualisation)
Right coronary	2–5	Hand (3–5)	RAO 30, LAO 20 + cranial 20, LAO 60
Left ventricle	35–40	10–15	RAO 30, possibly additional LAO 60
Aortogram	45–50	20	RAO 30 (assessment of aortic regurgitation), LAO 60 (best initial view of aortic anatomy)

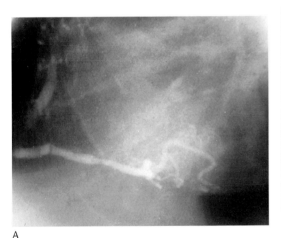

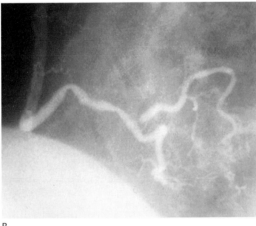

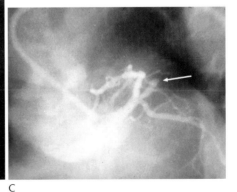

Fig. 13.10 Selective right coronary angiogram in the left anterior oblique projection. (A) The proximal portions of the posterior descending and left ventricular branches are foreshortened. (B) Addition of caudocranial angulation opens the bifurcations and reveals a stenosis at the origin of the left ventricular branch.

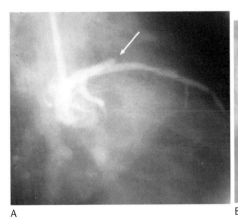

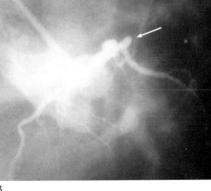

Fig. 13.11 Selective left coronary angiogram in a patient with occlusion of a large intermediate branch. (A) The right anterior oblique view shows overlapping (arrow) of the intermediate and left anterior descending branches. (B) The left anterior oblique view shows foreshortening (arrow) of the occluded branch. (C) Addition of craniocaudal angulation to the left anterior oblique view allows clear demonstration of the occluded branch (arrow).

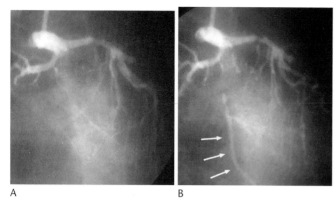

Fig. 13.12 Selective left coronary angiogram in the right anterior oblique projection. (A) An early frame shows no vessel lying between the upper left anterior descending branch and the circumflex branch. (B) A later view shows late collateral filling of an occluded obtuse marginal vessel (arrows).

two orthogonal planes showing either foreshortening or overlapping of vessels (Fig. 13.9). This is an essential principle of coronary angiography and it is the reason that the angiographic suspension must be capable of allowing steep craniocaudal or caudocranial angulation (Figs 13.10, 13.11). Without intelligent use of oblique and axial angulations, the full anatomy and pathological detail will not be revealed (Table 13.1).

In addition it is essential to ensure that the entire myocardial coronary supply is identified. There should be no 'gaps' in supply of the entire left ventricular myocardium; these gaps are potentially due to occluded vessels, anomalous anatomy or imperfect technique. Each ciné run must be of sufficient duration to allow late filling of occluded vessels by their collateral supply (Fig. 13.12). The possible routes of collateral supply and their vessels of origin should be fully understood; for example, the conus branch of the right coronary artery is an early branch to the right ventricular outflow tract that may supply collateral vessels to an occluded left anterior descending artery. If the catheter technique fails to opacify this branch, an important occluded vessel may be missed (Fig. 13.13).

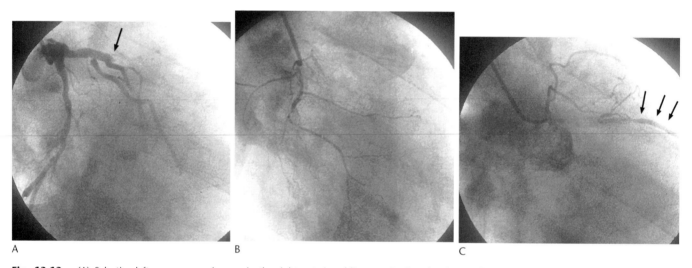

Fig. 13.13 (A) Selective left coronary angiogram in the right anterior oblique projection showing occlusion of the left anterior descending artery (arrow shows site of occlusion). (B) Selective right coronary angiogram of the same patient in the right anterior oblique projection—there is no evidence of collateral filling of the occluded vessel. (C) Repositioning of the catheter tip more anteriorly engages the ostium of the conus branch—collateral vessels to the occluded branch are revealed (arrows).

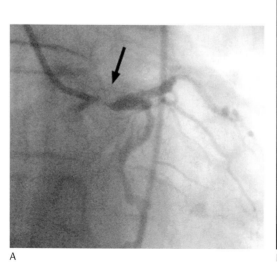

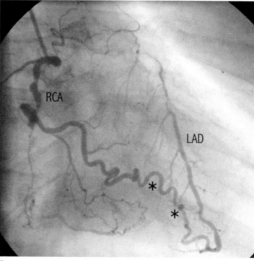

Fig. 13.14 (A) Selective left coronary angiogram in the right anterior oblique projection showing a severe left mainstem stenosis (arrow). (B) Right coronary angiogram in the same projection shows a large tortuous collateral (*) from the right coronary artery (RCA) to the distal left anterior descending artery (LAD).

The overall mortality rate should not exceed 0.3% and should normally be closer to 0.1%. These figures are from studies reported 20 years ago and the technique is nowadays likely to be much safer than this. The risk of mortality is predominantly confined to high-risk patients such as those with severely impaired left ventricular function or critical left mainstem stenosis. In all cases of selective coronary arteriography, the operator must be sensitive to the possibility of a stenosis of the left mainstem (Fig. 13.14). This lesion is associated with higher risks due to its proximal position in a large

vessel. If a catheter wedges in a left mainstem lesion, there can be very serious consequences.

Sometimes the coronary vessels may exhibit spasm during the investigation, either spontaneously or due to stimulation by the catheter tip. It is essential to distinguish this phenomenon from fixed lesions as the treatment is very different. The usual approach in the case of suspected spasm is a repeat angiogram after treatment with nitrates (sublingual or intracoronary) (Figs 13.15, 13.16). Another appearance that must be recognised is the 'muscle bridge'.

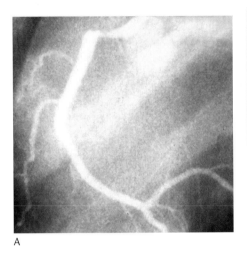

A

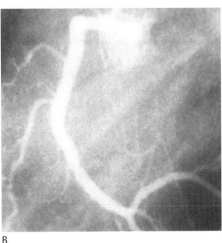

B

Fig. 13.15 Selective right coronary angiogram in the left anterior oblique projection. (A) There is spasm of the proximal vessel near the catheter tip. (B) The spasm is relieved after administration of nitrates.

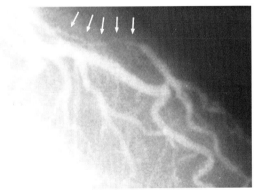

A

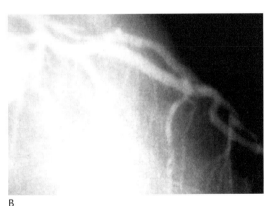

B

Fig. 13.16 Selective left coronary angiogram in the right anterior oblique projection showing severe spasm of the major diagonal branch (arrows) (A) and relief of the spasm after nitrate therapy (B).

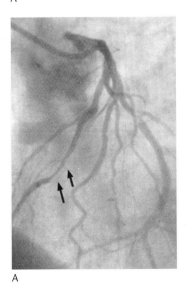

A

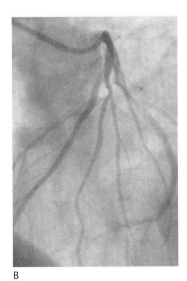

B

Fig. 13.17 Selective left coronary angiogram in the left anterior oblique projection with caudocranial angulation showing constriction of the mid part of the left anterior descending artery in systole due to a 'muscle bridge' (arrows) (A); there is no constriction in the diastolic frame (B).

The coronary arteries normally run over the external surface of the myocardium, usually covered by a layer of epicardial fat. In some cases, however, a short part of the course of the vessel lies intra-myocardially and this leads to systolic compression of the vessel (Fig. 13.17). This is usually of little clinical consequence as the dominant flow in the coronary arteries is in diastole. It is nevertheless important to recognise the phenomenon as it can have important significance for the cardiac surgeon.

The large demand for coronary arteriography has meant that in recent years there have been many more centres carrying out the examination, not all of which are supported by cardiac surgical or coronary angioplasty facilities. In general these centres should carry out elective procedures and those patients with known high risks should be studied in centres with maximal support.

In the majority of cases coronary angiography is a simple and straightforward procedure which need only take a few minutes to perform. It does not cause significant discomfort to the patient, particularly when non-ionic contrast media is used, and with small sized catheters and an atraumatic puncture it is possible to carry out the procedure as a day case. There will however be a number of situations in which coronary angiography can become much more complex. Abnormal aortic or vascular anatomy can make the passage of the catheter to the aortic root more torturous and difficult to manipulate. It will be much harder to engage a catheter satisfactorily within a dilated or aneurysmal aortic root (Figs 13.18, 13.19).

In cases where a patient has had previous coronary artery bypass grafting it is more difficult to engage the grafts and demonstrate their anatomy although with experience and knowledge of the usual graft sites it is normally possible to do this comprehensively (Figs 13.20, 13.21).

PATHOLOGICAL APPEARANCES OF THE CORONARY ARTERIES

Coronary heart disease is a condition with widespread manifestations. There can be very discreet localised narrowings in coronary arteries, there may be multiple lesions in a variety of branches or there may be diffuse disease affecting the majority of the coronary circulation. It is sometimes possible to clearly identify atheromatous plaques, sometimes with ulceration in them. Atheroma within the coronary arteries can take many forms and can produce irregular filling defects within the vessel or may be very diffuse and cause generalised lumenal narrowing. Interpretation of coronary anatomy and pathology requires considerable experience to evaluate the significance of the findings. Less commonly there will be other pathologies that can be identified by coronary angiography. Coronary fistula, coronary aneurysm and coronary dissection can all be identified from time to time. Even these conditions are frequently related to coronary atheroma.

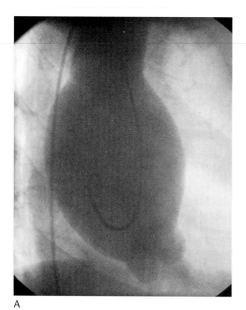

A

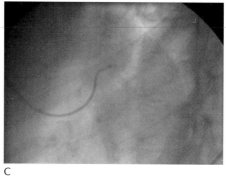

C

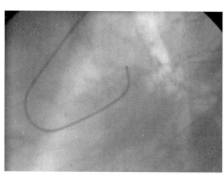

B

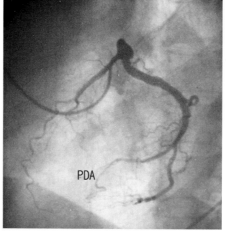

PDA

D

Fig. 13.18 (A) Ascending aortogram in the right anterior oblique projection showing a large fusiform aneurysm of the ascending aorta. (B) The left anterior oblique projection shows how a large size (JL6) Judkins left coronary catheter fails to engage the left coronary ostium. (C) A large size Amplatz curve (AL3) shows a good position. (D) The selective angiogram using the Amplatz catheter is of good quality. Note that the left coronary artery has a left dominant distribution with the posterior descending artery (PDA) arising from the circumflex vessel.

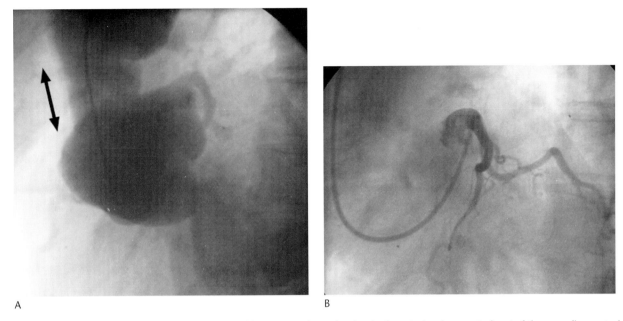

A   B

Fig. 13.19   (A) Ascending aortogram in the left anterior oblique view. The patient has had surgical replacement of part of the ascending aorta (arrow) after repair of a dissecting aneurysm. (B) A long-tip Sones catheter is used to selectively cannulate the left coronary artery. The curve of the catheter clearly demonstrates the large size of the aortic root. In this case the circumflex artery is non-dominant—compare with Fig. 13.18(D).

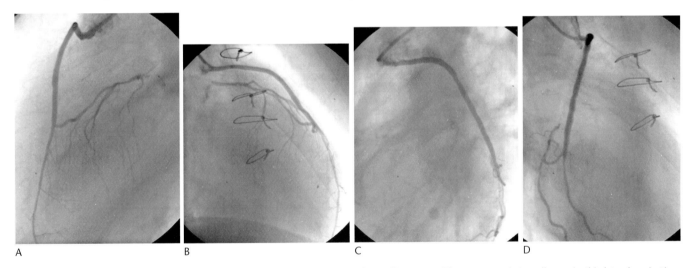

A   B   C   D

Fig. 13.20   (A) A saphenous vein graft from the aorta to the left anterior descending artery. The anastomosis is well seen in this lateral projection. (B) The graft shown in A seen in the right anterior oblique projection. (C) A second saphenous vein graft to the obtuse marginal vessel in the same patient—left anterior oblique projection. (D) The obtuse marginal graft shown in C in the right anterior oblique projection.

Anatomical variations of the coronary arteries are not uncommon and these must be recognised. There are variations in size and distribution of vessels but anomalous origins are important to detect. The commonest major anomaly is the origin of the circumflex artery from the proximal right coronary artery (Fig. 13.22). A 'single' coronary distribution is occasionally seen (Fig. 13.23).

Rarely a number of other conditions can affect the coronary arteries. Congenital coronary fistulas are occasionally seen and these are usually small and not of clinical significance. If the communication is large, the chronic high flow can lead to massive aneurysmal dilatation of the affected vessel (Fig. 13.24). Spontaneous dissection of the coronary artery can occasionally occur; this is often but not always associated with underlying coronary atheroma. Arteritis can rarely affect the coronaries, most commonly in Kawasaki's syndrome, which usually affects children. The syndrome, also termed mucocutaneous lymph node syndrome, is associated with aneurysmal dilatation of the proximal coronary arteries, which frequently resolves spontaneously.

Examination of the coronary arteries will of course include evaluation of any previous intervention such as coronary angioplasty or coronary artery bypass grafting. This type of examination requires more skill than conventional angiography as the origins of grafts have to be cannulated and the operator must have a good understanding of the previous procedure and its anatomical and pathological significance.

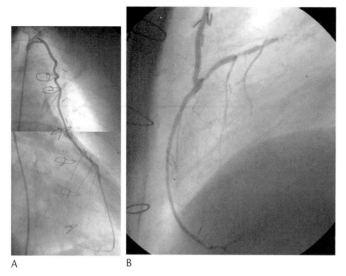

Fig. 13.21 (A) Right anterior oblique composite image showing the course of a left internal mammary graft to the left anterior descending artery. (B) The distal anastomosis of the same graft seen in the lateral projection.

AORTOGRAPHY

Although high-dose injection into the aortic root can give excellent anatomical demonstration of the anatomy of the aorta it is becoming less necessary to perform aortography in adult patients simply to determine the aortic anatomy. In most cases of aortic aneurysm or dissection it will be possible to evaluate the anatomy pathology by non-invasive imaging techniques. Aortography is however frequently employed in conjunction with coronary artery graft angiography if there is difficulty in identifying the site of origin of the grafts from the aortic root. Aortography is also useful in evaluation of regurgitation in the aortic valve.

RIGHT HEART CATHETERISATION

From time to time it is necessary to evaluate right-sided cardiac pressures and this is normally done by right heart catheterisation via the inferior vena cava and right atrium. Angiography is less often required for this study but occasionally pulmonary angiography is necessary to assess the pulmonary vasculature. The commonest indication for pulmonary angiography in adults is the assessment of possible pulmonary embolus. An angiographic suite is nevertheless an appropriate place to perform this type of examination as it is often carried out in conjunction with left heart catheterisation. All the safety backup facilities must be available and the imaging should be of adequate standard to visualise the catheter manipulation.

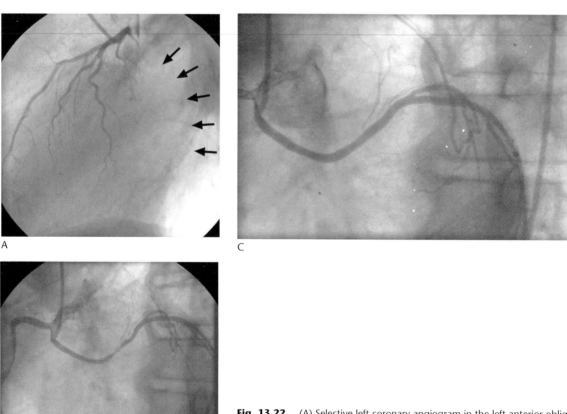

Fig. 13.22 (A) Selective left coronary angiogram in the left anterior oblique projection showing the left anterior descending artery—there is no opacification in the expected course of the circumflex artery (arrows). (B) Selective right coronary angiogram in the left anterior oblique projection showing the anomalous circumflex vessel branching early from the right coronary artery. This vessel passes posterior to the aortic root to reach the posterior left ventricular wall. The vessel has a localised stenosis. (C) The appearance after coronary angioplasty and stenting of the stenosis in the anomalous vessel.

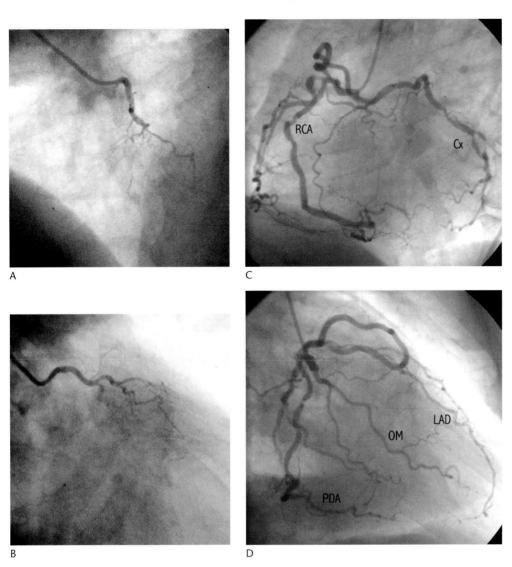

Fig. 13.23 (A) Selective left coronary angiogram in the left anterior oblique projection showing a recessive left coronary distribution. (B) The vessel shown in A in the right anterior oblique projection. (C) Selective right coronary angiogram in the left anterior oblique projection showing a 'single' coronary artery with a normal right coronary distribution (RCA) as well as a 'left coronary' vessel supplying left anterior descending and circumflex (Cx) branches. (D) The arteries shown in C seen in the right anterior oblique projection. LAD = left anterior descending artery; OM = obtuse marginal branch of the circumflex artery; PDA = posterior descending branch.

VASCULAR ACCESS

In the majority of cases percutaneous approach via the femoral route is concluded by simple compression to encourage closure of the arterial puncture. In most diagnostic catheterisation procedures anticoagulation is not used, as the single-use catheters and short duration of the procedure do not raise the risk of thrombus or embolus formation. In complex or prolonged cases heparinisation may be advisable. In some patients the femoral arterial puncture can be closed using special devices. These are most commonly based on a collagen plug. These devices add significant cost to a procedure and are not normally used in routine procedures unless there is a need for maintenance of anticoagulation or other reason to require rapid mobilisation of the patient.

There will however be situations where femoral access is difficult or impossible. In some patients with severe peripheral vascular disease or very tortuous arteries it may be unwise or impossible to approach from this route. The left heart can also be catheterised from the arm but whereas traditionally this was performed by cut-down technique to the brachial artery, this has been superseded more recently by percutaneous techniques. The brachial puncture

approach is quite practical and is performed just above the ante-cubital fossa at the point of maximum pulsation of the brachial artery; this is now less widely used because the radial technique has taken over a high proportion of studies which need to be carried out from the arm. The radial approach is ideal because the presence of an arterial arch in the hand minimises the risks to the perfusion of the hand (provided that there is adequate flow through the ulna artery as shown by the Allen test). The radial puncture is performed on a slightly extended wrist with a 20-gauge needle and a fine guide-wire is initially used to cannulate the artery. This wire can be used to introduce a fine dilator that can introduce a 5Fr or 6Fr arterial sheath without difficulty. Usually treatment to the radial artery is given by a small infusion of vasodilator to minimise the risk of spasm around the catheter. Most diagnostic and interventional techniques can now be performed through a 6Fr sheath. Closure of the radial puncture is easily performed by compression, as the vessel is very superficial and runs over a prominent bony area. Compression is usually carried out with a compression device mounted on a splint which holds the wrist immobile.

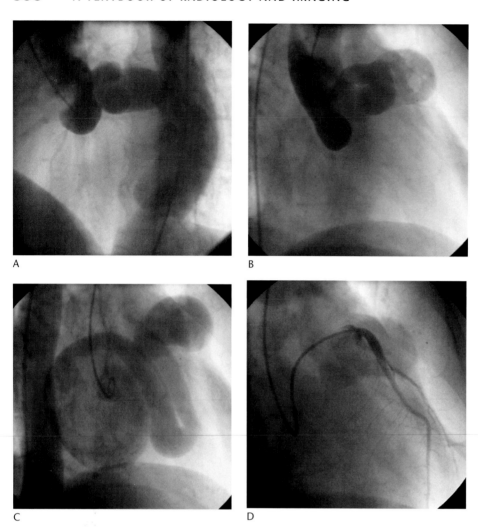

Fig. 13.24 A patient with a longstanding giant coronary artery fistula from the left coronary artery to the right atrium. (A) Aortic root injection in the left anterior oblique projection showing the tortuous proximal part of the vessel. (B) The vessel shown in A in the right anterior oblique projection. (C) A late frame in the right anterior oblique projection showing filling of the extensive distal aneurysmal portion of the vessel. (D) Selective angiogram of the normal size left anterior descending artery which arose from within the proximal part of the pathological vessel.

INTERVENTIONAL CARDIAC PROCEDURES

CORONARY ANGIOPLASTY

Percutaneous transluminal coronary angioplasty (PTCA) was first carried out in a human patient in 1977 and is now carried out in huge numbers throughout the developed world. In the UK approximately 500 procedures per million population are carried out per year but this is rapidly rising towards the 1200–1500 procedures per million per year carried out in some advanced European countries and the USA. Coronary angioplasty has now exceeded coronary artery bypass grafting as the most common procedure for coronary artery revascularisation.

The principle of coronary angioplasty is simple, namely the inflation of a balloon within a coronary artery which has been narrowed by atheromatous plaque. The balloon expansion ruptures and displaces the plaque to open the lumen of the vessel. However the pathophysiology of this technique is extremely complex, the plaque rupture releasing many complex substances which generate thrombosis and stimulate cellular response. In the years since its original introduction, the technology for coronary angioplasty has improved very considerably and now guide-wires, guide catheters and coronary balloons are extremely reliable and of very low profile, allow-

ing them to be passed very distally down tortuous vessels. The weak link of coronary angioplasty is the tendency towards restenosis and this can still complicate otherwise successful procedures in 15–20% of cases. Much work is being done to understand the mechanisms of restenosis and drug therapy and improvements in angioplasty technology have combined to slowly reduce, but not eliminate, this problem. The introduction of coronary artery stenting has made a major impact in the practice of coronary angioplasty. These balloon-mounted stents, usually made of stainless steel, are normally of a slotted tube design and they are crimped onto a low-profile balloon. Expansion of the balloon expands the stent into the wall of the artery, holding the vessel widely open and preventing prolapse of intima or atheromatous material back into the lumen. Many studies have shown that the use of coronary stents reduces early complications in the angioplasty procedure as well as reducing the incidence of coronary restenosis. Coronary stenting is now employed in the majority of angioplasty procedures, accounting for approximately 85% of coronary angioplasty procedures in the UK.

The technique of coronary angioplasty depends heavily on the highest quality of imaging possible. It is essential to visualise the exact nature of the lesion being treated and it is essential to visualise very clearly the equipment being used to carry out the procedure. A coronary angioplasty guide catheter is used to provide support at the ostium of the coronary artery and it is essential that

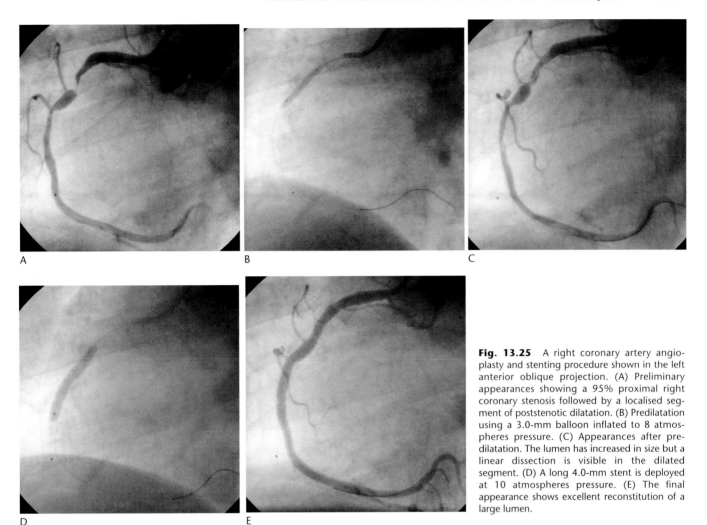

Fig. 13.25 A right coronary artery angioplasty and stenting procedure shown in the left anterior oblique projection. (A) Preliminary appearances showing a 95% proximal right coronary stenosis followed by a localised segment of poststenotic dilatation. (B) Predilatation using a 3.0-mm balloon inflated to 8 atmospheres pressure. (C) Appearances after predilatation. The lumen has increased in size but a linear dissection is visible in the dilated segment. (D) A long 4.0-mm stent is deployed at 10 atmospheres pressure. (E) The final appearance shows excellent reconstitution of a large lumen.

this fits well with good 'backup' from the aortic wall, so that if necessary a balloon or stent can be pushed along a torturous vessel or a narrowed artery. Once the guide catheter is in position a steerable fine guide-wire (0.014 in) is manipulated under fluoroscopic control into the distal portion of the vessel being treated. This guide-wire is then used to take the balloon catheter that has passed through the guide catheter down into the lesion. In some cases balloon dilatation alone is employed but commonly a predilation is performed with a balloon, after which stenting is carried out using a second balloon carrying a premounted stent (Fig. 13.25). In some cases 'primary stenting' is carried out, involving direct delivery of the stent to the lesion without any predilatation (Fig. 13.26).

A number of other devices are available to supplement coronary angioplasty but these are less commonly used. Atherectomy devices can be used to excise proliferative plaque, high-speed rotating burrs can be used to fragment plaque and thrombus suction catheters can be used to extract fresh thrombotic material. There are also a number of evaluation devices that can now be used within the coronary arteries and these include intracoronary ultrasound for direct intracoronary imaging and Doppler flow wires that can be used to evaluate the forward flow down the coronary artery. Coronary guide-wires incorporating tiny pressure transducers can also be used to calculate the fractional flow reserve by comparing the pressure of the coronary ostium with the distal pressure during tempo-

rary vasodilatation. This has been shown to be a highly accurate technique for evaluating adequate coronary artery function.

INTERVENTIONAL VALVE DILATATION

In a minority of situations it is possible to treat a stenotic valve in acquired heart disease by interventional approaches. The most common of these is percutaneous mitral balloon commissurotomy. A variety of techniques have been used for this but the Inoue approach is now widespread. This technique involves the use of a specially designed double-layer balloon that can be inflated in two stages to a predetermined size (Fig. 13.27). The technique involves transseptal puncturing of the interatrial septum from the inferior vena caval route. This is followed by deployment of the balloon into the left atrium using specially designed guide-wires. The balloon is passed through the stenotic mitral orifice using a steering device and inflation of the balloon is progressive, the distal portion inflating first to allow accurate seating in the valve followed by complete inflation which can lead to a maximum diameter of 30 mm (Fig. 13.28). In appropriately selected cases, when there is not too much calcification or fibrosis, and where transoesophageal echo has been used to exclude the presence of thrombus in the left atrium, the technique has been shown to be extremely effective and is comparable to surgical commissurotomy.

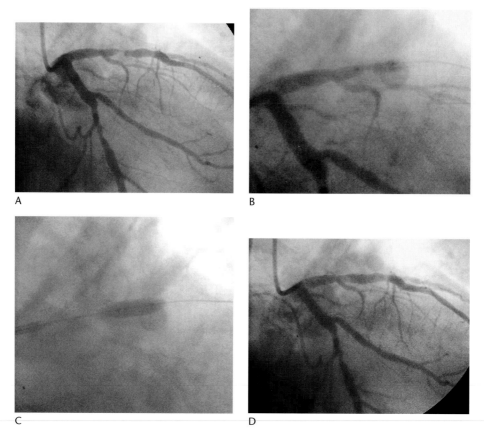

Fig. 13.26 Primary stenting procedure of a 90% stenosis in the proximal left anterior descending artery shown in the right anterior oblique projection. (A) Preliminary appearance of the stenosis. (B) Magnified view of stent positioning in the stenosis. (C) Deployment of a short 3.5-mm stent at 10 atmospheres pressure. (D) Final appearance showing full reconstitution of the lumen.

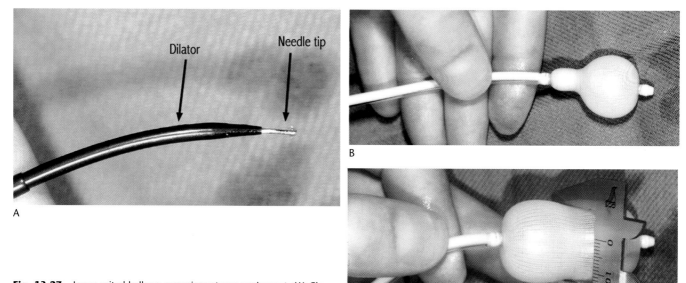

Fig. 13.27 Inoue mitral balloon commissurotomy equipment. (A) Close-up of the trans-septal needle and dilator. (B) Partial inflation of the distal portion of the balloon. (C) Measurement of the waist of the fully expanded balloon prior to use.

Dilatation of acquired aortic valve stenosis has proved to be much less useful. This technique is usually carried out as a retro-grade arterial approach (Fig. 13.29) (although an antegrade septal approach is also possible (Fig. 13.30)), but unfortunately in the majority of cases of acquired aortic valve stenosis the leaflets are far too thickened and calcified to respond adequately to balloon

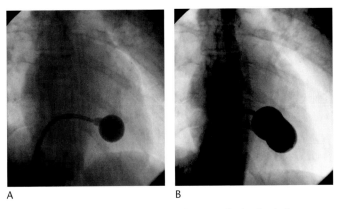

Fig. 13.28 Angiographic recording of Inoue mitral valve balloon commissurotomy in the PA projection. (A) The distal portion of the balloon is inflated in the left ventricle and pulled back to the mitral orifice. (B) The fully expanded balloon is shown with the waist seated in the mitral orifice.

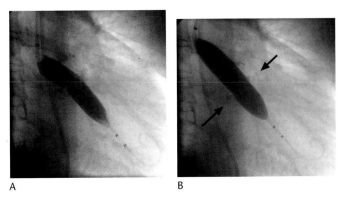

Fig. 13.29 Retrograde aortic valve balloon dilatation shown in the right anterior oblique projection. (A) Partially inflated balloon. (B) Fully inflated balloon—the calcified aortic valve is arrowed.

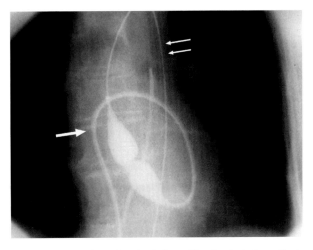

Fig. 13.30 Antegrade aortic valve balloon dilatation technique. The large arrow shows the trans-septal sheath passing into the left atrium. The small arrows show the distal guide-wire in the descending aorta.

dilatation. Early reports of this technique were encouraging but it was shown that initial improvement was rapidly lost and now the technique is only used for palliation or as a temporary treatment to allow clinical improvement before surgery is undertaken. The technique has much more application in paediatric cardiology.

OTHER INTERVENTIONAL TECHNIQUES

It is not uncommon to see displaced foreign bodies within the heart and circulation, no doubt due to the increasing use of interventional devices. This can be due to maldeployment of devices or fracturing of guide-wires or catheters. Retrieval of foreign bodies from the heart or adjacent vessels is now feasible via a number of techniques including basket retrieval and snaring (Fig. 13.31). These are specialised techniques but should be available in any interventional catheter unit.

From time to time critical emergencies will develop in the catheterisation laboratory that will demand cardiovascular support. Support may be given therapeutically but mechanical support may also be indicated, most usually with an intra-aortic balloon pump. This device has a rapidly inflating and deflating helium balloon that maintains diastolic aortic pressure in order to raise mean arterial pressure and preserve systemic perfusion. Aortic balloon catheters can be introduced on the ward but ideally they should be introduced in the catheterisation lab using interventional guide-wire techniques

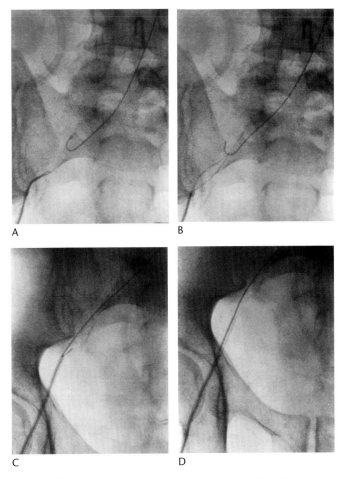

Fig. 13.31 Retrieval of a flexible guide-wire from the aorta using a simple wire snare. (A) The snare is enclosed in a catheter as it approaches the J-wire in the right common iliac artery. (B) The wire snare has looped over the J-wire. (C) The snare pulls the wire snugly back to the deployment catheter where it is firmly held. (D) The wire is pulled back out of the arterial sheath.

and fluoroscopy to ascertain the exact positioning in the descending thoracic aorta. Equipment and expertise for deploying aortic balloon pump devices should be available in all major catheter laboratories.

ANGIOGRAPHIC SCREENING OF PROSTHESES

In cases where prosthetic cardiac valves may be malfunctioning, it is useful to use the high-resolution pulsed acquisition of the angiographic suite to assess the movement of the valve components, particularly in the case of mechanical valves. This can sometimes show valve malfunction more clearly than echocardiography (Fig. 13.32).

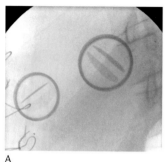
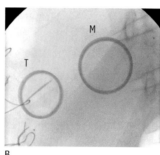

Fig. 13.32 A patient with bileaflet prosthetic mechanical valves in the mitral and tricuspid positions. The patient had progressive right heart failure. (A) Left anterior oblique pulsed acquisition showing leaflets of both valves open in diastole. (B) The systolic frame shows that the mitral leaflets (M) have both closed but one of the tricuspid leaflets (T) remains fixed in the open position.

REFERENCES

Kern, M. J. (1998) *The Cardiac Catherization Handbook 3E*. Mosby, Philadelphia.

Manning, W. J., Pennell, D. J. (2001) *Cardiac magnetic Resonance Imaging*. Churchill Livingstone, London.

Nienaber, C. A., Sechtem, U. (1996) *Imaging and Intervention in Cardiology*. Kluwer Academic Publishers.

Norell, M. S., Perrins, J. (2001) *Essential Intervention Cardiology*. W. B. Saunders, Philadelphia.

Otto, C. M. (1999) *Textbook of Clinical Echocardiography 2E*. W. B. Saunders, London.

Topol, E. J. (1999) *Textbook of Intervention Cardiology*. W. B. Saunders, London.

Walsh, C., Wilde, P. (1999) *Practical Echocardiography*. Greenwich Medical Media, London.

Zaret, B. L., Beller, G. A. (1999) *Nuclear Cardiology State of the Art and Future Directions*. Mosby.

14

CONGENITAL HEART DISEASE

Peter Wilde and Anne Boothroyd

INTRODUCTION

The incidence of congenital heart disease in live births is estimated at between 0.5 and 1.0% in various large series. Many of these recorded abnormalities are relatively simple, with only a small proportion of cases having very complex abnormalities. The common congenitally *bicuspid aortic valve* (2% incidence in the population) is not included in these figures, nor is the increasingly recognised *patent ductus arteriosus* in premature infants.

This relatively low incidence means that many radiologists will see only a small number of congenital heart disease cases each year, particularly if they are not working in a centre with special paediatric or cardiac interests. It is not possible for a general radiologist or even a general paediatric radiologist to be familiar with the detailed radiology of all forms of congenital heart disease. It is essential, however, that all radiologists are sufficiently well informed in this field to be able to recognise possible cardiac problems and guide further investigation. They should also be able to assist in basic medical management and be aware of the changing patterns of disease seen in the natural history or surgical management of many of these conditions.

Over the last three decades the progress in the treatment of congenital heart disease has been spectacular and, in particular, operative management has led to the survival of many patients who would previously have died from their congenital malformations. In many cases surgery is able to achieve complete or nearly complete anatomical correction of the abnormality, and in many other cases a high level of palliation can be achieved. An increasing number of patients will return for routine radiological assessment following surgery. Further evidence of this success is the increasing numbers of clinics being established for the review of adults with congenital heart disease. The treatment of congenital heart disease is generally undertaken in large specialist centres, and in these there will usually be a team approach to diagnosis and management. The best centres will have close cooperation between cardiac physicians, surgeons and radiologists. The specialist radiologist will be able to offer a range of investigations, particularly echocardiography and angiocardiography and, increasingly, MRI. More recently the radiologist has also had a role to play in the management of cases requiring interventional treatment, particularly balloon dilatation of stenotic valves and vessels and less commonly the embolisation and occlusion of abnormal communications and channels.

Radiologists may deal with congenital heart disease at various stages and in various ways. These include:

1. Recognition that congenital heart disease is present. A preliminary diagnosis or general diagnosis is frequently possible from the *chest radiograph*, but it is rare that the plain film will give a precise, accurate and reliable diagnosis of the intracardiac abnormality.

2. Detailed diagnosis by *echocardiography* with the possible addition of *transoesophageal echocardiography*, *MRI*, *cardiac catheterisation* and *angiography*.

3. Detailed evaluation of investigation results, usually at a joint case conference in which the full clinical picture is assessed and management is discussed.

4. Management, which can be continued medical management, palliative surgery, corrective surgery or *interventional catheter techniques*. The radiologist may well have an important role in the interventional techniques, as well as in monitoring management by the use of plain chest radiography and other non-invasive imaging techniques.

5. Follow-up, usually carried out jointly between the specialist centre and the referring centre. In many major centres there is now a clinic for 'grown-up congenital heart disease' (GUCH) patients who need to be managed throughout their adult life.

The two most obvious ways in which cardiac surgery has changed in recent years are the increasing number of total anatomical corrections that are possible and the decreasing age at which these operations are performed. In many large units a high proportion of congenital heart abnormalities are now completely corrected before the age of 1 year or even in the first few weeks of life. In some cases early palliative surgery precedes later definitive surgery. This has a particular effect on the practice of cardiac radiology, because the classical appearances of longstanding congenital heart abnormalities on the chest radiograph are becoming increasingly uncommon and their practical importance less.

Cardiac surgery is considered to include the heart and the great vessels, and can be divided into two major types: closed heart surgery and open heart surgery. In *closed heart surgery* the operation is performed while the heart continues to function, and for this

363

reason most closed heart operations are limited in terms of intra-cardiac repair. This type of procedure is most commonly carried out for abnormalities of the aorta and pulmonary arteries and palliation of other conditions. The procedures include *repair of coarctation*, insertion of a *systemic-to-pulmonary shunt* or *banding of the main pulmonary artery*.

Open heart surgery requires that the cardiac function must cease. During this time the patient is maintained on cardiopulmonary bypass or is cooled to low temperatures to facilitate a safe period of cardiac standstill. In this situation it is vital that the cardiac surgeon has full knowledge of the nature of the abnormality or abnormalities before undertaking the operation, so that the time taken for the repair is kept to an absolute minimum. This reduces the risks of operative mortality and morbidity, which increase progressively with the length of time the heart is taken out of circulation.

The practice of preoperative assessment has changed considerably in recent years. Nowadays the *clinical*, *radiographic* and, particularly, *echocardiographic* and *MRI* data are frequently adequate to make a complete diagnosis of the intracardiac abnormality. *Cardiac catheterisation* and *angiography* are still required in a significant number of patients with a full echo diagnosis, because additional details may be required for precise management decisions to be made. In some cases this detail is of a haemodynamic nature. It is often necessary to measure the pulmonary vascular resistance in patients with large left-to-right shunts to exclude the possibility of irreversible pulmonary damage. Certain pressure gradients and absolute intracardiac pressures are also needed if they are not obtained by Doppler echocardiography.

It is sometimes necessary to clarify anatomical detail by *angiocardiography*, often with a view to excluding known pitfalls that may be encountered by the surgeon. For example, coronary anatomy cannot adequately be assessed by echocardiography while it can be clearly assessed using ciné angiography. The pulmonary artery anatomy is often crucial to the management of many patients, and it is often not possible to visualise the left and right pulmonary arteries beyond their origins by echocardiography due to surrounding intrapulmonary air. There will also be cases where the echo study has been technically difficult for one reason or another and the angiogram is essential.

Finally, the cardiac catheterisation procedure is sometimes accompanied by an interventional procedure. These include *Rashkind balloon septostomy* for transposition of the great arteries (now sometimes performed under echocardiographic control), *dilatation of the pulmonary valve or coarctation* and, more recently, *ductal closure, occlusion of abnormal communications* and *vascular stenting*. These techniques are developing rapidly but require expert knowledge of intracardiac anatomy to ensure their success.

THE MORPHOLOGICAL APPROACH TO CONGENITAL HEART DISEASE

A number of different attempts have been made to classify congenital heart disease, but whichever approach is adopted there is a large array of differing conditions which must be recognised.

The first and most important requirement is for accurate description of what is being seen. It is therefore vital to recognise the morphological appearance of each cardiac chamber so that abnormal connections are unambiguously described. It is frequently helpful to use the phrase *morphologically left ventricle* to describe a ventricular chamber that has all the characteristics of the left ventricle irrespective of where it is in the patient and irrespective of which connections it makes. It is, for example, possible to have a morphologically left ventricle that lies on the right side of the body or to the right of the other ventricle.

The morphological features of important structures are here briefly reviewed.

Right atrium

The appearance of the atrial appendages is fundamental in the accurate determination of atrial morphology. It is not possible to determine this information from plain films, and it can be difficult to achieve using echocardiography. The right atrial appendage is broad based and triangular in shape and contains pectinate muscles. The inferior vena cava almost always enters the right atrium, and though this rule is not invariable, it is a clinically important guide. Angiocardiography or echocardiography can demonstrate the site of drainage of the inferior vena cava. The latter technique can also be very helpful in assessing the anatomy of the atrial septum to determine morphology; the septum secundum lies to the right of the septum primum and its lower margin forms the upper edge of the foramen ovale. This is frequently patent in early life, but even in later life the closed fossa ovale remains as a marker of the right side of the atrial septum.

Left atrium

This chamber can be defined most precisely by its atrial appendage, which is long and narrow, usually curling around the left side of the heart. The left atrium cannot reliably be defined by the presence of pulmonary veins as these can often be anomalous.

Right ventricle

This is rhomboid in shape and shows heavy bands of trabeculation throughout the chamber. There is often a prominent band crossing the main cavity of the ventricle, the 'moderator band'. The trabecular pattern is particularly suited to demonstration by angiocardiography, but can sometimes be deduced using echocardiography. In the assessment of trabecular pattern by any technique it is important to look comparatively at both ventricles because the typical patterns may be a little distorted in some complex cases.

The papillary muscles arise from multiple groups in the right ventricle, and there is usually some attachment of chordae to papillary muscle or muscles on the septum, which itself is heavily trabeculated. The atrioventricular valve of the right ventricle is by definition the tricuspid valve, and is inserted slightly more toward the apex of the heart than the atrioventricular valve of the left ventricle (mitral valve). This particular feature is very well demonstrated by echocardiography. There is normally an outflow muscular tube known as the conus or infundibulum which leads up to the exit semilunar valve. The semilunar valves (pulmonary and aortic) are named in accordance with the appropriate great artery, so the exit valve of the right ventricle is not necessarily the pulmonary valve.

Left ventricle

This is the ventricular chamber with a more symmetrical oval shape and fine lattice-like trabeculation. The basal half of the interventricular septum is smooth, without any trabeculation. There are normally two large papillary muscles in this ventricle, both of which arise from the free wall and not from the interventricular septum. Both papillary muscles give attachment to chordae from both mitral valve leaflets.

The atrioventricular valve entering the left ventricle is by definition the mitral valve, and the insertion of the mitral valve is further towards the base of the heart than the atrioventricular valve of the right ventricle, the tricuspid valve. In the left ventricle there is usually fibrous continuity between the inflow and outflow valves, although this is not always the case. The fibrous continuity is well demonstrated on the two-dimensional long-axis echocardiographic view, where the anterior leaflet of the mitral valve is seen arising from the posterior wall of the aortic root.

The pulmonary artery

This is the great artery which bifurcates into two branches after a short distance, each branch supplying one lung. If two great arteries are present then it is often easier to define the aorta first. It is also important to distinguish true pulmonary arteries arising from the pulmonary trunk from abnormal aortopulmonary vessels.

The aorta

This is the great artery which supplies branches to the head and neck. The aorta cannot be defined in terms of its connection to the heart (in transposition of the great arteries the aorta arises from the right ventricle) or the presence of coronary branches (anomalous coronary vessels can arise from the pulmonary artery).

CLASSIFICATION OF CARDIAC ABNORMALITIES

In recent years a reasonably standardised approach has been achieved in the description of congenital cardiac abnormalities. Although this is not necessarily used in the description of very simple abnormalities, it is invaluable in the description of complex abnormalities as it avoids confusion or ambiguity. This approach has five major descriptive steps:

1. Situs
2. Cardiac connections
3. Looping
4. Positions
5. Malformations.

These steps will be described in turn below.

Situs

The abdominal and thoracic viscera are asymmetrical, and for this reason normal situs can be recognised by obvious features such as the liver and inferior vena cava lying on the right side and the spleen and heart lying on the left side (Fig. 14.1). The very high association with the inferior vena cava draining into the right atrium has led to the development of the term *visceroatrial situs*. This essentially means that the atrial situs in almost all cases conforms to the situs of the upper abdominal viscera, irrespective of the situs or position of the remainder of the heart. A transverse upper abdominal ultrasound scan will allow definition of the visceroatrial situs by showing variations in position of the inferior vena cava, aorta and sometimes the azygos vein.

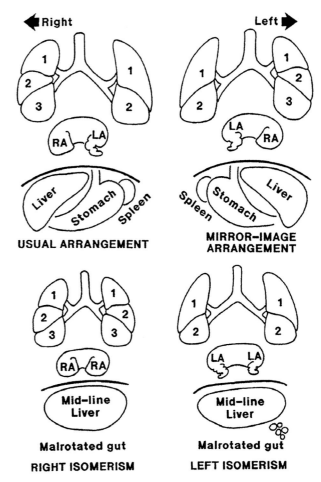

Fig. 14.1 Situs variations. The diagram shows the arrangement of bronchial, atrial and abdominal anatomy in the usual arrangement, mirror-image arrangement and right and left isomerism. (Courtesy of Professor R. Anderson.)

It is also important to recognise the presence of asymmetry in the lungs, which is usually apparent in the form of *bronchial situs*. The right main bronchus is shorter, wider and more vertically orientated than the left main bronchus, which is usually at least 1.5 times as long as the right from bifurcation to first major branch (Fig. 14.2). The bronchial situs nearly always corresponds to the

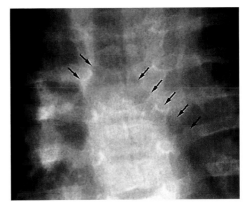

Fig. 14.2 Plain radiograph of the mediastinum showing normal bronchial anatomy. Arrows indicate the length of left and right bronchi.

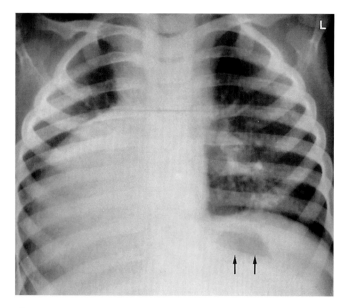

Fig. 14.3 Chest radiograph of a patient with visceroatrial situs solitus (gastric bubble arrowed) and isolated dextrocardia.

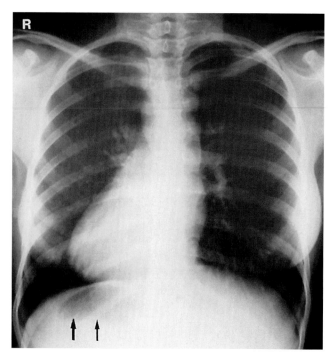

Fig. 14.4 Chest radiograph of a patient with total situs inversus (gastric bubble arrowed).

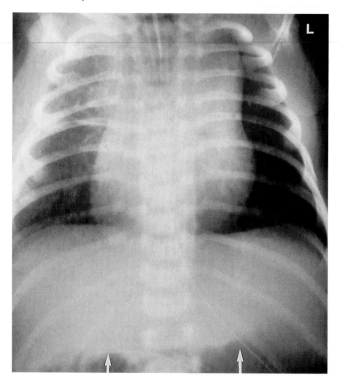

Fig. 14.5 Chest radiograph of an infant with situs ambiguous showing a centrally positioned cardiac apex and transverse liver (arrows). There were complex intracardiac anomalies.

visceroatrial situs. Special filtration techniques of chest radiography may be needed for the assessment of bronchial situs.

From time to time, situs abnormalities will occur, and it is important to describe variations accurately:

1. *Situs solitus* This describes the normal situation with normal visceroatrial situs (liver, inferior vena cava and right atrium on the right side) and normal bronchial situs. The 'position' of the cardiac mass and/or cardiac apex is not directly related to visceroatrial situs and may not correspond with it. The apex can occasionally be directed toward the right side even with normal visceroatrial situs, this sometimes being described as *isolated dextrocardia* or dextrorotation of the heart (Fig. 14.3).

2. *Situs inversus* In this condition there is complete reversal of the visceroatrial situs and the bronchial situs. The condition is not necessarily associated with any other cardiac abnormality. An example of this is shown in Figure 14.4. Meticulous technique in the use of radiographic side markers is of paramount importance. If films are marked up after processing, then cases of total situs inversus are almost certainly going to be marked wrongly. Once again the cardiac apex may not lie in the expected position. Thus, in most cases of situs inversus the cardiac apex lies on the right side, but occasionally it will lie on the left (*isolated levocardia*).

3. *Situs ambiguous* This describes a situation in which the left- and right-sided nature of abdominal or thoracic organs and the atria are not clearly distinct. A number of variations of this can be recognised. The first of these is most easily understood as '*bilateral right-sidedness*'. In this condition there is a midline liver running across the upper abdomen (Fig. 14.5), the spleen is absent, the stomach is usually centrally positioned, and the bronchial anatomy shows right-sided morphology of both major bronchi. Both atrial chambers have right-sided characteristics and, not surprisingly, there is a frequent association with abnormalities of pulmonary venous drainage. Often many other cardiac abnormalities are also associated with this condition. '*Bilateral left-sidedness*' is also associated with a midline liver, often smaller, but there is frequently

polysplenia and bilateral left atrial morphology, and the two main bronchi both show left morphology. There is, by definition, abnormal systemic venous drainage. Again, there is an association with major cardiac abnormality. The final form of situs ambiguous is one in which the morphological characteristics of the various structures are very hard to determine, and a left- or right-sided nature cannot easily be determined. In this case again many cardiac anomalies can be associated. The incidence of congenital heart disease with differing situs varies widely. The frequency is 1% in situs solitus with laevocardia (normal), 98% in situs solitus with isolated dextrocardia, 4% with situs inversus and dextrocardia (mirror image anatomy) and 100% in situs inversus with isolated laevocardia.

Cardiac connections

Once the cardiac chambers have been identified in morphological terms it should be possible to state which vessel or chamber is connected to which. For example, in transposition of the great arteries it can be stated that the aorta arises from the morphologically right ventricle and the pulmonary artery arises from the morphologically left ventricle. In this situation there is said to be *ventriculoarterial discordance*. From time to time there will be *atrioventricular discordance*, which will occur when the morphologically right atrium drains into the morphologically left ventricle and vice versa.

In some cases the connections will not be completely distinct, as, for example, in the *tetralogy of Fallot*, where the aorta partially overrides onto the right ventricle from its position above a large ventricular septal defect. Complete overriding of great arteries can occur in the presence of a ventricular septal defect, most typically in *double-outlet right ventricle*.

If there is a large ventricular septal defect lying between the atrioventricular valves there can also be partial or total override of the mitral or tricuspid valve. In such circumstances the 50% rule applies. If 50% or more of the valve opens into or arises from the ventricle it defines a connection. Double-inlet ventricle is thus a recognised occurrence. Although it is a simple matter to state that an atrioventricular valve is related to one or other or both ventricles, the diagnosis of the exact relationship may not be easy.

Looping (or topology)

This term relates to the ventricular loop which has been formed during cardiac development. If the heart is well enough developed to have two ventricles, each with an inlet and an outlet, and an interventricular septum lying between them, then it will be possible to define the loop. D-loop and L-loop configurations are stereoisomers (mirror images) of each other, the difference between the two types of loop being analogous to the difference between the left hand and right hand. Each hand is uniquely different, being defined by the relationship of the fingers and thumb with the palm and back of the hand. Whichever position a hand is in, it can always be distinguished as a right or left hand. Looping is also independent of cardiac situs or position.

The normal ventricular D-loop can be understood most simply by using the analogy of the right hand rule in which the morphological right ventricle is likened to a right hand. The inflow is represented by the thumb, the outflow is represented by the fingers, and the interventricular septum will lie on the palmar side of the hand. If, however, the morphologically right ventricle is configured in such a way that the relationship of inflow, outflow and interventricular septum can only be represented by a left hand, this infers that the ventricle is actually a stereoisomer of a normal D-loop ventricle, and is an L-loop ventricle (Fig. 14.6).

L-looping is most frequently seen in association with transposition of the great arteries in the condition known as anatomically corrected transposition or commonly just '*corrected transposition*.'

Position

Although the position of the heart in the chest is the first thing to be seen on a chest radiograph, the absolute position is of secondary importance in describing the fundamental nature of the congenital heart abnormality. The position is of course of practical importance in planning surgical procedures. If one imagines that the heart is a model made out of extremely flexible elastic material, then it is easy to see that the position of even a completely normal heart can be considerably distorted by twisting, stretching or turning various chambers into different positions, while the heart still maintains absolutely normal situs, cardiac connections and ventricular looping. Similarly, the presence of particular situs, connection or looping arrangements does not necessarily indicate what the final cardiac position will be.

A complex positional variation is the '*criss-cross*' heart. In this abnormality there is, in addition to any other abnormalities of situs or connection, an additional twist of the ventricular mass. This results in the ventricles lying in unexpected positions given the particular situs and connection. Sometimes the ventricles adopt a superoinferior relationship, but occasionally their positions can be completely reversed. The simplest example to understand would occur in a heart with normal situs and connections; in this case, twisting of the ventricular mass could lead to the morphologically left ventricle lying anterior to the posteriorly displaced morphological right ventricle.

It is important to note the position of the *aortic arch* relative to the trachea. The normal aortic arch is left-sided, but some congenital abnormalities are associated with a higher than normal incidence of right-sided arch. There are a number of variations in aortic branching patterns which will be considered later. The recognition of a right-sided aortic arch is of course important for surgical planning. A right-sided arch may also occur in isolation (Fig. 14.7).

Malformations

This refers to the specific deformities or abnormalities within the heart, such as *stenotic* or *atretic valves*, *abnormal communications* and *narrowed vessels*. These malformations are often the most

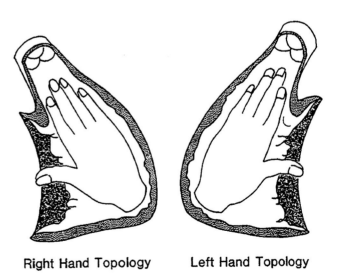

Right Hand Topology **Left Hand Topology**

Fig. 14.6 Diagram demonstrating the difference between right-hand topology (D-loop) and left-hand topology (L-loop). The two arrangements are mirror images of each other. (Courtesy of Professor R. Anderson.)

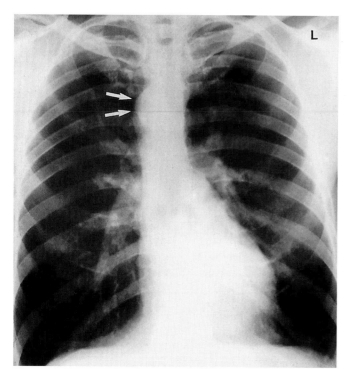

Fig. 14.7 Chest radiograph showing an isolated right-sided aortic arch (arrows indicate aortic knuckle).

obvious abnormality, and they are commonly used as the overall descriptive term for a particular abnormality (e.g. *ventricular septal defect, pulmonary atresia* or *coarctation of the aorta*). Some malformations are a little more complex, for example atrioventricular septal defects, and in some cases there are multiple associated malformations as in tetralogy of Fallot (ventricular septal defect and pulmonary stenosis).

In many cases the malformations are the only abnormality, and in this situation the full description of situs, connection, looping and position is omitted for simplicity in general discussion, the implicit assumption being made that all these other aspects are normal. This is acceptable in normal practice, provided that the full descriptive nomenclature is used as soon as the congenital heart abnormality is anything other than straightforward.

Malformations also occur commonly in association with the more complex abnormalities, and in fact they are frequently associated with major abnormalities of situs, looping or connection.

HAEMODYNAMIC AND FUNCTIONAL PRINCIPLES

A thorough understanding of the radiology of congenital heart disease must include not only structural abnormalities but also functional abnormalities. Normal cardiac anatomy and physiology must be understood before the developmental, functional and pathological consequences of the abnormalities can fully be appreciated.

DEVELOPMENTAL ASPECTS

Development of chambers and vessels

The blood flowing through a chamber or vessel is a powerful stimulus for the growth of the cavity. Conversely, if there is no flow then the structure will be hypoplastic or absent. It is the chamber size that is affected by flow, not usually the wall thickness (hypertrophy). This is seen most dramatically in the condition of *hypoplastic left heart*, in which the left ventricle fails to develop beyond a tiny size because there is aortic and/or mitral atresia that prevents normal flow through the left ventricle and aorta. It is also seen in some cases of *pulmonary atresia* when the low pulmonary blood flow predisposes to very small pulmonary arteries. The converse is also true, high flow leading to a large cavity size, as is seen in right heart dilatation with an atrial septal defect.

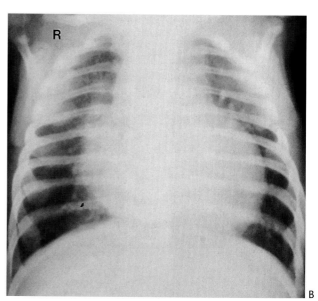

Fig. 14.8 (A) Chest radiograph of an infant aged 1 day. The heart is only slightly enlarged and the child was asymptomatic. (B) Chest radiograph of the same infant after 1 month. The heart size has increased and the pulmonary vasculature is now plethoric. The child had developed feeding difficulties, and a ventricular septal defect was diagnosed.

The pressure generated by a chamber stimulates the development of the muscular wall rather than the size of the cavity. Thus, in pulmonary atresia with an intact ventricular septum there is a high-pressure obstructed ventricle with very low flow through it. In this situation the chamber is usually very small but very hypertrophied. In tetralogy of Fallot, the right ventricle is subjected to high pressure and high flow (most of which passes down the aorta), and thus the chamber shows both dilatation and hypertrophy. Some surgical procedures are directed at increasing flow through structures in order to encourage their growth.

Physiological changes at birth

In fetal life the right-sided cardiac pressures and the pressure in the pulmonary artery remain high because the postnatal low-resistance pulmonary capillary bed has not yet developed. At birth, the first breath of the infant initiates the rapid decrease in pulmonary vascular resistance, which in turn leads to a rapid decrease in right-sided cardiac pressures. This causes the interatrial foramen to close by acting like a valve, and will also stimulate closure of the patent ductus arteriosus. Ductal closure is a complex phenomenon, and may take some hours or days or even weeks in premature infants. It is important to realise, however, that the consequential drop in pulmonary artery pressure can take several hours or days to be complete, and this will have important consequences on the clinical and radiological presentation of certain conditions in early life.

Signs and symptoms of left-to-right shunts will tend to increase in the early days and weeks of life as the pulmonary resistance falls (Fig. 14.8). However, some conditions (e.g. pulmonary atresia) are 'ductus dependent', and the closure of the ductus in early life will lead to progressive pulmonary oligaemia and consequent cyanosis.

PATHOLOGICAL CIRCULATIONS

Left-to-right shunt

In the normal postnatal situation the pressure in the right ventricle and pulmonary artery will be much lower than that on the left side because of the lower vascular resistance in the lungs. If any communication between the left and right side of the heart exists, there will be a left-to-right shunt. This can be measured by catheter oximetry, or non-invasively by radionuclide studies and Doppler techniques. The ratio of pulmonary to systemic flow (often called the Q_P/Q_S ratio) can vary from less than 2 : 1 (a small shunt) to 4 : 1 (a moderate shunt) or as much as 10 : 1 or over (a very large shunt). It is generally held that a shunt of 2 : 1 or less is difficult to detect on the chest radiograph by either pulmonary plethora or increased heart size.

If the left-to-right shunt is at the *atrial level* then the pressure in the left and right ventricles will not necessarily be affected. The right ventricle can tolerate a significantly increased flow of blood by increasing its cavity size and contractility while maintaining normal or slightly raised pressures. On the chest X-ray the lung fields will be *plethoric* (generalised enlargement of all the vessels), and the dilated right-sided chambers will manifest themselves as an increased heart size (Fig. 14.9). It is often possible to see 'end-on' vessels as prominent circular soft-tissue opacities in the central lung fields.

If this situation exists for many years the continuing large flow in the lungs can gradually damage the pulmonary circulation, and will eventually lead to a right-sided pressure increase and ultimately equalisation of left- and right-sided pressures. Thus, simple atrial septal defects do not often cause trouble in childhood or early adult life but may cause pulmonary hypertension or heart failure in middle age or later.

If the *ventricular septal defect* is small this will increase the flow through the lungs but will not necessarily raise the pressure on the right side. It is highly probable that small ventricular septal defects will close in the early years of life.

If there is a large ventricular septal defect, then the left and right ventricles will immediately be at the same pressure, and the lower resistance of the lungs will induce a large left-to-right shunt. In this situation the combination of increased flow and increased pressure in the lungs will produce progressive pulmonary vascular damage at a much earlier age than would occur with atrial mixing. Irreversible pulmonary damage will occur in this situation, and ultimately the right-sided pressure elevation will cause reversal of the shunt with the development of cyanosis (*Eisenmenger's syndrome*). The development of this condition is associated with a reduction in the left-to-right shunt with consequent reduction in the heart size and decreased pulmonary plethora. Thus the chest radiograph that is 'improving' or has returned to 'normal' may actually be showing the development of progressive irreversible damage. A similar situation can occur with any other high-pressure mixing situation such as might occur with a large *patent ductus arteriosus* or other *aorto-pulmonary connection*. The right-to-left shunting is occasionally demonstrated by radionuclide techniques (Fig. 14.10).

Circulation in transposition

Complete transposition of the great arteries with no other intracardiac abnormality is incompatible with life unless there is mixing of the two circulations at some point. It is useless to have a large amount of well-oxygenated blood returned to the left atrium if it is subsequently redirected to the left ventricle and then to the pulmonary artery and lungs again. There is usually a small amount of shunting across the foramen ovale, which sustains life in the early postnatal period, but it is essential to improve mixing at an early stage. In line with the principles outlined above, the obligatory shunting is best at an atrial level where the pressure is low, and it is thus common practice to perform a

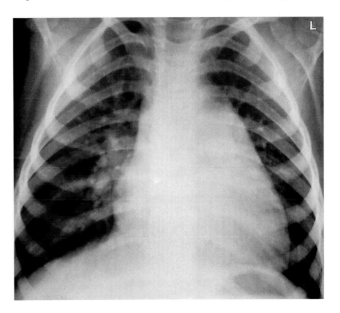

Fig. 14.9 Chest radiograph of a child with a moderately large atrial septal defect. The main pulmonary artery segment is large, and the lung vessels large.

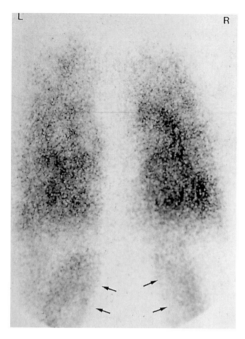

Fig. 14.10 Posterior view of a ⁹⁹ᵐTc-microsphere lung scan in a patient with Eisenmenger's syndrome. Renal uptake (arrows) is due to right-to-left shunting in the heart.

Rashkind balloon septostomy as soon as possible in cyanosed infants with transposition of the great arteries. This procedure ruptures the thin septum primum covering the foramen ovale, which facilitates increased atrial shunting (which must of course be in both directions). Although the total amount of shunting from left to right and right to left must be equal, there is overall much more blood flowing in the pulmonary circuit than the systemic circuit, so that the small proportion of this oxygenated pulmonary flow which passes across the atrial septum will be adequate to sustain the systemic requirements. The vessels in the lungs will consequently be enlarged.

Patients with complete transposition frequently have other communications between pulmonary and systemic circuits, common examples being ventricular septal defects and patent ductus arteriosus. These communications will be advantageous in increasing the mixing but disadvantageous in that they will predispose to high pulmonary pressures which might permanently damage the lungs.

Common mixing circulation

This can occur with a number of different conditions. A *common atrium* or *total anomalous pulmonary venous drainage* to the right atrium will produce this at the atrial level. An *atretic tricuspid valve* will lead to obligatory right-to-left shunting into the left atrium and consequent common mixing. At the ventricular level a very *large ventricular septal defect* or any of the 'single ventricle' variants will produce common mixing. At the great arterial level there will be common mixing in *pulmonary atresia* and *common truncus arteriosus*.

In all these situations the aorta and pulmonary artery will both be supplied with partially desaturated blood. The lungs will be at little disadvantage if they receive adequate flow (unless they are subjected to an excessively high pressure/flow combination) but the systemic supply will be significantly affected and the patient will be cyanosed, the degree depending on the particular haemodynamic details. If there is very rapid circulation through the lungs, then there will be a high proportion of saturated blood returned to the common mixing pool, and the cyanosis will be slight (as in truncus arteriosus). If pulmonary blood flow is low, then the common mixing pool will be very desaturated (e.g. in pulmonary atresia).

Pulmonary atresia

In many congenital cardiac abnormalities there is complete obstruction of the pulmonary artery or valve which may be associated with atresia or narrowing in the right ventricular outflow tract. In this situation no blood will enter the pulmonary circulation in the normal way, and the only flow in the pulmonary circuit will be that produced by *ductal flow* or by *systemic to pulmonary collaterals*, the latter being small or absent at birth.

In patients in this category, closure of the patent ductus arteriosus at birth can lead to rapid progressive cyanosis, and it is therefore necessary to increase the blood supply to the lungs. In the short term this is done by *medical therapy* to keep the patent ductus open, but as soon as practicable a *systemic-to-pulmonary shunt* is performed to improve the blood flow into the lungs. Patients surviving this early stage without surgical palliation will go on to develop *aortopulmonary collateral communications*. These vary considerably, and can enter the lungs in many sites. Some of these vessels may be of bronchial artery origin, but it is not always clear what their morphological origins are. Supply is most frequently from the descending aorta, but subclavian, internal mammary and intercostal arteries may give rise to collaterals.

Left-sided obstructions

Coarctation of the aorta and *aortic valve stenosis* are two common obstructive lesions which, if severe, can lead to left-sided heart failure in early life. This will be radiographically manifest as enlargement of pulmonary vessels (due to pulmonary venous hypertension, not plethora), possible interstitial or alveolar pulmonary oedema and cardiomegaly. Obstruction at the *mitral* or *left atrial* level is less common, but will give the pulmonary changes with less cardiomegaly because the left ventricle is not working against the obstruction.

Right-sided obstructions

Severe obstruction to the outflow into the lungs is usually a less serious problem than severe systemic outflow obstruction but it can still have important effects. Right ventricular failure can be caused by *very severe pulmonary stenosis*, but commonly this does not occur because a ventricular septal defect will also be present (e.g. tetralogy of Fallot) which will allow decompression of the elevated right-sided pressures by right to left shunting.

Birth asphyxia

Obstetric problems which lead to severe birth anoxia can have serious cardiac effects. These are most commonly manifest as heart failure with cardiomegaly and pulmonary changes. If resuscitation is achieved successfully, the chest radiograph may revert to normal over a few days.

IMPORTANT CONGENITAL CARDIAC ABNORMALITIES

A number of conditions will be discussed in detail, and are presented in order of frequency of occurrence as shown in Table 14.1. The data are taken from the Bristol Registry of Congenital Heart

Table 14.1 Incidence of congenital cardiac abnormalities*

Condition	Incidence (%)
Ventricular septal defect	36.1
Atrial septal defect	8.2
Patent ductus arteriosus	7.9
Pulmonary stenosis	6.9
Coarctation of the aorta	5.9
Aortic stenosis	5.7
Tetralogy of Fallot	4.6
Transposition of the great arteries	3.8
Atrioventricular septal defect	3.6
Pulmonary atresia	2.6
Single ventricle	2.2
Tricuspid atresia	1.5
Mitral valve abnormalities	1.4
Hypoplastic left heart syndrome	1.4
Cardiomyopathy	1.3
Anomalous pulmonary venous connection	1.2
Total	94.3

* Bristol Registry of Congenital Heart Disease, 1977–1987.

Disease, and represent all live births presenting with congenital heart disease to the centre in the period from 1977 to 1987. These figures have not changed significantly in recent decades and are essentially in line with published data from other centres.

The following conditions with a reported incidence of less than 1% are also discussed:

- Truncus arteriosus
- Ebstein's anomaly
- Sinus of Valsalva fistula
- Double-outlet ventricle
- Great arterial anomalies
- Coronary anomalies
- Arteriovenous malformations
- Cardiac tumours.

Systemic venous anomalies are also discussed. These are quite commonly associated with other forms of congenital heart disease, occurring in 10% of cases with diagnosed congenital heart disease.

VENTRICULAR SEPTAL DEFECT

This abnormality is the commonest of all, and can occur alone or be associated with other simple or complex congenital heart conditions. The interventricular septum has a complex curved shape, and defects can occur in any part of it. Various descriptive classifications have been proposed but the following classification (or a modification of it) is generally accepted.

Perimembranous defect This is the commonest type of ventricular septal defect (VSD), involving the membranous septum and adjacent muscular tissue below the aortic root and close to the upper margin of the tricuspid valve annulus. Sometimes this can be large and extend around toward the outlet part of the septum.

Muscular defects These can be grouped as follows:

1. *Inlet* or basal muscular defect lying in the muscular septum between the mitral and tricuspid valves.

2. Mid-muscular or *apical* defect between the main right and left ventricular chambers, sometimes called an apical trabecular defect.

3. *Outlet* defect, which involves either the high anterior trabeculated part of the septum or the band of muscle immediately below the pulmonary valve forming the conus of the right ventricle (the term 'conal' defect is sometimes used in the latter situation).

The distinction between these types has clinical importance because of the different position of the conduction pathway and the need to protect this during surgical repair.

It is possible for single or multiple VSDs to be present at any site throughout the large and complex shape of the interventricular septum. In diagnosis and investigation of this condition it is not only important to confirm the presence of interventricular communication but to localise the exact site and size of the communication and to determine if there are any additional communications. The latter point is essential if corrective surgery is to be successful.

If defects are of the large inlet or outlet type, it may be possible to override the inlet or outlet valves. The overriding aorta in the tetralogy of Fallot is a good example of this. The term *malalignment VSD* is sometimes used in this situation. Extreme forms of malalignment will result in such conditions as double-inlet (Fig. 14.11) or double-outlet ventricle; these will be considered elsewhere.

The *Gerbode defect* is a communication through the small portion of the basal septum that separates the left ventricular outflow tract from the right atrium (the atrioventricular septum). This defect is very rare and must be diagnosed with care, because it can easily be confused with a perimembranous defect and coexistent tricuspid regurgitation. There is some doubt as to whether this defect truly exists or whether it is always a complex of a small perimembranous VSD associated with tricuspid regurgitation.

Many other congenital heart defects are associated with a VSD, and these will be considered in the appropriate sections. Of particular importance is the association of VSD with *coarctation of the aorta*,

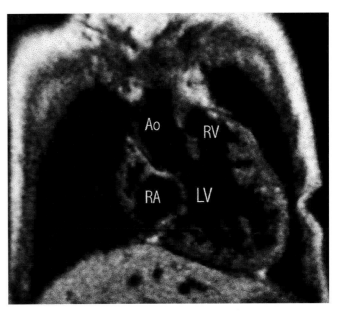

Fig. 14.11 Coronal spin-echo gated MRI scan showing a double-inlet left ventricle. The left ventricle is large and is seen connected to the inflow from the right atrium (RA). The right ventricle (RV) is rudimentary and lies in a superior position, filling directly from the left ventricle (LV) through a large VSD. Ao = aorta.

which can produce a particularly severe form of infantile cardiac failure. The remainder of this description will deal with the various forms of 'simple VSD', i.e. unassociated with other anomalies.

Clinical presentation

The presentation of this condition depends on the overall size of the interventricular communication. The condition does not normally present in the first few days of life unless the interventricular septal defect is very large. This is because the pulmonary vascular resistance drops markedly in the first days and weeks of life and thus prevents the early development of pulmonary plethora. The characteristic systolic murmur may take even longer to develop. Thus, even with large VSDs the patient may be asymptomatic, with a normal chest radiograph at birth. A large VSD will present after a few days or weeks, with breathlessness and feeding difficulties, and the chest X-ray will usually show moderate enlargement of the heart with prominence of the main pulmonary artery, the hilar pulmonary arteries and the peripheral pulmonary arteries. In severe cases there will be cardiac failure also.

With smaller VSDs, the presentation can be much later in life and may occur with the detection of an asymptomatic murmur. In these cases the chest X-ray can range from normal (if the communication is very small) to mild or moderate cardiac enlargement with mild or moderate pulmonary plethora.

In paediatric practice it is not an easy matter to distinguish VSD from other left-to-right cardiac shunts (e.g. patent ductus arteriosus, aortopulmonary communication or even a large atrial septal defect) on the basis of the chest X-ray alone, particularly in the young infant. Distinction becomes easier with increasing age, due to the differing natural histories of the conditions, but this is obviously of little immediate value in individual infants or children. It is important to point out, however, that a large VSD with a big shunt presenting early in life will inevitably lead to severe pulmonary damage and pulmonary hypertension in the first few years of life. It is thus essential to recognise the abnormality and treat the condition as soon as possible. *Echocardiography* is vital in the differential diagnosis of these conditions, and must be performed as soon as the condition is clinically or radiographically suspected.

Non-invasive imaging

The diagnosis of VSD can usually be confirmed on *two-dimensional echocardiography* (Fig. 14.12). It is most important that the full extent of the interventricular septum is examined in any case of suspected VSD. The examination will include, as an absolute minimum, the *parasternal long- and short-axis views* and the *apical four-chamber views* (Fig. 14.13). (Note: Orientation of echocardiographic images is variable, and paediatric cardiologists often present images in the

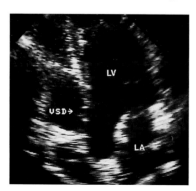

Fig. 14.12 Two-dimensional echocardiogram taken from the apex in a child with a small perimembranous ventricular septal defect (VSD). The margins of the defect act as distinct echogenic structures. LV = left ventricle; LA = left atrium.

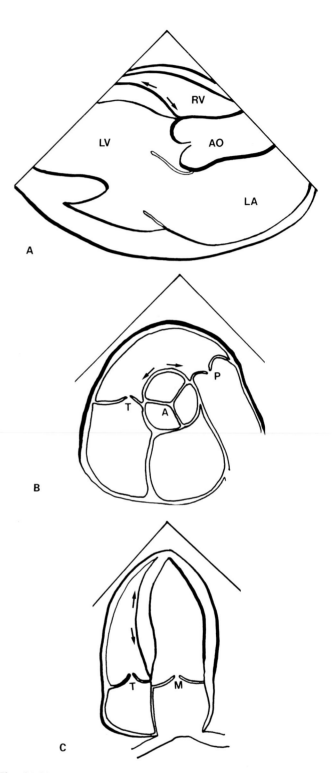

Fig. 14.13 (A) Parasternal long-axis echocardiogram. The arrows indicate the region for seeking a ventricular septal defect on Doppler examination. LV = left ventricle; RV = right ventricular outflow tract; AO = aortic root; LA = left atrium. (B) Parasternal short-axis echocardiogram at the level of the aortic root. The arrows indicate the area which should be examined just below the aortic valve to detect a perimembranous ventricular septal defect. T = tricuspid valve; A = aortic valve; P = pulmonary valve. (C) = Apical four-chamber echocardiogram. The arrows indicate where a muscular ventricular septal defect might be sought using Doppler techniques. T = tricuspid valve; M = mitral valve.

'inverted' position with the apex of the scan sector at the bottom of the image. In this chapter the conventional adult orientations are used as these are likely to be more familiar to the radiologist.) Each view will include a sweep along the heart in the particular plane being examined. Sometimes the defect is easier to identify because the edges of the septal hole act as strong ultrasonic reflectors and highlight the defect. In some parts of the septum the trabecular pattern will produce multiple reflections which can obscure small defects. In some cases of perimembranous VSD there is associated tissue in or near the defect which can partially obstruct it, the growth of this probably being one of the mechanisms of spontaneous closure of moderate or small defects. Sometimes there is prominent bulging of this tissue into the right ventricle, the so-called '*aneurysmal perimembranous VSD*'.

It may be necessary to use *Doppler flow assessment* to detect the presence of small defects, using the turbulent jet passing through the defect as a marker. Careful searching along the right ventricular surface of the septum with the pulsed Doppler sample volume will usually reveal any abnormal jet. In this situation the addition of *colour flow mapping* has been very valuable in speeding and simplifying the detection of small or multiple VSDs (Fig. 14.14), particularly in small restless children. Colour flow imaging will also show the direction of the jet, which is particularly important if a continuous-wave Doppler beam is to be aligned with the jet to measure the peak jet velocity and calculate the pressure drop across the VSD. This is an important non-invasive method for deducing the right ventricular pressure.

Mild tricuspid regurgitation is frequently associated with perimembranous VSDs, and Doppler techniques are particularly useful in detecting this, though care must be taken to avoid confusion with the VSD jet itself.

MRI has been used with success to demonstrate VSDs, but is cumbersome if used to detect small defects in uncommon positions. Defects cannot be visualised with any clarity using *nuclear medicine* techniques, but first-pass studies are occasionally useful in calculating pulmonary-to-systemic flow ratios, and in conjunction with echocardiography they can produce a non-invasive assessment of a VSD.

Cardiac catheterisation and angiography

Cardiac catheterisation is still frequently undertaken if there is any doubt about the intracardiac anatomy or about the nature of the pulmonary vascular resistance. Cardiac angiography must be performed in such a way that the interventricular septum is completely examined in its entirety. There is no such thing as 'the view that profiles the septum'; rather, there are many views that profile different parts of the septum, and they must be used in a logical fashion not only to locate the site of the known VSD but also to confirm or exclude the possibility of additional VSDs.

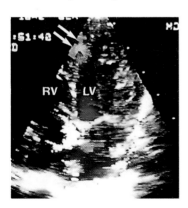

Fig. 14.14 Colour flow Doppler study taken in an apical four-chamber view. The arrows indicate the orange flow pattern (toward the transducer) of an apical muscular defect. LV = left ventricle. RV = right ventricle.

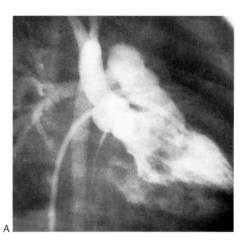

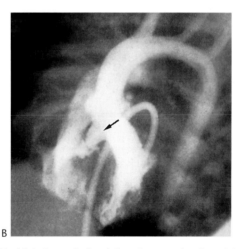

Fig. 14.15 (A) Left ventricular ciné angiogram taken in a right anterior oblique view. There is simultaneous filling of the aorta and pulmonary artery, indicating the presence of a ventricular septal defect which is not profiled in this projection. (B) Simultaneous view of the same angiogram but shown in the cranially angled LAO view. An aneurysmal perimembranous VSD is profiled (arrow).

If biplane ciné angiocardiography is available, the best two views to select for initial examination of the septum are:

1. 65° left anterior oblique (LAO) with a 20–25° cranial tilt
2. 30° right anterior oblique (RAO).

These two views will demonstrate the majority of the perimembranous, inlet and midmuscular septum (LAO view) and the high anterior and conal septum (RAO view) (Fig. 14.15). The outflow region will not be demonstrated adequately by the LAO view because the region will be obscured by contrast medium in the ventricle and aorta.

If the VSD demonstrated by these views is small and clearly localised then no additional view is necessary. If the VSD is large, however, it may be obscuring additional defects, and its dimension in the foreshortened plane may not be apparent. If multiple defects are shown, at least one additional view may be necessary to localise the defects precisely. With biplane studies the following additional two views may be helpful:

1. 55° LAO view with a 10–15° caudal tilt
2. 40° RAO view with a 15° caudal tilt.

The LAO view will distinguish high from low defects in this view, whereas the previous cranial tilt will distinguish basal from apical defects. The RAO view will profile the portion of the septum between the inflow and outflow portions.

The study of a VSD should not be concluded before consideration of the possible coexistence of a *patent ductus arteriosus*. A moderate or large VSD will give rise to simultaneous aortic and pulmonary opacification, and with some overlapping of structures it is not always possible to exclude a patent ductus with certainty. A separate aortogram (RAO 30°, LAO 60°) is thus required.

Large perimembranous VSDs can be associated with *aortic regurgitation* due to prolapse of the aortic root into the defect, and this is another reason for performing an aortogram in the complete assessment of a VSD.

Surgical treatment

Treatment of a VSD is most commonly surgical, but small defects may be left for some years (as long as there is no significant pulmonary hypertension) to see if spontaneous closure occurs. During this period, precautions must be taken against the development of infective endocarditis.

It has been common practice in the past to place a *band around the pulmonary artery* as a palliative operation in small infants with large VSDs, so that a definitive closure of the VSD can take place at a later age (often 3 or 4 years). This approach is rapidly giving way to earlier and earlier primary closure of the VSD, which is now performed under the age of 1 year in many cases, and in some cases in the first few weeks of life. *Primary closure* is a more complex operation in the very small infant but has the advantage that the pulmonary artery anatomy is not distorted and a second operation is not required.

Closure of the VSD is usually performed using a prosthetic patch, although sometimes the defect is closed by direct suture. Wherever possible the surgeon will close the defect from an approach via the right atrium and tricuspid valve. This avoids the need for any incision into the ventricle, but underlines the need for accurate diagnosis, because the entire septum cannot be inspected from this approach.

Recent studies using colour flow Doppler show that in the early postoperative period there is often leakage through the patch, which soon ceases as the patch endothelialises. The patch itself is usually easy to see in two-dimensional imaging as it is very echogenic.

ATRIAL SEPTAL DEFECT

This abnormality can be divided into two major categories, the *ostium* primum atrial septal defect (ASD) (which will be considered separately under the heading 'Atrioventricular septal defects') and the *ostium secundum* ASD, which is the more common type. The ostium secundum defect is usually at the level of the foramen ovale and does not involve the tissues of the septum primum or the atrioventricular valves. A third form of ASD is less common and is known as the *sinus venosus defect*. This is very high in the atrial septum near the insertion of the superior vena cava. This type of defect is often associated with some form of partially anomalous pulmonary venous drainage.

ASD must be distinguished from *patent foramen ovale*. The latter condition is a normal finding in small infants, because in the first few weeks or months of life the flap valve mechanism across the foramen ovale has not finally fused shut. In abnormalities where the atrial chambers are enlarged, this can cause stretching of the foramen ovale, which can sometimes regress after appropriate treat-

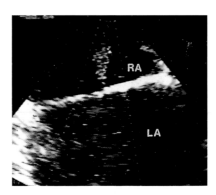

Fig. 14.16 Colour flow Doppler study taken from the subcostal position in an adult with mitral valve disease. The patent foramen ovale is seen as an orange jet (toward the transducer). This was an incidental finding. LA = left atrium; RA = right atrium.

ment. In practical terms, the patent foramen ovale is distinguished from a true ASD by the persisting interatrial pressure difference in the former condition. Echocardiographic features of a patent foramen ovale rather than an ASD are the presence of turbulence and a diameter of less than 3 mm. This can be detected in some adults as an incidental finding, particularly when using colour flow Doppler mapping (Fig. 14.16).

The low-pressure shunting that occurs with ASD is usually accommodated very well by the right ventricle, and patients with an isolated ASD very rarely present with significant problems in the early years of life. Presentation later in childhood or adolescence is quite common, when mild abnormalities are detected on routine medical examination or chest X-ray. The *chest X-ray* is usually normal if the pulmonary-to-systemic flow ratio is less than 2 : 1, but if it exceeds this level there will be pulmonary plethora and cardiac enlargement. The cardiac enlargement is mainly due to right atrial and right ventricular dilatation, both these chambers taking increased flow.

From time to time, ASD will present in the middle aged or elderly, when heart failure or pulmonary hypertension can finally develop and cause symptoms for the first time. In patients with

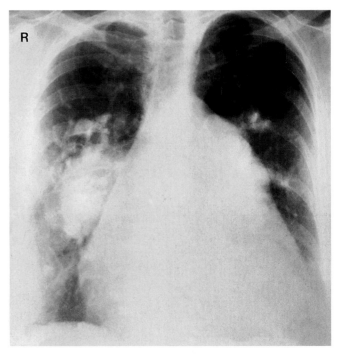

Fig. 14.17 Chest radiograph of an elderly women with an ASD and severe pulmonary hypertension. The main pulmonary artery and hilar pulmonary arteries are very large, with peripheral vascular attenuation.

significant pulmonary arterial hypertension (usually the elderly untreated patients), the chest X-ray will show dramatic appearances of centrally dilated pulmonary arteries and peripheral pulmonary vascular 'pruning' (Fig. 14.17). There is a risk of these patients with pulmonary hypertension having a paradoxical embolus from a systemic venous thrombosis. These patients may be inoperable.

ASD occurs quite commonly in association with many other cardiac abnormalities, and in some conditions it is an obligatory communication that sustains life, as in the case of tricuspid atresia or total anomalous pulmonary venous drainage.

Non-invasive diagnosis

Echocardiography is the cornerstone of diagnosis in this condition. Two-dimensional imaging will show the defect in almost all cases (Fig. 14.18). The typical *secundum defect* is best seen from the sub-costal view, which places the interatrial septum at a significant angle to the examining beam and reduces the chance of an artefactual false-positive diagnosis. The latter can occur in the apical view when the interatrial septum lies parallel to the beam and reflects poorly, causing 'drop-out' and an apparent defect. The characteristic dilatation of the right-sided chambers is well seen, and the dominance of the right

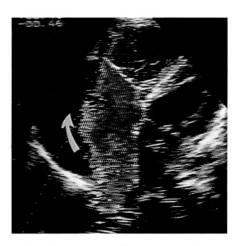

Fig. 14.20 Colour flow Doppler study in a patient with a secundum ASD septal defect in the same orientation as in Fig. 14.18. Flow through the defect toward the tricuspid valve is in red (toward the transducer).

ventricular volume overload will often be seen as 'paradoxical' septal motion (Fig. 14.19). This is an abnormal anterior movement of the interventricular septum during ventricular systole.

The *ostium primum defect* (also known as partial atrioventricular septal defect) is also well seen, as is atrioventricular valve anatomy. The less common *sinus venosus defect* is harder to visualise, as it lies high in the atrium near the termination of the superior vena cava. Transoesophageal studies are often used to demonstrate this difficult lesion. All studies of ASD must be accompanied by a thorough examination of the pulmonary and systemic venous connections, as these are quite often abnormal.

Doppler studies will often complete the diagnostic information. *Colour flow mapping* is particularly helpful in the diagnosis of the defect and any venous anomalies (Fig. 14.20). A short acceleration time in pulmonary artery flow can sometimes point to the presence of pulmonary hypertension, as will a high-velocity jet of tricuspid regurgitation. Pulmonary-to-systemic flow ratios can be calculated using Doppler techniques, but these are very time-consuming and are prone to error. Simpler and more accurate non-invasive assessment of the degree of left-to-right shunting can be achieved by first-pass *radionuclide studies*. Radionuclide 'first-pass' studies are also helpful in the older child with a suspected ASD in whom subcostal imaging is not diagnostic.

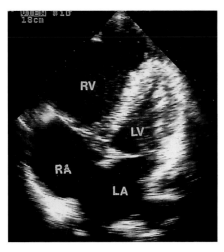

Fig. 14.18 Modified apical four-chamber echocardiogram of a patient with a secundum ASD. The right-sided chambers are considerably enlarged. LA = left atrium; RA = right atrium; LV = left ventricle; RV = right ventricle.

Cardiac catheterisation and angiography

A comprehensive echocardiographic diagnosis will often eliminate the need for invasive investigation, but there will be occasions when there is a need for catheterisation, either to calculate the shunt ratio accurately or to confirm or exclude some anatomical detail. A left atrial injection of contrast medium is occasionally helpful, but usually angiography is used to assess abnormal venous anatomy or to assess left ventricular function. ASD is of course commonly associated with other forms of congenital heart disease which might require cardiac catheterisation for diagnosis.

Treatment

The condition requires surgical closure in patients with a significant shunt. *Surgical treatment* is relatively straightforward, and so surgery for ASD is often also carried out in patients with relatively mild symptoms, because the operation has a very low mortality and complications in later life can be avoided. *Transcatheter occlusion*

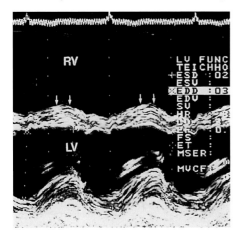

Fig. 14.19 M-mode echocardiogram of a patient with an ASD and right ventricular volume overload. There is 'paradoxical' motion of the interventricular septum (arrows). LV = left ventricle; RV = right ventricle.

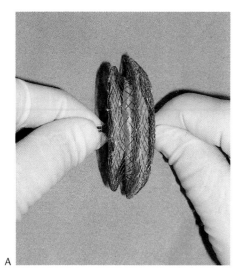
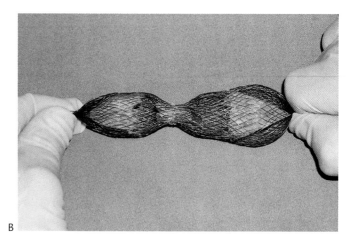

Fig. 14.21   (A) Photograph of a nitinol Amplatzer ASD occluder device in the unexpanded (deployment) position. (B) The same device partially stretched; full extension of the device allows deployment through a catheter delivery sheath.

of ASD is increasingly being performed with a variety of occlusion devices, the most commonly used device at present being the nitinol Amplatzer device (Fig. 14.21). Transoesophageal echocardiography has an important role in assessing the exact size of the secundum atrial septal defect and aids selection of an appropriately sized occlusion device. It is also invaluable in confirming a stable device position, assessing residual shunting and excluding any impingement on the atrioventricular valves (Fig. 14.22).

PATENT DUCTUS ARTERIOSUS

The patent arterial duct is a vital part of the fetal circulation, and this communication usually closes within the first few days of life. The ductus arteriosus often remains open rather longer in premature infants, but in the majority of cases it still closes spontaneously. If there is a persistent failure of closure of the duct, then the consequences will depend on the size of the communication. A tiny residual patent ductus arteriosus (PDA) can remain undiagnosed throughout life as it will produce minimal effects. A large PDA will

have similar effects to a large VSD, with pressure and volume overloading of the pulmonary circulation. In most diagnosed cases the PDA is closed surgically to avoid the risk of endocarditis, whether or not there is a large shunt. PDA is commonly associated with many other congenital cardiac abnormalities, and no investigation of congenital heart disease is complete without diagnosis or exclusion of a coexisting PDA.

The clinical sign of a continuous murmur is classically associated with a PDA, but *coronary artery fistulas* and a *ruptured sinus of Valsalva* can also give a continuous murmur, and must be distinguished from PDA by echocardiography or angiography.

The *chest X-ray* will show pulmonary plethora if the shunt is large, and there will be mild to moderate cardiac enlargement. The normally smooth outline of the aortic knuckle and upper descending aorta will often be interrupted by the 'bump' of the ductus, but this is often difficult to detect in young infants in whom the normal aorta is hard to visualise. In an older child or adult it is probably true to say that the presence of a well-defined aortic knuckle leading into a straight and uninterrupted descending aorta will

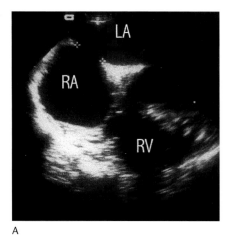
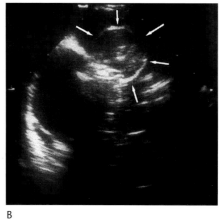
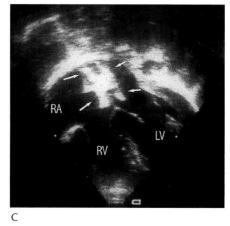

Fig. 14.22   (A) Transoesophageal echocardiogram showing an ASD prior to device closure. LA = left atrium; RA = right atrium; RV = right ventricle. (B) Balloon sizing of the defect is performed to determine the appropriate size of device to use; the balloon (arrows) lies in the left atrium. (C) The deployed nitinol Amplatzer device lies in a satisfactory position (arrows) occluding the ASD. (Courtesy Dr G. Stuart.)

almost certainly exclude the presence of a PDA. Later in life there may be some *calcification* present in a PDA. The ascending aorta and aortic arch carry greater flow than normal in this condition, and consequently the aortic knuckle is sometimes enlarged, but this cannot be regarded as a reliable sign.

The presence of a ductal communication can often be life-saving in neonates with pulmonary atresia. The physiological closure of the ductus will lead to increased cyanosis, and the use of *prostaglandin therapy* is directed toward maintaining ductal patency until a definitive palliative or corrective operation can be performed. In this situation the anatomy of the ductus arteriosus is different to normal, with the angulation of the communication being opposite to normal. This is due to the abnormal ductal flow, being from aorta to pulmonary artery in fetal life.

Non-invasive imaging

Echocardiography will show clearly the persistent communication on two-dimensional scanning in many cases. The best view for demonstration of the PDA is a modification of the parasternal short-axis view, sometimes called the '*ductus cut*'. The imaging plane in this view is orientated anatomically through the main pulmonary artery, the left pulmonary artery, the ductus itself and the descending aorta. A PDA can also be imaged from other views, particularly the suprasternal view, which will show the same structures (Fig. 14.23). The images can sometimes be misleading if there is particular prominence of the diverticulum at one or both ends of the ductus arteriosus. The aortic and pulmonary diverticula can both be large even when there is no actual continuity, and thus visualisation of complete continuity of the duct on the images is essential for a reliable diagnosis.

Doppler echocardiography is of great value in the diagnosis of this condition. Careful positioning of the pulsed Doppler sample volume in or near the duct will reveal the characteristic continuous turbulent signal of ductal flow. This can also be shown on continuous-wave Doppler (Fig. 14.24), and of course the flow can be mapped clearly using *colour flow imaging*. In older patients, imaging of the duct itself often proves difficult, and in this situation Doppler evaluation is of particular importance and is sometimes the only definite sign of the abnormality. Haemodynamic circumstances will affect the nature of ductal flow. *Aortopulmonary window* is a rare condition that can present similarly to a large

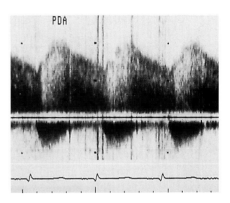

Fig. 14.24 Continuous-wave Doppler study taken from the parasternal position. Continuous flow through the PDA is shown above the baseline—toward the transducer. (Courtesy Dr R. Martin.)

PDA. There is usually a large direct communication from the ascending aorta to the pulmonary artery. Echocardiographers must be certain that the condition is not overlooked, and colour flow Doppler techniques will doubtless make this easier.

CT scanning and *nuclear medicine* studies have relatively little part to play in the assessment of the condition. *MRI* has an increasing role in the diagnosis of the condition, particularly in larger and adult patients in whom echocardiography may be difficult.

Cardiac catheterisation and angiography

Angiography is a reliable method of diagnosing the condition, and a well-placed aortic injection will show the abnormality. This is often achieved with an arterial catheter, but frequently the venous catheter can be passed via the right heart chambers to the pulmonary artery and then to the aorta via the actual patent ductus. Passage of the catheter through the communication can of course be diagnostic in itself but it is important to advance the catheter well down the descending aorta below the diaphragm to avoid confusion with a position in a lower-lobe pulmonary artery. This method does not show the size of the duct itself, and on occasion a catheter can be passed across the obstructed lumen of a recently closed ductus.

Standard cardiac oblique views, RAO 30° and LAO 60°, are usually best for the demonstration of the abnormality. Ideally, both views are recorded because each has its own advantages. The RAO view clearly separates the main pulmonary artery from the ascending aorta, and is excellent for the detection of very small shunts, but the view may foreshorten the duct itself. The LAO view will usually profile the duct well, but sometimes the superimposition of a large main pulmonary artery and the aorta can obscure detail. Angiographers must be careful not to miss an *aortopulmonary window*, as it can often be out of profile if inappropriate projections are selected and may not be shown at all if the ascending aorta is not opacified. *Coarctation of the aorta* is commonly associated with a PDA.

There are variations in the site of the ductus arteriosus which depend on variations in the development of the sixth arch. The ductus can be right-sided, and may occasionally form part of a vascular ring. There may be a bilateral ductus arteriosus in rare cases. Very rarely the ductus itself may become aneurysmal.

Treatment

In the majority of cases there is *spontaneous closure*, but in a few children there is a clinical need to close the communication. This is

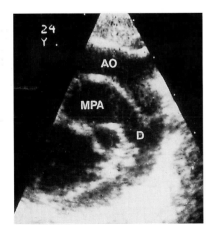

Fig. 14.23 Suprasternal echocardiogram of a patient with transposition of the great arteries and a PDA (D) The great arteries are parallel in this condition. AO = aorta; MPA = main pulmonary artery. (Courtesy Dr R. Martin.)

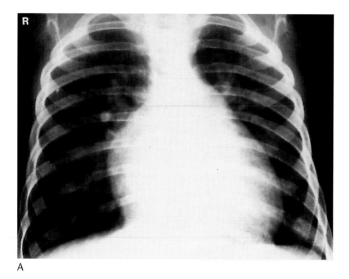

A

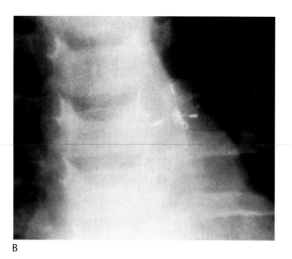

B

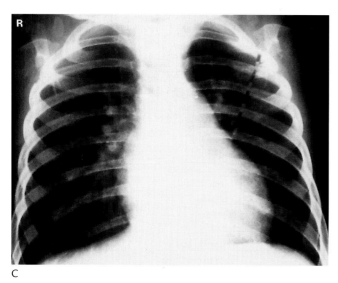

C

Fig. 14.25 (A) Chest radiograph of a child with a PDA immediately before closure. The heart is large, and there is pulmonary plethora. (B) Localised view of the Rashkind duct occluder in position in the same patient. (C) Chest radiograph in the same patient 24 hours after ductal occlusion. The heart has decreased considerably in size.

sometimes performed through a left thoracotomy incision, which allows the communication to be ligated and sometimes also divided. *Simple ligation* can sometimes be inadequate, with persistent communication being detectable in later life in a proportion of cases.

In recent years, transcatheter occlusion has become usual. Occlusion devices include the Rashkind and Amplatzer devices and embolisation coils (Fig. 14.25). Recognised complications include persistent shunting requiring insertion of a further device, projection of part of the device into the left pulmonary artery and rarely the displacement of the device.

PULMONARY STENOSIS

The most common form of pulmonary stenosis is *isolated pulmonary valve stenosis* in which there is fusion and thickening of the pulmonary valve leaflets. There may also be *infundibular stenosis* with right ventricular hypertrophy causing increased contractility and systolic narrowing of the outflow tract. *Distal pulmonary stenosis* involving the main pulmonary artery or its branches is also recognised (Fig. 14.26).

The severity of this condition varies greatly, and in mild cases the abnormality is of little clinical importance and may not present until late in life or not at all. Many cases of mild pulmonary stenosis present at routine medical examination with a heart murmur or with an abnormal chest radiograph or ECG.

More severe cases may present with tiredness and breathlessness, and the most severe cases may be associated with cyanosis and heart failure. In cases of moderate to severe stenosis, it is not reduction of cardiac output but the strain on the right side of the heart that causes problems. The *chest X-ray* often shows a prominent main pulmonary artery which is caused by poststenotic turbulence and consequent dilatation, and the proximal left pulmonary artery is also dilated in many cases because it lies in a direct line with the main pulmonary artery (Fig. 14.27). The right pulmonary artery is not usually so dilated because it branches quite sharply from the main pulmonary artery and turbulence from the stenotic valve is not carried down into it. Peripheral pulmonary vascularity is usually normal. In cases where infundibular stenosis predominates, the main pulmonary artery may not be recognised as abnormally

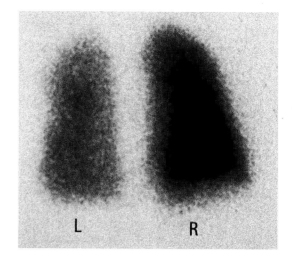

Fig. 14.26 Isotope perfusion study of a patient with left pulmonary artery branch stenosis. There is considerably less uptake of isotope in the left lung.

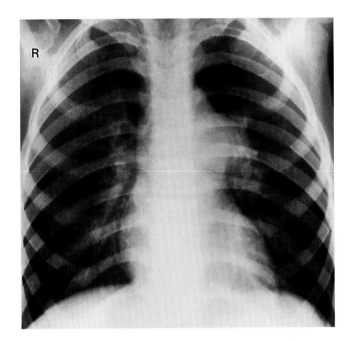

Fig. 14.27 Chest radiograph of a child with pulmonary valve stenosis. The main pulmonary artery and left pulmonary artery are considerably enlarged, but pulmonary vascularity is otherwise normal.

dilated on the chest X-ray because the turbulence caused by the obstruction is not carried into the main pulmonary artery. Conversely a very prominent pulmonary conus may be a normal finding in children and young adults and correlation with the clinical findings is required.

Peripheral pulmonary stenosis occurs occasionally as an isolated defect but more often this is secondary to surgical intervention with a shunt or to trauma from a malpositioned ductal closure device.

Non-invasive imaging

Diagnosis is usually possible by *echocardiography*, particularly if a Doppler examination with continuous-wave techniques is available. Two-dimensional imaging can be difficult, as the pulmonary valve lies partially behind the left sternal border, but turning the patient well to the left and keeping the transducer close to the sternum will frequently give a satisfactory short-axis view. Good-quality images are needed to distinguish simple leaflet fusion from a thickened and dysplastic valve. *Doppler studies* are the key to diagnosis, not only for detecting the high-velocity flow through the stenotic valve but also for quantifying the severity of the lesion. Infundibular stenosis (often dynamic with marked systolic narrowing) and pulmonary artery stenosis can both be diagnosed using echocardiography. The pressure drop or 'gradient' across the stenotic valve can be estimated using continuous-wave Doppler measurements.

Cardiac catheterisation and angiography

Contrast medium injection into the right ventricle will normally give an excellent demonstration of pulmonary valve anatomy, the best two views being the lateral projection and a steeply cranially tilted (20–25°) anterior view. The cranial tilt is necessary to minimise the foreshortening of the infundibulum and main pulmonary artery segment. Passage of the catheter across the valve will of course allow measurement of the pressure drop caused by the stenosis.

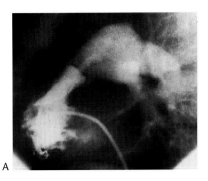
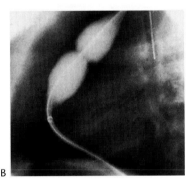

Fig. 14.28 (A) Lateral view of a right ventricular angiogram in a child with pulmonary valve stenosis. The doming of the stenotic valve and the central jet of contrast medium are seen. There is post-stenotic dilatation of the main pulmonary artery. (B) Lateral view of pulmonary valve dilatation in the same patient. The indentation in the balloon indicates that the valve is not yet fully dilated.

Treatment

Treatment has changed considerably in recent years. Mild forms of pulmonary stenosis (up to a pressure drop of approximately 40 mmHg) do not normally require surgery. More severe cases have traditionally had *pulmonary valvotomy* performed surgically, but recent interventional techniques have been very successful, and in most cases of pulmonary valve stenosis a *balloon dilatation* technique is now the treatment of choice (Fig. 14.28). Excellent results are obtained using this approach (Fig. 14.29). Occasionally the valve is too dysplastic (thickened, deformed and irregular) for balloon valvuloplasty to be indicated. Successful balloon valvuloplasty requires careful measurement of the pulmonary valve annulus from

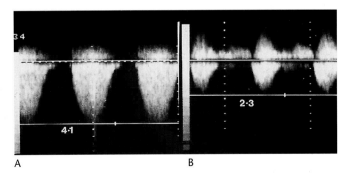

Fig. 14.29 Continuous-wave Doppler traces taken from a patient immediately before and after pulmonary valve dilatation. Peak velocity is indicated (in m/s), and can be used in the modified Bernoulli equation (pressure (in mmHg) = 4 × velocity (in m/s')) to show a predilatation pressure drop of 67 mmHg reduced to 21 mmHg.

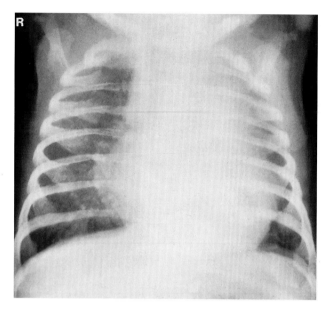

Fig. 14.30 Chest radiograph of an infant with coarctation of the aorta. There is cardiomegaly and evidence of left heart failure.

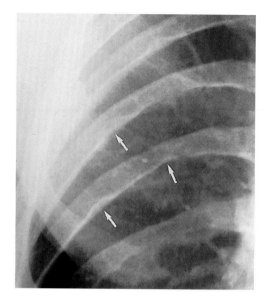

Fig. 14.31 Localised view of the ribs showing notching (arrows) in an adult patient presenting with coarctation of the aorta.

the preliminary angiogram and selection of an appropriate-sized balloon, usually slightly larger than the annulus itself. Pulmonary regurgitation may develop or increase after the procedure but it is rarely a problem.

COARCTATION OF THE AORTA

In this condition there is a characteristic shelf-like narrowing of the aorta which usually occurs just beyond the origin of the left subclavian artery. The severity of this narrowing can vary considerably and it is this severity which determines the age of presentation.

Severe coarctation of the aorta can present in the first few days or weeks of life with cardiac enlargement and cardiac failure (Fig. 14.30). Physiological closure of the PDA presents a potential hazard in severe coarctation in infancy, as it may impair renal and other vital perfusion.

Lesser degrees of coarctation may present later in life with abnormal physical signs or abnormality on the chest X-ray. The classic late appearances on the chest X-ray are a small or irregular contour of the upper descending aorta and rib notching, caused by the prominent intercostal collateral vessels which are bypassing the narrowing (Fig. 14.31). Rib notching is rare in the first 5 years of life, and it is increasingly common for the condition to be detected and treated before this age. There is an association with abnormalities of the aortic valve, in particular a *bicuspid aortic valve*, which can develop in later life to a stenotic aortic valve.

Coarctation of the aorta has numerous variations in severity, but the site of the coarctation itself can also vary. Occasionally the narrowing can occur between the left common carotid and the left subclavian artery, and in this situation the rib notching is likely to be unilateral, being generated only on the right side from the right subclavian distribution into the right intercostal vessels. Sometimes there is quite severe hypoplasia of the aortic arch, particularly between the left common carotid artery and the left subclavian artery.

Interruption of the aortic arch is the most severe variant of the condition. The interruption may occur at three sites: Type A distal to the left subclavian artery, Type B between the left common carotid and subclavian artery and Type C between the innominate artery and the left common carotid artery. The PDA supplies the lower half of the body, which becomes severely compromised as the ductus arteriosus closes. There may be a substantial gap between the two parts of the aorta.

Non-invasive diagnosis

In experienced hands, *echocardiography* is reliable in the diagnosis of the condition, but it becomes increasingly problematical in older patients because of difficult ultrasonic access from the suprasternal notch, the best site for imaging. Care must be taken to avoid misdiagnosis due to the aorta passing out of the plane of the scan. An associated PDA must always be sought. Doppler studies can help by demonstrating the abnormal persistent diastolic flow through the narrowing, but this also depends on good ultrasonic access. The 'gradient' across the coarctation can, in theory, be measured using Doppler techniques, but practical experience has shown this to be somewhat unreliable. *MRI* can be used very successfully to demonstrate coarctation (Fig. 14.32), both with regard to the coarctation itself and also the presence of any major collateral vessels. It is used increasingly for follow-up of coarctation post treatment.

In some cases the anatomy of the bypassing collaterals needs to be assessed for surgical planning. This is hard to achieve by echocardiography, and *angiography* is often necessary, although MRI is proving increasingly successful.

Cardiac catheter and angiography

Catheter access for an ascending aortic injection of contrast medium to demonstrate the aortic arch and coarctation can sometimes be a problem. A severe coarctation can prevent an arterial catheter from crossing from below, and in older patients without an ASD or VSD, access to the left side of the heart from the right heart chambers may not be possible. Left-sided access may be achieved by trans-septal puncture or by the brachial arterial approach, but these offer a higher risk of complications than usual.

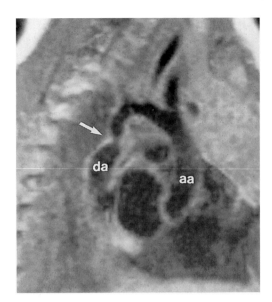

Fig. 14.32 Oblique sagittal gated spin-echo MRI scan of a child with coarctation of the aorta (arrow). aa = ascending aorta; da = descending aorta. (Courtesy of the Trustees of the Bristol MRI Centre.)

Alternative angiographic approaches may be used. A pulmonary artery injection may be followed through to the left side, and, with good equipment, excellent details of the coarctation and collateral vessels may be achieved. Digital subtraction angiography offers the opportunity for even better contrast enhancement in this situation (Fig. 14.33). Peripheral or central venous contrast injection causes considerable dilution of contrast medium, and images are not usually of satisfactory quality.

Treatment

There is a long-term risk of severe systemic hypertension in the upper body, and this is the indication for repair even in asymptomatic patients. In severely ill infants the operation is often carried out as an emergency, frequently following ultrasound diagnosis alone.

Surgical repair is carried out by various techniques, which include the incorporation of the left subclavian artery as a flap (Fig. 14.34) or direct anastomosis of the aorta after resection of the narrow segment. Occasionally, prosthetic patch material is incorporated into the repair. It should be noted, however, that surgical correction of coarctation carries a small but definite risk of paraplegia developing as an operative complication in older patients. Balloon dilatation and stent insertion are both used for restenosis following surgical repair of coarctation. In many centres balloon dilatation is used to treat native coarctation. Repair of aortic interruption is, of course, more complex, and it carries a higher mortality.

AORTIC STENOSIS

Congenital aortic stenosis has a variety of forms, varying from a simple malformation in which the leaflets of the aortic valve remain partially fused, to a complex dysplastic valve which may be bicuspid or even unicuspid. There are also various forms of *subaortic stenosis*, ranging from a simple diaphragm to more complex tubular narrowing or obstructive fibrous tissue in the left ventricular outflow tract. Distinctly different is the dynamic narrowing of the left ventricular outflow tract caused by *hypertrophic cardiomyopathy*.

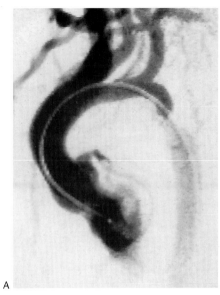

A

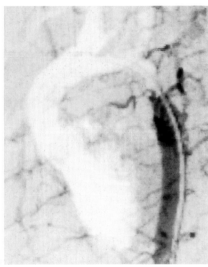

B

Fig. 14.33 (A) Digital subtraction study of a left ventriculogram in the LAO projection. A severe coarctation of the aorta is seen in the typical position. (B) Late image from the study in (A) shows delayed filling of the descending aorta by collaterals.

Supravalvular aortic stenosis occurs above the sinuses of Valsalva and is less common but can nevertheless be considered under the heading of congenital aortic stenosis. This most commonly occurs in *William's syndrome*, in which there is severe hypoplasia of the ascending aorta above the sinuses of Valsalva. The condition may be associated with vascular abnormalities elsewhere, including peripheral pulmonary artery stenosis and renal artery stenosis. Associated features are a typical '*elfin facies*' and vitamin D hypersensitivity. In suitable cases, surgery can enlarge the aorta at the point of stenosis.

The degree of obstruction in aortic stenosis is extremely variable, and the severity will determine the mode of presentation. *Severe cases* present in infancy with heart failure and left ventricular dilatation with impaired function. Severe aortic stenosis presenting in early infancy carries a high mortality, and early operation is required to divide the fused commissures. *Milder degrees* of aortic stenosis carry a better prognosis and can be operated on electively in childhood. Recently a number of critical cases have been detected by fetal echocardiography.

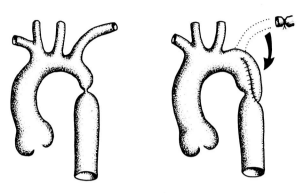

Fig. 14.34 Subclavian flap repair for coarctation of the aorta. (Reproduced from Jordan & Scott 1989, with permission.)

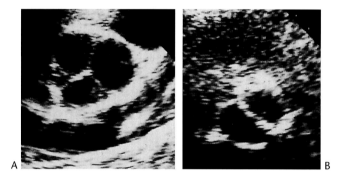

Fig. 14.35 (A) Short-axis echocardiogram of a normal aortic valve. showing three leaflets. (B) Short-axis echocardiogram of a bicuspid aortic valve.

The condition can be recognised on *chest X-ray* if there is a dilated ascending aorta due to poststenotic dilatation, but this is usually seen in older children only. Heart failure and cardiomegaly may be recognised in infancy, and in this situation there is little to distinguish the X-ray from that of severe coarctation or other forms of left ventricular failure.

Congenital bicuspid valves are not normally stenotic but they can lead to 'acquired' calcific aortic stenosis in adult life. They are present in up to 2% of the 'normal' population. The abnormality can be recognised clearly on *two-dimensional echocardiography* (Fig. 14.35). There is an association between coarctation of the aorta and congenital bicuspid aortic valve. There is also an increased incidence of 'left dominant' coronary circulation with bicuspid aortic valve.

Non-invasive diagnosis

The diagnosis of aortic stenosis can be made easily with *echocardiography*. Good-quality images of the left ventricle and aortic valve are usually possible from standard views. It is important to examine the subaortic and supra-aortic regions as carefully as the valve itself (Fig. 14.36). The most typical type of aortic stenosis shows thin (or only slightly thickened) leaflets that 'dome' in systole due to the narrow opening between the fused commissures. The presence of left ventricular hypertrophy should be noted as well as the overall contractility of the left ventricle. The aortic valve gradient can be measured using *continuous-wave Doppler studies*, the peak velocity of flow across the valve being used to calculate the peak pressure drop using the modified Bernoulli formula. *Colour flow Doppler examination* will show the stenotic jet, any subaortic obstruction and any coexisting aortic regurgitation.

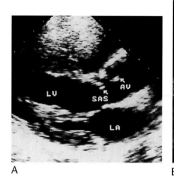
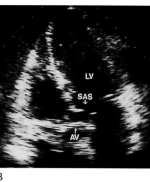

Fig. 14.36 (A) Parasternal long-axis echocardiogram showing an obstructive subaortic membrane. (B) Apical four-chamber echocardiogram of the same case showing the obstructive subaortic membrane. LV = left ventricle; AV = aortic valve; SAS = subaortic stenosis.

The detail of qualitative and quantitative information available from echocardiography means that surgery can often be performed on the basis of a good ultrasound study.

Cardiac catheterisation and angiography

This is still an important technique, and is used to measure valve 'gradient' and left ventricular pressures. Left ventricular angiography will allow assessment of ventricular function as well as assessing the function of the mitral valve. A supra-aortic injection is usually performed to detect or exclude coexistent aortic regurgitation.

Left ventriculography is best performed in RAO 30° projection and LAO 60° with 20° cranial tilt. The cranial tilt allows better profiling of the left ventricular outflow tract to exclude subaortic stenosis. Aortography is best performed in the same projections but without the cranial tilt.

Treatment

Minor degrees of stenosis can be observed for many years until there are signs of deleterious left ventricular effects. Echocardiography is useful as a routine check for early signs of left ventricular dilatation or impairment. Valve replacement is not practical in small infants and children as there are no suitable prostheses. Thus, severe cases in early life are usually treated by *surgical valvotomy*. This can be very successful, but will almost always be followed by *valve replacement* in later life. Transfer of the pulmonary valve to aortic position with the implantation of a homograft replacement in the pulmonary position is another surgical option. The introduction of *balloon valvuloplasty* has altered the management of some cases of congenital aortic stenosis, and the procedure has been life-saving in some critically ill infants. There are potential complications with the technique, however, one of which is the development of severe aortic regurgitation.

The surgical treatment of a localised diaphragm and a tubular hypoplasia of the outflow tract are substantially different and vary from case to case. Interventional techniques have played little part as yet in the treatment of subaortic stenosis.

TETRALOGY OF FALLOT

This abnormality is a complex of four related abnormalities which are part of a fundamental malformation of the heart. A large VSD (1) is associated with malalignment of the great arteries, such that the aortic root overrides the VSD (2) and is thus partly related to the right ventricle. There is associated stenosis of the right ventricular outflow tract (infundibulum) and pulmonary valve (3), together with a variable degree of hypoplasia of the pulmonary valve annulus and pulmonary arteries. The infundibular stenosis may have a dynamic component to the obstruction, being maximal in late systole. Finally there is right ventricular hypertrophy (4), which develops as a response to the systemic pressure in the right ventricle. In some cases the hypertrophied muscle bundles in the right ventricle can produce an additional intraventricular obstruction.

This abnormality is expressed in different ways, which depend mainly on the severity of the pulmonary stenosis. In mild cases of pulmonary stenosis the abnormality behaves much like a simple VSD, with possible benefit caused by the restriction of blood flow into the lungs (as in pulmonary artery banding). These patients form the *acyanotic* end of the spectrum. More typically, presenting cases are *cyanosed* because the pulmonary stenosis is sufficiently severs to restrict pulmonary blood flow. These children will present in childhood with varying degrees of cyanosis and fainting spells on exertion, which are usually caused by increasing infundibular obstruction to pulmonary flow with increasing cardiac work.

The most severe end of the spectrum is represented by critical pulmonary stenosis and severe pulmonary artery hypoplasia with very little flow into the lungs through the pulmonary valve. In this situation life must be sustained by alternative flow into the pulmonary vascularity, and this occurs by *ductal flow* or by *aorto-pulmonary collaterals* that develop in early life. The severe cases in this spectrum will present shortly after birth with progressive cyanosis as the ductus arteriosus closes. These babies will need urgent palliation by systemic shunting to maintain pulmonary blood flow or early primary correction.

Approximately 25% of patients with tetralogy of Fallot (or pulmonary atresia and VSD—a closely related condition) have a *right-sided aortic arch*. This type of right arch is usually associated with mirror imaging branching (i.e. left brachiocephalic, right common carotid and right subclavian in order of branching).

The *chest X-ray* is often not classical (see Fig. 14.37), but in the classical developed appearance there will be concavity in the left heart border in the region of the hypoplastic main pulmonary artery, upward prominence of the cardiac apex due to the distortion by the large right ventricle, pulmonary oligaemia, and in some cases a right-sided aortic arch (Fig. 14.37). While these signs are almost

diagnostic, many cases of tetralogy of Fallot have a nearly normal chest film.

Non-invasive imaging

Echocardiography is very useful in diagnosing the condition, and will show the VSD, the overriding aorta and the right ventricular hypertrophy very clearly. The pulmonary valve and pulmonary artery anatomy is often more difficult to assess by ultrasound, as these areas lie deeply and are partially surrounded by air, but it is still possible to measure the proximal parts of the vessels in many cases. The right ventricular outflow gradient and the pulmonary valve gradient can both be estimated using *Doppler techniques*, but there are many possible inaccuracies due to the many levels at which obstruction can occur. Right-to-left shunting across the VSD can be seen on colour flow Doppler examination (Fig. 14.38). Coronary anatomy cannot usually be assessed non-invasively.

Other non-invasive imaging techniques have little to add in most cases, but there are occasional applications, for example the occasional use of *thallium-201 scanning* to demonstrate the degree of right ventricular hypertrophy (Fig. 14.39).

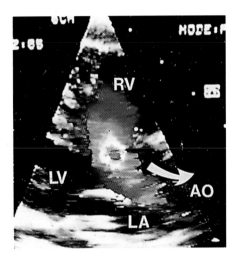

Fig. 14.38 Colour flow Doppler study in a child with tetralogy of Fallot. In the parasternal long-axis view here is right-to-left flow from the right ventricle (RV) to the aorta (AO) The majority of the flow is encoded blue (away from the transducer), but the fastest moving central flow shows aliasing (orange). LV = left ventricle; LA = left atrium.

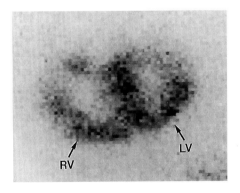

Fig. 14.39 Thallaum-201 scan in the left anterior view. In this adult patient with longstanding tetralogy of Fallot without complete correction there is marked right ventricular hypertrophy, with activity equalling that in the left ventricular wall.

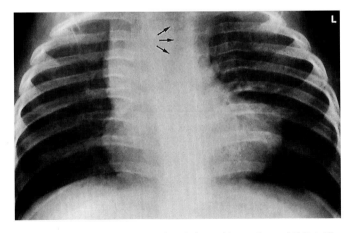

Fig. 14.37 Chest radiograph of an infant with tetralogy of Fallot. The trachea is indented by the right-sided aortic arch (arrows), the cardiac apex is angled upward, and the lung fields are oligemic.

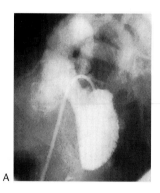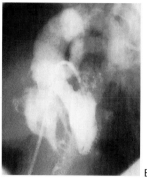

Fig. 14.40 (A) Cranially angled LAO left ventriculogram of a child with tetralogy of Fallot. There is early passage of contrast to the right ventricle across the VSD. Aortic override is seen. (B) Later image from the same study. The right ventricle is now well filled. The hypoplastic pulmonary arteries can be seen.

Cardiac catherterisation and angiography

This is often required in addition to echocardiography because precise assessment of anatomy is essential in surgical planning. The size of the pulmonary valve annulus as well as the size and anatomy of the more distal pulmonary arteries must be determined. The most common *coronary artery variant* occurring with tetralogy of Fallot is the anomalous origin of the left anterior descending coronary artery from the right coronary artery. This artery runs over the surface of the right ventricle just where the surgeon might make the incision to enlarge the right ventricular outflow tract, and so it is extremely important to detect this in advance, either by good-quality opacification of the aortic root or occasionally by selective coronary arteriography. Left ventricular angiography should be performed in views similar to those selected for a simple VSD (Fig. 14.40), but a steeper LAO view (e.g. 70°) is sometimes helpful, due to the rotation of the heart produced by the large right ventricle. Right ventriculography is best performed in a very steep LAO (e.g. 80–90°) and a cranially tilted (20°) anterior view to show the right ventricular outflow and pulmonary valve (Fig. 21.41). An aortogram performed in 30°

RAO and 60° LAO oblique views will show a patent ductus arteriosus, aortopulmonary collaterals, aortic arch anatomy, and brachiocephalic and coronary anatomy.

Treatment

Surgical treatment will depend on the severity of the condition, but the long-term aim will be total correction by closure of the VSD (using an oblique patch) and reconstruction of the right ventricular outflow tract and pulmonary arteries. In the latter situation a transannular patch may be incorporated into the repair to widen the outflow. In most cases the pulmonary valve function is destroyed by the reconstruction of the right ventricular outflow tract, but the pulmonary regurgitation that follows appears to be of little clinical significance.

In severe cases presenting in early life a palliative shunt may be performed if the child is too small or too ill for definitive repair. This is usually achieved with a *Blalock shunt* from the subclavian artery to the pulmonary artery. The classical procedure involves division of the subclavian artery and forming an end-to-side anastomosis with the ipsilateral pulmonary artery. The more recent 'modified Blalock' shunt uses an interposed prosthetic graft which allows continued patency of the subclavian artery (Fig. 14.42).

Postoperative appearances on the chest X-ray may be characteristic. Not only should the pulmonary oligaemia revert to normal, but also the right ventricular outflow tract and main pulmonary artery may look unusually large, due to the presence of an outflow patch. In cases palliated with a Blalock shunt there may be a difference in pulmonary blood flow in the two lungs, particularly if anatomical abnormalities prevent satisfactory central connection between the two pulmonary arteries. The Blalock shunt itself may cause troublesome narrowing of the pulmonary artery into which it is inserted and this can be recognised on angiography (Fig. 14.43). A confusing appearance is caused by the leakage of serous fluid through the walls of the modified Blalock shunt to form a seroma (Fig. 14.44). This may result in a prominent mediastinal mass, sometimes with calcification within its wall (Fig. 14.45).

Balloon dilatation of the pulmonary outflow tract and valve is performed in some centres as palliation prior to the definitive

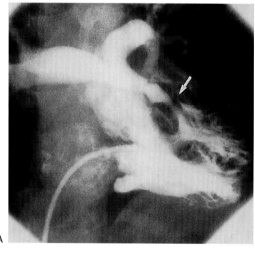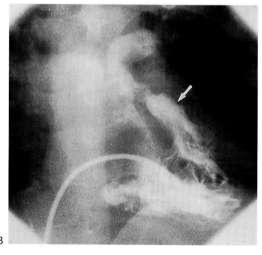

Fig. 14.41 (A) Cranially angled anterior view of a right ventriculogram of a patient with tetralogy of Fallot. Severe infundibular stenosis is seen in systole (arrows). The hypoplastic pulmonary annulus and main pulmonary artery can be seen. (B) Diastolic image from the same study. The right ventricular infundibulum is now much wider (arrow).

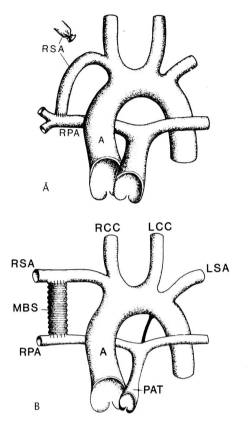

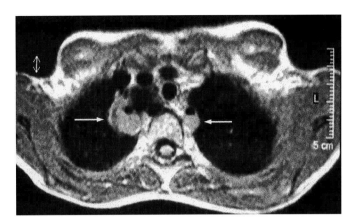

Fig. 14.44 Transverse spin-echo MRI scan of bilateral seromas (arrows) associated with bilateral modified Blalock–Taussig shunts.

TRANSPOSITION OF THE GREAT ARTERIES

D-loop transposition

The common form of this abnormality is D-loop transposition, in which the atrial and ventricular anatomy is normal. There is a simple reversal of connection of the great arteries, with the aorta arising from the morphologically right ventricle and the pulmonary artery arising from the morphologically left ventricle. The exact orientation of the great arteries varies, but the most common arrangement is with the aortic valve arising from a high anterior position from the right ventricle, and the pulmonary valve arising from the lower posterior position above the left ventricular outflow tract. There is loss of the normal arrangement where the right ventricular outflow twists around the left ventricular outflow. The two great arteries run parallel upward from their respective chambers (Fig. 14.46). This leads to the formation of a relatively narrow pedicle which can frequently be recognised on the chest X-ray.

These infants usually present in the first few weeks of life with cyanosis and breathlessness. Cyanosis depends on the exact degree of mixing at the atrial or ventricular level. Although the condition

Fig. 14.42 (A) The classic Blalock shunt. A = aorta; RPA = right pulmonary artery; RSA = right subclavian artery. (B) A modified Blalock shunt. MBS = modified Blalock shunt. RCC = right common carotid artery; LCC = left common carotid artery; LSA = left subclavian artery. PAT = pulmonary artery trunk. (Both diagrams reproduced from Jordan Scott 1989, with permission.)

surgical repair. It does not have the potential risk of inducing pulmonary branch stenosis as may happen with the Blalock shunt.

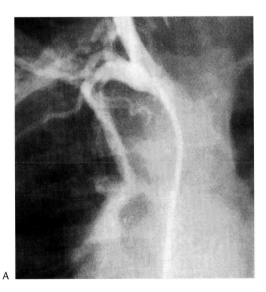

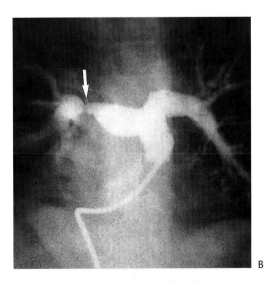

Fig. 14.43 (A) Anterior view of a selective angiogram of a right Blalock shunt. The right pulmonary artery is opacified. (B) Anterior view of a pulmonary arteriogram in the same patient. There is a severe stenosis at the site of insertion of the Blalock shunt.

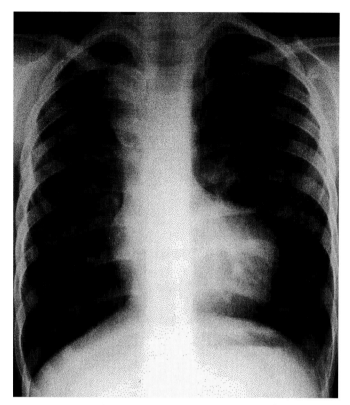

Fig. 14.45 Frontal chest radiograph showing a right-sided calcified seroma following a previous modified Blalock–Taussig shunt.

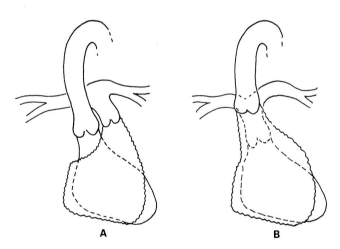

Fig. 14.46 (A) Normal great arterial connections in the anterior view. The morphological left ventricle (smooth outline) lies posteriorly to the morphological right ventricle (wavy outline) as shown by the interrupted line. (B) Connections in D-transposition of the great arteries in the anterior view. Compare with (A). The great arteries have an anteroposterior relationship, which gives the narrow pedicle.

can be diagnosed simply by echocardiography, cardiac catheterisation is commonly performed so that the Rashkind balloon septostomy can be performed at the same time. In this technique an inflated balloon is used to rupture the thin part of the septum primum covering the foramen ovale in order to improve the atrial mixing and thus allow a higher proportion of oxygenated blood to pass from the left atrium to the right atrium and right ventricle, and

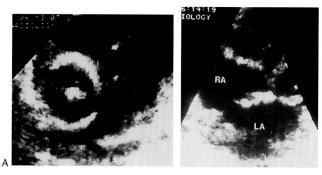

Fig. 14.47 (A) Subcostal echocardiogram showing a Rashkind balloon being drawn from the right atrium (RA) to the left atrium (LA) to rupture the atrial septum. (B) Echocardiogram of the same patient, taken immediately afterward, showing an ASD created by the balloon septostomy. (Courtesy Dr R. Martin.)

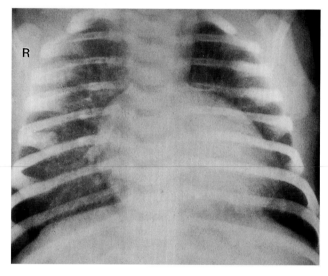

Fig. 14.48 Chest radiograph of an infant with D-transposition of the great arteries. The pedicle (mediastinum) is narrow, and there is cardiomegaly and pulmonary plethora.

then to the systemic circulation. This procedure has been performed under echocardiographic control (Fig. 14.47).

The *chest X-ray* is often, but not always, characteristic. The heart is slightly enlarged and rounded, and there is pulmonary plethora. The pedicle remains narrow because the main pulmonary artery is behind the aorta (Fig. 14.48). The condition may give a similar appearance on chest X-ray to truncus arteriosus, where there is again loss of the normal twisting arrangement of the main pulmonary artery around the aorta. There are many associated conditions, the most common of which are *VSD*, *PDA*, *coarctation of the aorta* and *pulmonary* (or *subpulmonary*) *stenosis*, the last being particularly important as it may preclude the arterial switch procedure.

L-loop transposition

This abnormality of the great arteries is distinctly different to the more usual D-loop transposition of the great arteries (TGA), but it still conforms to the morphological definition of transposition (or ventriculoarterial discordance). This condition is also known as '*anatomically corrected transposition*' or just '*corrected transposition*'. The

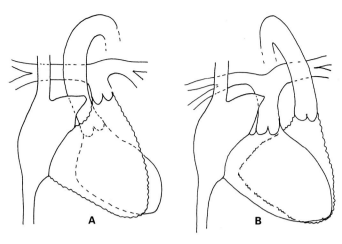

Fig. 14.49 (A) Normal cardiac connections in the anterior view. The morphological left ventricle (smooth outline) lies posterior to the morphological right ventricle (wavy outline) as shown by the interrupted line. (B) Connections in L-transposition of the great arteries ('corrected transposition'). The morphological right ventricle (wavy line) lies behind the morphological left ventricle (smooth line) as shown by the interrupted line. The aorta has a leftward origin, which accounts for the long curved left heart border seen in some cases.

cardiac apex is normally directed to the left, but the morphologically left ventricle lies anterior and to the right of the posterior ventricle, which is of right morphology. Visceroatrial situs is normal, which means that there is atrioventricular discordance as well as ventriculoarterial discordance (Fig. 14.49). Thus the abnormal connections result in a *physiologically corrected circulation*. Patients with this abnormality will usually have symptoms only if there is an associated abnormality, and the symptoms, treatment and prognosis will all depend on the nature of the additional malformations. Common

associations are *VSD* and *conduction abnormalities*. Right ventricular failure may develop later since this ventricle is not designed to support systemic pressures.

The *chest X-ray* may show a characteristic long curve to the left heart border due to the abnormal leftward origin of the aorta (Fig. 14.50), but this is not reliable in all cases as the positions of the great arteries are somewhat variable. A significant proportion of these patients have chest X-rays indistinguishable from normal.

Non-invasive imaging

Echocardiographic diagnosis is relatively straightforward in both types of TGA, but care must be taken to identify correctly the two parallel great arteries as they may not lie in typical positions. The aorta can be identified specifically if the vessel is traced up to the brachiocephalic artery origins. It is essential to avoid the pitfall of assuming which great artery is which simply by position. Two-dimensional imaging will show the smaller left ventricle in D-loop TGA, which pumps to the pulmonary circuit, and the reversed curve of the interventricular septum will usually be apparent (Fig. 14.51). Associated conditions must be sought. In the case of L-loop TGA, the reversal of the morphologically left and right ventricles can be demonstrated by the reversed insertions of the atrioventricular valves (Fig. 14.52). If this condition presents in adulthood it may cause difficulty unless the ventricular morphology is recognised.

Cardiac catheterisation and angiography
Angiography will show clearly the abnormal connections (Fig. 14.53) and will also be useful for clarifying details of anatomy

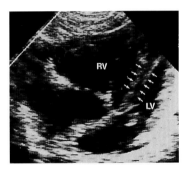

Fig. 14.51 Subcostal echocardiogram of a patient with D-transposition of the great arteries. The morphological right ventricle (RV) is much larger than the morphological left ventricle (LV), and the interventricular septum (arrows) is curved toward the left ventricle.

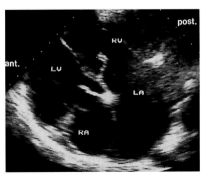

Fig. 14.52 Modified apical four-chamber view in a patient with L-transposition of the great arteries. The morphological left ventricle (LV) lies anteriorly and the morphological right ventricle (RV) lies posteriorly, as shown by the insertions of their respective atrioventricular valves. The tricuspid valve in the right ventricle is inserted more apically than the mitral valve. ant = anterior; post = posterior; RA = right atrium; LA = left atrium. (Compare the valve insertions with the diagrams in Figs 14.13C and 14.57A).

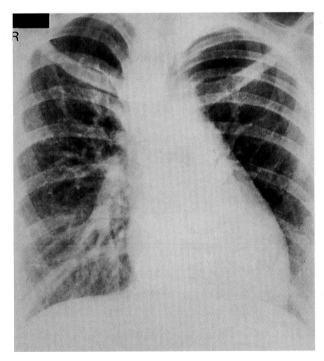

Fig. 14.50 Chest radiograph of a patient with L-transposition of the great arteries. There is a long smooth curve to the left heart border due to the abnormal leftward origin of the aorta.

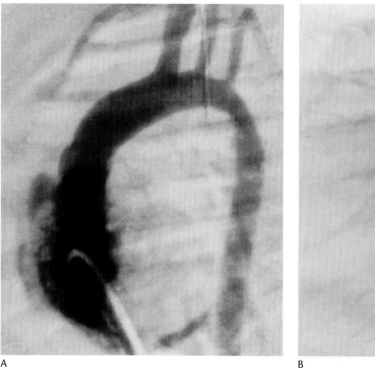
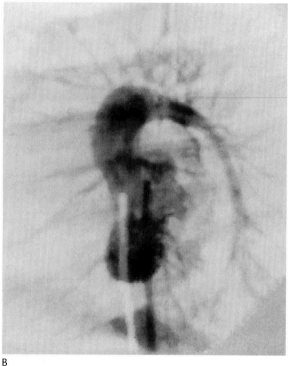

A   B

Fig. 14.53   (A) Digital subtraction angiogram of a right ventricular injection recorded in the left anterior oblique projection. The anteriorly placed morphological right ventricle gives rise to the aorta, indicating D-transposition of the great arteries. (B) Digital subtraction left ventriculogram of the same patient and in the same projection. The pulmonary artery arises from the morphological left ventricle.

concerning associated anomalies. It is again important to assess *coronary anatomy* for surgical planning, particularly when the great arterial switch procedure is being contemplated. Left ventriculography is probably best for assessment of possible VSDs, even though the cavity is usually at a lower pressure than the right ventricle. This is because of the relatively simpler contours of the morphological left ventricle. It is also essential to examine the left ventricular outflow to exclude obstruction which may preclude an arterial switch procedure. This is best achieved using a 20° cranially tilted LAO 60° projection which profiles the outflow well. Right ventriculography in standard oblique views (LAO 60° and RAO 30°) will confirm the diagnosis, show right ventricular function and demonstrate the coronary arteries. An aortic injection may be helpful to exclude a PDA and to show coronary anatomy in more detail.

Treatment

Initial palliation by *Rashkind septostomy* is frequently performed in the neonatal period as described above. Definitive surgical treatment is of two types. The more traditional approach has been to use an *atrial baffle operation* (Mustard or Senning) in which the venous returns are redirected at atrial level so that systemic venous return is directed to the left ventricle and pulmonary artery with pulmonary venous return being directed to the right ventricle and aorta via an intra-atrial conduit (Fig. 14.54). This operation provides a satisfactory physiological circulation but it leaves the right ventricle performing the systemic pumping function, and this can cause problems in later life. There are also problems with stenosis developing in the surgically formed systemic venous pathways, particularly in the earlier Mustard procedure in which a large prosthetic patch is incorporated into the atrial repair (Fig. 14.55). The Senning procedure makes better use of the native tissues.

Although the atrial baffle procedure is not commonly performed today, there are many adolescents and adults with this operative anatomy who may need further investigation or surgery.

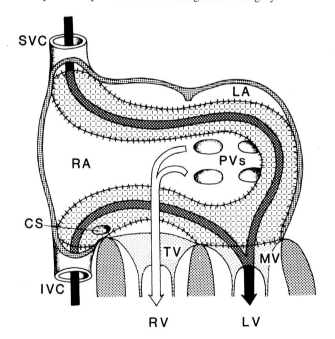

Fig. 14.54   Mustard procedure for D-transposition of the great arteries. A prosthetic intra-atrial conduit leads the systemic venous return from the superior vena cava (SVC) and inferior vena cava (IVC) to the left ventricle (LV) through the mitral valve (MV). Flow from the pulmonary veins (PVs) passes over the conduit to reach the right ventricle (RV) through the tricuspid valve (TV). RA = right atrium; LA = left atrium, CS = coronary sinus.

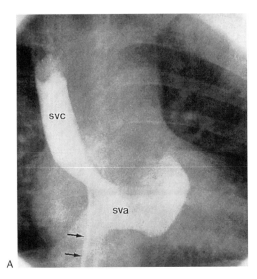
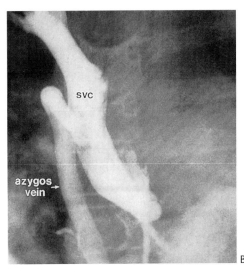

Fig. 14.55 (A) Anterior view of an angiogram performed with the venous catheter (arrows) passed to the superior vena cava (svc) in a patient with a previous Mustard operation. Contrast medium flows to the systemic venous atrium (sva) before its passage to the left ventricle. (B) Similar angiogram to that in (A), but there is severe postoperative narrowing at the point of entry of the superior vena cava to the systemic venous atrium. Flow bypasses the obstruction through a dilated azygos vein.

A more recent approach has been to use the *great arterial switch operation*. This is complicated by the need to transpose the coronary arteries as well as the great arteries themselves (Fig. 14.56). This procedure has superseded the atrial baffle procedure, with low operative mortality. The great arterial switch operation cannot be performed in patients where the morphologically left ventricle has become accustomed to functioning at low pressure over a long period. The procedure should thus be performed in the first few days or weeks of life or later in life in those patients with a large VSD and equalisation of the ventricular pressures. In cases where the left ventricle has adapted to a low pressure, some surgeons have 'trained' it by performing pulmonary artery banding some time before a 'switch' procedure.

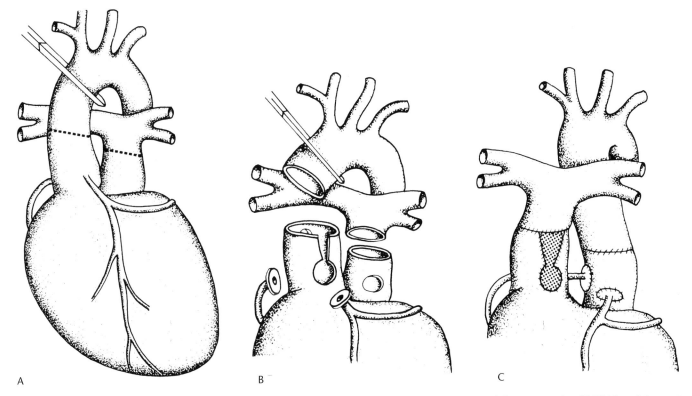

Fig. 14.56 (A) Cross-clamping of the aorta prior to the great arterial switch procedure for D-transposition of the great arteries. (B) Division of the great arteries and excision of the origins of the coronary arteries with a small 'button' of aortic wall. (C) Re-anastomosis of the great arteries and coronary arteries. Systemic arterial blood flows into the coronaries from the newly created 'aortic root', previously the main pulmonary artery. (Reproduced from Jordan & Scott 1989, with permission.)

If there is D-loop TGA with a large VSD, the *Rastelli procedure* may be indicated. In this operation the VSD is closed with an oblique patch, directing left ventricular flow to the aorta through the VSD. An external conduit, sometimes with a prosthetic or homograft valve, is used to connect the right ventricle to the main pulmonary artery. In this way, normal circulation is effectively reconstituted.

ATRIOVENTRICULAR SEPTAL DEFECT

This group of conditions has also been known as *atrioventricular canal defect*. All the variations of the condition have the same fundamental cardiac abnormality. The base of the interventricular septum in the region of the membranous septum is normally in continuity with the atrial septum primum. This central portion of the cardiac structure is missing in all types of atrioventricular septal defect (AVSD). The *partial* type of AVSD results in only an interatrial communication, and leads to the so-called 'ostium primum' ASD. The total AVSD leads to interventricular and interatrial communications with a large common atrioventricular valve. There is also an '*intermediate*' type in which the interventricular communication is relatively small, due to partial tethering of the common atrioventricular valve to the septal crest.

Figure 14.57 shows the difference between the normal heart, partial AVSD and complete AVSD, comparing them with a secundum ASD.

The atrioventricular valves are commonly malformed and produce regurgitation of varying degrees. This is not invariably present, but when it is, it will lead to exacerbation of any symptoms produced by left-to-right shunting. In the case of the partial defect (ostium primum ASD) the anterior leaflet of the mitral valve has a cleft, which can be an important cause of regurgitation.

There is an increased association of this condition with Down's syndrome. The presentation varies, depending on the precise nature of the abnormality, but tends to be earlier and more severe than with conventional ASDs and VSDs of similar size. There is no specific abnormality that can be detected on chest X-ray to differentiate these conditions from the more usual type of ASDs or VSDs, although the cardiac enlargement, pulmonary plethora, and cardiac failure are often all more prominent. The presence of only 11 pairs of ribs may be a clue to an underlying Down's syndrome aetiology.

Non-invasive diagnosis

Echocardiography is the key to diagnosis in this range of conditions. The atrioventricular valve anatomy can clearly be seen (Fig. 14.58), and the presence of a ventricular component to the defect is usually obvious. There is often considerable enlargement of the right-sided cardiac chambers, and the right atrium may be particularly large if there is accompanying atrioventricular valve regurgitation. *Doppler studies* will clearly demonstrate the presence of atrioventricular valve regurgitation, and this is particularly well seen on *colour flow studies*. This regurgitation is more commonly seen through the mitral valve in ostium primum ASD, and the regurgitant jet is often directed across the interatrial defect to the right atrium.

Cardiac catheterisation and angiography

Angiography is also capable of demonstrating the anatomy clearly. The most obvious abnormality seen on angiography is the absence of the usual left ventricular outflow tract. The mitral valve hinges directly from beneath the aortic root (Fig. 14.59), and when open creates a distinct appearance that has been likened to a '*gooseneck*', a misleading term that is open to misinterpretation; it does

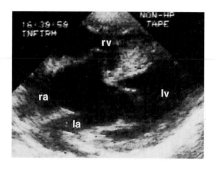

Fig. 14.58 Subcostal echocardiogram showing an ostium primum ASD defect lying between the left atrium (la) and the right atrium (ra). There is no ventricular septal defect between the left ventricle (lv) and the right ventricle (rv).

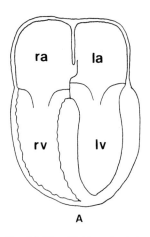 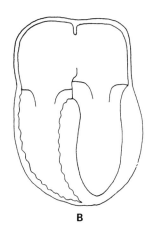 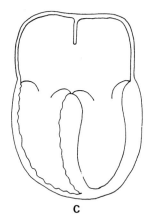 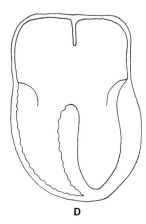

A	B	C	D

Fig. 14.57 (A) Normal relationships of the interventricular and interatrial septa with the atrioventricular valves. The atrioventricular valves are inserted into the septum primum (thin line). ra = right atrium; la = left atrium; rv = right ventricle; lv = left ventricle. (B) Ostium secundum ASD. The atrioventricular valves and left ventricular outflow tract are normal. (C) Ostium primum ASD. The septum primum is absent and the atrioventricular valves are inserted in a low position into the crest of the muscular interventricular septum. (D) Total AVSD. A large common valve separates the atrial cavities from the ventricular cavities. There is an ostium primum ASD and a large VSD in continuity.

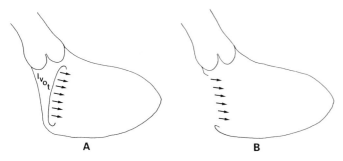

Fig. 14.59 (A) Normal left ventricular angiogram in the right anterior oblique projection. Diastolic inflow does not wash out contrast medium lying below the aortic root in the left ventricular outflow tract (Ivot). (B) Left ventricular angiogram performed in a patient with an AVSD. The normal left ventricular outflow region is missing due to the absent septum primum, and so the contrast medium in the subaortic region is washed out by the incoming mitral flow. This produces the frequently misinterpreted 'gooseneck' appearance.

not indicate narrowing of the left ventricular outflow tract in systole but merely reflects the washout of contrast medium during ventricular diastole as the abnormally positioned mitral valve is open.

Views can be the same as for assessing a straightforward VSD, but the large right-sided chambers may necessitate a more steeply angled LAO view to profile the basal septum. A conventional LAO view will show the common valve well as the non-opaque atrial blood passing through it, but a cranial tilt will aid in exclusion of additional defects and can help in detecting small interventricular communications in the 'intermediate' type. Both the cleft mitral valve and variable degrees of mitral prolapse are well shown on angiography. Atrioventricular valve regurgitation is well assessed by angiography, but it should be remembered that the catheter may have been passed into the left ventricle through the valve and so might itself produce regurgitation.

Treatment

Surgery in this condition is somewhat more complex than with conventional ASDs or VSDs, as the repair usually involves some form of reconstruction of the atrioventricular valves as well as patch closure of one or both septal defects. There is no place for interventional therapy in this condition at present.

PULMONARY ATRESIA

The presence or absence of a VSD with pulmonary atresia will markedly affect the expression of the condition.

Pulmonary atresia with VSD

In these circumstances the anomaly is essentially the same as a very severe form of tetralogy of Fallot. The obstructed outflow of the right ventricle, together with the usual override of the aorta, means that the right ventricle can empty into the aorta, although it must do this at the same pressure as the left ventricle. Flow thus continues through the right ventricle, and the chamber remains large and its walls become hypertrophied due to the systemic pressure in it. The pulmonary arteries are often very small, and they receive their blood supply from the PDA initially and then subsequently through aortopulmonary collateral vessels.

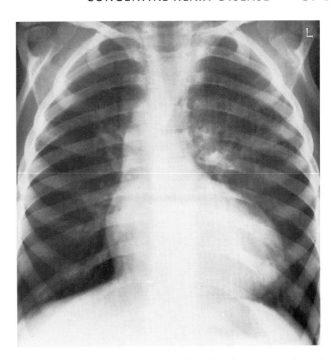

Fig. 14.60 Chest radiograph of a child with pulmonary atresia and a VSD. There is a right-sided aortic arch indenting the trachea which accentuates the concave pulmonary bay. The left heart border does not show an upturned apex as seen in Fig. 14.61.

The *chest X-ray* shows a slightly enlarged heart, often with a slightly upturned apex due to the right ventricular enlargement; the pulmonary bay is small and the lung fields are oligaemic. There is a right aortic arch in about 25% of cases (Fig. 14.60). In older patients the multiplicity of aortopulmonary collaterals can give a complex vascular pattern, particularly near the hilar regions, and this can sometimes be mistaken for pulmonary plethora. Palliation with various types of shunt is often required in early life, and this may give rise to uneven vascularity in the lungs (Fig. 14.61).

MRI is increasingly used in the assessment of the anatomy of the small central pulmonary arteries in this condition (Fig. 14.62).

Angiography is commonly required in the diagnosis of this condition because successful definitive surgery depends on careful planning of a reconstructed outflow from the right ventricle to the pulmonary arteries, which themselves often need reconstruction. It is usually not possible to determine all the details of the anatomy of the hypoplastic pulmonary arteries and the collaterals using echocardiography. A good-quality aortogram, together with a series of selective angiograms to different collaterals, is usually required. In difficult cases where there is very poor collateral flow to the pulmonary arteries it may be helpful to perform a wedged pulmonary venous injection to opacify the hypoplastic pulmonary arteries. It is important that comprehensive selective angiography is carried out as there may be many sites of origin of collaterals, both from the aorta and the brachiocephalic arteries.

Surgery may be similar to that required for a severe form of the tetralogy of Fallot, but this is only possible if there is a reasonably sized pulmonary artery. In some cases, complex reconstructions of hypoplastic pulmonary arteries are attempted, but often long-term palliation with multiple shunting procedures is the only option. In some cases a central pulmonary artery is reconstructed by 'unifocalization' of the distal pulmonary vessels. If the main pulmonary

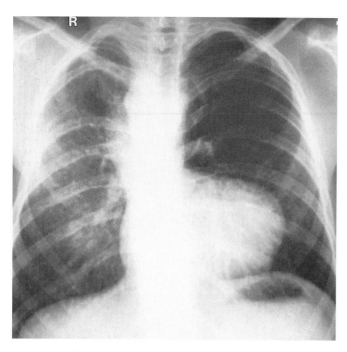

Fig. 14.61 Chest radiograph of an adult with long-term palliation of pulmonary atresia. There is a right-sided aortic arch and an upturned cardiac apex. The vascularity in the right lung is more prominent due to the presence of a right-sided shunt.

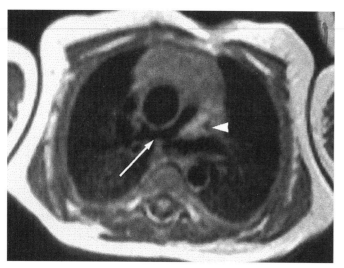

Fig. 14.62 Transverse spin-echo MRI image showing small pulmonary arteries (arrows) in a patient with pulmonary atresia.

artery is of good size, the VSD may be closed and an external conduit, usually with a valve, is placed from the right ventricle to the pulmonary artery, the *Rastelli procedure* (Fig. 14.63).

Pulmonary atresia with intact ventricular septum

In this situation there is no outlet for the right ventricle, and thus no way that it can decompress. The cavity is usually very small but often generates very high pressures (suprasystemic), especially if there is a small but functionally competent tricuspid valve. Under these circumstances the unusual problem of abnormal coronary

communications can occur. Blood may shunt from right to left through the abnormal vessels, and this can cause myocardial ischaemia and sometimes infarction. The *chest X-ray* will show a small pulmonary segment and pulmonary oligaemia, but the cardiac contour will show a more rounded left ventricular contour (as this chamber takes all the cardiac flow), often similar to that seen in tricuspid atresia. Imaging techniques are particularly important in this condition as the size and function of the right ventricle must be estimated in great detail.

Palliative shunting may be needed in early life, but a successful surgical correction is dependent on the degree of underdevelopment of the right ventricular cavity. If the right ventricle is extremely hypoplastic, then the condition must be considered as a form of 'single ventricle', but if there is reasonable development of the right ventricular cavity, a full correction might be possible, although this is often a high-risk procedure. Patients with very severe pulmonary valve stenosis are considered in a similar way.

Single ventricle (primitive ventricle)

There are many complex variants in this category and they must all be assessed carefully on their individual merits. The conditions are commonly referred to as 'single ventricle', but this is not always an easy description to understand, because often a second small or rudimentary ventricular chamber is present; however, according to accepted morphological classifications the small chamber may not be entitled to the name 'ventricle'. The second small chamber often acts, via a VSD, as an outlet chamber.

The following situations may lead to a 'single ventricle':

1. *Double-inlet ventricle*—both atrioventricular valves enter the same ventricle (Fig. 14.64) or there is considerable override of one valve across a VSD.

2. *Common inlet valve*—a single large atrioventricular valve enters a large ventricular chamber.

3. *Atresia of one atrioventricular valve, mitral or tricuspid*—may be indistinguishable from situation 2.

4. *Very large VSD* with little residual septal tissue, effectively a single chamber.

Multiple abnormalities are common, and nothing must be taken for granted in the assessment of the cases. Great arterial connections may be abnormal and must be assessed carefully. Atrial anatomy may be abnormal and there may be a single common atrium. The positions of the chambers may be distorted or twisted, and this must also be taken into careful consideration. Other malformations such as pulmonary stenosis, coarctation or PDA may well be present.

In all these cases there is common mixing of the pulmonary and systemic venous return in the heart, and the clinical presentation depends particularly on the presence or absence of *pulmonary stenosis*. If pulmonary stenosis is present, the patient may be cyanotic with pulmonary oligaemia, and if absent, the patient may have heart failure and pulmonary plethora.

There is no 'typical' *chest X-ray*, but the heart is often enlarged, with the pulmonary vascularity depending on the presence of other abnormalities. The size and position of the great arteries will help to determine the overall cardiac configuration. *Angiography* and *ultrasound* must be used, as appropriate for the circumstances, but in these complex cases it is often useful to assess the anatomy by both techniques to ensure maximum diagnostic accuracy. MRI is

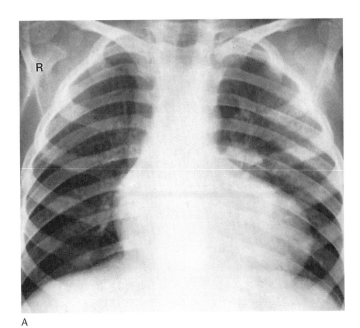

A

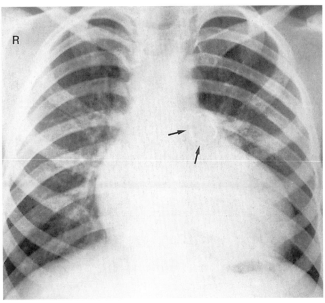

B

Fig. 14.63 (A) Chest radiograph of a child with pulmonary atresia and a left-sided aortic arch. (B) Chest radiograph of the same patient following closure of the VSD and insertion of an external valved conduit (arrows) from the right ventricle to the main pulmonary artery. (C) Lateral view of (B), showing the metallic frame of the prosthetic valve in the conduit.

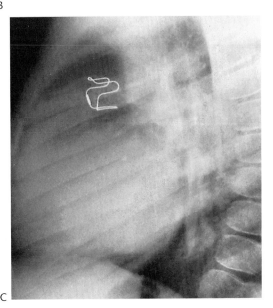

C

used when these modalities fail to demonstrate the complex anatomy entirely. This is particularly the case in older patients where detailed echo studies are more difficult.

In the presence of only one useful ventricle, surgical options are often palliative, using shunts or pulmonary artery banding, but reconstructive surgery using the single ventricular chamber is increasingly carried out. This is normally achieved by the use of the *Fontan procedure* or one of its variants such as total cavopulmonary connection (TCPC). This operation uses the single ventricle to pump systemic blood to the aorta while redirecting systemic venous return to the lungs without the use of a second ventricle. This is often achieved by the direct anastomosis of the right atrial appendage to the main pulmonary artery. The details of the technique will vary with individual cases, but the success of the procedure depends on a well-functioning systemic ventricle and low pulmonary vascular resistance. Occasionally, *cardiac transplantation* can be offered to these patients.

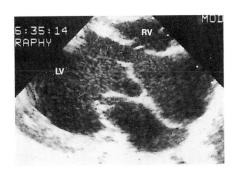

Fig. 14.64 Left parasternal echocardiogram of a patient with 'single ventricle'. Both atrioventricular valves enter the large left ventricle (LV) from two distinct atria. Outflow to the aorta is via a restrictive VSD and a small outflow chamber of right ventricular type (RV).

TRICUSPID ATRESIA

In this condition there is no tricuspid orifice, the valve having either fused leaflets or a mass of obstructive tissue in the expected valve plane (Fig. 14.65). There is obligatory flow of the systemic venous return across an ASD to the left atrium and the left ventricle. The left ventricle is large as it carries both pulmonary and systemic venous return. Some of the blood in the left ventricle then crosses a VSD to reach the right ventricle and the pulmonary artery, while the remainder passes out in the normal way through the aortic valve.

The VSD is often restrictive (small size with a pressure drop across it and a low-pressure right ventricle), and there may be associated pulmonary stenosis. The right ventricle is often so underdeveloped that the condition is considered as one of the 'single ventricle' group. There is often relatively low pulmonary blood flow, although this is not invariable, and the condition may be expressed in various ways, depending on the state of the VSD and right ventricular outflow.

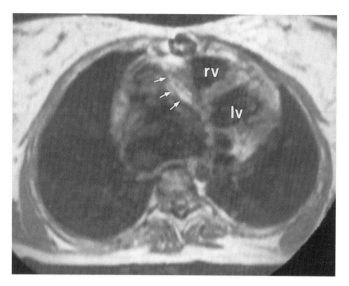

Fig. 14.65 Transverse gated spin-echo MRI scan of a patient with tricuspid atresia. A wedge-shaped segment of tissue (arrows) lies in the expected position of the tricuspid valve. rv = right ventricle; lv = left ventricle. (Courtesy of the Trustees of the Bristol MRI Centre.)

The *chest X-ray* commonly shows pulmonary oligaemia, a small pulmonary bay, and a moderately large heart with a rounded contour due to the downward and leftward enlargement of the left ventricle (Fig. 14.66). *Echocardiography* will show the anatomy clearly, with Doppler studies adding information about flow across the interatrial septum and the pressure drops across the VSD and the pulmonary valve.

Cardiac angiography will show the anatomy well. Left ventriculography should be modified by the use of a shallower than usual LAO projection (e.g. 40–50° LAO) to take account of the alteration of the position of the interventricular septum by the large left ventricle and small right ventricle.

Surgical treatment will depend on the details of the individual case. If the VSD is relatively small and the right ventricle is poorly developed, then correction can only be achieved by the use of a Fontan or TCPC procedure.

MITRAL VALVE ABNORMALITIES (including supramitral ring and cor triatriatum)

Obstructive lesions in or near the mitral valve include *congenital mitral stenosis*, *supramitral ring* and *cor triatriatum*. The first resembles rheumatic stenosis, with fusion of the valve leaflets and doming of the valve. A supramitral ring is an obstructive diaphragm lying very close to the mitral valve on the left atrial side. Cor triatriatum is a condition in which there is an obstructive membrane in the left atrium, which divides it into high- and low-pressure portions with a small and restrictive communication between the two (Fig. 14.67).

The *chest X-ray* is similar in all cases, showing a normal-size heart with increased pulmonary vessel size, due to pulmonary venous hypertension similar to that seen in the obstructed form of totally anomalous pulmonary venous drainage. There will often be pulmonary oedema. *Echocardiography* will show the obstructive detail well, often better than angiography. Doppler studies may indicate the degree of obstruction.

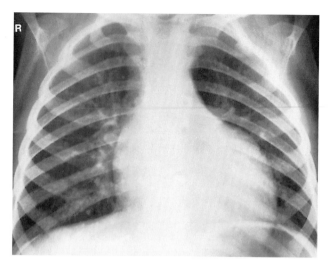

Fig. 14.66 Chest radiograph of a patient with tricuspid atresia. There is pulmonary oligaemia, a small pulmonary artery, and a prominent rounded left ventricular curve to the left heart border.

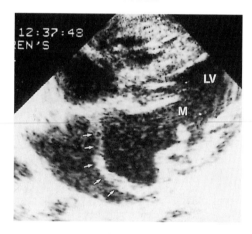

Fig. 14.67 Subcostal echocardiogram of a patient with cor triatriatum. A prominent membrane runs across the left atrium (arrows). M = mitral valve; LV = left ventricle.

Mitral regurgitation can form part of a complex abnormality such as AVSD, but it can also occur alone. In the latter case there may be abnormal papillary muscle formation such as a single papillary muscle giving a 'parachute' mitral valve. The chest X-ray will show signs of pulmonary venous hypertension and possibly pulmonary oedema. The heart will be larger than with obstructive mitral lesions because of the ventricular volume overload.

HYPOPLASTIC LEFT HEART SYNDROME (aortic atresia)

At the most severe end of the spectrum of aortic stenosis lies aortic atresia. If there is no flow through the aortic valve the left ventricle itself will not develop, being only a rudimentary slit-like cavity. The aortic atresia may also be associated with mitral atresia. This abnormality is known as hypoplastic left heart syndrome.

In this condition the right ventricle performs the entire systemic pumping function, with the systemic blood supply being directed through the ductus arteriosus. The brachiocephalic branches are supplied retrogradely, and the ascending aorta is diminutive in size, carrying only reverse flow from the PDA and aortic arch sufficient to fill the coronary arteries. The condition is almost uniformly fatal, and this probably explains why the condition appears relatively low on the list of incidence of congenital heart disease. Many cases probably die before being recognised at a paediatric cardiology referral centre. Patients with hypoplastic left heart are often born in good condition but deteriorate very rapidly in the first few days of life as the life-sustaining ductus closes.

In the case of hypoplastic left heart, the diagnosis can almost always be made by *echocardiography*. The key feature to identify is the diminutive ascending aorta and the single functional ventricle, because these are the features associated with the uniformly poor prognosis. *Cardiac catheterisation* may be required if high-quality echocardiography is unavailable. In this situation the best approach is to perform a normal catheter study from the venous approach, and pass the angiographic catheter to the pulmonary artery or, if possible, through the PDA to the descending aorta. An *angiogram* performed from either of these positions will immediately show the retrograde flow down the diminutive ascending aorta, and the diagnosis will be confirmed. The condition can now be recognised by *antenatal echocardiography*.

Some experimental approaches to surgery are being investigated at present, with radical multistage reconstructions being attempted in a few specialised centres. Some surgical successes have been achieved with *neonatal heart transplantation* in a small number of specialised centres.

ANOMALOUS PULMONARY VENOUS CONNECTION

This abnormality of cardiac connection can take various forms.

Partial anomalous pulmonary venous connection (PAPVC)

This can occur when one or more individual pulmonary veins drain to the right side of the atrial septum, either into the right atrium itself or into the superior or inferior vena cava. This abnormality is commonly associated with ASD, in particular the sinus venosus type of defect, and it is important to check pulmonary venous connections when performing echocardiographic or angiographic examination for ASD assessment. The anomalous veins can often be redirected correctly at surgery, providing the surgeon is aware of the problem.

Sometimes an anomalous pulmonary vein can drain down to the inferior vena cava below the diaphragm, more commonly on the right side (Fig. 14.68). This vein can sometimes be identified on the chest X-ray as a curved vessel in the right lower zone, widening as it approaches the right cardiophrenic angle (Fig. 14.69). This is sometimes referred to as the *scimitar syndrome*. The condition is frequently associated with hypoplasia of the right lung, and sometimes there is a shift of the heart to the right.

Total anomalous pulmonary venous connection (TAPVC)

This is a more serious condition which can take four forms, *supracardiac*, *cardiac*, *infracardiac* or *mixed*. In all four types the major

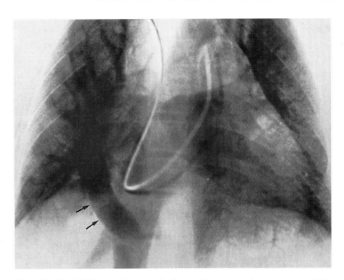

Fig. 14.68 Digital angiogram of a follow-through pulmonary artery injection in a patient with partial anomalous pulmonary venous drainage. A large vein (arrows) is seen draining from the right lung to the inferior vena cava below the diaphragm.

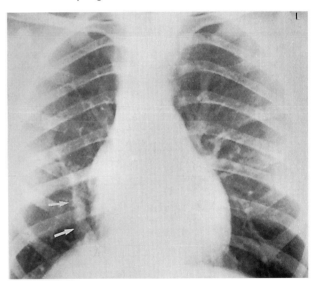

Fig. 14.69 Chest radiograph of the patient shown in Fig. 14.68. The anomalous vein (scimitar sign) is seen in the right lower zone (arrows).

pulmonary veins come to a confluence behind the left atrium but do not communicate directly with it (Fig. 14.70). In the case of *supracardiac TAPVC* there is a large ascending vein on the left side, which is a remnant of the embryological left superior vena cava. This connects into the left brachiocephalic vein, which then passes down the right-sided superior vena cava into the right atrium (Fig. 14.71). The *cardiac* type of abnormality drains into the right side of the heart, usually via the enlarged coronary sinus. In the case of *infracardiac TAPVC* the confluence of pulmonary veins drains downward in a descending vein which passes through the diaphragm, often obstructed at this point, into either the portal venous system or the inferior vena cava. The portal venous system is usually at a higher pressure than other venous systems, and this fact may also contribute to the 'obstruction' in this condition (Fig. 14.72). The pulmonary venous blood then returns to the right atrium through the inferior vena cava.

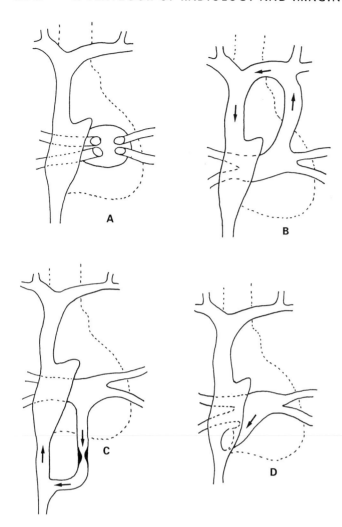

Fig. 14.70 (A) Normal pulmonary venous drainage to the left atrium. (B) TAPVC of the supracardiac type draining to a left-sided ascending vein and then to the left brachiocephalic vein. (C) TAPVC of the infracardiac type showing obstructed drainage to the inferior vena cava. (D) TAPVC of the cardiac type draining to the coronary sinus.

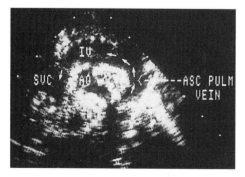

Fig. 14.71 Coronal suprasternal echocardiogram showing TAPVC of the supracardiac type draining as shown in Fig. 14.70B. IV = brachiocephalic vein or innominate vein; SVC = superior vena cava; AO = aorta. (Courtesy Dr R. Martin.)

In all of these conditions there is total cardiac mixing at the right atrial level, and the patient remains partially cyanosed. In the case of supracardiac or cardiac TAPVC the *chest X-ray* shows that the heart is enlarged and there is pulmonary plethora, which is obligatory due

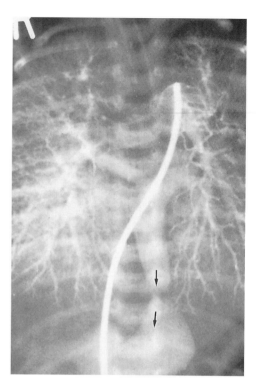

Fig. 14.72 Follow-through pulmonary arteriogram of a child with obstructed TAPVC of the intracardiac type draining past an obstruction at the diaphragmatic level (arrows) to a dilated vein connecting to the inferior vena cava.

to the need for a higher pulmonary flow in the mixed circulation (Fig. 14.73). The supracardiac TAPVC will often show wide mediastinum due to the left-sided ascending vein, and in long-established cases the classic *cottage loaf* heart will be evident. This will become less common because these cases are now usually diagnosed and

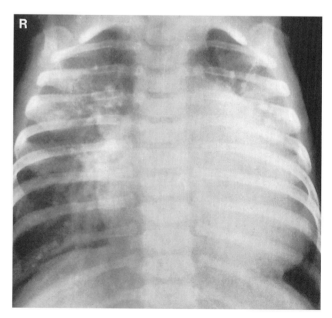

Fig. 14.73 Chest radiograph of a child with TAPVC of the cardiac type draining to the coronary sinus. There is marked cardiomegaly and pulmonary plethora but the upper mediastinum is not wide because the drainage is directly to the heart.

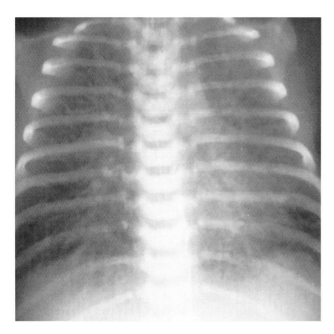

Fig. 14.74 Chest radiograph of a child with obstructed TAPVC of the infracardiac type. The heart borders are obscured by diffuse interstitial oedema but there is no significant cardiomegaly.

treated in infancy. The infracardiac type of abnormal drainage will often be associated with little or no cardiac enlargement, and the obstruction of the pulmonary circulation will lead to interstitial oedema and heart failure. The findings of a normal heart size with severe heart failure usually indicate infracardiac TAPVC (Fig. 14.74).

Non-invasive diagnosis

The types of TAPVC may be diagnosed by *echocardiography*, the abnormal venous confluence being visible behind the left atrium. The abnormal course of drainage can usually be traced although the infradiaphragmatic course may be difficult to define. The left atrium is usually small, and there is right-to-left flow across the atrial septal communication. The flow in the venous confluence and drainage channels can often be shown using *Doppler colour flow mapping*.

PAPVC can be diagnosed by the visualisation of the individual veins draining to the right atrium, but the diagnosis can be more difficult if the site of drainage is to the inferior or superior vena cava rather than to the right atrium. MRI can also be used to identify the anomalous veins.

Cardiac catheterisation and angiography

Angiography will also show these features, but it may not be necessary if high-quality ultrasound results are available. A large and rapid injection of contrast medium to the main pulmonary artery will opacify the pulmonary venous system well. The anterior view is the clearest for demonstrating the venous pathways. Infants presenting with this condition are often seriously ill, and the morbidity of catheterisation and angiography is significant.

The delineation of the individual pulmonary veins in PAPVC can be more difficult and may require separate injections to the left and right pulmonary arteries in oblique views. Sometimes the direct injection of contrast medium to the suspected abnormal veins can be diagnostic, but this approach can be surprisingly difficult to interpret as the contrast medium is rapidly diluted and the atrial

anatomy is often unclear. In either case, oblique views are preferable to posteroanterior and lateral views as they will separate the two atria more effectively.

Treatment

Surgery is directed toward reanastomosing the pulmonary venous confluence with the left atrium, dividing the abnormal connection and closing the ASD that is present. In spite of its apparently straightforward nature the operation carries a higher than average mortality. Surgical treatment of PAPVC usually consists of closing the associated ASD with a patch that incorporates all the pulmonary veins into the left atrium, but surgery may not be necessary at all for this condition.

TRUNCUS ARTERIOSUS

In this condition a single great artery arises from the heart, due to a failure of division of the embryonic common truncus arteriosus. The common truncus arises from above a large VSD (Fig. 14.75) and the pattern of division of the common truncus varies. A single common pulmonary artery with a well-developed main pulmonary artery segment may arise from the common truncus before it divides into left and right pulmonary arteries—*type 1 truncus arteriosus*. In *type 2 truncus arteriosus* the length of the main pulmonary artery segment is negligible, but the two pulmonary arteries arise close together just above the truncal valve. In *type 3 truncus arteriosus* the left and right pulmonary arteries arise independently from the main truncus at a higher level, usually one from each side of the main artery. Type 3 truncus is the least common form. Various intermediate forms have also been classified. Pulmonary atresia with large aortopulmonary collateral vessels has sometimes been called pseudotruncus, but this is misleading as the condition is developmentally quite different.

In all cases there is common mixing across the VSD, and the flow in the pulmonary arteries is very large, because it originates directly from the common truncus which is at systemic pressure. In many cases a fully developed main pulmonary artery segment does not develop in its usual position, and so the *chest X-ray* shows marked pulmonary plethora with a relatively narrow mediastinal

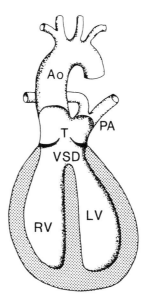

Fig. 14.75 Anatomy of truncus arteriosus. RV = right ventricle; LV = left ventricle; T = common truncus arteriosus; PA = pulmonary artery; Ao = aorta. (Reproduced from Jordan & Scott 1989, with permission.)

shadow (as in transposition of the great vessels). With truncus arteriosus there is also an increased incidence of *right-sided aortic arch*. In many patients the heart is moderately enlarged and there may be cardiac failure. *Echocardiographic* diagnosis is relatively straightforward (Fig. 14.76), which is helpful, as it is difficult to perform good angiography on these patients due to the very fast blood flow through the heart, which dilutes the contrast medium. The patients are often very ill, and catheterisation with angiography produces significant morbidity. There may still be difficulties in obtaining good detail of the truncal branching pattern, and MRI shows great promise in such cases.

Palliation by banding of the pulmonary artery is sometimes carried out, but the preferred operation is a complete correction with closure of the VSD. This will allow the left ventricle to empty through the truncal valve, and a separate prosthetic or homograft valved conduit must be placed from the right ventricle to the pulmonary arteries (Fig. 14.77).

EBSTEIN'S ANOMALY

This condition is an anomaly of the tricuspid valve. It has often been described as a displacement of the tricuspid valve toward the apex of the right ventricle which produces a larger right atrium and a smaller right ventricle. This is in effect what is present, although the more precise descriptions of cardiac morphologists detail a condition in which the tricuspid annulus is normally positioned and the

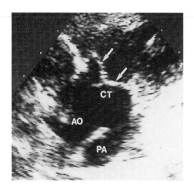

Fig. 14.76 Modified subcostal echocardiogram in truncus arteriosus. CT = common truncus; AO = aorta; PA = pulmonary artery. The truncal valve is arrowed.

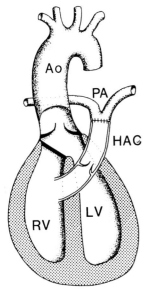

Fig. 14.77 Correction of common truncus arteriosus using the Rastelli procedure. RV = right ventricle; LV = left ventricle; Ao = aorta; HAC = homograft aortic conduit; PA = pulmonary artery. (Reproduced from Jordan & Scott 1989, with permission.)

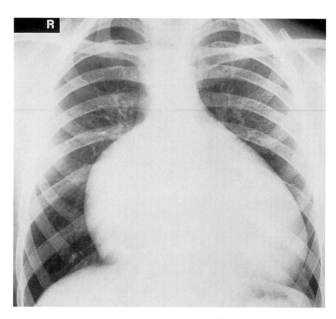

Fig. 14.78 Chest radiograph of a child with severe Ebstein's anomaly. There is marked globular cardomegaly and pulmonary oligaemia.

valve leaflets are larger and more redundant than normal, being adherent to the right ventricular walls, particularly the septum, for some distance into the ventricular cavity.

The result of this anomaly is a larger right atrium than normal (the so-called 'atrialised' portion of the right ventricle) and a relatively small right ventricle that is relatively ineffective when pumping blood to the lungs. There is often associated infundibular narrowing. The function of the tricuspid valve itself is variable, sometimes being normal, but often showing significant regurgitation. The clinical presentation varies considerably, severe cases presenting in infancy with right heart failure and poor forward flow to the pulmonary artery. The *chest X-ray* in these cases may show massive globular cardiomegaly with pulmonary oligaemia (Fig. 14.78). The mildest expression occurs in some adults who present with mild signs or symptoms and a virtually normal chest X-ray.

Ultrasound studies show the abnormal tricuspid valve as a very prominent feature (Fig. 14.79) and many of the functional aspects can be derived from Doppler studies. The need for catheterisation depends on the clinical severity and the quality of the echocardiogram.

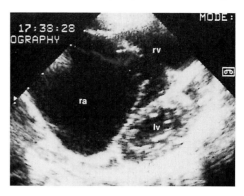

Fig. 14.79 Subcostal echocardiogram in a child with Ebstein's anomaly. The view shows the marked right atrial enlargement (ra) and the prominent tricuspid valve. In spite of the displacement of the valve, the right ventricle (rv) is still larger than the left ventricle (lv).

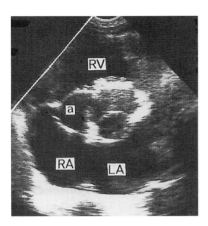

Fig. 14.80 Parasternal short-axis echocardiogram showing a sinus of Valsalva aneurysm. (a) RV = right ventricle; RA = right atrium; LA = left atrium.

SINUS OF VALSALVA FISTULA

In this condition there is usually enlargement of one of the sinuses of Valsalva in the aortic root, commonly the right sinus. This may rupture into the right ventricle and produce a left-to-right shunt. There will be continuous flow from the higher-pressure aorta to the right ventricle, and the murmur may be mistaken for a patent ductus arteriosus, a coronary fistula or the recognised association of VSD with aortic regurgitation.

The *chest X-ray* may show typical features of a left-to-right shunt, but the aneurysmal sinus itself is rarely visible on the cardiac contour. *Echocardiography*, particularly with colour flow Doppler mapping, will show the abnormality (Fig. 14.80). An aortic root *angiogram* will also show the lesion.

It is important to distinguish this condition from the *perimembranous ventricular defect*. The communications are in very similar positions, one above and one below the aortic valve. Besides visualisation of the defect, differentiation can be achieved using continuous-wave Doppler studies, which will show that there is prominent continuous flow through the aortoventricular defect, which is due to the persistent differential pressure between the two chambers.

The principles of surgical repair are relatively straightforward, but it may be complicated by aortic regurgitation due to the distortion of the aortic valve by the abnormality and the repair.

DOUBLE-OUTLET VENTRICLE

Double-outlet right ventricle is the most usual type of double-outlet ventricle. Once again each case must be assessed individually, but accurate anatomical assessment is vital. Corrective surgery is usually possible, but this depends on detailed knowledge of the intracardiac anatomy. There are usually two well-developed ventricles with a VSD, and so the positions of the great arteries and the septal defect must all be determined accurately. A double-outlet right ventricle with a large subaortic VSD can be corrected by closing the VSD with an oblique patch, allowing the left ventricle to empty to the aorta through the VSD. If the VSD is subpulmonary, a more complex procedure is required to redirect flow to the appropriate great arteries. The latter condition with a subpulmonary defect is often termed a *Taussig–Bing anomaly* (Fig. 14.81).

The chest radiograph will give clues about the nature of the anomaly, but echocardiography and cardiac angiography are both

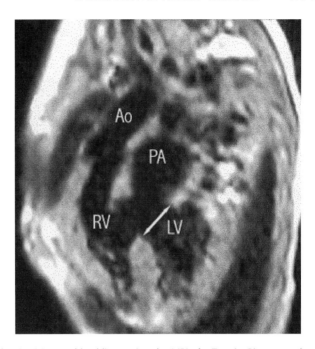

Fig. 14.81 Double oblique spin-echo MRI of a Taussig–Bing anomaly to demonstrate the intracardiac anatomy. There is a double-outlet right ventricle (RV) with the VSD (arrows) lying in a subpulmonary position. The aorta (Ao) is distant from the left ventricle (LV) and 'anatomical repair' by VSD closure is not possible. PA = pulmonary artery.

very important diagnostic techniques for the determination of the precise intracardiac anatomy. MRI may add invaluable information in selected cases.

GREAT ARTERIAL ANOMALIES (including vascular rings)

Anomalous right subclavian artery

The commonest major variation in the aortic arch and its branching is the anomalous right subclavian artery occurring with a normal left-sided arch. The right subclavian artery is the last brachiocephalic branch of the aorta, arising from the descending portion of the arch. The anomaly causes inconvenience for surgeons and those performing right brachial artery catheterisation, but it does not normally produce symptoms. The vessel runs obliquely behind the oesophagus, and its indentation can be recognised on the barium swallow.

Right-sided aortic arch

There are two common forms of right-sided aortic arch. The first is the so-called *mirror-image type*, with the brachiocephalic branches being the mirror image of normal. This type is the most usual form of right arch to be found in association with the various types of cyanotic heart disease (25% incidence in tetralogy of Fallot and pulmonary atresia). The second form of right arch is that with an *anomalous origin of the left subclavian artery*. This is almost the mirror image of the anomalous right subclavian type; in isolation this rarely causes symptoms, but when associated with a left-sided ductus arteriosus forms a vascular ring. In this circumstance the proximal portion of the aberrant vessel usually forms a prominent diverticulum known as the Kommerell diverticulum. Common aortic arch variations are shown in Figure 14.82.

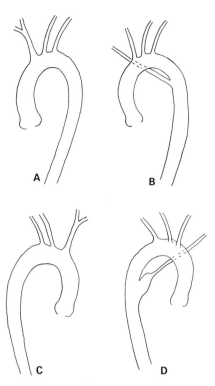

Fig. 14.82 (A) Normal left aortic arch branching. (B) Left aortic arch with an anomalous origin of the right subclavian artery. (C) Right aortic arch with 'mirror image' branching. This is the commonest type associated with cyanotic congenital heart disease. (D) Right aortic arch with an anomalous origin of the left subclavian artery arising from a posterior diverticulum. This is the commonest type of right aortic arch to occur as an isolated abnormality.

Double aortic arch

This anomaly is more serious as it forms a vascular ring that may compress the trachea or major bronchi and cause stridor in infancy. It can be diagnosed on the chest X-ray or barium swallow by evidence of bilateral compression on the trachea or oesophagus. Echocardiography may also be useful in making the diagnosis, but it can be difficult to identify with confidence the two separate arches. MRI or angiography are used for definitive confirmation of the anatomy (Fig. 14.83).

Anomalous origin of the left pulmonary artery (pulmonary artery sling)

This is another important cause of stridor in infancy. The left pulmonary artery arises as a branch of the right pulmonary artery and runs posteriorly to the right of the trachea, reaching its destination in the left hilum as it passes leftward behind the trachea. This is one of the few conditions where an abnormal vascular structure runs anterior to the oesophagus (between the oesophagus and trachea). This can occasionally be recognised as an abnormal soft-tissue structure on the lateral chest X-ray between the oesophagus and trachea and is the only aberrant vessel which produces an anterior indentation on the oesophagus. This condition is difficult to treat surgically as there may be distortion and narrowing of the trachea or bronchi.

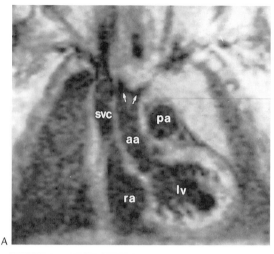

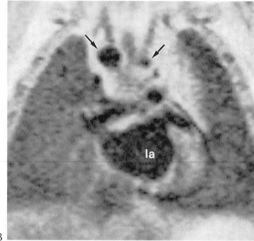

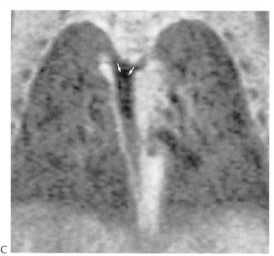

Fig. 14.83 (A) Coronal gated spin-echo MRI scan from a child with a double aortic arch. The ascending aorta (aa) bifurcates at its upper end (arrows). lv = left ventricle; pa = pulmonary artery; svc = superior vena cava; ra = right atrium. (B) A more posterior coronal section from the same study. The large right and small left arches are shown in cross-section (arrows) with brachiocephalic arteries arising from them. (C) A yet more posterior coronal section of the same study, showing confluence of the two arches to form the descending aorta. The findings were confirmed at surgery with no angiography being necessary. (Courtesy of the Trustees of the Bristol MRI Centre.)

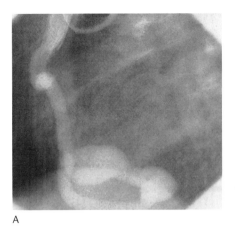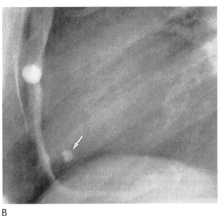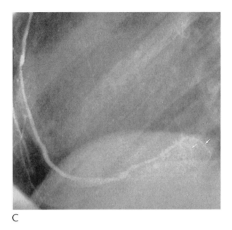

A   B   C

Fig. 14.84   (A) Selective right coronary arteriogram in the L → L AO projection in a child with an aneurysmal fistula to the right ventricle. (B) Angiogram, from the same patient, in the same projection immediately after embolisation with a detachable balloon (arrow). (C) Angiogram in the same projection taken 1 year later. The fistula remains closed, the right coronary artery has decreased in size, and the distal myocardial branches are now seen (arrows). (Courtesy of Dr G. Hartnell.)

Diagnosis may involve barium swallow and bronchography initially, but once again echocardiography may add more information. MRI or arteriography will produce the definitive diagnosis.

There are very many other vascular anomalies, some of which can cause tracheal compression. Sometimes a vascular ring is formed by *rudimentary vascular bands* which are not demonstrated angiographically, and this possibility must always be considered. Any vascular ring can potentially cause major airway obstruction, and thus stridor in infancy is a serious problem which must always be investigated thoroughly, usually with angiography (see Appendix at end of this chapter).

CORONARY ANOMALIES

There are many variants of coronary anatomy, and most cause no problems. The most common is the '*left dominant*' system in which the posterior descending artery arises from the circumflex artery rather than the right coronary artery, this occurring in 5–10% of the normal population. Numerous other variants in the course of the vessels have been documented. There is one anomalous course with theoretical clinical consequences, namely the left coronary artery which runs between the aorta and main pulmonary artery where it may be compressed, but it has been hard to document this problem precisely.

Clinically important abnormalities include *anomalous origin* of one or both coronary arteries *from the pulmonary artery*. This leads to desaturated coronary perfusion and/or reversed coronary flow, and can cause myocardial ischaemia, myocardial infarction or sudden death in infancy. Typically infants present at about 6 weeks of age when the pulmonary artery pressure has fallen, with evidence of distress on feeding presumed to be due to angina. Surviving infants can have marked cardiomegaly due to severe ischaemic cardiomyopathy.

Coronary fistulas to cardiac chambers or the pulmonary artery occur occasionally and often present asymptomatically with a continuous murmur. Ninety per cent drain to the right side of the heart, most often from the right coronary artery, and function as a left-to-right shunt. The shunt itself is often less of a worry in younger patients than the other potential complications such as coronary ischaemia (the 'steal' phenomenon) or endocarditis. In later life the

systemic-to-pulmonary shunting may become symptomatic. The fistulous communications can dilate to aneurysmal proportions with the development of unusually positioned bumps on the heart border seen on *chest X-ray*. The aneurysmal fistulas may calcify, and in theory they can rupture, but this latter has rarely been reported. These lesions may be diagnosed or suspected on *ultrasound examination*, but *angiography* is essential for precise evaluation. The communications are commonly closed surgically to prevent complications, but, more recently, interventional occlusion techniques have been employed to close them (Fig. 14.84).

ARTERIOVENOUS MALFORMATIONS (systemic and pulmonary)

Both types of arteriovenous malformation are uncommon.

Systemic arteriovenous malformations

These abnormalities may cause local problems but can also produce high-output cardiac failure. An intracranial arteriovenous malformation may result in a vein of Galen varix which, although rare, must be remembered when considering heart failure of unknown cause in infancy. The massively dilated vein can be readily identified on cranial ultrasound when clinically suspected.

Pulmonary arteriovenous malformations

These can sometimes be obvious on the chest X-ray, but this is not always the case as they may be obscured by other structures or they may be of the complex (plexiform) type with no large vessel or aneurysm present. These abnormalities can produce profound central cyanosis, and they require angiography for definitive diagnosis.

In some situations, systemic or pulmonary arteriovenous malformations are amenable to closure by transcatheter embolisation, but frequently surgical treatment is necessary. Follow-up after treatment may be carried out using lung perfusion scintigraphy with regions of interest over the kidneys to quantify any residual or recurrent right-to-left shunting.

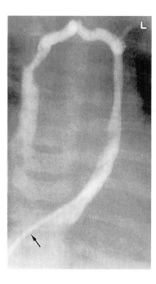

Fig. 14.85 Bilateral superior vena cava. A venous catheter (arrow) has been used for an angiogram in the left superior vena cava which drains to the coronary sinus. There is a large intercommunicating vein between the left and right venae cavae.

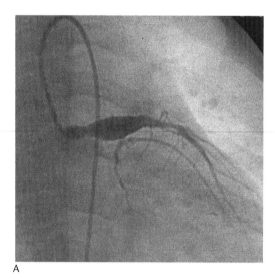

A

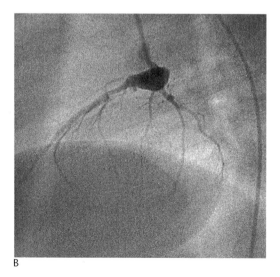

B

Fig. 14.86 Selective coronary angiograms showing Kawasaki's disease of the left coronary artery. There is a proximal fusiform aneurysm of the left anterior descending coronary artery. (A) Right anterior oblique projection. (B) Left anterior oblique projection.

SYSTEMIC VENOUS ANOMALIES

Bilateral superior vena cava

A bilateral superior vena cava is the commonest systemic venous anomaly, being present in about 10% of patients with congenital heart disease. Many of these are small left-sided connections, only about half being large enough to be of haemodynamic significance. In a proportion of cases there is an intercommunicating vein between the two venae cavae at the root of the neck (Fig. 14.85). The left superior vena cava usually drains into the coronary sinus. It is not normally of clinical importance, but is surgically important, as the venous connections need to be correctly placed in instituting cardiopulmonary bypass, and in some complex procedures the presence of a left-sided superior vena cava is a positive benefit for construction of the final repair.

The condition cannot be diagnosed easily on the plain chest radiograph but is generally recognisable on a good-quality *echocardiogram*. The condition is often signalled by an unusually large coronary sinus entering the right atrium. *Angiography* or *MRI* will provide a definitive diagnosis.

Interruption of the inferior vena cava

An uncommon anomaly is interruption of the inferior vena cava just before it reaches the heart. The venous drainage from the lower body continues into the azygos system, draining into the superior vena cava through the azygos vein on the right side. The hepatic veins usually drain directly to the right atrium. The abnormality rarely produces symptoms but can be very inconvenient if catheterisation is being performed via the inferior vena cava. It is often associated with ambiguous cardiac situs.

ACQUIRED HEART DISEASE IN CHILDHOOD

Although this chapter is entitled 'congenital heart disease' there are several causes of acquired heart disease which will present in childhood and these will be discussed briefly below.

KAWASAKI'S DISEASE

This is not a congenital abnormality but is acquired in childhood. It is probably infective in origin and has systemic features which give it the alternative name of '*mucocutaneous lymph node syndrome*'. A relatively mild illness in young children may be followed by the development of aneurysmal dilatation of the proximal coronary arteries (Fig. 14.86). These can often be seen on *echocardiography* and there is often no indication for angiography, because there is no specific therapy for the coronary abnormalities apart from general medical measures and observation. The coronary dilatations can resolve in many cases, but in a minority they can dilate and rupture or become stenotic.

CARDIAC TUMOURS

Cardiac tumours can occur occasionally in the newborn and have even been detected antenatally. The commonest tumour in children is the *rhabdomyoma*. This is usually histologically benign, a hamartoma, but can sometimes cause fatal obstruction within the heart. They are commonly multiple and are frequently associated with *tuberous sclerosis*. Surgery is best avoided as they do not grow with the heart and so become less of a problem as the child becomes older.

Teratomas and *fibromas* are occasionally diagnosed. The *myxoma* is a commoner tumour in the older child and has well-known features, particularly when it occurs in its commonest site, the left atrium. The presentation may be with a murmur, malaise and pyrexia, obstructive symptoms and signs, or with a systemic embolus. All tumours, but particularly the left atrial myxoma, are well suited to diagnosis by *echocardiography*, and the latter condition should always be treated by urgent surgical removal.

CARDIOMYOPATHY

Hypertrophic cardiomyopathy with left ventricular outflow obstruction can occur in infants and children, and is thought to be dominantly inherited in a proportion of cases. There are also associations with *Noonan's syndrome* and *maternal diabetes*, but in the latter circumstance the condition tends to resolve, whereas it tends to be progressive in the remainder. There is an association with arrhythmias and sudden death in a minority of cases. Diagnosis is classically made on the *echocardiogram*, which may show asymmetrical hypertrophy of the interventricular septum and obstruction of the left ventricular outflow tract by anterior motion of the mitral valve.

Dilated cardiomyopathies (alternatively called *endocardial fibroelastosis*) occur occasionally in infancy, and are most commonly related to intrauterine infections. Occasionally they are due to inherited factors or are secondary to valvular or coronary anomalies. The aetiology of the conditions is often hard to determine. The chest X-ray will show a large heart with pulmonary signs of cardiac failure (Fig. 14.87), and other imaging modalities will be capable of demonstrating the poor ventricular function. This is particularly clearly seen on two-dimensional echocardiography, which will also demonstrate the characteristic endocardial thickening. Occasionally the condition can be detected by fetal echocardiography. Surgery has little to offer in this condition apart from transplantation.

Endomyocardial fibrosis is a tropical condition in which there is endocardial thickening which leads to cavity obliteration.

ARRHYTHMOGENIC RIGHT VENTRICULAR DYSPLASIA

Arrhythmogenic right ventricular dysplasia (ARVD) is defined as a primary disorder of the right ventricle characterised by partial or total replacement of the myocardium by adipose or fibrous tissue. The diagnosis is important because of a high incidence of sudden death and requires the identification of specific anatomical and functional abnormalities of the right ventricle. The MRI features of ARVD are the presence of fat or extreme thinning in the infundibulum and inferior of diaphragmatic free wall of the right ventricle.

RHEUMATIC HEART DISEASE

New cases of rheumatic heart disease are now very rare in the UK. There is, however, a reported incidence of 7 cases per 1000 population in South Africa and the incidence is probably similar in most developing countries. Acutely, the carditis affects the mitral valve most frequently, producing mitral regurgitation. The aortic valve is the next most frequently affected valve. Mitral stenosis normally develops as a late complication due to scarring of the valve apparatus.

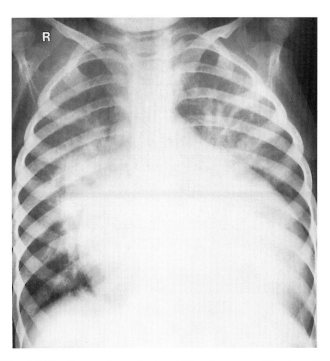

Fig. 14.87 Chest radiograph of a child with a severe dilated cardiomyopathy. There is marked cardiomegaly and left heart failure.

ONCOLOGY PATIENTS

Detailed assessment of left ventricular function is carried out in oncology patients who have received anthracyclines, particularly doxorubicin in the treatment of leukaemia and solid tumours. In addition radiotherapy may lead to coronary artery stenosis in the long term.

FETAL ECHOCARDIOGRAPHY

The routine 16–18-week antenatal ultrasound scan has now expanded considerably to include assessment of a wide range of organs. The heart can be clearly visualised at this stage with good equipment, and the 'routine' examination should include assessment of the '*four-chamber view*'. More detailed cardiac scanning starts with this view and includes other assessments as described below. This detailed cardiac assessment is only available in certain specialist centres at present, but the technique is becoming more widely available as experience develops.

Protocol for fetal cardiac scanning

- The transverse section of the fetal chest shows a four-chamber view with normal orientation of the cardiac apex to the left (Fig. 14.88). (The left side should be determined using the overall orientation of the fetus, not by comparison with adjacent organs, which might also be malpositioned.)
- The fetal heart should occupy about a third of the area of the thorax.
- Both ventricles should be of similar size (Fig. 14.89). Both atria should be of similar size.
- Mitral and tricuspid valves should be seen, in their normal offset relationship, the tricuspid valve being positioned slightly closer to the cardiac apex than the mitral valve.
- The valve of the foramen ovale should be visible as a thin mobile structure on the left side of the atrial septum.

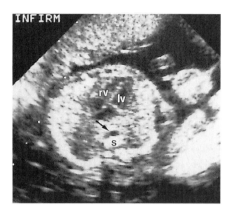

Fig. 14.88 Transverse echocardiogram of a 20-week-old fetus showing the 'four-chamber view'. rv = right ventricle; lv = left ventricle; s = spine. The descending aorta is arrowed.

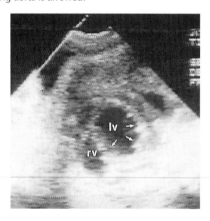

Fig. 14.89 Fetal echocardiogram in a fetus with a left ventricular cardiomyopathy due to critical aortic stenosis. The left ventricle (lv) is much larger than the right ventricle (rv), was visibly less contractile, and showed endocardial fibroelastosis (arrows) as an echogenic endocardium.

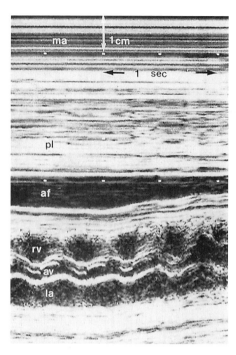

Fig. 14.90 M-mode echocardiogram across the normal aortic valve of a 20-week-old fetus. ma = maternal abdomen. pl = placenta; af = amniotic fluid; rv = right ventricle; av = aortic valve; la = left atrium. Depth and time markers are shown, indicating that the heart rate is 150 beats/min and the aortic root diameter is 4 mm.

• Adjustment of the transverse section should show normal connections of the pulmonary artery and aorta. M-mode tracings of cardiac valve movements can often be recorded (Fig. 14.90).

The schedule described above is possible in most cases and can be used to exclude most major structural abnormalities, depending on the experience of the operator. If abnormalities are detected, decisions regarding future management can be made, and these include termination of pregnancy, treatment of the mother with drugs (fetal cardiac failure) and referral to a specialist centre for delivery. Defects with minor anatomical derangements such as small VSD or isolated stenosis of the pulmonary valve cannot be detected reliably. Counselling of parents is a valuable part of the procedure.

The technique can be extended further. The long- and short-axis planes of the heart can be shown to confirm the anatomy and connections of the great arteries. The aortic arch can usually be visualised. Systemic and pulmonary venous connections can often be seen. Doppler studies can be used to confirm normal flow through valves and vessels, and this can sometimes demonstrate pathology such as a regurgitant valve.

Heart rate and rhythm, as well as more detailed assessment of ventricular function, can be derived from the fetal M-mode examination. The normal fetal heart rate is well in excess of 100 beats/ min (usually 150–180 beats/min at 18 weeks' gestation). Persistent bradycardia below 100 beats/min is associated with a high chance of structural cardiac abnormality. Transient periods of bradycardia, or even very brief periods of asystole, are of no prognostic significance.

Most patients scanned are mothers who have had a previous child with congenital heart disease. In this group there is a two- to three-fold increase in the chance of congenital heart disease in the fetus. This should be seen in the context of overall incidence, and even in these mothers the chance of congenital cardiac abnormality being present is still only 2–3%. Thus the great majority of scans are normal and are reassuring for the parents. There is a small but increasing group of parents with congenital heart defects in whom the risk of congenital heart disease in the fetus is slightly greater at 3–4%.

Referrals are also made in cases when a less experienced operator suspects an abnormality in a routine scan or a scan performed for another reason. It is not surprising to find that detailed cardiac scanning will reveal a much higher incidence of abnormality in this group, hence the importance of checking the four-chamber view as part of the protocol in the 'routine' antenatal scan. Detailed cardiac scans may also be helpful when other congenital abnormalities have been detected.

If a cardiac abnormality is detected it is essential to discuss the findings with the obstetrician and paediatric cardiologist so that proper advice can be given to the mother. In some cases of major abnormality, such as hypoplastic left heart syndrome, termination might be considered, but in other cases careful management of the pregnancy and early cardiological attention for the infant might be considered more appropriate. In many cases, detailed discussion of possible surgery and the prognosis will need to be discussed with the parents and paediatric cardiology or surgery specialists.

SUMMARY OF CHEST X-RAY APPEARANCES IN CONGENITAL HEART DISEASE

Particular points should be considered in the assessment of the chest film in the case of known or suspected congenital heart disease:

1. Note *abdominal* and *cardiac situs* at the start. If possible, assess the bronchial situs. Beware the handwritten side-marker: the radiographer may have been fooled too!

2. Note the overall *cardiac size*. It is generally unhelpful to read too much into this unless comparing serial films. Consider only normal, moderately enlarged or very enlarged.

3. Look at the *mediastinum*. Is the pulmonary artery segment absent, small, normal or enlarged? Is the aortic arch visible, is it normal in appearance, on which side is it? (Note tracheal indentation and descending aorta as part of this.) If a thymic shadow is present, then assessment can be difficult, particularly in the youngest infants.

4. Look at the *pulmonary vascularity*. First decide if the vessels are clearly visible or not. If not, consider heart failure (interstitial or alveolar pulmonary oedema), complex collateral vasculature or pulmonary disease. These are not always easy to distinguish. If vessels are distinct, are they:

   a. Definitely oligaemic
   b. Normal to oligaemic
   c. Normal
   d. Normal to plethoric
   e. Definitely plethoric.

(Abnormal vascular distribution within the lung is generally unhelpful in infants and small children unless very marked, e.g. unilateral plethora with a shunt.)

5. Is there any characteristic *unusual shape* to the heart contour that suggests a particular diagnosis?

6. Is there any *evidence of previous surgery* (e.g. thoracotomy, sternal wires or implanted prosthesis)?

7. *Note skeletal or other abnormalities* (e.g. 11 pairs of ribs suggests Down's syndrome, which in turn suggests AVSD).

Figure 14.91 summarises major patterns to be seen in a number of well-recognised congenital cardiac abnormalities. The recognition of these patterns will not lead to a definitive diagnosis in many cases but it will usually help to classify the type of abnormality present, often allowing the radiologist to highlight key functional and anatomical features which will be of vital importance in the further diagnosis and management of the patient.

SUMMARY OF IMAGING TECHNIQUES IN CONGENITAL HEART DISEASE

Plain chest radiograph

- Essential in initial assessment but not often fully diagnostic
- Essential in continuing management of patients
- Standard supine anteroposterior film in very small children and infants
- Standard erect posteroanterior film in older children and adults
- Localised view for bronchial anatomy.

Fluoroscopy

- Rarely needed for diagnostic purposes
- An essential part of diagnostic and therapeutic catheter techniques.

Barium swallow

- Very helpful in the initial assessment of vascular anomalies
- Otherwise superseded by other techniques.

Echocardiography

This is the most important non-invasive diagnostic technique. *Two-dimensional imaging* uses three main echocardiographic windows (left parasternal, apical and subcostal) to examine the heart in three main planes (long axis, short axis and four chamber). Modified views are also used as well as the suprasternal approach for assessing the great vessels.

M-mode imaging (one-dimensional imaging) is useful for accurate measurement of distances and timing within the heart.

Doppler echocardiography can be used in imaging congenital heart disease. *Pulsed Doppler interrogation* allows measurement of flow at a specific point selected within an image, but is limited in its ability to record high-velocity flow accurately, with aliasing being a common problem. Continuous-wave Doppler interrogation can be used to measure the highest velocities but has no depth resolution along the beam. The high velocities in pathological flows can be used to deduce pressure drops by means of the modified Bernoulli equation. *Colour flow mapping* is similar to pulsed Doppler examination, but the image as a whole is analysed, flow toward and away from the transducer being coded in different colours. Colour flow mapping is also limited in its ability to record high-velocity flow accurately.

Transoesophageal echocardiography can produce very high-resolution images, and is particularly suited to larger patients in whom good-quality imaging is hard to achieve. Paediatric-size transducers are now available. The technique has increasingly important applications in the operating theatre and intensive care unit.

Nuclear medicine

1. Myocardial perfusion:
   a. Infrequently used
   b. Occasional indications include postarterial switch and Kawasaki's disease.
2. First pass:
   a. Quantification or confirmation of pulmonary to systemic flow ratios.
3. Lung perfusion scintigraphy:
   a. Relative pulmonary perfusion
   b. Pre- and postintervention quantification useful on pulmonary arteries
   c. Screening for thrombi, especially post total cavo-pulmonary connection
   d. Quantification of right-to-left shunt.

CT

Helical CT with accurately timed contrast enhancement provides excellent images of the heart and great vessels and can provide excellent three-dimensional reconstructions of the entire pul-

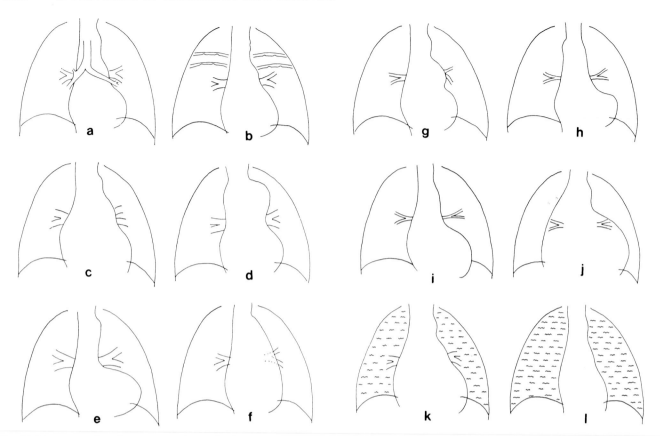

Fig. 14.91 **a** Normal cardiac contour and normal pulmonary artery size. Normal bronchial anatomy is superimposed. **b** Normal heart size and pulmonary vessels with a small and irregular aortic knuckle and rib notching. Established coarctation in an older child or adult. **c** Cardiomegaly and large pulmonary vessels. Left-to-right shunt, particularly ASD or VSD. Also consider PDA and partially or totally anomalous pulmonary venous connection of the cardiac type (draining directly to the heart). A left-to-right shunt alone rarely gives massive cardiomegaly. **d** Cardiomegaly and large pulmonary vessels with a very wide upper mediastinum. Totally anomalous pulmonary venous connection of the supracardiac type. A large thymus will widen the mediastinum also. **e** Moderate cardiomegaly and large pulmonary vessels with a small pulmonary artery segment. Pulmonary arteries must be anatomically abnormal, so consider D-transposition of the great arteries and truncus arteriosus. The latter is more likely if the aortic arch is right sided **f** Large smooth curve to the left heart border. L-transposition of the great arteries with an abnormal leftward position of the aorta. The appearance may also be due to other complex malpositions. L-loop TGA may occasionally have a virtually normal chest X-ray. **g** Prominent main pulmonary artery with normal or small pulmonary vessels. Pulmonary valve stenosis. The left pulmonary artery also may be dilated. The dilatation is not prominent in subpulmonary stenosis and is not invariably present in valvar stenosis. **h** Upturned cardiac apex, right-sided aortic arch, and small pulmonary vessels. This is almost diagnostic of tetralogy of Fallot, but can be seen in pulmonary atresia with a VSD and in a few cases of double outlet right ventricle similar haemodynamics). **I** Small pulmonary artery and pulmonary vessels with a large rounded left heart border. Tricuspid atresia. The condition is variable, and there can be normal or occasionally increased vascularity depending on the haemodynamics of the VSD and pulmonary valve. Sometimes pulmonary stenosis can give this appearance. **j** Very large heart with normal or small pulmonary vessels. Ebstein's anomaly, dilated cardiomyopathy (including anomalous coronary origin from the pulmonary artery), and pericardial effusion. There may be associated left heart failure with cardiomyopathy. **k** Cardiomegaly with large pulmonary vessels and pulmonary oedema. Left to right shunt with failure, left heart obstruction (aortic stenosis or coarctation), severe mitral regurgitation (alone or with other conditions) and cardiomyopathy. **I** Small heart with pulmonary oedema. Obstruction before the heart. Totally anomalous pulmonary venous connection of the obstructed intracardiac type, cor triatriatum or congenital mitral stenosis. Pulmonary conditions must be distinguished.

monary artery anatomy. The radiation dose and requirement for intravenous contrast are disadvantages compared to MRI but it has a role in patients in whom MRI has failed, for example those with ferromagnetic interventional devices causing artefact on MRI. Normal scan times are too slow to allow accurate recording of intracardiac detail although newer 'spiral' scanners are shortening scan times. In addition to this, contrast medium is needed to outline cardiac chambers. The technique is sometimes useful for the assessment of mediastinal masses, which may be close to the heart. A few very sophisticated fast scanners are in use in some specialist centres. These use an accelerator to produce an electron beam which can be moved very fast around the patient to give scan times of 50 ms or less.

MRI

MRI has a role chiefly in assessing areas where echocardiography is weak, such as extracardiac structures, or has failed to demonstrate intracardiac anatomy.

The advantages of cardiac MRI can be summarised as:

1. Short scan times or gating can 'freeze' cardiac motion.

2. Scans can be taken in transverse, coronal or sagittal planes, and complex combinations of these planes can also be achieved.

3. Cardiac chambers and walls can be distinguished clearly without the use of contrast media.

4. Blood flow patterns can be recognised. It may soon be possible to quantify stenotic and regurgitant lesions as well as volume flow (cardiac output, shunts, etc.).

5. Three-dimensional reconstructions of complex anatomy will soon be possible.

Cardiac angiography

It will be some time yet before cardiac angiography is superseded as one of the mainstays of cardiac imaging. As non-invasive techniques replace catheter techniques in more and more cases, there is a parallel increase in interventional therapies, which need the full resources of a catheterisation and angiography laboratory.

Many angiograms are still performed using 35-mm ciné film recording techniques from the image intensifier, although ciné has now been formally replaced as the recognised standard by the DICOM compatible method of digital storage. Equipment suspensions must allow a full range of oblique views, as well as cranial and caudal angulation, so that appropriate structures can be profiled. Biplane techniques are commonly in use in paediatric cardiology as they allow more views to be taken for smaller doses of contrast medium to the patient. Digital recording of images allows manipulation of contrast and other image detail and radiation doses can be reduced significantly. Every attempt to reduce the patient and operator dose should be made, as long interventional procedures in particular can be responsible for extremely high radiation doses. Digital recording of the radiographic image is the key requirement, subtraction of the digital image being only of secondary importance. Intravenous injections of contrast medium have not proved adequate, so digital techniques do not dispense with intracardiac catheters.

Contrast medium A major load can be put on the circulation of a sick child by contrast medium, and thus great care must be taken with its use. Nevertheless, it must be used properly, and inadequate volumes or rates of injection which produce poor angiograms are of no benefit to the patient. Ideally non-ionic media should be used, and iodine concentrations of 350–400 mg/ml are necessary. Lower concentrations are possible with good-quality digital equipment. Contrast medium should be administered fast enough to prevent unnecessary dilution, and catheter size must be selected appropriately for the anticipated injection. It is important to check that the catheter tip lies free in the ventricle on a test injection to avoid an intramyocardial injection. New non-ionic dimers are now being introduced which are isotonic at high iodine concentrations.

The following is a guide to contrast medium doses for use with non-ionic media of 370 mg iodine/ml when using conventional ciné film technique:

- Start with 1 ml/kg, suitable for a normal ventricle in a neonate.
- Reduce by 25–50% for hypoplastic chambers or a small aorta.
- Increase by 50–100% for large chambers with large flow or shunts.
- Also reduce progressively with increasing weight, as follows:

  2–10 kg, no change
  10–20 kg, reduce by 20%
  20–30 kg, reduce by 30%
  30–50 kg, reduce by 40%.

The contrast medium must be delivered in 1.5–2 cardiac cycles to avoid excessive dilution. Thus, neonates with heart rates of 150–180 beats/min will need it delivered in 0.5–0.7 s. This may not be possible if a relatively large dose is to be delivered through too small a catheter. If a child weighing 4 kg with a very large VSD and a heart rate of 180 beats/min is to be studied by left ventriculography, a dose of 8 ml of contrast medium should be delivered at 16 ml/s. This may not be achieved through a 5Fr catheter, and a 6Fr size must be used.

Total dose limits are hard to state with accuracy, as they depend on the condition of the child and the sequence of the injections; 4 ml/kg is a safe limit for divided doses of 370 mg iodine/ml non-ionic medium, provided the child is reasonably well and not dehydrated. With care and proper hydration this arbitrary limit can be exceeded. As with all diagnostic radiology, the potential benefits must be weighed against the potential hazards in any individual cases.

REFERENCES AND SUGGESTIONS FOR FURTHER READING

Elliott, L. P. (1991) *Cardiac Imaging in Infants, Children and Adults*. Philadelphia: J. B. Lippincott.
Freedom, R. M., Mawson, J. B., Yoo, S. J., Benson, L. N. (1997) *Congenital Heart Disease; Textbook of Angiocardiography*. London: Futura.
Higgins, C. B., Silverman, N. H., Kersting, S., Sommerhoff, B. A., Schmidt, K. (1990) *Congenital Heart Disease; Echocardiography and Magnetic Resonance Imaging*. New York: Raven Press.
Linker, D. T. (2000) *Practical Pediatric Echocardiography of Congenital Heart Disease*. Edinburgh: Churchill Livingstone.

Appendix: Vascular rings and anomalies of the aortic arch

Figures 14A.1 and 14A.2 are copied from the *Agfa Gevaert X-ray Bulletin* and are reproduced with kind permission of Dr Klinkhamer.

They illustrate the main congenital anomalies and the changes produced in the barium swallow which help in their diagnosis.

The very rare double aortic arch which may occur with either a left or a right descending aorta is not included in the illustrations.

Positive diagnosis of these anomalies is of course possible by angiography and is sometimes made as a chance finding at arch aortography or angiocardiography undertaken for the diagnosis of other lesions. The diagrams show how diagnosis can often be made or suggested by simpler radiological examinations and particularly by the oesophagogram.

The procedure is as follows:

1. A plain chest X-ray in the high kilovoltage range will visualise the trachea, the main bronchi and (in most instances) the descending aorta. This will give information of:
   a. The position of the aortic arch. A left-sided aortic arch gives a small impression in the left tracheobronchial angle. A right-sided aortic arch or an aberrant left pulmonary artery produces an impression in the right tracheobronchial wall. The arches of a double aortic arch are too small to produce impressions in the tracheobronchial walls of children and most adults. A bilateral impression is rarely seen in adults only. This differentiation is very useful, but not absolute. A double arch with arches of markedly unequal width can produce only one impression in the right or left tracheobronchial angle.
   b. The position of the descending aorta (on the left or on the right side of the vertebral column). Fluoroscopy can be helpful.

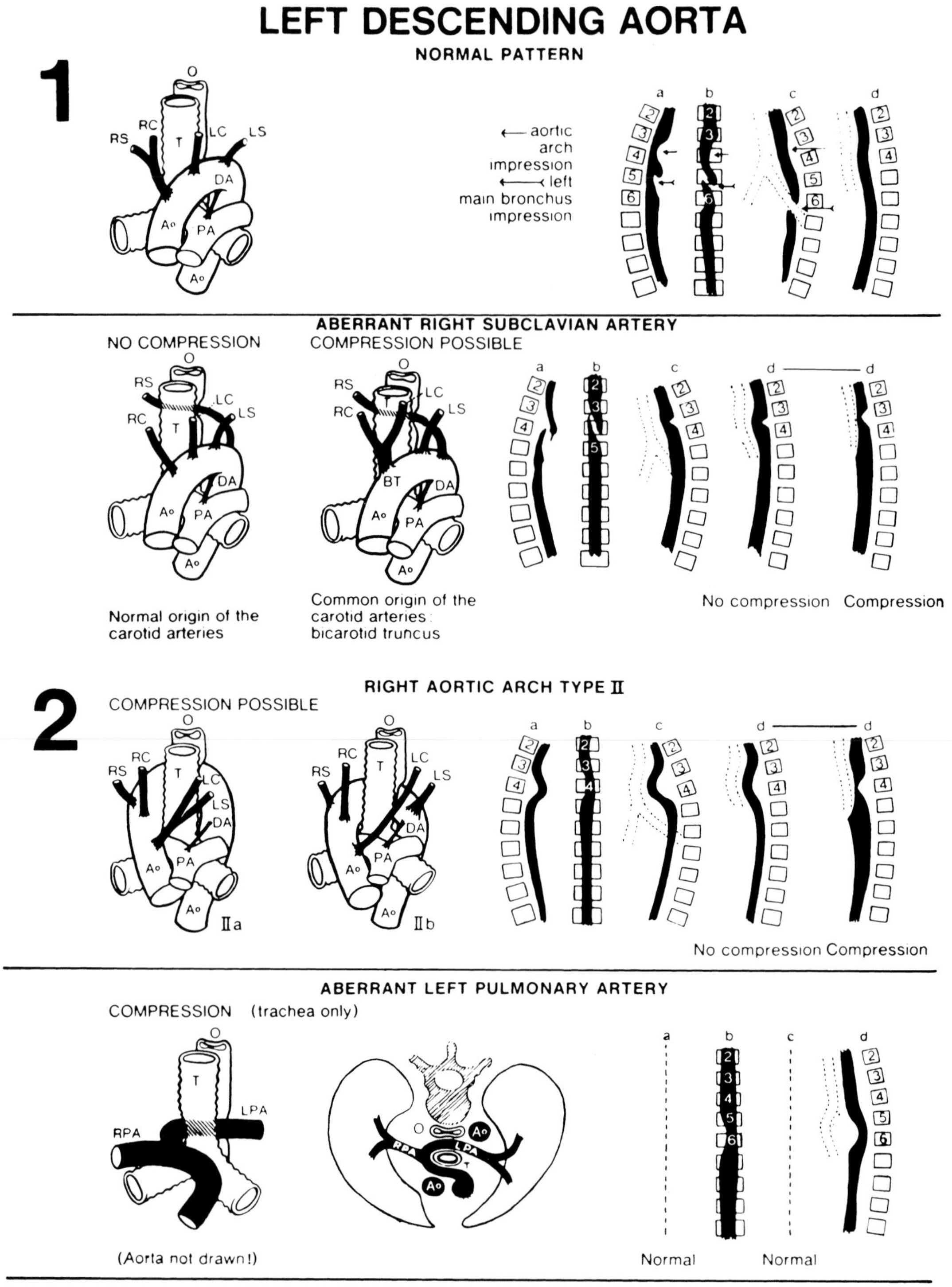

LEFT DESCENDING AORTA
NORMAL PATTERN

1

← aortic arch impression
←< left main bronchus impression

ABERRANT RIGHT SUBCLAVIAN ARTERY

NO COMPRESSION   **COMPRESSION POSSIBLE**

Normal origin of the carotid arteries

Common origin of the carotid arteries : bicarotid truncus

No compression   Compression

RIGHT AORTIC ARCH TYPE II

2

COMPRESSION POSSIBLE

IIa   IIb

No compression Compression

ABERRANT LEFT PULMONARY ARTERY

COMPRESSION   (trachea only)

(Aorta not drawn!)

Normal   Normal

Fig. 14A.1

2. Further differentiation must be made by means of the oesophagogram.
   a. The differentiation is based upon the impressions seen in the oesophagograms in oblique positions (a) and (c) and the PA view (b). The aberrant left pulmonary artery and the double aortic arch show a characteristic oesophagogram in the lateral view (d).

b. The lateral view (d) informs only of the presence or absence of tracheo-oesophageal compression. Lateral oesophagograms of the different anomalies producing compression are identical. The two exceptions are the aberrant left pulmonary artery and the double aortic arch.
3. Some types manifest themselves clinically by producing compression of the trachea and the oesophagus. In children,

RIGHT DESCENDING AORTA

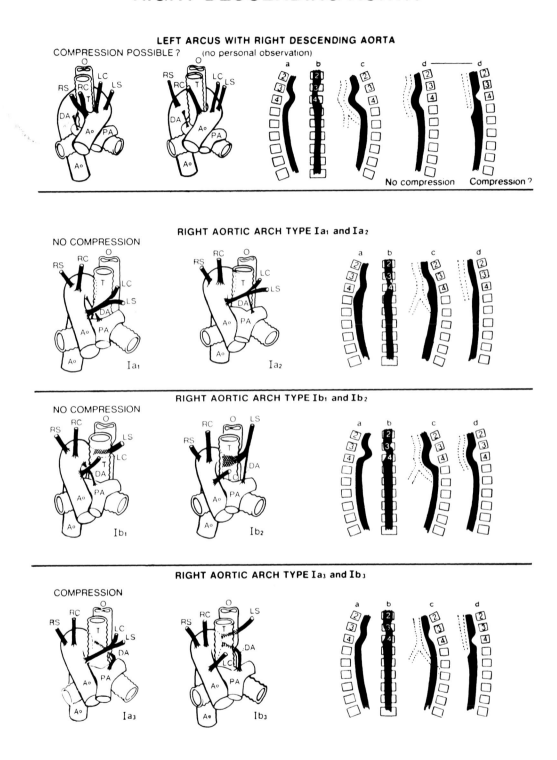

Fig. 14A.2

Key to Figures 14A.1 and 14A.2 T = trachea; O = oesophagus; Ao = aorta: PA = pulmonary artery; RPA = right branch of the pulmonary artery: LPA = left branch of the pulmonary artery; DA = ductus arteriosus; BT = bicarotid truncus; RC = right carotid artery; LC = left carotid artery; RS = right subclavian artery; LS = left subclavian artery. a = right anterior oblique view; b = postero-anterior view; c = left anterior oblique view; d = lateral view.

the tracheo-oesophageal compression will give rise mainly to respiratory signs (stridor, relapsing respiratory infections). In adults dysphagia is the principal complaint.

Classification of the right-sided aortic arch anomalies

The various types of right-sided aortic arch anomalies are classified as follows:

First, the anomalies are divided according to the course of the descending aorta.

Aorta descending on the RIGHT of the vertebral column—type I.

Aorta descending on the LEFT of the vertebral column column—type II.

Type I and type II are subdivided according to the branches of the aortic arch:

A. Left innominate artery, right carotid artery, right subclavian artery:

    type Ia   type IIa

B. Left carotid artery, right carotid artery, right subclavian artery:

    type Ib   type IIb

Type Ia and type Ib are finally subdivided according to the course of the ductus arteriosus:

1. Ductus arteriosus running from the right branch of the pulmonary artery to the right-sided aortic arch.

    type Ia_1 type Ib_1

2. Ductus arteriosus running from the left branch of the pulmonary artery to the left subclavian artery:

    type Ia_2 type Ib_2

3. Ductus arteriosus running from the left branch of the pulmonary artery retro-oesophageally to the right-sided aortic arch:

    type Ia_3 type Ib_3

15

ARTERIOGRAPHY AND INTERVENTIONAL ANGIOGRAPHY

David Sutton and Roger H. S. Gregson
with contributions from P. L. Allan and Jeremy P. R. Jenkins

Historical

It is a remarkable fact that the history of arteriography began only a few weeks after the discovery of X-rays. Roentgen announced his discovery of X-rays in December 1895, and the first arteriogram was produced within a month, when Haschek and Lindenthal in Vienna published the picture of the arteries of an amputated hand in January 1896 (Haschek & Lindenthal 1896).

Realising the enormous potential of Roentgen's work they had immediately begun experimenting with the injection of radiopaque substances into the arteries of amputated limbs. Even by today's standards of rapid communication this was an outstanding achievement. Unfortunately the absence of a safe intravascular contrast medium for in vivo work and the prolonged exposures then necessary (about 60 min) meant that this work could not be put into clinical practice.

It was to be another 27 years before the first successful in vivo arteriograms were achieved (Berberich & Hirsch 1923; Sicard & Forestier 1923; Brooks 1924). Soon afterwards, Moniz carried out his classical work on cerebral angiography which was first published in 1928 (Moniz 1931), and in 1929 Dos Santos described lumbar aortography (Dos Santos et al 1931).

Cardiac catheterisation was first carried out by Forssman in Germany in 1929 and in 1936 Amiaille first opacified the heart chambers by catheterisation. In 1937 Castellanos, Pereiras and Garcia described the use of right-heart angiocardiography in the diagnosis of congenital heart disease, and in 1941 Farinas first described retrograde catheter angiography.

Although all the basic work had now been done, it was not until the 1950s that arteriography became widely used in medicine. This was because arteriography was still an investigation that required surgical intervention, and Scandinavian workers did not develop percutaneous techniques of arteriography until the 1940s. The percutaneous technique of catheterisation was not developed until 1953 (Seldinger 1953). It was these innovations that, together with the development of organic iodinated contrast media, set the stage for the more widespread use of angiography.

James Bull introduced the technique of percutaneous carotid angiography to Britain at the National Hospital for Nervous Diseases in 1947. One of us was fortunate enough to acquire it from him in 1948 and later to work with Rob and Eastcott who were then pioneering the expansion of vascular surgery in Europe. In 1962 Sutton published the first British monograph on arteriography based on a personal experience of 10 000 cases. European workers extended the scope of percutaneous needle puncture to include most major vessels and even the vertebral artery (Sutton & Hoare 1951). At the same time percutaneous catheter techniques were developed further and became more versatile. By the 1980s catheter techniques had become generally accepted as the routine method for arteriography. Percutaneous catheter angiography also facilitated the development of new interventional techniques. Although percutaneous catheterisation was now well established it was still invasive and liable to complications from contrast media reactions and from trauma to vessel walls (see below). It also used quite high doses of X-rays. An ideal method should be completely safe and free of any hazard from technique, contrast or radiation. The goal of such an ideal method has drawn ever nearer as other imaging techniques have made technical advances.

Arterial imaging techniques

Direct arteriography by percutaneous needle or percutaneous catheterisation has been the standard method for most of the past half century, and has provided detailed images of high resolution that have set the standard for alternative techniques. Improvements in contrast media and in apparatus have helped to maintain its ascendancy. In the last decade however this has been seriously challenged by rival methods, some of which will be briefly noted here, and the more important of which will be discussed in depth at the end of this chapter.

Plain films

Normal blood vessels are not seen in the soft tissues on plain radiographs, but the presence of calcification in the wall of an artery

411

indicates arterial disease. Intimal calcification has an irregular amorphous appearance and is very common in elderly patients with atherosclerosis. It occurs in the thoracic and abdominal aorta and in the carotid, splenic, renal, iliac, femoral, popliteal and tibial arteries. A curvilinear form of this type of calcification indicates an aneurysm.

Medial calcification has a regular tubular appearance and is seen in diabetic patients with atherosclerosis, particularly in the tibial arteries and foot vessels. This type of calcification is also seen in patients with hyperparathyroidism due to chronic renal failure and in patients with premature ageing due to Werner's syndrome.

The presence of phleboliths in an unusual site indicates an arteriovenous malformation (AVM), which can also produce pressure erosion defects in an adjacent bone.

Ultrasound This is a non-invasive method of imaging the arteries. Real-time ultrasound has been used for many years in the diagnosis of abdominal aortic and peripheral aneurysms to measure their size, extent and rate of growth. It has also been used in screening studies for abdominal aortic aneurysms (AAA), because it is a safe, accurate and cost-effective test. (Fig. 15.1)

Duplex ultrasound is used in the diagnosis of arterial stenoses and occlusions in the carotid, renal and peripheral vessels to assess the severity of the stenosis and the length of the occlusion. It is also used in surgical graft surveillance studies to assess the development of graft stenoses and in the investigation of pulsating superficial masses in the neck, axilla, groin and popliteal fossa.

Echo-enhancing contrast media are now also available and are used to improve the colour Doppler signal in duplex ultrasound studies. The technique is discussed in detail below.

Intravascular ultrasound This is an invasive method of studying the arterial wall, but it is not widely available. It has been used in a research setting to look at atheromatous plaque morphology, the mechanism of angioplasty, thrombus characterisation and dissections in the arterial wall.

Angioscopy This is also an invasive method of studying the intimal surface of the arterial wall, by introducing an angioscope catheter containing optical fibres into the arterial system. By flushing away the blood, which obscures the field of view, the inner surface of both arteries and grafts, atheroma and thrombus can be directly visualised.

Radionuclide imaging

Radionuclide angiography is no longer performed but was able to demonstrate abdominal aortic aneurysms, arterial occlusions and

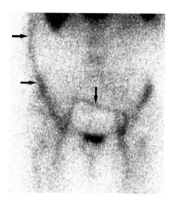
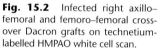

Fig. 15.2 Infected right axillo–femoral and femoro–femoral crossover Dacron grafts on technetium-labelled HMPAO white cell scan.

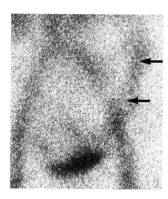

Fig. 15.3 Gastrointestinal bleeding into descending colon from a diverticulum on technetium-labelled red cell scan.

surgical graft patency. Radionuclide studies are however performed in arterial disease to confirm the diagnosis of an infected surgical graft by using ^{111}In-labelled white cells (Fig. 15.2) and to show the site of gastrointestinal bleeding by using ^{99m}Tc-labelled colloid or red cells (Fig. 15.3).

Venous angiography Venous angiography is also no longer performed but was able to demonstrate arterial patency or occlusion with the use of xeroangiography or a photographic subtraction technique using special types of film.

CT This is a non-invasive method of imaging the aorta and large arteries, which is generally performed following an intravenous injection of non-ionic intravascular contrast medium. The axial images produced show calcification in the wall of the aorta, contrast-enhanced flowing blood and unenhanced thrombus or atheroma within the vessel lumen (Figs 15.4–15.9).

The introduction of spiral or helical CT with its capability of imaging large columns of tissue very rapidly in a 20–30 s breath-hold has led to the development of CT angiography. This produces even higher quality axial images with better contrast enhancement than conventional CT and has the added advantage of being able to produce 2D coronal, sagittal, oblique and curved planar reconstructed images as well as the 3D maximum intensity projection (MIP) and shaded surface display (SSD) reconstructed images (Figs 15.10–15.14).

CT angiography is used in the assessment of thoracic and abdominal aortic aneurysms to see if they are suitable for endovascular repair and in the diagnosis of aortic dissection and pul-

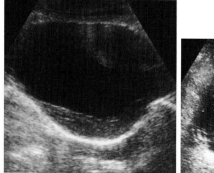
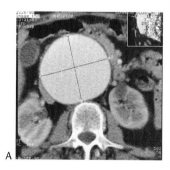

Fig. 15.1 (A,B) Ultrasound. Large 9-cm AAA containing thrombus.

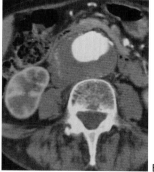

Fig. 15.4 CT. (A) Large 8.5-cm. AAA. (B) AAA containing thrombus.

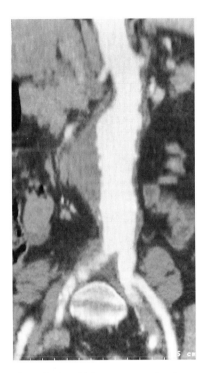

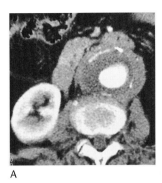
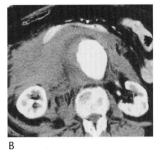
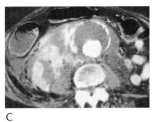

A   B   C

Fig. 15.6   CT. (A) Inflammatory AAA with calcification in its wall. (B) Leaking AAA with retroperitoneal haematoma. (C) Leaking AAA with active retroperitoneal bleeding.

Fig. 15.5   AAA on coronal planar reconstruction.

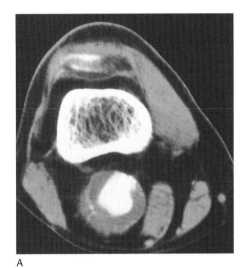

A

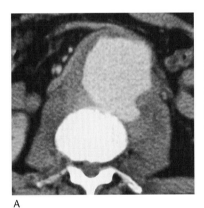
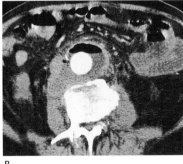

A   B

Fig. 15.7   CT. (A) AAA with contained leak into left psoas muscle. (B) Infected aortic bifemoral Dacron graft with gas–fluid level in the sac of the aneurysm.

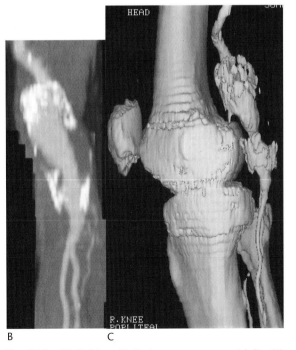

B   C

Fig. 15.8   CT. Right popliteal artery aneurysm on axial slice (A) and 3D MIP (B) and SSD (C) reconstructed images.

monary embolic disease. CT angiography is also used in the investigation of carotid, renal and peripheral vascular disease (see below and Chs. 29 and 55). The recent introduction of multislice spiral scanners has further enhanced the potential of CT vascular imaging (see Ch. 59).

MRI   This is a non-invasive method of imaging not only the aorta and large arteries without the use of a contrast medium, but also the smaller arteries, which is performed following an intravenous injection of a paramagnetic intravascular contrast medium.

On T_1-weighted spin-echo sequences flowing blood produces a signal void and appears black. The axial, coronal, sagittal and oblique images produced show no signal from flowing blood, but

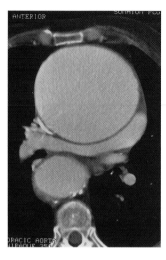

Fig. 15.9 CT. Large 9.5-cm ascending thoracic aortic aneurysm.

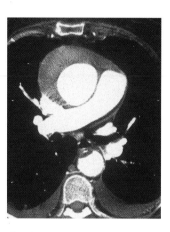

Fig. 15.10 CT. Type A dissecting aneurysm of ascending and descending thoracic aorta.

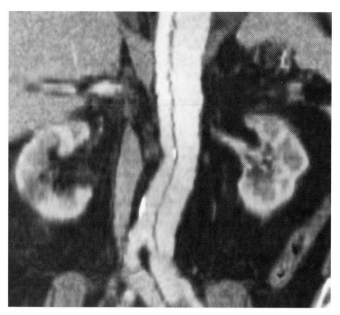

Fig. 15.12 CT. Type B aortic dissection in abdominal aorta and left common iliac artery on coronal planar reconstruction.

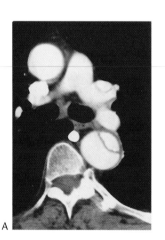

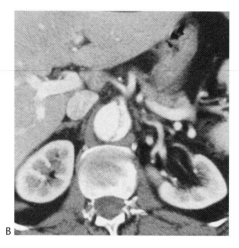

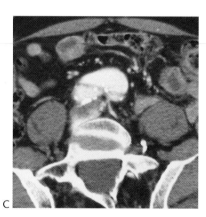

Fig. 15.11 (A–C) CT. Type B aortic dissection of descending thoracic and abdominal aorta and iliac arteries.

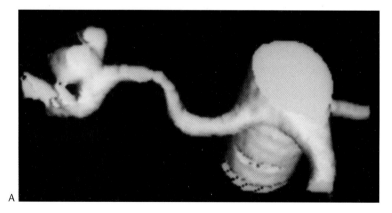

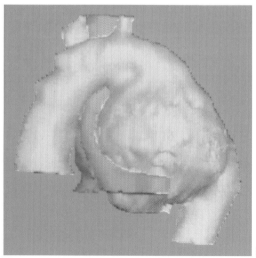

Fig. 15.13 (A) 3D spiral CT scan showing fibromuscular hyperplasia of right renal artery with poststenotic aneurysm at the bifurcation. (B) Computer-extracted 3D colour study of aortic aneurysm compressing the left main bronchus, which is shown in green. (Courtesy of Dr A. Al Katoubi.)

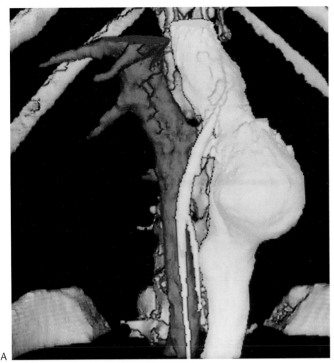

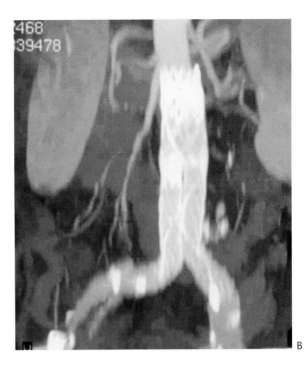

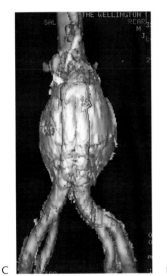

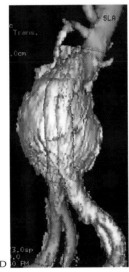

Fig. 15.14 (A) Spiral CT. 3D reconstruction showing abdominal aortic aneurysm. The inferior vena cava and hepatic veins are also well shown. (B) Spiral CT. 3D surface shaded study of prosthesis replacing aortic aneurym. AP view of double aorta–iliac graft in situ after transfemoral insertion. (Courtesy of Dr. A. L. Kutoubi.)

Digital subtraction angiography (DSA)

Arteriography is now generally performed as a digital subtraction technique and the conventional form of arteriography with the use of a film changer has become obsolete in most departments.

With DSA, a computer is used to subtract an initial image without contrast medium taken directly from the image intensifier from the subsequent angiographic images with contrast medium in the blood vessels. The bone, soft tissue and gas are removed leaving only the contrast-medium-filled blood vessels in the final subtracted arterial images, as long as no movement has occurred during the angiographic acquisition run.

DSA requires cooperative patients who can keep still and hold their breath, because any type of movement, such as body movement, cardiac pulsation, respiration and peristalsis, causes significant image degradation. Abdominal examinations are performed after an intravenous injection of 20 mg hyoscine butyl bromide (Buscopan) to prevent peristalsis and thoracic examinations can be done with ECG-triggered gating to prevent cardiac pulsation. With patients who are unable to keep still and hold their breath, it is sometimes better to obtain these digital images without subtraction. There are also various postprocessing facilities that can be used to enhance the image after it has been acquired but before it is printed on radiographic film.

The advantages of DSA over conventional arteriography are:

1. A reduction in both the volume and iodine concentration of the non-ionic contrast medium used for each run, because of the high contrast resolution of the imaging system.
2. A reduction in the length of the procedure due to the rapid image acquisition time for each run.

signal from thrombus in the vessel lumen and signal from the wall of the aorta, although calcification in the vessel wall cannot be demonstrated.

By using the 2D and 3D time-of-flight and phase-contrast fast-gradient echo sequences, flowing blood produces a high signal and appears white. These angiographic-type images show stenoses and occlusions in the vessel lumen. The paramagnetic agent, gadolinium DTPA is used as an intravenous contrast medium to increase the signal intensity of flowing blood (Figs 15.15–15.18).

MR imaging is used in the assessment of thoracic and abdominal aortic aneurysms and in the diagnosis of aortic dissection. MR angiography is also used in the investigation of carotid, renal and peripheral vascular disease.

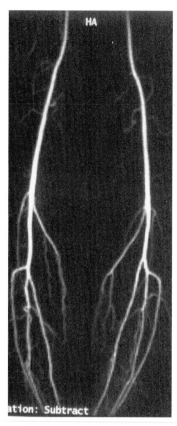

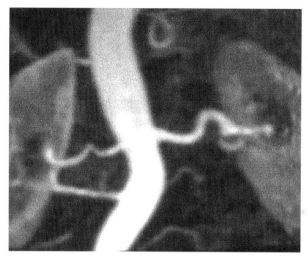

Fig. 15.16 MRA. Normal renal arteries and accessory artery to lower pole of right kidney.

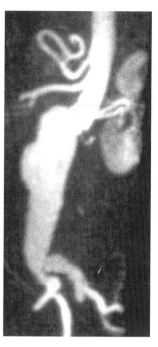

Fig. 15.18 MRA. Aneurysm of lower abdominal aorta.

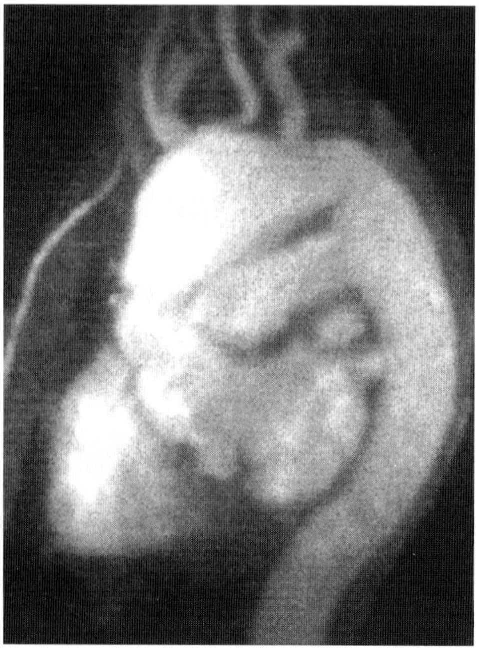

Fig. 15.15 MRA. Normal femoral, popliteal and tibial arteries.

Fig. 15.17 MRA. Aneurysm of thoracic aortic arch.

3. A reduction in the size of the catheters used from 6–8Fr down to 3–5Fr.
4. A reduction in the amount of radiographic film used.
5. A reduction in the radiation dose to the patient and angiographic staff.

The only disadvantage of DSA is that conventional arteriography has a better spatial resolution.

Intravenous DSA The high contrast resolution of the imaging system allows non-ionic contrast medium to be injected intravenously in order to produce arterial images in patients with no femoral pulses. A large volume of contrast medium is injected rapidly by a pump injector through a catheter positioned in the SVC or right atrium. The contrast medium is diluted as it passes through the lungs and into the left side of the heart and systemic circulation, but the images can be very good in cooperative patients with a normal cardiac output (Figs 15.19–15.23).

Carbon dioxide DSA The high contrast resolution of the imaging system even allows carbon dioxide to be used as an alternative arterial contrast medium in patients with a previous hypersensitivity reaction to non-ionic contrast media and in patients in renal failure. Carbon dioxide is very soluble and rapidly dissolves in the blood. It produces an image by displacing the blood in the artery and therefore needs to be injected by a pump injector, even though it is very compressible. Its use is contraindicated above the diaphragm in the coronary and cerebral circulations, but it is safe to use elsewhere in the body and the images are acceptable (Fig. 15.19).

Gadolinium-labelled DTPA can also be used as an arterial contrast medium in patients with a previous reaction to contrast medium, but it is very expensive.

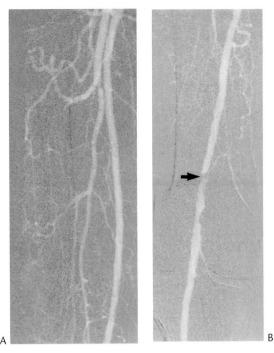

Fig. 15.19 (A, B) Normal right superficial femoral artery with stenosis (arrow) in right popliteal artery on carbon dioxide DSA.

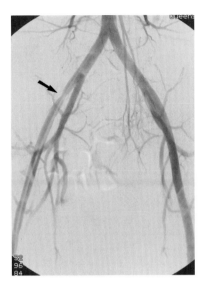

Fig. 15.20 DSA. Spasm (arrow) in right external iliac artery produced by the catheter in a child.

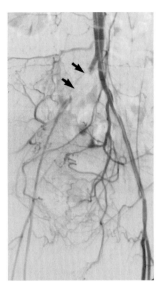

Fig. 15.21 DSA. Occlusion in right common iliac artery produced by a guide-wire dissection during cardiac catheterisation.

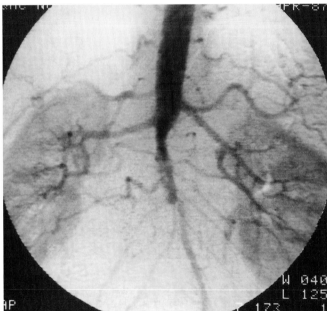

Fig. 15.22 Intravenous DSA image showing aortic thrombosis.

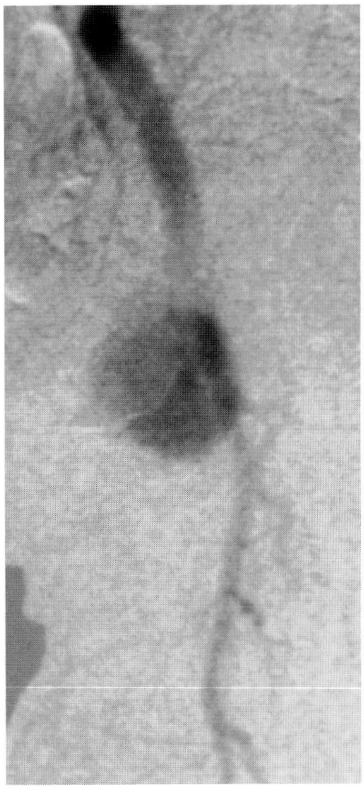

Fig. 15.23 Intravenous DSA image showing femoral false aneurysm following cardiac catheterisation.

CURRENT TECHNIQUES FOR IMAGING ARTERIES

Invasive and non-invasive are terms widely used in angiography. It was pointed out in Chapter 13 that different workers give different interpretations to these terms.

The following methods are currently used:

1. Non-invasive and radiation free—ultrasound, MRI

2. Mildly invasive and radiation free—MRI with IV gadolinium (CE MRI)

3. Mildly invasive plus radiation—multislice spiral CT with IV contrast

4. Invasive with radiation—percutaneous catheterisation

Ultrasound and MRI are discussed in detail at the end of this chapter. Multislice spiral CT is discussed in more technical detail in Chapter 59. Most diagnostic angiography is now carried out using non-invasive or mildly invasive methods. However, the development of interventional angiography has meant that the invasive technique of percutaneous catheterisation continues to be widely used, as does the fact that many hospitals, even in the developed world, still lack the sophisticated and expensive MR and CT equipment required.

Whilst ultrasound and MR are regarded as non-invasive and free of radiation hazard it should be noted that MR is still not generally accepted for obstetric imaging and that ultrasound is again being questioned.

Direct arteriography

It has been noted above that two basic techniques were used in the past for direct arteriography—direct needle puncture and direct catheterisation. Direct needle puncture had advantages of speed and simplicity, and many radiologists became very skilled in this technique, but it was less versatile than the catheter technique, which eventually supplanted it.

Percutaneous arterial catheterisation is based on the original work of Seldinger in Stockholm (Seldinger 1953). The use of a special needle and guide-wire permits the percutaneous introduction of a catheter into a superficial and palpable vessel such as a femoral artery. The basic technique is illustrated in Figure 15.24. The most useful sites for the insertion of catheters into the arterial tree are:

1. The femoral artery in the groin
2. The axillary artery in the axilla.

Catheters have also been inserted from the brachial artery just above the elbow, from the radial artery just above the wrist, from the common carotid in the neck, and from the abdominal using a translumbar approach. In practice, the femoral and axillary arteries permit investigations of most areas, and the other sites of insertion are little used except in special circumstances.

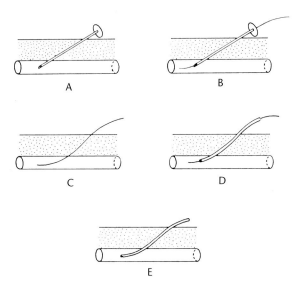

Fig. 15.24 Technique of percutaneous catheter insertion using the Selding–Sutton needle. (A) Needle inserted into artery. (B) Guide passed through needle into artery (C) Needle withdrawn leaving guidewire in artery. (D) Catheter passed over guide into artery. (E) Guide withdrawn leaving catheter in artery.

Selective and superselective arterial catheterisation

This is a refinement of the standard technique in which specially shaped catheters are introduced into branches or subbranches of the aorta. Arteries which are frequently catheterised include most major branches of the abdominal aorta (renal, coeliac axis, superior and inferior mesenteric arteries), major branches of the aortic arch (subclavian, innominate and left common carotid arteries and their major branches, including the vertebrals, and internal and external carotid arteries). Superselective catheterisation is frequently performed on branches of the coeliac axis, including the splenic, hepatic, and gastroduodenal arteries, and on branches of the external carotid such as the internal maxillary.

Most catheterisations are now performed with relatively small catheters, usually of 5 Fr gauge, or less. Superselective catheterisation is sometimes achieved, particularly with intracranial vessels, by passing very fine catheters (2 or 3 Fr) through a larger catheter (5 or 6 Fr, thin walled).

Technique of percutaneous catheterisation

A simplified Seldinger technique routinely used by the author is illustrated in Figure 15.24, and consists of the following consecutive steps:

1. The artery (usually the femoral and less commonly the axillary) is punctured by a thin-walled needle as described above.
2. Once the needle tip is firmly in the vessel lumen the connecting tubing is detached, allowing blood to spurt back (Fig. 15.24A). The guide-wire is then immediately passed through the needle into the vessel, and its tip advanced 5–8 cm along the lumen (Fig. 15.24B). Holding the guide-wire firmly in position, the needle is then withdrawn along it and off the guide-wire (Fig. 15.24C). Meanwhile, firm manual pressure is maintained with gauze swabs at the puncture site to prevent oozing of blood and haematoma formation.
3. The catheter, with a two-way tap attached to its hind end, is now passed along the guide-wire and into the artery. The guide-wire is longer than the catheter and protrudes from its back end once the catheter tip reaches beyond its front end (Fig. 15.24). It can then be removed, leaving the catheter safely in the artery (Fig. 15.24E). Saline can now be perfused through the catheter exactly as with needle puncture.

The catheter can now be pushed along the artery to any desired level. In tortuous or atheromatous arteries it may be necessary to use special guides with more flexible tips in order to advance catheters through difficult areas.

Saline infusion of the catheter is maintained either by slow hand injection or by an automatic drip system. Unless contraindicated for clinical reasons, heparinised saline is routinely used to counteract any tendency to clot formation in or around the catheter tip.

Anaesthesia

Most angiographic procedures can be carried out under local anaesthesia, but basal sedation may be necessary with the more complex investigations. Some drugs such as pethidine are more likely than others to produce a hypotensive reaction and must therefore be used with caution, particularly if arterial stenosis is suspected. Hypotension can precipitate thrombosis in such patients.

General anaesthesia is usually necessary with children, and may be required with difficult or very nervous patients or those unable to cooperate. Besides prolonging the investigation and increasing its cost, it undoubtedly adds to the hazards because, apart from the added complications of general anaesthesia, the patient is unable to react to misplaced injections or other mishaps. With a conscious patient, symptoms and untoward reactions are at once apparent, and the procedure can be stopped immediately.

Contrast media

The earliest vascular contrast media mentioned above were far from ideal. They included lipiodol injected into veins in small quantity (Sicard & Forestier 1923), and strontium bromide (Berberich & Hirsch 1923) and sodium iodide (Brooks 1924), which were the first contrast agents injected into arteries. Thorium dioxide (Thorotrast) was used by Moniz (1931) and became the standard medium in the 1930s. Unfortunately it was retained indefinitely by the reticuloendothelial system, and being radioactive gave rise to delayed malignancy. Abdominal films taken years after injection showed a characteristic stippling in the spleen resembling miliary calcification.

Organic iodide preparations stemmed from the work of Swick (1929), who developed uroselectan (Iopax) (containing one atom of iodine per molecule) as a reliable agent for intravenous urography. Later, organic iodines were developed, first with two and then with three atoms of iodine per molecule. The standard media widely used in the 1970s and 1980s were Hypaque, Conray and Triosil.

It was estimated that over 50 million doses of iodinated contrast media per annum were currently used worldwide in radiological practice, and they represented a major item in the operating expenses of most radiological departments.

The ideal contrast medium should be completely non-toxic and completely painless to the patient in the high concentrations used for angiography. A further advance toward this ideal was the introduction in the 1980s of *low-osmolality* contrast media. These agents are relatively painless, compared with their high-osmolar predecessors, and are claimed to produce fewer toxic side-effects. Both these benefits are related to the low osmolality, which is closer to that of normal plasma than was that of their predecessors. At an iodine concentration of 280 mg/ml the osmolality measures about 480 mmol/kg H_2O. This compares with 1500 mmol/kg H_2O for the equivalent Conray (high-osmolar) preparation and 300 mmol/kg H_2O for plasma (Table 15.1).

Further low-osmolality contrast media introduced in recent years include the non-ionic monomers Ultravist (iopromide) from Schering; and Iomeron (iomeprol) from Bracco (Italy). Also recently introduced are Isovist (iotrolan) by Schering, a dimeric non-ionic low-osmolar contrast medium, and Visipaque (iodixanol)—also an isotonic non-ionic dimer—from Nycomed.

Osmolality is proportional to the ratio of iodine atoms to the number of particles in solution. In the older hyperosmolar contrast media, this ratio was 3 : 2, whereas the new low-osmolar agents have a ratio of 3 : 1 and do not ionise in solution. Ioxaglate, which is a monoacid dimer, does ionise in solution but has a similar iodine : particle ratio (6 : 2 or effectively 3 : 1) and therefore enjoys the same benefits of low osmolality. To date the only drawback to the new media is that they cost a good deal more than their predecessors, and this remains an important factor inhibiting their more widespread use.

Dosage

Peripheral and smaller arteries As a general principle, the dose of contrast medium injected is related to the flow rate in the vessel being injected. Small vessels with low flow rates require small amounts at low pressures, while large vessels with high flow rates require larger volumes at high pressures. The recommended doses for different smaller arteries are listed in Table 15.2, and in most

Table 15.1 Low osmolar non-ionic contrast media

Product	Iodine atoms : particles in solution	Iodine conc. (mg/ml)	Osmolality (mOsm/kg)	Viscosity at 37°C (mPa/s)
Iopamidol (Niopam, Bracco)	3 : 1	150		
		200		2.7
		300		4.7
		340		
		370		8.6
Iohexol (Omnipaque, Nycomed)	3 : 1	140	290	1.5
		180	360	2.0
		240	510	3.3
		300	640	6.1
		350	780	10.6
Iopromide (Ultravist, Schering)	3 : 1	150	340	
		240	480	
		300	620	
		370	780	
Iomeprol (Iomeron, Bracco)		150		
		200		
		250		
		300		
		350		
		400		
Iodixanol (Visipaque, Nycomed)	6 : 1	150	290	1.7
		270	290	5.8
		320	290	11.4
Iotrolan (Isovist, Schering)	6 : 1	240	270	
		300	320	

Table 15.2 Contrast media doses

Type of examination	Contrast medium conc. (mg/ml)	Volume (ml)	Rate (ml/sc)
Thoracic aorta	350–370	40	20
Abdominal aorta	350–370	30	15
Lumbar aorta	300	25	7
Femoral artery	300	10	Hand
Subclavian artery	300	15	Hand
Carotid artery	300	10	Hand
Renal artery	300	10	Hand
Coeliac artery	300	30	5
Sup. mesenteric artery	300	30	5
Inferior mesenteric artery	300	10	Hand
Other arteries	300	2–5	Hand
IV DSA	350–370	40	20

Note: Ionic contrast media, including ioxaglate (Hexabrix) should no longer be used.

arteries the recommended dose can safety he repeated after a short interval. In each case the injection is made in about 1–2 s.

Of the high-osmolar contrast media, we regarded Urografin 310 as the best for cerebral angiography and Triosil 370 as preferable for coronary angiography, as there is experimental evidence that these agents are less toxic than other high-osmolar products at these sites. The quantity used for coronary artery injections varies from 4 to 8 ml, depending on the state of the patient and the flow rate in the individual vessel.

As already explained, the new low-osmolar contrast media are preferable to the older high-osmolar products, and should be used routinely whenever cost is not a major inhibiting factor.

Larger arteries

1. **Arch aortography** For injections into the aortic arch, which has the highest flow rate in the body, 40 ml of high-concentration contrast medium is injected by a pressure machine at 20 ml/s. Triosil 370 or 440 and Conray 420 were high-osmolar products widely used for this purpose, though they have now been replaced by the new low-osmolar agents such as iopamidol 370, and iohexol 350.

2. **Abdominal aortography** Whether performed by catheter or by lumbar injection, 30 ml of a high-concentration contrast medium (Iopamidol or iohexol 350), delivered in 1.5–2 s, is regarded as a safe dose for high aortic injection, i.e. above the renal arteries, and provided both kidneys are functioning normally. However, if there is severe renal impairment or only one kidney functioning, caution should be observed, and the dose reduced to a maximum of 20 ml. A similar precaution is necessary if there is an aortic thrombosis present which would result in a higher dose to the kidneys.

For a low aortic injection, i.e. below the renal arteries, 25 ml injected in 1.5 s is usually adequate.

The normal coeliac axis and superior mesenteric arteries both have high flow rates and can tolerate injections of 30 ml of Hypaque 350 or equivalents at one injection. Some workers recommend doses as high as 50 ml where it is desirable to show the portal circulation. Speed of injection, however, is relatively low at 8 ml/s.

As already noted, doses can be substantially reduced for arterial DSA, not IV DSA. These have now largely taken over from direct arteriography, except with interventional techniques.

Contrast medium reactions

Reactions to the intravascular injection of contrast media, whether intravenous or intra-arterial, are not uncommon (about 12% in one major intravenous series using high-osmolar contrast media). Fortunately, the vast majority are trivial or of minor importance. Reactions can be classified as mild, intermediate or severe. The severe complications are in some cases potentially fatal, but formed less than 0.26% of the series just quoted.

The mechanism of these reactions is debated, though many factors have been postulated, including anxiety, histamine and serotonin release, antigen–antibody formation, activation of the complement and coagulation systems, and interruption of the blood–brain barrier.

Mild reactions include sneezing, mild urticaria, nausea and vomiting, conjunctival injection, mild pallor or sweating, limited urticaria or itchy skin rash, feelings of heat or cold, tachycardia or bradycardia, and arm pain following intravenous injections. Recovery is rapid and requires no treatment except reassurance.

Intermediate reactions include widespread urticaria, bronchospasm and laryngospasm, angioneurotic oedema, moderate hypotension, faintness, headache, severe vomiting, rigors, dyspnoea, chest or abdominal pain. Immediate treatment is required but response is rapid.

Severe reactions are rare but can be fatal. They include cardio-pulmonary collapse with severe hypotension, pulmonary oedema, refractory bronchospasm and laryngospasm. Also seen are myocardial ischaemia, tachycardia, bradycardia, other arrhythmias, cardiac arrest, severe collapse, loss of consciousness and oedema of the glottis.

The mortality from hyperosmolar intravenous contrast medium injections is estimated at 1 case per 40 000 injections. Arterial injections probably carry a similar risk.

The risk from the newer low-osmolar media appears to be significantly lower for minor and intermediate reactions (about 3% as against 12%); it also appears to be significantly lower for severe reactions, but is not yet accurately quantified for fatal reactions, where the evidence remains inconclusive.

Risk factors

Major risk factors associated with the use of contrast media include:

1. Allergy, especially asthma
2. Extremes of age (under 1 year and over 60 years)
3. Cardiovascular disease
4. History of previous reactions to contrast medium.

Minor risk factors include diabetes mellitus, dehydration, impaired renal function, haemoglobinopathy and dysproteinaemia. *Drug risks* include β-blocker therapy (predisposes to bronchospasm and other severe reactions), adrenal suppression (patients on steroids require additional steroids before contrast administration) and interleukin-2 therapy (may cause contrast hypersensitivity).

Previous minor reactions to contrast medium are not a contraindication to a repeat examination, but patients with previous severe reactions should be examined by other means. Patients with previous intermediate reactions should be carefully assessed and the examination abandoned or, if essential, only repeated under careful control. This implies pretreatment for 3 days with oral prednisone (50 mg) 8-hourly. Ephedrine (25 mg) and diphenhydramine (50 mg) are also given 1 h before the examination, and only a low-osmolar contrast medium should be used.

Pretesting for allergy with small doses of contrast medium was once widely performed but has now been abandoned as completely unreliable. Fatalities have occurred after previous negative test doses, and test doses have themselves resulted in fatalities.

Treatment

Emergency drugs and equipment should be immediately available wherever contrast media are used. Intermediate and severe reactions usually involve hypotension, which is treated by elevation of the legs and may require rapid intravascular fluid. Oxygen may also need to be administered, and it is essential to distinguish a vaso-vagal reaction (characterised by hypotension with bradycardia) from an allergic or anaphylactoid reaction (characterised by hypotension with tachycardia). The former requires atropine, 0.6–1.2 mg IV, whilst the latter requires epinephrine (adrenaline).

Iodism The radiologist should be aware that free iodine present in contrast media will interfere with the performance of radioactive iodine tests of thyroid function. Salivary gland enlargement ('iodine mumps') may follow several days after the injection, and hyperthyroidism may be induced. Minor skin rashes may also be seen several days after contrast medium administration.

Nephrotoxicity Intravascular contrast media may have a nephrotoxic effect. The pathogenesis is debated but may be multifactorial due to vasoconstriction, a direct toxic effect on tubular cells, and cast formation in tubules with intrarenal obstruction. Acute renal failure due to nephrotoxicity is claimed to occur in 5% of patients with chronic renal failure but in less than 1% of patients with normal function. Clinically the patient may be asymptomatic with rapid recovery, may show non-oliguric renal dysfunction or, rarely, show severe oliguric renal failure.

Risk factors include large doses of contrast medium, dehydration, diabetes mellitus, pre-existing renal insufficiency and multiple myeloma. Caution in administering contrast media is desirable in diabetic patients with impaired renal function, in multiple myeloma patients with Bence Jones proteinuria, and in hyperuricaemic patients. Dehydration is definitely contraindicated in patients at risk.

Pharmacoangiography

In the past the injection of drugs to improve the resolution of vascular tumours was widely used. These were either vasoconstrictors like epinephrine (adrenaline) or vasodilators like tolazoline. Improvements in technique such as DSA and progress in CT and MRA have rendered this procedure obsolete. However the administration of chemotherapeutic drugs and fibrinolysis are still practised by catheter injection.

Hyperventilation can be used in cerebral angiography to produce similar effects, since normal cerebral vessels react to hyperoxaemia and hypocapnia by vasoconstriction while tumour vessels are unaffected. Hyperventilation was performed by the anaesthetist in cerebral angiograms conducted under general anaesthesia.

Complications

Many complications have resulted from arteriography, and these are summarised in Box 15.1. This formidable list of complications emphasises that arteriography should not be undertaken lightly and that it is best performed by radiologists with considerable training and experience in this field. The complication rate is also significantly lower at centres where large numbers of arteriograms are routinely performed than at centres where they are only occasionally seen.

A full discussion of the complications of arteriography will be found in specialist monographs, but attention is drawn below to some of the more important complications.

Damage to arterial walls This may result from a traumatic needle or catheter puncture. Local subintimal stripping may result, particularly if contrast medium or saline is accidentally injected subintimally. In small vessels this can result in actual occlusion and thrombosis (see below). The use of short bevelled needles, together with skill and experience, is the main means of preventing these accidents.

Perivascular injection of contrast medium can also occur, but is relatively harmless apart from local pain and discomfort to the patient being examined under local anaesthesia.

Thrombosis of arteries As just noted, this can result from trauma to the arterial wall at arterial puncture, or from subintimal stripping

---

Box 15.1	Complications of contrast arteriography

A. *General*
1. Contrast reactions
   a. Severe life-threatening
   b. Intermediate
   c. Minor (coughing, sneezing, mild, urticaria)
2. Embolus
   a. Catheter clot
   b. Cholesterol
   c. Cotton fibre
   d. Air
3. Septicaemia
4. Vagal inhibition

B. *Local*
1. Puncture site
   a. Haemorrhage and haematoma
   b. False aneurysm
   c. Arteriovenous fistula
   d. Perivascular or subintimal contrast injection
   e. Local thrombosis
   f. Local infection
   g. Damage to adjacent nerves
2. Damage to target or other organs due to
   a. Excess of contrast
   b. Catheter clot embolus
3. Fracture and loss of guide-wire tip
4. Knot formation in catheters
5. Embolisation accidents (see below)
6. Angioplasty accidents (see below)

---

from injections of contrast medium or saline with formation of a local dissecting aneurysm. Another well-documented mechanism is formation of clot at the end of a catheter. This is then stripped off as the catheter is withdrawn through the puncture hole and forms a focus for local thrombosis. Another causative or contributory factor is a severe hypotensive reaction (see below). Whatever mechanism or combination of mechanisms is responsible, there is also a direct relationship with the experience of the operator and with the adequacy of the patient's cardiovascular system. Patients with cardiovascular insufficiency and severely atheromatous vessels are at greater risk, and should only be examined by experienced operators.

Systemic heparinisation This is generally recommended to counter catheter clot formation and thrombosis. As soon as the catheter has been passed into the aorta, 3000 units of heparin are injected. The procedure is useful in prolonged catheterisation procedures, and rarely causes any problem. If there is excessive oozing from the puncture site at completion, heparinisation can be reversed by injecting 10 mg of protamine sulfate per 1000 units of heparin used.

Allergy The minor allergic contrast reactions (see above) rarely give rise to concern, and patients can be reassured that sneezing, coughing or urticaria will rapidly subside. However, radiologists must be aware of the danger of the very rare major hypersensitivity reaction, and be prepared for its prompt treatment. This requires dexamethasone 10–20 mg IV, and if necessary artificial respiration with positive pressure and oxygen. For oedema of the glottis, 0.5 mg of epinephrine (adrenaline) subcutaneously or intramuscularly is recommended, together with slow intravenous injection of an antihistamine. Arrangements should also be ready beforehand for the emergency treatment of such catastrophies as cardiac arrest, ventricular fibrillation and collapse with circulatory insufficiency.

Hypotension Severe hypotensive reactions may occur with any arteriographic procedure, but particularly with complex or prolonged investigations. Blood pressure should be monitored, and it should be remembered that patients with vascular disease, particularly atheromatous stenosis, may have lesions in many vessels and that hypotension can precipitate a thrombosis. Coronary infarction or hemiplegia from a carotid thrombosis are potential complications.

Hypotension has also been recorded several hours after a major procedure and the patient must be monitored on the ward for several hours after arteriography.

Catheter clot embolus Clot may form in and around the tip of a catheter, particularly during a prolonged procedure, and such a clot may be detached by a contrast medium injection. The main danger is with catheters lying in or proximal to the cerebral vessels, when detached clot may be directed to the brain. Left ventriculography, coronary arteriography, arch aortography and 'headhunter' catheterisation of the cerebral and subclavian vessels are all procedures that carry this risk. The use of small catheters and speedy and skilled angiography help to minimise the risk, as does systemic heparinisation.

Cholesterol embolisation This may occur spontaneously in patients with severe atheromatous disease. It may also occur after surgery, and is occasionally precipitated by arterial catheterisation. A large shower of cholesterol crystals can produce disastrous results, particularly if vital organs are involved. Postmortem studies suggest that minor degrees of cholesterol crystal embolism are commoner than is generally appreciated.

Air embolus Undoubtedly air embolus has been a cause of fatalities in the past, particularly when large steel syringes were used for major injections. Air could easily enter a large opaque syringe and could be injected without the operator being aware of the mishap, especially if the nozzle was horizontal or pointing upwards. Even with the translucent plastic syringes now in general use, great care must be taken not to include air when loading with contrast medium or saline solution, and all injections should be made with the nozzle pointing down.

Haematomas and false aneurysms The occurrence of these at the puncture site should be relatively uncommon, provided small needles are used and the tips of larger catheters are well tapered. They are seen most frequently with hypertensive patients. After an arterial puncture, firm manual pressure transmitted through gauze swabs should be maintained on the puncture site until all oozing has stopped. The puncture site should also be inspected before the patient leaves the department (an hour or two later) and the following morning, and the patient warned to report immediately if there is any further swelling or oozing.

False aneurysms (pulsating haematomas) will require surgical treatment.

It is important to ensure that any patient is taken off anticoagulant drugs before arteriography and that the prothrombin time has fallen to normal before the investigation.

Damage to nerves Transaxillary catheterisation carries the particular risk of damage to branches of the brachial plexus since the artery is closely related to its distal part. This can result in severe disability. Most of the reported cases were due to nerve compression by haematomas or false aneurysms, though direct damage by needle puncture may be responsible in some cases. Transaxillary catheterisation should only be undertaken by senior and experienced angiographers, and observation for signs of haematoma or nerve damage should be maintained for 24 h after the investigation. If symptoms of paresis appear and progress, they are usually due to compression by a haematoma, and urgent surgical decompression of the neurovascular sheath is essential if permanent paralysis is to be prevented.

Femoral nerve palsy is a much rarer complication of femoral artery puncture, though transient pain or paraesthesia in the cutaneous distribution of the femoral nerve is not uncommon but is usually resolved within 24 h.

Vagal inhibition This may occur after a major contrast medium injection, and has been encountered after intravenous urography and intravenous cholangiography. It is characterised by collapse of the patient with bradycardia. This helps to distinguish it from circulatory collapse in acute allergy, which is usually associated with tachycardia. The distinction is of vital importance, since the latter is often treated with epinephrine (adrenaline), a drug which is contraindicated in vagal inhibition, where atropine is the drug of choice and may be life-saving.

Damage to organs Because angiography often targets vital organs, including the heart, brain, kidneys and bowel, it is not surprising that damage to such organs can result, followed by death or serious morbidity. In most cases the cause has been arterial thrombosis from the causes mentioned above, or organ damage from an excessive dose of contrast medium.

Non-fatal brain damage has resulted in hemiplegia, both transient and permanent. Cortical blindness—occasionally permanent, but fortunately in most cases transient—has resulted from vertebral angiography.

Spinal cord damage is a rare and tragic complication of arteriography, usually due to an excessive dose of contrast medium entering a main artery of supply to the spinal cord. Thus, paraplegia has been recorded after both lumbar and abdominal aortography, presumably from injection of the artery of Adamkewicz which supplies the cord from T8 downward and arises from one of the upper lumbar or lower intercostal arteries.

Tetraplegia has resulted from vertebral angiography and from thyroid axis angiography. In the latter case, an excess of contrast medium has entered the deep cervical artery which supplies the cervical cord. It has been suggested that such cases should be treated by replacement of cerebrospinal fluid with isotonic saline and by systemic steroids, though others doubt the value of this.

Coronary angiography This carries the special dangers of vagal inhibition, ventricular fibrillation, cardiac systole and myocardial infarction. All of these are potentially fatal unless immediate treatment is at hand.

Embolisation and angioplasty These carry special hazards which are discussed later in this chapter.

Indications for arteriography
Vascular lesions

The vascular lesions investigated by angiography will be discussed under the following headings:

1. Congenital
2. Aneurysms
3. Stenoses and thromboses
4. Arteritis
5. Trauma
6. Embolus
7. Angiomatous malformation
8. Arteriovenous fistula
9. Haemorrhage
10. Masses and tumours.

Trauma may lead to aneurysm, thrombosis or arteriovenous fistula. Arteritis can also lead to aneurysm or thrombosis.

Congenital

Congenital anomalies of the arterial system are not uncommon. Those involving the aortic origin and the ascending aorta have been described in Chapter 14. The major coronary abnormalities are also discussed in the cardiac chapter (see Ch. 13). Anomalies of the great vessels are noted in the neuroradiology chapter (see Ch. 55), as are the commoner anomalies of the cerebral arteries. Anatomical variations of the peripheral arterial system are well described in anatomical texts, but some of those with clinical implications will be noted here.

The brachial artery occasionally divides into its radial and ulnar branches at a high level, and this had some practical importance when brachial arteriography was more widely practised. In the lower limb the popliteal artery sometimes divides into its anterior and posterior tibial branches above the knee joint. The femoral artery, which normally arises from the external iliac, may occasionally be replaced by a large branch of the dilated hypogastric artery passing through the greater sciatic notch and behind the femoral neck, the so-called persistent *primitive sciatic artery*. In these cases the true femoral artery is hypoplastic and may terminate in the profunda femoris. Congenital anomalies of the renal supply are very common, and some 25% of kidneys have an accessory artery supplying them. For this reason arteriography is performed on live renal donors to check that the proposed kidney is suitable for grafting. Occasionally three renal arteries are found, but four arteries are very rarely seen. Horseshoe and ectopic kidneys frequently have accessory arteries, often arising from the aortic bifurcation or iliac artery.

Anomalies of the arterial supply to the liver are also frequently seen. The classical anatomical description of the common hepatic artery arising from the coeliac axis and dividing into right and left hepatic arteries is only seen in some 50% of cases. Some 20% have a right hepatic artery or an accessory right hepatic arising from the superior mesenteric artery. A further 20% have a left hepatic or accessory left hepatic artery arising from the left gastric artery. In about 2% of patients the common hepatic artery arises from the superior mesenteric.

Other major branches of the coeliac axis, i.e. the splenic and left gastric arteries, may sometimes arise directly from the aorta.

The bronchial arteries which arise on the anterior surface of the aorta just below the level of the carina are double on the left in 60% of cases and on the right in 30%.

Coarctation of the aorta *(Fig. 15.25)* The condition has been described above, in Chapter 14. Poststenotic aneurysm occurs as a complication in some 4% of cases (see Fig. 15.38). In addition, it should be realised that the condition may occur at more distal sites

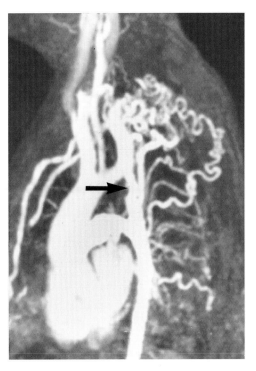

Fig. 15.25 MRA. Coarctation of the descending thoracic aorta distal to the left subclavian artery (arrow) with hypertrophied collateral vessels in the chest wall.

than the classic level in the distal arch, and can involve the lower thoracic or abdominal aorta. So-called abdominal coarctation usually affects the upper abdominal aorta, and may involve a short or long segment. Splanchnic vessels and the renal artery origins may also be involved in the lesion (Fig. 15.26).

Pseudocoarctation Pseudocoarctation or lateral buckling of the aortic arch is an unusual condition which can simulate a rounded mass in the region of the aortic knuckle. There is a sharp kink in the aorta at the junction of the arch and descending aorta in the region of the ligamentum arteriosum. Buckling of the aorta may also occur in the mid-arch, and this is best identified in the lateral view.

Hypoplasia of the aorta This is sometimes encountered as a chance finding. It may be associated with Marfan's syndrome, where there is a mesodermal defect and medial degeneration of the aorta. However, in Marfan's syndrome the aorta will eventually dilate because of the medial defect, and dissecting aneurysms may develop, particularly in the ascending aorta.

Aneurysms

Aneurysms can be classified on an aetiological basis as follows:

1. Congenital
2. Infective
3. Degenerative
4. Traumatic
5. Dissecting
6. Necrotising vasculitis
7. Poststenotic.

Congenital aneurysms These are commonest in the intracranial vessels, where they have in the past been termed 'congenital berry aneurysms'. While these aneurysms are basically due to a defect in

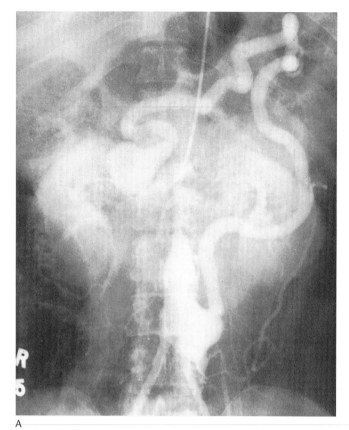

A

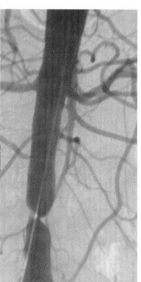

B

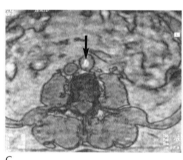

C

Fig. 15.26 (A) Abdominal coarctation with involvement of the superior mesenteric origin. There is a collateral circulation through the artery of Drummond from the left colic branch of the inferior mesenteric to the middle colic branch of the superior mesenteric. Owing to the increased flow, aneurysms have developed at both ends of the collateral. (Courtesy of Dr R. Eban.) (B and C) DSA and 2D time of flight MRI showing lower abdominal aortic stenosis.

the muscular coat at points of arterial bifurcation, it is clear from clinical experience that other factors such as age, atheroma and hypertension are also important in their pathogenesis, as is the fact that they usually arise where the arteries lie in the subarachnoid space unsupported by surrounding soft tissues. They are discussed in more detail in Chapter 55. Congenital aneurysms have been described elsewhere in the body but are relatively rare, a fact which supports the importance of the local cerebral anatomy in their aetiology.

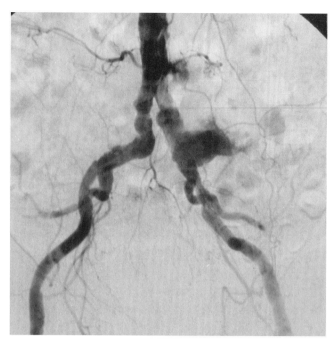

Fig. 15.27 Mycotic aneurysm of left common iliac artery in a patient with salmonella septicaemia.

Infective aneurysms Infective aneurysms may be classified as mycotic or syphilitic. *Mycotic aneurysms* are nearly always secondary to bacterial endocarditis. They may involve any artery in the body, and we have encountered examples in the abdomen and pelvis, in the brain and in the limbs (Fig. 15.27). They can grow in size very rapidly and usually require urgent surgery to prevent rupture. Mycotic aneurysms are occasionally secondary to involvement of the arterial wall by an adjacent infection such as a pyogenic or tuberculous abscess.

Syphilitic aneurysms were once extremely common, but with the advent of antibiotics they are now rarely seen in developed countries. They can involve arteries in any part of the body but are commonest in the ascending aorta and arch, where they can reach a large size (Fig. 15.28). Angiography is usually required as a prelude to surgery with most mycotic aneurysms, though the diagnosis can be made with non-invasive imaging in most areas. CT or MRI will characterise large thoracic aneurysms, which can simulate mediastinal masses at simple radiography.

Degenerative aneurysms Degenerative aneurysms result from atheroma. They are commoner in males, and are seen most frequently in the abdominal aorta (see Fig. 15.14). Other common sites are the iliacs and the popliteal arteries (Figs 15.29, 15.30A,B). They are also becoming more frequent in the thoracic aorta, where they have replaced syphilis as the main type of aneurysm in developed countries. Degenerative thoracic aneurysms affect mainly the descending aorta and distal arch, and rarely involve the ascending aorta. Atheromatous aneurysms may also occur in the splenic artery, in the renal artery, and in cerebral arteries, including the internal carotid and basilar arteries, where they can be fusiform or saccular. Atheroma is also thought to be a major contributory factor to the development of the smaller so-called 'congenital' berry aneurysms.

Degenerative aneurysms are often fusiform, resulting in generalised dilatation of the artery, but they may become saccular, particularly in the sites of election mentioned above. Such saccular

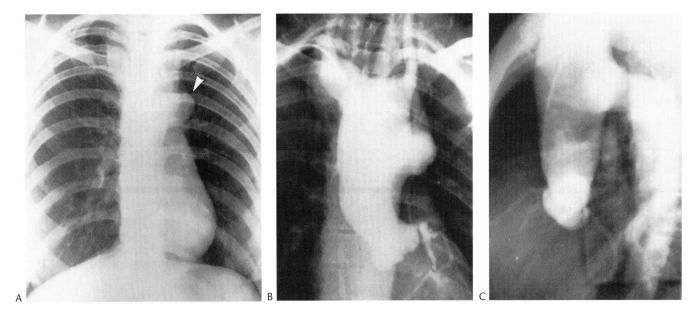

Fig. 15.28   (A) Chest film showing aortic knuckle (arrow) apparently displaced downward by a supra-aortic mass. (B,C) Angiograms showing that this is due to an aneurysm of the arch and innominate artery.

aneurysms may rupture with disastrous or even fatal consequences. They may also form a nidus for intraluminal clot which can embolise to more distal vessels.

Imaging *Simple radiography* often shows characteristic curved linear calcification in the wall of large aortic aneurysms or of atheromatous aneurysms at other sites.

Ultrasound is the simplest method of confirming a suspected diagnosis of abdominal aortic aneurysm (see Fig. 15.1) and monitoring any growth. It can also be used to diagnose popliteal and other peripheral aneurysms.

CT has the advantage of showing both the lumen and the extent of any intraluminal clot. It can also show evidence of leakage and the important relationship of the renal arteries to the upper limit of an abdominal aneurysm. Direct measurement of the aneurysm in all planes is possible. CT can also characterise the so-called 'inflamma-

tory aneurysm' (see Figs 15.3–15.10) or perianeurysmal fibrosis. This has a thickened irregular and enhancing wall, probably due to slow periarterial haemorrhage, and should be differentiated from retroperitoneal fibrosis.

MRI can also easily define large aneurysms and their relationships as well as imaging them in all planes.

Traumatic aneurysms

These can occur wherever an arterial wall is subject to injury (Fig. 15.30C). Such aneurysms are commonest in the limbs, but can occur in the thorax, abdomen, and head and neck. They may follow direct penetrating injury from a knife, missile or foreign body, or they may result from closed injury. Trauma to the femoral artery in the groin is a well-recognised occupational hazard in the butchering trade.

Traumatic aneurysm of the aortic arch is a frequent and potentially fatal result of chest injury in automobile accidents. It can easily be missed, with disastrous results, if not specifically suspected and looked for, as many of these patients have multiple injuries. The shearing effect of an acute deceleration injury usually involves the distal arch in the region of the ligamentum arteriosum. In most cases the injury is rapidly fatal, but some 20% of cases survive the acute episode by the formation of a periaortic haematoma and false aneurysm or because the adventitia has not yet ruptured.

It is vital to recognise these cases because secondary rupture will follow within 24 h in 30%, and within a week in most of the remainder. Only 2% will survive to chronic aneurysm formation, according to a study of 262 cases at the American Armed Forces Institute of Pathology.

Imaging *Simple chest X-ray* may show broadening of the mediastinum, but this will be difficult to assess on portable or emergency films. *CT* may show periaortic haemorrhage.

Aortography will show the false aneurysm, usually near the isthmus (Figs 15.31, 15.32), but the signs may be more subtle,

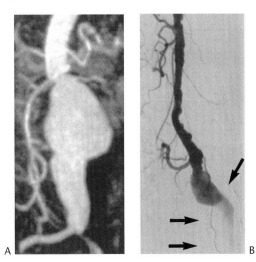

Fig. 15.29   (A) MRA. AAA and left common iliac artery stenosis. (B) DSA. Right popliteal artery aneurysm.

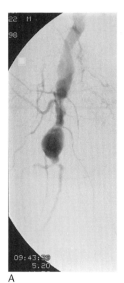
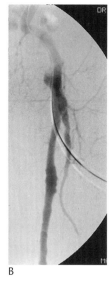
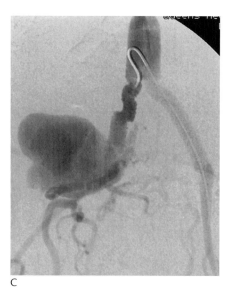

A   B   C

Fig. 15.30 DSA. (A,B) Bilateral common femoral and right deep femoral artery aneurysms and occlusion of right superficial femoral artery. (C) Aorto–bi-iliac Dacron graft with false aneurysm at distal anastomosis of right limb and occlusion of right external iliac artery.

consisting merely of an intimal flap or mural irregularity at the site of the tear. A small ductus diverticulum may occur near this site but should be differentiated by its smooth wall and inferomedial position.

Dissecting aneurysms

Dissecting aneurysms are mainly encountered in the aorta, and hypertension is the main predisposing cause. The incidence in the USA has been estimated at 5–10 cases annually per million population. Men are mostly affected, usually aged between 50 and

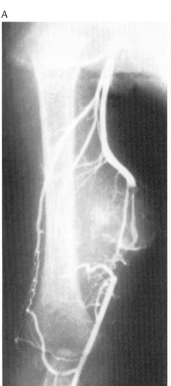

A

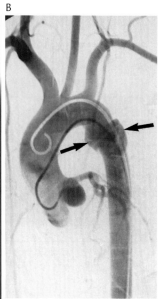

B

Fig. 15.31 (A) Traumatic false aneurysm with rupture of the brachial artery in a child, following a fall while carrying a glass milk bottle. (B) Traumatic false aneurysm of aortic arch.

70 years. Only 5% of cases are under 40 years, and these are usually associated with rare causes such as Marfan's syndrome or, in women, with pregnancy. Other rare associations are with coarctation, aortic stenosis and bicuspid aortic valves.

Dissections usually commence in the aortic arch or ascending aorta and extend distally. De Bakey has classified them into three groups (Fig. 15.33). Type I commences in the ascending aorta and extends through the arch and descending aorta to the iliacs. Type II commences in the ascending aorta but does not extend beyond the arch. Type III commences in the distal arch and extends down to the iliacs.

Type II is the least common and is often associated with Marfan's syndrome. It forms 10% of the cases, with types I and III representing 45% each.

From the surgical viewpoint a more practical classification is into two groups: type A, including all cases involving the ascending aorta (i.e. type I and II above), and type B, including those not involving the ascending aorta (i.e. type III above); the former are best treated surgically and the latter medically (see below).

The clinical features in classical cases are well known, and include sudden agonising pain in the chest. It is important to realise, however, that many cases are atypical and easily missed or misdiagnosed, as symptoms may vary considerably depending on the aortic branches involved. Hemiplegia and vertebral symptoms may result from involvement of great vessels and their cerebral branches. Paraplegia can follow occlusion of intercostal or lumbar arteries supplying the cord. In the abdomen the coeliac axis and mesenteric arteries can be affected, giving rise to abdominal pain, mesenteric ischaemia or pancreatitis. Renal artery occlusion may precipitate acute hypertension or anuria. The iliac vessels may be obstructed with lower-limb ischaemia. Retrograde spread of the dissection in the ascending aorta can lead to coronary involvement, causing cardiac ischaemia or rupture into the pericardium with cardiac tamponade.

Dissecting aneurysms carry a grave prognosis: 30% are fatal within 24 h and a further 50% of sufferers die in the next few days or weeks. Only 20% are likely to survive beyond 6 weeks, and half of these will die later from rupture of the aneurysm. Some of the late survivals are associated with a large re-entry of the dissection into the true lumen in the lower abdominal aorta, giving rise to the

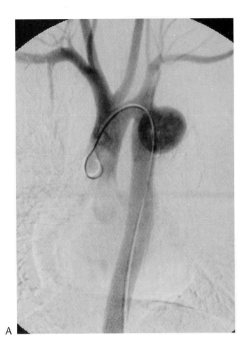
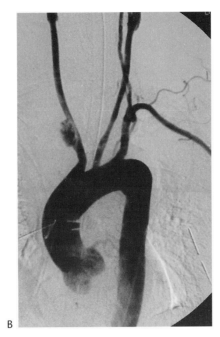
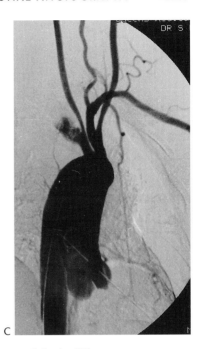

Fig. 15.32 DSA studies. (A) Traumatic false aneurysm of the arch following RTA. (B,C) Ruptured innominate artery following RTA.

so-called 'double-bore' aorta. We have diagnosed cases of this type by aortography, where the true diagnosis was completely unsuspected by the referring physician.

The best prognosis rests with type III cases not involving the ascending aorta, and present opinion favours medical treatment in these, since the survival rate is not significantly affected by surgery. However, surgery is recommended for types I and II or group A, which involve the ascending aorta. In one series of group A cases treated surgically, survival was 64% as against a medically treated survival rate of 22%. There is thus some urgency in establishing the diagnosis and case type as rapidly as possible.

Imaging *Simple radiographs* of the chest may show widening of the mediastinum, though this may be difficult to assess on portable films. More characteristic is localised dilatation of the aortic

knuckle and upper descending aorta, which may give rise to a prominent 'hump' sign due to lateral projection of the knuckle. Lateral and anterior displacement of the trachea has also been described, and the descending aorta often bulges to the left and is sometimes lobulated. A recent chest film, if available, is most helpful, as a change in contour then becomes obvious. Medial displacement of the calcified intima at the aortic knuckle has been described but is rarely clear cut, and a pleural effusion (haemothorax) is present in about 20% of cases. In patients with Marfan's syndrome, localised bulging of the ascending aorta to the right may be recognised.

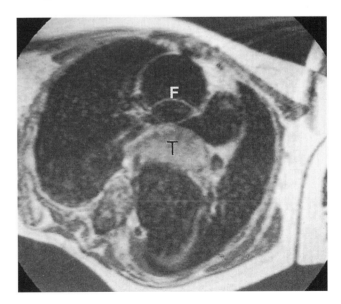

Fig. 15.34 Axial MRI section of thorax shows a dissecting aneurysm. In the ascending aorta both lumens are patent and separated by an intimal flap (F). In the descending aorta the false lumen contains thrombus (T). (Courtesy of Dr Peter Wilde and Bristol MRI Centre.)

I II III

Fig. 15.33 Types of dissecting aneurysms (see text).

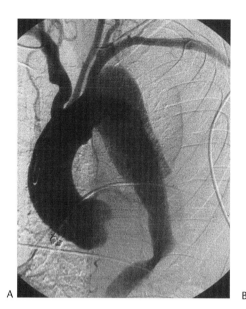
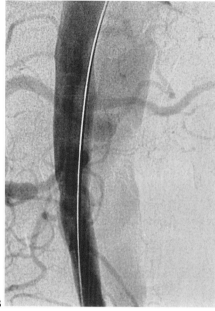
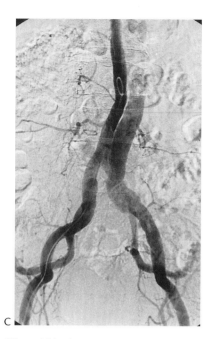

Fig. 15.35   DSA. (A–C) Type B dissecting aneurysm of descending thoracic and abdominal aorta with filling of false lumen in aortic arch and left common iliac artery and occlusion of left renal artery.

Arteriography   Arteriography has been widely used in the past to confirm the diagnosis of dissecting aneurysm (see previous edition). However modern CT and MR apparatus can provide diagnostic angiograms using minimal invasive techniques (Fig. 15.34; see also Figs 15.10, 15.11). MRI can also provide coronal sagittal and oblique longitudinal views of a dissection (see Figs 25.000 and 25.000). Modern CT apparatus can provide similar images (Fig. 15.12).

Another alternative which is less invasive than direct catheterisation is DSA as in Figure 15.35.

The thoracic aorta is the commonest site for dissection but the lesion is occasionally encountered in more peripheral vessels. We have encountered examples in the abdominal aorta, the iliacs and the renal arteries. Localised dissection in the internal carotid artery is also well documented (See Ch. 55).

Iatrogenic arterial dissection as a complication of angiography has been mentioned above. Such events are usually minor in degree and resolve spontaneously, particularly where they are produced by retrograde catheterisation so that blood flow flattens rather than fills the intimal flap.

Necrotising vasculitis

The mysterious disease *polyarteritis nodosa* is associated with necrotising vasculitis. The process involves the walls of small vessels, and as the disease progresses these weaken and aneurysms develop. The nodose lesions have a predilection for arterial bifurcations, but can occur anywhere along the artery. Any artery in the body may be involved, including the vasa vasorum, which accounts for the protean clinical manifestations.

The kidneys are very frequently involved and hypertension is seen in 70% of cases. Multiple small aneurysms may be identified at angiography and are characteristic, though not always seen (Fig. 15.36). The small aneurysms can rupture, giving rise to perirenal haematomas. Aneurysms of other splanchnic vessels can also rupture, leading to retroperitoneal or other abdominal haemor-

rhages. The demonstration of multiple small aneurysms is almost diagnostic, so that renal and visceral angiography is a valuable tool.

Other rarer causes of similar small aneurysms are *Wegener's granulomatosis* and *systemic lupus erythematosus. Atrial myxoma* embolisation can also give rise to small peripheral aneurysms, as can necrotising arteritis resulting from abuse of drugs, particularly *metamphetamine. Acute pancreatitis* may involve small vessels adjacent to the pancreas and lead to aneurysms which can rupture with serious consequences (Fig. 15.37).

Aneurysm of a coronary artery is a well-recognised complication of *Kawasaki's disease.* This mysterious condition first characterised

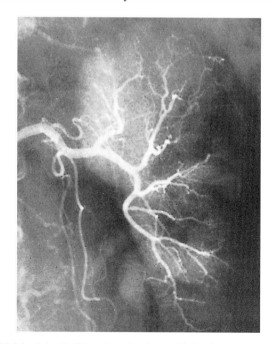

Fig. 15.36   Polyarteritis nodosa showing multiple microaneurysms.

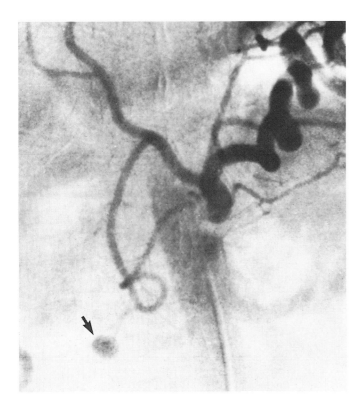

Fig. 15.37 Aneurysm of the pancreaticoduodenal arcade (arrow) secondary to acute pancreatitis (subtraction film).

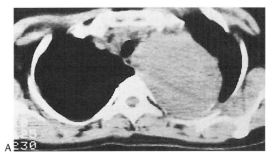

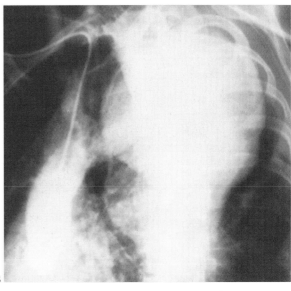

Fig. 15.38 (A) CT of a large mediastinal mass presenting in a young woman. (B) Transaxillary aortogram confirms giant poststenotic aneurysm and previously unrecognised mild coarctation.

in Japan is now being increasingly diagnosed in America and Europe. It presents in young children with pyrexia, a rash, conjunctivitis, and later swollen hands and feet with sloughing of the palms and soles. Early diagnosis is vital as treatment with gamma-globulin in the first 10 days can prevent the development of aneurysms.

Poststenotic aneurysms

These are probably due to turbulence and eddy flows affecting the vessel wall distal to the arterial stenosis. They are a well-recognised complication of coarctation, occurring in some 4% of cases (Fig. 15.38). They may also be seen in the subclavian artery in the thoracic inlet syndrome (see below), and in the renal artery with fibromuscular hyperplasia. They can also complicate atheromatous stenosis in any artery.

Stenoses and thromboses

Congenital stenoses Congenital stenoses of major arteries as in thoracic and abdominal coarctation of the aorta have been described above. Abdominal coarctation may also involve the origins of splanchnic or renal arteries. Congenital stenoses have also been described in other vessel, including the pulmonary arteries.

Extrinsic pressure Pressure from tumours, cysts or other masses can also involve arteries and obstruct flow; in these cases the cause is usually obvious. Less commonly, localised arterial obstruction is due to a fibrous band, as may sometimes occur in the thoracic inlet syndrome, in renal artery stenosis or in the coeliac compression syndrome. An anomalous tendon can obstruct the popliteal artery in popliteal entrapment, as can a developmental cyst in the popliteal wall (see below).

Arteritis Arteritis of inflammatory or unknown aetiology may also lead to arterial stenosis, as in Takayasu's disease.

Atheroma This is far and away the commonest cause of arterial stenosis and thrombosis in clinical practice, and, depending on the site, can give rise to a variety of clinical syndromes. It is found most often in males, though females are also frequently affected, particularly in the older age groups. Lesions of the greatest clinical importance involve:

1. Internal carotid and vertebral origins, giving rise to transient ischaemic attacks and cerebrovascular insufficiency (see Ch. 55)
2. Coronary artery lesions causing cardiac ischaemia (see Ch. 13)
3. Renal arteries, with resulting hypertension
4. The abdominal aorta
5. Iliac and femoral arteries.

Intermittent claudication is the cardinal symptom of stenosis and thrombosis of the aorta, iliacs and femorals. Atheromatous stenosis also involves the major vessels to the upper limb, but is of less clinical significance because of the excellent collateral circulation.

Atheromatous stenosis of the abdominal aorta is frequently seen, as is its successor aortic thrombosis (Leriches' syndrome). Lesions usually commence near the aortic bifurcation, and thrombosis

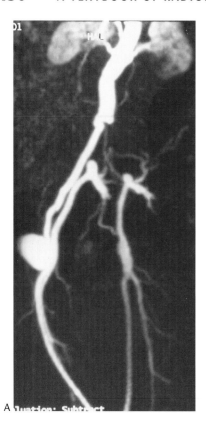

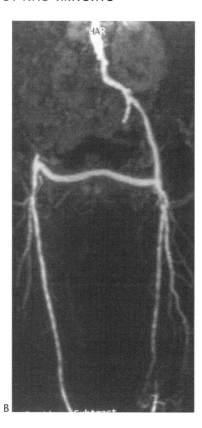

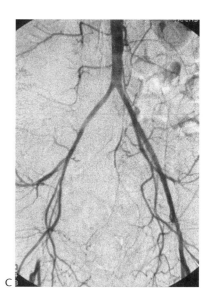

Fig. 15.39 (A) Aorto–bifemoral Dacron graft with occlusion of left limb and false aneurysm at distal anastomosis of right limb (MRA). (B) Occlusion of right common and external iliac arteries and patent left to right femoro–femoral Dacron crossover graft (MRA). (C) Occlusion of right external iliac and common femoral artery following the use of a device to seal the arterial puncture site after a cardiac catheter (DSA)

extends upward, but usually stops short of the renal arteries (see Fig. 15.22). Occasionally the origin of a renal artery is involved, with secondary hypertension ensuing.

The iliacs are among the commonest sites for atheromatous stenosis and thrombosis (Fig. 15.29), as are the femoral and popliteal arteries.

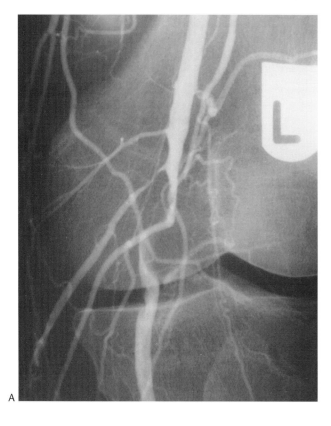

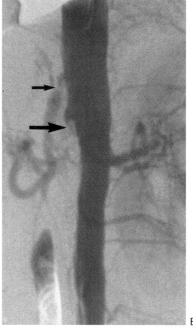

Fig. 15.40 (A) Localised defect in the popliteal artery due to a popliteal cyst. (B) DSA. Coeliac artery stenosis (top arrow) and superior mesenteric artery occlusion (lower arrow).

Dacron grafts are used to replace thrombosed iliacs. Figure 15.39 illustrates bypass and crossover grafts shown by MRA. Figure 15.39A also shows a false aneurysm at the graft junction with the right femoral artery. Iatrogenic trauma is a not uncommon cause of false aneurysms. A true aneurysm retains the outer coat of the vessel wall as boundary. A false aneurysm has ruptured the vessel wall and the haematoma has developed a new capsule being in effect a pulsating haematoma.

So-called 'primary popliteal thrombosis' occurs in young males, and though atheroma at a young age is occasionally responsible, most cases are due to rare congenital anomalies, namely popliteal cysts and popliteal entrapment.

Popliteal cysts These usually present with calf claudication in men with an average age of 36 years. Angiography shows a healthy smooth-walled femoral artery and either a smooth narrowing suggesting external compression or a localised thrombosis in the popliteal artery (Fig. 15.40A). The cyst secretes mucin, and lies in the wall of the artery. It is claimed to be due to developmental inclusion of mucin-secreting synovial capsular cells from the knee joint. Similar lesions have been described in other vessels including the iliac, radial and ulnar arteries. The diagnosis has been made by CT of the popliteal artery, and could also be suggested by ultrasound or MRI.

Popliteal entrapment This also occurs mainly in young males, and may present in boys or adolescents either with calf claudication or, more commonly, acute popliteal thrombosis. The condition is due to an anomalous tendon of the medial head of gastrocnemius passing over and trapping the artery. Angiography shows either a characteristic linear external compression or thrombosis of the popliteal.

Coeliac or superior mesenteric stenoses These stenoses resulting from atheroma are quite common, particularly at the origins of these arteries (Fig. 15.40B). Other causes include fibromuscular hyperplasia and involvement by arteritis as in Takayasu's disease, or by congenital coarctation or external coeliac compression. Such lesions have been cited as causing dyspepsia and other gastrointestinal symptoms. However, it should be realised that the collateral circulation between the splanchnic vessels is so good that even total occlusion of two of the three main vessels (coeliac axis, superior and inferior mesenteric) can be easily tolerated (Fig. 15.41), and the inferior mesenteric is usually occluded in Leriches' syndrome without referrable symptoms.

Coeliac compression syndrome is the term used for gastrointestinal symptoms associated with narrowing of the coeliac at its origin by external compression. This is due either to the median arcuate ligament of the diaphragm or to coeliac plexus fibrosis. As implied above, this is more likely to be a chance association than a true syndrome.

Coronary stenosis and *thrombosis* due to atheroma and their investigation and treatment have been discussed in the cornary chapters.

Renal artery stenosis This is an important and sometimes remediable cause of renal ischaemia and hypertension. Atheroma is the

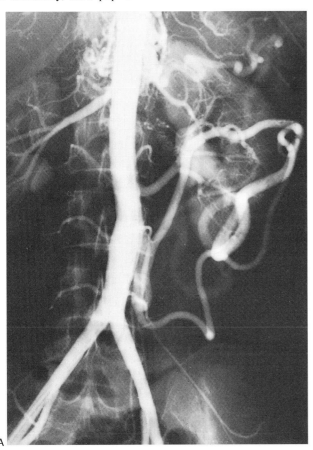 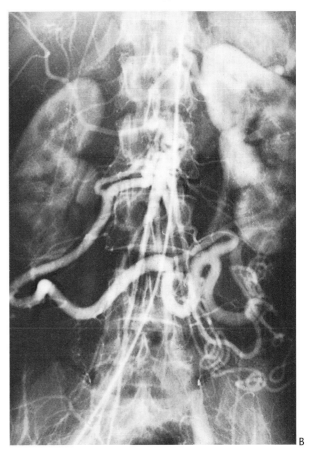

Fig. 15.41 (A) Occlusion of coeliac and superior mesenteric arteries. Separate origin of splenic artery. Artery of Drummond arising from inferior mesenteric. (B) Artery of Drummond supplies the superior mesenteric origin and then the hepatic artery through pancreatic arcades.

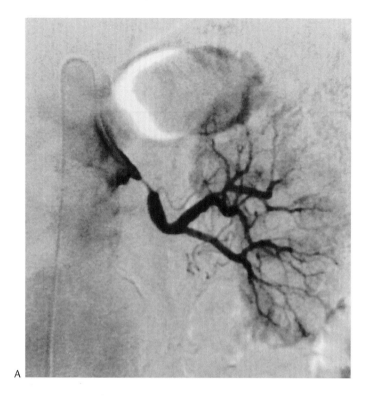

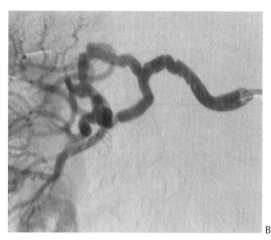

Fig. 15.42 (A) Renal artery stenosis due to atheroma. (B) DSA. Renal artery stenosis due to fibromuscular dysphasia.

main aetiological cause (Fig. 15.42A), but in younger, mainly female, patients fibromuscular hyperplasia is also important (Fig. 15.42B). This is a rare disease of unknown aetiology leading to irregular beading of the vessel; it is discussed further below. Other rare causes of renal artery stenosis include extrinsic pressure by fibrous bands or sympathetic chain fibres, neurofibromatosis, and arterial stretching or compression by tumours. Aortic involvement by abdominal coarctation or by arteritis can also affect the renal artery, as can aortic thrombosis.

Whatever the cause of the renal ischaemia, secondary hypertension may result, and the kidney can develop changes recognisable at both plain X-ray and urography. The affected kidney becomes smaller than normal but remains smooth in contour, unlike the irregular contour of the small kidney of chronic pyelonephritis. At

urography, the excretion of contrast medium is slightly later than from the normal side, but as the investigation proceeds, contrast becomes denser on the affected side and shows small spindly calices.

The radiological treatment of renal artery stenosis by percutaneous angioplasty has been discussed below. The anatomy of renal artery stenosis is best shown by catheter arteriography, but screening for the condition can be accomplished on an outpatient basis by intravenous DSA, spiral CT or MRA.

Subclavian stenosis Compression of the subclavian artery at the root of the neck is seen in the thoracic inlet syndrome, and may be associated with various congenital anomalies. Some, such as cervical rib or an anomalous first rib, will be readily diagnosed on a

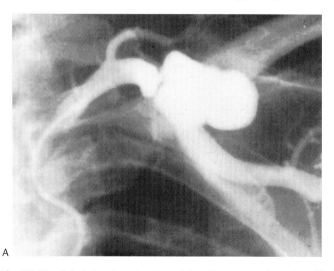

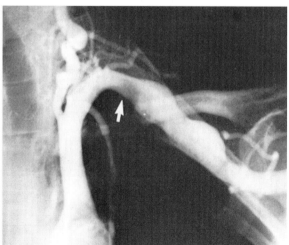

Fig. 15.43 Subclavian stenosis with poststenotic aneurysm formation. (A) Saccular. (B) Fusiform aneurysm.

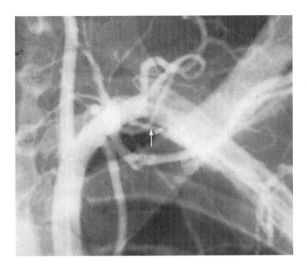

Fig. 15.44 Subclavian thrombosis (arrow).

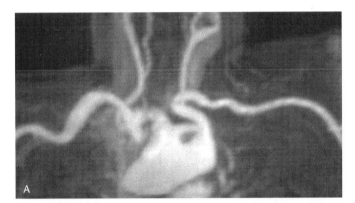

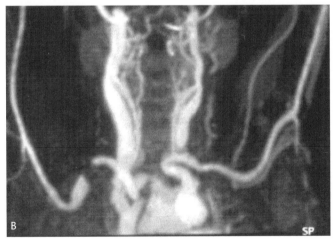

Fig. 15.45 MRA. (A,B) Right subclavian artery aneurysm with arms down, but occlusion due to compression in the thoracic outlet with arms up.

plain film, but others, such as fibrous bands or compression by the scalenus anticus muscle, will only be manifest at angiography.

Clinically these patients may present with ischaemic hands, with Raynaud's phenomenon, or with digital emboli. The latter derive from clot arising at the level of the lesion or in a poststenotic aneurysm. These are a frequent complication and are usually fusiform, though they can also be saccular (Fig. 15.43). Thrombosis of the subclavian artery can also result (Fig. 15.44).

Arteriography In these patients arteriography may appear normal or equivocal with the arm in neutral position, and Adson's manoeuvre may be necessary to confirm the lesion. This consists of fully abducting the arm with the head fully turned to the opposite side. These patients can also be investigated less invasively by intravenous DSA or MRA (Fig. 15.45).

Raynaud's phenomenon

This frequently occurs in normal healthy individuals as an abnormal response to cold. In these cases it appears to be purely due to a spastic response of the small vessels. Apart from this primary type, the condition may also be secondary to a variety of conditions which impair blood flow and includes major and minor vascular lesions. Box 15.2 lists the numerous diseases which have been associated with digital ischaemia and Raynaud's phenomenon.

Atheromatous lesions in the subclavian, axillary and brachial arteries are quite common, but are often asymptomatic because of the excellent collateral circulation at the root of the neck, shoulder and elbow. Thus thrombosis of the first part of the subclavian artery is often encountered by chance during arch or headhunter angiography, when the vertebral artery on the affected side is demonstrated to supply the distal subclavian by reversed flow (subclavian steal) (Fig. 15.46; see also Ch. 55). Atheromatous occlusions are also encountered in the distal vessels of the upper limb. In the digital vessels they can give rise to severe localised ischaemia which may require amputation. In elderly men, most cases of localised digital ischaemia are due to atheroma (Fig. 15.47).

Generalised digital ischaemia is usually due to a generalised disease such as scleroderma.

Buerger's disease

This has remained a controversial subject since the condition was first described in 1908. The diagnosis of Buerger's disease or 'thromboangitis obliterans' was once widely applied to a variety of vascular thromboses including the first cases of internal carotid thrombosis described by Moniz, as well as to the lower limb lesions

---

Box 15.2   Digital ischaemia and Raynaud's phenomenon

Lesions of major vessels (often with small-vessel emboli)
Atheroma
Takayasu's disease
Non-specific arteritis
African idiopathic aortitis
Thoracic inlet syndrome
Buerger's disease
Fibromuscular hyperplasia

Collagen disorder
Scleroderma
Rheumatoid arthritis
Polyarteritis nodosa

Blood disorders
Polycythaemia
Sickle-cell disease
Cryoagglutination
The contraceptive pill
PVC poisoning

Specific conditions
Raynaud's phenomenon (spastic type)
Vibrating tools
Ergotism

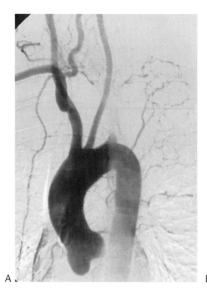

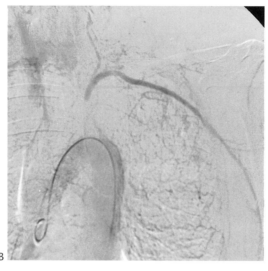

Fig. 15.46 DSA. (A,B) Left subclavian artery steal syndrome.

originally described. As a healthy reaction to the overdiagnosis of Buerger's disease, pathologists have pointed out that most of the cases examined by them were indistinguishable pathologically from atheromatous disease with thrombosis. This led some to the view that Buerger's disease was a myth and that most cases were in fact due to atheromatous disease.

Angiographic studies show that whatever the pathological nature of the lesions, Buerger's disease does appear to be a separate clinical entity. It occurs in a much younger age group than typical atheromatous vascular disease, the patients being mainly in their twenties or early thirties. It also has a much higher male sex incidence than has atheroma, female patients being extremely rare; and there is a much

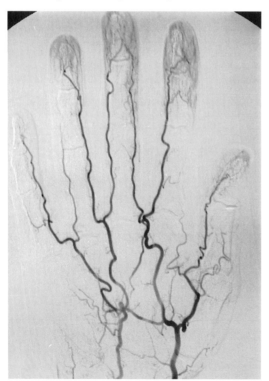

Fig. 15.47 DSA. Digital artery occlusions due to thoracic outlet syndrome.

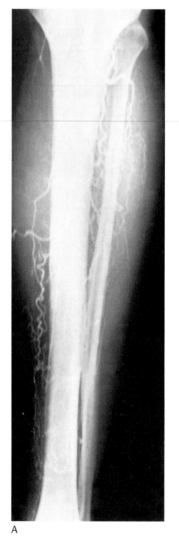

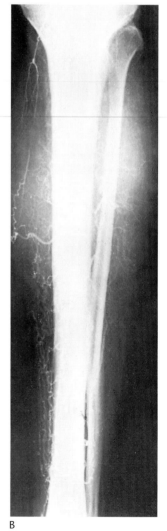

Fig. 15.48 Buerger's disease. Femoral arteriography showed normal smooth-walled femoral and popliteal arteries, but occlusion of the calf vessels with collaterals.

stronger association with heavy cigarette smoking, the patients usually showing strong addiction, sometimes maintained despite the threat of amputation. Unlike atheroma, the major vessels (aorta, iliacs and femorals) usually appear smooth walled and healthy, and the disease starts in the foot vessels and spreads retrogradely up the calf vessels. The typical angiographic appearance is of healthy femoral and popliteal arteries, with the calf vessels largely occluded and replaced by fine collaterals (Fig. 15.48). Long tortuous collaterals following the course of the occluded anterior and posterior tibial or peroneal arteries are sometimes seen and may represent hypertrophied vasa vasorum.

Spasm

Ergot poisoning may occur in migraine patients who have overdosed themselves with ergotamine tartrate, of which there are several proprietary preparations. This results in peripheral vascular spasm, presenting as ischaemic lower limbs. Such patients are easily misdiagnosed unless an adequate history is obtained, and we have been asked to perform angiography on several such patients without the referring physician suspecting the true diagnosis. The angiographic appearances are unusual but are diagnostic, consisting of spastic contraction of the vessels below the common femoral (the superficial femoral, popliteal and peripheral vessels), which are uniformly narrowed, so that they appear more like narrow threads than normal vessels. Upper-limb vessel involvement has also been described, as has spasm of splanchnic and renal vessels. If the condition is correctly diagnosed, withdrawal of the offending drug brings a rapid reversal of the spasm.

Localised spasm of peripheral arteries may be induced at angiography, usually in small vessels with a prominent muscular coat, either by the guide-wire or catheter tip or by a local high concentration of contrast medium. It may be observed on the angiogram just distal to the tip of the catheter, and should not be mistaken for a local stenosis. Any doubt can be resolved by repeating the contrast injection with the catheter tip withdrawn to a more proximal position. *Beaded spasm* is a term used for an unusual appearance usually seen in the femoral and popliteal arteries and less commonly in other arteries such as the iliacs and splanchnics. The condition has also been referred to as 'standing' or 'stationary arterial waves' or 'arterial beading'. Its nature remains controversial but it is generally thought to represent a physical phenomenon due to arterial pressure waves. In our experience it has been seen most frequently in the femoral arteries of patients with Buerger's disease and high peripheral resistance from obliterated calf vessels. The regular and perfectly symmetrical nature of the beading has been likened to a chain of pearls, and helps to distinguish it from the asymmetrical and less regular beading of fibromuscular hyperplasia.

Fibromuscular hyperplasia

This is an unusual arterial disease first described in the renal arteries as a rare cause of renal artery stenosis and occurring mainly in young women. The diagnosis is made by angiography, which shows an irregular beaded appearance of the affected artery (Fig. 15.42B). The lumen of the artery, when examined pathologically, exhibits both stenoses and sacculations, and the latter may become aneurysmal (Fig. 15.13).

The lesions are presumably congenital, though usually presenting in early adult life, and they have been described in many other arteries but they are commonest in the renals. We have encountered examples in the iliac and splanchnic arteries as well as in the inter-

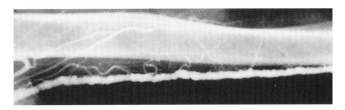

Fig. 15.49 Fibromuscular hyperplasia of the brachial artery in a woman of 50 years presenting with digital ischaemia.

nal carotid artery, which is now a well-recognised site for the lesion.

This disease appears to be extremely rare in limb vessels, though we have previously reported a case in the brachial arteries of a middle-aged woman (Fig. 15.49).

Arteritis

Takayasu's arteritis This is a rare condition first described in Japan in 1908 but now recognised to have a worldwide distribution. It manifests mainly in young women aged 20–30 years, and the incidence in the USA is 0.11%. The aorta is attacked by a granulomatous inflammation of the media proceeding to fibrosis and atheroma-like changes with involvement of the main branches, which can become thrombosed. The main pulmonary artery and its major branches may also be involved. The aetiology is unknown, but an autoimmune mechanism has been postulated by some workers.

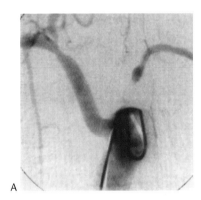

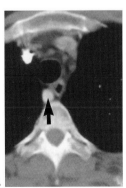

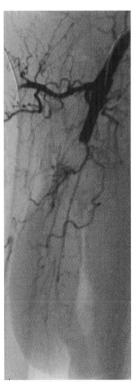

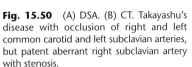

Fig. 15.50 (A) DSA. (B) CT. Takayashu's disease with occlusion of right and left common carotid and left subclavian arteries, but patent aberrant right subclavian artery with stenosis.

Fig. 15.51 DSA. Occlusion of right brachial artery due to supracondylar fracture of right humerus.

Clinical manifestations depend on the major aortic branches most affected and include upper-limb ischaemia, ocular and cerebral symptoms, renovascular hypertension, coronary disease and lower-limb ischaemia. The *aortic arch syndrome* of progressive occlusion of the great vessels of the arch is a common complication (pulseless disease).

Angiography shows a surprising irregularity of the aorta, which resembles that of an elderly atheromatous person, together with stenoses or occlusions of the origins of the major branches (Fig. 15.50).

Giant cell arteritis This is a vasculitis affecting people above the age of 50 or 60 years and usually involving smaller or middle-sized arteries. It is not clear whether the cause is inflammatory or whether an autoimmune mechanism is involved. Temporal arteritis is common, as is involvement of intracerebral vessels, and blindness is a complication in some 10% of cases. Large-vessel vasculitis is very uncommon but is occasionally seen, and can give rise to lower-limb ischaemia or an aortic arch syndrome. Angiography of the temporal artery may show irregular stenotic areas with intervening normal areas (skip lesions).

Trauma Damage to arteries may follow direct trauma as in open wounds from stabbing or missiles. It may also be iatrogenic following arterial catheterisation. Closed injuries can occur in crush injury to the chest as in an automobile accident. The damage to the arterial wall can result in aneurysm as described above. These can be true or false aneurysm or dissecting aneurysm. The damage can also lead to arterial rupture with haemorrhage or to arterial thrombosis (Figs 15.51, 15.52).

Other causes of thrombosis Damage to arteries and thrombosis may also result from frostbite or radiation which can be accidental or following radiotherapy. Thrombosis can also occur from blood diseases such as protein C deficiency, protein S deficiency, antithrombin III deficiency and polycythaemia. Arterial thrombosis is also common in advanced malignant disease.

Embolus Major embolus to the systemic arterial system is most commonly cardiac in origin, being seen in patients with atrial fibrillation and intra-atrial clot, or following clot formation in the left ventricle after cardiac infarction. Another cardiac cause is clot forming on prosthetic valves after cardiac surgery.

Embolus may also follow clot formation in a large aneurysm, which is then detached and carried distally.

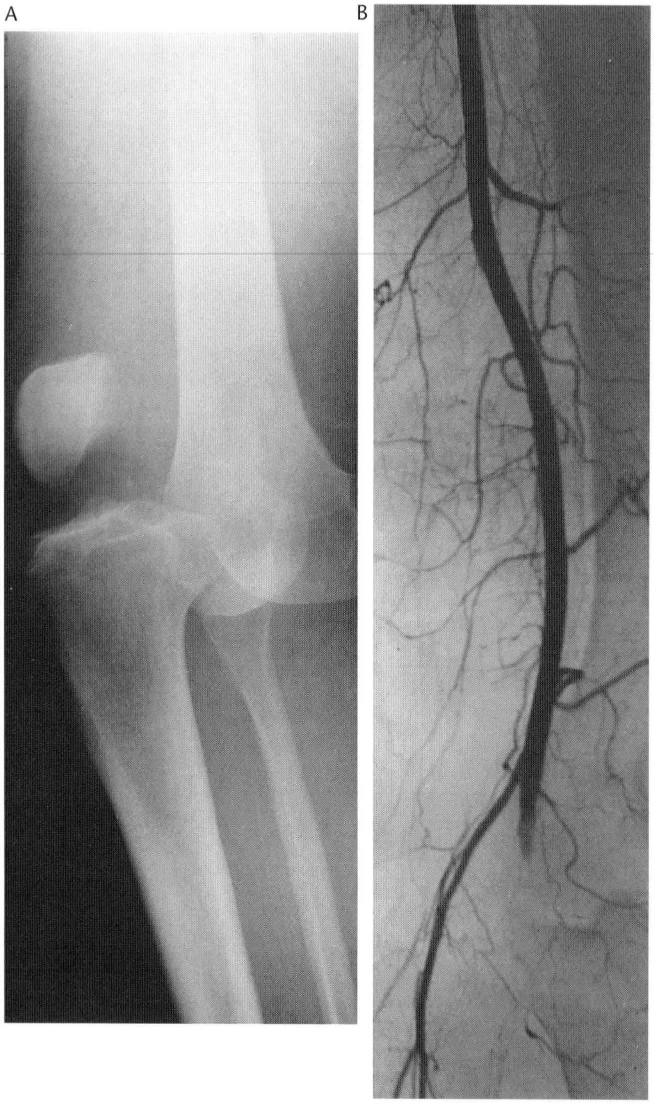

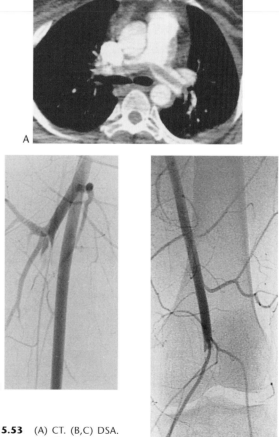

Fig. 15.53 (A) CT. (B,C) DSA. Pulmonary emboli with right deep femoral and left popliteal artery paradoxical emboli.

Fig. 15.52 (A) Plain film. (B) DSA. Occlusion of left popliteal artery due to dislocation of left knee.

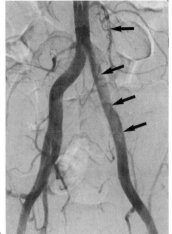

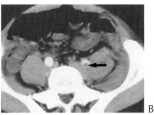

Fig. 15.54 (A) DSA. (B) CT. Left common iliac and inferior mesenteric artery emboli (arrows).

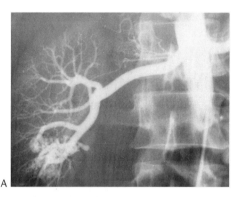

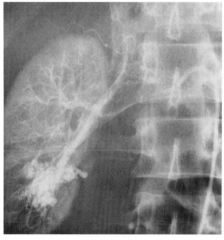

The rare paradoxical embolus is carried from the venous system through a patent foramen ovale. This is present in one-third of the population but remains closed unless right atrial pressure exceeds left atrial pressure, as in chronic lung disease or pulmonary embolus, when clots may pass through to the left heart and systemic circulation.

Ulcerated atheromatous plaques in major vessels can also give rise to emboli from cholesterol showers or debris, which being smaller lodge in small peripheral vessels in the limbs and are usually less serious. However, when they affect the brain they can give rise to transient ischaemic attacks or more serious strokes (see Ch. 55).

Finally, clot embolus is a well-recognized complication of catheter angiography, as previously described.

Seventy-five per cent of large emboli lodge at the aortic bifurcation, iliac bifurcation or major vessels of the lower limb. The clinical diagnosis is usually obvious from the acute onset of pain,

Fig. 15.56 (A,B) Arteriogram. High-flow angiomatous malformation in right kidney.

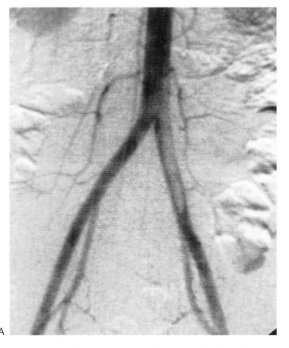

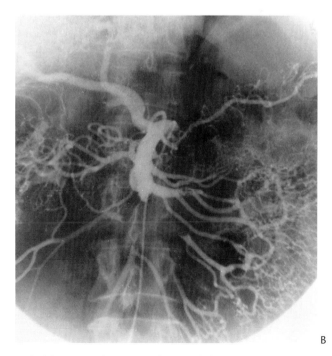

Fig. 15.55 (A) Embolus of the aortic bifurcation with clot defect extending into the left common iliac. DSA study. (B) Embolus of the superior mesenteric artery.

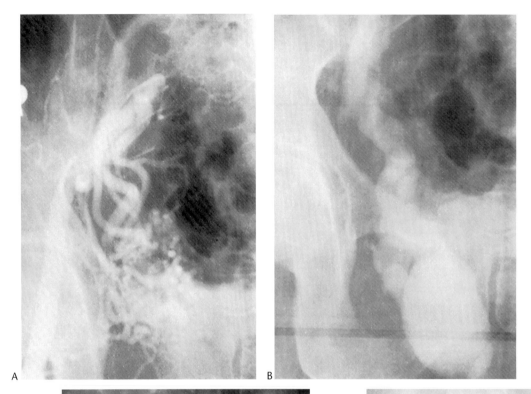

A

B

Fig. 15.57 Angioma of the pelvis, presenting as vulval swelling. Aneurysmal dilatation of draining vein.

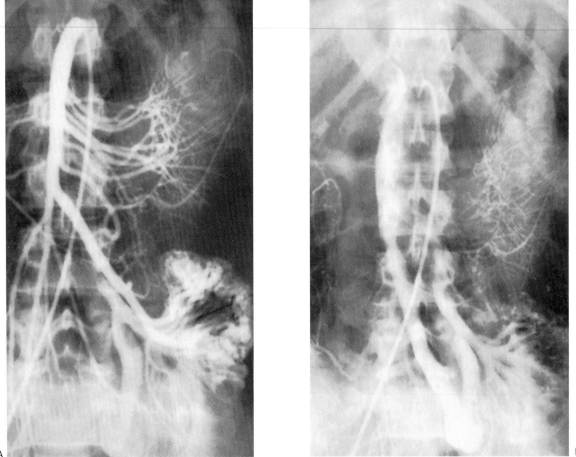

A

B

Fig. 15.58 Angioma of the small bowel with high-volume shunting into the portal system in a woman of 24 years with repeated attacks of melena. In the previous 10 years she had had four barium enemas and five barium follow-throughs with negative findings. Large angiomas like this are unusual in the bowel, small areas of dysplasia being more common.

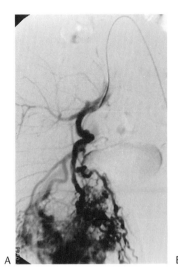
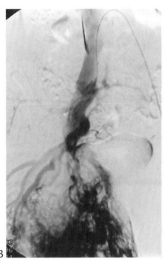
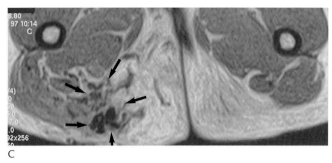

Fig. 15.59 (A,B) DSA. (C) Proton-density MRI. High-flow angiomatous malformation in right buttock (arrows).

numbness, pallor and coldness, with loss of peripheral pulses in the context of cardiac disease, aneurysm or previous cardiac surgery. If, however, the onset is more insidious it may be difficult to differentiate from arterial thrombosis.

Angiography shows a sharp cut-off at the point of occlusion (Fig. 15.53) with sometimes a characteristic convex upper margin (meniscus sign). Larger emboli (Figs 15.54, 15.55) affecting the aortic, iliac or femoral bifurcation are usually removed surgically with a Fogarty balloon catheter. They should be treated as surgical emergencies since a delay of more than 24 h leads to a significantly higher amputation rate. Smaller and more distal emboli and those in the arm have a better prognosis, but if the limb is at risk, treatment by intra-arterial thrombolysis may be attempted as described below. Mesenteric embolism should be suspected in patients with acute abdominal pain and coexisting atrial fibrillation, mitral stenosis or a recent cardiac infarction.

Angiomatous malformations

These lesions, also referred to as angiomas and congenital arteriovenous fistulas, represent direct communications between arterioles and venules without the interposition of a capillary bed. They are presumably congenital but often present in adults, probably due to increasing size after adult blood pressure is established. They are common in the cerebral circulation (see Ch. 55), but can present anywhere in the body. They should be distinguished from acquired communications between arteries and veins—arteriovenous fistulas—which are described below.

Figures 15.56–15.59 show the angiographic appearances in lesions presenting in the kidney, vulva, bowel and buttock respectively. In all cases there are hypertrophied arteries leading to the lesion and hypertrophied veins draining it, their size depending on the degree of shunt present. Both arteries and veins fill rapidly, and before contrast medium has passed through normal capillaries in the adjacent regions. Some smaller angiomas and those at very fine vessel level are more difficult to demonstrate and may require superselective angiography of the feeding vessels to show their full extent. Treatment by angiographic embolisation is discussed below.

Arteriovenous fistula

This term is best limited to the condition where there is a single communication between an artery and a vein, and is mainly of traumatic origin, particularly following gunshot or other pene-

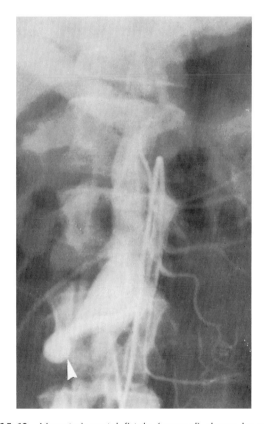

Fig. 15.60 Mesenteric-portal fistula (arrowed) shown by selective superior mesenteric injection. There is rapid filling of dilated superior mesenteric and portal veins. The lesion followed a crush injury to the abdomen.

trating wounds. Occasionally it may result from a closed injury (Fig. 15.60). Traumatic fistulas may occur anywhere in the body, and we have encountered cases in all anatomical sites from the scalp to the foot.

Spontaneous arteriovenous fistula is also occasionally encountered, resulting from rupture of an aneurysm into an adjacent vein (Fig. 15.61). A site of election for this is the cavernous sinus, where rupture of an aneurysm can give rise to pulsating exophthalmos (see Ch. 55). Another well-documented site is the abdominal aorta, where rupture of an aneurysm into the inferior vena cava leads to

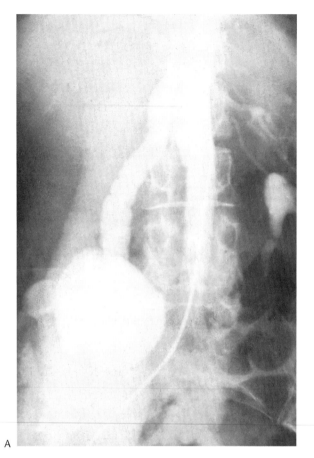
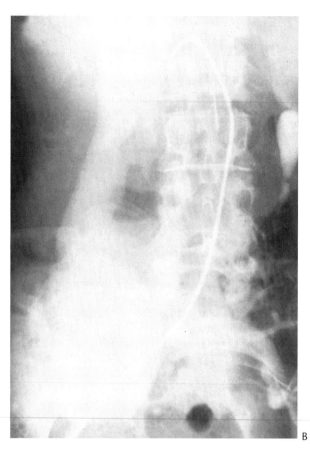

A   B

Fig. 15.61   Giant renal arteriovenous fistula, possibly due to rupture of an aneurysm associated with fibromuscular hyperplasia. The patient presented with heart failure and a pulsating mass clinically thought to be pelvic because of ptosed kidney. (A) Arterial phase. (B) Venous phase showing a dilated inferior vena cava.

aortocaval fistula (Fig. 15.62). These intra-abdominal cases can give rise to difficult diagnostic problems, and the larger shunts can give rise to high-output cardiac failure without the true cause being suspected.

So-called congenital arteriovenous fistulas are sometimes seen in infants and children, but it is usually difficult or impossible to exclude trauma in these cases.

Iatrogenic arteriovenous fistulas, apart from those deliberately induced for dialysis, can arise from many procedures, particularly orthopaedic operations on the hip, ankle and spine. Aortocaval and ilioiliac fistulas have followed lumbar disc operations when the rougeur has been passed through the anterior spinal ligament, and renal arteriovenous fistula is a common complication of renal biopsy. Arteriography has given rise to arteriovenous fistula at the site of puncture, usually of small arteries (brachial and vertebral), but it has also been recorded in the femoral artery. Because of the grossly hypertrophied drainage veins carrying arterial blood, a fistula may be very difficult to locate at surgery, and prior angiography with localisation of the fistula is essential. As with angiomas, the dilated feeding artery fills early, as do the dilated drainage veins, and large amounts of contrast medium with rapid serial films are necessary to clearly define the anatomy and the site of the fistula.

A large arteriovenous fistula throws an extra burden on the heart because of the large amount of shunt, and can result in cardiac failure from high cardiac output unless successfully treated. As noted below, many fistulas, particularly smaller ones, are now treated successfully by embolisation.

Haemorrhage

Arteriography can be extremely useful in the diagnosis and treatment of internal haemorrhage. Serious or life-threatening haemorrhage can be due to many causes, including trauma, peptic ulceration, ruptured aneurysms, neoplasms or inflammatory lesions involving blood vessels, radiation and blood disorders. In many situations previously requiring surgical intervention, percutaneous catheterisation and embolisation as described below offers a simpler and safer alternative to surgery.

Upper gastrointestinal tract haemorrhage   The common causes are oesophageal varices, Mallory–Weiss tears, gastritis, gastric ulcer and duodenal ulcer. Endoscopy is now widely used for both diagnosis and treatment, and angiography and embolisation have played a diminishing role in recent years.

Haemorrhage from the small bowel is much less common and more difficult to diagnose. Scintigraphy, as described below, may be useful in demonstrating the site, and arteriography will occasionally demonstrate rare causes such as angioma (Fig. 15.58). Other rare causes are jejunal diverticulum, Meckel's diverticulum, neoplasms and typhoid enteritis (Fig. 15.63).

Lower gastrointestinal tract haemorrhage   Radionuclide scintigraphy is the technique of choice for the investigation of acute lower gastrointestinal tract bleeding. ^{99m}Tc-labelled sulphur colloid or ^{99m}Tc-labelled red cells may be used to localise the approximate source of the haemorrhage, provided the patient is still bleeding (see Ch. 21).

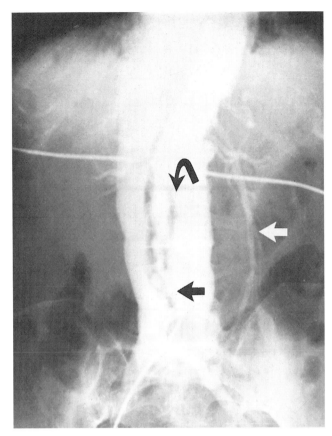

Fig. 15.62 Aortocaval fistula following spontaneous rupture of an abdominal aortic aneurysm. The superior mesenteric is displaced by the aneurysm containing mural thrombus (white arrow). The fistula into the inferior vena cava is marked by the black arrow. The curved arrow suggests an intimal flap in the aneurysm. (From Gregson et al (1983) by permission of the editor of Clinical Radiology.)

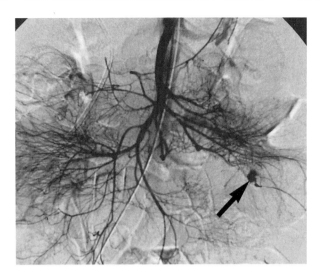

Fig. 15.63 DSA. Active bleeding (arrow) into the small intestine due to lymphoma.

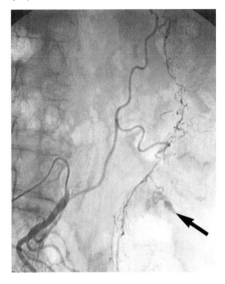

Fig. 15.64 DSA. Active bleeding (arrow) into the descending colon from a diverticulum.

Diverticulosis is the commonest cause and, rather surprisingly, most bleeding diverticula lie in the ascending colon, though diverticula are much less common here than in the sigmoid and descending colon (Fig. 15.64). *Angiodysplasia*, the second commonest cause, also involves mainly the caecum or ascending colon, and these lesions can be multiple.

Colonoscopy is less successful in identifying these lesions than arteriography, which is often necessary. Bleeding from colonic diverticula can be controlled by vasopressin, though success may only prove temporary. Some cases have been controlled by embolisation, though this requires difficult superselective catheterisation.

The alternative of emergency colectomy carries a high mortality, and even temporary control may permit a later elective colectomy. Angiodysplasias are often small and require high-quality angiograms for their demonstration, as bleeding is less severe than with diverticula. Arteriovenous shunting with early venous filling should raise suspicion. These lesions are usually treated surgically.

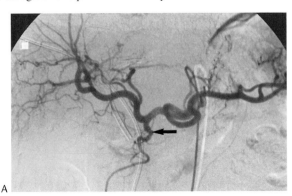
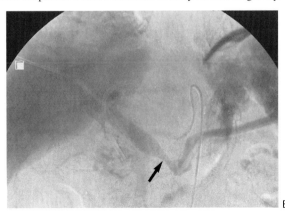

A   B

Fig. 15.65 (A,B) DSA. Vascular encasement of gastroduodenal artery and hepatic portal vein by a carcinoma in the head of the pancreas.

Neoplasms and mass lesions

Arteriography was once widely used for the characterisation of tumours, cysts and other mass lesions but with the advent and constant improvement of the non-invasive techniques of ultrasound, CT and MRI the method has become largely obsolete as a purely diagnostic tool. Where angiography is still used, its purpose is either to complement the non-invasive investigations by providing anatomical information to the surgeon about the vascularity and blood supply of a tumour, or in some cases to permit embolisation of inoperable tumours or of highly vascular tumours prior to surgery. In rare cases it may be used to help establish the correct diagnosis where ultrasound and CT have proved equivocal or inconclusive.

The value of angiography in tumour diagnosis arose from three facts. First, tumours often have circulations different from those in the tissues in which they arise. This results in abnormal or 'pathological' vessels being outlined by contrast and thus localising and characterising the neoplasm. Arteriovenous shunting with early opacification of drainage veins is a frequent feature of the more malignant neoplasms, which tend to be more vascular than benign tumours. Second, the growth of the tumour may displace and stretch the normal vessels at its margins, thus enabling less vascular tumours to be located. Third, tumours may actually involve adjacent arteries, leading to 'cuffing' (Fig. 15.65) or irregular narrowing of the affected arteries.

Renal masses

Hypernephromas are usually highly vascular tumours, and the demonstration of typical pathological vessels in a renal mass is diagnostic (Fig. 15.66). Occasionally these tumours are so vascular that they simulate angiomatous malformations. Conversely, they are also occasionally non-vascular, simulating cysts. However, such cases will sometimes show tortuous or irregular vessels entering the periphery of the mass, a feature not seen with cysts.

Renal cysts are typically rounded avascular masses best shown in the nephrogram phase. The cortex at the margin of the cyst is compressed and displaced, producing a pointed projection of opacified cortex, the so-called 'beak sign'. Further, the normal arteries at the margins of the cyst are stretched and displaced.

Carcinoma of the renal pelvis is much less vascular than hypernephroma, but high-quality angiograms will show one or more abnormal fine tortuous vessels leading to the tumour, and similar appearances may be seen in carcinoma of the ureter.

Wilms' tumour (nephroblastoma) occurs in children below the age of 5 years, though occasionally presenting at an older age and even in an adult. These tumours can reach a very large size, and 10% are bilateral. At angiography they may show only limited neovascularity.

Angiomyolipoma (hamartoma) is a benign tumour, but the angiogram shows a vascular lesion which can be mistaken for a carcinoma. Such tumours are common in tuberous sclerosis, when they may be multiple. *Xanthogranulomatous pyelonephritis* is a chronic inflammatory condition which can also produce a vascular abnormality resembling that of a malignant tumour.

Renal oncocytomas have been described as rare benign tumours resembling hypernephromas but that are well encapsulated and sometimes showing a 'spoke-wheel' pattern at angiography. The existence of this entity remains controversial, and they are considered by some to be low-grade hypernephromas.

Benign tumours of the kidney are rare but important in differential diagnosis. *Adenomas* are usually small and subcapsular in situation. A rare form of giant benign renal adenoma has been described which at angiography is well circumscribed and separate from adjacent normal renal tissue. There is no arteriovenous shunting or other feature to suggest malignancy.

The rare *renin-secreting juxtaglomerular cell tumour* is found in hypertensive patients. At angiography it shows as a small cortical defect in the nephrogram phase, resembling a small cyst. A few fine vessels to the tumour may be identified, as may the slight bulge in

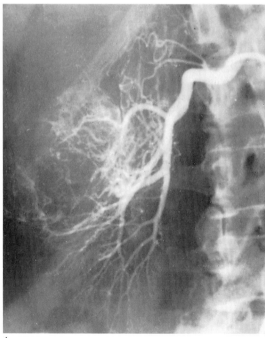

A

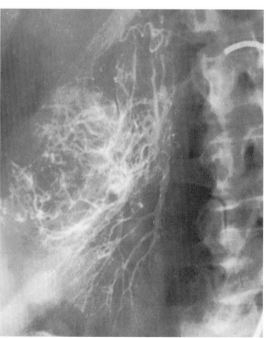

B

Fig. 15.66 Renal carcinoma showing pathological vessels.

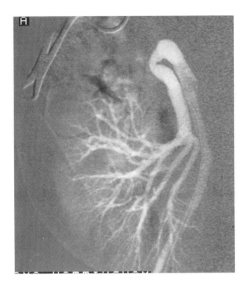

the surface of the kidney. Renin assay from the renal veins helps to confirm the diagnosis by demonstrating higher concentrations on the affected side.

Renal angiography has also been used in the past to confirm such benign conditions as *pseudotumours* (e.g. enlarged column of Bertin, dromedary hump, congenital polar enlargement, suprahilar and infrahilar lips, and areas of compensatory hypertrophy).

Renal graft angiography Multiple arteries occur in 25% of kidneys, and it is therefore necessary to perform angiography on live kidney donors to ensure that the proposed kidney has only one artery of supply. The grafted kidney is usually placed in the right iliac fossa with its artery anastomosed to the patient's internal iliac artery.

The commonest cause of failure of a transplant kidney is renal rejection, which can be early or delayed. Sometimes it is difficult to differentiate clinically between rejection of the graft and other complications affecting renal function.

A graft arteriogram will show whether the kidney is perfusing normally and will demonstrate such complications as stenosis at the anastomosis (Fig. 15.67). Generalised small-vessel occlusions, which are usually due to rejection, will be shown, as will thrombosis of the main artery or impaired perfusion. Kidney transplant arteriography can be performed by injection of a large bolus of contrast medium into the common iliac artery (20 ml of iopamidol 300 or equivalent of other contrast media). Selective angiography of the internal iliac artery will give better resolution, and intra-arterial DSA will permit low doses of contrast medium.

Hepatic tumours

The primary investigation of liver masses is by ultrasound, with scintiscanning, CT and MRI all able to provide further help in characterising lesions. Angiography now has little place in such diagnostic studies, but it can still be used for therapeutic purposes such as intra-arterial chemotherapy or embolisation or for the elucidation of the occasional problem case (see Ch. 25). Selective hepatic angiography can demonstrate both primary and secondary carcinoma of the liver. Such malignant tumours usually show a well-marked pathological circulation (Fig. 15.68), but are occasionally poorly vascularised and difficult to differentiate from benign masses. The latter tend merely to displace and stretch branches of the hepatic artery, though some are more vascular.

Haemangioma is the commonest benign tumour of the liver to show an abnormal circulation. These lesions are sometimes multiple, and can then be suspected as deposits at ultrasound or other non-invasive investigations. Differentiation is possible on the angiogram as the lesions, though vascular, show a typical sluggish circulation, with persistence of contrast medium in the venous phase (Fig. 15.69). This is quite unlike the rapid arteriovenous shunting seen in malignant tumours.

Hepatic adenomas may also occur, and have been described as a complication of hormonal treatment with contraceptive pills or with androgens. At angiography they are vascular tumours, but their vascular pattern is more regular than that of a malignant

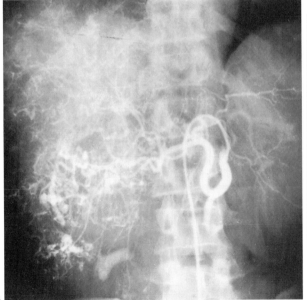
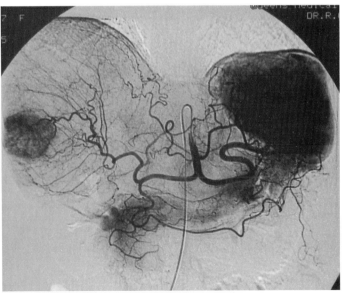

Fig. 15.68 (A) Selective hepatic arteriogram. A large vascular tumour is shown in the lower part of the right lobe of the liver. Histology: primary hepatoma. (B) Selective hepatic angiogram shows solitary vascular deposit from colonic carcinoma.

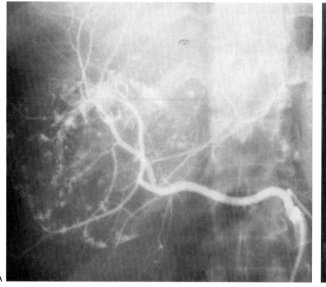

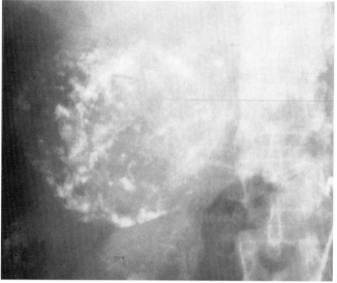

Fig. 15.69 (A) Vascular lesion simulating tumour in the liver. Haemangioma. (B) Note absence of drainage veins or arteriovenous shunting and persistence of contrast medium in the late phase.

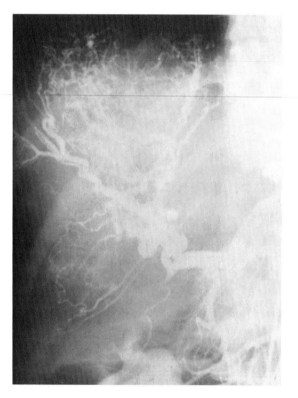

Fig. 15.70 Angiogram showing a large vascular mass with a smaller mass in the lower part of the right lobe.

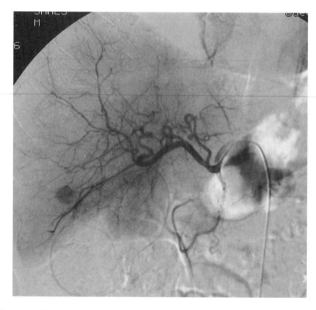

Fig. 15.71 DSA. Small hepatocellular carcinoma in the right lobe of the liver in haemochromatosis.

tumour, and they stand out as encapsulated tumours in the hepatogram phase (Fig. 15.70). Figure 15.71 shows a small hepatocellular carcinoma. Figure 15.72 shows a large vascular tumour in a child.

Pancreatic tumours

Ultrasound, CT and endoscopic retrograde cholangiopancreatography (ERCP) are now the methods of choice for the diagnosis of pancreatic tumours. Angiography, once widely used for this purpose, is now obsolete except for the elucidation of suspected small endocrine tumours.

Pancreatic *carcinoma* is relatively avascular, and tumours were recognised by displacement of vessels supplying the pancreas or by invasion of their walls with cuffing or occlusion.

Cystadenoma of the pancreas, however, can be highly vascular, and shows a florid pathological circulation (Fig. 15.73).

Islet cell adenomas of the pancreas may be quite small and difficult to diagnose by non-invasive imaging techniques. At superselective angiography, however, they can be identified as a rounded blush of contrast in the venous or capillary phase (Fig. 15.74). Large islet cell adenomas are occasionally seen and can be highly vascular.

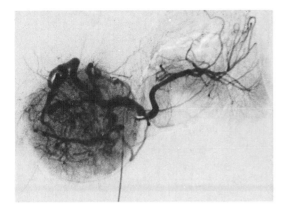

Fig. 15.72 DSA. Large tumour in the liver in a child due to focal nodular hyperplasia.

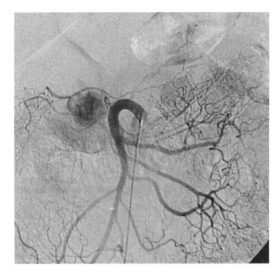

Fig. 15.74 DSA. Insulinoma in the head of the pancreas.

Malignant bone tumours are usually highly vascular, and the angiographic appearances are pathognomonic. Prior to the advent of CT, angiography was widely used to demonstrate the extra-osseous spread of such tumours. Secondary deposits in bone vary in their vascularity, ranging from the highly vascular to the relatively non-vascular. Hypernephroma and thyroid metastases have been amongst the most vascular encountered, and such deposits in the soft tissues can simulate pulsating aneurysms.

Sarcoma of the soft tissues, when highly malignant, usually shows abundant pathological vessels, but low-grade fibrosarcomas may be relatively non-vascular.

Chromaffinoma (chemodectoma)

These tumours are most frequently found at the carotid bifurcation, where they are known as *carotid body tumours*. They are extremely vascular and show a characteristic appearance at angiography (Fig. 15.75). Occasionally they are familial, when they can also be bilateral. Clinically they have been mistaken for local aneurysms, and, conversely, rare aneurysms at this site have been mistaken for carotid body tumours.

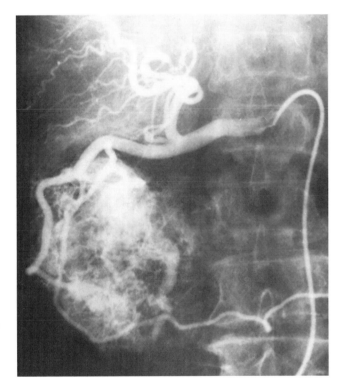

Fig. 15.73 Pancreatic cystadenoma showing florid pathological circulation in the head of the pancreas.

Pancreatic hormone-producing tumours can also be identified by venous blood sampling and assay from the pancreatic drainage veins. The samples are obtained by transhepatic portal vein catheterisation as described below (see Ch. 26).

Adrenal tumours Angiography is no longer used for the diagnosis of adrenal tumours and CT is now the primary imaging method (see Ch. 27).

Tumours of bone and soft tissue

The newer imaging techniques, particularly CT and MRI, are now the investigations of choice for tumours involving bone and for soft-tissue tumours in all parts of the body. Angiography is now rarely undertaken in these cases except for embolisation or other therapeutic purposes.

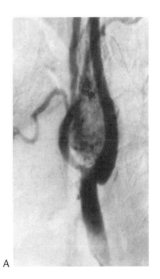
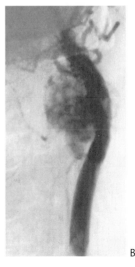

A B

Fig. 15.75 Carotid body tumour (A) Lateral projection. (B) A.P. projection.

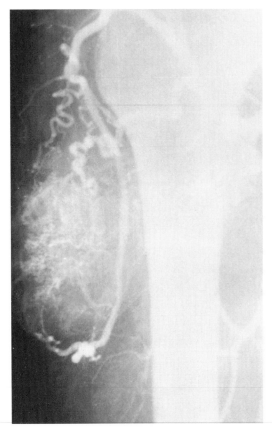

Fig. 15.76 Haemangiopericytoma. Patient presented with a lump in the right thigh. The vascular tumour was highly malignant and metastasised rapidly.

of the external carotid feeding branches may be required to show their full extent or for embolisation, which may be required prior to surgery or in inoperable cases (see Ch. 47). The *glomus tympanicum tumour* lies in the middle ear, and will require high-quality subtraction films for its demonstration.

These tumours occur less commonly in other sites, but the angiographic appearances are similar. The *glomus vagale tumour* lies between the carotid body and glomus jugulare sites, while the *aortic body tumour* lies in the mediastinum above the aortic arch. Pelvic tumours are also described.

Nasopharyngeal angiofibroma (juvenile angiofibroma)

These highly vascular tumours present as swellings arising from the nasopharynx of adolescent boys. They may invade the antrum and produce swelling of the cheek. They are best shown by CT, which is now the primary investigation of choice (see Ch. 47), but they are also well shown by superselective angiography of the external carotid artery. Surgery, which may otherwise be hazardous, can be aided by prior embolisation of the main feeding vessels.

Haemangiopericytoma These rare tumours of small blood vessels may occur anywhere in the body where there are capillaries, but are mainly seen in the soft tissues. They may be benign but they can also be highly malignant. In our experience the latter type are very vascular (Fig. 15.76), and malignancy may be related to the degree of vascularity. Specific diagnosis, however, depends on biopsy, and is made by the histopathologist.

Another common site for chromaffinoma is the glomus jugulare at the base of the skull (*glomus jugulare tumour*). Here they are also very vascular, and the angiographic appearance is similar to that of the carotid body tumour. Careful superselective angiography

INTERVENTIONAL VASCULAR RADIOLOGY

Interventional vascular radiology has developed from diagnostic angiography and now plays a central role in the management of patients with vascular disease. These therapeutic angiographic procedures are often simple, effective and efficient and have a low

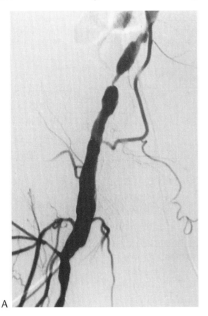
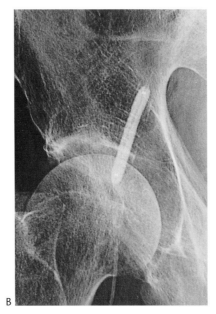
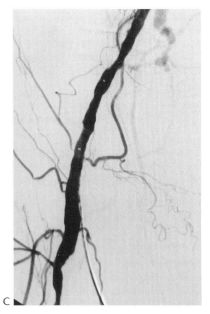

Fig. 15.77 (A) Arteriogram showing 75–90% stenoses in the right external iliac artery and occlusion of the right superficial femoral artery before angioplasty. (B) Balloon catheter in the external iliac artery during the angioplasty. (C) Angiographic result in the external iliac artery after angioplasty.

morbidity and mortality. They have therefore not only increased the number of treatment options available to patients by enabling a percutaneous endovascular procedure to be performed instead of a conventional surgical one, but have also increased the range of treatment available by offering procedures to patients, who are either unfit for surgery or whose symptoms do not merit its risks.

Interventional vascular radiology includes transluminal angioplasty and vascular stent insertion, therapeutic embolisation, vascular infusion therapy and the insertion and retrieval of intravascular foreign bodies. The scope and complexity of these procedures, however, continues to grow and patients undergoing interventional vascular procedures need to have their management explained to them so that they can give informed consent. This includes the diagnosis and prognosis of their condition, the treatment options available for their condition and an explanation of the proposed procedure including its risks and benefits.

Transluminal angioplasty

The technique of percutaneous transluminal angioplasty (PTA) was initially performed in 1964 by Dotter and Judkins, who used coaxial catheters to dilate arterial stenoses. However, it was the development of the polyvinyl chloride balloon catheter by Gruntzig and Hopff in 1974 that led to the widespread use of this technique, which is the commonest interventional vascular procedure performed in the world today.

The basic technique of PTA involves passing a guide-wire and catheter across a stenosis or through an occlusion in a blood vessel. A balloon catheter is then positioned across the diseased segment and dilated up to the same size as the adjacent lumen, in order to increase the blood flow through the artery or vein (Fig. 15.77).

The mechanism of how PTA works was originally thought to be due to compression and redistribution of the soft atheromatous material along the arterial wall, but histopathological studies with electron microscopy have now shown that the balloon splits the atheromatous plaque producing clefts in the intima, which extend into the media but not the adventitia. Platelets then aggregate on the damaged surface, and healing of the intima and media occurs over several weeks by the formation of intimal hyperplasia and fibrosis with retraction of the plaque, resulting in an improved arterial luminal diameter (Fig. 15.78).

In patients with vascular disease atherosclerosis is by far the commonest cause of an arterial stenosis or occlusion that is suitable for treatment by PTA, but stenosis due to other pathological conditions such as fibromuscular dysplasia, arteritis, intimal hyperplasia, radiation damage and trauma are also amenable to treatment with PTA.

Angioplasty in peripheral vascular disease

Many patients undergoing investigation for peripheral vascular disease with symptoms of intermittent claudication, rest pain, ischaemic ulceration and gangrene are suitable for PTA. This can be performed in symptomatic patients as an alternative to a surgical bypass graft or in combination with surgery to improve the inflow or outflow in the adjacent arteries. It is also used to treat patients with intermittent claudication, whose symptoms limit their lifestyle but are not severe enough to require reconstructive surgery, and to try and prevent amputation in patients with rest pain, ulceration and gangrene, who are unfit for surgery (limb salvage angioplasty).

PTA is therefore indicated in symptomatic patients with arterial stenoses or short occlusions on angiography of the lower limbs. The contraindications to PTA include the presence of fresh thrombus in the arteries, which should be treated by either thrombolysis or aspiration thrombectomy, a total aortic occlusion and long occlusions in the iliac, femoral or popliteal arteries, although even these can now occasionally be treated successfully. The ideal lesion for PTA is a short, smooth, central 50–90% stenosis in a large artery, such as the common or external iliac artery in a patient with normal distal arteries, because the technical and clinical success rates are very high (Fig. 15.79). Patients undergoing PTA should be started on treatment with an antiplatelet drug such as aspirin, dipyridamole,

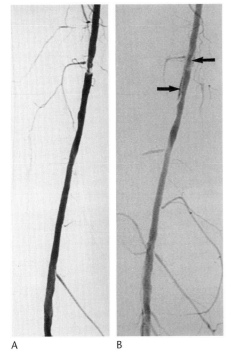

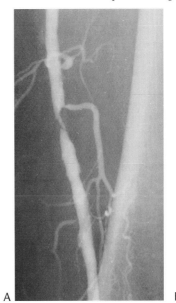

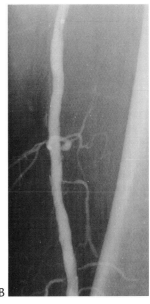

Fig. 15.78 (A) Arteriogram showing 75% stenosis in right superficial femoral artery before angioplasty. (B) Angiographic result (arrows) with intimal clefts after angioplasty.

Fig. 15.79 (A) A suitable lesion for PTA-arteriogram showing 75% stenosis in the distal left superficial femoral artery. (B) Arteriogram after angioplasty.

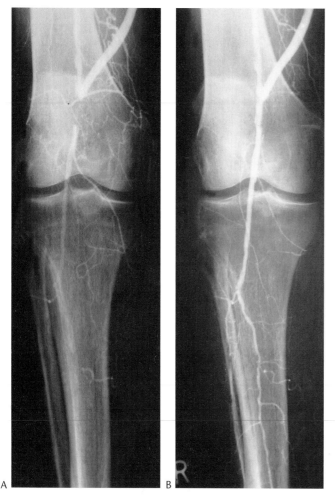

Fig. 15.80 (A) Arteriogram showing a short 2 cm occlusion in the right popliteal artery, below the distal anastomosis of a femoropopliteal vein graft. (B) Arteriogram after angioplasty.

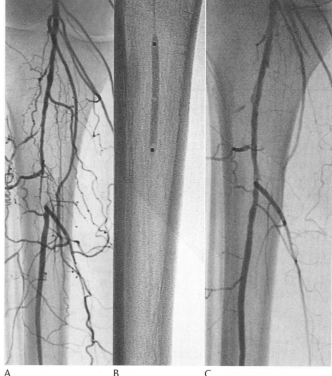

Fig. 15.81 (A) Arteriogram showing short occlusion in right tibio-peroneal trunk before angioplasty. (B) Balloon catheter in tibioperoneal trunk during angioplasty. (C) Angiographic result after angioplasty.

clopidogrel or ticlopidine 24 h before the procedure and this should be continued for at least 3–6 months after the procedure and possibly for life. Increased exercise and stopping smoking should also be encouraged. During the procedure patients should receive 3000–5000 units of heparin intra-arterially. After the procedure some patients are treated with warfarin.

Iliac artery stenoses and short occlusions up to 5–7 cm in length are usually approached from below following a retrograde catheterisation of the ipsilateral common femoral artery (Fig. 15.77). This can be punctured even if there is no femoral pulse, with the help of palpation, fluoroscopy, ultrasound or DSA. Iliac artery lesions can also be approached across the aortic bifurcation following catheterisation of the contralateral common femoral artery or following catheterisation of the axillary or brachial artery, usually in the left arm. Stenoses in the internal iliac, common femoral, proximal superficial and deep femoral arteries are often approached across the aortic bifurcation. Distal superficial femoral and popliteal artery stenoses and short occlusions up to 10–15 cm in length are usually approached from above following an antegrade catheterisation of the ipsilateral common or superficial femoral artery (Fig. 15.80). Femoral artery lesions can also be approached from below following catheterisation of the ipsilateral popliteal artery with the patient lying prone. Stenosis of the lower abdominal aorta and tibial artery stenoses and short occlusions up to 3–5 cm in length are also suitable for PTA. (Fig. 15.81). Long occlusions up to 20–30 cm in length in the superficial femoral and popliteal arteries can be treated by the technique of subintimal angioplasty, where a guide-wire is used to deliberately dissect the artery above an occlusion and then re-enter the lumen below it. The subintimal channel is then dilated with a balloon. Long occlusions in the iliac and tibial arteries can also be treated by this technique.

The size of the balloon should be similar to the size of the artery undergoing PTA, because a balloon that is too small produces an inadequate dilatation and a balloon that is too big can rupture the artery. The size of the balloon used in iliac artery PTA is usually about 6–10 or 12 mm in diameter and in superficial femoral and popliteal artery PTA it is usually 4–6 mm in diameter. The tibial arteries require 2–3 mm diameter balloons and the aorta either a large single 12–16 mm diameter balloon or two 8–10 mm diameter balloons. Lesions at the aortic bifurcation also require the simultaneous use of two 6–10 mm diameter balloons (kissing balloon technique). The balloons are usually 4 cm in length, but range from 2 to 10 cm long.

The initial technical success of the procedure is usually based on haemodynamic pressure measurements and/or angiographic appearances, depending upon the site of the PTA. The intra-arterial pressure is measured above and below the lesion before aortic or iliac artery PTA. A pressure gradient of 15–20 mmHg or greater at rest is a significant drop, but a pressure gradient of up to 10 mmHg at rest is not. In patients without a significant drop in pressure, injection of a vasodilator such as papaverine, tolazoline or glyceryl trinitrate through the catheter simulates the effect of exercise. An increase in the pressure gradient to more that 20 mmHg then indicates that the stenosis is significant and requires angioplasty. The ideal haemo-dynamic result following PTA is no residual pressure gradient at all, but this is not always attainable.

The intra-arterial pressure is not usually measured in femoral, popliteal or tibial artery PTA, because the measurements are not so accurate in these smaller arteries with the catheter positioned in an antegrade direction. Arteriography is performed before and after angioplasty in femoral, popliteal and tibial artery PTA and the ideal angiographic result is no residual stenosis at all, but slight narrowing of the arterial lumen is often acceptable if the blood flow is good. Endovascular ultrasound and angioscopy have also been used to assess the initial technical success of PTA, but Duplex ultrasound is used to assess the patency rate of the vessel following PTA.

The technical success rate in iliac artery PTA is 90–95% for stenoses and 80–90% for occlusions with a patency rate of 65–95% at 2 years and 50–85% at 5 years. The technical success rate in femoral and popliteal artery PTA is 85–95% for stenoses and 60–90% for occlusions with a patency rate of 45–85% at 2 years and 20–70% at 5 years. In comparison the patency rate for aorto-bifemoral bypass surgery is 70–85% at 5 years with an operative mortality of 2–5% and the patency rate for femoro-popliteal bypass surgery is 40–80% at 5 years with an operative mortality of 1–2%. The procedure-related mortality for angioplasty is negligible at 0.1%, but the 30-day mortality following angioplasty is 1% due to the co-morbidity in most patients.

The complication rate for PTA is 2–5% with complications occurring at the arterial puncture site, the angioplasty site, distal to the site of the angioplasty and in the systemic circulation.

Complications at the arterial puncture site are similar to those in diagnostic arteriography and include haemorrhage and haematoma formation, subintimal dissection and thrombosis, the development of a false aneurysm or an arteriovenous fistula, nerve trauma and local infection (see Fig. 15.23). A high antegrade catheterisation of the common femoral artery above the inguinal ligament may produce a retroperitoneal haemorrhage, which can be fatal. A false aneurysm can be treated by injecting thrombin into the false aneurysm under ultrasound guidance or by using the ultrasound probe to compress and occlude the neck of the false aneurysm in order to thrombose it, whilst maintaining flow in the adjacent artery.

Complications at the angioplasty site include flow limiting subintimal dissection, thrombosis and perforation. Subintimal dissection may produce occlusion of the artery, particularly in an antegrade direction where the flow of blood tends to open the flap, whereas in a retrograde direction the flow of blood tends to close the flap (see Fig. 15.21). Subintimal dissection can be treated by further angioplasty or the insertion of a vascular stent. Perforation of the femoral or popliteal artery within an occlusion is not usually significant, but rupture of an iliac artery produces a retroperitoneal haemorrhage, which can be fatal. Arterial rupture can be treated by the insertion of a covered vascular stent at the site or by inflation of the angioplasty balloon at the site prior to surgery. Acute occlusion at the site of the angioplasty due to thrombosis is one of the indications for thrombolysis. Rupture of the balloon also occasionally occurs, but is not usually significant.

Complications distal to the site of the angioplasty include arterial spasm and embolisation. Spasm in the popliteal and tibial arteries can be treated with nifedipine, isosorbide dinitrate or tolazoline, which are best given prophylactically. Distal embolisation of thrombus or atheromatous debris can be treated by aspiration thrombo-embolectomy or thrombolysis.

Systemic complications include a vasovagal reaction, hypotension, myocardial infarction, cerebrovascular accident, cholesterol crystal embolisation, renal failure and septicaemia.

Restenosis and chronic re-occlusion are detected on follow-up with duplex ultrasound and can be treated by repeat angioplasty or the insertion of a vascular stent. Recurrent stenoses can also be treated by brachytherapy.

Subclavian, axillary and brachial artery stenoses and short occlusions up to 3–5 cm in length are also suitable for PTA in patients with an ischaemic arm or a subclavian steal syndrome and are usually approached from below following catheterisation of the femoral artery (Fig. 15.82). Subclavian and axillary artery lesions can also be approached from above following a retrograde catheterisation of the brachial artery. The size of balloon used in subclavian and axillary artery PTA is usually 6–10 mm in diameter. The technical success rate in subclavian artery PTA is 80–95%, with a patency rate of 75% at 4 years. The complication rate is 5% and this includes cerebral infarction.

Coronary angioplasty Coronary artery PTA and other cardiac interventional vascular procedures such as balloon valvuloplasty of the pulmonary, aortic and mitral valves, atrial septostomy, balloon dilatation of aortic coarctation and closure of a patent ductus arteriosus are discussed in Chapters 7 and 17.

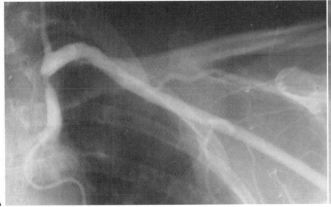 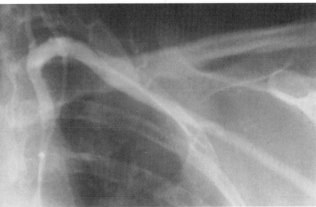

Fig. 15.82   (A) Arteriogram showing 75% stenosis in left subclavian artery before angioplasty. (B) Angiographic result with filling of internal mammary artery after angioplasty.

Renal angioplasty Many patients with hypertension undergo investigation in the search for a treatable cause for their raised blood pressure, but only 4–5% of them have renovascular hypertension due to a renal artery stenosis. This may be due to either atherosclerosis or fibromuscular dysplasia.

Renovascular hypertension is the main indication for renal artery PTA, but its use in patients with deteriorating renal failure due to renal artery disease is becoming increasingly important. Renal artery stenoses and short occlusions up to 1–2 cm in length are usually approached from below following catheterisation of the femoral artery, but can be approached from above following catheterisation of the left axillary or brachial artery, if there is a very acute angle between the aorta and renal artery. The size of balloon used in renal artery PTA is usually about 4–6 mm in diameter.

The technical success rate in renal artery PTA is 90% for stenoses and 50% for occlusions. Long-term results show that 95% of patients with fibromuscular dysplasia benefit from PTA with 60% cured of their hypertension and 35% improved, whereas 70% of patients with non-ostial atheroma benefit from PTA and of these only 30% are cured and 40% improved. About 40% of patients with renal failure show an improvement in serum creatinine following renal artery PTA. Ostial atheromatous stenoses and restenosis after PTA should be treated with a vascular stent (Fig. 15.83). The complication rate for renal artery PTA is 5–10% and this includes renal infarction.

Renal transplant artery stenoses are also suitable for PTA and are usually approached across the aortic bifurcation following catheterisation of the contralateral femoral artery. Stenoses on the venous side of an arteriovenous fistula occur in patients on haemodialysis and can be treated by PTA.

Carotid angioplasty Innominate, carotid and vertebral artery stenoses, but not occlusions, can be treated by PTA in patients with transient ischaemic attacks or vertebrobasilar insufficiency and are approached from below following catheterisation of the femoral

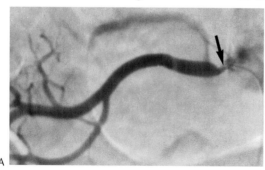
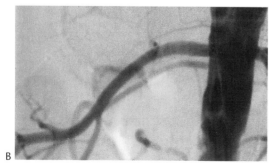

Fig. 15.83 (A) Arteriogram showing 75% osteal stenosis (arrow) in right renal artery before angioplasty. (B) Angiographic result after angioplasty and insertion of a vascular stent.

artery. The size of balloon used in innominate and common carotid artery PTA is usually 8–10 mm in diameter, but it is 5–6 mm in diameter for internal carotid artery PTA and 3–4 mm in diameter for vertebral artery PTA. Internal carotid artery PTA should be performed with a cerebral protection device in place to prevent embolic complications. Atheromatous stenoses in the internal carotid artery are also treated with vascular stents. The technical success rate in carotid artery PTA is 90–95%. The complication rate for carotid artery PTA is 5–10%, with a stroke rate of 1–3% and a procedure-related mortality of 0.3%.

Mesenteric angioplasty Coeliac and superior mesenteric artery stenoses and even occlusions can be treated by PTA in patients with chronic mesenteric ischaemia and are usually approached from below following catheterisation of the femoral artery, but can be approached from above following catheterisation of the left axillary or brachial artery. The size of balloon used in mesenteric artery PTA is usually 5–7 mm in diameter. The technical success rate in mesenteric artery PTA is 90%. Vascular stents have also been used in the coeliac and superior mesenteric arteries.

Adjunctive techniques to angioplasty

There are also a number of other devices and techniques available for use in the treatment of patients with peripheral vascular disease. These have been developed to improve the initial technical success and long-term patency rates of PTA and include mechanical rotational devices, atheroma removal devices and intravascular stents.

Mechanical rotating devices are used to recanalise complete occlusions, where conventional catheter and guide-wire combinations have failed. The recanalised channel still requires balloon dilatation, if the recanalisation is successful. The Rotational Transluminal Angioplasty Catheter System (ROTACS) is a low-speed battery-driven catheter that rotates at about 100 rpm and produces a recanalisation rate of 80%. The Kensey catheter is a high-speed electric-motor-driven catheter, that rotates at 10 000–20 000 rpm and produces a recanalisation rate of 70–90% with a long-term patency rate of 50–70% at 2 years. The Rotablator is a very high-speed gas-turbine-driven catheter that rotates at 100 000–200 000 rpm and produces a recanalisation rate of 90%, but it has a long-term patency rate of only 25–40% at 2 years. These mechanical rotating devices produce microparticles with distal embolisation but they are rarely used now.

Atheroma removing devices are also used to recanalise complete occlusions, where conventional catheter and guide-wire combinations have failed, but can be used to treat stenoses. Subsequent balloon dilatation is again required.

The Transluminal Endarterectomy Catheter (TEC) cuts through the atheroma, which is then aspirated through the catheter by a vacuum producing a technical success rate of 80–90%. The Simpson atherectomy catheter slices off the atheroma, which is then collected in a small chamber producing a technical success rate of 80–90%. The small capacity of the chamber limits its use to eccentric stenoses. Both these atherectomy devices have high restenosis rates of 15–45% and are only occasionally used.

Laser-assisted angioplasty uses a hot-tip metal probe or a sapphire-tipped hybrid probe, coupled to a continuous- or pulsed-wave argon or neodymium : yttrium aluminium garnet laser generator, to recanalise complete occlusions. The recanalised channel is produced by direct heat from the hot-tip metal probe, which reaches a temperature of about 400°C, or direct heat and laser energy from the sapphire-tipped hybrid probe, which allows 10% of the laser energy to exit directly through a window in the tip of the probe. Balloon dilatation of the recanalised channel is required. Laser-assisted angioplasty has a primary recanalisation rate of 70–90% with a long-term patency rate of 60–70% at 2 years, but a high risk of arterial perforation of up to 20%. Laser-assisted angioplasty is rarely used now.

Intravascular stents

Arterial stents

Intravascular stents are used to maintain the lumen of a vessel by a mechanical supporting effect on its wall. Intravascular stents are used mainly in the iliac, coronary and renal arteries, but have been used in the aorta, and the femoral, popliteal, subclavian and carotid arteries. The types of vascular stent available include the self-expanding Wallstent, Memotherm and Gianturco Z stents and the balloon expandable Palmaz, Strecker and Bridge stents. The indications for the insertion of a vascular stent in the arterial system are to prevent an acute occlusion developing after an intimal flap has been produced by angioplasty, to abolish the pressure gradient across a significant residual stenosis after angioplasty, to treat recurrent stenoses, and stenoses in the aorta, renal osteal (Fig. 15.83) and carotid arteries and occlusions in the iliac, coronary and renal arteries (Fig. 15.84). The long-term patency rate in the iliac arteries is 90–95% at 2 years. The complication and mortality rates for arterial stents are similar to angioplasty in the same vessel.

Covered stents such as the Jostent have been used to treat ruptures in the iliac artery after angioplasty and false aneurysms or arteriovenous fistulas in the peripheral arteries in the arms and legs (Fig. 15.85).

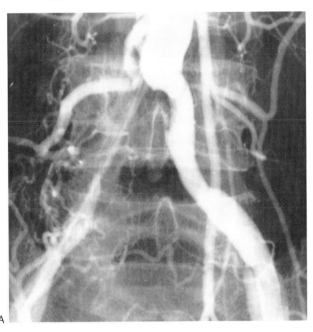
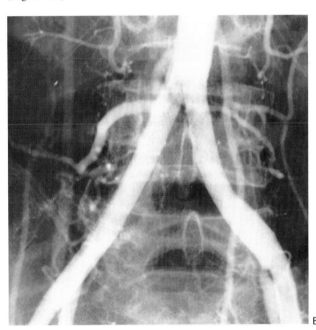

Fig. 15.84 (A) Arteriogram showing a short 4 cm occlusion in the right common iliac artery. (B) Arteriogram after insertion of Wallstens in both common iliac arteries.

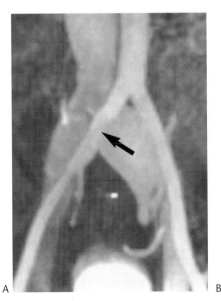
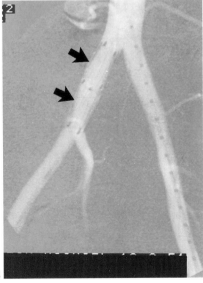

Fig. 15.85 (A) Traumatic AV fistula (arrow) between right common iliac artery and left common iliac vein produced by lumbar disc surgery on MRA. (B) Angiographic result after insertion of a covered stent (arrows).

Endovascular aneurysm repair

The first endovascular repair of an abdominal aortic aneurysm (EVAR) was performed by Parodi in Argentina in 1990 and since then endovascular grafts have developed from simple devices to commercially available systems, which are now used for the treatment of abdominal and thoracic aortic aneurysms and iliac, subclavian and popliteal artery aneurysms.

Endovascular grafts consist of a series of metal stents covered by a surgical graft material. The three basic types of graft available for the endovascular repair of abdominal aortic aneurysms are the aorto–biiliac system, the aorto–uniiliac system (which also needs the use of an occluding device in the contralateral common iliac artery and a femoro–femoral crossover graft) and the straight aorto–aortic system, which is also used for the endovascular repair of thoracic aortic aneurysms and dissections.

In patients being considered for EVAR, it is essential to obtain a series of measurements on the aorta and iliac arteries using CT or MR angiography, so that an endovascular graft of the appropriate length and diameter can be used (Fig. 15.86). These large-calibre systems require a femoral arteriotomy for insertion (Figs 15.87, 15.88) but smaller-calibre systems for the treatment of iliac or popliteal artery aneurysms can be used percutaneously.

The complications of EVAR include rupture of the iliac arteries or aortic aneurysm during insertion of the endovascular graft, renal artery occlusion during insertion of the endovascular graft, distal embolisation during the procedure, renal failure after the procedure, development of an endoleak from the proximal or distal ends of the graft (type 1) (Fig. 15.89) from a patent lumbar or inferior mesenteric artery (type 2) or from a defect in the graft system (type 3), thrombosis of the graft or one of its limbs, graft migration into the sac of the aneurysm and rupture of the aneurysm as well as typical surgical complications.

Venous stents Intravascular stents are also used in the venous system, particularly in the management of patients with SVC obstruction due to bronchial carcinoma or other mediastinal

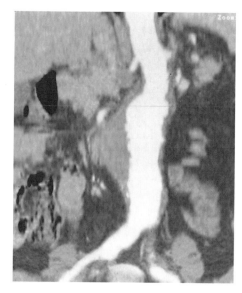

Fig. 15.86 CT showing coronal planar reconstruction of AAA.

tumours. The stents most commonly used are the Wallstent and the Gianturco Z stent and they are positioned in the SVC and brachiocephalic veins following catheterisation of the basilic vein, internal jugular vein or femoral vein. Initial thrombolysis may also be required if the SVC obstruction is complicated by the presence of thrombus.

Intravascular stents have also been used in patients with IVC obstruction due to hepatic or retroperitoneal tumours and to treat stenoses in the hepatic, iliac and subclavian veins and renal dialysis access shunts.

Inferior vena caval filters There are a large number of permanent and temporary filters available for insertion into the IVC and these include the Greenfield titanium filter, the Cardial steel filter, the

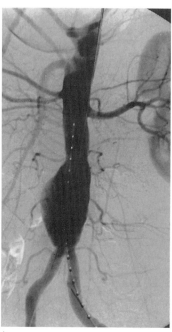

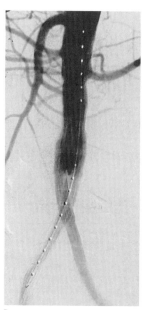

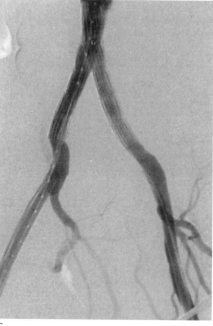

Fig. 15.87 (A) Arteriogram showing infrarenal AAA suitable for EVAR. (B,C) Angiographic result after insertion of aortobiiliac stent.

A

B

C

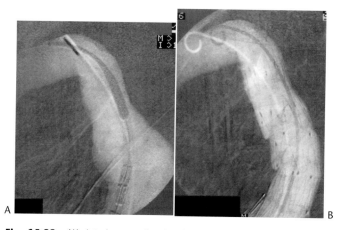

Fig. 15.88 (A) Arteriogram showing fusiform aneurysm of descending thoracic aorta. (B) Angiographic result after insertion of straight aortic stent.

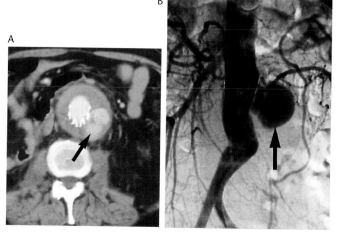

Fig. 15.89 Type 1 endoleak after early EVAR on CT (A) and arteriogram (B).

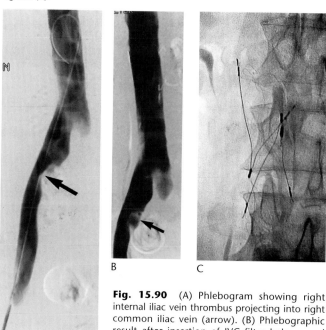

Fig. 15.90 (A) Phlebogram showing right internal iliac vein thrombus projecting into right common iliac vein (arrow). (B) Phlebographic result after insertion of IVC filter below renal veins. (C) Birds nest IVC filter.

Gianturco-Roehm bird's nest filter, the Gunther tulip filter, the Simon nitinol filter, the LGM Venatech filter and the Antheor filter. The indications for the insertion of an IVC filter are recurrent pulmonary emboli in patients despite good anticoagulation, pulmonary emboli or deep vein thrombosis in patients with a contraindication to anticoagulation, deep vein thrombosis in patients with pulmonary arterial hypertension and as prophylaxis against pulmonary emboli in high-risk patients.

IVC filters are ideally positioned below the renal veins (Fig. 15.90) following catheterisation of the femoral or internal jugular vein, but can be positioned in the suprarenal IVC if there is thrombus in the renal veins or infrarenal IVC. Most IVC filters are permanent insertions, but the Gunther tulip filter is retrievable from the IVC for up to 2 weeks and the Antheor filter is a temporary filter on a catheter, which can be used during venous thrombolysis. IVC filters reduce the rate of recurrent pulmonary emboli from 20% to 4% and the associated mortality from 10% to less than 2%. The complications of insertion of a filter include thrombosis of the femoral or internal jugular veins, caval thrombosis, central migration of the filter and structural failure of the filter.

Transjugular liver biopsy A transjugular liver biopsy is performed in patients who are at risk of bleeding from the liver following a percutaneous biopsy. The indications for a transjugular liver biopsy are therefore patients with abnormal clotting studies, thrombocytopenia or ascites, but it can be performed in patients who also require portal pressure studies.

The biopsy is obtained from the right lobe of the liver, by positioning a guiding catheter in the right hepatic vein following catheterisation of the right internal jugular vein under ultrasound guidance. A sample of tissue is obtained in almost all cases and any bleeding is contained within the liver or passes straight into the hepatic vein, although it is still possible to bleed into the peritoneal cavity if the biopsy is close to the liver capsule.

Transjugular intrahepatic portosystemic shunt The first successful transjugular intrahepatic portosystemic shunt (TIPS) was performed by Richter in Germany in 1988. The procedure involves creating a tract between the hepatic vein and the portal vein to reduce the portal venous pressure. The indications for a TIPS procedure are recurrent gastrointestinal bleeding in patients with varices despite endoscopic sclerotherapy or banding, intractable ascites in patients with chronic liver disease and the Budd–Chiari syndrome.

The tract is produced in the right lobe of the liver by passing a needle from the right hepatic vein into the right portal vein through a guiding catheter introduced from the right internal jugular vein under ultrasound guidance, after initially confirming the position of the hepatic portal vein by either arterioportography or wedged hepatic venography. This tract is then dilated with an angioplasty balloon and an intravascular stent positioned across the hepatic tissue from the portal vein to the hepatic vein. The portal venous pressure is measured before and after the shunt has been created and should ideally be reduced to 10–15 mmHg. Gastric varices can also be embolised with steel coils (Fig. 15.91).

The technical success rate for a TIPS procedure is about 90%, but there is a procedure-related mortality of 1–3% and a 30-day mortality of about 15%. The complications of a TIPS procedure include hepatic encephalopathy and thrombosis of the shunt due to intimal hyperplasia.

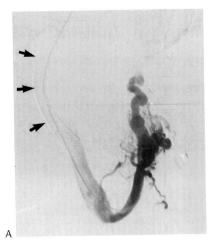
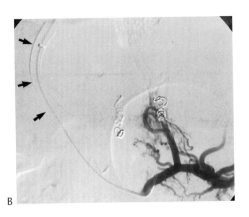
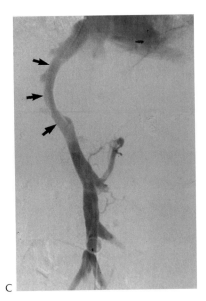

Fig. 15.91 (A) Phlebogram showing gastric varices during a TIPS with vascular stent in the liver. (B) Phlebographic result after embolisation with metal coils. (C) Phlebographic result after successful TIPS. Guide has passed through the hepatic vein and liver to reach (arrows) a portal vein.

Central venous catheters Central venous catheters are frequently used in the management of patients who are seriously ill for venous pressure measurement, fluid replacement, antibiotics, chemotherapy and parenteral nutrition. They include the Swan–Ganz catheter, the Hickman catheter and the Groshong catheter, but there are many other types of single, double and triple lumen catheters available.

Catheters for short- or long-term use are usually introduced via the internal jugular or subclavian veins under ultrasound guidance and positioned with the tip of the catheter in the SVC. Catheters for long-term use pass through a subcutaneous tunnel, but can also be totally implanted if they are connected to a subcutaneous port reservoir. Central venous catheters can also be introduced via the common femoral, median basilic and cephalic veins and even the IVC.

The complications of insertion of a central venous catheter include pneumothorax, mediastinal haematoma, catheter fracture, subcutaneous infection, septicaemia, catheter-induced thrombosis and pulmonary embolus.

Retrieval of vascular foreign bodies A variety of diagnostic, monitoring and therapeutic lines, catheters, wires and other foreign bodies such as embolisation coils are introduced into the arterial or venous systems of an increasing number of patients during their clinical management. Occasionally small or large fragments of these catheters or wires are broken off during their insertion or removal and are lost within the vascular system, usually on the venous side. Foreign bodies in the veins migrate centrally and may lodge in the right atrium, right ventricle and main pulmonary arteries or their branches, whereas foreign bodies in the arteries are carried peripherally and tend to lodge at a vessel bifurcation.

Intravascular foreign bodies produce a high complication rate of 70% with a mortality rate of 40% if they are not removed. These complications may occur immediately or be delayed for weeks, months or years and include cardiac arrhythmias, myocardial perforation, endocarditis, pulmonary emboli, septicaemia and mycotic aneurysms.

A venous foreign body is retrieved following catheterisation of the femoral or internal jugular vein and an arterial foreign body via the femoral artery. A vascular sheath, large enough to accommodate the foreign body, is placed in the femoral vein or artery. The foreign body is then grasped by a loop snare, stone retrieval basket or biopsy forceps and withdrawn into the sheath for removal, although it may initially need to be dislodged by a catheter to get it into a better position.

Vascular infusion therapy

The purpose of vascular infusion therapy is to deliver a small dose of a drug to an organ system, at a higher concentration than can be obtained by systemic administration, via a catheter selectively positioned in the artery supplying that particular vascular bed. The drugs that have been used in therapeutic pharmacoangiography include vasoconstrictors, vasodilators, cytotoxic and fibrinolytic drugs.

Vasoconstrictors, such as vasopressin, epinephrine (adrenaline) and norepinephrine (noradrenaline) can be used in the treatment of acute gastrointestinal haemorrhage. After localising the site of the bleeding by selective arteriography, an intra-arterial infusion of vasopressin at 0.1–0.2 units/min for 20 min is used to control it, by causing vasoconstriction of the blood supply to the gastrointestinal tract. If repeat arteriography after 20 min no longer shows extravasation of contrast medium, the infusion is continued for 12–24 h and then the dose is reduced for a further 12–24 h, but if bleeding is still occurring the dose is increased before being gradually reduced. A vasopressin infusion into the left gastric artery is effective in controlling bleeding from oesophageal mucosal tears and erosive gastritis in 80% of patients, although recurrent bleeding occurs in 20% of patients. An infusion into the superior or inferior mesenteric artery is also effective in controlling bleeding from colonic diverticula in 90% of patients, but once again there is recurrent bleeding in 30% of patients. This type of treatment is much less effective for chronic peptic ulcers and gastrointestinal tumours.

The complications of vasopressin include hypertension, cardiac arrhythmias, myocardial infarction, lower limb and mesenteric ischaemia and infarction due to its vasoconstrictor effect as well as oedema and electrolyte imbalance due to its antidiuretic effect.

The use of vasodilators, such as isosorbide dinitrate or glyceryl trinitrate, nifedipine and tolazoline to prevent arterial spasm in patients undergoing popliteal, tibial and coronary artery PTA has already been discussed. Vasodilators, such as papaverine, tolazoline, reserpine and the prostaglandins E_1 and $F_{2\alpha}$ have also been used in the treatment of Raynaud's disease, frostbite, trauma and mesenteric ischaemia.

A variety of cytotoxic drugs have been used as intra-arterial infusions in the treatment of both primary and secondary tumours. An infusion of 5-fluorouracil and mitomycin C or cisplatin over 5 days into the hepatic artery in patients with hepatic metastases from colorectal carcinoma produces response rates ranging from 45% to 60%, after several cycles of chemotherapy, but an infusion of cisplatin and vinblastine in patients with hepatic metastases from breast carcinoma only produces a response rate of 20–30%. The use of 5-fluorouracil, doxorubicin and mitomycin C produces a response rate of 60% in patients with hepatocellular carcinoma, but when used in combination with Lipiodol and gelatin sponge fragments to embolise the hepatic artery response rates of up to 90% are produced. This technique is called chemoembolisation. Various other tumours including bronchial, renal and bladder carcinoma, gynaecological malignancies and bone tumours have also been treated by selective intra-arterial infusions of cytotoxic drugs. The commonest complication of this type of treatment is thrombosis of the artery supplying the tumour, as the catheters remain in position for several days.

Thrombolysis

Fibrinolytic therapy has been used in the treatment of various thrombotic diseases, such as acute myocardial infarction, acute lower limb ischaemia and acute pulmonary embolism over the past 30 years. The technique of thrombolysis in lower limb ischaemia was described in 1974 by Dotter, who used a catheter with its tip in the acute occlusion to deliver an intra-arterial infusion of a low dose of streptokinase into the thrombus, in order to reduce the haemorrhagic complications produced by the systemic fibrinolytic effect of the high-dose intravenous infusions that had been previously tried.

Thrombolysis can be performed in patients with acute critical lower limb ischaemia as an alternative to an embolectomy or a surgical bypass graft, as these patients tend to have a poor clinical outcome.

The indications for intra-arterial thrombolysis are therefore distal arterial thrombosis or embolus involving the popliteal and tibial arteries, thrombosis of a surgical graft, thrombosis at the site of a recent angioplasty and proximal arterial thrombosis involving the iliac and femoral arteries in a high-risk patient. Surgery is still indicated for proximal arterial embolus or thrombosis involving the aorta, iliac and femoral arteries, particularly if the ischaemia is very severe. The contraindications to intra-arterial thrombolysis include a cerebral infarct within the previous 3 months due to the risk of developing a cerebral haemorrhage, recent major surgery or trauma within the last month, active bleeding from any site, a bleeding diathesis, pregnancy, diabetic retinopathy and muscle necrosis due to the risk of developing acute renal failure from the release of myoglobin.

Thrombolysis is usually performed at the time of the diagnostic arteriography by positioning the tip of the catheter within the thrombus. Iliac and proximal femoral artery occlusions are approached across the aortic bifurcation following catheterisation of the contralateral femoral artery. Distal femoral and popliteal artery occlusions are approached following catheterisation of the ipsilateral femoral artery. With the low-dose infusion technique, streptokinase at 5000 units/h, urokinase at 50 000 units/h or recombinant tissue plasminogen activator at 0.5 mg/h is injected into the thrombus and the degree of lysis monitored by arteriography over 24–48 h. Higher doses of these fibrinolytic drugs reduce the lysis time to 6–18 h. Any underlying stenosis revealed as the lysis progresses requires PTA. More recently accelerated thrombolytic regimens have been developed to shorten the lysis time still further and in pulse spray pharmacomechanical thrombosis, the fibrinolytic drug is injected throughout the thrombus via multiple holes or slits in the catheter resulting in a lysis time of 1–3 h. The complications of thrombolysis include groin haematoma, retroperitoneal haemorrhage and bleeding from other sites, pericatheter thrombolysis, distal embolisation of thrombus, acute renal failure and a cerebrovascular accident. Thrombolysis results in limb salvage in 70–80% of patients with a critically ischaemic limb, an amputation rate of 5–10% and a 30-day mortality rate of 10%.

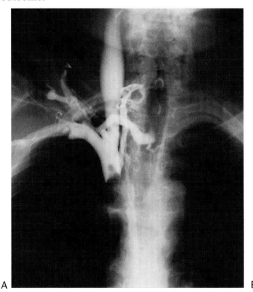
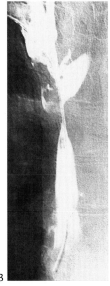
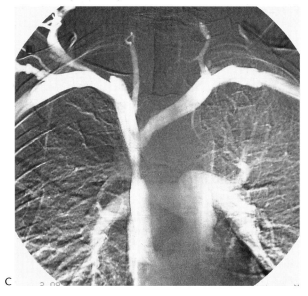

A   B   C

Fig. 15.92 Venograms showing complete occlusion of the superior vena cava due to thrombus (A) before thrombolysis and (B) a pulse spray catheter in the superior cava during the lysis with tissue plasminogan activator. (C) Angiographic result in the superior vena cava and brachiocephalic veins after thrombolysis and the insertion of a Wallstent.

Thrombolysis has also been used in the treatment of acute critical upper limb ischaemia, thrombosed haemodialysis access grafts, renal artery occlusions, SVC obstruction, deep vein thrombosis in the legs and hepatic vein thrombosis (Fig. 15.92). In the technique of aspiration thrombectomy, small fragments of fresh thrombus can be aspirated through a catheter with a large internal lumen. Large amounts of fresh thrombus can be removed by mechanical thromboembolectomy devices such as the Amplatz thrombectomy device which uses an impeller driven by an air turbine at speeds of 150 000 rpm to fragment the thrombus or the Hydrolyser catheter which uses a jet of fluid to produce the Venturi effect, which fragments and aspirates the thrombus.

Therapeutic embolisation

The basic technique of therapeutic embolisation involves the injection of embolic material through a catheter selectively positioned in an artery or vein in order to deliberately occlude the artery, vein or vascular bed of an organ by the formation of thrombus in the blood vessels.

A large number of different solid and liquid materials have been used for therapeutic embolisation over the past 30 years. The properties of the ideal embolic material are that it should be thrombogenic, but not toxic, and produce a permanent vascular occlusion. It should also be easy to inject through an angiographic catheter and available in a wide range of shapes and sizes, that are both sterile and radiopaque.

The most commonly used embolic agents today include solid particulate materials, such as gelatin sponge fragments (Gelfoam or Sterispon) and polyvinyl alcohol particles (PVA or Ivalon), mechanical devices, such as spiral metal coils and detachable balloons, sclerosing liquids, such as ethanol and sodium tetradecyl sulphate (SDS or Sotradecol), and tissue adhesives, such as butyl-cyanoacrylate (Bucrylate). All these embolic materials produce a permanent vascular occlusion, except Gelfoam, which only produces a temporary occlusion that recanalises within a month. None of them however are the ideal embolic agent, and they are often used in combination to produce occlusions at various levels in the vascular tree. The gelatin sponge is not radiopaque and has to be cut up into small 1–3 mm fragments, which are then suspended in contrast medium before injection. The PVA particles are also not radiopaque, but are available in a range of sizes from 150–250, 250–600 and 600–1000 mm particles, which also need to be suspended in contrast medium before injection.

The metal coils are made of stainless steel or platinum and are available in a range of sizes and lengths with a spiral diameter of 1–20 mm or larger. The stainless steel coils have threads of wool, silk or Dacron attached to them to increase their thrombogenicity. Metal coils are radiopaque and are delivered by being pushed through the catheter with a guide-wire. The detachable balloons are made of latex or silicone and are available in 1 and 2 mm sizes, which can be inflated up to 4 and 8 mm in diameter. The balloons are not radiopaque and have to be filled with contrast medium before being detached from their microcatheter. Ethanol, Sotradecol and hypertonic 50% dextrose solution are mixed with contrast medium before injection, but the tissue adhesive Bucrylate is mixed with tantalum powder or ethiodol before injection, which makes it radiopaque and prolongs its polymerisation time. Lyophilised dura mater fragments should no longer be used because of the potential risk of transmission of Creuzfeldt–Jakob disease and tungsten coils have been withdrawn because they degrade to produce raised serum tungsten levels in the body.

Embolisation is generally performed as an alternative to a surgical procedure, particularly if the patient is unfit for surgery and the operation carries a high risk, but it may be the optimal method of treatment for the patient. Embolisation is also performed in combination with surgery, generally to reduce the blood loss during an operation and thus shorten the procedure.

The indications for arterial embolisation include the management of acute haemorrhage, the management of tumours, the treatment of arteriovenous malformations (AVM), arteriovenous fistulas and aneurysms as well as the ablation of function of an organ. The indications for venous embolisation are the treatment of gastro-oesophageal varices, the treatment of testicular varicocoeles and the ablation of function of the adrenal gland.

Embolisation in the management of acute haemorrhage

Embolisation is used in the management of patients with bleeding from the gastrointestinal, genitourinary and respiratory tracts and in bleeding following trauma.

In patients with severe and continuing or recurrent bleeding from the upper or lower gastrointestinal tracts mesenteric angiography should be performed, when endoscopy and colonoscopy have failed to identify its site. It should also be performed after a positive radionuclide scan using either ^{99m}Tc-labelled sulphur colloid or labelled red blood cells have demonstrated gastrointestinal haemorrhage. Active bleeding from mucosal ulcers, tumours and following trauma of the stomach, duodenum or rectum can be stopped by embolisation of the left gastric, gastroduodenal or superior rectal arteries with Gelfoam and metal coils in patients who are not suitable for surgery. The stomach, duodenum and rectum all have a dual blood supply, unless there has been previous gastrointestinal surgery and the risk of infarction and perforation is therefore low. Active bleeding from the small intestine, caecum and colon has been treated by embolisation with Gelfoam and metal coils, but the risk of infarction and perforation is high because of the single blood supply to these structures. A vasopressin infusion can be used to control bleeding in these patients.

Active bleeding from a false aneurysm in the pancreas due to recurrent pancreatitis or following trauma can be treated by embolisation of the gastroduodenal or splenic arteries with metal coils and active bleeding from a false aneurysm in the liver due to hepatic metastases or following liver biopsy, blunt trauma or hepatobiliary surgery can be treated by embolisation of the appropriate branch of the right or left hepatic arteries with metal coils.

In patients with severe and continuing or recurrent bleeding from the kidney or bladder, renal or pelvic angiography should be performed. Haematuria can be controlled by embolisation of the renal artery using Ivalon, Gelfoam, ethanol and metal coils in patients with renal cell carcinoma, who are unsuitable for surgery (Fig. 15.93). Active bleeding from a false aneurysm in the kidney following renal biopsy or trauma can be treated by embolisation of the appropriate branch of the renal artery with metal coils. Embolisation with metal coils is also the treatment of choice in patients with a renal AVM. Embolisation of both internal iliac arteries with Gelfoam and metal coils is also used to control haematuria in patients with bladder tumours, who are unsuitable for surgery, and to treat patients with vaginal bleeding from gynaecological tumours. Continuing post-traumatic internal haemorrhage following pelvic fractures, which has not responded to external fixation, can be treated by embolization of the appropriate branch of the internal iliac artery with metal coils.

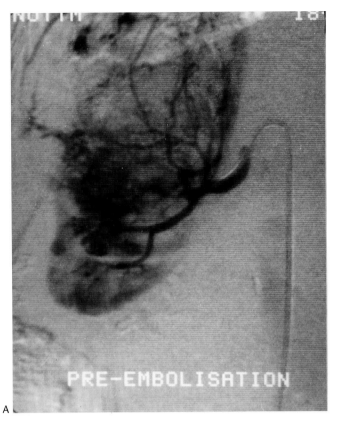
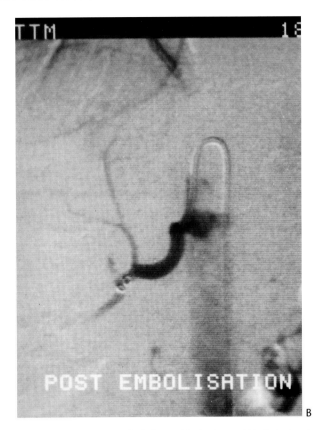

Fig. 15.93 (A) Renal arteriogram showing a large renal cell carcinoma. (B) After embolisation of the right kidney with absolute ethyl alcohol, gelatin sponge fragments, and spiral metal coils.

Embolisation of the bronchial arteries with Gelfoam and Ivalon is also effective in controlling massive haemoptysis and embolisation of the internal maxillary arteries with Gelfoam has been used in the treatment of life-threatening epistaxis.

Embolisation of gastro-oesophageal varices with metal coils is usually performed during a TIPS procedure, but can also be carried out following a percutaneous transhepatic catheterisation of the portal venous system.

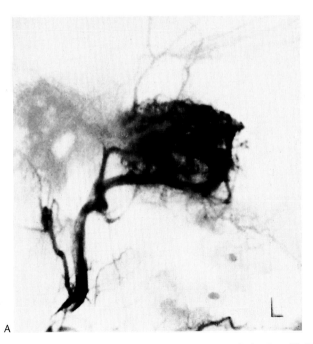
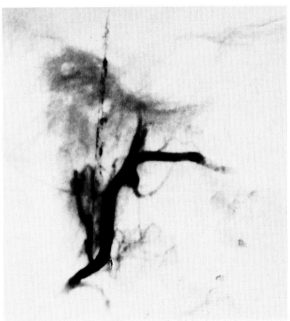

Fig. 15.94 Nasopharyngeal angiofibroma. (A) Before embolisation. (B) After embolisation.

Embolisation in the management of tumours

Embolisation is used in the management of patients with neoplastic disease as a preoperative technique to reduce blood loss during surgery, as a palliative technique to alleviate symptoms and occasionally as a definitive procedure instead of surgery.

Preoperative embolisation of a neoplasm is done to reduce blood loss during the surgery and to decrease tumour size, thus making the surgery much easier. This type of embolisation was frequently performed several days before nephrectomy in patients with renal cell carcinoma, but this can in fact make the surgery more difficult as the inflammatory response that develops affects the tissue planes around the kidney. Preoperative embolisation is still performed for renal cell carcinoma, but the timing of the procedure should ideally be only a few hours before the surgery. A balloon occlusion catheter can also be effectively used for this purpose. Other tumours that may require preoperative embolisation include intracranial meningiomas, nasopharyngeal angiofibromas (Fig. 15.94), chemodactomas, primary bone tumours and primary hepatic tumours.

Palliative embolisation is performed to alleviate symptoms such as bleeding, pain and the metabolic effects of endocrine tumours. This type of embolisation is usually performed in patients with hepatic metastases. The liver has a dual blood supply and normally receives 75% of its blood from the hepatic portal vein and only 25% of its blood from the hepatic artery. Tumours however tend to receive 90% of their blood supply from the hepatic artery, but only 10% from the portal venous system. Hepatic artery embolisation is therefore contraindicated if the portal vein is occluded.

Embolisation of the hepatic artery with Gelfoam and metal coils is used to control haemobilia in patients with a false aneurysm from hepatic metastases and to reduce pain from stretching of the liver capsule in patients with hepatomegaly from a primary tumour or hepatic metastases by reducing the size of the liver. Embolisation of the liver is effective in controlling the symptoms of flushing and diarrhoea produced by 5-hydroxytryptamine in patients with the carcinoid syndrome, by ablating the functioning capacity of the hepatic metastases. Symptomatic relief can also be produced in patients with hepatic metastases from insulinomas, glucagonomas and vipomas. Chemoembolisation using doxorubicin mixed with Lipiodol has also been used in the treatment of multifocal hepatocellular carcinoma and hepatic metastases (Fig. 15.95).

Therapeutic embolisation has been performed as the definitive procedure in the treatment of benign bone tumours, benign hepatic tumours and ectopic parathyroid tumours in the mediastinum. Recently embolisation of the uterine arteries with Ivalon has been used in the treatment of fibroids. Embolisation of adrenal tumours by venous infarction has also been performed in patients with both Cushing's syndrome and Conn's syndrome.

Embolisation in the treatment of vascular abnormalities

Embolisation is used in the treatment of AVMs, arteriovenous fistulas and aneurysms.

Patients with AVMs in the head, neck, and upper and lower limbs, are difficult to treat surgically because the operative field is readily obscured by blood from the large number of arteries and veins in the malformation, the surgery often needs to be extensive to remove the malformation and they have a tendency to recur if incompletely excised. Embolisation alone is therefore often the optimal method of treatment but it can also be used in a preoperative capacity. Small AVMs can be treated by embolising the feeding arteries and the nidus of the lesion in one procedure, but large AVMs may require several procedures. AVMs with a significant arteriovenous component are most suited to embolisation with Bucrylate or ethanol and AVMs with a significant capillary–venous component can be treated by a direct venous approach using Sotradecol or ethanol. Post-traumatic arteriovenous fistulas (Fig. 15.96) and both true and false aneurysms can be embolised with large occluding devices such as metal coils or balloons or treated with covered stents (Figs 15.97, 15.98). Embolisation with metal coils is also the treatment of choice in patients with pulmonary AVMs.

Patients with impaired fertility due to a left testicular varicocoele can be treated by embolisation of the left gonadal vein with metal coils and Sotradecol. Successful treatment results in an improved sperm count and quality.

Embolisation to ablate organ function

Embolisation is used not only to ablate the functioning tissue in adrenal and parathyroid adenomas and hepatic metastases from carcinoid tumours, insulinomas and glucagonomas, but also the spleen

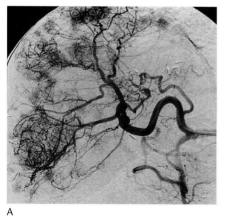
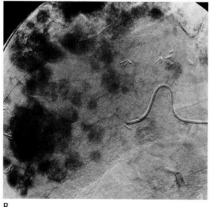
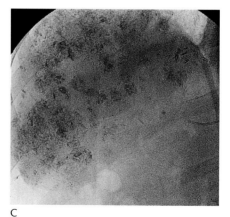

A   B   C

Fig. 15.95 (A,B) Arteriogram showing hypervascular multifocal hepatocellular carcinoma in the liver. (C) Lipiodol and doxorubicin in the liver after chemoembolisation.

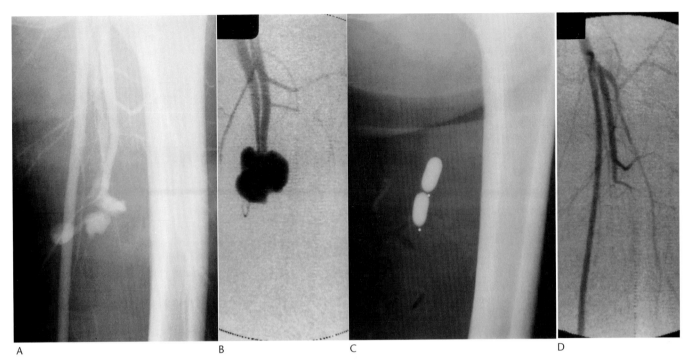

A　　　　　　　　　　B　　　　　　　　C　　　　　　　　　　D

Fig. 15.96 (A,B) Arteriograms showing an arteriovenous fistula between the left deep femoral artery and vein with false aneurysm formation due to a stab wound. (C,D) After embolisatin with the balloons.

in patients with hypersplenism. Embolisation of the spleen with Gelfoam, Ivalon and metal coils is occasionally performed in patients who are unsuitable for surgery, and is best undertaken in several stages as there is a high risk of abscess formation in the infarcted splenic tissue. Embolisation of the internal pudendal artery with Gelfoam is also effective in treating patients with priapism.

Complications of embolisation

The complications of embolisation include the complications of both the arteriography and the use of contrast media, the post-embolisation syndrome and the specific complications of the procedure.

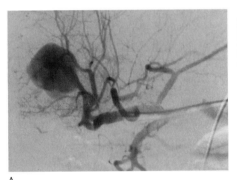

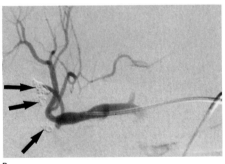

A　　　　　　　　　　　　　　B

Fig. 15.97 (A) Arteriogram showing false aneurysm of anterior branch of right hepatic artery at the site of the hepatojejunostomy. (B) Angiographic result after embolisation with metal coils (arrows).

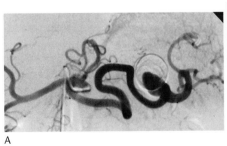

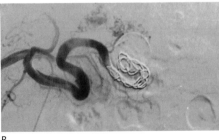

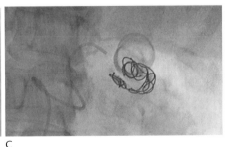

A　　　　　　　　　　B　　　　　　　　　C

Fig. 15.98 (A) Arteriogram showing splenic artery aneurysm. (B) Angiographic result after embolisation with metal coils. (C) Embolisation coils proximal and distal to the neck of the aneurysm.

The postembolisation syndrome usually occurs within 24–48 h of the procedure and lasts for 3–7 days after the procedure. It is characterised by pain at the site of the embolisation, nausea and vomiting, malaise, fever, leucocytosis and raised inflammatory markers and is more severe when a large volume of tissue has been embolised. The development of an abscess can however occur in the infarcted tissue and it is important not to confuse this with the postembolisation syndrome. Prophylactic antibiotics are therefore required in patients undergoing embolisation of solid organs and strict aseptic technique is essential during the procedure. The presence of gas within the necrotic tissue is a normal finding after embolisation and does not necessarily indicate the presence of a developing abscess. A more extensive volume of tissue infarction than planned may occur due to retrograde extension of thrombus in the embolised vessel and accidental tissue necrosis may be produced in adjacent critical organs due to either reflux of solid embolic material into their arterial supply or permeation of liquid embolic material into their capillary bed.

Pulmonary emboli can occur when small particulate embolic material passes through arteriovenous communications in either vascular tissue or systemic AVMs, but this is not usually clinically significant. Similarly systemic emboli can occur during the treatment of a pulmonary AVM. Large embolic devices such as metal coils and detachable balloons can be retrieved from the vascular system if they become misplaced. Release of metabolically active substances from functioning endocrine tissue occurs after embolisation of hepatic metastases from carcinoid tumours and insulinomas.

Prophylactic pharmacological blocking agents are therefore required in these patients. Release of toxic radicals also occurs after embolisation of any tissue and this can lead to renal failure if large volumes of tissue are infarcted. Dehydration and the large doses of contrast medium used during an embolisation also contribute to the development of renal failure.

The overall complication rate for most embolisation ranges from 3–10% with a procedure-related mortality of 1–2%, but splenic embolisation has a complication rate of nearly 20% and a mortality rate of 7%.

DOPPLER ULTRASOUND OF THE PERIPHERAL ARTERIES AND ABDOMINAL VESSELS

Paul Allan

Doppler ultrasound techniques are based on the Doppler equation, which was described by Christian Johann Doppler in 1842. The underlying principle is that when sound or light waves are moving between a transmitter and a receiver which are stationary in relation to each other then the receiver will register the same frequency as the transmitter emitted. If there is relative movement toward each other then the receiver will register a slightly higher frequency (shorter wavelength) than was transmitted; conversely, if there is relative motion apart, then the receiver will register a slightly lower frequency (longer wavelength). These small changes in frequency are known as Doppler shifts and can easily be measured by modern ultrasound equipment through direct comparison of the returning frequency with the transmitted frequency.

The derivation of the Doppler equation used in medical ultrasound is

$$F_d = F_t - F_r = \frac{2F_t v \cos\theta}{c}.$$

F_d is the frequency or Doppler shift, F_t is the transmitted frequency, F_r is the received frequency, v is the velocity of the reflector (usually blood in the vessels), θ is the angle between the direction of the ultrasound beam and the direction of flow of the blood and c is the mean velocity of sound in the tissues, 1540 m/s. Using modern ultrasound equipment, the only variable which is unknown is the velocity of the reflecting blood cells, this can therefore be calculated as

$$v = \frac{F_d c}{2F_t \cos\theta}.$$

The basic information obtained with Doppler is quite limited. It shows if there is moving blood present, which way it is going and how fast it is moving. Some information on the character of flow can be deduced, such as the presence of turbulent flow and decreased diastolic flow. Doppler shifts are given in units of frequency—kilohertz (kHz). The velocity of flow in metres or centimetres per second can only be calculated and displayed if an angle correction is applied using a cursor on the image of the vessel.

TYPES OF DOPPLER EQUIPMENT

Continuous-wave Doppler (CW Doppler)

This is the simplest type of equipment. The probe contains two transducer crystals: one transmits continuously, the other receives continuously. The Doppler shift is calculated and 'displayed' as an audio signal. It is fortuitous that the conditions of medical Doppler result in Doppler shifts that are conveniently located within the range of human hearing. CW Doppler equipment is simple and cheap, but the main disadvantage is that anything moving in the line of the ultrasound beam contributes to the Doppler signal and localising the source of the shift is therefore not possible. This type of equipment is used in vascular clinics to locate arterial pulses, measure perfusion pressures, test for venous reflux, etc.

Duplex Doppler

These machines combine real-time imaging with pulsed Doppler. This allows the operator to identify a specific segment in a particular vessel and to place the gate, or sample volume, at a specific location so that the source of the Doppler signal is known. The time taken by the pulses of ultrasound to travel to and from the blood vessel means that, for deeper vessels, the pulse repetition frequency is limited, as the system has to wait for a pulse to return before transmitting the next pulse. This in turn means that the magnitude of Doppler shifts that can be measured is limited and detection of higher shifts in deeper vessels may not be possible in some circumstances, as this requires higher pulse repetition frequencies. When the pulse repetition frequency is inadequate for the Doppler shift being measured, then the phenomenon of aliasing occurs. In spectral Doppler this results in the peak frequencies being cut off at the top of the display and being registered just above the baseline (Fig. 15.99). In addition to transmitting the Doppler information as an audio signal, it can also be displayed as a spectral trace, or waveform, scrolling across the screen.

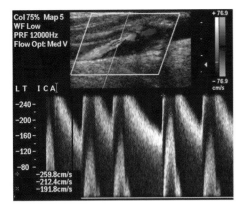

Fig. 15.99 Colour and spectral Doppler of the origin of the internal carotid artery. The colour Doppler shows a high-velocity jet at the site of an hypoechoic plaque with aliasing of the colour Doppler information; the spectral display also shows aliasing of the Doppler signal, a rough estimate of the peak velocity can be obtained by adding the two systolic components together: 260 + 212 = 472 cm/s.

Vessels have different waveforms, or Doppler 'signatures', which depend primarily on the size of the vessel and the type of capillary bed they are supplying. For example, the internal carotid artery supplies the relatively low-resistance cerebral circulation and therefore has high diastolic flow in comparison to the external carotid artery, which supplies the higher-resistance circulation of the scalp and face, resulting in significantly lower diastolic flow (Fig. 15.100). The waveform characteristics can change significantly in response to physiological stimuli, as shown by the increased diastolic flow that is seen in the femoral arteries on exercising the leg muscles (Fig. 15.101).

Colour Doppler

In duplex Doppler equipment, Doppler sampling is restricted to the small area within the sample volume. In colour Doppler systems the pulses along each scan line are divided on return to the transducer, some are used to provide imaging information and the rest are used to calculate the mean Doppler shift within small pixels of the image. This mean shift information is then coded on a colour scale and displayed as a colour map over the greyscale image. The choice of colours is arbitrary: usually shades of blue and red are used to represent flow towards and away from the transducer, with paler shades of the colour representing higher velocities. The advantage of this technique is that areas of normal and abnormal flow can be identified and localised rapidly, although pulsed Doppler ultrasound is still required to obtain useful velocity information, such as peak systolic velocity (Fig. 15.99).

Power Doppler

The intensity of the Doppler signal depends on the volume of blood reflecting the sound pulses and the amplitude of the signal depends on the velocity at which the blood is travelling. Small volumes of blood moving slowly produce a weak signal, which is difficult to define from background noise. One way to improve this situation is to integrate the energy from all the shift information in both directions together, thus increasing the overall power of the Doppler information and sensitivity of the system, but at the expense of losing directional and velocity information (Fig. 15.102). Power Doppler techniques are therefore good for showing areas of flowing blood, particularly when it is moving slowly, or in small vessels. Because of its higher sensitivity, it is more prone to movement arte-

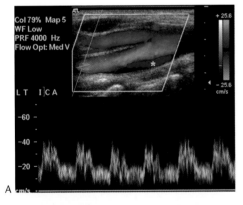

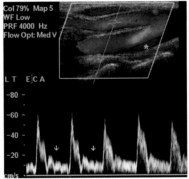

Fig. 15.100 The carotid bifurcation showing (A) higher diastolic flow in the internal carotid artery compared with (B) the external carotid artery; the normal region of reversed flow in the bulb is also seen (*). In addition, the external carotid waveform shows fluctuations (arrows) induced by tapping the superficial temporal artery. A branch artery can also be seen arising from the external carotid artery.

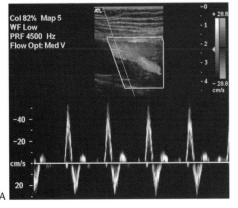

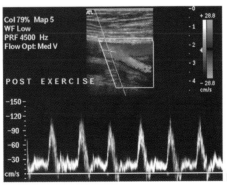

Fig. 15.101 The common femoral artery waveform at rest (A) and after moderate exercise (B).

fact from respiratory motion, or bowel activity, although modern signal-processing techniques reduce this problem significantly compared with earlier techniques. Some manufacturers provide Doppler imaging using a combination of power Doppler for sensitivity associated with colour Doppler for directional information.

ECHO-ENHANCING AGENTS

The signal-to-noise ratio for many Doppler applications is very poor. In order to improve this, echo-enhancing agents were developed. The first compounds were too large to pass through the pulmonary capillaries and were therefore restricted to use in the right heart, or for ultrasound hysterosalpingo-contrast sonography (HyCoSy). Subsequently, second-generation agents were developed. These are generally less than 8–10 μm in diameter and can therefore pass through the pulmonary capillaries into the systemic circulation. The first of these to be released commercially was based on small crystals of galactose, stabilised with palmitic acid, which trap small amounts of air in cavities. The agent is injected into a peripheral vein. It can then be visualised as it passes through the systemic circulation and it continues to produce appreciable enhancement of the Doppler signal for up to 3–4 min after injection (Fig. 15.103). Insonating blood containing echo-enhancing agents in an appropriate manner can produce echoes at the second and third harmonic frequencies, as well as the fundamental frequency; by tuning the receiver to the second harmonic frequency it is possible to filter out echoes returning at the fundamental frequency, and thus much of the noise and clutter associated with Doppler ultrasound. The information gathered from the second harmonic frequency therefore has a much better signal-to-noise ratio for signals returning from the echo-enhancing agent in the blood.

Newer echo-enhancing agents have been released and these, together with new signal processing techniques, have significantly widened the role of these agents. The microbubbles of an echo-enhancing agent can respond in one of four ways to ultrasound, depending on the intensity of the ultrasound pulse. At low intensity levels they act as simple backscatterers of sound. A moderate increase in intensity will cause the microbubbles to resonate and produce linear backscatter. A further increase in intensity produces non-linear oscillation and backscatter. Finally, at high intensities, the bubbles rupture, producing a short intense burst of energy which is received by the transducer as a very strong momentary signal. This provides an opportunity to either image echo-enhancing agents at relatively low intensities (signified by a low mechanical index, or MI), which will not destroy the agent and will allow regions of blood flow to be identified more easily; or at

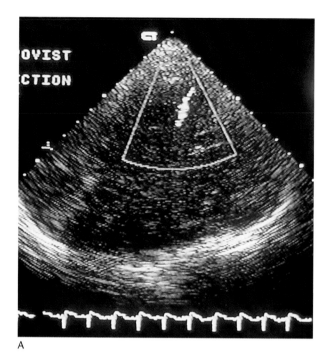

A

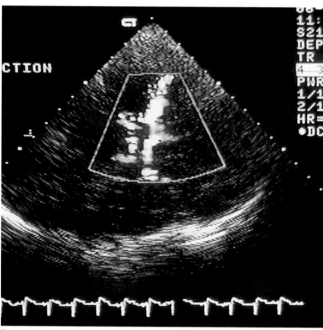

B

Fig. 15.103 Transcranial colour Doppler images of the circle of Willis before (A) and after (B) an injection of the echo-enhancing agent Levovist. Before the Levovist injection only the middle cerebral artery is seen; after the injection all the major components of the circle of Willis are visible.

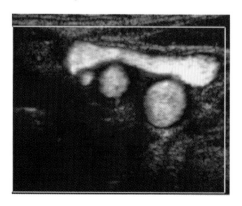

Fig. 15.102 Transverse view of the right carotid bifurcation using power Doppler ultrasound. It is not possible to distinguish the direction, or velocity of flow in the two branches of the artery from the more superficial internal jugular vein.

higher power which will destroy the microbubbles but will show clearly areas of tissue containing the agent and areas without the agent. Furthermore, sweeping the beam intermittently through a volume of tissue at high intensity with destruction of agent at each sweep allows some quantification of the rate of re-accumulation of echo-enhancing agent between sweeps and hence some assessment of blood flow.

MEASUREMENT OF A STENOSIS

In simple haemodynamic terms, blood flows from regions of high energy to regions of lower energy; in practice this means from areas of greater pressure to areas of lower pressure. Energy is normally lost as blood travels from the heart to the capillaries, but if there are stenoses in the vessels, this energy loss is increased and there is a reduction in the distal pressure, resulting in impaired tissue perfusion.

Stenoses can be assessed using two aspects of the ultrasound examination. First, if the stenosis can be seen adequately, a direct measurement of the degree of stenosis may be made. This situation is usually restricted to larger arteries, such as the carotid or common femoral arteries. Alternatively, the increase in velocity that occurs as blood passes through a stenosis can be used to help quantify the stenosis. In addition, some information on the type of plaque may be apparent. In the carotid arteries, smooth echogenic plaque is less likely to be associated with symptoms than irregular hypoechoic plaque.

The difference between a haemodynamically significant stenosis and a clinically significant stenosis must be distinguished. A 50% diameter stenosis is said to be haemodynamically significant as the volume of blood flowing along the vessel starts to fall above this degree of stenosis. A clinically significant stenosis is more difficult to define. In carotid examinations it is usually taken to be at, or above, a 70% diameter reduction, as this is the level above which symptoms and signs are strongly associated with carotid disease. In the lower limbs and other territories it is less easy to define clinical significance as the presence of symptoms is highly dependent on the development and efficiency of any collateral channels that may be present.

Direct measurement

Two main measurements can be made: diameter reduction or cross-sectional area reduction. It is important to distinguish between the two, as a 50% diameter reduction is equivalent to a 75% area reduction; there is, therefore, the potential for significant misunderstanding in the interpretation of examination results if the terms are not defined. Area measurements are a little more accurate and take account of asymmetrical distribution of plaque around the circumference of the vessel; however, they take a little longer to perform accurately. Diameters are a little easier to measure, but the vessel should always be examined both longitudinally and transversely in order to determine the most appropriate diameter to measure, usually the shortest.

In many cases the details of the plaque may be difficult to define, but in some cases the plaque will be seen clearly enough to identify certain characteristics which may be relevant to the patient's symptoms. Smooth, echogenic plaques are likely to be fibrotic and stable, whereas irregular, hypoechoic plaques are more likely to be unstable and act as a source of emboli from adherent thrombus, or plaque contents. Sometimes obvious ulceration may be seen but care should be taken not to misinterpret a space between two adjacent plaques as an ulcer.

Doppler criteria

These criteria are usually based on peak systolic and end-diastolic velocities, in some cases, the ratio of the peak velocity at the stenosis to the peak velocity proximal to the stenosis may be of value, the internal carotid/common carotid (IC/CC) ratio in carotid examinations. These velocity measurements are useful in situations where the residual vessel lumen cannot be visualised well enough to perform a direct measurement of the stenosis. In addition, examination of the spectral display may show changes in the waveform that are associated with stenoses or occlusions in adjacent segments of the vessel, such as spectral broadening, delayed acceleration and damping of the waveform.

Other Doppler-based indices have been developed to quantify changes in the waveform, these are the resistance index (RI), the pulsatility index (PI) and the systolic–diastolic ratio (Fig. 15.104). These have the advantage that they can be used in situations where accurate angle correction and thus velocity estimation, are not possible. The RI and PI reflect the degree of distal resistance, so that with increased peripheral resistance, as may occur with acute vascular rejection of a renal transplant, the RI tends toward a value of 1.0, whereas the PI tends toward values of 1.0 or more.

The acceleration time (AT) is the time taken, in seconds, for the peak systolic velocity to be reached. The acceleration index (AI) relates the acceleration time to the peak systolic velocity achieved. The application of these various indices will be discussed in relation to their value in specific clinical situations in the following sections.

CAROTID AND VERTEBRAL ARTERIES

Disease in the carotid arteries is associated with cerebral vascular events, and for severe disease of more than 70% diameter reduction it has been shown that surgery is beneficial in symptomatic patients who have a stenosis of more than 70% diameter reduction, as subsequent significant vascular events occurred in 16.8% of the non-operative group, compared with only 2.8% of the operative group. The main indications for carotid ultrasound are therefore patients with transient ischaemic attacks (TIAs) or reversible ischaemic neurological deficits (RINDs), who may benefit from carotid

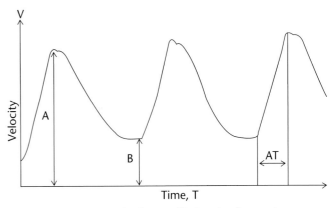

Fig. 15.104 Definition of indices used in Doppler ultrasound.

Peak systolic velocity: A

End diastolic velocity: B

Time-averaged mean velocity: TAMean

Time-averaged maximum velocity: TAMax

Resistance index (RI): $\dfrac{A - B}{A}$

Pulsatility index (PI): $\dfrac{A - B}{TAMax}$

Systolic/diastolic ratio: $\dfrac{A}{B}$

Accelearation time: AT

Acceleration index: $\dfrac{A}{AT}$

endarterectomy surgery. It is not usually indicated in patients with established and completed strokes, unless these are milder, resolving strokes in younger patients who might be considered suitable for surgery. Patients with asymptomatic bruits will not normally be considered for surgery at present, several trials have looked at the benefit of endarterectomy in these patients but the results are not conclusive and depend on the surgical unit having a low perioperative morbidity and mortality. A recent Cochrane Review of these trials concluded that there was some evidence favouring surgery slightly but that this was barely significant and 50 patients would need to be operated upon to prevent one of them having a stroke. Other indications for carotid ultrasound include atypical symptoms which may be due to carotid disease; postendarterectomy patients; those in whom arteriography is technically impossible, or contraindicated; and the assessment of pulsatile cervical masses, including possible carotid body tumours.

The carotid vessels are scanned from low in the neck to high behind the mandible, the level and orientation of the bifurcation are noted, together with any obvious areas of disease. The vessels are then scanned using colour Doppler ultrasound, and any abnormal areas of flow identified for subsequent assessment using spectral Doppler ultrasound. It should be remembered that there is normally a region of reversed flow in the carotid bulb (Fig. 15.100) and that this does not signify the presence of disease; in fact, its absence is strongly suggestive of a disturbance in blood flow. The external carotid artery can be distinguished from the internal carotid artery by four features: (i) it is usually more anterior than the internal carotid artery; (ii) it has visible branches, the internal carotid artery does not have any branches in the cervical region; (iii) it has less diastolic flow than the internal carotid artery; and (iv) tapping the superficial temporal artery as it passes over the zygoma induces fluctuations in the waveform of the external carotid artery but not the internal carotid artery (Fig. 15.100B). If no areas of significant disease are seen, it is common practice to take peak systolic velocity readings from the upper common, the internal carotid and the external carotid arteries. If areas of disease are seen they are assessed by direct measurement, or by Doppler criteria such as peak systolic velocity and related measurements (Fig. 15.99). It is important to realise that the precise criteria vary depending on the type of equipment used and other technical factors relating to the examination: it is therefore important for each department to develop its own specific values which allow reliable identification of the key stenosis levels of 50% and 70% diameter reduction. The criteria used in our institution are listed in Table 15.3. Plaque morphology may be apparent in the carotids and different types of plaque may be identified. Type 1 plaques have a thin rim over the surface but are predominantly anechoic (Fig. 15.105A); type 4 plaques are predominantly echogenic (Fig. 15.105B); type 2 plaques have <25%

echogenic components, whereas type 3 plaques have <25% hypoechoic components. The presence of irregular, hypoechoic or ulcerated (Fig. 15.105C) plaques should be noted, as these may be relevant to symptoms, even if the stenosis is not particularly great.

Occlusion of the internal carotid artery must be diagnosed with care on ultrasound. At high degrees of stenosis (>90% diameter reduction) there is only a small volume of blood flowing through the residual lumen and it is also flowing relatively slowly. The machine must therefore be reset to look for this low-volume, slow flow and not the much higher velocities that might have been expected. The greater sensitivity of power Doppler ultrasound is of value here (Fig. 15.106) and echo-enhancing agents will also contribute to confirming the diagnosis of occlusion, or identifying a small residual lumen, which is still potentially an operative candidate.

Pulsatile neck lumps can be identified rapidly with colour Doppler ultrasound. They may be due to adjacent lymph nodes, cysts or other masses. Carotid body tumours have a characteristic location between the internal and external carotid arteries, appearing as a predominantly hypoechoic mass splaying the arteries (Fig. 15.107) and relatively vascular on colour Doppler ultrasound. Aneurysms of the carotid may occur spontaneously, as a result of penetrating neck trauma or hyperextension injuries; ultrasound will show the nature of these masses and the involvement of the various carotid segments.

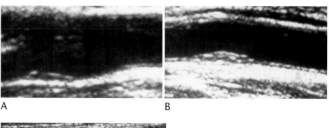

A   B

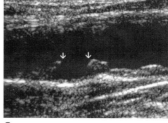

C

Fig. 15.105 (A) Type 1 plaque showing a thin rim over the surface of a predominantly hypoechoic plaque. (B) Type 4 plaque showing a predominantly echogenic plaque with a smooth surface. (C) An ulcerated plaque (arrows).

Table 15.3 Diagnostic criteria for Doppler diagnosis of stenoses of 50 and 70% diameter reduction

Diameter stenosis (%)	Peak systolic velocity, ICA (m/s)	Peak diastolic velocity, ICA (m/s)	ICA/CCA systolic ratio
50	>1.5	>0.5	>2
70	>2.3	>0.75	>3

From Robinson et al (1988). Am. J. Roentgenol. 151: 1045–1049
CCA, common carotid artery; ICA, internal carotid artery.

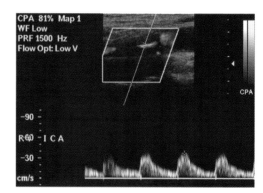

Fig. 15.106 Power Doppler image of a critical ICA stenosis showing the narrow residual lumen.

Dissection of the carotid artery can occur as an extension of an aortic dissection, spontaneously within the carotid itself, or as a result of trauma. Ultrasound may show one of several appearances. Rarely two patent channels separated by a flap may be seen, and Doppler ultrasound will show significantly different flow patterns in the two channels. More frequently, the false channel will thrombose, producing a characteristic, tapering stenosis (Fig. 15.108) or occlusion of the vessel. Recanalisation of dissected vessels over a period of 6–8 weeks may be seen in 50–60% of cases.

Measurement of the *intima-medial thickness* (IMT) is feasible with today's high-resolution ultrasound machines. When the ultrasound beam is at right angles to the carotid walls, two white lines will be seen in normal vessels, particularly on the posterior wall. The first corresponds to the blood/intima boundary; the second to the outer media/adventitia region. Normally this is less than 0.8 mm (Fig. 15.109), but several studies have shown that this increases significantly in patients with evidence of atheroma in other areas, such as the coronary arteries. The IMT increases slowly with age, but it may provide a useful tool in the assessment of patients with arterial disease in order to measure both the prevalence of disease and the progression, or regression, of disease over a period of time, depending on the treatment regimens employed.

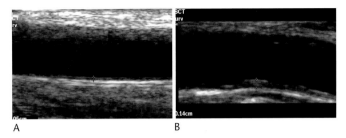

Fig. 15.109 (A) The normal appearance of the intimal line with an IMT of 0.5 mm. (B) A thickened intimal line in a patient with an IMT of 1.4 mm.

The *accuracy of carotid Doppler ultrasound* has been well established over recent years. One study reviewed 16 spectral Doppler studies with a total of 2146 Doppler/arteriogram comparisons: duplex Doppler ultrasound had an overall sensitivity of 96%, a specificity of 86%, a positive predictive value of 89%, a negative predictive value of 94% and an accuracy of 91% for the diagnosis of a stenosis diameter greater than 50%. Subsequently, further studies have confirmed the value of colour Doppler ultrasound with similar or better levels of accuracy, and also its value in improving diagnostic confidence, clarifying difficult situations and reducing examination times.

The vertebral arteries

These can be visualised using colour Doppler ultrasound. They may be examined in three segments of their course: most commonly in the vertebral canal as they pass cranially through the foramina transversaria; in the lower neck as they pass from the subclavian artery towards C6; and in the upper neck as they wind around the lateral masses of the atlas and enter the foramen magnum. There is often asymmetry in the diameter of the two vessels, in which case the left is usually the larger, and in up to 10% of individuals one of the vertebral arteries will have significant segments of atresia. The main items of information that can be gathered on these vessels include the fact that both are present, the direction of flow in them, and whether the flow is normal or damped; occasionally a stenosis in the artery may be demonstrated. A stenosis, or absent segment, in one vessel is not usually of clinical significance as the basilar circulation can be maintained from the other artery. If reversed flow is demonstrated, it is a sign of an occluded, or severely stenotic, subclavian artery (subclavian steal syndrome) (Fig. 15.110). In some patients, exercise of the ipsilateral arm muscles may be required to produce reversed flow.

TRANSCRANIAL DOPPLER ULTRASOUND

The use of ultrasound to examine the neonatal brain through the fontanelles and thin calvarial bones has been established for many years, but transcranial ultrasound in adults was limited by the marked attenuation of the ultrasound beam by the skull bones, which can be up to 60 dB both on the way in and the way out. Transcranial Doppler ultrasound has been possible using pulsed Doppler ultrasound without imaging since 1982, but developments in transducers and imaging processing now mean that useful colour Doppler images and spectra can be obtained in adults. The advantages include an ability to identify specific segments of the main cerebral arteries and to appreciate rapidly the direction of flow within these; in addition, more accurate and reproducible angle-corrected velocity estimations can be made.

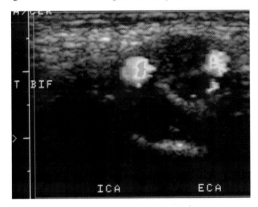

Fig. 15.107 Transverse view of a carotid bifurcation with an hypoechoic carotid body tumour splaying the two major branches.

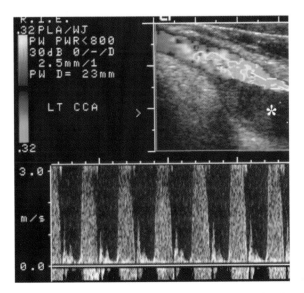

Fig. 15.108 A dissection of the common carotid artery, showing the thrombosed channel posteriorly (*) and the tapered stenosis anteriorly.

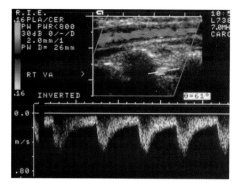

Fig. 15.110 Colour Doppler image of the neck showing the common carotid artery (orange) with the vertebral artery between the lateral processes of the cervical spine. The blue of the vertebral artery shows that it is flowing in the opposite direction to the carotid; this is confirmed by the spectral display.

The main access point for transcranial Doppler ultrasound is the thin squamous temporal bone in front of the ear. Careful scanning will locate the best acoustic window, although in 10% of subjects no suitable window will be found; problems are more likely in females, patients with black-coloured skin and the elderly. The ultrasound system should be set to high sensitivity and, when the bone window is located, colour Doppler ultrasound is used to identify the ipsilateral middle cerebral artery, which can then be traced centrally to locate the circle of Willis and its branches. A complete circle is only found in 25–30% of subjects, and many variations of the anatomy exist. The use of echo-enhancing agents has further improved the strength of the signal obtained, and these agents will certainly be of value in these examinations (Fig. 15.103). The foramen magnum can be used to examine the upper vertebral arteries and the lower basilar artery; the orbit can be used to examine the upper internal carotid artery and the anterior cerebral artery, although attention must be paid to the power output of the transducer as the beam will not be attenuated by bone at these sites and passes through sensitive structures, such as the retina.

The cerebral veins and the major venous sinuses are less easy to examine because of their orientation in relation to the scan plane and the slow flow within them.

The main indications for transcranial colour Doppler ultrasound include monitoring of spasm and flow after strokes and subarachnoid haemorrhage, the assessment of intracranial collateral pathways, and the detection of significant stenoses (>65%) of the main cerebral arteries. Cerebral artery aneurysms more than 5 mm in diameter can be detected using transcranial power Doppler in the majority of cases. It is also valuable in research into the changes in blood flow induced by drugs and physiological changes.

THE PERIPHERAL ARTERIES

The arteries of the limbs can be examined with ultrasound in patients with claudication in order to identify segments of stenosis, or occlusion. In the lower limb the arteries are followed from the groin distally to the calf, and segments of abnormal flow identified with colour Doppler ultrasound. These can then be assessed using spectral Doppler ultrasound; the normal waveform is triphasic due to the relatively high distal resistance in the resting lower limb, which reflects the pulse pressure wave. A velocity of more than 4 m/s at a stenosis, or a fourfold increase in velocity in relation to the velocity above the abnormal segment, is compatible with a stenosis of 70% or more (Fig. 15.111). The main indication for ultrasound of the peripheral arteries is to identify patients who may benefit from angioplasty, and to distinguish these from patients who require distal bypass grafts.

The iliac arteries are more difficult to visualise in some patients but, with care and attention, they can often be examined adequately. If this is not possible, changes in the waveform at the groin, such as damping or spectral broadening, may indicate significant disease proximally.

There are three types of *bypass graft* procedure used by surgeons: synthetic grafts, in situ and reversed autologous vein grafts. These can be monitored with colour Doppler ultrasound. Graft occlusion occurring in the first 4–6 weeks after operation is usually due to technical factors, and failure after 2–3 years is usually caused by recurrent atheroma. Graft failure during the intervening period is usually the result of neointimal hyperplasia, which occurs most frequently at the origin of the graft, the distal insertion, or at the sites of inadequately ablated valves and communicating veins in cases of autologous vein grafts. Of all graft failures, 80% occur during this interim period. If problems with the graft can be identified on colour Doppler ultrasound as part of a surveillance programme before graft failure occurs, the secondary patency rate can be improved from 70% to 90%. The criteria used for assessing graft stenoses are similar to those for arterial stenosis: peak systolic velocities of more than 3.5 m/s are associated with stenoses of more than 70% diameter reduction, as is a velocity ratio of more than 2.5 (Fig. 15.112). It should be remembered that a physiological stenosis will occur if there is a significant mismatch in calibre between the graft and the native artery; this should not be mistaken for a pathological stenosis. If the maximum graft velocity is less than 0.45 m/s

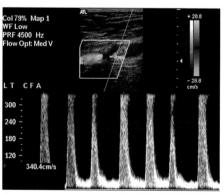

A

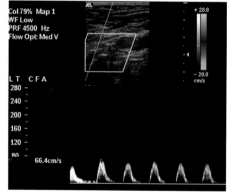

B

Fig. 15.111 A high-grade stenosis of the common femoral artery showing aliasing and a peak velocity in excess of 3.4 m/s (A), compared with a prestenosis velocity of 0.66 m/s (B), producing a velocity ratio of more than 5 : 1 indicating a severe stenosis.

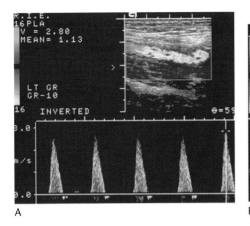
A

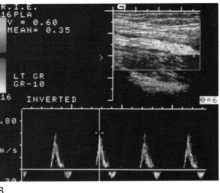
B

Fig. 15.112 An in situ vein graft showing a stenosis on colour Doppler ultrasound with a peak velocity of 2.8 m/s (A), compared with a prestenosis velocity of 0.6 m/s (B), producing a velocity ratio of 4.6:1 consistent with a severe stenosis.

along more than half the length of the graft, there is a high association with subsequent graft failure (Fig. 15.113).

Arteriovenous fistulas may occur, particularly with in situ vein grafts, if any perforator veins or superficial communicating veins are missed at operation.

False aneurysms

These can occur after femoral catheterisation, especially if larger catheters are used, or multiple catheter exchanges performed; anticoagulation following angioplasty is also a factor. Rates of occurrence from 0.6% to 6.0% have been reported. Colour Doppler ultrasound provides a reliable method for the diagnosis of false aneurysms and monitoring their progress (Fig. 15.114). Spectral Doppler traces taken from the neck of the false aneurysm show a characteristic to and fro pattern as blood flows in and out of the false aneurysm during the cardiac cycle. Many false aneurysms will thrombose spontaneously; a few will increase in size.

Thrombosis can be encouraged by ultrasound-guided compression. The transducer is used to press on the false aneurysm, and pressure is applied to stop flow in the lumen of the aneurysm and the channel linking it to the artery, but not within the artery itself. This pressure is maintained for 15 min, then released gradually. If flow is still present, pressure is reapplied for a further 15 min, and these cycles are repeated until thrombosis occurs. The procedure is uncomfortable and may be painful for the patient, so that some analgesia is often required. Most false aneurysms can be treated in this way, but the presence of infection and inability to apply adequate compression are contraindications; false aneurysms which are more than 7–10 days may take a little longer to thrombose. In some

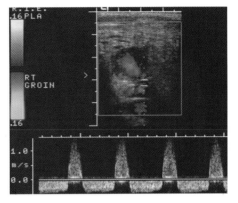

Fig. 15.114 A false aneurysm of the common femoral artery following arteriography. Colour Doppler ultrasound shows the blood in the false aneurysm and the spectral trace shows the characteristic to and fro flow of blood in and out of the aneurysm during the cardiac cycle.

centres, preparations of fibrinogen are available and this can be injected directly into the aneurysm lumen under ultrasound control. This usually results in rapid and complete thrombosis of the false aneurysm.

Arteries of the upper limb

Stenosis and occlusion of the arteries in the upper limb can be assessed with ultrasound. Compression syndromes can be investigated by imaging the subclavian artery while moving the arm to different positions, and the point of compression accurately identified.

Dialysis grafts

Haemodialysis grafts may occlude, or develop a stenosis or a false aneurysm, and these can be examined using colour Doppler ultrasound. It is important to check the venous side of the fistula proximally to the subclavian vein as some stenoses that affect fistula function can occur in these proximal veins. The flow in the fistula is best assessed by measuring the flow in the brachial artery above the fistula, assuming that most of the blood flowing in the brachial artery will flow through the fistula. The flow can be roughly estimated by measuring the cross-sectional area of the artery and multiplying this by the time-averaged mean velocity and then by a factor of 60 to give the volume flow in millilitres per minute (Fig. 15.115). Flows under 400 ml/min are inadequate for satisfactory dialysis;

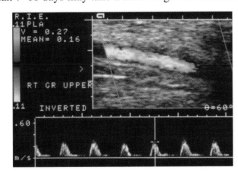

Fig. 15.113 Image of an upper segment of a femoto-popliteal graft showing damped flow of low velocity (27 cm/s), which is strongly suggestive of a graft at risk of failure.

conversely, flows over 1200 ml/min are excessive and problems may occur with cardiac output and reserve. Dialysis is best performed with fistula flows of 500–800 ml/min.

ABDOMINAL VESSELS

In the abdomen, Doppler ultrasound can provide useful information about many of the major arteries and veins. The conditions for examination are a little more challenging than for the peripheral arteries and carotids as the vessels lie deeper, respiratory motion is present, and bowel gas interferes with the image. The examinations are best performed with the patient breathing quietly, only holding his or her breath for a short time whenever necessary. Colour and power Doppler ultrasound are frequently used during an abdominal examination simply to identify structures as arteries or veins and to distinguish vessels from cysts or dilated ducts.

The liver

The normal fasting diameter of the *portal vein* is less than 13 mm, but this will increase after eating. The patency of the portal vein can be confirmed and cavernous transformation identified: tumour invasion of the major portal branches in patients with hepatocellular carcinoma can also be assessed. The direction of blood flow in the portal vein and its major tributaries can be demonstrated in patients with portal hypertension and, if surgical or transjugular shunts have been created, these can be monitored using Doppler ultrasound for the development of stenosis (Fig. 15.116), or occlusion. In patients

with intestinal ischaemia, gas bubbles may be seen in the vein, or heard on Doppler ultrasound, as they pass up into the liver (Fig. 15.117). Following liver transplantation, flow in the portal vein and hepatic artery is monitored as thrombosis or stenosis, particularly of the artery, are significant complications.

The hepatic artery normally arises from the coeliac axis, but the right hepatic artery may have a separate origin from the superior mesenteric artery in some patients; this variation may be apparent on ultrasound and is of some importance if a patient is being considered for transplantation. Flow in the hepatic artery increases in patients with portal hypertension and also in patients with liver tumours; it is also significantly increased following transplantation after which thrombosis of the artery, or one of its major branches, is a serious complication. Following liver transplantation the hepatic artery flow on colour and spectral Doppler can be overshadowed by the prominent portal vein flow (Fig. 15.118), therefore it is important to search carefully for the arterial signal at the porta, as well as in the right and left lobes of the liver. Aneurysms of the artery can occur spontaneously but are also seen following penetrating trauma

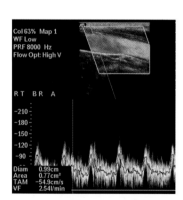

Fig. 15.115 Colour and spectral Doppler of the brachial artery in a patient with a dialysis fistula; the calculated flow volume is 2.54 L/min.

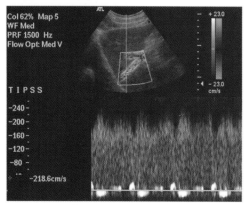

Fig. 15.116 A TIPS in a patient with portal hypertension. Spectral Doppler ultrasound shows evidence of a degree of stenosis with flow in excess of 2 m/s.

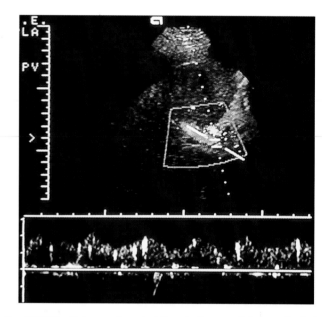

Fig. 15.117 Colour and spectral Doppler images of the portal vein in a patient with ascites. The spectral display shows intermittent strong signals from gas bubbles.

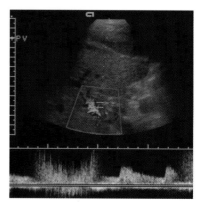

Fig. 15.118 Spectral Doppler trace showing the hepatic artery frequency shifts to be less than those from the portal vein and illustrating how the arterial signal can be swamped by the portal vein signal.

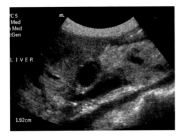

Fig. 15.119 An aneurysm of the hepatic artery in a transplant patient, colour Doppler showed arterial flow within the lumen.

(including liver biopsy) and at the anastomosis following transplantation (Fig. 15.119).

The hepatic veins drain into the IVC. They normally show pulsatile flow predominantly towards the heart, which reflects the pressure changes in the right atrium over the cardiac cycle (Fig. 15.120). If the liver becomes less compliant through cirrhosis, or other causes of portal hypertension, these pulsatile changes are reduced or lost completely. Budd–Chiari syndrome can be diagnosed using colour Doppler ultrasound, which shows absence of the normal veins, together with abnormal collateral channels, some of which show flow out towards the capsule of the liver (Fig. 15.121). In some patients the changes are only partial, affecting some of the veins, or affecting a segment of a vein. Doppler ultrasound will not diagnose microscopic veno-occlusive disease. Following transplantation, stenosis of the veins, or of the IVC at the anastomosis, may result in abnormal flow or thrombosis.

It had been hoped that patterns of flow and vascularity on Doppler ultrasound would help in the diagnosis of *benign* and *malignant tumours*. Unfortunately, although some characteristics of a malignant type of circulation can be defined, the discrimination between types of tumour remains poor and inadequate. Malignant circulation with high shifts, multidirectional flow, arteriovenous shunting and abnormal vessels has been described in 50–80% of hepatocellular carcinomas, but many of these changes are also seen in 30–40% of metastases. Similarly, patterns of vascularity such as central disposition in a lesion, or distribution around the margin, do not allow distinction of tumour type. However, the newer techniques for imaging blood flow using low output (low mechanical index) techniques allow much better visualisation of blood flow distribution in lesions and may improve the value of ultrasound in these circumstances.

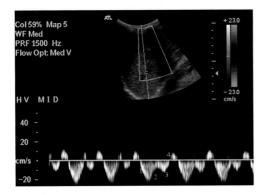

Fig. 15.120 (A) Normal hepatic vein spectral display showing variation in flow during the cardiac cycle. (B) The cardiac variations reflect the pressure changes in the right atrium during the cardiac cycle. 1 = Forward flow into the atrium during diastolic relaxation; 2 = reverse flow during tricuspid valve closure and ventricular systole; 3 = forward flow as tricuspid valve opens; 4 = reverse flow during atrial systole.

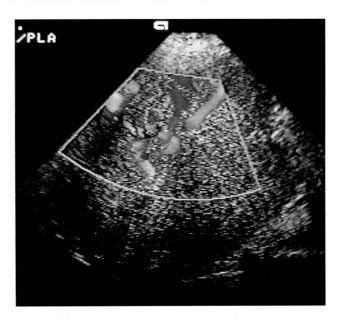

Fig. 15.121 Colour Doppler image of the liver in a patient with Budd–Chiari syndrome. Instead of the normal regular pattern of hepatic veins, there is a complex network of abnormal collaterals.

THE KIDNEYS

The renal arterial circulation has a distinctive waveform with high diastolic flow, reflecting a relatively low peripheral resistance. Various diseases produce changes in the waveform, which may be bilateral or unilateral. Unfortunately, these changes tend to be nonspecific, so they are not as useful as it had first been hoped.

Renal artery stenoses

These can be diagnosed if the stenotic segment is visualised directly; a velocity of over 1.8 m/s or a ratio of over 3.5 between the velocities in the renal artery and the aorta (the RAR) is diagnostic of a stenosis of more than 60% diameter reduction. Unfortunately, the proximal renal arteries cannot be visualised directly in a number of patients, which reduces the value of the technique as a screening test for renal artery stenosis.

The parenchymal arteries can be demonstrated in most patients, and it has been shown that significant proximal stenoses (>70%) produce changes in the waveforms in these vessels. The acceleration time is the time interval for the systolic acceleration period, an increase in this above 0.1 s is associated with a significant stenosis (Fig. 15.122). Changes to the waveform shape with loss of the early systolic complex also reflect a proximal stenosis. The overall changes produced by a significant proximal stenosis result in a waveform with slow acceleration and a reduced peak frequency known as a tardus parvus waveform.

Renal vein thrombosis

This may be demonstrated directly, if the main renal veins are visible. Sometimes they are obscured, or thrombosis affects the smaller intrarenal veins. In these cases the diagnosis may be suggested by a significant reduction in diastolic flow in the renal artery as a result of increased intrarenal vascular resistance (Fig. 15.123), or even reversed diastolic flow.

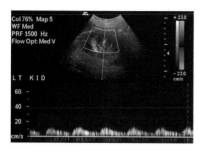

Fig. 15.122 Intraparenchymal Doppler examination of a patient with renal artery stenosis shows a damped waveform with a prolonged acceleration time of 0.18 s.

The changes in the waveform in different *diffuse parenchymal diseases* are non-specific, but an RI of over 0.7 is indicative of parenchymal change (Fig. 15.123), although it is not possible to discriminate between different types of disease and avoid the necessity for biopsy.

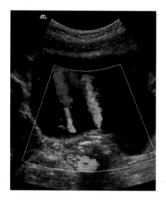

Fig. 15.124 Transverse colour Doppler view of the bladder showing a pair of normal ureteric jets.

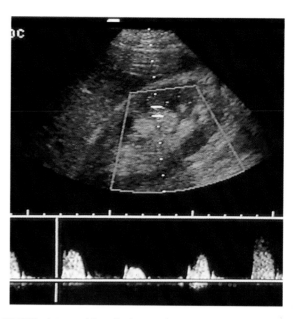

Fig. 15.123 Intrarenal Doppler image of a patient with acute renal failure shows no significant diastolic flow R.I. = 1.0. This pattern may also be seen in patients with renal vein thrombosis.

Ureteric obstruction

This results in increased intrarenal pressure, which is reflected in an increase in the RI in the renal arteries. An RI of more than 0.7, or a difference between the sides of more than 0.1, is suggestive of

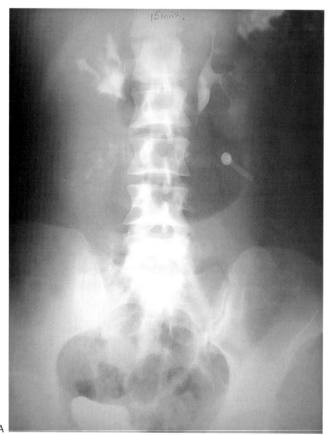

A

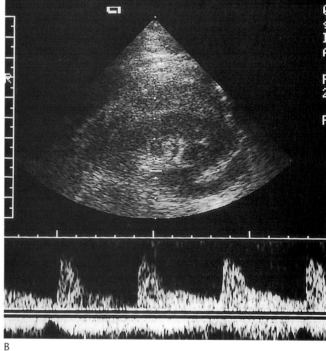

B

Fig. 15.125 (A) A film from an intravenous urography examination in a patient who sustained right renal trauma in a road traffic accident: there is only minimal excretion of contrast from the lower fragment. (B) Spectral Doppler ultrasound shows both arterial and venous flow in this fragment.

obstruction in the appropriate clinical circumstances; these changes can be of value in the distinction between non-obstructive dilatation and obstructive dilatation in pregnant patients. Some care is needed as the changes can take several hours to develop, and underlying renal disease must also be considered; the RI in the kidneys of children under 5 years of age is normally slightly higher than in older patients. Colour Doppler may be used to identify the ureteric jets as urine enters the bladder at the vesico-ureteric junctions (Fig. 15.124) in patients with an obstructed ureter the jets on the affected side will be less frequent, or absent.

Renal trauma and tumours

Demonstration of arterial and venous flow in the renal fragments resulting from severe **renal trauma** allows assessment of the viability of the kidney (Fig. 15.125). Arteriovenous fistulas caused by penetrating trauma or biopsy result in increased, pulsatile venous flow; flow in the supplying artery may be increased, and colour Doppler ultrasound may show the tissue vibrations which produce an audible bruit. **Renal tumours** may show typical changes of a malignant circulation, but 20% may be relatively avascular, and little or no flow is demonstrable.

Renal transplants

Renal transplants may suffer from various vascular complications, and the relatively superficial location of the kidney makes ultrasound assessment straightforward. Stenosis of the main artery at the site of the anastomosis can be identified on colour Doppler ultrasound, or because of abnormal shifts on spectral Doppler ultrasound. Distinction between acute vascular rejection, acute tubular necrosis and cyclosporin toxicity is not reliable, although rejection tends to produce higher resistance indices than the others. An RI of over 0.7 is a sign of abnormally high peripheral resistance, and serial measurement can be used as an indicator of improving or deteriorating renal function. Care must be taken not to compress the transplant parenchyma with excessive transducer pressure as this can result in an artefactual increase in the RI (Fig. 15.126).

PELVIS

The female pelvis

The organs of the female pelvis can be examined both transabdominally through the full bladder, or transvaginally; this second approach allows the transducer to be positioned close to the major vessels supplying the ovaries and the uterus. The blood flow to the ovaries and uterus varies during the menstrual cycle, with increased flow and decreased pulsatility near ovulation; these changes can also be used to monitor patients undergoing *infertility* treatment and pharmacological induction of ovulation. Uterine flow is increased in cases of *trophoblastic disease*, with a low RI; return of the RI and waveform to normal correlates well with successful treatment. In *ovarian tumours* there is an increase in blood flow in the ovarian arteries but, as in the liver, the changes are not sufficiently specific to allow accurate distinction between different tumours. *Ovarian torsion* results in a significant decrease in ovarian blood flow, although some flow may still be present in a torted but salvageable ovary. Absence of flow suggests a non-salvageable gonad.

In patients with *ectopic pregnancy* the presence of active trophoblastic tissue can be demonstrated on colour and spectral Doppler ultrasound as a region of increased vascularity with a low RI (<0.6). In addition, there is increased flow to the uterus and ovaries, although this is less marked than with an intrauterine pregnancy.

An increase in the uterine artery RI during an established pregnancy is a sign of increased resistance in the placenta, which may reflect developing *intrauterine growth retardation*; however, the changes are not sufficiently diagnostic for use as a screening technique, and need to be assessed in conjunction with other parameters. In the fetal circulation, flow to the developing brain is dominant and protected if intrauterine growth retardation develops; this is reflected in an increased RI in the abdominal aorta and branches compared with the carotids, as the cerebral circulation is maintained at the expense of the lower body.

The male pelvis

In patients with an acutely tender scrotum, differentiation of acute epididymo-orchitis from torsion may be aided by colour Doppler ultrasound. In *epididymo-orchitis* the testis and the epididymis show increased flow, which may be generalised or focal in distribu-

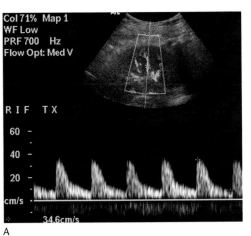

A

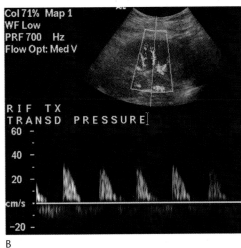

B

Fig. 15.126 (A) Colour and spectral Doppler from a transplant kidney with a moderately elevated RI of 0.79. (B) The effect of transducer pressure over the transplant with a decrease in diastolic flow to zero.

tion. In cases of *testicular torsion* there is absent or markedly reduced flow to the affected side; comparison should be made with the other side if there is any doubt. After several hours increased flow in the peritesticular tissues is seen.

The perfusion of *testicular tumours* is variable and does not allow definitive diagnosis of benign from malignant lesions. *Varicoceles* are seen as multiple serpiginous cystic areas in the epididymis, more marked on standing and coughing. If confirmation of their vascular nature is required, colour Doppler ultrasound can be used in conjunction with getting the patient to cough, or to perform a Valsalva manoeuvre.

In prostatic disease there is increased flow on transrectal colour Doppler ultrasound in areas of *prostatitis*, but this can also be seen in *prostatic carcinoma*. The presence of abnormal colour Doppler findings indicates disease, but this must be considered in the light of other clinical information, and biopsy of abnormal areas performed if malignancy is a possibility. Colour Doppler ultrasound can subsequently be used to monitor the response of both conditions to appropriate treatment.

Impotence

This may be due to psychological causes or vascular disease. The vascular responses during the development and maintenance of an erection can be monitored with Doppler ultrasound after the cavernosal injection of papaverine (40–80 mg). A normal response shows an immediate, marked increase in penile arterial flow; as the erectile pressure increases, the diastolic flow decreases, becoming zero as a full erection is obtained. Peak systolic flow should then be over 0.35 m/s with a well-defined waveform of short duration. Arterial inflow disease results in a lower peak systolic velocity and a damped waveform; whereas venous leakage produces a continual high level of flow in diastole, despite a good arterial response; psychogenic or neurological impotence patients show a normal response to this test.

AORTA AND INFERIOR VENA CAVA

The most common indication for examining the *abdominal aorta* is for the diagnosis and assessment of aneurysms, Doppler ultrasound is not usually required for this. However, if a dissection is suspected, both colour Doppler and spectral Doppler ultrasound can be used to demonstrate patency or thrombosis of the channels and the arteries which they supply. The *coeliac axis* and its major branches can be examined as they arise from the upper aorta. The *superior mesenteric artery* also arises at this level and runs inferiorly to the left of the superior mesenteric vein; occasionally the right hepatic artery arises from the superior mesenteric artery rather than the coeliac artery. The *inferior mesenteric artery* is more difficult to demonstrate, as it is smaller and more likely to be obscured by bowel gas; in suitable subjects it is best found by scanning trans-

versely up the aorta from the bifurcation; it normally arises 3–4 cm above the bifurcation and runs inferiorly on the left of the aorta (Fig. 15.127).

The waveforms in the vessels supplying the bowel vary with food, having relatively high pulsatility with low diastolic flow in fasting subjects, and higher diastolic flow following food. Stenosis of the coeliac axis and superior mesenteric artery may be identified on ultrasound: peak systolic flows of over 1.8 m/s correlate with 50% stenosis, and velocities of over 2.8 m/s with stenosis of 75% or more. If both vessels are seen to be significantly narrowed, or occluded, this supports a diagnosis of *intestinal ischaemia* in the appropriate clinical situation; unfortunately, the status of the inferior mesenteric artery and its contribution to bowel blood flow is difficult to assess in most patients. Other, indirect, signs of ischaemia may be seen on ultrasound, including dilated, oedematous, or hypoperistaltic bowel and gas in the portal vein.

The IVC and congenital variations of this can be examined with colour Doppler ultrasound. The main indications are assessment for the possible extension of thrombosis or tumour from the legs or renal veins, diagnosis of compression from masses, assessment of caval filters (Fig. 15.128), and following liver transplantation.

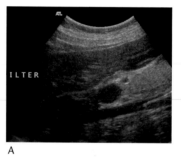
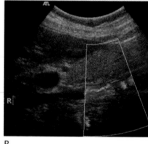

A   B

Fig. 15.128 (A) A caval filter inserted for recurrent pulmonary emboli. (B) Colour Doppler ultrasound confirms the patency of the cava at the level of the filter. The change in colour from red to blue reflects the relative change in the direction of flow in relation to the transducer as the blood flows through the sector.

MAGNETIC RESONANCE ANGIOGRAPHY

Jeremy P.R. Jenkins

MRI is sensitive to the detection of flow, and applications in the non-invasive assessment of vascular structures are increasing. This has been brought about by the development and implementation of multiplanar data acquisitions, sophisticated radiofrequency (RF) pulse sequences, faster 3D scanning techniques with breath-hold facility, and post-processing of data into two- and three-dimensional display formats (Fig.15.129). The ability to acquire not only morphological but also functional information non-invasively is an important advantage. Contrast-enhanced magnetic resonance angiography (CE-MRA), utilising a bolus intravenous injection of gadolinium-chelate (concentration of 0.1 or 0.2 mmol/kg body weight—so-called single or double dose techniques), combined with a breath-hold 3D *time-of-flight* sequence, has further extended its role competing with conventional X-ray angiography in spatial and contrast resolution (Fig.15.130).

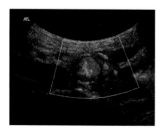

Fig. 15.127 Transverse colour Doppler image of the lower abdominal aorta showing the inferior mesenteric artery lying to the left of the aorta (orange), the inferior mesenteric vein is seen further laterally (blue).

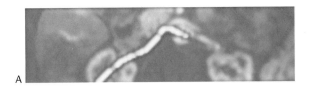

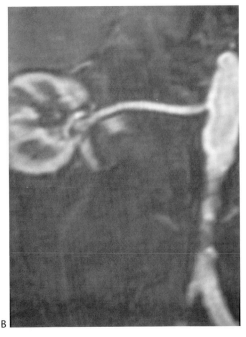

Fig. 15.129   Reformatting of post-processed data in order to straighten out a curved structure — in this case a normal renal artery. (A) Raw data image. (B) Reformatted 3D CE-MRA image.

An understanding of the basic processes involved in flow phenomena is required in order to interpret the MRA images obtained. Only a brief review will be given. The appearance of flowing blood is essentially a balance between those effects that produce a decrease or an increase in signal intensity. A decrease in the inten-

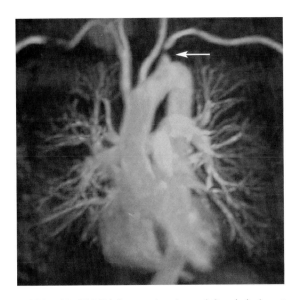

Fig. 15.130   3D CE-MRA image showing a left subclavian stenosis (arrow).

sity of flowing blood can be achieved by *saturation*, *dephasing* and *washout* effects, whereas an increase occurs with *flow-related enhancement* and *rephasing* of spins.

Protons exposed to repeated RF pulses become saturated (have a low magnetisation) and produce a low signal. Unsaturated (i.e. fully magnetised) protons give a high signal when excited by an RF pulse. The *saturation* effect relates to the longer T_1 (and thus lower signal intensity) of blood compared with adjacent tissue. With appropriate T_1-weighting the intraluminal signal would be expected to be lower than that from the surrounding tissues. In conventional spin-echo imaging this saturation effect is often opposed by the *flow-related enhancement* or *entry* phenomenon. This results from fresh blood (unsaturated protons) entering the imaging volume and producing a high intraluminal signal. In a multislice sequence this enhancement is more pronounced in sections nearest the entry point of the vessel into the imaging volume.

The most important process leading to a reduction in intraluminal signal is the *washout* effect. In order to generate a spin-echo signal protons must receive both the 90° and 180° RF pulses. Because these pulses are usually 'slice selective' their effect is limited to the image sections. Blood flowing at above a certain velocity will have passed through the plane of section in the interval between the 90° and 180° RF pulses, and thus produce a signal void. For this to occur the average velocity within the vessel has to be equal to or greater than the slice thickness of the section divided by the time interval between the two RF pulses echo time (TE). In conventional spin-echo imaging, rapidly flowing (arterial) blood is usually demonstrated as a *signal void* with slow-flowing (venous) blood as a *high signal*.

Another cause of intraluminal signal loss, particularly for inplane flow, is the spin *dephasing* effect. The moving spins in flowing blood are subjected to magnetic field gradients, which lead to phase differences that are constantly changing relative to adjacent stationary spins. The greater the flow the larger the phase differences, which are also dependent on the strength and duration of the magnetic field gradients. There is thus a direct relationship between flow velocity and phase shifts which can be exploited to allow precise measurements of the former. Dephasing effects can reduce the intraluminal signal sufficiently to mask any flow-related enhancement that might be present.

Under certain circumstances, the phase differences induced by blood flowing through magnetic field gradients can be partially corrected, leading to an increase in signal from flowing blood. This *rephasing* effect is termed even-echo rephasing (gradient-refocused echo imaging) and allows both the display and quantification of flow.

From the preceding discussion, it is clear that the signal intensity appearance of flowing blood is complex and dependent on several factors. These include flow velocity, repetition time (TR), echo time (TE), type of echo produced, slice thickness and position of the section in the multislice set. Although the TE for the MRA sequence should be as short as possible to minimise flow-related dephasing of spins, it is often desirable to increase the TE to produce an out-of-phase image (i.e. with the fat and water protons opposed, which for a 1.5 T magnet system would be 6.9 ms) in order to reduce the signal from fat.

A number of MRA methods, that have exploited the above-mentioned phenomena are currently being used for the display and quantification of blood flow. The two techniques most widely studied are *time-of-flight* and *phase contrast*. Each has advantages

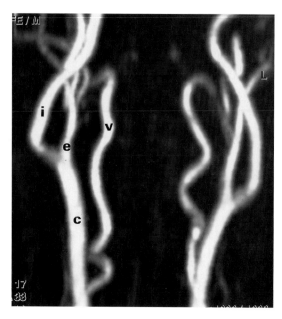

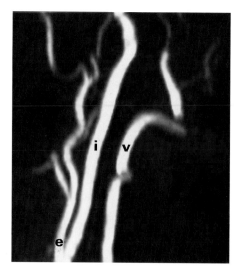

Fig. 15.132 Lateral MIP image of a two-dimensional time-of-flight MRA targeted to show the right neck arteries (same key as in Fig. 15.131.

Fig. 15.131 Coronal maximum intensity projection (MIP) image of a two-dimensional time-for-flight MR angiogram showing normal bilateral neck arteries. c, common carotid artery; e, external carotid artery; i, internal carotid artery; v, vertebral artery.

and disadvantages, and can be implemented in either a two- or three-dimensional mode. Different techniques will be required for specific applications. In the *time-of-flight (saturation)* method the blood is modified by a selective RF pulse which then enters the region of interest. The effect is dependent on the T_1 relaxation rate of blood, which is short. This technique is thus best suited for studies of defined regions containing tortuous vessels with fast-flowing blood, such as the carotid arteries and the circle of Willis (Fig. 15.131). *Phase contrast (gradient refocused)* methods rely on velocity-induced phase differences to discriminate flowing blood from surrounding stationary tissue. These techniques are sensitive to the detection of slow flow in small vessels and produce a more efficient suppression of the stationary background tissue. A further advantage of the phase-sensitive methods is that a precise measure of blood flow velocity can be made. *Subtraction* techniques (analo-

gous to DSA) can be used to provide high signal from blood with the elimination of the background signal from stationary tissue. The use of *saturation RF pulses* allows tagging of particular vascular areas in order to visualise venous and arterial anatomy separately.

The source MRA data collected are computed to form projection angiograms using the maximum intensity projection (MIP) method. For each ray in the projected set only the maximum value is extracted, as it is assumed that the blood in the vessel represents the highest signal in the data set. MR angiograms thus formed can be imaged as either 'black blood' or 'white blood', the former producing an image akin to DSA. Post-processing techniques also allow for improved visualisation of separate vessels without overlap, for instance the targeting of the internal carotid artery branches of one side separate from the contralateral side. (Fig. 15.132)

It should be remembered, as with all techniques, that there are potential pitfalls in interpretation. Respiratory and cardiac motion can cause ghosting as well as variation in flow velocity profiles. Surgical clips can lead to signal voids which can be easily recognised on the original source MRA image, but can be mistaken on the MIP image

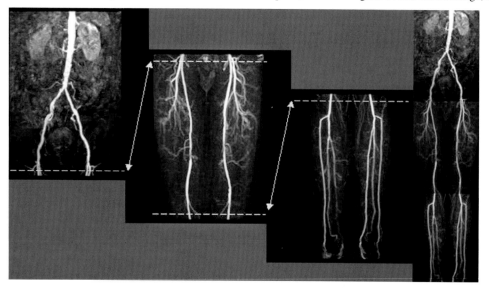

Fig. 15.133 Peripheral 3D CE-MRA performed in sections with tracking of the contrast bolus using set prescribed table movements, with slight overlap, to demonstrate the aortic bifurcation and peripheral vessels including the run-off. The final image is a composite to show the whole study. (Courtesy of Philips Medical Systems.)

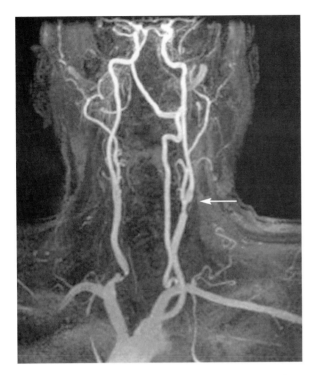

Fig. 15.134 Bilateral carotid arteries with a left common carotid stenosis (arrow) with no venous enhancement on a 3D CE-MRA image using elliptical centric view ordering of the data (see Ch. 59). (Courtesy of IGE Medical Systems.)

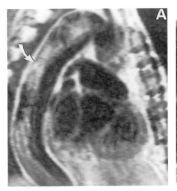
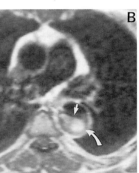

Fig. 15.135 Chronic descending aortic dissection on (A) sagittal and (B) transverse gated T$_2$-weighted spin echo (TE 2b ms.). Note the signal from the slow-flowing blood in the false lumen (curved arrow), and the itimal flap (straight arrows).

for a stenosis, thrombus or slow flow. It is thus imperative that the original source data set is reviewed in every case. Flow voids can occur due to turbulence (e.g. at the renal ostia on *phase contrast* MRA, or at the confluence of two tributaries such as the superior mesenteric and splenic veins). Low-signal structures can be lost using the MIP method, leading to an apparent loss of part of a vessel or overestimation of a stenosis.

First described by Prince in 1993, 3D CE-MRA, which combines gadolinium-chelate administration with a 3D breath-hold time-of-flight sequence, is the preferred technique in the assessment of the arterial tree, including renal arteries, pulmonary and peripheral circulation. The gadolinium-chelate shortens the T$_1$ of blood, increasing flow-related enhancement over a large field of view, improving visualisation of smaller arteries, overcoming the problems described above for the non-contrast techniques. Timing of the MRA sequence is vital for optimum imaging, with the centre K-space (which provides image contrast) of the sequence coinciding with the peak enhancement from the contrast administration. The use of rapid 3D acquisitions allows the data to be acquired during the first pass of the contrast bolus, thereby reducing the effects of dilution from recirculation, and minimising enhancement of venous structures (Figs. 15.133, 15.134). It can also be used in patients with poor renal blood flow and renal insufficiency. This technique is now preferred in many vascular centres as the method of choice in the assessment of the peripheral arterial tree. The aid of a moving table to follow the arterial contrast bolus allows visualisation of the whole of the pelvic and leg arteries

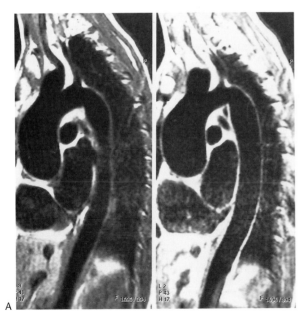
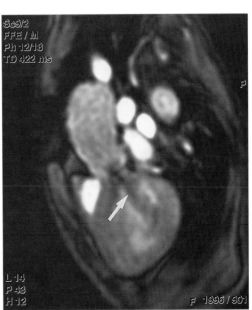

Fig. 15.136 (A) Moderate degree of aneurysmal dilatation of the ascending aorta extending into the proximal part of the innominate artery on contiguous parasagittal T$_1$-weighted spin echo (SE 750/15) image. (B) A sagittal-oblique phase contrast gradient echo (GE 750/7/40°) sequence in th same patient through the outflow tract shows a jet of signal void in the left ventricle (arrowed) consistent with aortic regurgitation.

including popliteal–tibial arteries, collateral vessels and run-off (Fig.15.133). Indeed, the demonstration of the collateral and small vessels is better demonstrated on CE-MRA compared with conventional X-ray arteriography. The current contrast media available are extracellular space agents, but several agents limited to the intravascular space are due for release.

THORACIC AORTA

One of the major applications of vascular MRI is in the assessment of the thoracic aorta. MRA (using conventional ECG-gated spin-echo T_1-weighted and multiphase gradient echo refocused sequences) has significant advantages over X-ray angiography and

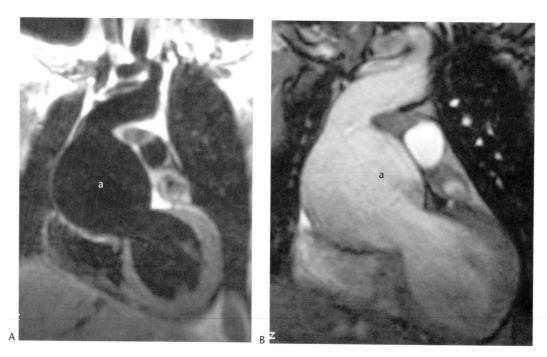

Fig. 15.137 Flask-shaped dilatation (a) of the aortic root and ascending aorta characteristic of Marfan's syndrome, on coronal-oblique ECG-gated (A) T_1-weighted spin-echo and (B) phase-constrast gradient-echo image.

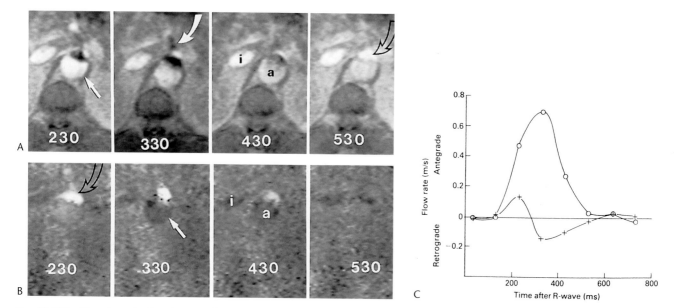

Fig. 15.138 Chronic aortic dissection on: (A) a set of four transverse cine gradient refocused (TE 28 ms) MR angiograms through the upper abdomen at the same anatomic level; (B) flow velocity maps derived from the angiograms in part (A) and (C) a plot of the maximum flow rates in the true and false lumens at different times in the cardiac cycle, showing reversal of blood flow in the false lumen (o, true lumen; t, false lumen) (Same patient as in part A, images have been taken at 100 ms intervals from the R-wave of the patient's ECG (indicated by the number on each image). There is a high signal within the false lumen (straight arrow) of the aorta (a) and inferior vena cava (i). Note signal loss in the true lumen (curved open arrow) and superior mesenteric artery (curved closed arrow) during systole due to high flow rates, with a return of signal at 530 ms as the flow rate reduces. In part B, flow direction and velocty can be derived. Antegrade flow appears as light grey, absence of flow as mid-grey (similar to background), and retrograde flow as dark grey. The true lumen (curved arrow) shows antegrade flow during systole, whereas false lumen (straight arrow) shows initial antegrade flow with flow reversed at 330 ms (see part C). Flow in the inferior vena cava (i) is consistently caudocranial. (Reproduced with permission from Mitchell et al 1988).

CT in the evaluation of aortic aneurysms and dissection, detecting aortic dilatations and differentiating an aortic aneurysm from solid masses (Figs 15.135, 15.136). Advantages of MRA include capability of topographic overview of the aorta and surrounding structures in any plane, together with visualisation of the origin of arch vessels. The size of the thoracic aorta can be accurately assessed using well-defined imaging planes and true short-axis views. The following are the normal dimensions of the thoracic aorta in a young adult (each with a range of ±4 mm): at the level of the sinus of Valsalva, 33 mm; midpart of the ascending aorta, 30 mm; transverse part of the aortic arch, 27 mm; descending aorta, 24 mm. Progressive aortic dilatation producing a typical flask-shaped appearance, as occurs in Marfan's syndrome (Fig. 15.137), is easily demonstrated on follow-up MRI examinations.

The use of phase-contrast methods allows clear separation between the true and false lumens, and assessment of the re-entry site can be made in aortic dissection (Fig. 15.138). Small entry sites between true and false lumens, however, are more accurately demonstrated by transoesophageal echocardiography. Knowledge of normal anatomy (e.g. location of the left brachiocephalic vein and superior pericardial recess) and awareness of artefacts that can mimic aortic dissection are important in order to avoid any possible misinterpretation. MRI is superior to CT and transoesophageal echocardiography in the assessment of the postoperative patient, and is without significant signal artefact in the majority. Postsurgical complications include haemorrhage, haemopericardium, pseudo-aneurysm formation, infection, graft occlusion or arteriovenous fistula. In the surgically treated patient, assessment of the arch vessels and anastomoses is easily achieved by MRI, but with difficulty on transoesophageal echocardiography.

The precise location, extent and severity of *aortic coarctation* can be assessed with MRI, providing information equivalent to that from X-ray angiography. The whole of the thoracic aorta can usually be demonstrated by oblique sagittal scanning along the line of the aortic arch (Fig. 15.139). In some instances the aorta is more tortuous, and multislice imaging is required for complete assessment. On MRI, the degree of stenosis of the coarctation segment, compared with the normal, correlates well with measurements made on X-ray angiography. A precise measurement of the pressure gradient and velocity across the coarctation segment can be obtained using MRA techniques (Fig. 15.140). A pressure gradient can be calculated from the measured peak flow velocity at the stenosis using the modified Bernoulli equation. Collateral vessels, including the internal mammary, intercostal and posterior mediastinal arteries, can be visualised (Fig. 15.139). The evaluation of the descending aorta below the isthmus, which can be difficult on two-dimensional echocardiography, is also important in the preoperative assessment and can be well demonstrated on MRI. If detail is limited using the conventional MRI/MRA techniques, a CE-MRA study can be performed to demonstrate the vascular abnormality (Fig.15.141).

PULMONARY ARTERIES

The normal dimensions of the main pulmonary arteries can be well shown on transverse and coronal ECG-gated spin-echo and gradient-refocused images. High signals can be seen in peripheral small branching pulmonary arteries on gated spin-echo images due to slow blood flow towards end-diastole. Similar high signals can be seen in the main pulmonary arteries and aorta. These signals clear with the onset of systole. Abnormal persistence of signal in the pulmonary arteries during systole, on gated spin-echo images, has been used to identify patients with pulmonary arterial hypertension.

On gradient-refocused images the normal pulmonary arteries are characterised by a rapid increase in intraluminal signal intensity and diameter in systole, with a consequent decrease in diastole. In addition, branch vessels down to the subsegmental level and beyond can be delineated, extending the range of pulmonary vessels accessible to examination. By using 3D CE-MRA techniques it is possible to visualise up to the fifth and sixth branch order in the pulmonary tree. In contrast to the appearance of normal pulmonary arteries, the normal *pulmonary veins* have a distinctive signal intensity peak in both systole and diastole. These different appearances allow distinction to be made between pulmonary arteries and veins. In *pulmonary arterial hypertension* there is reduction in the normal compliance, with loss of the pulsatile systolic increase and diastolic decrease in diameter and signal intensity of the proximal pulmonary arteries.

MRI is gaining acceptance as the preferred technique for assessing pulmonary arteries in patients with pulmonary artery *atresia* or *obstruction* (Fig. 15.142). In neonates and infants, thin sections

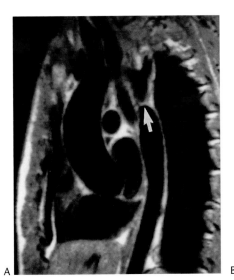
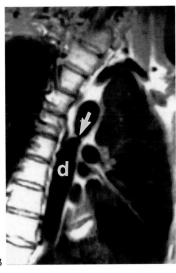

Fig. 15.139 Post-ductal coarctation of the aorta showing a narrowed diaphragm (arrowed) on (A) sagittal-oblique and (B) coronal-oblique intermediate-weighted ECG-gated spin echo (SE 1000/21) scans. Note the dilated collateral vessels supplying the descending aorta (d) beyond the coarctation.

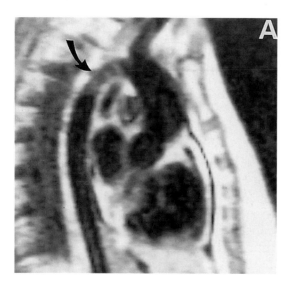

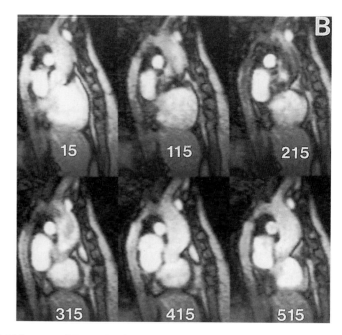

Fig. 15.140   Coarctation of the aorta, arrowed, previously repaired. (A) Oblique gated T_1-weighted spin echo scan (TE 26 ms). (B) A set of six cine gradient refocused echo (TE 12 ms) MR angiograms at the same anatomic level, spaced at 100 ms intervals from 15 ms from the R-wave of the ECG. At peak flow rates during systole there is some signal reduction at the repaired coarctation site (arrowed), indicating turbulence. Velocity maps (not shown) were performed at this site, giving a peak velocity (v) of 2 m/s (pressure gradient = $4v^2$, making a calculated gradient of 16 mmHg). This compared favourably with the value of 20 mmHg obtained from Doppler ultrasound.

(< 5 mm) are required. Gated spin-echo imaging can clearly demonstrate hypoplastic pulmonary arteries to the level of the first hilar branch. The use of MRA techniques extends the range for assessment of more peripheral branches, overcoming the limitation of two-dimensional echocardiography in depicting distal pulmonary artery branch stenoses (Fig. 15.142). Important clinical determinants in the management of patients with right ventricular outflow obstruction are the size of the pulmonary artery and the presence or absence of a pulmonary confluence. Assessment of pulmonary artery growth following correction surgery is required to monitor and detect any developing stenoses. It should be noted that calculating vessel diameters from the intraluminal high signal obtained by MRA techniques could lead to an underestimate of true vessel size, because of magnetic susceptibility effects between the vessel wall

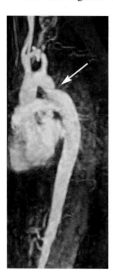

Fig. 15.141   Coarctation of the aorta (arrow) on a 3D CE-MRA image in the sagittal-oblique plane.

and adjacent lung, which may lead to signal loss at the edge of the vessel. The combined use of gated spin-echo imaging should overcome this problem. Difficulties in evaluating pulmonary arteries in patients with obstructive lesions have been encountered with both cine angiocardiography and two-dimensional echocardiography, and MRI should have a useful role here.

Pulmonary emboli as small as 3 mm in diameter can be detected experimentally on spin-echo imaging, but may be difficult to interpret due to flow-related artefacts and poor differentiation between thrombus and areas of atelectasis or endobronchial mucous plugs. In addition, this technique does not allow acute and chronic pulmonary emboli to be distinguished. In a study of 10 patients with pulmonary embolic disease, acute and chronic emboli were distinguished using MRA techniques. On gradient-refocused echo imaging, acute pulmonary embolus was recognised as a persistent low-signal intraluminal filling defect (due to the magnetic susceptibility effect of haemosiderin) with a curvilinear capping by the high-signal intensity vascular column. Abrupt vessel cut-off without capping or the presence of webs or a narrowed and irregular vessel were interpreted to be due to a chronic pulmonary embolus. No emboli distal to lobar branches, however, were demonstrated. The use of CE-MRA would be of benefit in these cases (Figs 15.143, 15.144). MRA techniques may have a limited useful future role in the assessment of pulmonary embolic disease, particularly in those individuals allergic to iodinated contrast medium, with the advent of multislice CT.

CAROTID ARTERIES

The normal carotid bifurcation can be reliably imaged on MRA (Fig. 15.131). Both carotid bifurcations can be imaged simultaneously in less than 10 min by using a multislab three-dimensional

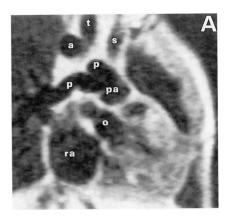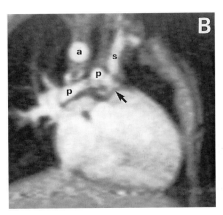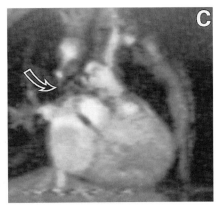

Fig. 15.142   Congenital branch pulmonary artery stenosis in a 11-year-old child with corrected Fallot's tetralogy and persistent pulmonary artery hypertension. (A) Oblique–coronal gated T₁weighted spin echo (TE 26 ms) image (B,C) Gradient-refocused echo (TE 12 ms) MR angiograms at the same anatomic level. (B) End-diastole. (C) In systole, showing signal loss, due to turbulence, in the right pulmonary artery (curved arrow). a, right-sided aortic arch; o, outflow tract of the left ventricle; p, right and left pulmonary arteries; pa, main pulmonary artery; ra, right atrium; s, left-sided superior vena cava; t, trachea; straight arrow in part B, position of the pulmonary valve.

sequence. Subsequent images can be reformatted in multiple orientations to optimise the demonstration or show both bifurcations. Patients who have undergone recent carotid endarterectomy can also be evaluated non-invasively. As indicated in the assessment of aortic coarctation, short TE values are essential to demonstrate carotid artery stenoses. In severe stenosis there may, however, be profound signal loss mimicking occlusion. Recent developments with the use of 3D CE-MRA should help to resolve this problem (Fig.15.134). In order to demonstrate the circle of Willis, images are usually acquired in the transverse plane, where detail of the basal arterial tree and small branches can be obtained.

On MRA, aneurysms and arteriovenous malformations (including intraspinal angiomas) can be visualised together with the relative flow contribution of the individual feeding vessels, allowing improved treatment planning.

ABDOMINAL VESSELS

The normal short-axis diameter of the suprarenal abdominal aorta is approximately 25 mm, tapering down to its bifurcation, where it measures 15 mm. The indications for MRA of the abdominal aorta include patients with known iodinated contrast allergy or renal insufficiency, and those with difficult vascular access due to severe aortoiliac occlusive disease. MRA can also be used to demonstrate arteriovenous malformations. The relationship and effect of

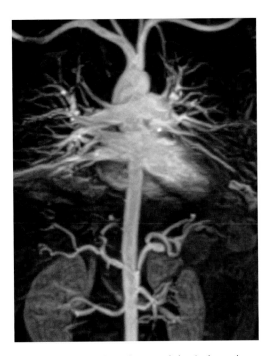

Fig. 15.143   Normal thoracic and upper abdominal vessels on a 3D CE-MRA in the coronal plane.

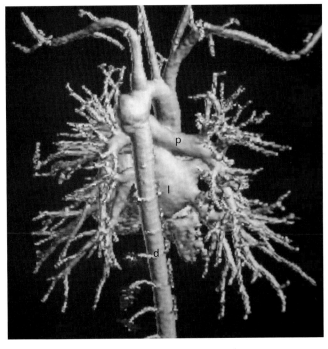

Fig. 15.144   Posterior view of a surface-rendered reformatted image of a CE-MRA study showing normal thoracic vessels. d = descending aorta; p = pulmonary artery; l = left atrium (Courtesy of GE Medical Systems).

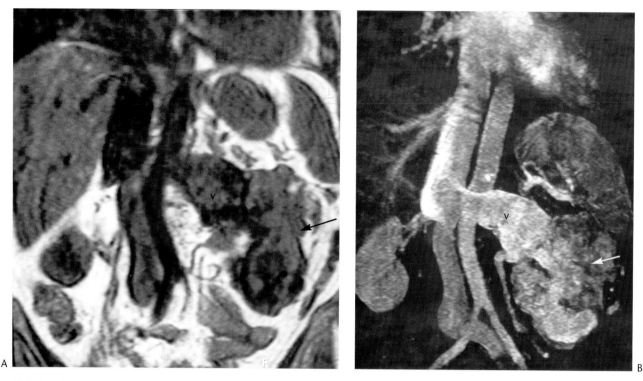

Fig. 15.145 Clear cell renal carcinoma (arrow) with dilatation and tumour infiltration of the left renal vein (v) on coronal (A) T₁-weighted spin-echo and (B) 3D CE-MRA studies.

tumours on adjacent vascular structures can be more easily appreciated than with conventional spin-echo imaging (Fig.15.145).

RENAL ARTERIES

Both renal arteries originate at approximately the same level, 2 cm below the origin of the superior mesenteric artery. An accessory renal artery occurs in a fifth of individuals, being commoner on the left below the level of the main renal vessel. The calibre of the renal arteries varies between 5 and 10 mm, and is dependent on the total renal blood flow indirectly reflecting renal function.

The clinical signs of renal artery stenosis include renovascular hypertension and azotaemia. Renovascular hypertension is believed to be the cause of 1–5% of all cases of hypertension. Approximately 70% of cases of renal artery stenosis (Fig.15.146) are due to atherosclerosis occurring in older individuals, with the remainder due to fibromuscular dysplasia (Fig.15.147), which more often affects younger patients. Atherosclerotic renovascular lesions typically (85%) involve the proximal main renal arteries or the ostium, whereas those due to fibromuscular dysplasia are usually in the more distal and segmental parts of the renal artery, limiting the role of phase contrast and/or time-of-flight in ruling out renovascular hypertension in the younger individual.

MRA of the renal arteries poses particular problems related to cardiac, respiratory and bowel motion artefacts, overlapping renal veins and inferior vena cava, renal vessel tortuosity, and complex flow patterns with disparate flow velocities between the aorta and renal arteries. Phase-contrast and/or time-of-flight MRA can be used for detecting stenoses of the main renal artery. On *phase-contrast MRA*, false ostial stenosis can be demonstrated due to loss

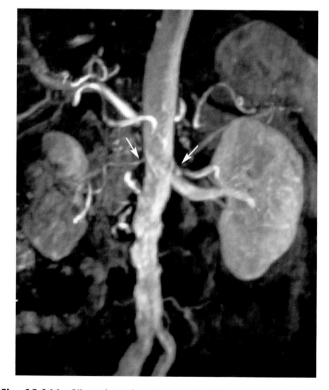

Fig. 15.146 Bilateral renal artery stenosis (arrows) on a coronal 3D CE-MRA image.

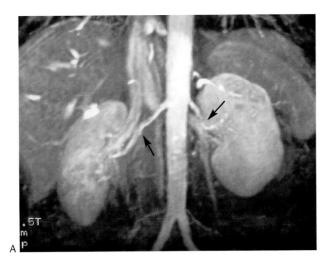

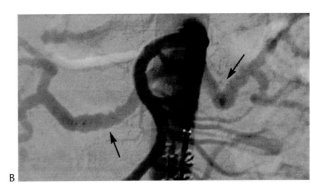

Fig. 15.147 Bilateral fibromuscular dysplasia (arrows) in a 39-year-old woman on (A), 3D CE-MRA confirmed on subsequent (B) conventional arteriography.

of signal at the origin of the renal arteries from dephasing due to normal non-laminar flow at vessel origins. Using *time-of-flight MRA* the proximal renal artery is well visualised, but visualisation of the vessel more distally is hampered mainly by saturation of spins leading to fading away of the signal in the vessels with slow flow.

CE-MRA has particular advantages overcoming the problems using conventional MRA techniques (Figs 15.146, 15.147). In screening for stenosis of the main renal arteries, and differentiation from fibromuscular dysplasia, the use of 3D CE-MRA provides the optimum method for its detection, and allows the demonstration of small accessory renal arteries and segmental branches (Fig.15.148).

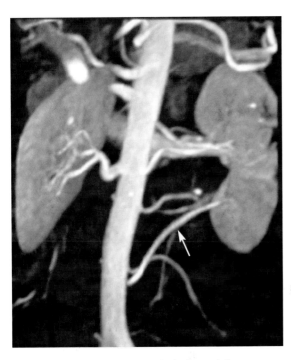

Fig. 15.148 Normal renal arteries, including a left accessory vessel (arrow), on a CE-MRA image showing scarring to the left kidney (Courtesy of GE Medical Systems).

PERIPHERAL VESSELS

The absence of physiological motion in the extremities makes them ideal areas for vascular study with MRI. The advent of CE-MRA combined with a moving table facility provides a clear demonstration of the normal and diseased peripheral arterial tree with advantages over conventional X-ray technique (Figs 15.133, 15.149). No provision for an intra-arterial catheter is required, and the collateral vessels and run-off into the more distal vessels is more clearly shown. In many vascular centres 3D CE-MRA has replaced conventional X-ray angiography in the assessment of the peripheral arterial circulation.

SAFETY OF MR CONTRAST AGENTS

Gadolinium-based MR contrast agents are extremely safe but, as with any drug administration, their use does carry the risk of a severe anaphylactic reaction and death. There are a number of risk factors including a history of asthma or other hypersensitivity disorders. Epileptic fits have been reported after MR contrast injection. The incidence of such severe reactions has been estimated in the region of 1 in 400 000 although a study has suggested that this may be an underestimate (2 severe reactions occurred in a series of 21 000 patient records reviewed (0.01%)).

Studies have shown a low incidence of minor side-effects comparable to a placebo injection of saline (0.4% nausea and vomiting, local warmth and pain, 0.3% headache, and 0.1% paraesthesia and dizziness). Moderately severe reactions (including bronchospasm, laryngospasm, facial oedema, arrhthymias and urticaria) have been estimated to occur in about 1 in 5000 cases.

Gadolinium compounds can be used safely in patients with renal impairment, and can be eliminated from the body by haemodialysis. The use of non-ionic gadolinium contrast agents has a theoretical advantage over the ionic compounds. A potential cause for concern is in relation to the dissociation of the gadolinium ion from the chelate leading to free gadolinium, which is toxic. In individuals with normal renal function the rate of dissociation is slower than the renal clearance preventing its occurrence. In patients with renal

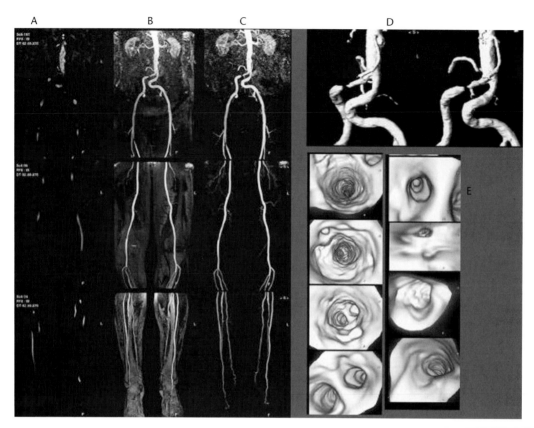

Fig. 15.149 Right iliac stenosis on a peripheral 3D CE-MRA study showing: (A) reference image; (B) postcontrast study during the arterial phase; (C) subtraction of A and B; (D) 3D surface-rendered image; (E) intraluminal navigator images. (Courtesy of Philip Medical Systems.)

impairment, however, the MR contrast excretion is delayed allowing the contrast to remain longer in circulation, and there is increased competition for the chelate from copper and zinc ions in the intravascular space. In order to eliminate this potential hazard the contrast can be dialysed with over 95% of the agent being removed by the third dialysis treatment. The use of an MR contrast agent is safer, however, than administering a standard regime of an iodine-based contrast medium.

MR contrast agents are well tolerated in neonates, infants and children with no evidence of any enhanced risk. It should be noted, however, that neonates and young infants have lower glomerular filtration and renal clearance rates compared with older children and adults. These effects lead to a delay in excretion with a longer biological half-life for the gadolinium contrast agent. In the neonate the half-life for gadolinium compound is about 6.5 hours, and this can increase to 9 hours in the premature infant. This delayed excretion allows for a wider MR post-contrast imaging window in these cases. By about 2 months of age the half-life approach that in adults (1.5 hours). The routine adult dose regime (0.1 mmol/kg body weight) should still be used in neonates and young children despite the prolonged half-life for the compound due to a greater (x2) extracellular fluid volume in proportion to their body weight compared with adults. Therefore, in a neonate and young infant given a routine injection of MR contrast medium the blood concentration of gadolinium compound after equilibration will be approximately half that of an equivalent dose administered to an adult. Clinical experience has shown, however, that adequate enhancement using a routine adult dose regime can be achieved in these cases.

There is no data available to assess the potential risk to a foetus of gadolinium compounds given to a woman during pregnancy, as it is known that the contrast agent does cross the placenta. A conservative approach is to not administer any gadolinium compound to a pregnant patient unless the potential benefit outweighs any potential risk to the foetus. During lactation it has been shown that gadolinium-chelate does cross into the breast milk. If a gadolinium contrast agent is administered to a nursing mother she should avoid breast feeding for 36–48 hours after the injection to prevent any contrast being absorbed by the child.

REFERENCES

See end of Chapter 16.

16

PHLEBOGRAPHY

David Sutton and Roger H. S. Gregson
with contributions from Paul L. Allan and Jeremy P. R. Jenkins

Contrast phlebography* has been the main imaging method for investigating disorders of veins for many decades. In recent years this pre-eminence has been increasingly challenged by improved CT techniques, and without radiation exposure by ultrasound and MRA. The two latter methods are discussed in detail at the end of this chapter. Contrast phlebography by direct venous injection is nevertheless still widely used. The types of contrast phlebography used in clinical practice include:

1. Phlebography of the lower limb
2. Pelvic phlebography and inferior vena cavography
3. Hepatic, renal and gonadal vein phlebography
4. Venous sampling for endocrine tumours
5. Percutaneous transvenous interventional procedures
6. Phlebography of the upper limb and superior vena cava
7. Portal phlebography.

Intraosseous phlebography and spinal phlebography were once fairly widely practised in the past, but are now obsolete.

The investigations listed use direct contrast phlebography. Indirect phlebography can be achieved by serial filming following arteriography. The latter method is the one routinely used for the demonstration of the cerebral veins following cerebral angiography and commonly for the demonstration of the renal veins following selective renal arteriography. It is also used for portal phlebography following selective coeliac or splenic arteriography—so-called *arterioportography*.

CT
CT, particularly spiral CT, will demonstrate the major veins well, but usually requires contrast injections for the confirmation of such lesions as caval thrombosis or portal thrombosis. The latest types of CT scanner (multislice spiral) can image large areas of venous drainage in excellent 3D detail; they can also produce double-phase (arterial and venous) vascular images, or abdominal triple-phase (arterial, portal and venous) from a single intravenous injection of contrast (see Fig. 16.29) MR provides no radiation hazards but will show veins as well as arteries and can provide double and triple – phase images just as well (Fig. 16.44).

Digital subtraction angiography (DSA)
This technique is limited in the area that can be examined at one time but will reduce contrast medium dosage in areas where it can be used, as well as producing images free of bone or other superimposed structures.

THE LOWER LIMB

Indications
Phlebography of the lower limb is practised at most medical centres for the following purposes:

1. To demonstrate deep venous thrombosis (DVT) in the calf, thigh, pelvis or inferior vena cava.
2. To show suspected venous obstruction by tumour or extrinsic pressure.
3. To investigate secondary or recurrent varicose veins thought to be associated with an abnormality of the deep-venous system such as post-thrombotic destruction of valves and associated incompetent perforators, or with inadequate surgery.
4. To investigate swollen legs where the differential diagnosis between lymphoedema, cellulitis and venous incompetence (or obstruction) is not clear.
5. To investigate varicose ulcers in the post-thrombotic syndrome.
6. To outline venous malformations.

Suspected DVT is the commonest cause for patient referral, and in most cases there is strong clinical evidence for the lesion. In some cases, however, for example in patients with repeated pulmonary emboli but no obvious source, the investigation may be undertaken to exclude the lower limb as a source of emboli.

C-reactive protein assay
This is a simple blood test which has been shown to have a sensitivity of 100% and a specificity of 52% in DVT. A normal result

---

* Phlebography is preferred to the alternative venography, because it is etymologically correct (Gk) while venography is a hybrid (Gk & L).

483

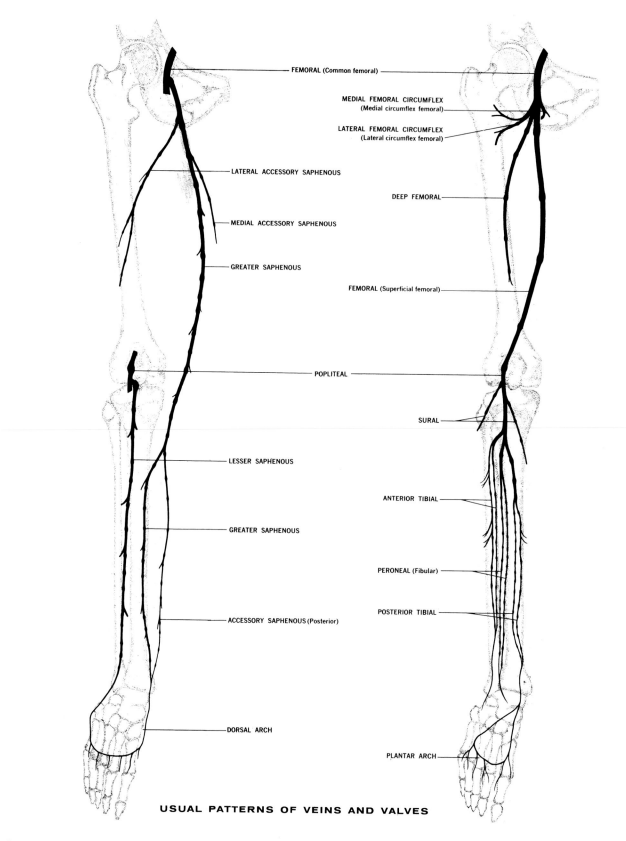

FEMORAL (Common femoral)

MEDIAL FEMORAL CIRCUMFLEX
(Medial circumflex femoral)

LATERAL FEMORAL CIRCUMFLEX
(Lateral circumflex femoral)

LATERAL ACCESSORY SAPHENOUS

DEEP FEMORAL

MEDIAL ACCESSORY SAPHENOUS

GREATER SAPHENOUS

FEMORAL (Superficial femoral)

POPLITEAL

SURAL

LESSER SAPHENOUS

ANTERIOR TIBIAL

GREATER SAPHENOUS

PERONEAL (Fibular)

POSTERIOR TIBIAL

ACCESSORY SAPHENOUS (Posterior)

DORSAL ARCH

PLANTAR ARCH

USUAL PATTERNS OF VEINS AND VALVES

Fig. 16.1 Diagram of the deep and superficial veins of the lower limb. (Copyright Eastman Kodak Co. Reprinted by courtesy of the Health Sciences Division, Eastman Kodak Co.)

can therefore exclude DVT and prevent further unnecessary investigation.

Normal anatomy

The venous drainage of the lower limb can be divided into two separate systems, the deep veins and the superficial veins. These are connected by the communicating veins (Figs 16.1, 16.2).

The *deep veins* in the calf follow the same distribution as the main arteries but are usually double, forming the anterior tibial, posterior tibial and peroneal veins. The calf veins, or sural veins, arise in calf muscles and emerge from them to join the peroneal, posterior tibial or popliteal veins.

The *communicating veins* are usually small and paired and connect the superficial and deep veins. Normally they are extremely narrow, but they can become quite large when hypertrophied. They are valved so that blood only flows from the superficial to the deep veins. Under pathological conditions they can become incompetent, permitting reverse flow from the deep to the superficial veins (Fig. 16.3). They are most numerous and important in the calf, though there is usually one in the mid-thigh and sometimes two or three at different levels (Fig. 16.4).

The popliteal vein is a smooth large vessel lying behind the knee and passing up into the femoral vein, which follows the course of the femoral artery. The femoral vein is sometimes double, or the profunda vein, which usually lies in the upper two-thirds of the thigh, may connect in its lower part with the femoral or popliteal vein. Perforating or communicating veins in the thigh are normally

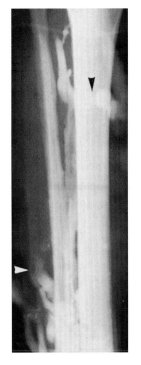

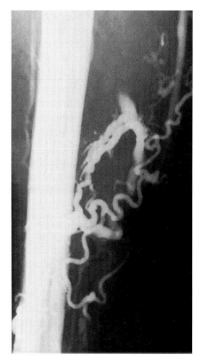

Fig. 16.3 Incompetent perforating veins in the calf (arrows).

Fig. 16.4 Incompetent perforating veins in the thigh.

small, but if incompetent may be demonstrated connecting the superficial and deep veins (Fig. 16.4).

The *superficial leg veins* drain into the saphenous veins. The short saphenous vein passes up the lateral side of the leg to the knee, where it passes deeply to join the popliteal vein. The long saphenous vein passes up the medial side of the calf and thigh and then joins the femoral vein below the groin.

The venous system can be regarded as a blood reservoir, and normally contains some two-thirds of the body's blood, largely in the lower limbs. Flow to the heart depends on the pressure gradient between the veins and right atrium, and is assisted by the muscle contractions, particularly in the calf, acting as a pump. The veins themselves can also actively contract and help onward flow of blood. In addition, the valves are of great importance in preventing retrograde flow, and their destruction or damage by thrombosis has serious haemodynamic consequences leading to venous incompetence.

Technique

Ascending phlebography

A large number of different techniques have been described in the literature. No standard technique has been generally accepted. The technique used by us has been modified over the years, and is as follows. A small needle is inserted percutaneously into a vein on the dorsum of the foot. Occasionally this may prove impossible, and the needle may have to be inserted by cut-down. If the foot is swollen or oedematous, prior bed rest with the foot elevated is desirable to reduce the swelling. Once the needle is in position, compression is applied just above the ankle and also just above the knee by tourniquets or by inflatable cuffs. The pressure used is just

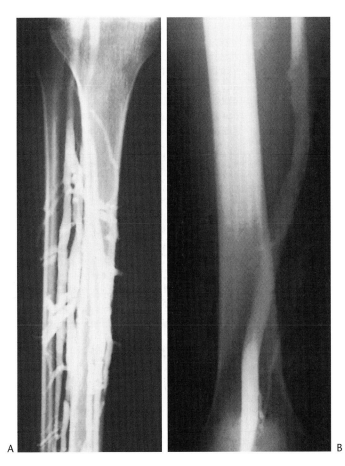

Fig. 16.2 (A,B) Normal ascending phlebogram of the deep veins.

sufficient to occlude the superficial veins completely without affecting the patency of the deep veins.

Contrast medium (40–50 ml) is then injected by hand pressure. In some cases more may be required to obtain adequate filling of the femoral and iliac veins, but it should rarely be necessary to use more than 80–100 ml. In the past, 65% Hypaque or an equivalent other medium has been used. However, the newer contrast media with low osmolality are now regarded as mandatory (see Ch. 15), and these are better tolerated by the patient and less likely to produce complications.

Usually the foot veins punctured with small butterfly needles (21 British standard wire gauge) therefore the injection can take 20–30 s. Flow is monitored by observation with an image intensifier, and films obtained at appropriate moments as the veins are sequentially filled. While some workers conduct the examination with the patient supine, others insist that the patient should be tilted on the table into a 30–60° feet-down position. This is mainly to prevent layering of contrast medium posteriorly, which gives rise to artefactual filling defects, and to ensure mixing of blood and contrast medium. The foot and leg should be medially rotated to separate the tibia and fibula and the deep veins of the calf. The weight should not be borne by the foot being injected, so that the calf muscles remain relaxed and their veins can be filled with contrast.

Descending phlebography

This is less frequently practised but is occasionally used, with the patient supine on a tilting table and the feet against the footrest. The femoral vein is punctured at the groin. The catheter tip is advanced 5 cm into the artery and the catheter strapped down to the skin. The patient is then tilted to the erect or near-erect position, and contrast medium injected. If the patient performs the Valsalva manoeuvre, contrast medium will reflux down an incompetent femoral vein into the popliteal vein. It has been claimed, however, that contrast will sometimes flow past competent valves, though it is usually possible to assess the degree of true incompetence and show the valves clearly, particularly when they are competent (Fig. 16.5).

Complications

With the older contrast media, a few patients tolerated the procedure badly and complained of pain and discomfort in the calf with ascending phlebography. Nausea, vomiting and minor allergic reactions were also occasionally seen, as with all contrast media. The new low-osmolality contrast media should be better tolerated and give rise to little discomfort.

Care should be taken to ensure there is no contrast medium extravasation at the site of puncture, as this can be quite painful, and with a large volume of extravasation the consequences, particularly in an ischaemic or oedematous foot, can be serious. Skin necrosis has been recorded to result from this accident.

Phlebitis and postphlebography venous thrombosis can occur where large volumes of high-concentration contrast are used. This should be guarded against by flushing out residual contrast agent with saline at the end of the procedure, and by using the new low-osmolality contrast media.

Radiological findings

In the normal patient the deep veins of the calf are outlined by contrast at ascending phlebography with cuffs inflated; three paired

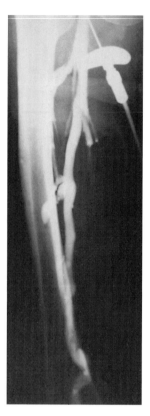

Fig. 16.5 Descending phlebogram showing incompetent valves and reflux down to the popliteal vein.

veins accompanying the peroneal, posterior and anterior tibial arteries can be recognised, the last being smaller than the others. There is no filling of the superficial or communicating veins (Fig. 16.2), but with progressive injections of contrast medium there will be varying degrees of filling of the soleal muscle veins, which are typically large and valveless and drain into the peroneal and posterior tibial veins. There may also be filling of the gastrocnemius veins, which are valved and usually multiple, running a downward course from their points of entry into the upper popliteal vein.

The popliteal vein is single and commences near the knee joint, passing upwards to become the femoral vein. Views of the calf are usually obtained in both anteroposterior and lateral projections. Valves are usually obvious in the distended veins but can be accentuated by the patient performing the Valsalva manoeuvre.

A good-quality ascending phlebogram will also demonstrate the iliac veins and inferior vena cava, but these are best shown by releasing the tourniquet and manually compressing the calf to improve the upward flow of contrast medium at the same time as the pelvic exposure is made. This ensures a good bolus of contrast medium entering the iliac veins. If the suspected lesion affects only the pelvic veins or inferior vena cava, direct pelvic phlebography is to be preferred (see below).

Deep vein thrombosis

Venous thrombosis appears to be multifactorial in origin, and is associated with slowing of the blood flow and an increased liability to blood coagulation. Conditions known to predispose include malignant disease, age, obesity, trauma and surgery, as well as prolonged immobilisation, myocardial infarction and congestive heart failure. A rare but frequently fatal condition is Hughes–Stovin syndrome, usually seen in young boys, where recurrent DVT is associated with haemoptysis from a ruptured segmental pulmonary aneurysm.

The risk of DVT is particularly high after abdominal and pelvic surgery, and even higher after operations on the hip, knee or femur. It becomes even greater if there is associated myocardial infarction or congestive heart failure. The thrombosis may be bilateral in some 30% of patients.

Clinically, symptoms are present only if there is significant obstruction or inflammation produced by the thrombosis, and it is claimed that 50% or more of cases are silent and symptomless.

The main danger is pulmonary embolus, and the incidence in the USA of this complication is over 500 000 cases per annum. The mortality in different series ranges from 10% to 30%. The vast majority of these emboli arise from the leg veins. As already noted, half the cases show no prodromal leg symptoms before the embolus occurs.

Acute thrombosis

Acute thrombosis of the deep veins appears as filling defects within the veins, the defect often being outlined by a marginal layer of contrast. Views in more than one plane may show that the clot is adherent to the vein at some point in one or other plane. Upward extension of the clot may be seen lying more freely in the lumen, and such a floating tail is likely to embolise. Adherent clot is regarded as relatively less dangerous. Clot may be identified in calf veins only, or involving the popliteal and femoral veins, or in the iliac veins and inferior vena cava (Figs 16.6–16.9).

True clot defects should be distinguished from:

1. Artefacts due to layering
2. Streaming from the entry of large non-opacified tributary veins
3. Turbulence around valves.

Films in more than one plane, the Valsalva manoeuvre and multiple films all help in this respect, as do large doses of contrast medium and the semierect position.

Acute thrombosis is later followed by clot retraction, thrombolysis and recanalisation, but the venous valves are damaged and destroyed so that the vein becomes irregular and incompetent. Some veins are severely stenosed or occluded, and in these cases venous return is largely by dilated collaterals. In either case a *post-thrombotic syndrome* may develop, characterised by swelling and pain in the affected leg. Eventually this may lead to induration and ulceration. This is usually on the medial aspect of the ankle, but is occasionally lateral in position. This is related to the fact that the medial aspect of the lower third of the leg just above the ankle is the site for a group of communicating veins, usually three in number. As these are at the most dependent part of the limb the increased pressure from incompetence and partial obstruction is greatest here and is accentuated by the pressure from calf muscle contractions.

Phlebography in patients with post-thrombotic states will show involved veins to be irregular and incompetent. In severe cases the major veins may be occluded in whole or in part and replaced by numerous collateral veins.

Recurrent varicose veins

The recurrence of varicose veins after surgery is a frequent clinical problem and may occur several years later. In these patients a useful

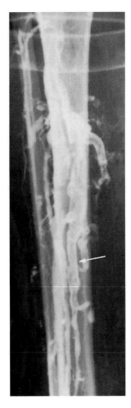

Fig. 16.6 Phlebogram showing venous thrombosis in deep veins of the calf. The clot shows as a central filling defect with marginal contrast (arrow).

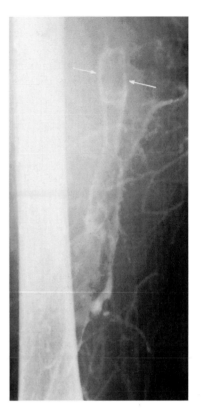

Fig. 16.7 Phlebogram showing venous thrombosis in the femoral vein. The clot shows as a central filling defect with marginal contrast (arrows).

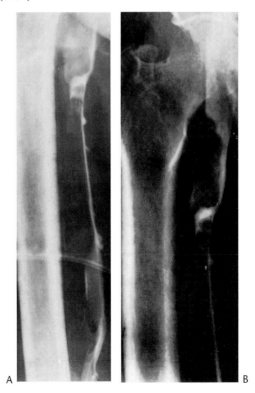

A   B

Fig. 16.8 (A,B) Extensive clot in the femoral vein adherent in part.

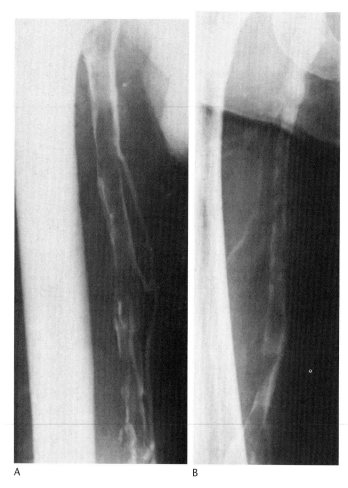

A   B

Fig. 16.9 (A,B) Extensive clot in the femoral vein.

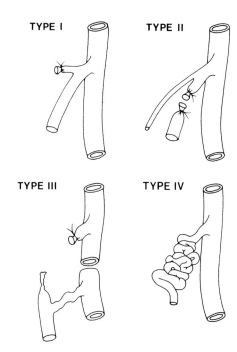

Fig. 16.10 The four types of recurrence in the thigh are shown diagrammatically. More than one type may apply in a given patient. (Reproduced from Starnes et al (1984), with permission.)

procedure is direct injection of one or more of the superficial thigh varicose veins to demonstrate their distribution and the pattern of recurrences at the groin following the previous high ligation of the long saphenous vein. There are several mechanisms, but the most usual is a tortuous leash of recanalised vein and not a missed tributary of the long saphenous or a missed perforating vein (Fig. 16.10). The procedure may have the additional bonus of sclerosing the recanalised trunk and producing a clinical cure.

CONGENITAL ANOMALIES

Duplication

Duplication of the popliteal or femoral vein or of both is not infrequent, as is duplication of the long saphenous vein. Congenital *absence* of the posterior tibial veins is another anomaly that is not infrequent. In this case veins are usually seen passing laterally above the ankle to drain into the peroneal veins.

Congenital absence of the venous valves

This is described in the major veins giving rise to venous stasis (*primary deep-venous insufficiency*) and should be considered when

children or teenagers present with varicosities or chronic leg swelling. However, such a diagnosis should be made with caution as previously unrecognised DVT with recanalisation cannot always be excluded. It is claimed that such recanalisation can sometimes result in apparently normal-looking veins without the usual irregularities seen in the post-thrombotic syndrome.

Klippel–Trenaunay syndrome

This is characterised by a naevus with hypertrophy of bones and soft tissues of affected limbs, usually legs, though arms may also be affected. There is venous dysplasia, and the normal venous return is replaced by persistence of a more primitive system, usually a large lateral venous channel in the leg, or a single large medial venous channel in the arm (Fig. 16.27). These can be associated with superficial varicosities. The large drainage vein is often valveless and shows very sluggish flow. Abnormal large drainage veins also occur in the penis, resulting in erectile dysfunction and impotence.

Ehlers–Danlos syndrome

This may cause the development of large venous aneurysms.

Other anomalies

A large *varix* or venous aneurysm can occur anywhere in the venous system. Such lesions are not uncommon at the termination of the long or short saphenous veins. Superficial or deep-venous varices or *venous angioma* are sometimes seen, such lesions having no obvious connection with an arterial lesion. Their anatomy is well shown by simple phlebography.

THE PELVIS AND ABDOMEN

As noted above, the iliac veins and IVC are quite well shown by good-quality ascending phlebograms from the foot, and their demonstration should be part of all such investigations. However, they can be more constantly and clearly demonstrated by direct femoral phlebography, which is the technique of choice where the lesion is known to be intra-abdominal. The method is also used in the occasional cases where ascending phlebography from the foot has failed to clearly exclude or confirm clot in the iliacs or IVC because of poor contrast for technical or other reasons.

The lesions shown by pelvic and inferior caval phlebography include:

1. Acute thrombosis with recent clot, or post-thrombotic sequelae with partial obstruction and collateral circulation.

2. Obstruction by neoplastic or glandular masses, usually by extrinsic pressure, but also by tumour invasion as in hypernephromas.

3. Extrinsic pressure from large benign tumours or other lesions, e.g. lymphocoele, aneurysms, retroperitoneal fibrosis, haematoma.

4. Obstruction of the left common iliac vein by pressure from the right common iliac artery (so-called 'lymphoedema praecox').

5. Post-traumatic or radiotherapy venous damage.

6. Pelvic varicosities.

7. Congenital anomalies.

Technique

The iliac veins and IVC are well shown by direct injection into the femoral veins of 30–40 ml of contrast medium on each side. Both veins are injected at the same time, unless only one iliac vein is obstructed and it is desired to show collateral and bypass drainage pathways clearly (Fig. 16.16). A unilateral injection will also suffice if only the inferior vena cava is under examination. The injection is made through a large cannula inserted into the femoral vein at the groin, or after percutaneous insertion of a catheter which is passed 5–8 cm up the vein.

To obtain good filling, contrast medium is injected rapidly as a bolus, taking 2–4 s for the 40 ml volume on each side. Serial films of the abdomen are obtained at the rate of 1 per second for 5 s as normal flow is rapid. Better and more prolonged filling can be obtained if the patient performs the Valsalva manoeuvre. A catheter inserted on one side can also be manipulated to the other side. (Fig. 16.11A), allowing both iliacs to be injected separately.

Radiographic appearances

The normal external and common iliac veins and IVC are valveless and appear as large contrast-filled tubes. There may be a slight extrinsic pressure defect at the termination of the left common iliac where it is crossed by the overlying right common iliac artery. Occasionally the artery can partially obstruct venous flow (see below). The internal iliac veins do contain valves and are not normally demonstrated. The Valsalva will manoeuvre fill their terminations and sometimes provides better filling, but this is unusual. Streamlining by non-opacified blood may be seen where large veins such as the renal veins enter the inferior vena cava. Figure 16.11B illustrates the normal inferior vena cava and its connections.

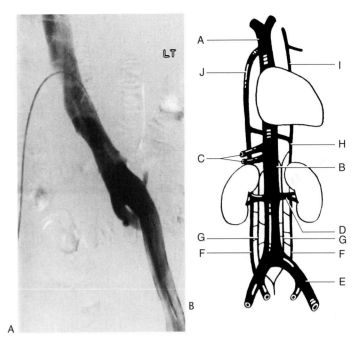

Fig. 16.11 DSA. (A) Normal left iliac veins, shown by catheter from right iliac both sides shown by injection from right side. (B) Venous drainage and connections of the IVC. A = superior vena cava; B = inferior vena cava; C = hepatic veins; D = renal veins; E = iliac veins; F = ascending lumbar veins; G = vertebral venous plexus; H = hemiazygos vein; I = ascending hemiazygos vein; J = azygos vein.

Congenital anomalies

Anomalies of the IVC occur in less than 1% of patients, but the incidence is higher in patients with congenital heart disease.

Left-sided inferior vena cava is the commonest of these anomalies. In these cases the left-sided vena cava terminates in the left renal vein, which then usually drains into a normally sited terminal segment of the IVC (Fig. 16.12A,B). Less frequent is a *double inferior vena cava* with the right larger than the left, or both equal in size (Fig. 16.13). The left vena cava again terminates in the left renal vein (Fig. 16.12C). Occasionally a left IVC may drain into the lumbar and hemiazygos systems, the coronary sinus, or the left atrium. The suprarenal segment of a normal or abnormal infrarenal inferior vena cava occasionally drains into the azygos vein and hemiazygos vein instead of passing through the liver. This anomaly has been recognised on CT, when the dilated veins are shown behind the diaphragmatic crura adjacent to the aorta as it enters the thorax.

Both *agenesis* and *hypoplasia* of the IVC have been described. In these cases blood from the pelvis and lower limbs drains mainly into the lumbar, hemiazygos and azygos veins, which act as collaterals.

Thrombosis

Thrombosis of the iliacs or IVC in the acute phase shows similar appearances to those described above in lower-limb thrombosis, i.e. clot defect occupying most of the lumen with attachment to the vein wall (Fig. 16.14A), or, more dangerously, with a tail of clot extending into the lumen. In the latter case, surgery may be indicated to prevent emboli passing to the lung. In the past this consisted of plication of the IVC, an operation superseded by the transvenous insertion of filters (see below). Collateral bridging vessels will be seen, dependent on the site and extent of obstruction.

Complete thrombosis of the inferior vena cava is occasionally seen, and there is then a collateral circulation utilising a wide variety of collaterals including the lumbar and azygos veins, the vertebral plexus, the anterior abdominal wall veins, and the retroperitoneal or even mesenteric veins (Figs 16.14B, 16.15). Such complete thrombosis usually extends to the level of the renal veins,

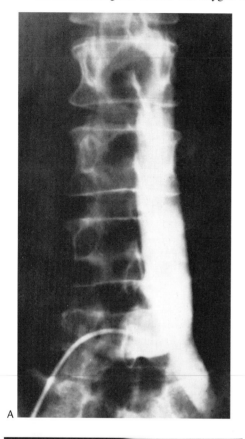

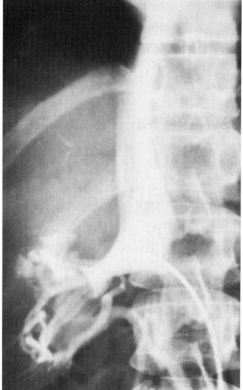

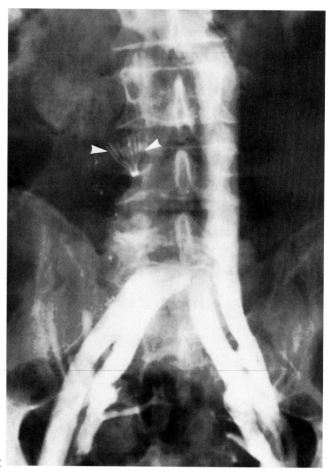

Fig. 16.12 (A) Left-sided IVC as a chance finding in a patient undergoing renal vein catheterisation. (B). The catheter has passed over to the right renal vein through the left IVC where it joins the left renal vein; the upper part of the IVC is normally sited. (C) Double inferior vena cava. A Mobin–Uddin umbrella (arrows) has been inserted in the normal right-sided IVC. The postoperative phlebogram shows an unsuspected double IVC with the right side now occluded.

which remain patent. The upper limit can be demonstrated by retrograde phlebography from above, a catheter being passed from the arm through the right auricle to the upper inferior vena cava.

Recanalisation of the iliac veins and IVC may occur after complete thrombosis, when the vessels will appear smaller and more irregular with evidence of collateral vessels (Fig. 16.16).

Lipoma

Lipoma of the deep central veins is a rare intravascular tumour usually found in the IVC and occasionally in the SVC. Though it can be large enough to occupy most of the lumen, it only rarely produces obstruction, and most are diagnosed as incidental findings on CT or MRI.

Other primary tumours are rare but have been recorded in the ilacs or IVC. They include leiomyoma, leiomyosarcoma, endothelioma and enchondroma and usually present with venous obstruction.

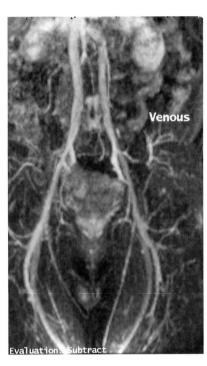

Fig. 16.13 Two-phase MRA. Normal iliac veins with duplication of IVC.

Glandular and neoplastic masses

These can produce considerable distortion of the iliac veins and IVC. Large benign masses can produce marked displacement with little obstruction when only the IVC is affected (see Fig. 27.37), but the iliacs are more easily obstructed by extrinsic pressure (Fig. 16.17). In the past, inferior vena cavography was widely used to assess para-aortic glandular involvement in reticulosis in conjunction with lymphangiography, but with the development of CT and ultrasound this is no longer indicated.

Renal vein invasion by hypernephroma is quite common, and tumour may then spread into the IVC. Such tumour spread is well shown by inferior vena cavography (Fig. 16.18A) or by CT. The iliac veins may also be invaded by malignant tumours (Fig. 16.18B–D). Hepatic tumours may spread into a hepatic vein and extend into the IVC.

Inferior vena caval webs (congenital mucosal folds) have been demonstrated in the terminal segment of the IVC in association with the Budd–Chiari syndrome.

Spontaneous iliac vein rupture

This is a very rare condition which has been reported in patients with proximal iliac obstruction (several by the common iliac artery). In one fatal case the rupture was precipitated by straining at

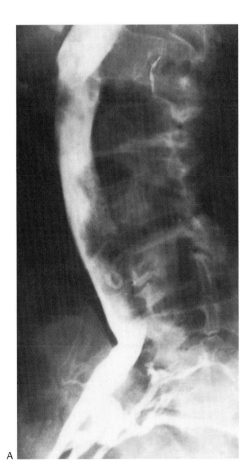
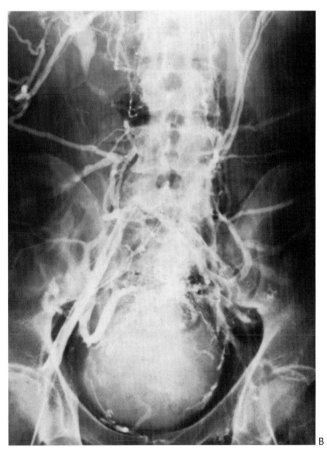

A   B

Fig. 16.14 (A) Recent clot obstructing the left common iliac and partially obstructing the lower IVC. (B) Thrombosis of the IVC and common iliacs with collateral circulation. There is some irregular recanalisation of the common iliacs.

stool. The patient presented with severe groin pain and circulatory collapse from the internal haemorrhage. Ruptured calf veins with haematoma formation are also well documented.

Therapeutic interruption of the inferior vena cava

Pulmonary embolus is a major cause of death. It is estimated that there are 630 000 cases per annum in the USA with some 200 000 deaths. In untreated cases the recurrence rate is said to be 60% with a significant further mortality rate (22%). Most cases are treated by anti-coagulation, with thrombolysis by streptokinase or pulmonary embolectomy indicated in cases of massive pulmonary embolus. If anticoagulation is contraindicated, or fails to prevent recurrence, or if the patient has severe cardiac or pulmonary disease, then caval interruption should be considered, since over 90% of emboli arise from the leg veins.

Therapeutic interruption of the IVC to prevent further pulmonary emboli was first practised in 1945 by operative occlusion. Later, operative partial interruption was practised by suture partition, bead compression and external fenestrated clipping. Because of the risks involved to seriously ill patients from general anaesthesia and laparotomy, these operations were gradually replaced by a simpler technique. This involved transvenous insertion of devices from the right internal jugular vein after operative cutdown under local anaesthesia. The devices used included:

1. The Mobin–Uddin umbrella filter (1967) (Fig. 16.12C)
2. The Kimray–Greenfield filter (1973)
3. The Hunter detachable balloon (1975).

A preliminary inferior vena cavogram is necessary to confirm patency, to demonstrate possible anomalies, and to show the level of the lowest renal vein. The device is passed down below the renal veins before being detached and stabilised. In some cases, filters can be introduced percutaneously from a femoral vein approach, for example the 'bird-nest filter' (Cook Inc.) devised by Roehm and coworkers. This can be introduced through a sheath and an 8Fr. It consists of four stainless steel wires 0.18 mm wide and 2.5 cm long. The filter has two fine wire hooks at each end which can be fixed to the caval wall. The whole procedure can be rapidly performed by a radiologist, but requires preliminary phlebography to ensure that the iliacs and IVC are free of clot.

There are now a wide variety of filters which can be introduced percutaneously from a transfemoral or transjugular approach, and these are listed in Chapter 15. Complications are also discussed in Chapter 15.

Miscellaneous abdominal conditions
Vulval varices

These are seen in pregnancy in 1 or 2% of patients, and persist in a small proportion, some of whom complain of discomfort requiring surgery. In some cases, phlebography by direct injection of the varix

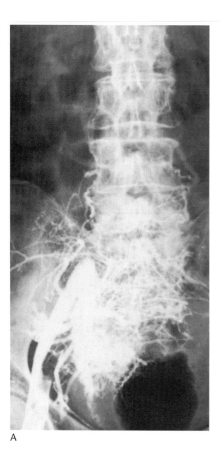 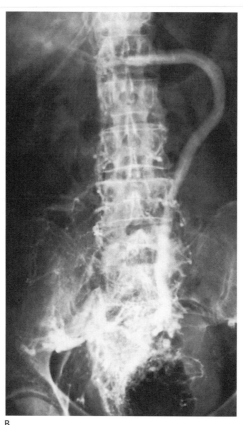 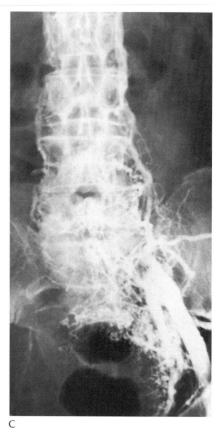

A   B   C

Fig. 16.15 (A,B) Thrombosis of the IVC and common iliacs. Collateral drainage from the right leg via internal iliacs and haemorrhoidal plexus ← inferior mesenteric vein ← portal vein. (C) Same patient. Collateral drainage from the left leg mainly via ascending lumbar veins and vertebral venous plexus.

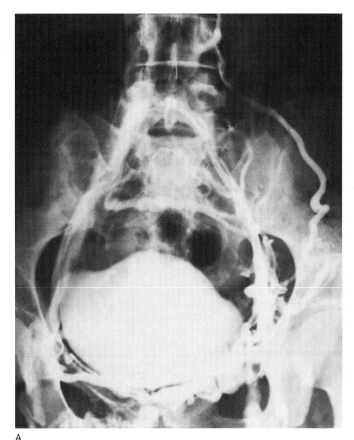

A

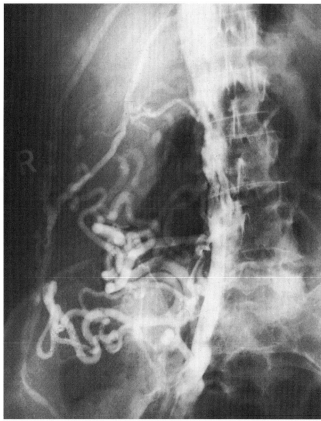

B

Fig. 16.16 (A) Thrombosis of left iliac veins with partial recanalisation and drainage of the left leg mainly by collaterals to the right iliacs via pubic veins. (B) Thrombosis of the IVC with recanalisation and collateral circulation.

will be required to show the anatomy and drainage. This is mainly into the internal pudendal and obturator veins and thence to the internal iliac, but there may be partial drainage to the external pudendal and femoral veins.

Lymphedema praecox

This was the term used for swelling of the left leg, usually occurring in young females and sometimes associated with partial obstruction of the left common iliac vein by the right common iliac artery passing over it (Fig. 16.17A).

Pelvic varicosities in the uterovaginal plexus

Also occurring in the broad ligament, these are said to be fairly common, and have been cited as a cause of the *'pelvic congestion syndrome'*. They can also be associated with vulval varices. High-dose bilateral femoral phlebography with simultaneous compression of the IVC has been recommended to demonstrate these pelvic varicosities, but is not always successful. Bilateral selective internal iliac arteriography with follow-through to the venous phase is a more reliable technique for demonstrating these lesions.

Gonadal veins (ovarian and testicular veins)

The right gonadal vein crosses in front of the ureter at the level of L4 as it passes up and medially to enter the IVC below the right

renal vein. When hypertrophied, the ovarian vein can cause obstruction to the ureter, giving rise to the so-called *ovarian vein syndrome*. This remains a controversial subject, and the existence of this entity is not generally accepted.

The left gonadal vein usually drains into the left renal vein. Both gonadal veins can be demonstrated by passing a catheter into their upper ends from a transfemoral vein approach and injecting contrast medium. *Varicoceles*, which occur mainly on the left side, have been treated by percutaneous embolisation of their drainage vein. Considerable success has been claimed for this procedure in the treatment of varicocele associated with male infertility. Another rare indication for the procedure is the localisation of an *ectopic testis* which the non-invasive techniques of ultrasonography, CT and MRI have failed to locate.

Hepatic vein obstruction (Budd–Chiari syndrome)

Following the passage of a catheter into the upper part of the IVC, the hepatic veins can often be demonstrated by a forced injection of contrast medium, particularly if the patient performs the Valsalva manoeuvre during injection. Failure to fill the hepatic veins provides some evidence of thrombosis as occurs in Budd–Chiari syndrome. On inferior vena cavography, the upper IVC may be seen to be compressed or obstructed (Fig. 16.19) when a tumour is responsible.

Direct *hepatic phlebography* is performed by passing a catheter from the arm through the right auricle and into a hepatic vein. Alternatively a transfemoral vein approach is possible. In Budd–

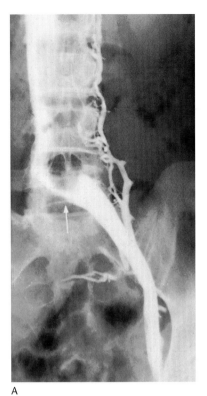
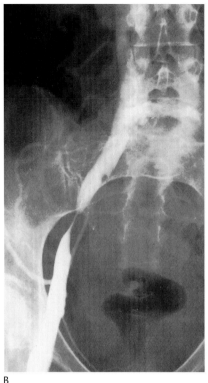
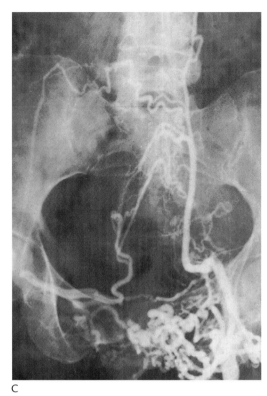

A   B   C

Fig. 16.17 (A) Obstruction of the left common iliac vein by pressure from the right common iliac artery (arrow). Note collateral circulation via the ascending lumbar vein. (B) Iliac vein obstruction by a glandular mass. (C) Obstruction of the left iliac veins in a patient with carcinoma of the cervix treated by radiotherapy.

Chiari syndrome due to small-vessel disease the normal wedged hepatic vein pattern is replaced by fine collateral vessels ('spider's web network'), or actual occlusions may be shown (Fig. 16.20B; see also Fig. 25.45).

Budd–Chiari syndrome is due to complete or partial obstruction of the venous drainage of the liver. This may be thrombotic or non-thrombotic (Box 16.1), and may involve the small intrahepatic vessels, the main hepatic veins, or the intrahepatic and suprahepatic inferior vena cava, or combinations of all three. The clinical features include pain, hepatomegaly, ascites, and the development of portal hypertension and collateral circulation. Acute cases carry a high morbidity, and 86% die within 6 months unless successfully treated by surgery or interventional radiology (see Ch. 25). In Europe and North America the commonest type is idiopathic, while membranous occlusion of the vena cava (MOVC), though rare in the west, is common in Japan, Asia and South Africa. The diagnosis can be confirmed by ultrasound and/or phlebography. Colour-coded duplex Doppler ultrasound is most helpful in assessing hepatic venous patency (see Ch. 25). The intra- and extrahepatic portal vein can be assessed at the same time for patency and direction of flow.

Surgical treatment in the past has been mainly by portosystemic shunting or by orthoptic liver transplantation. More recently, interventional radiology has provided less hazardous alternatives. These include transfemoral thrombolysis via infusion of the hepatic artery in patients with acute venous thrombosis and normal hepatic function. In other cases, venous recanalisation is attempted first by a transfemoral or transjugular approach, or, if this is not possible, by a transhepatic approach. Balloon dilatation and vein stenting can also be used if recanalisation is successful, as can the tips procedure. Balloon dilatation is also used with MOVC cases.

Renal phlebography

The renal veins can be selectively catheterised using the Seldinger percutaneous technique. A forced injection of 10 ml of contrast medium will show the venous drainage of most of the kidney and will thus confirm or exclude a renal vein thrombosis (Fig. 16.21A,B). The renal veins can also be shown by serial films taken after selective renal arteriography. The normal renal veins usually show well by this method. If they do not and a collateral venous drainage is also shown, this is good presumptive evidence of main renal vein occlusion.

It is important to realise that there may be more than one renal vein on either side, and attempts should always be made to identify and catheterise accessory veins. On the left side, 7% of individuals have a lower accessory vein which is smaller than the normal upper vein and is retroaortic in position. The two veins form a circumaortic ring with the lower one usually entering the inferior vena cava at L3–4 (Fig. 16.21C).

Renal vein thrombosis

This has also been investigated by inferior vena cavography. In the normal inferior vena cavagram, 'streamlining' effects are usually visible when the large renal veins enter the IVC. Absence of this normal streamlining effect is thought to be very suggestive of renal vein thrombosis, particularly when unilateral. Direct renal phlebography will prove the diagnosis conclusively.

Renal vein thrombosis is common in dehydrated infants with diarrhoea. It also occurs in adults in association with IVC thrombosis, or thrombotic disease elsewhere. Occasionally, it is seen with pyelonephritis or other renal disease. The affected kidney is usually

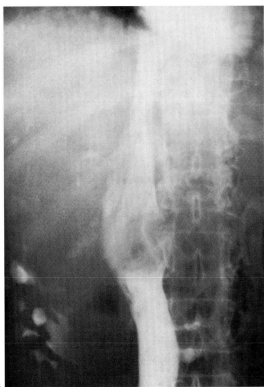

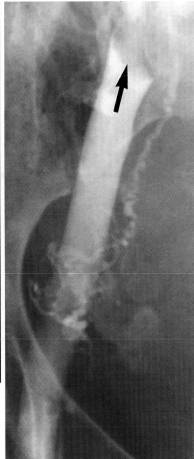

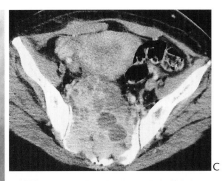

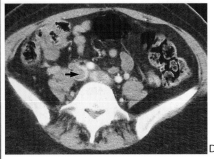

Fig. 16.18 (A) Invasion of the IVC by hypernephroma spreading up the right renal vein. (B) Tumour envasion (arrow) of right common iliac vein from giant cell tumour of the sacrum. (C,D) CT scans of lesion.

enlarged from venous engorgement, and the nephrotic syndrome may result. The vein itself is narrowed and irregular, and the small peripheral veins may be occluded.

As noted above, hypernephroma frequently involves the renal vein, and tumour may extend into the IVC (Fig. 16.18). The renal vein may also be occluded or compressed by extrinsic tumour masses, by aneurysm, or by retroperitoneal fibrosis.

Renal vein renin

In cases of renal artery stenosis or suspected renal ischaemia it is helpful to assay the renin in the renal venous blood from the suspected kidney. This is obtained by percutaneous catheterisation of the renal veins using the Seldinger technique. Samples are obtained from an arm vein at the same time so that comparisons can be made with peripheral venous blood. A renal vein–renin ratio greater than 1.5 : 1 is usually significant.

Adrenal vein phlebography

The adrenal veins can be selectively catheterised using special catheters. Small tumours have been demonstrated by this means when other methods have failed. In our experience the method has proved of most value in the diagnosis of small Conn's tumours in primary hyperaldosteronism. The method is discussed in greater detail in Chapter 27 (See Fig. 27.31), but has now been superseded

by CT and MRI. The technique is sometimes used for deliberate infarction of adrenal tumours.

Venous sampling

Endocrine tumours can be difficult to localise, but identification may be assisted by assay of the hormone concentration in the veins draining from the possible sites of the tumour. The method has proved useful for some adrenal tumours, for example, a small adenoma may be functional or non-functional in Conn's syndrome, and in Cushing's syndrome larger but ectopic phaeochromocytomas may be difficult to localise, and in these cases systemic venous sampling may identify the ectopic site in the pelvis or the thorax (see Ch. 27). Islet cell tumours of the pancreas have also been identified by venous sampling of pancreatic drainage veins. In these cases the portal system is entered by a percutaneous transhepatic approach (see Ch. 25). Parathyroid tumours may be difficult to localise, either because they are small and not identifiable even at surgery on the thyroid, or because they are ectopic in the mediastinum. Venous sampling of the thyroid veins draining into the internal jugular and innominate veins and of the thymic and upper intercostals is performed by a transfemoral approach. Some investigators have reported good results but most have a high failure rate. Small pituitary adenomas in Cushing's syndrome have been lateralised by sampling the petrous sinus blood obtained from a transjugular approach after transfemoral catheterisation.

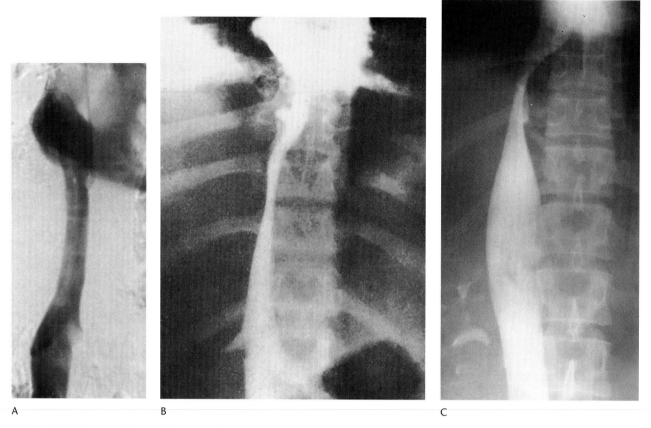

A   B   C

Fig. 16.19 (A) DSA. Normal suprarenal IVC. (B) Obstruction of hepatic veins with compression and distortion of the upper IVC by liver neoplasm resulting in Budd–Chiari syndrome. The patient was performing the Valsalva manoeuvre. Note reflux filling of the renal veins, but not the hepatic veins. (C) Another patient with Budd–Chiari syndrome and thrombosed hepatic veins.

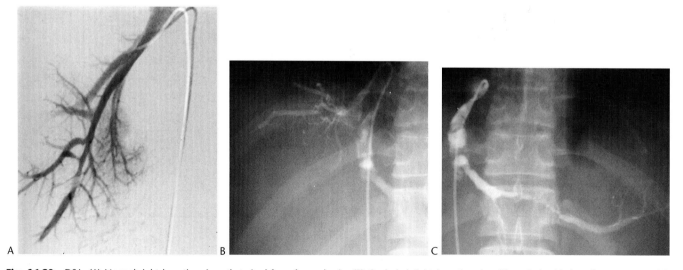

A   B   C

Fig. 16.20 DSA. (A) Normal right hepatic vein catheterised from femoral vein. (B) Occluded right hepatic vein with typical spider's web appearance. (C) Thrombosis in left hepatic vein. B and C are from same patient as in Fig. 16.19C.

Transvenous interventional procedures

There are now a wide variety of interventional procedures performed in veins or by transvenous access. Some are dealt with in the preceding chapter, for example vena cava filter insertion and transvenous embolisation. Others are described in or mentioned in other sections, for example TIPS (See Ch. 25) and transvenous embolisation of adrenal adenomas (see Ch. 27). Some are performed by cardiologists or other specialists, but the radiologist should be familiar with most of them. The list below classifies the commonest procedures but is by no means exhaustive.

1. *Vein stenting*: SVC, IVC, peripheral veins, TIPS, haemodialysis shunts
2. *Venous access*: central (via subclavian or internal jugular) or peripheral (via arm or leg)

3. Venous embolisation: varices; varicocele; AV fistula; vascular malformation; adrenal
4. Vena caval filter
5. Thrombolysis
6. Transvenous dilatation.

UPPER LIMB AND SUPERIOR VENA CAVA

The usual indications for investigation of the venous drainage of the arm and SVC are:

1. Oedema of the upper limb thought to be associated with venous thrombosis or obstruction, in order to demonstrate the site of obstruction, in either the axillary, subclavian or innominate veins
2. Superior vena caval obstruction
3. Demonstration of the full anatomy of venous angiomas or varices
4. Demonstration of congenital venous anomalies as in Klippel–Trenaunay syndrome.

Technique

A vein at the elbow is catheterised and a catheter advanced several centimetres up the arm. This can be done percutaneously in most cases, though occasionally a cutdown exposure may be necessary. It is best to use the median basilic vein, since this will make it possible to opacify the axillary vein. Use of the median cephalic vein will of course bypass the basilic and axillary veins, since the

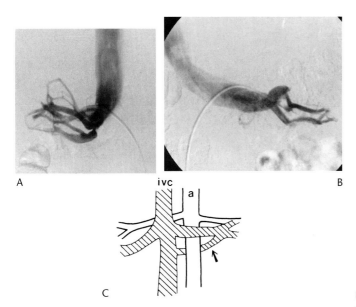

Fig. 16.21 Selective right renal (A) and left renal (B) vein phlebograms. (C) Circumaortic ring formed by renal veins. A = aorta; IVC = inferior vena cava.

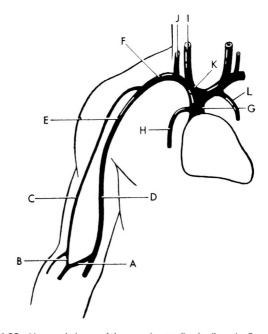

Fig. 16.22 Venous drainage of the arm. A = median basilar vein; B = median cephalic vein; C = cephalic vein; D = basilic vein; E = axillary vein; F = subclavian vein; G = superior vena cava; H = azygos vein; L = internal jugular vein; J = external jugular vein; K = innominate vein; L = hemiazygos vein.

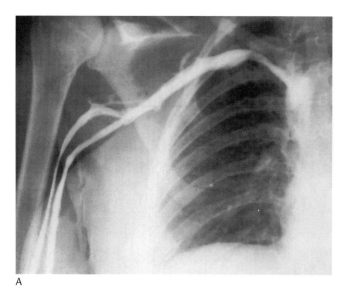

A

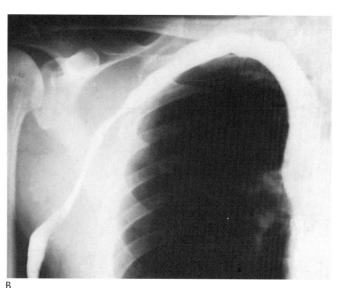

B

Fig. 16.23 Arm phlebogram showing normal appearances.

cephalic vein does not join the subclavian vein until it has pierced the clavipectoral fascia (Fig. 16.22).

Some 30 ml of contrast medium is injected within 2 s, using a pressure injector if necessary. A rapid rate of injection is essential, since otherwise the contrast will fail to show the SVC well. It is rapidly diluted in the thorax by the large blood flow from the head and neck and contralateral upper limb.

Serial films are taken at speeds of one or two films per second.

Another technique which can be used where percutaneous puncture of an elbow vein proves difficult is similar to that used for ascending phlebography of the lower limb. A vein on the dorsum of the hand is percutaneously punctured with a fine needle of the type routinely used by anaesthetists (SWG 21 or 23).

A tourniquet is applied just above the elbow, and some 30 ml of contrast medium injected. The tourniquet is then released, and the forearm massaged to ensure that a good bolus of contrast medium is delivered to the large veins in 2 s.

Radiographic appearances

The normal findings are illustrated in Figure 16.23.

Left-sided superior vena cava is an important congenital anomaly in which the SVC lies on the left and drains into the coronary sinus. It may occur alone or in association with congenital heart disease. Occasionally there is a *double superior vena cava*, the right draining normally to the right auricle, and the left into the coronary sinus (Fig. 16.24).

Where a localised thrombosis is present in a major drainage vein, such as the axillary or subclavian vein, the blockage is usually well shown, together with the collateral circulation which develops to bypass the lesion.

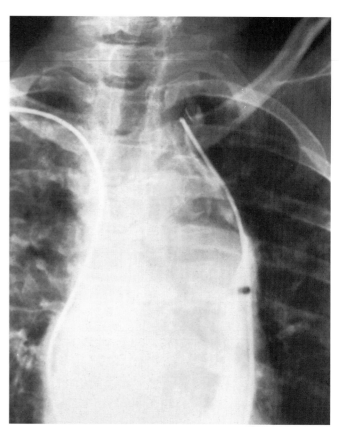

Fig. 16.24 Double SVC. A catheter has been passed from the right arm for pulmonary angiography. Instead of entering the ventricle it has passed through the dilated coronary sinus and into the left SVC draining into it, as evident on contrast injection. Note the widened mediastinum.

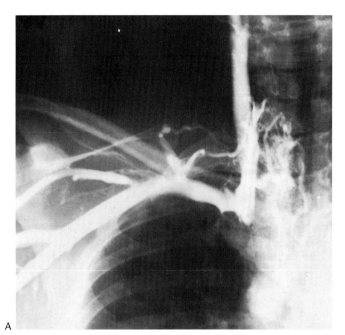

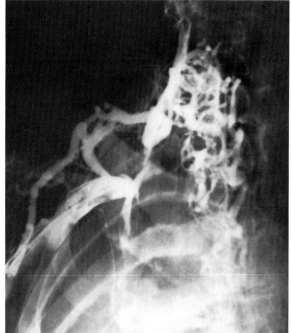

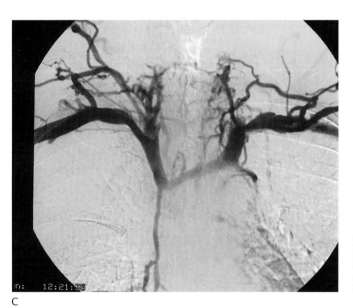

Fig. 16.25 (A) Right arm phlebogram confirms malignant occlusion of the innominate and SVC with reflux up the right internal jugular, and vertebral collaterals. (B) Occlusion of the SVC and innominate, and termination of the right subclavian vein. Collaterals are seen to the vertebral plexus. (C) SVC obstruction due to a central bronchial carcinoma.

Superior vena caval obstruction

This is characterised by venous engorgement of the head, neck and arms. The involvement of the SVC by malignant glands can be recognised well before clinical evidence of SVC obstruction is seen. In these cases, extrinsic pressure defects on the vein will be seen. In the past, superior vena cavography has been used to assess the suitability of cases of bronchial carcinoma for surgery, and to exclude clinically silent mediastinal glandular involvement. However, CT now provides a less invasive method of assessing mediastinal glandular involvement. DSA will also enable the SVC to be checked using only a small amount of low-concentration con-

trast medium. Radioisotope scanning can also confirm caval obstruction.

The majority of patients (over 95%) with SVC obstruction are suffering from *malignant neoplasm* (Fig. 16.25). Of these, about 80% have carcinoma of the lung and about 20% are suffering from lymphomas.

The small group of patients with *benign SVC obstruction* are usually suffering from *fibrosing mediastinitis* (Fig. 16.26). These patients present with a relatively slow onset, permitting the development of multiple collaterals. The aetiology is either unknown (idiopathic) or it is granulomatous. In the UK the latter cases are usually *tuberculous*, but in North America *histoplasmosis* is also a

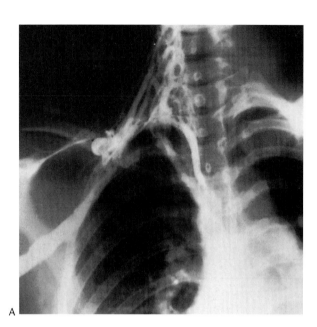
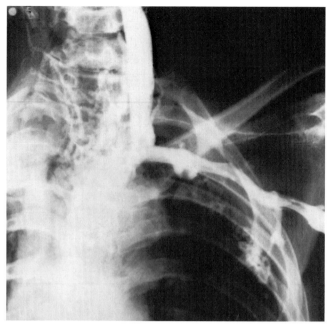

Fig. 16.26   (A). Right arm phlebogram in fibrosing mediastinitis with involvement of the SVC and the right innominate vein. (B) Left arm phlebogram in a patient with fibrosing mediastinitis (tuberculous). Note the kinked trachea. The SVC and left innominate are occluded. Collateral circulation via the left internal jugular and vertebral plexus.

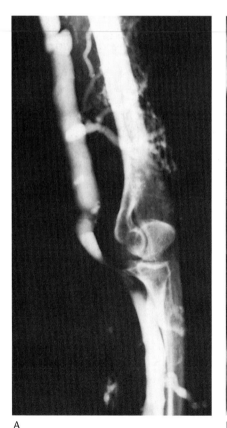
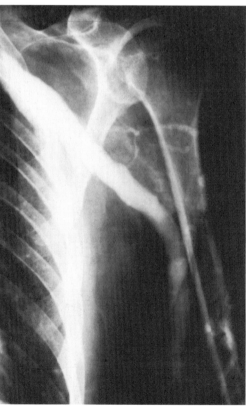

Fig. 16.27   (A,B) Klippel–Trenaunay syndrome involving the left arm. Drainage is via a single medial vein which appears valveless with very sluggish flow.

cause of the syndrome. Very rarely, thrombosis of the SVC is seen as a complication of ventriculoatrial shunts. Compression of the SVC may also be occasionally seen with aneurysm and other non-malignant mediastinal masses.

Klippel–Trenaunay syndrome has been noted above. The appearances in the affected upper limb of a patient with this condition are illustrated in Figure 16.27. Multiple phleboliths were present in addition to the venous dysplasia.

PORTAL PHLEBOGRAPHY

Imaging of the portal system, which is illustrated diagrammatically in Fig. 16.28, is mainly requested in the investigation of portal hypertension and its complications. The causes of portal hypertension are listed in Box 16.2, and are usually classified into prehepatic, intrahepatic and posthepatic obstruction to the portal circulation.

Imaging methods should be non-invasive where feasible (ultrasound, MRI) or minimally invasive (spiral CT), and the invasive techniques should only be used as a prelude to surgery or adjunct to interventional radiology (see Ch. 15). Fig. 16.29 and 16.38 show patent portal veins imaged by spiral CT and MRI, respectively. Invasive techniques widely used in the past but now obsolete included operative mesenteric portography and percutaneous splenic puncture and injection. Arterioportography is still used because it can show the

Box 16.2 Causes of portal hypertension
Prehepatic
Portal vein thrombosis
Portal vein compression by tumour or glandular mass
Splenomegaly
Intrahepatic
Cirrhosis
Veno-occlusive disease
Portal tract obstruction
Parasites
Lymphoma
Myeloproliferative disorders
Sarcoid
Hepatitis
Felty's syndrome
Posthepatic
Budd–Chiari syndrome
Constrictive pericarditis
Cardiac failure

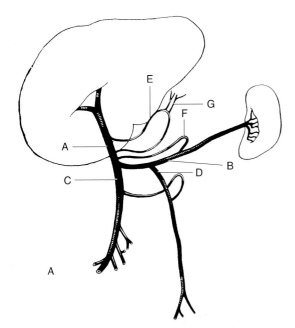

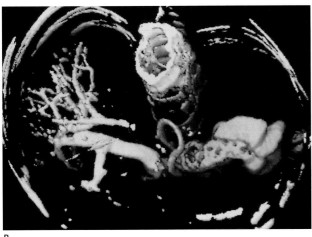

Fig. 16.28 (A) Portal circulation. A = portal vein;, B = splenic vein; C = superior mesenteric vein; D = inferior mesenteric vein; E = left gastric vein; F = gastroepiploic vein; G = oesophageal vein. (B) Spiral CT reconstruction showing a patent portal vein. (Courtesy of Dr A. Al-Kutoubi.)

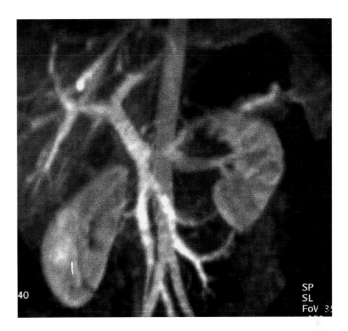

Fig. 16.29 Normal superior mesenteric, portal and hepatic veins shown by three-phase MRA.

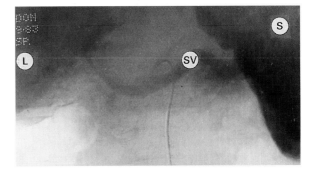

Fig. 16.30 Arterioportography—subtraction film. Venous phase of selective splenic angiogram. The portal vein is compressed by a mass of malignant glands. The spleen is grossly enlarged. SV = splenic vein; L = liver; S = spleen. (Courtesy of Dr Janet Murfitt.)

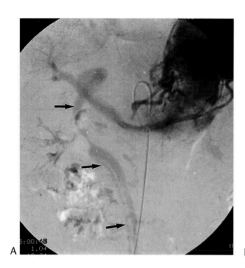

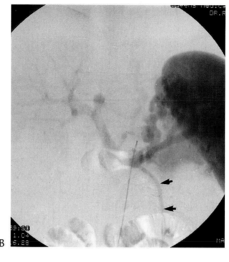

Fig. 16.31 DSA. (A) Gastro-oesophageal varices and patent left umbilical vein containing some thrombus filling from left portal vein. (B) Gastric varices and patent inferior mesentric vein filling from splenic vein.

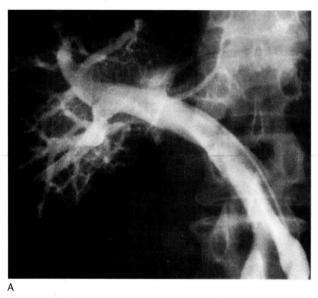

A

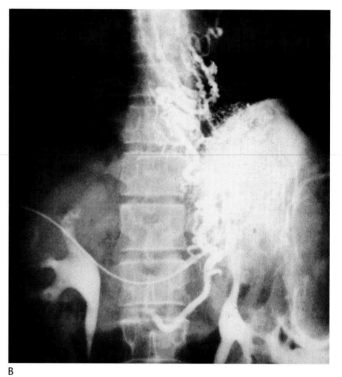

B

Fig. 16.32 (A) Transhepatic portal phlebogram showing the main portal vein and mesenteric tributaries. (Courtesy of Dr Janet Murfitt.) (B) Gastric and oesophageal varices demonstrated by transhepatic portal vein catheterisation.

arterial and systemic venous as well as the portal anatomy. Transhepatic portography is also used for interventional procedures and for blood sampling in the investigation of islet cell tumours of the pancreas.

Arterioportography *(Fig. 16.30)*

Advocates of this method prefer it because it obviates the dangers of direct splenic puncture and because the information obtained comprises both arterial and venous phases and can show the whole portal system. It can also contribute to the planning of shunt surgery. The normal technique is to catheterise the coeliac axis and then inject from a superselective position of the catheter tip in the splenic artery. A 30–50 ml volume of contrast medium is injected at a rate of 5 ml/s, and serial films obtained in the arterial and venous phase. If the patient's condition permits, the common hepatic artery

can also be injected to show the state of the liver and pancreas, with late films to demonstrate any possible hepaticofugal flow in the portal veins. If required, the left gastric artery can be injected to show varices and the superior mesenteric artery can also be injected to demonstrate the superior mesenteric vein. It may be essential to show this if mesocaval shunting is being considered.

DSA considerably improves the definition of arterioportography. It also permits adequate visualisation with much smaller doses of contrast medium (Fig. 16.31).

Transhepatic portal phlebography *(Fig. 16.32)*

The main collateral venous supply of gastro-oesophageal varices may be visualised by percutaneous transhepatic catheterisation of the portal vein (Fig. 16.31). Apart from being demonstrated by injection through the percutaneous catheter, the varices can be selectively catheterised and obliterated by embolisation. The major indication was severe cirrhosis in patients in whom surgery was contraindicated. After successful obliteration of varices, surgery may be performed electively or deferred.

The method of transhepatic portal phlebography has also been used for the purpose of obtaining venous samples for assay from the pancreatic drainage veins into the splenic and superior mesenteric veins. These assays are helpful in the localisation of pancreatic hormone-producing tumours. The method is discussed in greater detail in Chapter 26.

DOPPLER ULTRASOUND AND THE PERIPHERAL VEINS

Paul L. Allan

The indications for venous ultrasound of the lower limb veins include the diagnosis or exclusion of DVT, the assessment of chronic venous insufficiency and mapping of veins to be used in

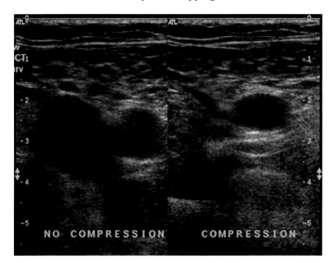

Fig. 16.33 Normal compression of the left common femoral vein. The vein is seen in the left image on the left side of the artery. On compression the vein lumen disappears and only the vein walls are visible.

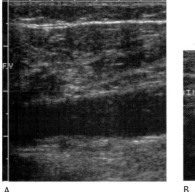
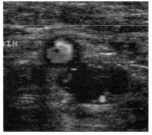

Fig. 16.34 (A) Predominantly hypoechoic thrombus expanding the common femoral vein. (B) A transverse view showing the thrombus occupying most of the vein lumen, with only a small amount of flow around the periphery.

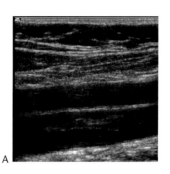
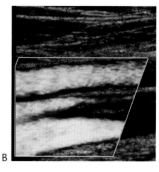

Fig. 16.35 (A) A tail of fresh thrombus extending up a superficial femoral vein. (B) The same thrombus on power Doppler.

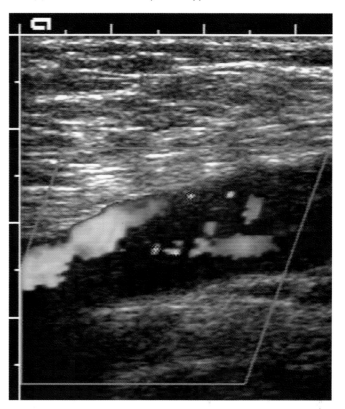

Fig. 16.36 Moderately echogenic thrombus in a superficial femoral vein. A small amount of blood flow is seen posteriorly.

graft procedures. In the upper limb and neck the indications include the diagnosis of venous thrombosis, venous stenosis in dialysis fistulas and locating patent veins for central line insertion.

DEEP VEIN THROMBOSIS

Three aspects of the ultrasound examination are used in the diagnosis of DVT: compressibility of the vein; flow on Doppler ultrasound; and visible thrombus in the lumen. A normal vein is compressible so that the lumen is obliterated with only light or moderate pressure from the transducer (Fig. 16.33), whereas thrombus will hold the vein walls apart. Care must be taken, as fresh thrombus is partially compressible and may be overlooked. Normally flow in the lower limb veins is spontaneous, showing respiratory variation; a quick squeeze of the calf muscles, or getting the patient to plantarflex their foot, should result in a rapid, brief augmentation of the flow. In the

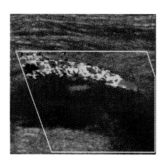

Fig. 16.37 Longitudinal view of the popliteal vein with a popliteal cyst immediately deep to the vessel.

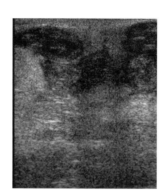

Fig. 16.38 Echogenic thrombus in a long saphenous vein.

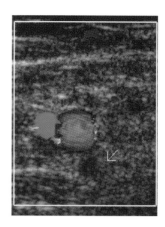

Fig. 16.39 Transverse view of the superficial femoral vessels. The artery is seen in the middle with a patent vein on the left but a thrombosed vein lying inferiorly.

presence of thrombus there will be no flow in the thrombosed segment; if there is occlusive, segmental thrombus elsewhere in the main veins of the limb, then augmentation will be damped as a result of the increased resistance and proximal thrombus will remove the respiratory variations normally seen in patent veins. The normal vein lumen should be anechoic and colour Doppler ultrasound, or power Doppler ultrasound, should show complete fill-in across the lumen of the vein. Fresh thrombus is relatively anechoic and tends to expand the vein lumen slightly (Fig. 16.34). In acute thromboses, a tail of thrombus may be seen extending up the vein (Fig. 16.35). Although some have concern that compression manoeuvres may dislodge fresh thrombus, in practice this is exceedingly unlikely and the patient is more at risk from walking around. As it matures it contracts and becomes increasingly echogenic (Fig. 16.36). Following DVT the veins usually recanalise with the lumen clearing completely but residual wall thickening and irregularity may persist. In some 25% of patients significant segments may remain obstructed with collaterals forming around these occluded segments.

An advantage of ultrasound is that it may show causes for the patient's symptoms other than DVT, such as a ruptured popilteal or Baker's cyst (Fig. 16.37), a muscle haematoma or superficial thrombophlebitis (Fig. 16.38); it can also show pelvic masses which may have predisposed the patient to develop a DVT. Problems can occur if visualisation of the veins is poor, as may well be the case in obese or oedematous legs. Approximately 15% of the population have a dual segment of superficial femoral vein, which may cause problems if one component is thrombosed while the other is patent and the situation is not recognised (Fig. 16.39). Non-occlusive thrombus may also be missed if the failure of the colour signal to fill the lumen is not appreciated. In the later stages of pregnancy the enlarging uterus may compress the iliac veins in the supine position and therefore affect the flow in the leg veins; this problem can be overcome if the patient is examined in the decubitus or vertical position, when the uterus will be shifted off the iliac vein. If there is doubt about a segment of vein a venogram can be arranged, or a repeat scan performed 2–3 days later in order to see if any thrombus has extended from an occult point of origin into the larger, proximal veins.

Providing care and attention is taken with the examination, ultrasound has been shown to be highly accurate in the diagnosis of symptomatic DVT, with a sensitivity and specificity of over 95% and 100%, respectively, for proximal thrombus in the common femoral, superficial femoral and popliteal veins. Flow can usually

be demonstrated in the major calf veins, if these are patent. However, it is more difficult to exclude reliably small segmental calf vein thrombi, or thrombi in the muscle venous sinuses. This is not usually a problem as ultrasound can provide a clear positive or negative result in 80–85% of cases. If there is any doubt concerning the adequacy of the ultrasound examination, or if there is a problem area, then subsequent venography can concentrate on the particular segment concerned. In some patients, ultrasound will be negative but there is a strong clinical likelihood of DVT, or the patient's symptoms deteriorate over a few days; in these patients, a repeat ultrasound can be performed to see if any thrombus has extended from an occult site into one of the main veins. In many hospitals, ultrasound has become the primary examination for the confirmation or exclusion of DVT, with venography being reserved for those cases where ultrasound does not give sufficient information for management decisions. However, ultrasound has a sensitivity of only 60% for asymptomatic thrombus and so is of lesser value in detecting thrombus in asymptomatic patients at risk of DVT.

Varicose veins and chronic venous insufficiency

Varicose veins are a common problem, and colour Doppler ultrasound is not usually required in the diagnosis unless there is a possibility of previous DVT damaging the deep veins, in which case

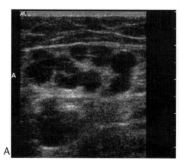
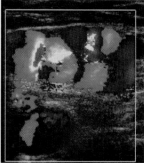

Fig. 16.40 (A) The left saphenofemoral junction in a patient with recurrent varicose veins. The upper long saphenous vein is replaced by multiple irregular channels, compatible with recanalisation after surgery. The colour Doppler image (B) shows abnormal flow patterns.

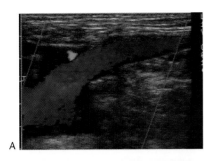

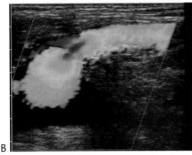

Fig. 16.41 (A) The saphenofemoral junction on colour Doppler showing flow upwards (orange), followed by (B) reflux downwards (blue).

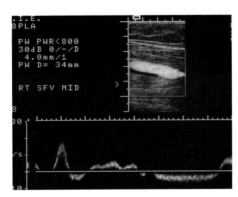

Fig. 16.42 Colour and spectral Doppler trace showing significant reflux of approximately 3 s.

removal of the superficial veins may have a major effect on the venous drainage of the limb. Most cases of primary varicose veins will be sorted out using hand-held continuous-wave Doppler ultrasound in the vascular clinic, but some patients may have atypical anatomy with unusual locations for the saphenopopliteal and saphenofemoral junctions; colour and power Doppler techniques can rapidly clarify these situations.

Recurrent varicose veins

These may show one of three patterns of recurrence: the saphenofemoral junction appears intact, suggesting that the original operation was inadequate; it may be abnormal in shape (Fig. 16.40) or show collaterals linking the saphenous vein below the point of surgical interruption to the common femoral vein; or there may be collaterals draining into other veins in the pelvis, perineum, or around the hip and buttock. Colour Doppler ultrasound will allow these channels to be identified and the patterns of reflux established so that appropriate surgery can be planned.

Chronic venous insufficiency

This can develop after DVT, or without any history of previous thrombosis. In this condition the venous valves are damaged; this leads to venous reflux, stasis and increased hydrostatic pressure in the tissues of the lower limb. This results in leg swelling, skin changes and ulceration. Patients are examined standing in order to demonstrate the reflux. Manual compression of the calf forces blood up the veins and, if the valves in any particular segment are incompetent, the blood subsequently falls back; this effect is seen on colour Doppler ultrasound as a change of the colour image from one colour to the opposite colour (Fig. 16.41), or on spectral Doppler ultrasound as flow above and below the baseline (Fig. 16.42). A little reflux of short duration (<0.5 s) is not significant, but more persistent reflux should be noted and the pattern of incompetent segments explored; in addition to the superficial and deep-vein systems, outward flow in incompetent perforator veins linking these may be seen. Other methods of inducing reflux include pneumatic pressure cuffs and getting the patient to perform a Valsalva manoeuvre. However, a Valsalva will only show incompetence down to the first competent valve in the thigh, so that incompetence below this level may not be appreciated unless other measures are undertaken.

Saphenous vein mapping

The long saphenous vein is frequently used as a conduit for bypass operations, usually for coronary artery or lower-limb arterial bypass. If there is any doubt about the suitability of one or both veins they can be examined using colour Doppler ultrasound so that the length and calibre of suitable segments can be assessed. The course of the vein is marked out with an indelible marker pen, the sites of major branches and perforators are also indicated on the skin; this is particularly important if an in situ femoral bypass graft is being considered as arteriovenous shunts will result if any connections are left intact. The vein should be at least 4 mm in minimum diameter for most of its length, but must be at least 2 mm at the ankle if a long femorodistal graft is being planned. The measurements are best done with the patient standing in order to obtain maximum distension; in addition, care should be taken not to compress the vein with the transducer.

MRI OF VEINS

Jeremy P. R. Jenkins

An understanding of the flow phenomena and MRI methodology (given in detail in Ch. 15) are applicable to the MRI study of veins. The detection and assessment of venous obstruction or thrombus is an accepted MRI technique. Thrombi in abdominal and pelvic veins can be identified on T_1- and T_2-weighted spin-echo sequences (Fig. 16.43). Phlebograms, using magnetic resonance angiography (MRA) techniques can be used to assess the deep-venous system, but are more time consuming and often add little information compared with standard spin-echo and gradient-echo techniques.

A number of MRI studies in the assessment of DVT of the *pelvis* and *lower extremities* have shown a high sensitivity and specificity (greater than 95%) in the detection of thrombus, equivalent to that of X-ray phlebography. An advantage of MRI over X-ray phlebog-

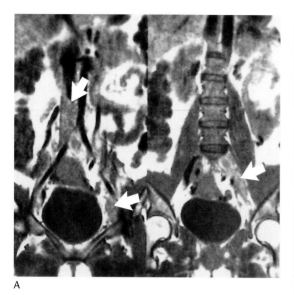

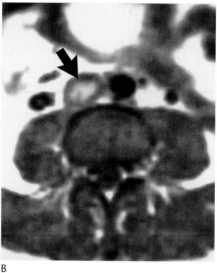

A   B

Fig. 16.43 Acute thrombosis (arrow) within the IVC and left iliac veins on (A) coronal and (B) transverse T₁-weighted spin-echo images (SE 560/25).

raphy is in the demonstration of thrombus within deep pelvic veins, a location where phlebography and ultrasound are ineffective. There are, however, problems with MRI in differentiating turbulent flow from thrombus. Also lack of visualisation of a vein is not sufficient to diagnose an acute thrombosis, as an adjacent mass can produce venous compression without intraluminal thrombus. Phlebography remains the standard technique in the demonstration of calf DVT. MRI can, however, identify other lesions which mimic the symptoms of a DVT such as calf haematoma, ruptured popliteal cyst or compartment syndrome.

The presence of acute thrombus on gradient-echo sequences results in a filling defect with low to almost absent signal intensity. The vessel is distended with thrombus, and there may be some high signal from flowing blood surrounding a portion of the thrombus. On spin-echo imaging, an acute thrombus shows signal intensity where normally there should be a signal void (Fig. 16.43). The distinction between acute and chronic thrombus can be difficult, although a homogeneous signal is indicative of an acute clot; heterogeneity in appearance with a lower peripheral and higher central signal is in keeping with thrombus of greater age. Non visualisation of the vein, small lumen, or an irregular wall thickening in conjunction with prominent collateral vessels suggests a chronic DVT.

Improved visualisation of the *calf veins* on MRI can be achieved in the majority of individuals by utilising mechanical flow-enhancing measures. Magnetic resonance venography of the calf can be performed with the placement of a tourniquet around the thigh which, when subsequently released and combined with termination of a Valsalva manoeuvre by the patient, results in a transient increase in venous blood flow in the leg. Due to its expense and limited availability, MRI is unlikely to become the primary means of assessing DVT in the near future. In those individuals who are allergic to iodinated contrast medium or with limited venous access, Doppler ultrasound is recommended if the region of clinical suspicion is in the thigh. If it is suspected that a pelvic rather than a calf vein thrombosis, or other lesion, is the cause of the patient's symptoms, then MRI is an alternative technique.

In the assessment of abdominal vessels there are technical difficulties due to respiratory motion with resultant reduced signal-to-noise ratio. For venous imaging, two-dimensional *time-of-flight*

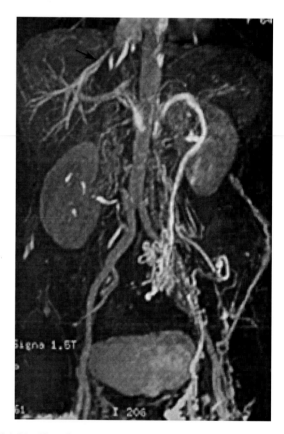

Fig. 16.44 Thrombotic obstruction of the IVC and common iliac veins in a 64-year-old woman with contrast outlining a collateral venous circulation, on a 3D CE-MRA study using the left pedal vein as the injection site. Note the normal hepatic vein (arrow) draining into a patent portion of the IVC adjacent to the right atrium. Contrast is seen in the abdominal aorta.

angiography has advantages over *phase-contrast angiography* in terms of speed and flexibility. Sequential two-dimensional *time-of-flight imaging* can be used to acquire several overlapping slices in the same breath-hold. Improved signal-to-noise and spatial resolution can also be achieved by the use of a torso phased array coil combined with the three-dimensional contrast-enhanced MRA (CE-MRA) technique (Fig. 16.44; see Ch. 15).

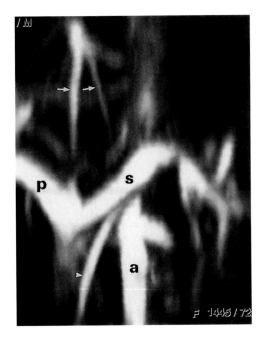

Fig. 16.45 Coronal plane maximum intensity projection (MIP) of a 2D phase-contrast MRA showing normal hepatic veins (short arrows). P = portal vein; s = splenic vein; a = aorta; arrowhead = superior mesenteric artery.

MRA is an accurate and reproducible technique for imaging the *portal vein*. The main indications for imaging are to confirm patency, show thrombus or detect tumour invasion of the portal vein, and, in portal hypertension, to show patency of the porto-systemic shunts, varices and collateral vessels. The presence and age of thrombus can be assessed by routine spin-echo imaging as indicated above, with the differentiation of thrombus from tumour with gadolinium-chelate administration. MRA, with its wide field of view, has a particular advantage over Doppler ultrasound in depicting varices and portosystemic vessels in patients with portal hypertension, which is important information in the surgical planning prior to liver transplantation. Not only can MRI provide information relating to the vascular anatomy, patency and anomalies, but also it can show the hepatic parenchyma and surrounding tissues using conventional sequences.

The *major hepatic veins* are well visualised on MRA (Fig. 16.45). In liver cirrhosis the IVC and hepatic veins can appear compressed and distorted, producing a similar picture on MRA as occurs in Budd–Chiari syndrome. Comma-shaped collateral vessels which produce a 'spider-web' appearance of the collateral vessels around the obstructed vein, as depicted on X-ray contrast venography, can be demonstrated on MRA, and is suggestive of Budd–Chiari syndrome rather than cirrhosis.

MRI has been shown to be useful in assessing the patency of the thoracic inlet and mediastinal venous system. *SVC obstruction* or patients with unilateral upper extremity swelling and pain can be assessed with spin-echo, gradient-echo and CE-MRA techniques with advantages over contrast-enhanced CT.

REFERENCES AND SUGGESTIONS FOR THE READING

Historical interest
Berberich, J., Hirsch, S. (1923) Die roentgenographische Darstellung der Arterien und Venen am lebenden Menschen. *Klinische Wochenschrift*, 2226–2228.

Brooks, B. (1924) Intra-arterial injection of sodium iodide. *Journal of the American Medical Association*, **82**, 1016–1019.

Castellanos, A., Pereirao, R., Garcia, A. (1937) La angiocardiografia radio-opaqua. *Arch de la Socec de la Eshudios de la Habana*, **31**, 523–596.

Doby, T. (1976) *Development of Angiography*. Littleton, MA: Publishing Sciences Group.

Dos Santos, R., Lamas, A. C., Caldas, J. P. (1931) *Arteriographie des Membres et de la Aorte Abdominale*. Paris: Masson.

Farinas, P. L. (1941) A new technique for the arteriographic examination of the abdominal aorta and its branches. *American Journal of Roentgenology*, **46**, 641–645.

Forssman, W. (1929) Die Sondierung der rechten Herzens. *Klinische Wochenschrift*, **8**, 2087–2089.

Gruntzig, A. (1978) Transluminal dilatation of coronary artery stenosis. *Lancet*, **i**, 263.

Gruntzig, A. et al, (1978) Treatment of renovascular hypertension with percutaneous transluminal dilatation of a renal artery stenosis. *Lancet*, **i**, 801.

Haschek, E., Lindenthal, T. O. (1896) Ein Beitrag zur praktischen Verwerthung der Photographie nach Röntgen. *Wiener Klinische Wochenschrift*, **9**, 63–64.

Moniz, E. (1931) *Diagnostic des Tumeurs Cérébrals et Epreuve de l'Encephalographie Artérielle*. Paris: Masson.

Orrin, H. C. (1920) *X-ray Atlas of the Systemic Arteries of the Human Body*. London: Baillière Tindall & Cox.

Seldinger, S. (1953) Catheter replacement of the needle in percutaneous arteriography. *Acta Radiologica*, **39**, 368–376.

Serbinenko, F. A. (1974) Balloon catheterization and occlusion of major cerebral vessels. *Journal of Neurosurgery*, **41**, 125–145.

Sicard, J. A., Forestier, J. (1923) Injections intravasculaires d'huile iodée Sous contrôle radiologique. *Comptes Rendus de la Société de Biologie*, **88**, 1200.

Sicard, J. A., Forestier, J. (1932) *The Use of Lipiodol in Diagnosis and Treatment*. London: Oxford University Press.

Sutton, D. (1962) *Arteriography*. Edinburgh: Livingstone.

Sutton, D., Hoare, R. (1951) Vertebral angiography. *British Journal of Radiology*, **211**, 589.

Swick, M. (1929) Darstellung der Niere und Harnwege. Durch intravenöse Einhingung eines Kontraststoflas des Uroselectans. *Klinische Wochenschrift*, **8**, 2087–2089.

General
Abrams, H. L. (ed.) (1997) *Angiography*, 4th edn. Boston: Little Brown.

Allan, P. L., Pozniak, M. A., Dubbins, P. A., McDicken, W. N. (eds) (2000). *Clinical Colour Doppler Ultrasound*, London, Churchill Livingstone.

Ansell, G., Wilkins, R. A. (eds) (1996) *Complications in Diagnostic Radiology*, 3rd edn. Oxford: Blackwell.

Becker, D. M., Philbrick, J. T., Bayne Selby, J. (1992) Inferior vena cava filters. Indications, safety, effectiveness. *Archives of Internal Medicine*, **152**, 1985–1994.

Bell, A. M., Cumberland, D. C. (1989) Percutaneous atherectomy. *Clinical Radiology*, **40**, 122–126.

Belli, A-M. (1998) Thrombolysis in the peripheral vascular system. *Cardiovascular Interventional Radiology*, **21**, 95–101.

Bluth, E. I., Stavros, A. T., Marich, K. W., et al (1988) Carotid Duplex sonography: a multicenter recommendation for standardized imaging and Doppler criteria. *Radiographics*, **8**, 487.

Carr, D. H. (ed.) (1988) *Contrast Media*. Edinburgh: Churchill Livingstone.

Chuang, V. P., Wallace, S. (1981) Hepatic artery embolization in the treatment of hepatic neoplasms. *Radiology*, **140**, 51–58.

Chung, J. W., Park, J. H., Han, J. K., et al (1996) Hepatic tumours: predisposing factors for complications of transcatheter oily chemoembolization. *Radiology*, **198**, 33–40.

Debrun, G., Legre, J., Kasbarian, M., et al (1979) Endovascular occlusion of vertebral fistulae by detachable balloons with conservation of vertebral blood flow. *Radiology*, **130**, 141–147.

Ekelund, L., Gerlock, J., Ogoncharenko, V. (1978) The epinephrine effect in reneal angiography revisited. *Clinical Radiology*, **29**, 387–392.

Gregson, R. H. S., Sutton, D., Brennan, J., et al (1983) Spontaneous aortocaval fistula. *Clinical Radiology*, **34**, 683–687.

Hemingway, A. P., Allison, D. J. (1988) Complications of embolization: analysis of 410 procedures. *Radiology*, **166**, 669–672.

Henderson, M. J., Manhire, A. R. (1990) Cholesterol embolisation following angiography. *Clinical Radiology*, **42**, 281–282.

Herlinger, H. (1978) Arterioportography. *Clinical Radiology*, **29**, 255–275.

Johnston, K. W. (1992) Femoral and popliteal arteries: reanalysis of results of balloon angioplasty. *Radiology*, **183**, 767–771.

Johnston, K. W. (1993) Iliac arteries: reanalysis of results of balloon angioplasty. *Radiology*, **186**, 207–212.

Kerns, S. R., Hawkins, I. F., Sabatelli, F. W. (1995) Current status of carbon dioxide angiography. *Radiological Clinics of North America*, **33**, 15–29.

LaBerge, J. M., Ring, E. J., Gordon, R. L., et al (1993) Creation of transjugular intrahepatic portosystemic shunts with the Wallstent endoprosthesis: results in 100 patients. *Radiology*, **187**, 413–420.

Lang, E. K. (1981) Transcatheter embolization of pelvic vessels for control of intractable haemorrhage. *Clinical Radiology*, **35**, 85–93.

Lea Thomas, M. (1982) *Phlebography of the Lower Limb*. Edinburgh: Churchill Livingstone.

Lee, P. H., Kellet, M. J., Bailey, J., Prior, J. P. (1996) Klippel–Trenaunay syndrome as a cause of erectile dysfunction. *Clinical Radiology*, **51**, 596–597.

Lunderquist, A., Vang, J. (1974) Transhepatic catheterization and obliteration of the coronary vein in patients with portal varices. *New England Journal of Medicine*, **291**, 646–649.

Mandell, V. S., et al (1985) Persistent sciatic artery. *American Journal of Roentgenology*, **144**, 245–249.

Matsi, P. J., Manninen, H. I. (1998) Complications of lower limb percutaneous transluminal angioplasty. *Cardiovascular Interventional Radiology*, **21**, 361–366.

May, J., White, G. H., Waugh, R., et al (1999) Endovascular treatment of abdominal aortic aneurysms. *Cardiovascular Surgery*, **7**, 484–490.

Miller, D. C., Stinson, E. G., Oyer, P. E., et al (1979) Operative treatment of aortic dissections: experience with 125 patients. *Journal of Thoracic and Cardiovascular Surgery*, **78**, 365.

Murphy K. J., Brunberg, J. A. & Cohan, R. H. (1996). Adverse reactions to gadolinium contrast media: a review of 36 cases. *American Journal of Roentenology*, **167**, 847–849.

Murray, D., Platts, A. D., Watkinson, A. F. (2000) Imaging and intervention of vascular retroperitoneal pathology. *Imaging*, **12**, 61–81.

O'Halpin, D., Legge, D., MacErlain, D. P. (1984) Therapeutic arterial embolisation: report of five years experience. *Clinical Radiology*. **35**, 85–93.

Okesendal, A. N. & Hals, P. A. (1993). Biodistribution and toxicity of MR imaging contrast-media. *Journal of Magnetic Resonance Imaging*, **3**. 157.

Oudkerk, M., Kuijpers, T. J. A., Schmitz, P. I. M., et al (1996) Self-expanding metal stents for palliative treatment of superior vena cava syndrome. *Cardiovascular Interventional Radiology*, **19**, 146–151.

Prince, M., Grist, T. M. & Debatin, J. F. 3D Contrast MR Angiography, Springer, Berlin, 1999, (2ⁿᵈ Ed.).

Royal, S. A., Callen, P. W. (1979) CT evaluation of anomalies of the IVC and left renal vein. *American Journal of Roentgenology*, **132**, 759–763.

Rubin, G. D., Dake, M. D., Semba, C. P. (1995) Current status of 3-dimensional spiral CT scanning for imaging the vasculature. *Radiological Clinics of North America*, **33**, 51–70.

Starnes, H. F., Vallance, R., Hamilton, D. N. H. (1984) Recurrent varicose veins: a radiological approach to investigation. *Clinical Radiology*, **35**, 95–99.

Thomas, E. A., Cobby, M. J. D., Rhys Davies, E., et al (1989) Liquid crystal thermography and C-reactive protein in detection of deep venous thrombosis. *British Medical Journal*, **299**, 951–952.

Thorogood, S. V., Maskell, G. F. (1996) Case report: intravascular lipoma of the superior vena cava. *British Journal of Radiology*, **69**, 963–964.

Viamonte, M., Jr, Pereiras, R., Russell, E., Le Page, J., Hudson, D. (1977) Transhepatic obliteration of gastro-oesophageal varices. *American Journal of Roentgenology*, **129**, 237–241.

Wallace, S., Chuang, V. P., Swanson, D., et al (1981) Embolization of renal carcinomas: experience with 100 patients. *Radiology*, **138**, 563–570.

Wells, I. P., Hammonds, J. C., Franklin, K. (1983) Embolization of hypernephromas: a simple technique using ethanol. *Clinical Radiology*, **34**, 689–692.

Whitehouse, G. H. (1990) Venous thrombosis and thrombo-embolisms. *Clinical Radiology*, **41**, 77–80.

Wilbur, A. C., Woelfel, G. F., Meyer, J. P., Flanigan, D. P., Spigos, D. G. (1985) Adventitial cystic disease of the popliteal artery. *Radiology*, **155**, 63–64.

Ultrasound

Allan, P. L., Pozniak, M. A., Dubbins, P. A., McDicken, W. N. (eds) (2000) *Clinical Colour Doppler Ultrasound*. London: Churchill Livingstone.

Strandness, D. E., Jr (1993) *Duplex Scanning in Vascular Disorders*, 2nd edn. New York: Raven Press.

Taylor, K. J. W., Burns, P. N., Wells, P. N. T. (eds) (1995) *Clinical Applications of Doppler Ultrasound*, 2nd edn. New York: Raven Press.

Wolff, K. J., Fobbe, F. (eds) (1995) *Color Duplex Sonography: principles and clinical applications*. Stuttgart: Georg Thieme.

MRI

Bradley, W. G. (1999) Flow phenomenona. In: Stark, Bradley (eds) *Magnetic Resonance Imaging*, 3rd edn, pp. 231–255. St Louis: Mosby.

Fenlon, H. M., Yucel, E. K. (1999) Advances in abdominal, aortic, and peripheral contrast-enhanced MR angiography. *Magnetic Resonance Imaging Clinics of North America*, **7**, 319–336.

Hartnell, G. G. (1993) Magnetic resonance imaging of systemic thoracic and abdominal veins. *Magnetic Resonance Imaging Clinics of North America*, **1**, 281–294.

Holtz, D. J., et al (1996) MR venography of the calf: value of flow-enhanced time-of-flight echoplanar imaging. *American Journal of Roentgenology*, **166**, 663–668.

Krinsky, G. (ed.) (1998) Body MR angiography. *Magnetic Resonance Imaging Clinics of North America*, **6**, 223–439.

Mittal, T. K., Evans, C. Perkins, T., Wood, A. M. (2001) Renal arteriography using gadolinium enhanced 3D MR angiography—clinical experience with the technique, its limitations and pitfalls. *British Journal of Roentgenology*, **74**, 495–502.

Murphy, K. J., Brunberg, J. A., Cohan, R. H. (1998) Adverse reactions to gadolinium contrast media: a review of 36 cases. *American Journal of Roentgenology*, **167**, 847–849.

Okesendal, A. N., Hals, P. A. (1993) Biodistribution and toxicity of MR imaging contrast-media. *Journal of Magnetic Resonance Imaging*, **3**, 157.

Prince, M. R., Yucel, E. K., Kaufman, J. A., Harrison, D. C., Geller, S. C. (1993) Dynamic gadolinium-enhanced three-dimensional abdominal arteriography. *Journal of Magnetic Resonance Imaging*, **3**, 877–881.

Prince, M., Grist, T. M. Debatin, J. F. (1999) 3D Contrast MR Angiography, 2nd edn. Springer: Berlin.

Prince, M. R., Narasimham, D. L., et al (1996) Three-dimensional gadolinium-enhanced MR angiography of the thoracic aorta. *American Journal of Roentgenology*, **166**, 1387–1397.

Ruehm, S. G., Goyen, M., Barkhausen, J., et al (2001) Rapid magnetic resonance angiography for detection of atherosclerosis. *Lancet*, **357**, 1086–1091.

Scott, S. (1995) Basic concepts of magnetic resonance angiography. *Radiologic Clinics of North America*, **33**, 91–113.

Shellock, E. G., Kanal, E. (1999) Bioeffects and safety. In: Stark, Bradley (eds) *Magnetic Resonance Imaging*, 3rd edn, pp. 291–308. St Louis: Mosby. www.mrisafety.com.

Spritzer, C. E. (1993) Venography of the extremities and pelvis. *Magnetic Resonance Imaging Clinics of North America*, **1**, 239–251.

Whitehouse, G. H. (1990) Editorial—venous thrombosis and thromboembolism. *Clinical Radiology*, **41**, 77–80.

REFERENCES AND SUGGESTIONS FOR FURTHER READING

Allan, P. L., Pozniak, M. A., Dubbins, P. A., McDicken, W. N. (eds) (2000). *Clinical Colour Doppler Ultrasound*, London, Churchill Livingstone.

Murphy, K. J., Brunberg, J. A. & Cohan, R. H. (1996). Adverse reactions to gadolinium contrast media: a review of 36 cases. *American Journal of Roentgenology*, **167**, 847–849.

Okesendal, A. N. & Hals, P. A. (1993). Biodistribution and toxicity of MR imaging contrast-media. *Journal of Magnetic Resonance Imaging*, **3**, 157.

Prince, M., Grist, T. M. & Debatin, J. F. 3D Contrast MR Angiography. Springer, Berlin, 1999, (2ⁿᵈ Ed.).

Shellock, F. G .& Kanal, E. Bioeffects and safety. In: Magnetic Resonance Imaging (Stark & Bradley, Eds). Chapter 14; 291–306. Mosby, 1999 (3rd Ed). www.mrisafety.com/

17

THE LYMPHATIC SYSTEM

Graham R. Cherryman and Bruno Morgan

In this chapter the structure, function and methods of imaging the lymphatic system are discussed. Benign and malignant conditions affecting the lymphatic system are reviewed with emphasis on the lymphomas. As lymphoma can involve any tissue and any part of the lymphatic system, experience in this condition is helpful for determining the lymph node status of any malignant disease.

STRUCTURE AND FUNCTION OF THE LYMPHATIC SYSTEM

The presence of a functioning lymphatic system is essential to health for two reasons: (i) it provides an important pathway for drainage of fluid from cells and tissues back to the bloodstream and (ii) it is a vital part of the immune system. The lymphatic system consists of a network of lymphatic capillaries that commence in the body tissues, freely anastomose and eventually drain back into the venous system via larger lymphatic trunks. Aggregates of lymphatic tissue are interspersed as *lymph nodes* in this matrix and elsewhere, in the *spleen*, *thymus* and *gastrointestinal tract*. There are lymphatics within most body tissues except avascular tissues such as articular cartilage. Lymphatics are also not present in brain, spinal cord, bone marrow and splenic pulp. Within these tissues there are microscopic clefts that have a similar function to lymphatics but, in contrast to lymphatic capillaries, lack an endothelial lining.

The characteristic endothelial wall seen in lymphatic capillaries is permeable to larger molecules that cannot pass through the endothelial lining of vascular capillaries. This allows the lymphatic system to absorb proteins and particulate matter including cells and cell debris and microorganisms as well as excess extracellular tissue fluid. This is vital for haemostasis with up to 50% of circulating proteins passing through the lymphatic system in one day. The lymphatics draining the gut are also known as *lacteals*. Following a meal the lymph (chyle) within these gut lymphatics appears milky white due to the presence of fat chylomicrons being transported away from the gut wall.

In the body the larger lymphatic trunks accompany the arteries and veins. Almost all lymph in the body eventually passes into the thorax and re-enters the vascular space through either the thoracic duct or the right lymphatic duct. In the retroperitoneum the para-aortic lymphatic trunks empty into the cisterna chyli at the level of the second lumbar vertebra. The cisterna chyli may be recognised on CT sections (Fig. 17.1). Typically the cisterna chyli is a saccular structure about 5 cm long, passing up through the diaphragm to become the thoracic duct, which is smaller in diameter than the cisterna chyli and not normally identified on CT examination. The thoracic duct may opacify after lymphography (Fig. 17.2).

The thoracic duct receives all the lymph flow from below the diaphragm as well as that from the left side of the thorax and neck. Typically the thoracic duct terminates by anastomosing with the left subclavian vein. On the right a smaller right lymphatic trunk drains lymph from the right side of the thorax and neck into the right subclavian vein. There are a number of variations in the anatomy of the larger lymphatic ducts.

Valves within the lymphatics allow movement of lymph in one direction only. The combination of filtration pressure in the interstitial spaces, movement of the limbs and muscles propel lymph through the lymphatic system aided by the contraction of the smooth

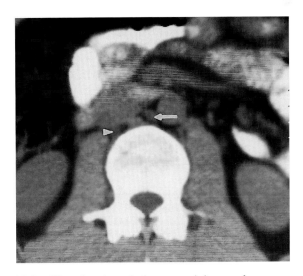

Fig. 17.1 CT section through the upper abdomen of a young male patient shows the cisterna chyli as a small (0.5 cm) low-attenuation structure lying between the aorta and IVC (arrow). The cisterna chyli may be seen on CT examination in almost all patients providing there is sufficient retroperitoneal fat. A smaller lymphatic duct may be seen behind the IVC (arrowhead).

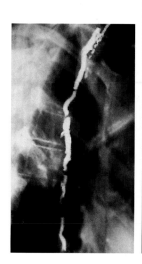

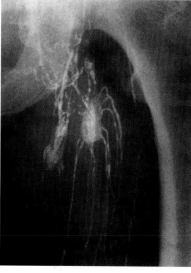

Fig. 17.2 Early phase lymphogram film with contrast medium outlining the thoracic duct.

Fig. 17.3 Early phase lymphogram film with opacification of both lymph nodes and lymph vessels. There are several afferent lymphatics feeding into each lymph node. The single efferent lymphatic always leaves the lymph node through the hilum.

muscle fibres found within the walls of the larger lymphatic trunks. Lymph drainage is about 2.5 L/day.

Lymph from almost all parts of the body traverses one or more lymph nodes before reaching the venous circulation. Lymph nodes are encapsulated aggregates of lymphatic tissue, normally small and bean shaped and situated in the path of the lymphatic vessels (Fig. 17.3), they are variable in size from microscopic to *ca.* 2 cm, and number approximately 600. A fibrous capsule covers the outer surface of the lymph node. Fibrous tissue extends into the lymph node in the form of trabeculae arising from the undersurface of this capsule, so that the lymphoid tissue within the lymph node is supported by a fine meshwork of fibrocellular elements. A slight depression on one side of the lymph node is termed the hilum, and it is through the hilum that blood vessels enter and leave the lymph node. A single efferent lymphatic also leaves from the hilum.

Internally the lymph node contains a central medulla and a peripheral cortex although the line of demarcation between the two is often indistinct. The cortex is deficient at the hilum so that the efferent lymphatic derives its lymph from the medulla. Afferent lymphatics are usually multiple and pass through the capsule into the cortex. Lymph enters a lymph node through one of these afferent vessels and passes onward into a subcapsular lymphatic plexus. From here the lymph passes into the sinuses of the cortex, then through the sinuses of the medulla, before leaving the lymph node through the efferent vessel. The flow of lymph in the sinuses is slightly retarded, and this encourages the deposition of particulate matter. This enables phagocytes to filter off particulate antigenic and other noxious matter from the lymph prior to drainage of lymph in the venous circulation.

The lymph node has a number of other functions, including a role in both the cellular and the humoral immune responses. Lymphocytes and other antibody-producing cells are generated in the lymph node, usually within the cortex, where densely packed cells form follicles, often with their own germinal centre. The

number and size of the follicles vary and at times of great antigenic stimulation may increase to such an extent that the lymph node itself enlarges. In these circumstances the enlarged lymph node is termed reactive.

TOPOGRAPHY OF THE LYMPHATIC SYSTEM

The radiologist should have an understanding of the major lymphatic pathways of the body, especially those of the head and neck, thorax, abdomen and pelvis.

LYMPHATIC DRAINAGE OF THE HEAD AND NECK

There are approximately 300 lymph nodes in the average adult neck, loosely arranged into several groups (Som 1987). Understanding lymph drainage is important as lymph node resection may prove curative for early involvement in head and neck cancer and may improve prognosis in more advanced cancer. However there is free communication between all the lymph node groups and chains in the neck and metastatic involvement of cervical lymph nodes may occur along apparently illogical pathways, accounting for 'skip lesions'. Lymphatics and lymph nodes of the neck make up a collar of lymphoid tissue around the skull base consisting, from posterior to anterior, of *occipital, mastoid, parotid* (intra- or extra-glandular), *submandibular, facial, submental* and *sublingual* lymph nodes. It is important to recognise the deep and impalpable *retropharyngeal* lymph nodes (Fig. 17.4) found in the neck lateral to the longus colli and longus capitis muscles that drain lymph from the nasopharynx, oropharynx, sinuses and middle ear. Pathology in the retropharyngeal region may be associated with abnormalities of the 9th–12th cranial nerves.

Drainage is complex but can be simplified to three main routes with variable terminology. Most deep structures eventually drain to the *jugulodigastric* lymph node, which is located behind the angle of the mandible just above where the posterior belly of the digastric

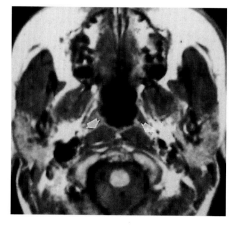

Fig. 17.4 Axial T_1-weighted MRI examination of the neck. Bilateral retropharyngeal nodes may be identified (arrows). On T_1-weighted sequences, lymph nodes appear darker than the surrounding fat. Note the flow void phenomenon—the great vessels of the neck appear black.

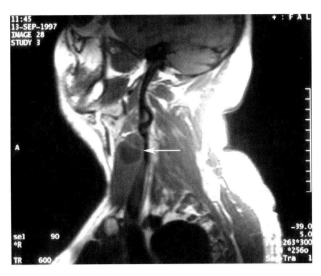

Fig. 17.5 T_1-weighted sagittal MRI scan demonstrating a malignant lymph node in the deep cervical chain invading the jugular vein (as shown by flow void).

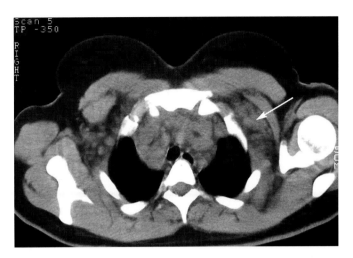

Fig. 17.7 CT examination showing supraclavicular and superior mediastinal lymph nodes.

muscle crosses the jugular vein. This is at the apex of the *deep cervical (internal jugular)* nodal chain. This pathway extends down the internal jugular vein, just behind the anterior border of the sternocleidomastoid muscle. The lymph nodes lie outside the carotid sheath, but on CT and MRI are seen to be close to the structures within the carotid sheath (Fig. 17.5). This chain can be divided into upper, middle and lower groups by the landmarks of the hyoid and cricoid cartilage as seen on CT scan. Drainage is into nodes in the lower neck, often called the lymph nodes of *Virchow* or *Trosier*, that drain into the venous system directly or via the thoracic duct or right lymphatic duct. The posterior nodal groups drain into the *spinal accessory (posterior triangle)* nodal chain that runs in the posterior triangle of the neck deep to the sternocleidomastoid muscle. The lymph nodes of this group typically lie within fat, and as a consequence are well seen on CT and MRI scans (Fig. 17.6). The

spinal accessory chain joins the *transverse (supraclavicular)* nodal pathway again to link with the lymph nodes of *Virchow* or *Trosier*. Superficial and anterior neck structures may drain into the *anterior, superficial cervical (external jugular)* nodal groups including the *pretracheal, prelaryngeal* and *paratracheal* nodal chains. As well as draining into the lower neck nodes these nodal groups can drain to the *upper mediastinal* lymph nodes. The '*Delphian node*' is a prelaryngeal midline lymph node that can signal subglottic malignancy. Isolated enlargement of the lower neck lymph nodes may be secondary to breast, thoracic or subdiaphragmatic primary tumour or lymphoma (Fig. 17.7).

Along cancer staging guidelines these nodes can be divided into groups or levels. Level I includes the submandibular and submental nodes, levels II, III and IV the upper, middle and lower deep cervical chain, level V the spinal accessory and transverse chains, level V1 the anterior chains and level VII the upper mediastinal nodes.

LYMPHATIC DRAINAGE OF THE THORAX

The lymph nodes of the mediastinum consist of a *posterior mediastinal group* of lymph nodes found below the level of the pulmonary veins and in close relationship to the aorta and oesophagus and extending inferiorly to the diaphragm. Above the posterior mediastinal lymph nodes are the *paratracheobronchial* lymph nodes. These consist of a subcarinal lymph node group, the lymph nodes of the pulmonary root, the lymph nodes between the trachea and the bronchi, and the paratracheal lymph nodes. Above these lymph nodes are the lymph nodes of the *aorto-pulmonary window* and the *anterior mediastinum* (Glazer et al 1985, Kiyono et al 1988). These latter lymph nodes are found in front of the great vessels. In addition, enlargement of the *internal mammary* and *diaphragmatic* lymph nodes (Fig. 17.8) should be recognised on CT examination.

The lymphatic drainage of the lungs does not strictly follow the lobar boundaries. The right upper lung drains to the right paratracheal lymph nodes, the right middle lung drains to both the right paratracheal and right subcarinal lymph nodes, while the lymphatic drainage from the right lower lung goes to the right paratracheal, subcarinal and posterior mediastinal lymph nodes. The upper portion of the left lung drains to the paratracheal lymph nodes,

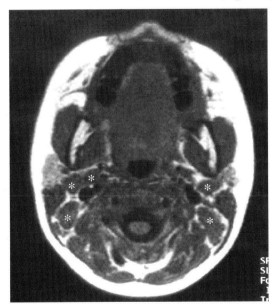

Fig. 17.6 T_1-weighted axial MRI examination of a patient with Hodgkin's disease demonstrating anterior and posterior triangle nodes as small areas of low signal within the relatively bright signal of fat.

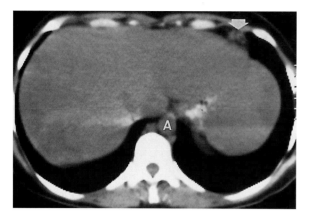

Fig. 17.8 CT scan showing enlargement and almost certain involvement of a diaphragmatic lymph node. The enlargement of a diaphragmatic or paracardiac lymph node is of great importance in patients with Hodgkin's disease considered for mantle irradiation. Normal-sized lymph nodes in this area are not seen on CT examination. A = aorta.

while both the mid and lower portions of the left lung drain to the paratracheal and subcarinal lymph nodes.

LYMPHATIC DRAINAGE OF THE ABDOMEN AND PELVIS

Lymph from the *inguinal* nodes drains into the *external iliac* nodal chain. The *external* and *internal iliac* and *obturator* lymph nodes drain into the *retroperitoneal para-aortic* nodal chains. The lymph node pathways from the legs are shown well by lymphogram (Fig. 17.9) (Harrison & Clouse 1985). Large and non-homogeneous lymph nodes in the groin are usually opacified. These are difficult to evaluate radiologically as they are frequently enlarged as a result of previous infection/reaction and often contain numerous fibrofatty filling defects. Pathological enlargement of the groin lymph nodes may be seen on CT sections, but in such cases the diseased lymph nodes are usually palpable (Fig. 17.10). In the pelvis, lymphographic contrast agents will opacify the *external iliac* and *common iliac* lymph nodes. The *internal iliac* and *obturator* lymph nodes drain the pelvic viscera into the retroperitoneal nodes and are usually only seen on lymphography if there is derangement of the normal flow pattern, for example secondary to surgery, but these nodes, if enlarged, may be seen on cross-sectional imaging studies.

In the retroperitoneum the lymph nodes as high as L2 typically opacify at lymphangiography. There are lymph nodes between the aorta and inferior vena cava (Fig. 17.11). Abdominal viscera generally drain into the *mesenteric* lymph nodes (Fig. 17.12) and then into the *preaortic* nodes around the coeliac axis and superior and inferior mesenteric arteries. The lymph nodes around the stomach and pancreas as well as those closest to the porta hepatis and renal and splenic hila may be seen on cross-sectional imaging, but these fail to opacify at lymphography (Fig. 17.13).

Drainage around the stomach and pancreas is complicated and diverse. Surgical treatment of gastric cancer has been improved by radical resection of wide areas of lymph node groups to attempt to cover all drainage pathways (Otsuji et al 2000). Drainage is ultimately to the cisterna chyli and thoracic duct.

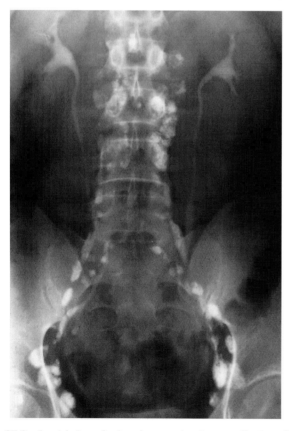

Fig. 17.9 Frontal view of a lymphogram showing opacification of the pelvic and retroperitoneal lymph nodes.

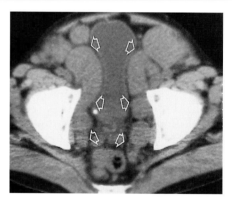

Fig. 17.10 CT section through the pelvis showing bilateral pelvic and groin lymph node enlargement in a patient with non-Hodgkin lymphoma.

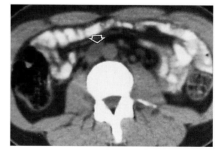

Fig. 17.11 Contrast-enhanced CT study showing enlargement and involvement of an interaorticocaval lymph node (arrow) in a patient with a right-sided testicular malignancy. Right-sided testicular tumours frequently spread to the interaorticocaval lymph nodes. This is extremely uncommon when the testicular primary is on the left.

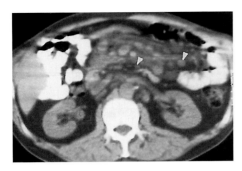

Fig. 17.12 CT section showing mesenteric lymph node involvement (arrowheads) in a patient with non-Hodgkin's lymphoma. This is common in non-Hodgkin's lymphoma, but seen in fewer than 5% of patients with Hodgkin's disease.

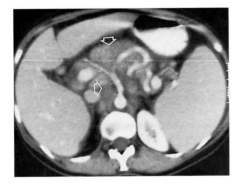

Fig. 17.13 Contrast-enhanced CT scan showing considerable enlargement of upper abdominal, peripancreatic and portal lymph nodes (arrows). The superior mesenteric artery and the hepatic artery are outlined by contrast.

Drainage of the anterior abdominal wall can drain widely and even into *axillary* nodes. The anal canal drains to the inguinal nodes and this area should be imaged in staging studies.

IMAGING THE LYMPHATIC SYSTEM

Clinical examination is the first step in the evaluation of the lymphatic system. Enlargement of neck, axillary and groin lymph nodes may be palpable, and large abdominal nodal masses may also be palpated. Smaller volume enlargement of abdominal and pelvic lymph nodes, together with any enlargement of lymph nodes within the thorax, is impalpable. The determination of tumour extent and bulk within the body is only possible after the appropriate imaging tests have been performed. The presence of adenopathy may be seen on plain-film examination (Fig. 17.14) and inferred from displacement of normal structures. The chest radiograph remains the most important radiological window into the thorax. Enlargement of mediastinal and hilar lymph nodes has a characteristic appearance. In many instances the information available from a chest radiograph is sufficient to plan further management of the patient. Radiographs of the abdomen are less helpful, as only large masses can be confidently recognised and the nodal nature of these masses is difficult to establish. The addition of a contrast medium (especially an intravenous pyelogram (IVP)) to opacify the ureters is an historical but limited method of demonstrating mass effect and the

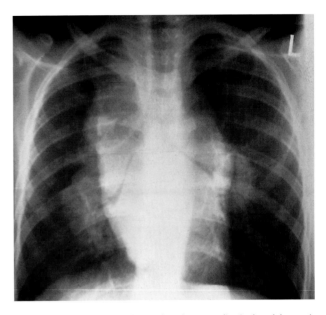

Fig. 17.14 Frontal chest radiograph. A large mediastinal nodal mass in a patient presenting with Hodgkin's disease is seen compressing the major airways.

displacement of normal abdominal structures by a large abdominal mass (Fig. 17.15). Radiological examination of the lymphatic system may concentrate on the lymphatic ducts or the lymph nodes. Developments in cross-sectional imaging changed the emphasis to imaging of lymph nodes, especially as clusters of lymph nodes often correspond well to numbers of afferent lymphatics.

IMAGING LYMPHATIC DUCTS

Lymphography

For many years bipedal lymphography was the standard test for the non-surgical demonstration of lymphadenopathy affecting the abdominal and pelvic lymph nodes. Lymphography is a sensitive test that studies the lymphatic ducts and the internal architecture of nodes. It may on occasion demonstrate micrometastases in normal-sized lymph nodes and can be used for follow-up imaging of nodal diseases as the contrast persists in lymph nodes for 6–12 months. Lymphography is only moderately specific however, and false-positive findings are not infrequent, especially in the elderly, in whom fibrofatty deposits within the lymph nodes may be incorrectly considered metastatic foci. Lymphography only examines lymph nodes and ducts in the drainage pathway from the legs or arms. This limits the value of the lymphogram technique, particularly in the staging of pelvic malignancies.

Successful lymphography is a difficult procedure for patient and operator and depends on several sequential steps. Contraindications include allergies to contrast agents, vital dyes, and local anaesthesia; cardiovascular or pulmonary disease, especially heart failure, angina, pulmonary fibrosis or emphysema; and previous pulmonary irradiation. The last is a significant risk factor as the arteriovenous shunts opened up at pulmonary irradiation predispose to systemic oil embolism. Lymphography is often considered an outpatient procedure, but observation for 24 h in hospital is prudent (MacDonald 1987). The small lymphatic ducts in the foot must be cannulated using a cut-down procedure; oily contrast media is then slowly

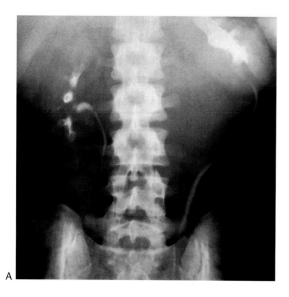

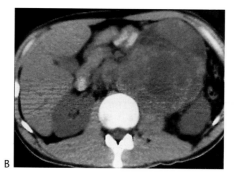

Fig. 17.15 (A) The opacified ureters are seen on intravenous urography to be displaced around a large central abdominal mass. (B) The presence of this mass is confirmed on the CT section. The final diagnosis was testicular teratoma.

injected and radiographs taken, both immediately after the procedure, to demonstrate the lymphatics, and again after at least 24 h delay to demonstrate the lymph nodes. Contrast medium will then remain in the lymph nodes for months, and during this time follow-up films can be used to demonstrate changes within the opacified lymph nodes. This procedure is well described elsewhere (Cherryman 1996).

The vast majority of previous indications for lymphography involved diagnosis of lymph node disease. This has been effectively replaced by cross-sectional imaging, such as CT, which can study all nodes in the body at greater ease for the radiology department and patient.

Lymphoscintigraphy

There is still occasionally a need for studying the lymphatic drainage system as well as just lymph nodes. Indications would include investigation of the primary lymphoedemas and the study of major drainage nodes for tumours (sentinel node imaging/mapping). As the lymphatic system is the only mechanism of transporting macromolecules from tissues, intradermal injection of a macromolecule such as ^{99m}Tc-radiolabelled serum albumin will preferentially outline the drainage lymphatics and nodes. The technique is straightforward and can be performed in most nuclear medicine departments (Witte et al 2000; Fig. 17.16).

As this technique does not rely on cannulating a lymphatic duct it can be performed at any site including studying the lymphatic drainage of a tumour in any part of the body. This may be done with gamma camera imaging or using a probe intraoperatively to identify nodes for immediate histology using frozen sections (Yudd et al 1999).

IMAGING LYMPH NODES

Ultrasound

As lymph node drainage may be diverse and staging of tumours may require inspection of lymph nodes at many distant sites, ultrasound is rarely used as a primary imaging strategy. Furthermore nodal groups in the mediastinum, retroperitoneum and deep pelvis

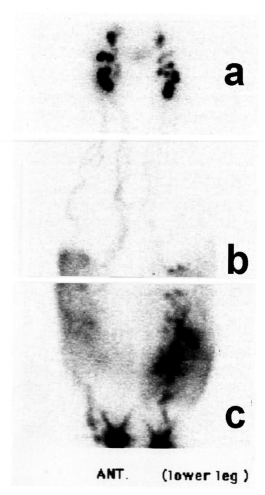

Fig 17.16 Lymphangioscintigram demonstrating lymphoedema with poor lymph drainage in the left leg. Letters a, b and c correspond to groin nodes, the knees and ankles, respectively.

may be difficult to see. Ultrasound can be useful in investigating nodal masses particularly as an aid to biopsy. Head and neck nodal staging may use ultrasound in combination with fine needle aspiration cytology. Endoscopic ultrasound can provide high-resolution imaging to detect locoregional lymphadenopathy in oesophageal, pancreatic and rectal carcinoma.

CT and MRI

Today the formal staging of malignant disease in patients is undertaken largely using CT, supplemented by MRI and ultrasound examinations. Furthermore CT observation of lymph node groups in the inguinal regions may be helpful in the investigation of lymphoedema. CT is generally the method of choice, providing a direct and reproducible demonstration of normal and abnormal lymph nodes. MRI has potential to replace CT in the assessment of nodal disease, although at higher cost. Radiation dose issues make MRI a potentially important option in the follow-up of nodal disease in remission. Lymph node enlargement is the imaging hallmark of metastatic involvement and a series of size criteria for normal and abnormal lymph nodes have evolved in the different areas of the body (see below). Care should be taken when comparing lymph node sizes that standard window settings are used and that the correct measurement is made, typically the maximum diameter perpendicular to the longest diameter (maximum short-axis diameter). Enlargement of the lymph nodes above this criterion is suggestive but not diagnostic of malignant involvement. The images should always be interpreted in the light of the clinical findings and the known behaviour of the particular tumour. For example, a slightly enlarged right paracaval lymph node is unlikely to be involved in a patient with a left-sided testicular teratoma, but a similarly sized para-aortic lymph node on the left may be the site of metastatic disease following spread of disease from a right testicular tumour. This is because cross-flow in the lymphatic drainage of the retroperitoneum is far more likely to occur from right to left across the midline than from left to right (Dixon et al 1986).

Increasing specificity for malignant involvement can be obtained using contrast media. Both CT with iodinated contrast media and MRI with gadolinium chelates can demonstrate rim enhancement of a necrotic lymph node that, in the absence of apparent infection, is a specific sign of malignancy. Specific lymph node contrast media are being developed for CT and MRI including the ultrasmall supraparamagnetic iron oxides (USPIO) in MRI (Bellin et al 2000). USPIOs are opsonised by normal lymph nodes reducing their normal high signal on T_2 (or particularly T_2^*). Although time consuming, requiring re-imaging on the next day, this may prove useful in tumour staging where lymph node biopsy is difficult such as retroperitoneal nodes in prostate cancer. Analysis of dynamic contrast enhancement characteristics has also proved useful for predicting malignant involvement but this is currently limited to individual lymph node groups and therefore has limited clinical potential (Laissy et al 1994).

Radionuclide techniques

Sentinel node imaging using ^{99m}Tc-labelled human serum albumen has already been discussed in the lymphatic section. Other injected radiopharmaceuticals may collect in lymph vessels and nodes (McKusick 1985). Circulating radionuclides may be taken up by metastatic lymph nodes. This is best recognised with gallium-67, which is a tumour-avid isotope taken up by tumours arising from the lymphatic system, liver or lung. Different cell types will take up the isotope differentially. The technique has been applied to patients

with lymphoma. The sensitivity of the test to the presence of active lymphoma tissue is related to the volume of the tumour, the location injected, the dose and the instrumentation. Gallium-67 imaging is sensitive to the presence of lymphoma in patients but has proved less effective than CT in determining the extent of disease site by site within individual patients. Approximately 5% of positive results with gallium-67 imaging are incorrect, usually as a result of concomitant or unsuspected infection. At present the clinical role of gallium-67 scanning in lymphoma is best limited to the follow-up of patients with initial positive scans (Fig. 17.17).

Positron emission tomography scanning

This is a functional imaging technique. The most common usage of positron emission tomography (PET) is for lymph node imaging using the glucose analogue 18-FDG, (2-[F-18]fluoro-2-deoxy-D-glucose). This detects increased metabolism in tumour-bearing nodes and is therefore potentially more sensitive and specific than CT. Furthermore PET images can be superimposed on CT images to give anatomical and metabolic information together. PET may prove even more useful in the follow-up of disease where it may distinguish recurrent disease from reactive or residual scarring in enlarged lymph nodes. As 18-FDG has a longer half-life than other positron emitters it is more practical to use, as a cyclotron is not required on site. Potentially dual-headed SPECT gamma cameras can also be converted to acquire PET images. PET however does not specifically image malignancy but increase in metabolism, and there is therefore scope for false-positive results. Also it is still not capable of excluding the microscopic tumour involvement that histology can show. It is therefore a complimentary technique at increased cost that can be very useful in certain cases. Whether PET comes into widespread routine use remains to be seen.

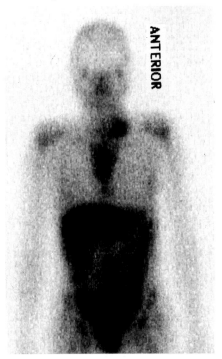

Fig. 17.17 Gallium-67 radioisotope scan in a patient with nodular sclerosing Hodgkin's disease affecting supraclavicular and mediastinal nodes. Note the normal uptake in the liver.

DISORDERS OF THE LYMPHATIC DUCTS

These may be directly opacified at lymphography. The injection of water-soluble radiological contrast media is an acceptable and safe alternative to the injection of oily contrast media but will not opacify the lymph nodes (O'Donnell & Clouse 1985). The technique of lymphography in the oedematous leg is difficult, and prior elevation of the limb for 48–72 h may help reduce the amount of limb oedema. In most cases lymphography can be replaced by lymhangioscintigraphy (Witte et al 2000).

Allen et al (1946) divided the lymphoedemas into primary and secondary. The primary type may be further subdivided into *congenital, praecox* (before the age of 35 years) and *tarda* (after the age of 35 years). On the basis of the lymphographic appearances the lymphoedemas may be divided into the *aplasias* with no demonstrable lymphatics, the *hypoplasias* with a reduced number of lymphatics, and the *hyperplasias* with an increase in the number of lymphatics present.

Primary lymphoedema

This is a vascular dysplasia often associated with arterial and venous malformations in the same limb and other congenital defects. Most patients have aplasia or severe hypoplasia of the lymphatics. The oedema may be precipitated by minor trauma or surgery. Peak incidence is seen in girls at puberty and typically involves the left leg. The term *Milroy's disease* is loosely applied to primary lymphoedema, but should be limited to those few cases that are both congenital and familial.

The advent of CT has also reduced the need for lymphographic evaluation of the lymphatics, as the size and number of lymph nodes parallel the size and number of lymphatics. CT assessment of the size and number of the lymph nodes can objectively classify patients into aplasia, hypoplasia and hyperplasia of the lymphatic system.

Secondary lymphoedema

This is more common than primary lymphoedema, and indicates the presence of obstruction to the normal forward passage of lymph. This may be due to previous surgery or irradiation but may also result from recurrent tumour. Uncommon causes of secondary lymphoedema include infection, especially with *filariasis* (Fig. 17.18). In patients with secondary lymphoedema, CT is again the most useful investigation, especially when looking for new or recurrent tumour.

DISORDERS OF THE LYMPH NODES

Malignant involvement of a lymph node typically results in the enlargement of the affected lymph node. This may be considered to involve four stages. First, the deposition of a malignant cell within

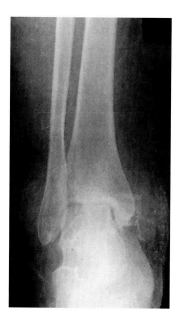

Fig. 17.18 Early phase lymphogram film. The limb is swollen, and when lymphography was attempted, lymphatics filled poorly. This is an example of secondary lymphoedema due to filariasis.

the lymph node and subsequent cell division, resulting in the presence of a micrometastasis within the affected lymph node. At this stage the lymph node remains of normal size and shape and will appear normal on CT and MRI examination (Fig. 17.19). Surgical staging, with either lymph node sampling or formal lymphadenectomy, will demonstrate malignant involvement of lymph nodes before either the CT/MRI scan or the lymphogram become abnormal. Surgery and careful histology is the present 'gold standard' for evaluating lymph node involvement in patients with malignant disease. This is seen, for example, in the axillary staging of patients with breast cancer.

There is a period in which lymphography might demonstrate the presence of a micrometastasis while the lymph node itself remains of normal size. This accounts for the slightly greater sensitivity of lymphography over CT and/or MRI in evaluating the retroperitoneal lymph nodes, and is most useful in evaluating slower-growing tumours where this stage is likely to persist longer. The CT demonstration of a micrometastasis within a lymph node is more difficult but may be possible in the neck (Fig. 17.20). A CT density measurement is required to differentiate a small metastasis within a lymph node from a focal deposit of fat. In the neck the incidence of fibrofatty foci within normal-sized lymph nodes is less than in the abdominal, pelvic and axillary lymph nodes, making this a valid technique.

Eventually an involved lymph node will enlarge and become recognisable clinically and/or with cross-sectional imaging. Some tumours result in discrete lymph node metastases, while other

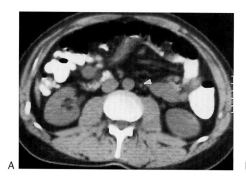

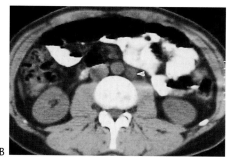

Fig. 17.19 (A) Staging CT on this patient with a testicular primary shows no significant adenopathy. Note the 0.25 cm node in the left retroperitoneum (arrowhead). (B) Seven months later this lymph node has enlarged (arrowhead), indicating the presence of an occult primary in the lymph node at the time of original staging.

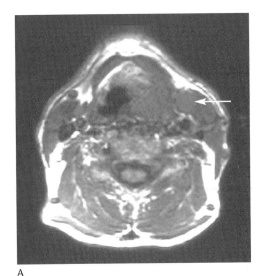

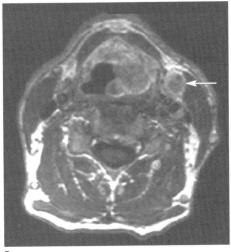

A B

Fig. 17.20 T$_1$-weighted axial MRI showing lymph node involvement from a supraglottic SCC (arrows) pre contrast (A), and demonstrating rim enhancement secondary to central necrosis post contrast (B).

tumours rapidly pass onto the next phase, in which the outline of the tumour becomes blurred due to the presence of tumour extending into the perinodal tissues (Fig. 17.21). The final or fourth stage of malignant spread of tumour to a lymph node results in a large amorphous tumour mass with infiltration of the tissue planes. At this time it is impossible to identify any residual nodal outline.

Benign conditions affecting the lymph nodes

These are important radiologically as they may result in lymph node enlargement, which may be confused with malignant involvement. Mycoplasma pneumonia can present with mediastinal and hilar lymphadenopathy on a chest radiograph in a similar manner to lymphoma. Benign focal lesions within the lymph nodes can also be mistaken for deposits.

Acute inflammation will enlarge lymph nodes. On lymphograms the texture of the lymph node will become more foamy, an appearance usually associated with lymphoma (Fig. 17.22). Central defects within the lymph node may also be seen. Typically it is the granulomatous or

abscess-forming inflammations that produce filling defects in the lymph nodes similar to those seen in secondary deposits (Fig. 17.23). Lymph nodes may be seen to enlarge in a number of granulomatous diseases, including sarcoid and tuberculosis.

Reactive hyperplasia usually associated with a proliferation of histiocytes is another frequent cause of lymph node enlargement. This may be related to recent surgery (Fig. 17.24).

Fibrofatty deposits are seen within the lymph nodes of older patients, and these are most commonly seen in the pelvis. They may be considered a normal finding in the inguinal region, but in the remainder of the pelvis they are a source of confusion, as they may be incorrectly interpreted as secondary deposits in patients with a primary pelvic neoplasm.

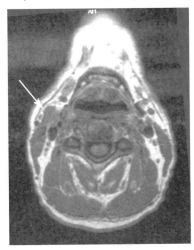

Fig. 17.21 T$_1$-weighted axial MRI showing extra-capsular tumour spread from lymph node demonstrated by ill defined lymph node margins and abnormal signal in the surrounding fat.

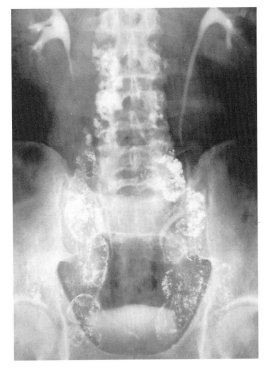

Fig. 17.22 The lymph nodes are generally enlarged and appear foamy in a patient with lymphoma.

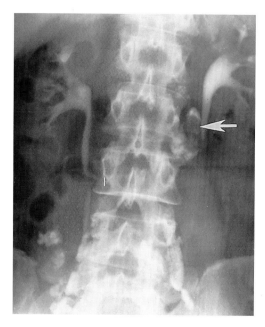

Fig. 17.23 A single focal deposit is seen within the enlarged and opacified lymph node medial to the left ureter (arrow) in this patient with an endometrial cancer.

Malignant conditions affecting the lymph nodes

Tumours spread by three mechanisms, local invasion, lymph node and haematogenous (metastatic) spread. The mechanism of spread depends on the particular tumour subtype and location. For example testicular seminomas virtually always spread by logical lymph node progression to the para-aortic nodes yet testicular teratomas undergo metastatic spread much more commonly. In the naso-pharynx squamous cell carcinomas (SCC) present with lymph node involvement in 80–90%, yet this is less than 10% for SCC of the glottis.

There are many conventions for the staging of different tumours, and all methods reflect the bulk and distribution of tumour tissue within the body. This is of some prognostic and therapeutic significance, although in many tumours the histology diagnosis and

grading is of paramount importance. The TNM system (UICC 1987) is the most widely accepted staging system, although it is inappropriate for patients with lymphoma.

If it is assumed that a primary neoplasm starts as a single malignant cell that has the capacity to replicate itself, then it will take approximately 30 cell divisions for a tumour mass to reach a diameter of 1 cm and become radiologically visible. The doubling time of a tumour varies greatly, and may be a few days for a rapidly growing malignancy, or several months for a slow-growing tumour type. From this it may be seen that all tumours will take months or years to become radiologically detectable. For most of their life all tumours are subclinical. Once past the 30-cell division barrier it will require only a few further cell divisions for the tumour burden to become overwhelming and the untreated patient to succumb. Malignant neoplasms may metastasise at the subclinical level. In such patients, by the time the primary tumour has become apparent the patient is already incurable by local methods (surgery and radiotherapy), as these will not treat the distant tumour spread. Metastases result from lymphatic and/or vascular invasion followed by the dissemination of tumour cells within blood or lymph vessels throughout the body. Although tumours can create their own blood supply by the process of angiogenesis, they do not have their own lymphatic drainage and spread is initially by local invasion of surrounding lymphatics. Malignant cells may also be scavenged directly from the interstitial tissues by surrounding lymphatics. Malignant cells may then drain into regional lymph nodes prior to any direct vascular invasion by the tumour. Most of these cells will die but some may have the ability to survive and grow in the new environment. This depends on the underlying cell properties and the genetics of the particular tumour type. If the cells survive tumour growth will occur in the lymph node, which may then progress to subsequent drainage nodes. The tumour may also locally invade beyond the lymph node capsule. Once a lymph node is completely invaded by tumour the usual lymph node drainage of that region will be disrupted. The detection of metastatic lymph nodes is an important component of tumour staging and is always a poor prognostic indicator and may change management. The demonstration of nodal disease in the neck of patients with a primary tumour of the head and neck reduces survival by 50% for ipsilateral adenopathy, and by a further 50% for contralateral adenopathy. Extranodal spread of malignancy is associated with a further significant reduction in prognosis.

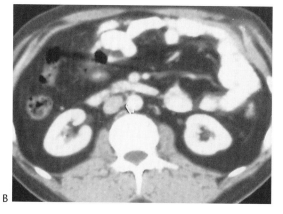

Fig. 17.24 (A) Staging CT scans in a patient with a recently resected right-sided testicular tumour showed prominent lymph nodes between the aorta and inferior vena cava (arrow). (B) One month later these have resolved without treatment. Reactive enlargement of lymph nodes is a possible source of error if patients are scanned too close to the date of their surgery. It is better to wait 3–4 weeks.

STRATEGIES FOR IMAGING THE LYMPHATIC SYSTEM IN MALIGNANT DISEASE

DIAGNOSIS AND T AND M STAGING

Imaging will demonstrate malignant disease within a body structure or viscus as a change in shape and/or a change in attenuation of the affected area. It is possible to propose, from the clinical details and the pattern of disease dissemination seen on CT scanning, the likely primary sites in a patient presenting with lymphadenopathy, but this speculation should never replace formal histological investigation. On occasion the radiologist may help by providing material for pathological examination from percutaneous biopsy.

Radiological investigation, generally using CT or MRI, is essential in the TNM staging of malignant tumours and may provide information in those tumours (e.g. lymphomas) that are staged by other conventions. The size and location of any primary tumour should be assessed clinically and radiologically. Whenever possible, objective measurements should be taken. These measurements are invaluable in assessing response. There are recognised criteria for primary tumour or T-staging of most common tumours (UICC 1987). Knowledge of the site and extent of the primary tumour mass are valuable in predicting the likely routes of lymphatic and vascular spread.

The M-stage of malignancy recognises the spread of tumour to distant organs. This is a result of haematogenous dissemination, and the most common sites for such involvement are the lungs, liver and brain. These may be diagnosed in several ways, but the overall information available from CT examination, often allowing a TNM (tumour, nodes and metastases) stage to be assigned to a patient at the one examination, makes this technique supreme.

Lymph node involvement (N-staging)

Similarly, criteria have evolved to determine the extent of lymph node involvement at the time of diagnosis (Table 17.1). The regional lymph nodes for the common malignancies have been defined and stages of involvement recognised (UICC 1987).

Consider a young man presenting with a testicular teratoma. The primary tumour is removed at orchidectomy, and the specimen assessed for evidence of complete resection of the primary tumour and for lymphatic and/or vascular invasion. Teratoma typically spreads initially to the para-aortic lymph nodes, and these then represent the first-echelon lymph nodes for testicular malignancies. Enlargement of the para-aortic lymph nodes increases the overall staging to stage II. The subscripts A, B and C reflect the disease bulk in terms of the cross-sectional diameter of the retroperitoneal nodal mass as seen on CT. 'A' represents a cross-sectional diameter less than 2 cm (Fig. 17.25), 'B' a cross-sectional diameter of between 2 and 5 cm and 'C' a cross-sectional diameter of more than 5 cm (Fig. 17.26). The disease may then progress cephalad through the lymphatic system to involve the lymph nodes of the mediastinum (stage III disease), although more frequently involvement of the mediastinal lymph nodes with testicular teratoma is associated with evidence of vascular dissemination of tumour to the lungs. The presence of pulmonary or other extranodal metastases would automatically make the disease stage IV. A further attempt is made to quantify the tumour bulk in the lung fields in terms of both the size and the number of pulmonary metastases.

Treatment planning

A patient with a fully treated primary tumour and no evidence of metastatic disease may require no further treatment unless there is evidence of disease relapse. In most circumstances, patients are watched clinically and with simple investigations such as serial chest radiographs, but there are certain tumours in which a more

Table 17.1 Cotswold modification of the Ann Arbor staging of lymphoma

Stage	Area of Involvement
I	One lymph node region or extra lymphatic site
II	Two or more lymph node regions on the same side of the diaphragm
III	Lymph node regions on both sides of the diaphragm
IIIa	Involves spleen, Splenic hilar, coeliac or portal nodes
IIIB	Nodes inferior into renal vessels, including mesenteric
IV	Diffuse involvement of one or more extra nodal organs

Qualifiers:	
A	No symptoms
B 'symptoms'	Unexplained weight loss of more than 10% body weight in the preceding 6 months
	Unexplained fever above 38.4°C, and/or night sweats.
E	Localised extranodal site
X	Bulk disease
CS	Clinical stage
PS	Pathological stage (laparotomy)
S	Spleen
H	Liver
M	Bone marrow
P	Lung
O	Cortical bone

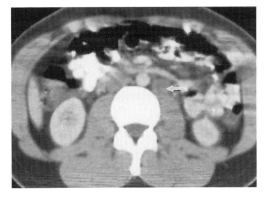

Fig. 17.25 Small-volume (<2 cm) retroperitoneal metastatic disease in a patient with a left-sided teratoma. Left-sided testicular primary teratomas almost always spread initially to a retroperitoneal lymph node under the left renal vein (arrow).

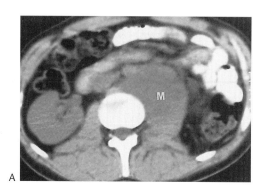
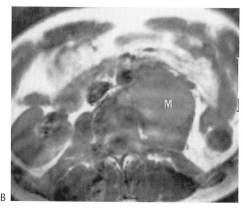

Fig. 17.26 Large retroperitoneal metastasis (M) arising from an ipsilateral testicular teratoma seen both on CT (A) and MRI (B).

aggressive surveillance policy is rewarding. These are usually those tumours for which curative or salvage chemotherapy is available, and this includes testicular teratoma. Apparently stage I teratoma patients may have occult disease. As treatment is available early detection of occult disease is important. Patients can therefore be placed on a surveillance protocol, which includes regular clinical examination, serum marker estimation, chest radiograph and 3-monthly CT examination of the chest, abdomen and pelvis for 2 years (90% of relapses will occur in the first year). Another strategy when chemotherapy and targeted radiotherapy are likely to be successful is to automatically treat all cases after surgery in case of occult disease. This adjuvant therapy may involve overtreatment of many patients but will reduce relapse rates.

Radiotherapy planning

For cases considered curable by radiotherapy, accurate staging is essential before embarking on a course of treatment. For example, the presence of abdominal adenopathy would preclude the possibility of a cure if the pelvis were to be irradiated for a pelvic primary tumour. The demonstration of the position, size and extent of a localised primary tumour on CT examination may be used to plan radiotherapy fields. This is usually accomplished with special software packages, and allows dose to the tumour to be maximised while vital structures, e.g. the spinal cord or kidneys, may be partly protected. The superior soft-tissue contrast of MRI compared to CT, especially when evaluating soft-tissue spread of tumour (e.g. in muscle) and the CNS, makes MRI potentially useful in planning radiotherapy treatment fields.

The operability of tumours or residual masses may also be assessed at CT or MRI examination, and in particular the proximity of vessels and other vital structures to the tumour mass may be determined.

Response to treatment

The treatment of any cancer is limited by the ability of the normal body tissues to withstand the treatment. There is morbidity and mortality associated with any treatment. Imaging is an important part of treatment evaluation. A rapid and complete response to treatment may allow a reduction in the number of treatments required, which reduces both the possible side-effects and complications (Oliver et al 1983). Alternatively, a poor or absent response

to first-time treatment could lead to either a change of treatment or to a change of approach from a curative to a palliative one. The objective recording of a response to a particular treatment is also important in the evaluation of treatments and comparative treatment studies. It must be appreciated that like must be compared with like, and CT-staged patients in one arm of the study must be imaged according to the same convention in the other arm of the study. Guidelines have been made on how to measure response in clinical trials. WHO criteria state a reduction in tumour size on CT of greater than 50% of the product of its diameters in the axial plane is a partial response (PR), while the objective disappearance of tumour should be regarded as a complete response (CR). In both cases the response should be confirmed at imaging at least 4 weeks later. Progressive disease is an increase of more than 25% or the detection of new lesions. As new lesions, such as new lymphadenopathy, are often small imaging technique is important. A new protocol for follow-up of tumours on trials (RECIST) stipulate imaging protocols (such as use of IV contrast and narrow collimation for CT) as well as tumour measurement criteria (Therasse et al 2000). On occasion a tumour may enlarge on treatment and yet still be responding (Fig. 17.27).

The addition of a more sophisticated imaging modality to the initial staging protocol of a particular tumour type may also appear to alter the outcome. Previously occult metastases will be demonstrated, altering the staging typically from stage I (no metastases) to stage IV (distant metastases). This will have the effect of improving survival rates in stage I disease in the survey, as some patients with metastases are now excluded from this group. The survival rate of the group of patients with stage IV disease will also apparently improve, as some of them now will have very small volume metastatic disease. However, the overall survival for the group will not change. This can occur between all disease stages and is known as 'stage migration'. This is a further reason why imaging criteria for staging and restaging needs to be standardised.

Residual masses

The radiologist may be asked to comment on the possible malignant potential of any residual mass following treatment of a malignancy (Lewis et al 1982). At present it is not possible to deduce residual malignant potential from the appearances. PET may provide the best imaging strategy with future possible strategies using radionuclides targeted to the specific cell types. If MRI scans show residual

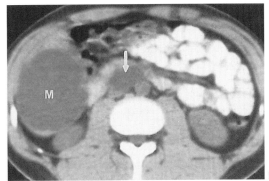

Fig. 17.27 (A) CT scan through the abdomen of this patient with metastatic teratoma. (B) CT scan showing an increase in tumour size, along with a decrease in attenuation following treatment, for a testicular teratoma. This almost always indicates differentiation of the tumour into a benign variant. The residuum is excised to protect the patient in the future. Note both the residual interaorticocaval lymph node (arrow) and the liver metastasis (M), both of which enlarge on treatment.

tumour masses as low signal intensity on T_2-weighted images, especially when the pretreatment images showed high signal, these are likely to be dormant (Fig. 17.28). Unfortunately the converse, that high signal on T_2-weighted sequences equals activity, is not true. In many cases the most pragmatic approach is surveillance with early repeat imaging.

THE LYMPHOMAS

These are primary neoplasms of the immune system and arise within lymphoid tissue (Neumann et al 1985). Lymphomas account for approximately 4% of the newly diagnosed malignant tumours in the UK. The incidence is rising and this is only partly due to the emergence of AIDS. In children, lymphoma is the third most frequent malignancy, following behind leukaemia and central nervous system neoplasia.

Lymphomas commonly present as enlargement of one or groups of lymph nodes causing painless rubbery lumps under the skin. Disease can also present in extranodal lymphatic tissue and mimic a multitude of other diseases in these tissues. As a group the lym-

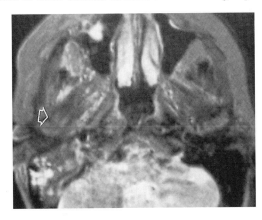

Fig. 17.28 Long-term reassessment of a patient who had previously had a parotid malignancy resected, now with clinical suspicion of recurrence, shows considerable distortion of the architecture, but the low signal intensity on T_2-weighted MRI sequences suggested the scar tissue (arrow) to be benign. This was confirmed at subsequent re-exploration.

phomas vary enormously in outlook, but all will reduce life expectancy if untreated. Treatment for lymphoma has been transformed by refinement of histology, staging and radiotherapy techniques but particularly by the advent of combination chemotherapy (De Vita et al 1970). This has a large impact on radiology, with imaging being used over large periods of time to finesse management. This is particularly important in the case of Hodgkin's disease where 15–20 years after treatment the cumulative mortality from the complications of treatment is greater than the disease itself. Therefore it is becoming increasingly important to reduce the complications of all stages of management including radiology (Mauch et al 1995).

The lymphomas are a heterogeneous group of diseases with variable manifestations and prognosis. The histological subtype and the anatomical extent of disease at the time of diagnosis have prognostic significance. A practicable histological classification is the key to the appropriate investigation and management of patients with lymphoma (Callihan et al 1980). The first and most important distinction is between Hodgkin's disease and the non-Hodgkin lymphomas (NHLs). This is important as Hodgkin's disease has particular characteristics primarily presenting as nodal or splenic disease and generally involving contiguous nodal sites rather than skipping from one group to another. This has a profound effect on management and therefore treatment.

HODGKIN'S DISEASE

Hodgkin's disease accounts for approximately 25% of newly diagnosed lymphomas. The disease may present at any age, but characteristically has a peak incidence in young adulthood, with a second peak incidence in old age. The disease is slightly more common in males. The aetiology of Hodgkin's disease is obscure but diagnosis rests on the identification of the neoplastic binucleated Reed–Sternberg cell or its mononucleated variant, the Hodgkin cell. Although these cells may only make up 1% of the total cellular content they are considered to be the pathological cell type. These cells are not pathognomonic and should be assessed in the presence of the surrounding cytological and architectural background (Gupta & Lister 1995). The histological diagnosis is therefore difficult, and the radiologist should not hesitate to question the diagnosis if the radiological findings are atypical. Fine-needle aspiration cytology is rarely helpful, and every effort should be made to obtain an adequate specimen for histological review. This usually requires the surgical excision of enlarged lymph nodes.

After a time the disease begins to spread by contiguity through the lymphatic system. Hematogenous dissemination is a late phenomenon and almost invariably follows splenic involvement. The orderly spread of disease through the lymphatic system has important therapeutic considerations. Localised disease may be irradiated and cure anticipated. The radiation portals may be chosen to include both the obvious disease sites and the adjacent lymph node groups, which may in turn be the site of occult involvement. This is known as extended field irradiation, and differs from the more standard involved field techniques commonly employed in other tumours. The use of the extended field technique in Hodgkin's disease is an example of how knowledge generated by clinical, radiological and surgical mapping of disease can be used to modify treatment successfully.

Lymph nodes involved with Hodgkin's disease will enlarge, and eventually disease will spread extranodally into the adjacent tissues. The four stages of nodal involvement described above may be recognised. True tumour invasion of surrounding organs and structures is a late phenomenon in patients with Hodgkin's disease. CT scanning will initially demonstrate contiguity between the enlarged lymph nodes and adjacent structures, but early tumour invasion of contiguous structures is difficult to recognise radiologically.

The histopathological classification of Hodgkin's disease, now widely accepted, was developed by Lukes et al (1966) and subsequently accepted at the Rye Conference. In essence there are four subgroups of Hodgkin's disease. Three of these are related—at least in part—to the strength of the host reaction *lymphocyte-predominant* (LP) indicating a strong host response *lymphocyte-depleted* (LD) indicating a very weak response, and *mixed-cellularity* (MC) indicating an intermediate group with an intermediate and moderate immune response (Castellino 1986).

Patients with the LP form almost invariably present with a localised disease, often with palpable supraclavicular lymph nodes. This variety is most frequently seen in young asymptomatic males. On histologicl review of the excised lymph nodes, the characteristic Reed–Sternberg cells are scanty. This form of Hodgkin's disease has an excellent prognosis, and may be treated with local rather than systemic therapy.

The typical patient with the LD form of Hodgkin's disease is older, usually polysymptomatic, and on investigation will be found to have advanced disseminated disease. Histological review of excised lymph nodes will show numerous Reed–Sternberg cells. The prognosis is very poor. Both lymphocyte-depleted and lymphocyte-predominant subtypes may be reclassified as B-cell non-Hodgkin's lymphomas (Gupta & Lister 1995).

MC Hodgkin's disease is the most frequently seen of these three histopathological subtypes. It may be seen in every age group, but is especially frequent in young adults. Patients with MC disease are often symptomatic and are more likely to have abdominal disease than the nodular sclerosing subtype. Patients presenting with lymphoma may have many symptoms. Pruritis is not uncommon but is not related to prognosis. Three specific signs and symptoms in patients with Hodgkin's disease, known as the *B symptoms*, are related to prognosis, and are unexplained weight loss of more than 10% body weight in the preceding 6 months, unexplained fever above 38.4°C and/or night sweats. B symptoms suggest that the disease may involve abdominal lymph nodes and/or the spleen. The

prognosis of MC Hodgkin's disease lies between that of LP and LD disease. LP or MC variants may progress to LD or even to a NHL.

The fourth histological subtype of Hodgkin's disease is *nodular sclerosing* (NS). This is the only subgroup more common in female patients. Typically patients present in adolescence or early adulthood, and almost invariably the mediastinal and supraclavicular lymph node groups are involved. Histologically, lymph nodes involved with NS Hodgkin's disease will show a thick fibrous rim. Recent attention has focused on the contents within this connective tissue reaction, and it is now felt that there are subgroups within NS Hodgkin's disease. These subgroups can be divided into type I with a strong host response and a good prognosis, and type II with a weak host response and a poor prognosis. Most patients with NS Hodgkin's disease will have a good prognosis, and unlike the LP and MC subtypes, NS Hodgkin's disease rarely progresses to a stage with a less favourable histology.

The presence of fibrous stroma around the lymph nodes is important radiologically. Patients with NS Hodgkin's disease typically have large lymph nodes at presentation. These slowly reduce in size on successful therapy, and it is not uncommon for residual soft-tissue masses to persist. Interpretation of radiological findings at this time may be difficult. The temptation to overdiagnose poor response to treatment and/or residual active disease should be resisted. A surveillance strategy can therefore be used with early repeat scanning. If the original staging showed bulk disease then radiotherapy can be added to a chemotherapy protocol. Other imaging strategies would include gallium-67 scan or PET imaging to investigate for any active disease.

Hodgkin's lymphoma virtually always presents as nodal disease that progresses contiguously to adjacent nodal groups. Prognosis therefore depends on the anatomical extent of disease at the time of presentation. Furthermore treatment can concentrate on affected sites rather than systemic disease, such as using radiotherapy as opposed to chemotherapy. Staging for Hodgkin's disease therefore takes this into account. The Ann Arbor staging system has been accepted for many years (Carbone et al 1971). In this system, lymph nodes are considered part of clearly defined lymph node groups, for example left neck and left axilla. Involvement of one or more lymph nodes within a group is considered to represent involvement of that group. This system was modified in 1989 to take account of the increasing use of CT for staging and therefore clinical staging rather than the pathological staging using laparotomy, splenectomy and lymph node sampling (Lister et al 1989). The Cotswold modification also introduces the concept of bulk disease (stage X) to describe bulk nodal disease of greater than 10 cm or greater than one-third chest diameter on CXR at T5. (Table 17.1, Fig. 17.29)

This classification makes a distinction between localised extranodal involvement (stage 1, 2 or 3 E) and disseminated extranodal involvement stage 4. Local involvement is either lymphoma originating in the extranodal lymphatic tissue of the organ such as localised gastric lymphoma (stage 1E) or direct spread from involved nodes into extranodal sites such as mediastinal nodal disease spreading into lung (in the presence of neck nodes, stage IIE). Disseminated involvement of extranodal sites implies haematogenous (or metastatic) spread and is therefore systemic disease. The B symptoms listed are an important prognostic marker and increase the likelihood of disseminated disease.

Stage 3 and 4 Hodgkin's lymphoma are treated with chemotherapy, normally ABVD (doxorubicin (previously Adriamycin), bleomycin,

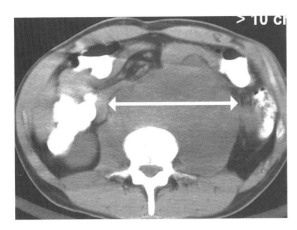

Fig. 17.29 CT examination of the abdomen demonstrating bulk retro-peritoneal lymph node disease (stage X).

vincristine and dacarbazine). The increasing use of chemotherapy in early-stage disease has made accurate staging less important. This means the radiologist must be aware of the potential treatment strategies to be used. It should be noted that diagnosis of splenic disease is difficult without laparotomy, with only one-third of enlarged spleens being involved and one-third of splenic involvement not causing enlargement. Also nodal disease in Hodgkin's lymphoma may be small and discrete. Occult abdominal disease may therefore be missed. Treatment can therefore take two strategies. First, those patients with good prognosis disease, such as type I nodular sclerosing Hodgkin's lymphoma, with no B symptoms, are unlikely to have more advanced disease and may have extended field radiotherapy. Second, if occult disease manifests itself later in a few patients they can be successfully salvaged with chemotherapy.

NON-HODGKIN LYMPHOMAS

NHLs are a much more heterogeneous group of malignant tumours than the Hodgkin's lymphomas (Bragg et al 1986). They are most frequently seen in the elderly. They differ from Hodgkin's disease in that nodal disease is not contiguous, extranodal presentation and spread is common and the disease normally presents as stage 3 or 4 (often with bone marrow involvement).

The origin and subtypes of the NHLs may be considered as follows. In fetal life T- and B-lymphocyte precursors are formed: T cells migrate to the thymus and eventually mature into helper T cells or suppressor/cytotoxic T cells, and leave the thymus to circulate around the body. The T cell antigens on these cells may be recognised by monoclonal antibody techniques. After circulating around the body, T cells accumulate in the lymph nodes and in the spleen. B cells are formed in the liver and migrate to bone marrow. Subsequently they may also be found in lymph nodes, but the T cells and the B cells are found in different parts of the lymph node. The T cells remain paracortical while the B cells are found within the lymphoid follicles. Depending on their nuclear morphology, two subgroups of B-cell types within the follicle may be recognised: B cells with large round nuclei are known as centroblasts (non-cleaved), while those with irregular nuclei are known as centrocytes or cleaved cells. B cells may be found within the circulation, where they are known as plasma cells. Monocytes from the circulation may lodge in the body tissues, where they are known as histiocytes. Histiocytes are thought to be a third possible cell of origin for the NHLs, but *histiocytic lymphomas* account for fewer than 5% of the NHLs.

The majority of NHLs arise from the follicular cells within the lymph node follicle, and may consist of cells that appear cleaved, non-cleaved, or a mixture of the two. Although most NHLs are of B-cell origin and have a tendency to form follicles, they do not all form typical follicles. In practice, many show tumour infiltration throughout the affected lymph node. From this simple observation two important subgroups may be recognised—those that tend to remain in the follicles and are *follicular* (or *nodular*) and those that show the diffusion of tumour cells into the remainder of the lymph node and are called *diffuse*. On occasion, both diffuse and follicular features may be seen within the same excised lymph node, or within two lymph nodes excised from the same patient at the same time. Finally, follicular lymphomas may evolve into diffuse large cell forms as part of their natural history.

Follicular lymphomas are usually low grade while diffuse lymphomas are generally intermediate or high grade. T-cell lymphomas (10% of the total) are found in the skin and thymus from peripheral T cells.

NHLs frequently present as painless enlargement of lymph nodes, but the disease may also develop at a number of extranodal sites, leading to a wide variety of presenting features.

There have been many attempts to classify the pathological appearances of the tumour, but the terminology unfortunately remains confusing. Probably the greatest difficulty in understanding the nomenclature of NHLs is the lack of a normal cellular counterpart (such as squamous cell carcinoma, etc.). The National Cancer Institute Working Party (NCI 1981) considered all the contemporary classifications and proposed a working formulation, dividing the NHLs into low-, intermediate- and high-grade groups. Classification and understanding of lymphomas is improving and becoming more reproducible with the use of immunophenotyping and genetic techniques. New entities are being discovered such as the low-grade lymphoma of mucosa-associated lymphoid tissue (MALT). With this expanding knowledge there will be a divergence of the classic low-grade/high-grade distinctions with more individual histological subtypes having different prognoses and treatment protocols. A recent classification taking this information into account is the REAL classification (Harris et al 1994). Radiologists (along with most clinicians) may find this artificial and still prefer to divide their patients into two groups, the low-grade nodular or *follicular lymphomas* and the high-grade *diffuse lymphomas*.

Nodal presentations of the NHLs

The most common site is the neck, and, unlike Hodgkin's disease, the lymphoid tissue of Waldeyer's ring is usually involved. The patient will frequently have nodal enlargement at a number of palpable and radiologically obvious sites. These are often non-contiguous, and if the lymph nodes are followed up without treatment they may be found to spontaneously fluctuate in size. A patient with NHL is much more likely to present with enlarged lymph nodes in unusual sites, for example those of the elbow or knee, than a patient with Hodgkin's disease. The secondary effects of lymph node enlargement such as limb swelling or superior vena cava obstruction are not uncommon. Backache is suggestive of retroperitoneal lymph node involvement, and constitutional symptoms, especially weight loss, fever and anorexia, are typical.

The Ann Arbor approach to staging may be used for the NHLs, however the majority of patients, especially those with follicular lymphomas, will have widespread disease (stage III or IV) at presentation. Stage will therefore have little impact on prognosis, which depends primarily on histology, disease bulk, plasma lactate dehydrogenase level (LDH) and the presence of B symptoms.

Only about one-third of patients will have clinically localised disease at presentation. Of these, fewer than one-half will still have limited disease by the time they have been fully staged radiologically. This small subgroup (about one-sixth of the total) is important if local radiotherapy is to be considered as a curative option. With true stage I diffuse lymphoma there is a 90% chance of long-term disease-free survival. With stage II disease the proportion of patients free of relapse at 5 years falls to 40%. For this reason, chemotherapy is usually given in stage II disease unless the patient is elderly or there is some contraindication to its use. In early-stage follicular lymphomas local radiotherapy will achieve symptomatic control, and over 70% of patients may well be alive after 10 years. But patients with a follicular lymphoma will relapse and cannot ever be regarded as cured. Unlike Hodgkin's disease, where there is an orderly spread of disease by contiguity through the lymph nodes, the spread of NHL does not follow a contiguous pattern, and there is no clinical advantage in planning extended rather than involved field irradiation. Palliative local radiotherapy is important, especially in the elderly, and good short-term local control is to be expected. In such patients extensive investigation is not warranted.

Most patients with NHL will have extensive disease and qualify for chemotherapy. In such instances the finer nuances of radiological staging are no longer required for treatment planning. However, some idea of tumour extent and bulk is important in assessing response to chemotherapy and for comparison of results. In most patients with diffuse NHL, combination chemotherapy is required. Currently standard treatment regimens are based around the 'CHOP' regimen (cyclophosphamide, doxorubicin, vincristine and prednisolone). There are many newer regimens being studies with an emphasis not only on efficacy for remission induction but also short- and long-term toxicity. All will produce a complete response in approximately 75% of patients; of these, three-quarters will still be alive after 5 years. The prognosis is worse in men, in patients with large abdominal nodal masses and in those with hepatic or marrow involvement. The proportion of complete responders is greatest in those with stage II disease, and falls to 60% in those with stage III disease, and to 35% in those patients with stage IV disease. The prognosis for incomplete responders is poor, and almost all these patients will be dead in 2 years. Recent attention has focused on early use of ultra-high-dose therapy with autologous bone marrow grafting for both Hodgkin's and NHLs in relapsed or poorly responding disease.

Advanced *follicular (low-grade) lymphomas* are often treated expectantly, as there is little evidence that any treatment alters the outcome. Patients are usually treated symptomatically either with local irradiation and/or chemotherapy. The younger patient may occasionally be given combination chemotherapy, more in the hope than anticipation of cure. Long-term chemotherapy has been advocated for low-grade lymphomas. Unfortunately, this approach may lead to bone marrow depression and drug resistance. This may be important if the disease progresses to the diffuse form, and intensive chemotherapy then offers the only hope of disease control.

The majority of *T-cell lymphomas* are seen in younger patients, often with large mediastinal masses. The tumours are aggressive, with short histories, constitutional symptoms, bone marrow involvement and, frequently, central nervous system spread with leptomeningitis, nerve palsy, root compression and increased intracranial pressure. The prognosis is poor, and systemic treatment is required.

Extranodal presentations of the NHLs

Extranodal sites of disease are commonly found on detailed staging of patients with a primary nodal presentation (Glazer et al 1983). Previously treated nodal disease may relapse extranodally. The NHLs may also present at an extranodal site without clinically obvious nodal disease. These patients may be difficult to diagnose and to treat. Histology demonstrates that in advanced NHL extranodal disease is considerably more common than is recognised on imaging.

GASTROINTESTINAL LYMPHOMA

The *small bowel* and *stomach* are the most frequent sites of involvement. In the small bowel the disease is believed to originate within the lymphoid tissue of the mucosal lining. For this reason it is most frequently seen where there is the most lymphoid tissue present. The incidence increases from the duodenum through the jejunum to the ileum. The disease may be single- or multifocal, and grows eventually to ulcerate through the mucosal bowel wall and serosa. Ultimately the regional lymph nodes are involved. The disease may progress to bowel obstruction and perforation. Most patients have *diffuse high-grade NHL of B-cell origin*. Patients with longstanding coeliac disease may develop *T-cell lymphomas*, and these respond poorly to treatment. The incidence of gastrointestinal lymphoma has increased sharply over the past few years, especially those cases associated with immunosuppression (Turowski & Basson 1995).

The clinical presentation of the bowel lymphomas is varied. Many patients present acutely with abdominal pain and have urgent surgery. The diagnosis may be made after an often incomplete resection and exploration of the abdomen. Complete resection of the tumour with no evidence of spread beyond the bowel is associated with a significantly better prognosis. NHL of the gut may present subacutely, and the diagnosis is then suggested at barium examination or CT scanning. Blackledge et al (1979) suggested a simple staging system for gastrointestinal lymphoma that is useful prognostically. Treatment of gut NHL depends on histology, stage and the presence or absence of residual disease. The present therapeutic trend is toward the use of combination chemotherapy unless the tumour is both low grade and of limited extent. Small-bowel lymphoma is the most common paediatric bowel tumour, almost invariably involves the terminal ileum, and is of intermediate or high grade.

Stomach lymphomas often mimic adenocarcinomas clinically, with nausea and weight loss being the usual presentation symptoms (Fig. 17.30). The diagnosis may be suggested by the CT appearances (Doyle & Dixon 1994). For local disease treatment is surgical, followed by combination chemotherapy.

A further gastric lymphoma is the low-grade lymphoma of mucosa-associated lymphoid tissue (MALToma). These lymphomas

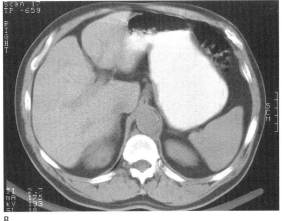

Fig. 17.30 CT scans through the abdomen of a patient with gastric NHL showing thickening of the gastric wall and prominence of the rugal folds, with associated nodal disease, (A) before (B) and after treatment.

have been linked to *Helicobacter pylori* infection and stage 1E disease can be cured by *H. pylori* eradication therapy. Accurate staging is therefore crucial (Ferreri et al 1998).

CENTRAL NERVOUS SYSTEM LYMPHOMA

Primary NHL represents about 1% of primary brain tumours (Fig. 17.31). The incidence is highest in immunocompromised patients, especially those with AIDS or renal transplants or on long-term immunosuppression for some other reason. Patients rarely develop systemic lymphoma, either at the time of diagnosis or later. Detailed systemic staging is superfluous. Treatment is primarily irradiation, and the prognosis is poor. Primary Hodgkin's disease of the brain is rare.

Secondary central nervous system lymphoma is not uncommon. It is most frequently seen in high-grade tumours, especially in children and those with T-cell disease. Approximately 50% of these patients with central nervous system involvement will develop cord compression, while the other 50% will show evidence of lymphomatous meningitis with nerve and root lesions, raised intracranial pressure and mental confusion. Central nervous system involvement is also a feature of testicular, orbital head/ neck primary sites. At all times when CT or MRI scanning any patient with a known lymphoma, the *paravertebral tissues* should be closely examined; involvement here may portend cord compression (Fig. 17.32). *Orbital lymphomas* (Fig. 17.33) almost always disseminate systemically. This is especially true if the disease is bilateral and/or involves neck lymph nodes. CT of the head and neck is the single most useful staging investigation.

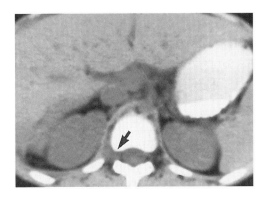

Fig. 17.32 CT scan showing normal fat and soft-tissue densities in the left paravertebral area. On the right the fat in the paravertebral area is obliterated by lymphoma tissue (arrow), which is closely applied to the nerve root exit foramen. The paravertebral tissues should be systematically reviewed when CT scanning any patient with malignant disease, so that lesions may be detected and treated prior to the onset of cord compression.

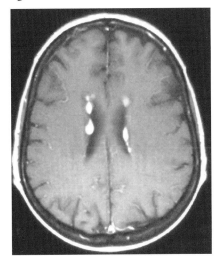

Fig. 17.31 T$_1$-weighted contrast-enhanced axial MRI of the brain showing periventricular enhancing nodules in disseminated mantle cell lymphoma.

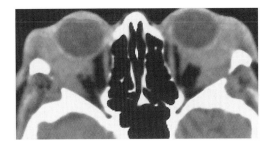

Fig. 17.33 CT scan through the orbits of a patient presenting with orbital NHL. Diffuse thickening of the tissues is seen bilaterally.

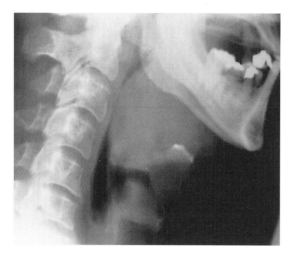

Fig. 17.34 Lateral soft-tissue radiograph of the neck showing abnormal soft tissue from a primary NHL of the neck arising in the epiglottis and presenting with dysphagia.

HEAD AND NECK LYMPHOMA

Primary nodal lymphomas arising in the head and neck do not require CT staging of the neck. An experienced clinician should be able to palpate enlarged lymph nodes within the neck. Abdominal CT staging is useful, as the disease often relapses outside the head and neck, typically in the gastrointestinal tract. Extranodal NHL of the head and neck is usually associated with disease dissemination in the body and a poor prognosis (Fig. 17.34).

THORACIC LYMPHOMA

Involvement of the lungs is a common feature of both NHL (Fig. 17.35) and Hodgkin's disease. In high-grade NHL, pulmonary involvement may be extensive and explosive, the radiological appearances often mimicking those seen in infection. Low-grade NHL may also involve the lungs. Typically, many of these low-grade tumours are indolent, often in the past being described as pseudolymphomas. Some of these arise in the bronchus-associated lymphoid tissue.

In patients with more typical variants of NHL, thoracic involvement of the lungs and mediastinum is less common than for Hodgkin's disease and is normally associated with disease elsewhere.

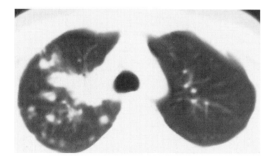

Fig. 17.35 CT scan showing pulmonary involvement in a patient with NHL. A mass of tumour tissue is seen around the right hilum. In addition, a number of ill-defined intrapulmonary nodules are seen on the right.

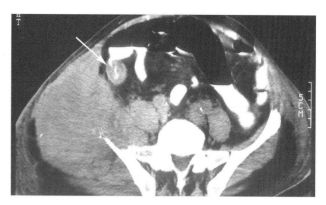

Fig. 17.36 Abdominal CT examination of a patient with NHL showing secondary involvement of the iliac bone. Note also the involvement of the terminal ileum demonstrated by the use of oral contrast.

BONE LYMPHOMA

Bone marrow involvement is commonly found in the NHLs (Fig. 17.36). On occasion a patient will present with an apparent primary bone NHL. These are most common in younger patients, and involve the appendicular skeleton, especially in the metaphyseal region. Radiologically, the most common appearance is a permeative destructive lesion. Pathologically, the lesions are typically high grade. Full radiological staging of the abdomen and chest should be undertaken, and a high percentage of patients will prove to have disseminated disease. Recent work has suggested that while MRI and CT are comparable in their ability to detect lymphadenopathy, MRI is significantly better than CT in demonstrating occult marrow infiltration (Hoane et al 1994), and this may eventually make MRI the preferred imaging modality for the staging of lymphoma.

TESTICULAR LYMPHOMA

Testicular lymphomas occur in middle-aged and elderly men. Twenty-five per cent will be bilateral. Testicular NHL is aggressive, high grade, and tends to spread not only to the regional lymph nodes in the abdomen but also to lung, the central nervous system, and in the neck to Waldeyer's ring.

CROSS-SECTIONAL IMAGING IN LYMPHOMA

THORAX

CT is the current 'gold standard' for evaluating the extent of thoracic involvement in patients with Hodgkin's disease and, when required, for those with NHL. The pattern of lymphomatous involvement is different for Hodgkin's disease and NHL. In addition, the therapeutic implications of any positive findings in these two conditions also differ.

Intravenous contrast is helpful in assessing the mediastinum, and is crucial to the complete CT evaluation of the lung hila. This is less important in follow-up imaging. The presence of intravenous contrast medium is not detrimental to the imaging of the lung fields, and when it is to be used, precontrast studies are not warranted.

Normal mediastinal structures, in particular blood vessels, should be routinely identified. Normal-sized lymph nodes may on occasion be seen within the mediastinal fat, but this would appear to be a less common observation in the UK than in the USA. CT sections through the mediastinum of a patient with lymphoma should clearly demonstrate the extent of adenopathy. CT identifies abnormal lymph nodes by an abnormal increase in the cross-sectional diameter of the lymph nodes. Typically, mediastinal lymph nodes more than 1 cm in diameter are interpreted as being involved. Hilar nodal enlargement usually follows mediastinal involvement, at least in Hodgkin's disease. Micrometastases occurring in normal-sized mediastinal lymph nodes cannot be diagnosed on CT, and, equally, nodal enlargement for non-malignant reasons may not be discriminated from malignant enlargement. Care should be taken to recognise any aberrant vessels that may mimic adenopathy, particularly on non-contrast-enhanced scans. The superior pericardial recess may also be confused for adenopathy but normally has lower density and a concave anterior border.

HODGKIN'S DISEASE

The anterior mediastinum is the focus from which Hodgkin's disease of the chest appears to spread (MacDonald et al 1987). It is extremely uncommon to have disease at other sites within the thorax in the absence of anterior mediastinal involvement. Recognition of adenopathy at this site is the first step to successful CT scan interpretation. The typical CT appearance of a nodal mass in a patient with Hodgkin's disease is usually that of a homogeneous soft-tissue mass with sharply defined and often lobulated borders. Occasionally the centre of the nodal mass contains an area of decreased attenuation due to necrosis. If intravenous contrast medium has been given, the lymph node may enhance. It should be noted that in many cases CXR actually gives all the information needed to manage the patient. However, conventional radiographs will only recognise an abnormality in this region when the contour of the mediastinum and its pleural reflections is altered. In general, enlarged lymph nodes on the right side of the mediastinum are easier to identify on plain chest radiography than those on the left side, where the overlying shadow of the aortic arch makes small-volume adenopathy more difficult to recognise. Castellino et al (1986) reviewed the contribution that CT scanning of the thorax made in their Hodgkin's disease practice. From their study it is clear that CT will demonstrate abnormal lymph nodes more readily than conventional X-ray techniques within the thorax. Furthermore, as CT is increasingly available and is necessary in the abdomen the extra information available from CT of the thorax should be obtained.

Primary Hodgkin's disease is managed by chemotherapy or radiotherapy or a combination of both. The most profound impact on management might be expected in those patients being considered for radiotherapy. CT demonstration of the extent of disease at a particular site may influence the size of the proposed fields, and CT demonstration of disease at previously unsuspected sites, particularly in the posterior mediastinum and diaphragmatic area, may lead to a change in management from radiotherapy to chemotherapy. Thus, mediastinal CT in Hodgkin's disease is of most value when a high proportion of patients are being considered for radiotherapy. When the patient is to have chemotherapy from the start, then the more precise demonstration of disease extent within the thorax is of no immediate consequence. The value of CT scanning of the mediastinum in these patients is limited to baseline studies for the monitoring of response and assessment of residual changes. In any institution the proportion of patients considered for radiotherapy will vary, and it is this that accounts for differing opinions on the impact of mediastinal CT on the management of patients with Hodgkin's disease. Studies from different institutions confirm that the value of mediastinal CT in patients with Hodgkin's disease is maximal in those who are being considered for radiation therapy.

A decrease in size of previously enlarged lymph nodes also serves as an indicator of response to chemotherapy. In many instances this can be adequately assessed on serial chest radiographs but—especially when the chest radiograph has returned to normal—the CT scan may show residual adenopathy. Interpretation of this residual adenopathy may be difficult. Serial MRI and/or gallium-67 studies beginning before treatment commences may help distinguish active from inactive disease following chemotherapy. This is of potential value in tailoring the chemotherapy regimen (and toxicity) to the individual (Abrahamsen et al 1994).

CT scanning of the lungs may show evidence of Hodgkin's disease. The most characteristic finding is the presence of one or more nodules within the parenchyma. They are most frequently seen near the lung bases and/or the pulmonary hila, suggesting a haematogenous spread. The demonstration of these would classify the case as stage IV according to the Ann Arbor convention. As with other small pulmonary nodules, CT has a small advantage over conventional chest radiographs in the demonstration of smaller pulmonary lesions. In lymphoma these small focal changes are often poorly defined.

Lymphoma may involve the lung fields in a variety of other ways. These include patchy pulmonary shadowing, pulmonary consolidation and lobar collapse. Pulmonary involvement is uncommon in the patient with newly diagnosed Hodgkin's disease, being seen at most in 10% of patients. Parenchymal lesions in newly presented patients who have no mediastinal or hilar adenopathy are best considered not to represent Hodgkin's disease. Pulmonary disease is a feature of recurrent Hodgkin's disease, where it may be confused not only with infection but also with the effects of treatment. These include pulmonary consolidation and fibrosis following radiotherapy, drug reactions, and opportunistic infections during or following systemic chemotherapy.

A frequent concern to the clinician is the possibility of early tumour infiltration from enlarged hilar lymph nodes into the surrounding lung tissue. This is well recognised and indicated in the Ann Arbor staging system as, for example, stage IIE disease. Although this is a frequent indication for requesting thoracic CT, in practice it is exceptional to detect this infiltration on CT unless the chest radiograph is abnormal.

CT may be helpful in assessing the patency and diameter of airways, especially in children. Over half the children presenting with Hodgkin's disease show significant airway obstruction on CT examination, and occasionally this may require emergency treatment.

CT is ideally suited to demonstrating pleural and pleurally based lesions. These include *solid plaques* of tumour tissue and *pleural effusions*. It is important to remember that most pleural effusions seen in patients with Hodgkin's disease are benign, and are thought to be a consequence of lymphatic obstruction secondary to mediastinal and hilar lymph node involvement and enlargement.

NON-HODGKIN LYMPHOMAS

The contribution that thoracic CT scanning might make in the management of patients with NHL is less certain, for several reasons. NHL is more likely than Hodgkin's disease to be widespread and require systemic therapy, the mediastinum is a less frequent site of disease, and in many instances the presence of mediastinal involvement will be recognised on a routine chest radiograph. Lung involvement is uncommon, and is seen in fewer than 5% of patients at diagnosis. The presence of a pleural effusion in NHL usually reflects the presence of pleural tumour. This is a reflection of the lower incidence of mediastinal adenopathy seen in NHL than in Hodgkin's disease.

A survey concluded that the addition of CT scanning to the diagnostic work-up of patients presenting with a new NHL may occasionally show additional sites of disease but does not result in a change in management.

ABDOMEN

CT is now the standard method of imaging the abdomen in patients with lymphoma. In one study of 168 patients presenting with a NHL (Pond et al 1989), 29% had abdominal disease detectable only on CT scanning. Protocols depend on equipment used. Adequate opacification of bowel with oral contrast media is essential (Fig. 17.37). Intravenous contrast is helpful at staging to detect extranodal disease although it is less important in follow-up scanning. A good knowledge of vascular anatomy and variants is important in diagnosing lymphadenopathy (Fig. 17.38). Abnormal lymph nodes may be recognised by an increase in size. Retroperitoneal nodes greater than 1.5 cm in diameter are considered abnormal. Particular attention should be paid to the retrocrural region (Fig. 17.39) (where nodes greater than 0.6 cm in diameter are regarded as pathological), the retroperitoneum, the pelvic lymph nodes and (especially in patients with NHL) the mesenteric lymph nodes. Involvement of the spleen or liver is often difficult to detect. On occasion, focal deposits may be seen in the spleen or liver (Fig. 17.40); more typically, lymphomatous involvement results in an increase in the size of the affected organ. This may be obvious, but in many cases early involvement is especially difficult to diagnose. In addition, in patients with Hodgkin's disease the spleen may enlarge in the absence of direct involvement, leading to possible radiological overstaging.

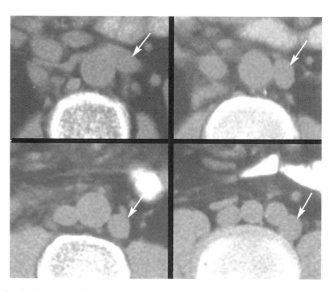

Fig 17.38   Left-sided IVC (arrows) draining into the left renal vein. This may be mistaken for lymphadenopathy. Although intravenous contrast was not used the correct diagnosis was made due to knowledge of anatomy and its variants.

HEAD, NECK AND SPINE

Enlarged lymph nodes in the neck are usually palpable. CT may demonstrate non-palpable lymph node enlargement and/or central necrosis within the lymph node, the latter being a certain sign of a pathological condition. In addition, CT imaging may show that a

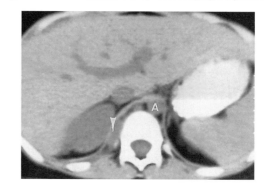

Fig. 17.39   CT scan on a patient with NHL shows enlargement of the retrocrural lymph nodes (arrowhead). A = aorta.

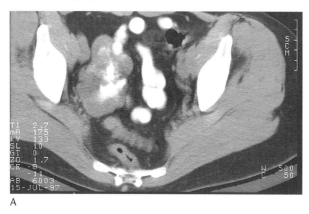

A

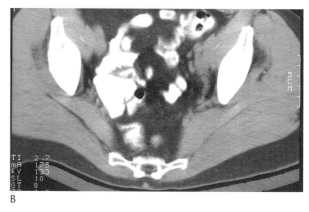

B

Fig. 17.37   (A) Possible terminal ileal lymphoma in a symptomatic patient with previous abdominal radiation. (B) Adequate bowel opacification shows this to be caecum. (See also Fig. 17.38)

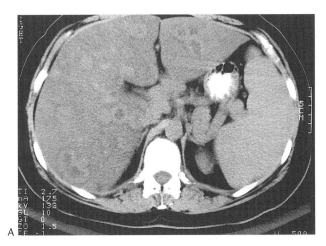
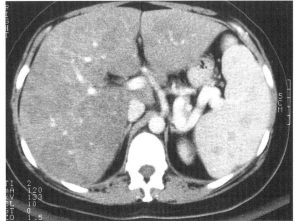

Fig. 17.40 (A,B) Adult T-cell lymphoma presenting with liver and spleen disease. Although in this case the use of intravenous contrast demonstrated splenic involvement it did not change patient management.

single palpable mass consists of a conglomerate mass of several enlarged lymph nodes, an observation that may alter staging and prognosis of primary head and neck cancers. CT examination of the neck is usually performed during the dynamic infusion of intravenous contrast medium, which allows all the vascular structures to be highlighted, and in addition may demonstrate ring enhancement of lymph nodes with metastatic squamous carcinomas. With MRI, intravenous contrast medium is not required to identify the vessels, and this may be of value in patients who are sensitive to iodine. The MRI characteristics of enlarged lymph nodes are non-specific and do not allow the cause of the enlargement, or whether the underlying pathology is benign or malignant, unless central necrosis is recognised by central high signal on T_2 (or low signal on T_1) or contrast-enhancement characteristics.

The main criterion for abnormality when imaging the neck with CT and/or MRI is an increase in the size. Normally the lymph nodes high in the neck are larger than those lower in the neck, presumably due to benign enlargement secondary to previous recurrent throat infections. It is generally accepted that lymph nodes larger than 1 cm in diameter are abnormal, unless the lymph node is in the jugulodigastric region, where 1.5 cm is a more reasonable upper limit of normal cross-sectional diameter. Using these criteria, approximately 80% of the lymph nodes considered abnormal at CT and/or MRI examination will, under the appropriate clinical conditions, contain tumour.

MRI is the investigation of choice for CNS and spine imaging. MRI provides a more complete picture of the compressive lesion than may be obtained with myelography. MRI may also prove of value in the assessment of bone marrow involvement and complement the information available from bone marrow aspirate and trephine. Lymphoma in the CNS has numerous manifestations and imaging protocols are similar to other CNS indications covered elsewhere in this book.

IMAGING THE COMPLICATIONS OF DISEASE AND THERAPY

The primary purpose of imaging all tumours is to establish the extent of disease along accepted staging frameworks to decide on and monitor treatment and advise on prognosis. However at all stages in this pathway the radiologist should be alert to potential complications of the disease or treatment that do not fit into the direct staging classifications. Lymphoma can invade extranodally to cause a variety of complications, and particular care should be taken in all cases to check for spinal invasion from nodal or extranodal disease as treatment is not as effective once symptoms present (Fig. 17.41).

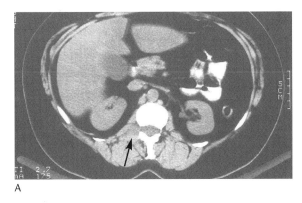
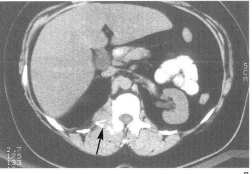

Fig. 17.41 CT scans showing lymphoma in the left paravertebral area (arrows) (A). On follow-up (B) there has been progression with destruction of the transverse process and encroachment on the nerve root exit foramen.

Diffuse extranodal involvement of abdominal organs surprisingly rarely results in functional impairment but lymph node enlargement can obstruct any drainage system. This is seen in biliary dilatation and jaundice due to portal nodes and hydronephrosis secondary to retroperitoneal nodes or bladder lymphoma (Fig. 17.42). If renal function is impaired by ureteric obstruction this can be considered a 'critical organ' to successful therapy. Good renal function is vital for successful chemotherapy, because fast response, as can occur in high-grade lymphomas and leukaemias, can lead to a tumour lysis syndrome and subsequent renal failure.

Anaesthetists should be alerted if there is bulk mediastinal disease prior to any surgical procedure, such as mediastinal biopsy, as this may affect the airway.

Treatment itself can cause a variety of complications. In many cases this is difficult for the radiologist who must be aware of the many causes of acute shadowing on chest radiograph or CT including atypical infections, recurrent disease, haemorrhage and graft versus host disease (Fig. 17.43). Specific chemotherapy agents have different complications including doxorubicin affecting cardiac function, bleomycin and cyclophosphamide causing lung fibrosis, and vincristine causing neuropathy and ileus.

Radiation changes can cause fibrosis in both the chest and abdomen (Fig. 17.44). It should be noted that fibrosis caused by bleomycin is compounded by radiation and this effect can occur months after ceasing bleomycin therapy.

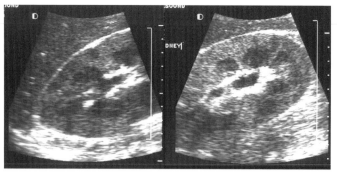

Fig. 17.42 Lymphoma deposits in the kidney as shown by echo-poor areas on ultrasound. These rarely affect renal function but there is early hydronephrosis due to retroperitoneal lymph node disease. If bilateral this should be treated by stents or nephrostomy prior to chemotherapy.

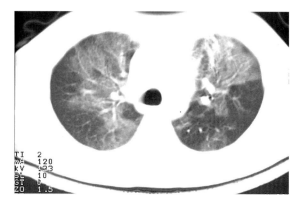

Fig. 17.43 CT examination showing interstitial pulmonary shadowing in an immunosuppressed patient on chemotherapy. In this case the diagnosis was varicella pneumonia.

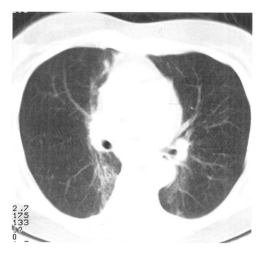

Fig. 17.44 CT examination showing midline fibrosis with linear borders secondary to mediastinal radiotherapy.

REFERENCES AND SUGGESTIONS FOR FURTHER READING

Abrahamsen, A. F., Lien, H. H., Aas, W., et al (1994) Magnetic resonance imaging and (67) gallium scan in mediastinal lymphoma: a prospective pilot study. *Annals of Oncology*, **5**, 433–436.

Allen, E. V., Barker, N. W., Hines, E. A. (1946) *Peripheral Vascular Diseases*. Philadelphia: Saunders.

Amendola, M. A. (1986) CT staging of lymphoma. In: Glazer, G. M. (ed.) *Staging of Neoplasms*, pp. 147–189. New York: Churchill Livingstone.

Bellin, M.F., Beigelman C, Precetti-Morel, S. (2000) Iron oxide-enhanced MR lymphography: initial experience. *European Journal Radiology*, **34**, 257–164.

Blackledge, G., Bush, H., Dodge, O. G., Crowther, D. F. (1979) A study of gastrointestinal lymphoma. *Clinical Oncology*, **5**, 209–219.

Blake, P. R., Carr, D. H., Goolden, A. W. G. (1986) Intracranial Hodgkin's disease. *British Journal of Radiology*, **59**, 414–416.

Bragg, D. G., Colby T. V., Ward J. H. (1986) New concepts in the non-Hodgkin lymphomas: radiological implications. *Radiology*, **159**, 289–304.

Callihan, T. R., Berard, C. W. (1980) The classification and pathology of the lymphomas and leukemias. *Seminars in Roentgenology*, **15**, 203–218.

Carbone, P. P., Kaplan, H. S., Musshoff, K., Smithers, E. W., Tubiana, M. (1971) Report of the Committee on Hodgkin's Disease Staging. *Cancer Research*, **31**, 1860–1861.

Castellino, R. A. (1986) Hodgkin's disease: practical concepts for the diagnostic radiologist. *Radiology*, **159**, 305–310.

Castellino, R. A., Blank, N., Hoppe, R. T., Cho, C. (1986) Hodgkin disease: contributions of chest CT in the initial staging evaluation. *Radiology*, **160**, 603–605.

Cherryman, G. R. (1996) Lymphatic system In: Whitehouse, G. H. Worthington, B. S. (eds) *Techniques in Diagnostic Imaging*, 3rd edn, pp. 236–241. Oxford: Blackwell Science.

Chou, C. K., Chen, L. T., Sheu, R. S., Yang, C. W., Jaw, T. S., Lui, G. C. (1994) MRI manifestations of gastrointestinal lymphoma. *Abdominal Imaging*, **19**, 495–500.

De Vita, V. T., Serpick, A. A., Carbone, P. P. (1970) Combination chemotherapy in the treatment of advanced Hodgkins disease. *Annals of Internal Medicine*, **73**, 891–895.

Dixon, A. K., Ellis, M., Sikora, K. (1986) Computed tomography of testicular tumours: distribution of abdominal lymphadenopathy. *Clinical Radiology*, **37**, 519–523.

Dooms, G. C., Hricak, H., Moseley, M. E., Bottles, K. Fisher, M., Higgens, C. B. (1985) Characterisation of lymphadenopathy by magnetic resonance times: preliminary results. *Radiology*, **155**, 691–697.

Doyle, T. C. A., Dixon, A. K. (1994) Pointers to the diagnosis of gastric lymphoma on computed tomography. *Australasian Radiology*, **38**, 176–178.

Ferreri, A. J., Ponzoni, M., Cordio, S., et al (1998) Low sensitivity of computed tomography in the staging of gastric lymphomas of mucosa-associated lymphoid tissue: impact on prospective trials and ordinary clinical practice. *American Journal of Clinical Oncology*, **21**, 614–616.

Glazer, H. S., Lee, J. K. T., Balfe, D. M., Mauro, M. A., Griffith, R, Sagel, S. S. (1983) Non-Hodgkin lymphoma: computed tomographic demonstration of unusual extranodal involvement. *Radiology,* **149**, 211–217.

Glazer, G. M., Gross, B. H., Quint, L. E., Francis, I. R., Bookstein, F. L., Oninger, M. B. (1985) Normal mediastinal lymph nodes: number and size according to American Thoracic Society Mapping. *American Journal of Roentgenology,* **144**, 261–265.

Gupta, R. K., Lister, T. A. (1995) Hodgkin's disease. In Price, P., Sikora, K (eds) *Treatment of Cancer,* 3rd edn, pp. 851–879. London: Chapman and Hall.

Harris, N. L., Jaffe, E. S., Stein, H., et al (1994) A revised European–American classification of lymphoid neoplasms: a proposal from the international lymphoma study group. *Blood,* **84**, 1361–1392.

Harrison, D. A., Clouse, M. E. (1985) Normal anatomy. In: Clouse, M. E., Wallace, S. (eds) *Lymphatic Imaging,* 2nd edn, pp. 15–94. Baltimore: Williams and Wilkins.

Heron, C. W., Husband, J. E., Williams, M. P., Cherryman, G. R. (1988) The value of thoracic computed tomography in the detection of recurrent Hodgkin's disease. *British Journal of Radiology,* **61**, 567–572.

Hoane, B. R., Shields, A. F., Porter, B. A., Borrow, J. W. (1994) Comparison of initial lymphoma staging using computed tomography (CT) and magnetic resonance (MR) imaging. *American Journal of Hematology,* **47**, 100–105.

Jack, C. R., O'Neill, B. P., Banks, P. M., Reese, D. F. (1988) Central nervous system lymphoma: histological types and CT appearance. *Radiology,* **167**, 211–215.

Kaplan, H. S. (1980) *Hodgkin's Disease,* 2nd edn. Cambridge, MA: Harvard University Press.

Khoury, M. B., Godwin, J. C., Halvorsen, R. A., Hanun, Y., Putman, C. E. (1984) The role of thoracic CT in non-Hodgkin's lymphoma. *Radiology,* **158**, 659–662.

Kiyono, K., Sone, S., Sakai, F., et al (1988) The number and size of normal mediastinal lymph nodes: a postmortem study. *American Journal of Roentgenology,* **150**, 771–778.

Laissy, J. P., Gay-Depassier, P., Soyer, P., et al (1994) Enlarged mediastinal lymph nodes in bronchogenic carcinoma: assessment with dynamic contrast-enhanced MR imaging. Work in progress. *Radiology,* **191**, 263–267.

Lewis, E., Bamardino, M. E., Salvador, P. G., Cabanillas, F. F., Barnes, P. A., Thomas, J. L. (1982) Post therapy CT detected mass in lymphoma: is it viable tissue? *Journal of Computer Assisted Tomography,* **6**, 792–795.

Lister, T. A., Crowther, D., Sutcliffe, S. B., et al (1989) Report of a committee convened to discuss the evaluation and staging of patients with Hodgkin's disease: Cotswolds meeting. *Journal of Clinical Oncology,* **7**, 1630–1636.

Lukes, R. J., Butler, J. J., Hicks, E. B. (1966) Natural history of Hodgkin's disease as related to its pathological picture. *Cancer,* **19**, 317–344.

MacDonald, J. S. (1982) Lymphography in lymph node disease. In: Kinmonth, J.B. (ed.) *The Lymphatics: Surgery, Lymphography and Diseases of the Chyle and Lymph Systems,* pp. 327–370. London: Edward Arnold.

MacDonald, J. S. (1987) Lymphography. In: Ansell, G., Wilkins, R.A. (eds) *Complications in Diagnostic Imaging,* pp. 300–309. Oxford: Blackwell.

MacDonald, J. S., McCready, V. R., Cosgrove, D. O., Cherryman, G. R., Selby, P. (1987) Radiological and other imaging methods. In: Selby, P., McElwain, T. J. (eds) *Hodgkin's Disease,* pp. 126–160. Oxford: Blackwell.

McKusick, K. A. (1985) Radionuclide lymphography. In: Clouse M. E., Wallace, S. (eds) *Lymphatic Imaging,* 2nd edn, pp. 95–111. Baltimore: Williams and Wilkins.

Mauch, P. M., Kalish, L. A., Marcus, K. C., et al (1995) Long term survival in Hodgkin's disease: relative impact of mortalility, second tumours, infection and cerebrovascular disease. *Cancer Journal from Scientific American,* **1**, 33–42.

Meyer, J. E., Linggood, R-M., Lindfors, Y. K., McLoud, T. C., Stomper, P. C. (1984) Impact of thoracic computed tomography on radiation therapy planning in Hodgkin disease. *Journal of Computer Assisted Tomography,* **8**, 892–904.

NCI (National Cancer Institute Sponsored Study of Classification of Non-Hodgkin's Lymphomas) (1981) Summary and description of a working formulation for clinical usage. *Cancer,* **49**, 2112–2135.

Neumann, C. H., Parker, B. R., Castellino, R. A. (1985) Hodgkin's disease and the non-Hodgkin lymphomas. In: Bragg, D. G., Rubin, P., Youker, J. E. (eds) *Oncologic Imaging,* pp. 477–501. New York: Pergamon Press.

O'Donnell, T. F., Jr, Clouse, M. E. (1985) Abnormal peripheral lymphatics. In: Clouse, M. E., Wallace, S. (eds) *Lymphatic Imaging,* 2nd edn, pp. 142–179. Baltimore: Williams and Wilkins.

Oliver, T. W., Bernardino, M. E., Sones, P. J., Jr (1983) Monitoring the response of lymphoma patients to therapy: correlation of abdominal CT findings with clinical course and histological cell type. *Radiology,* **149**, 219–224.

Otsuji, E., Toma, A, Kobayashi, S., et al (2000) Long-term benefit of extended, lymphadenectomy with gastrectomy in distally located early gastric carcinoma. *American Journal of Surgery,* **180**, 127–132.

Pond, G. D., Castellino, R. A., Homing, S., Hoppe, R. T. (1989) Non-Hodgkin lymphoma: influence of lymphography, CT, and bone marrow biopsy on staging and management. *Radiology,* **170**, 159–164.

Sandrasegaran, K., Robinson, P. J., Selby, P. (1994) Staging of lymphoma in adults. *Clinical Radiology,* **49**, 149–191.

Shiels, R. A., Stone, J., Ash, D. V., et al (1984) Priorities for computed tomography and lymphography in the staging and initial management of Hodgkin's disease. *Clinical Radiology,* **35**, 447–449.

Som, P. M. (1987) Lymph nodes of the neck. *Radiology,* **165**, 593–600.

Therasse, P., Arbuck, S. G., Eisenhauer, E. A., et al (2000) New guidelines to evaluate the response to treatment in solid tumors. *Journal of the National Cancer Institute,* **92**, 205–216.

Turowski, G. A., Basson, M. D. (1995) Primary malignant lymphoma of the intestine. *American Journal of Surgery,* **169**, 4333–4341.

UICC (International Union Against Cancer) (1987) *TNM Classification of Malignant Tumours,* 4th edn. Berlin: Springer-Verlag.

Williams, M. P., Cherryman, G. R., Husband, J. E. (1989) Magnetic resonance imaging of spinal cord compression. *Clinical Radiology,* **40**, 286–290.

Witte, C. L., Witte, M. H., Unger, E. C., et al (2000) Advances in imaging of lymph flow disorders. *Radiographics,* **20**, 1697–1719.

Yudd, A. P., Kempf, J. S., Goydos, J. S., Stahl, T. J., Feinstein R. S. (1999) Use of sentinel node lymphoscintigraphy in malignant melanoma. *Radiographics,* **19**, 343–353. (See discussion in *Radiographics,* **19**, 354–356.)

18

THE SALIVARY GLANDS, PHARYNX AND OESOPHAGUS

A. H. A. Chapman

with contributions from John A. Spencer, J. Ashley Guthrie and Philip J. A. Robinson

THE SALIVARY GLANDS

ANATOMY

The parotid gland is located behind the angle of the mandible, with the anterior part of the gland lying on the masseter muscle. It has a large single duct (Stenson's) that runs forwards crossing the masseter muscle, turning inwards at its anterior border to pierce the buccinator muscle and then opening into the mouth on a papilla opposite the second upper molar tooth. The gland is divided into superficial and deep parts and at its anterior margin there is a small separate accessory part which lies between the duct and the zygomatic arch.

The submandibular gland is located below the mandible and has a superficial part that lies on the mylohyoid muscle and a deep part that extends deep to the posterior border of this muscle. A single duct (Wharton's) emerges from the deep surface of the gland, turns around the posterior border of the mylohyoid muscle and runs deep to that muscle to open on a papilla at the side of the frenulum beneath the tongue.

The sublingual gland lies anteriorly in the floor of the mouth and opens into the mouth through a number of ducts. Ducts within all of these glands are evenly distributed and gently tapered (Fig. 18.1).

CT and MRI anatomy

The parotid and submandibular salivary glands are well demonstrated in most patients by both CT and MRI. The parotid glands have variable amounts of fatty stroma and thus have lower CT attenuation (−25 to +15 HU) than adjacent muscles, lymph nodes and vessels (Fig. 18.2). The higher density of the gland in childhood should not be misinterpreted as pathology. Conversely, in some adults the attenuation of the parotid glands approaches that of muscle, and in these dense glands MRI is superior in detection of

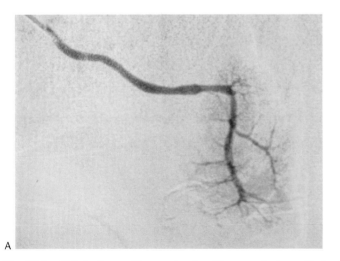
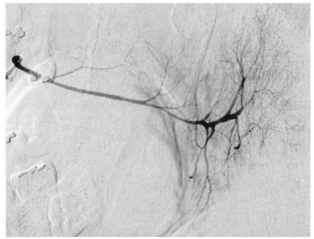

Fig. 18.1 Digital subtracted images showing (A) a normal submandibular sialogram and (B) a normal parotid sialogram. (Courtesy of Dr P. Chennels.)

533

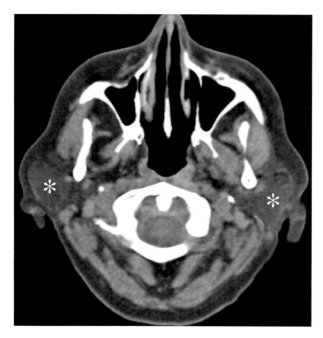

Fig. 18.2 Fatty change in the parotids of an adult—note the low attenuation of the parotid glands (asterisks). (Courtesy of Richard W. Whitehouse.)

mass lesions. The submandibular glands have higher attenuation than the parotid glands but are still easily distinguished from the adjacent musculature. The sublingual salivary glands and minor (accessory) salivary glands which line the upper aerodigestive tract are not routinely visualised. The minor salivary glands may give rise to masses in the parapharyngeal space.

The parotid space lies deep to the subcutaneous fat in the pre-auricular region, encompassed by the superficial layer of the deep cervical fascia, which splits around the parotid gland (Fig. 18.3). The gland extends from the external auditory canal down to or just below the angle of the mandible. The parotid gland is divided into deep and superficial lobes by the facial nerve, but this structure cannot be routinely identified on CT or MRI so the plane between the back of the mandibular ramus and the retromandibular vein is used instead. Also within the parotid space is the external carotid artery, which lies in the deep lobe medial to the retromandibular vein. The deep lobe extends medially to reach the lateral margin of the parapharyngeal

space, and there may be difficulties in distinction between parapharyngeal and deep parotid pathology. There are between 20 and 30 lymph nodes within the parotid gland, making it a site for metastatic disease from the scalp, external auditory canal and face.

The parapharyngeal space lies medial to the parotid space and is bounded anteriorly by the masticator space, posteriorly by the carotid space, and medially by the pharyngeal mucosa (Fig. 18.3). It extends from the skull base to the superior cornu of the hyoid bone and is routinely identified as a triangle of fat on axial CT images. Although it includes the minor salivary glands, primary pathology of this space is unusual but extension of pathology from the parotid space is not uncommon. In view of this, any soft-tissue abnormality identified within this space should be critically assessed to determine whether it has arisen from an adjacent anatomical space (Figs 18.4,18.5).

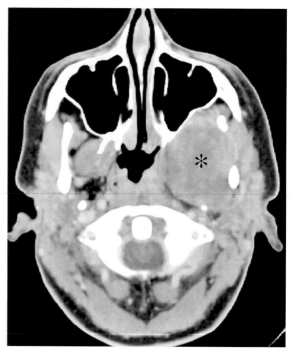

Fig. 18.4 Heterogenous mass (asterisks) filling the parapharyngeal space and displacing all the adjacent spaces. This was a Vth nerve neurofibroma extending down through the skull base into the parapharyngeal space. (Courtesy of Dr J. E. Gillespie.)

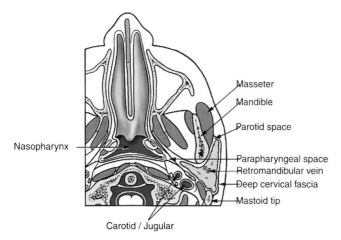

Fig. 18.3 Anatomy of the parotid and parapharyngeal spaces.

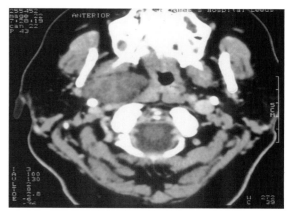

Fig. 18.5 Pleomorphic adenoma in a minor salivary gland resulting in a right-sided parapharyngeal mass.

The submandibular and sublingual glands lie within their respective spaces; they are separated by the mylohyoid muscle anteriorly but the spaces are continuous with each other posteriorly where the posterior part of the sublingual gland and the deep part of the submandibular gland lie in close proximity. The submandibular space is encircled by the superficial layer of the deep cervical fascia and contains the superficial part of the submandibular gland together with submandibular and submental lymph nodes. The sublingual space contains not only the sublingual gland and duct but also the deep portion of the submandibular gland and duct. Masses arising in the submandibular space tend to remain within that space but masses in the sublingual space may extend to the submandibular space. Parotid tail lesions occasionally present as masses at the angle of the mandible and may be mistaken for submandibular masses.

TECHNIQUES

Plain films

Anteroposterior (normal and soft-tissue exposure), tangential, lateral and lateral oblique plain radiographs are useful for showing calculi and soft-tissue swelling of the parotid gland.

The submandibular gland is best shown on a lateral oblique view. This is supplemented by a lateral view obtained with the patient's finger in the mouth, depressing the tongue and pushing the submandibular gland into sight beneath the mandible. Stones in the anterior part of the duct are best demonstrated by placing an occlusal film in the mouth and using a submentovertical type of projection (Fig. 18.6).

Sialography

Sialography can be performed on the parotid and submandibular glands. An initial series of plain films is necessary to identify radio-opaque stones. The examination is usually performed with the

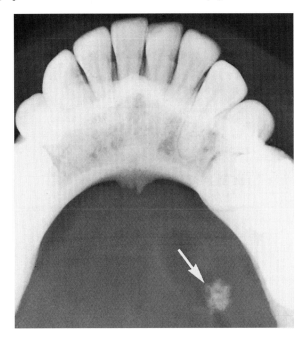

Fig. 18.6 Stone in submandibular duct shown on intraoral view. (Courtesy of Miss Ruth Donaldson.)

patient lying supine on the X-ray table. The appropriate duct orifice is located and intubated by means of either a blunt-tipped, slightly angulated, metal cannula, or a fine thin-walled polythene catheter with a tapered end. In cases of difficulty, a sialogogue such as lemon juice or citric acid can be given, the duct orifice can be dilated or a fine guide-wire can be introduced into the duct, over which a catheter can be advanced. Approximately 0.5–1.5 ml of contrast medium (Lipiodol Ultra Fluid or a water-soluble medium) is slowly injected by hand until the duct system is filled. The injection should stop if the patient experiences discomfort, as trauma from catheterising the duct may result in extravasation of contrast medium into the local tissues; water-soluble contrast media are therefore sometimes preferred as they are rapidly absorbed. However, water-soluble contrast media are quickly washed out of the duct, so the catheter should be left occluding the duct while films are taken. A series of radiographs matching the controls is taken, or subtracted images can be obtained with digital X-ray equipment. To complete the examination, a few drops of lemon juice or citric acid are given for the patient to rinse around the mouth to stimulate salivation. A further film is then taken after an interval of 10 min and normally this postsialogogue film will show most of the contrast medium to have cleared from the ducts.

Sialography is used to diagnose stones, chronic inflammation and tumours in the parotid and submandibular glands. The examination is contraindicated in acute sialadenitis for fear of exacerbating the condition.

Ultrasound

The parotid and submandibular glands are examined using a 7.5 MHz or higher frequency linear array transducer with the patient's chin turned away from the side being examined (Fig. 18.7). Both glands have a homogenous echo pattern with scattered echogenic streaks produced by branch ducts converging to join the main duct. In the parotid gland the external carotid artery and retromandibular vein can both be seen, allowing the position of the facial nerve to be inferred. Small hypoechoic lymph nodes with an echogenic hilum are seen within the parotid gland and adjacent to the margin of the submandibular gland.

CT

Examination with CT is usually in the axial plane. Coronal images may be helpful and can be obtained directly, with the patient prone or supine (in the hanging head position), or indirectly, from reconstruction of data acquired axially. Volume acquisition of data with spiral or helical CT facilitates multiplanar reconstruction. The parotid duct will be demonstrated on thin sections taken parallel to the hard palate. The gantry angulation should be adjusted to avoid dental fillings. The scan should extend from the skull base to the level of the hyoid bone, to demonstrate the facial nerve canal and to ensure that the parotid tail and the high deep cervical and jugulodigastric lymph nodes have been included. Dynamic examination

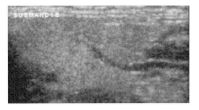

Fig. 18.7 Longitudinal oblique sonogram of submandibular gland showing the main (Wharton's) duct.

during intravenous contrast enhancement increases the conspicuity of salivary masses and affords some prediction of their nature. Direct ductal injection of a non-ionic contrast medium (CT sialography) is an alternative method of increasing conspicuity of salivary gland masses but the technique is invasive and is not widely practised as MRI is generally more appropriate.

MRI

The intrinsic contrast advantage of MRI is less than in other areas of the body, but the multiplanar imaging capability is valuable. A major advantage is the reduced artefact from dental amalgam, which can significantly degrade some CT examinations. The inability of MRI to demonstrate calcification is a disadvantage (Fig. 18.8); its presence is important both in the diagnosis of pleomorphic adenoma and calculus-related disease. Masses in the salivary glands have lower signal on T_1-weighted images, particularly contrasted against the fatty stroma of the parotid gland (Fig. 18.9). Contrast enhancement with gadolinium-based compounds may actually reduce the conspicuity of some masses (Fig. 18.10). Most salivary pathologies result in increased T_2 signal. Fat-suppressed T_2-weighted sequences are superior in determining the extent of invasion of surrounding tissues, features also well shown on STIR images. MR sialography has also been described using very heavily T2-weighted images, which contrast the ductal fluid against the stroma. Early experience suggests that small calculi may be missed by this technique and that it also fails to show the fine detail of smaller ducts necessary to diagnose sialectasis.

CT and MRI examinations of the salivary glands are usually requested to evaluate a mass in the region of a salivary gland. The requirement of imaging is to determine whether the mass arises in the gland and is contained within it, and, when it extends beyond the gland, its relationship to adjacent structures. The margins of the mass may be smooth or infiltrative; its nature solid, cystic, necrotic or haemorrhagic. While most benign lesions have smooth margins, some low-grade malignancies also have this characteristic (Fig. 18.11) and some haemorrhagic and inflammatory benign lesions can simulate high-grade cancers. The value of CT and MRI is more in the detection, anatomical placement and demarcation of masses than in their characterisation.

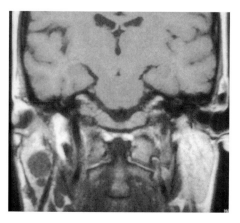

Fig. 18.9 Unenhanced coronal T_1-weighted MR image through the parotid glands showing a well circumscribed bilobed mass in the right superficial lobe. Diagnosis: pleomorphic adenoma.

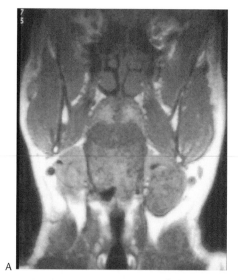

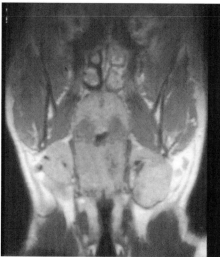

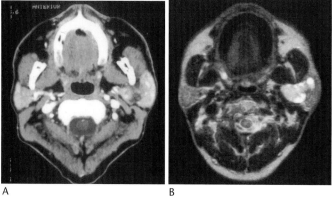

Fig. 18.8 Pleomorphic adenoma. (A) Axial contrast-enhanced CT through the parotid glands showing expansion of the left deep lobe and superficial lobe calcifications. (B) Axial T_2-weighted MR image through the parotid glands showing expansion of the left deep lobe by a high-signal mass and cystic change in the superficial lobe but no evidence of the calcifications.

Fig. 18.10 (A) Unenhanced coronal T_1-weighted MR image through the submandibular glands showing a poorly defined mass expanding the left gland. Diagnosis: poorly differentiated carcinoma. (B) Enhanced coronal T_1-weighted MR image through the submandibular glands showing reduced conspicuity of the mass expanding the left gland. Diagnosis: poorly differentiated carcinoma.

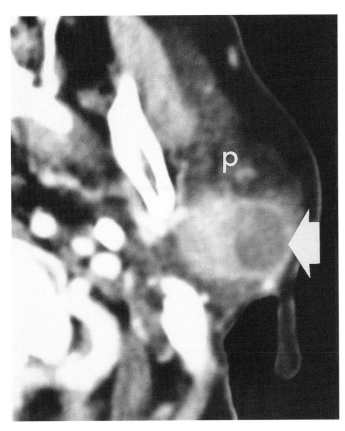

Fig. 18.11 Axial contrast-enhanced CT image of the left parotid gland (p) showing a mixed cystic/solid enhancing mass (arrow). Diagnosis: low-grade carcinoma.

SALIVARY GLAND LESIONS

Sialolithiasis

Salivary gland calculi may be solitary or multiple; 80% develop in the submandibular glands because these produce a more alkaline and viscous saliva and the ducts take an uphill course. Calculi form as a result of stasis or infection, and once formed predispose to further infection and stone formation. The majority are radio-

opaque and may be seen on plain radiographs. Multiple calculi are more frequent in the parotid glands. Sialography can identify and locate opaque and non-opaque calculi and the associated strictures that often develop in the duct system. When a stone is large enough to produce obstruction (generally when it exceeds 3 mm in a main duct), dilatation of the proximal ducts occurs (Fig. 18.12A) and if there is secondary infection small cavities may form within the gland (sialectasis). Calculi may also be demonstrated with ultrasound (Fig. 18.12B), although CT is the most sensitive of all the techniques. Unenhanced scans should be obtained to show stones and then intravenous contrast medium can be given if an abscess is suspected. Thin-section T_2-weighted MIP MR imaging (MR sialography) will also show the ductal system but is less satisfactory for identifying small calculi because of associated signal void. MR sialography is certainly useful for assessing the ducts when there is acute sialadenitis and conventional sialography is contraindicated.

Patients with duct calculi present with pain and swelling of the gland that is related to meals. Calculi in the distal parotid and submandibular ducts can be surgically removed transorally, by incising the duct, removing the calculus and repairing the duct. Stones can sometimes be removed under X-ray guidance by cannulating the duct and deploying a small stone retrieval basket through the cannula. Stones more proximally situated often necessitate resection of the gland. The sublingual glands rarely become inflamed; if they do, the obstruction generally causes the formation of a small retention cyst. Sialolithiasis may lead to *chronic sclerosing sialadenitis* with fibrosis and atrophy of the gland and intraglandular calcifications. This most frequently affects, and is the commonest disease of, the submandibular glands. Clinically the patient complains of recurrent pain and swelling of the gland. It is generally associated with sialolithiasis and resolves after removal of the stone but in 20% symptoms persist and the gland has to be removed.

Acute parotitis

After mumps, sialolithiasis is the most frequent cause of acute parotitis. Staphylococcal and streptococcal infections may develop in debilitated, dehydrated patients with poor oral hygiene. Other causes of acute parotitis include tuberculosis, candidiasis and cat scratch disease. CT features of parotitis are a swollen gland, increased enhancement, surrounding inflammatory stranding and

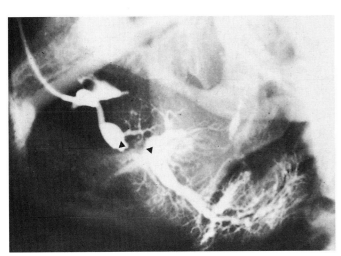

A

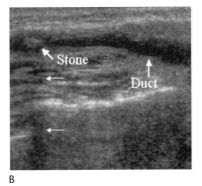

B

Fig. 18.12 (A) Obstructive sialectasis. Parotid sialogram demonstrating a non-opaque calculus in the main duct (between the arrowheads). The stone is causing obstruction, and the main duct is dilated. (Courtesy of Dr G. J. S. Parkin.) (B) Parotid duct stone and dilated main duct demonstrated by ultrasound.

local lymphadenopathy. MR shows an increased signal on T$_2$-weighted images. Parotitis may be complicated by abscess formation, which is seen as an area of non-enhancement on contrast-enhanced scans with an irregular enhancing rim. Deep parotid infection may extend to the parapharyngeal space (Fig. 18.13).

Sialosis

Sialosis refers to a recurrent non-inflammatory enlargement of the parotid gland and causes include alcoholism, malnutrition and radiotherapy. The gland appears generally enlarged on imaging.

Strictures

Strictures usually result from a combination of obstruction and infection. Strictures involving the main parotid or submandibular duct may be single or multiple (Fig. 18.14A). They are often sited at the orifice of a parotid or submandibular duct as a result of trauma from ill-fitting dentures. Cheek biting may also affect the orifice of the parotid duct. Small stones may pass spontaneously but leave duct strictures. Ducts proximal to a stricture dilate and

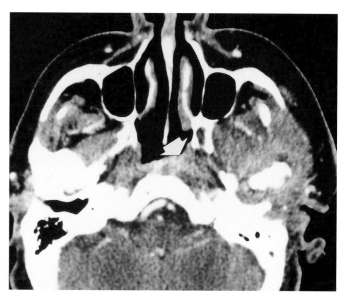

Fig. 18.13   Axial contrast-enhanced CT image of the left parotid gland showing a diffuse enlargement of the deep lobe with loss of the fat planes around the pterygoid muscles and effacement of the left side of nasopharynx (arrow). Diagnosis: deep parotid infection.

contrast medium is retained on the postsialogogue film. Localized strictures can be dilated using a guide-wire and a small balloon catheter (Fig. 18.14B–D).

Sialectasis

Sialectasis refers to a change in calibre of the salivary ducts and is most often caused by a stricture or stone. The small ducts within the parenchyma of the gland may be involved if there has been a past infection in childhood or if there is *Sjögren's syndrome, rheumatoid arthritis, scleroderma* or *systemic lupus erythematosis.* Sialectasis varies in severity: *punctate* sialectasis consists of punctate glandular collections (less than 1 mm in size) (Fig. 18.15A); *globular* sialectasis consists of collections of 1–2 mm in size with intraglandular ducts that are irregular, deformed and sparse (Fig. 18.15B); *cavitating* sialectasis results from coalescence of the globules into cavities; and in *destructive* sialectasis contrast medium extravasates into large cavities (Fig. 18.15C).

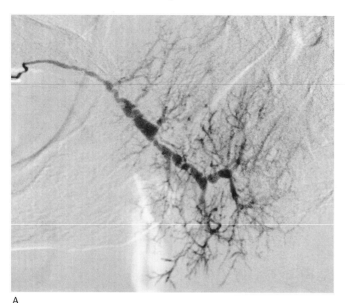

A

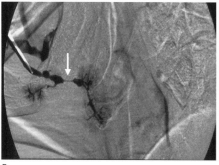

B

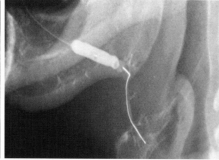

C

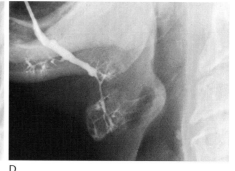

D

Fig. 18.14   Parotid sialogram. (A) Multiple strictures in the main and in some of the branch ducts. Digital subtraction image. (B) Parotid sialogram shows an inflammatory parotid duct stricture (arrow) secondary to stone disease. Digital subtracted image. (C) Balloon dilatation of the stricture. (D) Postprocedure sialogram. (B–D courtesy of Dr F. Carmichael.)

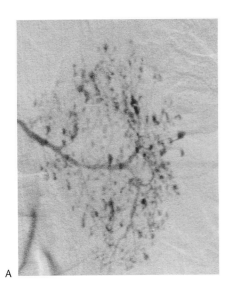

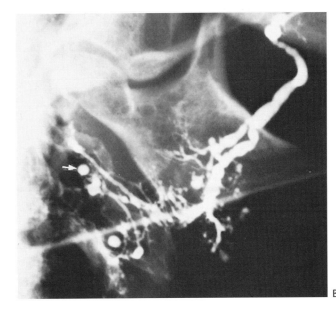

A

B

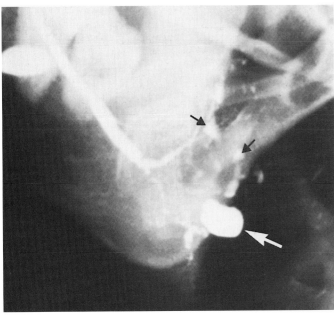

C

Fig. 18.15   (A) Parotid sialogram showing punctate sialectasis. There are numerous small collections of contrast medium evenly distributed throughout the gland. Digital subtraction image. (Courtesy of Dr P. Chennels.) (B) Parotid sialogram showing globular sialectasis. Collections of contrast medium 1–2 mm in diameter are evenly distributed throughout the gland (one has been identified with an arrow). The intraglandular ducts are stunted, irregular and sparse. (C) Parotid sialogram showing cavitating and destructive sialectasis. There is a large cavity indicated by the white arrow. There are also numerous small irregular collections of contrast medium (some indicated by black arrows) throughout the gland, almost entirely replacing the normal intraglandular duct system. (Courtesy of Dr G. J. S. Parkin.)

sialadenitis and mucosa-associated lymphoid tissue (MALT) lymphoma is difficult for the histologist to make. Sarcoidosis may also involve the salivary glands and produce a similar CT appearance to myoepithelial sialadenitis, with a honeycomb of low-density foci in a generally enhancing gland. Parotid enlargement from lymphoid hyperplasia is a feature of HIV infection prior to the development of AIDS. Proliferation of ductal epithelium leads to the formation of multiple cysts reminiscent to that seen in myoepithelial sialadenitis but there is usually associated cervical lymphadenopathy.

Myoepithelial sialadenitis (benign lymphoepithelial lesion, Mikulicz's disease)

This disease generally involves the parotid glands (85%) and occasionally the submandibular glands (15%). It is characterised histologically by lymphocytic infiltration, parenchymal atrophy and myoepithelial islands. The glands swell and pain may be experienced. Most patients will have Sjögren's syndrome, an autoimmune disease involving lacrimal as well as salivary glands, causing keratoconjunctivitis sicca and xerostomia. Sjögren's syndrome may be primary, or secondary when associated with other connective tissue diseases—most frequently rheumatoid arthritis. Patients with myoepithelial sialadenitis have an increased risk of developing lymphoma but sometimes the distiction between myoepithelial

Malignant lymphoma

Malignant lymphoma accounts for approximately 15% of malignant tumours of the major salivary glands. It is often difficult to determine if parotid lymphoma has a nodal or extranodal origin. Most are extranodal non-Hodgkin's lymphomas arising de novo (Fig. 18.16). Six per cent of patients with Sjögren's syndrome develop non-Hodgkin's lymphoma and it is thought that the benign lymphoid infiltrates of myoepithelial sialadenitis progress to lymphoma. In myoepithelial sialadenitis tumours often arise from lymphoid tissue that is similar to MALT. MALT-type lymphomas, wherever they arise, are relatively indolent and often cured by local treatment, although a small proportion may transform to higher grade disease.

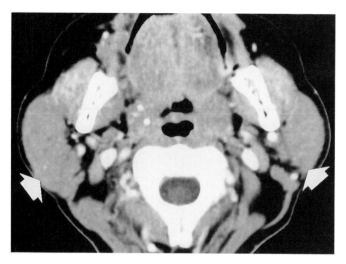

Fig. 18.16   Axial contrast-enhanced CT image of the parotid glands showing diffuse enlargement of both glands, which are of increased attenuation (arrows). Diagnosis: infiltration with non-Hodgkin's lymphoma.

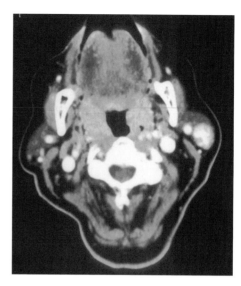

Fig. 18.18   Axial contrast-enhanced CT through the parotid glands showing a well-circumscribed dense mass in the left superficial lobe with calcifications. Diagnosis: pleomorphic adenoma.

Salivary gland tumours

Eighty per cent of salivary gland tumours are found in the parotid glands. The most common tumour is the pleomorphic adenoma, the majority of which are benign (Fig. 18.17). Carcinomas are rare but the probability of a salivary gland tumour being malignant is greatest for masses arising in the smaller salivary glands.

Benign tumours (Table 18.1)

The typical CT appearance of the *mixed (pleomorphic) adenoma* is that of a smoothly marginated mass which is of higher attenuation than the surrounding gland (Fig. 18.18) and shows no significant contrast enhancement. Larger masses may be lobulated or show necrosis, haemorrhage and calcification (Figs 18.8, 18.19). They show inhomogeneity of texture on MRI (Fig. 18.8), haemorrhage being manifest as high signal on T_1-weighted sequences. Displaced,

stretched ducts are features of a benign tumour mass at sialography (Fig. 18.20).

The second most common benign tumour is the *adenolymphoma (Warthin's tumour)*, typically located in the superficial part of the parotid gland. This is a mass of heterotopic salivary gland tissue within parotid lymph nodes. It may be bilateral in up to 15% of cases. These are well-marginated lesions which commonly cavitate, leading to a cystic appearance on CT (Fig. 18.21). They are thus of lower attenuation than the pleomorphic adenoma and more homogeneous on MRI. They may be multifocal. Non-neoplastic benign masses of the salivary glands include *development cysts* and lesions of the *haemangioma/ lymphangioma* spectrum (Fig. 18.22), which are the most common salivary tumours of childhood. *Parotid haemangiomas* present in infancy and show marked contrast enhancement. *First branchial cleft cysts* are rare but may occur superficial to, within, or deep to the parotid gland. These cystic lesions have a

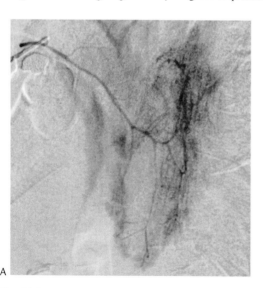

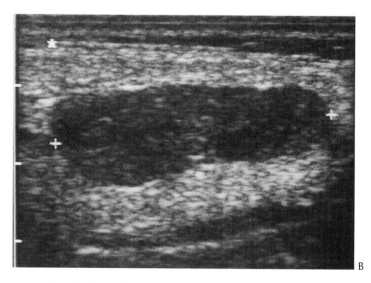

A   B

Fig. 18.17   (A) Parotid sialogram showing a deficiency of branch ducts deep within the gland. (B) Ultrasound scan showing a hypoechoic mass within the parotid gland. Diagnosis: pleomorphic adenoma. (Courtesy of Dr P. Chennels.)

Table 18.1   Pathology of salivary gland neoplasms*

Neoplasm	Approx.	Features
Adenomas (65%)		
Pleomorphic adenoma (mixed parotid tumour)	50	Benign but may recur if incompletely excised; 80% parotid but still commonest benign submandibular and sublingual gland tumour.
Adenolymphoma (Warthin's tumour)	10	May be multiple; 15% bilateral. Generally parotid gland. Increased risk in smokers. Can concentrate technetium pertechnetate
Basal cell (monomorphic) adenoma	3	Parotid and submandibular glands
Myoepithelioma	1	Parotid and submandibular glands
Oncocytoma	1	Generally parotid gland. Diffuse nodular oncocyte hyperplasia produces a generalised enlargement of the gland
Carcinomas (35%)		
Mucoepidermoid tumour	15	Squamous and mucous cells 50% in parotid gland.
Adenocarcinoma	7	Arises from a major gland in 60% (of which 90% are parotid) and a minor gland in 40%. Variable degree of malignancy
Adenoid cystic carcinoma	3	Commonest submandibular and sublingual carcinoma, although most frequently seen in the parotid gland. Tendency to local invasion. Metastasises late
Acinic cell carcinoma	6	Low grade
Carcinoma in mixed tumour	3	Variable degree of malignancy
Undifferentiated carcinoma	1	Highly malignant. Often difficult to differentiate from metastases

From Chandrasoma, P., Taylor, C. R. (1998) *Concise Pathology*; 3rd edn, p. 479. Stamford, CT: Appleton & Lange; Ellis, G. L., Auclair, P. L. (1995) *Atlas of Tumour Pathology. Tumours of the Salivary Glands*. Washington, DC: American Registry of Pathology, Armed Forces Institute of Pathology.

variable wall thickness if there have been previous episodes of infection.

Malignant tumours (Table 18.1)

Malignant tumours account for 20% of parotid masses (Fig. 18.23), 50% of submandibular masses and 70% of sublingual gland masses, so the smaller the gland the higher the risk of malignancy. Malignant tumours of the salivary glands are less common than benign lesions, and are usually mucoepidermoid carcinomas. Mucoepidermoid carcinoma is also the commonest malignant parotid tumour in children. On imaging, they may be poorly defined, relating to the histological grade of the lesion. Parotid adenoid cystic carcinoma is unusual in its perineural spread, and

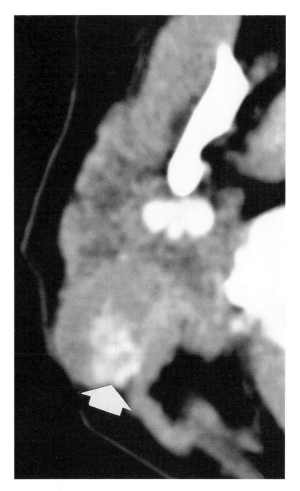

Fig. 18.19   Axial contrast-enhanced CT image of the right parotid gland showing a higher attenuation non-enhancing mass containing calcification (arrow). Diagnosis: pleomorphic adenoma.

recurrent disease may even enter the skull (Fig. 18.24). Malignant transformation may occur in a pleomorphic adenoma and this rapidly growing, poor-prognosis tumour is suggested when the benign calcifications of the adenoma are seen elsewhere within the gland (Fig. 18.25). Neurological involvement (facial nerve paralysis and V_3 involvement) strongly suggests malignancy; assessment of the facial nerve canal in the adjacent skull base is important as perineural extension of malignant tumours occurs and may result in the widening of the bony canal

The value of CT and MRI is in the detection and demarcation of masses and not their characterisation. Some haemorrhagic and inflammatory benign lesions can simulate high-grade cancers. Rapid growth, pain, regional lymphadenopathy and facial palsy suggest malignancy. Masses in the deep lobe of the parotid need to be differentiated from parapharyngeal pathologies such as *carcinoma*, *sarcoma* and *neural tumours*.

Metastatic and lymphomatous involvement of the parotid gland may occur due to the presence of intraparotid lymph nodes, a feature not seen in the other salivary glands. Metastases are usually secondary to skin neoplasms, such as malignant melanoma and squamous cell carcinomas of the face, external auditory meatus and scalp, and squamous cell carcinomas of the nasopharynx.

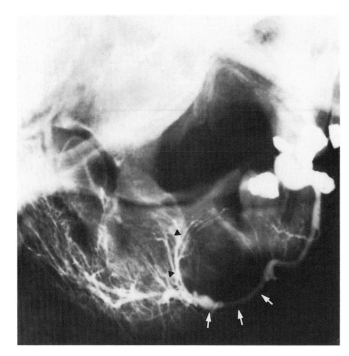

Fig. 18.20   Parotid sialogram showing a 2.5 cm benign salivary tumour in the anterior part of the gland, which is displacing the main duct (white arrows) downward and the intraglandular ducts (black arrows) backward. The site of the tumour is devoid of ducts.

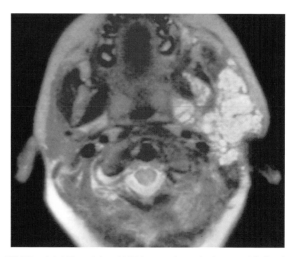

Fig. 18.22   Axial T$_2$-weighted MR image through the parotid glands showing a diffuse high signal mass expanding the left gland and involving the adjacent parapharyngeal and masticator spaces. Diagnosis: lymphangioma.

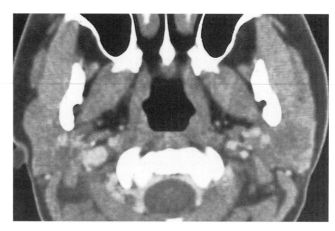

Fig. 18.23   Left parotid adenocarcinoma—heterogeneously enhancing mass within the left parotid gland. (Courtesy of Richard W. Whitehouse.)

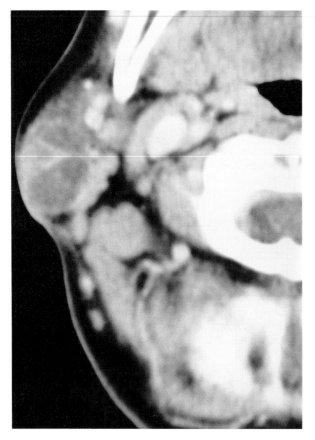

Fig. 18.21   Axial contrast-enhanced CT image of the right parotid gland showing a septated cystic lesion with a thin smooth wall. Diagnosis: haemorrhagic adenolymphoma (Warthin's tumour).

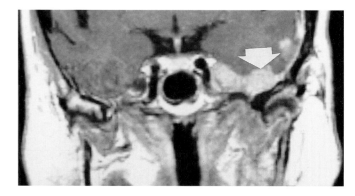

Fig. 18.24   Contrast-enhanced coronal T$_1$-weighted MRI scan of the parotid glands showing enhancing recurrent tumour (arrow) in the middle cranial fossa. Diagnosis: recurrent adenoid cystic carcinoma demonstrating perineural intracranial invasion.

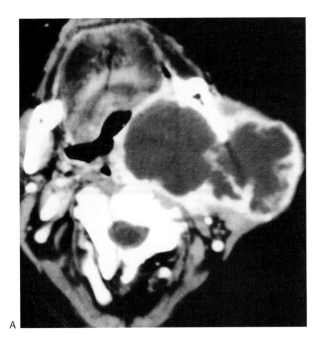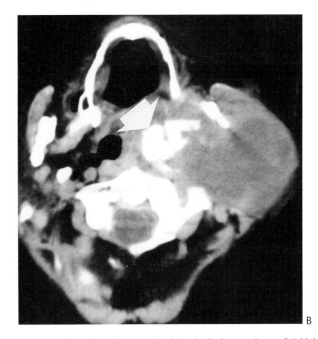

Fig. 18.25   (A) Axial contrast-enhanced CT image of the left parotid gland showing a complex enhancing mass involving both deep and superficial lobes. (B) Unenhanced axial CT image revealing a large calcification (arrow). Diagnosis: carcinoma ex pleomorphic adenoma.

Following parotidectomy, the surgical void fills with fat and scar tissue. Recurrent tumour is best diagnosed with MRI, where distinction between scar and tumour can be made because tumour shows greater contrast enhancement.

Fine needle aspiration cytology

FNAC will correctly predict a benign or malignant process in approximately 90% of cases and make a specific diagnosis in 70%. Enthusiasm for FNAC of salivary gland masses varies. It tends to be used in situations where the clinical picture and imaging suggest a benign diagnosis and long-term follow-up is planned, when a metastasis or a mass secondary to a systemic disease such as lymphoma is suspected, or when a patient is considered unfit for surgery.

THE PHARYNX AND OESOPHAGUS

ANATOMY

The pharynx

The oropharynx begins at the back of the oral cavity at the anterior faucal pillars and ends at the level of the hyoid bone (or tip of epiglottis) in the hypopharynx. It is separated from the nasopharynx by the soft palate. The constrictor muscles form the posterior and lateral walls and the base of the tongue forms the lower anterior wall. The hypopharynx extends from the level of the hyoid bone to the lower border of the cricopharyngeal muscle. Anteriorly lie the epiglottis and larynx. The valeculae are pockets that lie between the epiglottis and the back of the tongue. The pyriform fossae are lateral recesses.

The oesophagus

The oesophagus begins at the upper oesophageal sphincter at the level of C6 and finishes at the lower oesophageal sphincter at the level of T11 and is approximately 25 cm long. It has an inner circular and an outer longitudinal muscle coat. These muscle layers comprise predominately striated muscle in the upper third of the oesophagus and predominantly smooth muscle in the lower two-thirds, with the transition occurring at the level of the aortic knuckle. The mucosa of the oesophagus is stratified squamous epithelium and this changes to columnar epithelium along an irregular horizontal line (Z line) in the region of the gastro-oesophageal junction. The aortic arch indents the left wall of the oesophagus and immediately below this point the left main bronchus produces an indentation on the left anterolateral wall. After passing through the diaphragmatic hiatus the oesophagus extends for approximately 2 cm before joining the fundus of the stomach. Lymphatic drainage of the upper oesophagus is to cervical nodes, the midoesophagus is to preaortic nodes and the lower oesophagus drains to coeliac and left gastric nodes.

CT anatomy

The oesophagus is divided into four anatomical segments for staging purposes. The cervical oesophagus extends from the cricoid cartilage to the sternoclavicular joint. The upper thoracic oesophagus extends from the thoracic inlet to the carina (approximately 24 cm from the upper incisor teeth). The middle and lower thirds of the thoracic oesophagus are the proximal and distal halves of the part of the oesophagus that lies between the carina and the gastro-oesophageal junction. Each of these two segments are approximately 8 cm in length. The normal oesophagus is surrounded by fat and has a well-defined outer margin with a maximal mural thickness of 3 mm. The principal anterior relations of the thoracic oesophagus are the trachea, the left main bronchus, the right pulmonary artery and the pericardium. The posterior relations are the thoracic duct, azygous vein and descending aorta. The fat plane surrounding the oesophagus is often thin, particularly around the mid-third segment. It may be absent between the oesophagus and the left main bronchus, descending aorta, pericardium of the left atrium and crus of the diaphragm. The muscularis and other histological layers cannot be resolved. The cervical oesophagus is usually devoid of luminal gas, but gas can be seen in the normal thoracic oesophagus. The presence of an air–fluid level or a fluid-filled lumen of more than 1 cm usually indicates the presence of functional or mechanical obstruction. The gastro-oesophageal junction is a difficult area to evaluate with CT. The gastric fundus may be difficult to distend particularly in the presence of an oesophageal stricture and the combination of the oesophagus running oblique to the scan plane and non-distended gastric mucosal folds results in a pseudotumour appearance. The situation may be further compounded by the presence of a hiatus hernia.

EUS anatomy

Endoscopic ultrasonography (EUS) utilises the combined technology of videoendoscopy and high-frequency ultrasound. The most frequently used diagnostic system is manufactured by Olympus and has a radial transducer array. An alternative linear array system is marketed by Hitachi and allows the performance of biopsies, cyst drainages and transgastric stent placements. The frequency range is 7.5–12 MHz, although in Japan systems using frequencies up to 30 MHz are available and are used to evaluate early cancers. The ultrasound endoscope measures 13 mm in diameter and, as it is wider, it will not pass through some strictures that have been traversed with an optical endoscope. The system is forward-oblique viewing and has a water-filled balloon to provide mucosal contact. A narrower blind scope is also available which relies on ultrasound for guidance and can be passed over a guide-wire so it is used when a stricture prevents the passage of the larger videoscope.

Scanning at 7.5–10 MHz shows five layers to the wall of the gastrointestinal tract. The first layer results from the echo rebounding from the surface of the mucosa and is hyperechoic. The second layer corresponds to the mucosa and muscularis mucosa and appears as a thick dark band. The third layer is hyperechoic and corresponds to the submucosa, and the fourth is a further dark band produced by the muscularis propria. The fifth layer is hyperechoic and produced by the junction between the muscularis propria and adventitia or serosa (Fig. 18.26). Disruption of the tissue planes delineated by these boundary echoes is vital to the diagnosis and staging of gastrointestinal tract cancer.

PHARYNGEAL MOTILITY

Dysphagia (difficulty in swallowing), odynophagia (pain on swallowing), aspiration (choking) and the sensation of 'a lump in the throat' are all symptoms of swallowing disorders. Patients with dysphagia are frequently poor at localising the site of obstruction, often believing that the problem lies either at the top or bottom of the oesophagus. Patients suffering from aspiration may complain of difficulty swallowing, so barium studies in elderly patients or those with neurological problems should be started cautiously. A small mouthful of barium should be taken and the pharynx screened in

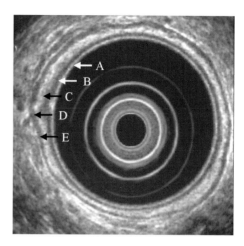

Fig. 18.26 Endoscopic ultrasound of the oesophagus showing the layers of the bowel wall. A = mucosa; B = muscularis mucosa; C = submucosa; D = muscularis propria; E = adventitia. (Courtesy of Dr K. Harris.)

the lateral position to check for aspiration. Once satisfied the patient is not aspirating, the barium swallow can commence. Swallowing starts in the mouth and finishes in the stomach, so the whole mechanism should be examined. A patient with reflux oesophagitis and a hiatus hernia may have a peptic lower oesophageal stricture and impaired cricopharyngeal relaxation. Bread or a marshmallow soaked in barium can be swallowed to establish which narrowing is clinically significant.

Technique of examination

The risk of aspiration needs to be considered before embarking on a barium swallow, as deep aspiration of barium into the lungs plugs bronchi and predisposes to pneumonia (Fig. 18.27). A history of coughing after swallowing suggests aspiration, but such a history cannot be relied upon as the patients most at risk are those with an absent cough reflex. When aspiration is considered likely, a study of the pharynx should first be made with the patient swallowing a teaspoonful of a non-ionic contrast medium (e.g. Gastromiro), which

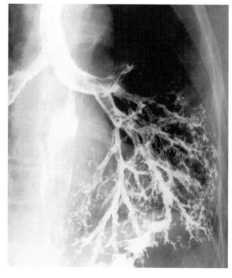

Fig. 18.27 Deep aspiration of barium into the left lower lobe and lingula.

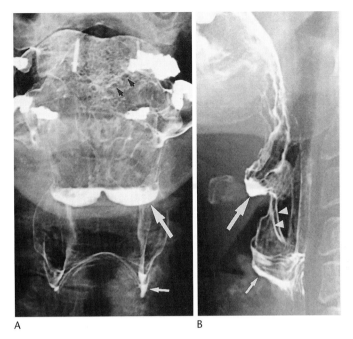

Fig. 18.28 (A) Frontal and (B) lateral views of the normal hypopharynx after a mouthful of barium has been swallowed. The large white arrow indicates a valleculum, and the lower white arrow points to the inferior recess of the pyriform sinus. Arrowheads mark the aryepiglottic folds. Circumvallate papillae (black arrows). There are a number of dental fillings.

is readily absorbed if it enters the lungs. If the risk of aspiration is considered small, a thin barium preparation may be used (100% w/v), as this strength will clearly demonstrate pharyngeal motility without obscuring the epiglottis. A video (or cine) recording of pharyngeal motility, taken with the patient in the lateral position, will show aspiration. At least three swallows are normally recorded because there can be some variability from one swallow to the next.

It is important that the first swallow is recorded, as patients with a tendency to aspirate are most likely to do so during this swallow. Patients sometimes develop trick movements to avoid aspiration and it may be that, as a result of anxiety, these are forgotten during the first swallow. Once a patient has aspirated it is more difficult to determine the timing of aspiration as the larynx is already coated with barium. Should aspiration occur to the level of the carina, the examination is terminated for safety.

The pharynx is normally examined in the lateral and AP projections. A slightly oblique lateral projection is also useful if the shoulders are obscuring the upper cervical oesophagus. The lateral swallow is the most useful and so should always be recorded first. When making video or cine recordings the image intensifier is kept still and the cones adjusted so that bolus movement can be observed in the mouth as well as the pharynx and cervical oesophagus (Fig. 18.28).

Patients suspected of aspirating often have severe neurological problems, so a lateral video of the pharynx is recorded with the patient sitting on the footrest of the table or in a special chair attached to the footrest. Patients too disabled for this can be examined with a C-arm, lying supine or semierect. Large boluses and thinner fluids are more likely to be aspirated than smaller boluses and thicker fluids. To determine if a patient is aspirating, a small volume (teaspoonful) of a contrast medium of thin fluid consistency, such as Gastromiro or dilute barium, is given. If this is swallowed without aspiration, larger volumes are tried by giving the fluid from a tablespoon, and then asking the patient to swallow from a cup. Examining the patient in this way is safe but suction equipment should be available, and, in the unlikely event of significant aspiration, physiotherapy should be arranged.

The normal swallow

When fluid is taken into the mouth it is initially held in the front of the mouth, above or below the tongue. An upward and backward movement of the tongue propels the bolus into the oropharynx (Fig. 18.29A) at the same time as the soft palate moves upward and backward to close off the nasopharynx. The adjacent posterior pharyngeal wall bulges forward (Passavant's cushion) to meet the soft palate to ensure complete closure. This bulge is produced by contraction of the superior constrictor muscle. The peristaltic wave starts at this point and runs down the pharynx, producing a bulge of the posterior and lateral side walls. The hyoid bone, larynx and pharynx elevate as the epiglottis inverts to cover the aryepiglottic folds. At the same time these folds move upward and inward to close the laryngeal opening (Fig. 18.29B,C).

A wave of relaxation precedes the peristaltic wave of contraction, relaxing the cricopharyngeus muscle, which is situated at the top end of the oesophagus. Sometimes there is a slight delay in relaxation of this muscle or it contracts a little early, to produce a posterior bulge into the head or tail of the barium column. In the AP

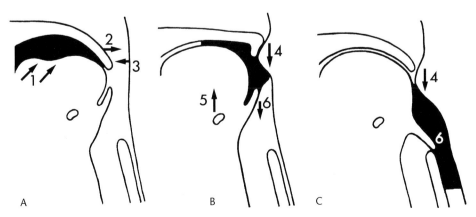

Fig. 18.29 (A) The normal swallow: 1, tongue propels bolus to oropharynx; 2, soft palate moves up and back to close nasopharynx; 3, posterior pharyngeal wall bulges forward to meet the soft palate. (B,C.) 4, peristaltic wave runs down pharynx; 5, hyoid bone elevates; 6, epiglottis inverts.

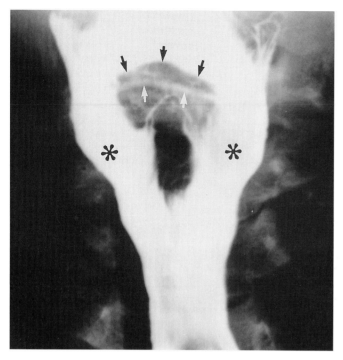

Fig. 18.30 Barium swallow showing the hypopharynx. Frontal view. The epiglottis is outlined by barium (arrows). The epiglottis and aryepiglottic folds protect the larynx and in so doing bulge into the pharynx, separating the bolus of barium so that it runs down two lateral food channels (asterisks).

projection the epiglottis and aryepiglottic folds divide the barium column into two lateral food channels, between which the inverted epiglottis is seen as a filling defect (Fig. 18.30). Peristalsis produces an inverted-V shape to the tail of the barium column as it passes down the pharynx and oesophagus.

Poor lip seal causes leakage from the front of the mouth, whereas poor apposition of the tongue to the soft palate, as may occur when the soft palate or tongue is weak, results in leakage into the pharynx, and is a cause of early aspiration. Failure of epiglottic inversion exposes the larynx, and may lead to aspiration in mid swallow. On the frontal view, asymmetry of movement of the epiglottis may be observed when one side of the pharynx is paralysed or when epiglottic movement is impeded, as may occur if the epiglottis

impinges on a particularly prominent cervical osteophyte. Weakness of the pharyngeal constrictor results in failure of clearance of barium from the pharynx, with pooling in the vallecula and piriform fossa and the attendant risk of spillage into the larynx when respiration is resumed (late aspiration). More severe paralysis results in a complete loss of the peristaltic wave. When paralysis is unilateral, the contracting normal side of the pharynx pushes the bolus toward the paralysed side so that it runs down the food channel on that side. The patient's head must be facing directly forward for this AP swallow, as turning the head to either side occludes the food channel on that side.

The soft palate may be seen to compensate for tongue weakness by a more pronounced downward and forward movement (Fig. 18.31A). Poor soft-palate movement may be compensated for by pronounced upward movement of the back of the tongue or excessive superior pharyngeal constrictor activity, producing a particularly prominent Passavant's cushion (Fig. 18.31B,C), but if the latter compensation mechanism fails, nasopharyngeal reflux will occur. The back of the tongue moves in conjunction with superior constrictor to propel the bolus, so a weak constrictor muscle leads to a more pronounced posterior movement of the back of the tongue (Fig. 18.31D). If the back of the tongue is weak, the superior constrictor muscle may compensate and a prominent bulge may be seen running down the back wall of the pharynx (Fig. 18.31E).

The cricopharyngeus muscle produces a prominent posterior bulge on the back of the pharynx at the level of C7. A persistent bulge during a swallow is an abnormal finding: it can result from failure of the muscle to relax; weakness of the pharyngeal constrictors, which push the bolus through this segment; or impaired laryngeal elevation, as may result from surgical scarring or radiotherapy (Fig. 18.32).

A prominent cricopharyngeal bulge and prominence of the posterior pharyngeal wall peristaltic wave may be seen if there is a distal oesophageal obstruction. Failure of cricopharyngeal relaxation can give the sensation of a lump in the throat (globus sensation), and, if severe, result in a functional obstruction with retention of barium in the pyriform fossa, and even overflow aspiration. In symptomatic patients, failure of cricopharyngeus relaxation may respond to balloon dilatation or cricopharyngeal myotomy.

In patients with hiatus hernias and gastro-oesophageal reflux, a cricopharyngeal bar may result from failure of the muscle to relax; as this may protect against aspiration, careful assessment is required before proceeding with any therapeutic measure to

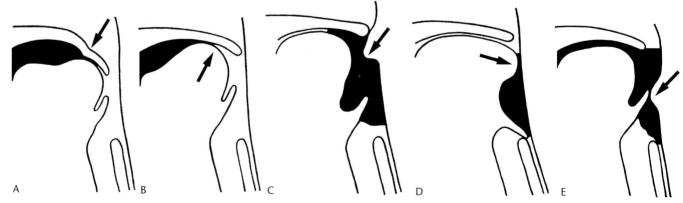

Fig. 18.31 (A) Pronounced soft palate movement compensates for weakness of the tongue. (B) Pronounced tongue movement or (C) superior pharyngeal constrictor activity compensates for weakness of the soft palate. (D) Pronounced movement of the back of the tongue compensates for weakness of the pharyngeal constrictor muscles. (E) Pronounced pharyngeal constrictor activity compensates for weakness of the tongue.

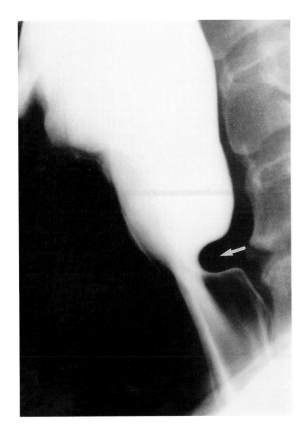

Fig.18.32 Barium swallow showing the cervical oesophagus. Lateral view. The posterior impression (arrow) is produced by failure of the cricopharyngeus muscle to relax.

render the muscle incompetent. Impaired cricopharyngeus relaxation, by causing a degree of obstruction, may elevate pharyngeal pressure and cause a pulsion diverticulum to develop at a site of weakness of the posterior pharyngeal wall between the horizontal and oblique fibres of the inferior constrictor muscle. The resulting

posterior pharyngeal diverticulum (*Zenker's diverticulum, posterior pharyngeal pouch*) may retain food, which can stagnate and cause halitosis. A large diverticulum will displace the oesophagus forward so that the swallowed bolus directly enters the diverticulum and then overflows into the oesophagus (Fig. 18.33A,B). The diverticulum may compress the oesophagus producing dysphagia or causing fluids to overflow back into the pyriform fossa, risking overflow aspiration. Sometimes a transient pouch is observed, which disappears when the oesophagus is distended. This does not retain the bolus, although it may in time develop into a permanent diverticulum. *Lateral pharyngeal pouches* result from weakness of the thyrohyoid membrane. These bulges of the lateral hypopharyngeal side wall are transient and usually bilateral. Occasionally they retain a little of the bolus, to cause late aspiration. Glass blowers and players of wind instruments, by increasing their pharyngeal pressure, may produce a diverticulum at this site, in which case overflow aspiration is more likely, and occasionally a food-filled mass is palpable in the neck.

A weakness of the anterolateral oesophageal wall immediately below the cricopharyngeus muscle may result in a transient pouch or permanent *lateral cervical oesophageal diverticulum* (*Killian–Jamieson diverticulum*; Fig. 18.33C). Although rare, this diverticulum may also produce symptoms from food retention or overflow aspiration.

When aspiration is known to be a clinical problem a therapeutic swallow may be performed in conjunction with a speech therapist. The purpose of this examination is to find a volume and consistency of fluid or food that can be swallowed without aspiration and to see whether changing the patient's method of swallowing is helpful (Table 18.2). As the patient is known to aspirate, the study is started with semisolids, as these are cohesive and least likely to be aspirated. The patient then progresses to thick and finally thin fluids. Even when an adequate oral fluid intake cannot be maintained and a gastrostomy is required, patients derive considerable psychological benefit by being able to maintain some oral intake.

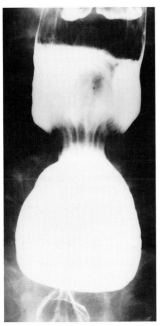

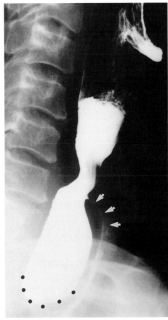

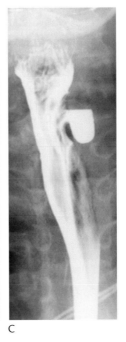

Fig. 18.33 Posterior pharyngeal diverticulum. (A) Frontal view. (B) Lateral view. Barium fills the diverticulum and then spills over into the anteriorly displaced oesophagus (arrows). (C) Lateral cervical oesophageal diverticulum (Killian–Jamieson diverticulum).

A   B   C

Table 18.2   Methods commonly used to modify swallowing

Problem	Method
Early swallow aspiration (premature leak from mouth to pharynx)	Thickened fluids
Midswallow aspiration (poor epiglottic movement and laryngeal closure)	Semisolid bolus
Late swallow aspiration (weak pharyngeal muscles—pooling in pyriform sinuses)	Thin fluids
Weak tongue—difficulty moving bolus to pharynx	Elevate chin
Premature leak of bolus from mouth or poor epiglottic movement	Chin tuck
Unilateral pharyngeal palsy—diverts food away from the paralysed food channel	Chin turn
Aspiration	Supraglottic swallow (breathe in, hold breath, swallow and exhale)

Patients who still aspirate and have sufficient cognitive function may be helped by changing the chin posture during swallowing or by certain swallowing manoeuvres, such as the supraglottic swallow (Table 18.2).

On occasion it is pharyngeal morphology and not function that needs to be demonstrated, and for this good barium coating of the pharynx is required. The pharynx should be dry, so the patient should not smoke, eat or drink for at least 3 h prior to the study. Distension of the pharynx is achieved by asking the patient to whistle or blow into closed lips and AP and lateral images of the pharynx are obtained.

Oesophageal webs

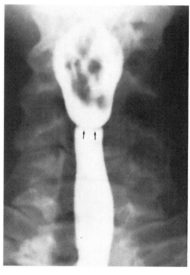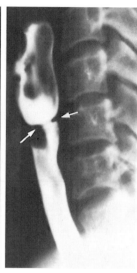

Fig. 18.34   A concentric upper oesophageal web seen in both the frontal and lateral projections (arrows). The way in which the web narrows the lumen is well seen in the lateral view.

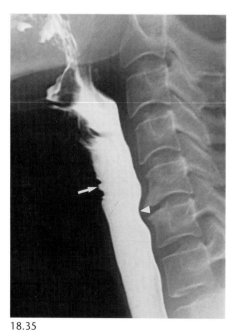

18.35

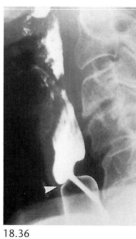

18.36

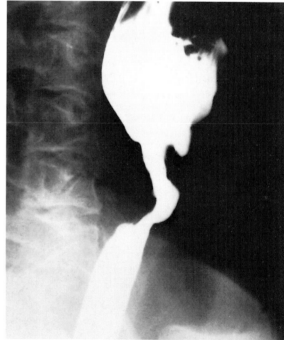

18.37

Fig. 18.35   Barium swallow showing the cervical oesophagus. Lateral view. The small irregular anterior indentation (arrow) is caused by a venous plexus. Osteophytes at the C5–6 disc space produce an impression on the back of the barium column (arrowhead).

Fig. 18.36   Postcricoid web. Lateral view showing typical thin anterior web (arrowhead). The lumen is also restricted by cricopharyngeal spasm posteriorly helping to produce a barium jet phenomenon.

Fig. 18.37   Postcricoid carcinoma. Lateral view showing irregular narrowing.

These shelf-like 1–2 mm thick infoldings of the mucosa protrude into the lumen from the anterior wall of the cervical oesophagus (Fig. 18.34). They are generally semicircular but may form a complete ring. Webs may be multiple and occasionally develop in the mid- and lower oesophagus. They may only be seen on one frame of a cine or video recording, and are best shown in the lateral projection with the oesophagus fully distended with barium. Webs must be differentiated from the slight infolding of the mucosa of the anterior wall of the cervical oesophagus that produces an irregularity to the anterior margin of the barium column at the level of the cricoid cartilage. This is a normal finding and is caused by laxity of mucosa at this site (Fig. 18.35). Similar small mucosal indentations in the cervical oesophagus may also be produced by islands of ectopic gastric mucosa. It is thought that these represent residual rests of embryonic columnar epithelium, and are not usually of clinical significance.

Webs are common incidental findings, especially in middle-aged women, and may be seen in up to 8% of barium swallows. Occasionally a web narrows the oesophagus enough to cause dysphagia. The oesophagus may balloon above a web, and when a complete ring has formed a jet of barium may be seen passing through it (Fig. 18.36). Webs can occur when the oesophagus is involved by epidermolysis bullosa or the benign form of bullous pemphigoid. An association with the Plummer–Vinson syndrome of iron-deficiency anaemia, dysphagia, stomatitis, glossitis and koilonychia has been described. There may be an increased risk of developing pharyngeal and cervical oesophageal carcinomas (Fig. 18.37) with this syndrome. Webs may also be an ageing phenomenon or result from oesophageal reflux. They are fragile and often break down with the passage of an endoscope, although occasionally balloon dilatation is required.

OESOPHAGEAL MOTILITY

Oesophageal *manometry* is used to evaluate motility, but when it is unavailable the barium swallow provides a useful alternative. Motility often varies from one swallow to the next, so at least five single prone swallows should be recorded for proper evaluation. Radionuclide imaging of the oesophagus is reserved for patients in whom the first-line tests of endoscopy and barium swallow produce unexpected or inconclusive results, and those in whom the initial tests are negative. Scintigraphy has the advantages of using physiological fluids or solids, producing quantifiable results, and being highly sensitive in the early detection of motility disorders.

Peristalsis

Primary oesophageal peristalsis is initiated by the act of swallowing. When barium is swallowed, the tail end of the peristaltic wave has the shape of an inverted 'V' as it passes down the oesophagus. Peristalsis starts in the pharynx with contraction of the superior constrictor muscle. As the inner circular muscle contracts and narrows the lumen of the oesophagus, the outer longitudinal layer contracts and shortens the oesophagus, drawing the oesophagogastric junction up into the chest. During a normal swallow the oesophagogastric junction may be pulled above the diaphragmatic hiatus by as much as 2 cm. The primary peristaltic wave runs the length of the oesophagus and consists of a wave of relaxation followed by a slightly slower wave of contraction. Should a patient take

a second swallow immediately after the first, then the fast relaxation wave of the second swallow will catch up with the slower contraction wave of the first swallow and stop its progress. It is for this reason that when peristalsis is being assessed the patient should only take single swallows. A secondary peristaltic wave is initiated by luminal distension or mucosal irritation, and acts as an important protective mechanism, quickly returning refluxed acid to the stomach. The upper oesophageal sphincter (cricopharyngeus muscle) relaxes as the peristaltic wave passes, but remains in a state of tonic contraction at other times to prevent inhaled air entering the oesophagus or refluxed acid reaching the pharynx. Should the upper oesophageal sphincter fail, then oesophageal reflux may result in aspiration, which is prone to occur at night and is a cause of nocturnal asthmatic attacks.

Abnormal motility

Tertiary contractions are non-propulsive and uncoordinated and their non-peristaltic nature means they move the bolus up as well as down the oesophagus. They are seen as intermittent ripples along the wall of the oesophagus lasting only a few seconds, as multiple simultaneous contraction rings (Fig. 18.38A), or as a segmented barium column producing a corkscrew appearance (Fig. 18.38B).

The variability of oesophageal motility makes it necessary to observe at least five single prone swallows. If two or more of the five swallows are abnormal, the patient is considered to have a motility disorder. In young adults 95% of swallows will be entirely normal but with age the proportion of abnormal swallows increases. Primary and secondary waves become weak, failing to clear the oesophagus of the bolus, the peristaltic wave may fail to run the complete length of the oesophagus, tertiary contractions

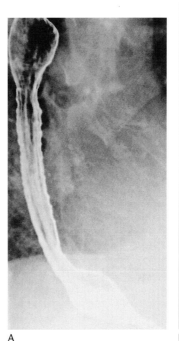
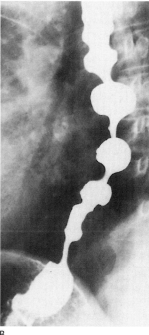

A   B

Fig. 18.38 Tertiary contractions of the oesophagus seen as (A) a rippling of the oesophageal wall or (B) a series of indentations resembling a corkscrew (hence the description 'corkscrew oesophagus').

become more frequent and the lower oesophageal sphincter may on occasions fail to relax. When primary peristalsis is observed to fail, there is proximal escape of some of the bolus from the inverted 'V' of the peristaltic wave. This tends to occur at the level of the aortic knuckle because there is normally a reduction in amplitude of the pressure of the peristaltic wave in this region of the oesophagus. Tertiary contractions are most frequent in the lower two-thirds of the oesophagus.

Striated muscle coats the pharynx and upper 4 cm of the oesophagus, while the lower half of the oesophagus has a smooth muscle coat; between the two, striated and smooth muscle intermingle. The transition from smooth to striated muscle is at the level of the aortic knuckle. Disorders involving striated muscle, such as motor neurone disease and myasthenia gravis, will only affect the pharynx and upper third of the oesophagus, whereas disorders of smooth muscle, such as scleroderma, affect the lower two-thirds of the oesophagus.

Diffuse oesophageal spasm

Diffuse oesophageal spasm is a condition in which episodes of pronounced abnormal motility occur without cause, and these spasms may be associated with severe intermittent chest pain, dysphagia and even food impaction. The intermittent nature of the disorder makes it difficult to diagnose by barium studies or routine oesophageal manometry: 24 h manometry may be required. Even then, when abnormal motility is observed it may not coincide with the time of the patient's chest pain, making results difficult to interpret.

Nutcracker oesophagus

This is a manometric diagnosis in which patients with non-cardiac chest pain have primary peristaltic waves with pressures in excess of 180 mmHg (normally 100 mmHg). The barium swallow and oesophageal scintigram show normal peristalsis and cannot therefore be used to diagnose this condition.

Hypertrophic lower oesophageal sphincter

This again is a manometric finding in which the resting lower oesophageal sphincter pressure is 40 mmHg or more.

Non-specific oesophageal motility disorder

This term is used to describe the remaining abnormalities of motility, such as loss of peristalsis, incomplete lower oesophageal relaxation and solitary abnormal contractions (triple peaked on manometry).

Presbyoesophagus

Abnormal motility in the elderly is referred to as presbyoesophagus, although an underlying cause, for example diabetes, can often be identified in such patients. Elderly patients with severely disordered motility may become symptomatic with chest pain or dysphagia.

These disorders of motility may be primary or secondary to a wide variety of diseases, including oesophagitis, diabetes, alcoholism, and collagen, endocrine and neuromuscular diseases. Calcium channel blockers can be useful for treating primary motility disorders.

Non-cardiac chest pain

Primary motility disorders may cause chest pain but oesophagitis is a more frequent cause and is easier to treat. It can be diagnosed by endoscopy or a good-quality double-contrast barium swallow. Sometimes it is convenient to observe motility at the end of a double-contrast barium meal with single-contrast barium swallows. However, it is best to wait 30 min for the effect of the Buscopan (hyoscine butylbromide) to wear off before assessing motility in this way. Clinicians suspecting oesophageal reflux as the cause of chest pain may request oesophageal scintigraphy to detect reflux, perform 24 h pH monitoring, or just embark on a therapeutic trial of an H_2 antagonist or proton pump inhibitor.

The transit test

The transit test is used to detect abnormal oesophageal motility, and to assess the severity of established motility disorders and the response to treatment. Scintigraphic tests have been shown to be more sensitive than endoscopy, radiography and manometry in the identification of patients with motility problems. This includes patients with atypical chest pain (pain of cardiac type with normal ECG and enzymes), patients with dysphagia but normal endoscopy/barium studies, and patients with suspected muscular or neuromuscular dysfunction (systemic sclerosis, diabetes and autonomic neuropathy, oesophagitis, columnar-lined oesophagus, postoperative or postsclerotherapy dysphagia).

The transit test demonstrates oesophageal function by visualising the passage of a swallowed bolus into the stomach. The labelled material may be prepared in either liquid or solid form – for example, orange juice labelled with ^{99m}Tc-DTPA, or scrambled egg labelled with ^{99m}Tc colloid. Minor motility disorders are more likely to be detected if the examination is carried out with the patient supine, but patients with major motility disorders are best examined in the sitting position so that gravity can assist the clearing of the oesophagus. Each swallow consists of one mouthful (8–10 ml) of the labelled material and is swallowed in a single gulp, the patient being asked not to swallow again for the next 30 s, during which time the image acquisition is made. It is helpful to rehearse the technique with the patient using unlabelled material first. Because transit through the oesophagus is rapid, it is necessary to acquire images at 2–4 frames per second. The images can then be displayed as a cine loop, and time–activity curves derived for the upper third, middle third, lower third and whole oesophagus. A convenient way of displaying the entire study is to use a functional image, with distance on the vertical axis and time on the horizontal axis. Effectively this is done by compressing each frame of the acquisition to a single vertical profile and stacking the profiles from left to right (Fig. 18.39). Because swallowing patterns and transit times vary from minute to minute in some individuals, it is important to obtain several separate swallows on each patient. Typically, three consecutive swallows may be obtained in the supine position, and a further three swallows in the sitting position. Between each

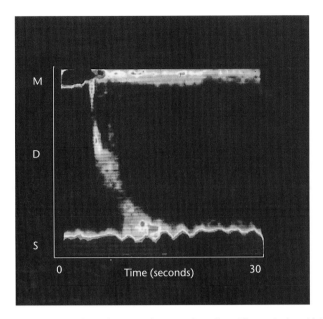

Fig. 18.39 Condensed image of a normal swallow. Timescale (*x* axis) is 30 s, *y* axis corresponds to the length of the oesophagus with the mouth at the top and gastric fundus at the bottom. M = mouth; D = distance; S = stomach.

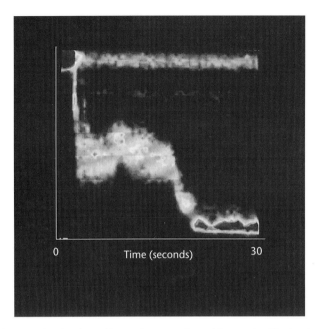

Fig. 18.41 Condensed image from a patient with oesophagitis showing a 'step–delay' pattern with transient hold up of the bolus in the middle third of the oesophagus.

swallow the oesophagus is rinsed with an unlabelled drink in order to clear residual activity.

The results can be expressed either qualitatively, or by using a grading system, or by measurement of the mean transit time between mouth and stomach. Transit through the upper third of the oesophagus usually takes about 1 s, through the middle third about 2 s, and through the lower third about 6 s, giving a transit time through the whole oesophagus of 8–10 s. Grading systems take into account the degree of delay in transit time, the severity of disruption of the transit pattern, and the frequency of the abnormality in repeated swallows. Qualitatively, several different patterns can be recognised:

- *Normal.* The bolus traverses the oesophagus in a single wave of peristalsis in 8–10 s or so, with no delay, no fragmentation of the bolus, and no reflux (Fig. 18.39).

- *Transfer dysphagia.* Once initiated, transit shows a normal progression but there is delay in initiating swallowing, and sometimes fragmentation of the bolus in the pharynx (Fig. 18.40).

- *'Step–delay' pattern.* The initial peristaltic wave dies out in the

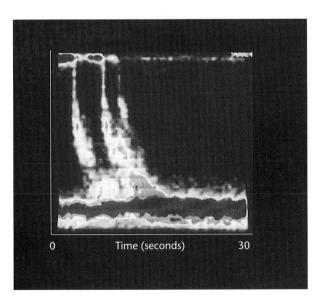

Fig. 18.40 Condensed image in a patient with pharyngeal incoordination leading to transfer dysphagia, showing fragmentation of the initial swallowed bolus but normal rate of transit through the rest of the oesophagus.

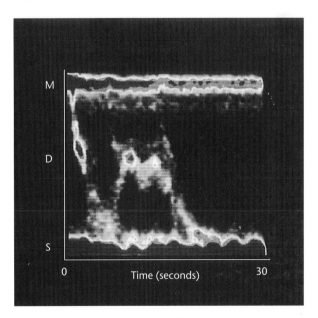

Fig. 18.42 Condensed image showing intraoesophageal reflux—retrograde motion of part of the swallowed bolus from the lower end to the middle third, with later clearing by a second swallow. M = mouth; D = distance; S = stomach.

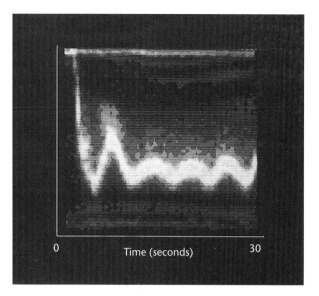

Fig. 18.43 Condensed image in a patient with achalasia showing stasis of the swallowed bolus in the middle third of the oesophagus, with to-and-fro movement caused by respiratory excursion.

middle third of the oesophagus and the bolus then remains stationary until it is stripped down the lower third by the next peristaltic wave (Fig. 18.41).

- *Intraoesophageal reflux.* The swallowed bolus proceeds normally to the lower third, then part or all of it refluxes back to the middle third, before being cleared by further peristalsis (Fig. 18.42).

- *Incoordinate.* After swallowing, the bolus is immediately fragmented by dystonic contractions, and no peristaltic wave develops.

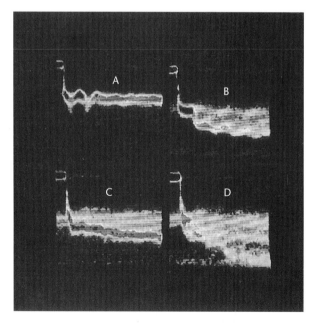

Fig. 18.44 Condensed images of sequential swallows in a patient with achalasia, obtained with the patient supine (A) then with the patient semierect (B,C) and sitting (D), showing improving clearance as the patient was brought from the supine to the erect position.

- *Adynamic.* Swallowing is initiated normally, but peristalsis is weak or absent and bolus remains in the middle third of the oesophagus if the patient is supine, or clears only very slowly from the lower oesophagus if the patient is sitting (Fig. 18.43).

Patients with diffuse oesophageal spasm, frequent tertiary contractions, or presbyoesophagus typically show an incoordinate pattern with delayed transit. Patients with **autonomic neuropathy** associated with diabetes, and those with **systemic sclerosis** involving the oesophagus, typically show delayed clearance with adynamic patterns. About half of all patients with reflux oesophagitis have abnormal motility. It is well established that delay in clearance of material refluxed from the stomach is an important contributory factor in the pathogenesis of oesophagitis, so its likely that minor motility disorders predispose to oesophagitis in refluxing patients. However, it is also possible that oesophagitis itself may impair motility. Both intraoesophageal reflux and the step–delay patterns are associated with reflux oesophagitis. Patients with achalasia show an adynamic pattern with marked prolongation of transit times. A swallowed bolus may remain in the oesophagus indefinitely if the patient lies supine, and even clearing in the erect position may be severely delayed (Fig. 18.44). After medical or surgical treatment of achalasia, the delay may be less marked but the abnormality still persists.

Achalasia

Achalasia is a motor disorder of the oesophagus generally occurring in the 35–50 year age group. It is caused by degeneration of neurones of Auerbach's plexus, which is situated between the longitudinal and circular muscle coats. Primary and secondary peristalsis initially fails, tertiary contractions develop, and there is a failure of relaxation of the lower oesophageal sphincter. Unlike strictures of the oesophagus, which initially cause dysphagia for solids but allow liquids to pass, achalasia causes dysphagia for both solids and liquids. If the patient presents early, pronounced tertiary contractions may be seen (*vigorous achalasia*) with only modest dilatation, and the patient may complain of severe chest pains identical to those of patients with *diffuse oesophageal spasm*. These two conditions have been considered to be at different ends of the same disease spectrum, and sometimes diffuse oesophageal spasm may be observed to progress to achalasia.

A barium swallow will show the gastro-oesophageal junction failing to open fully and tapering to a rat tail or bird beak appearance. Intact mucosal folds can be traced through this narrowed segment (Fig. 18.45A), which at times opens briefly to allow a little barium to spurt into the stomach. In the absence of peristalsis, this occurs when the hydrostatic pressure in the oesophagus exceeds that of the lower oesophageal sphincter. Inhalation of amyl nitrate causes prompt relaxation of the lower oesophageal sphincter, and may be used as a diagnostic test. With time, tertiary peristalsis becomes less evident, and the oesophagus dilates, lengthens and becomes tortuous. The dilatation may involve the entire length of the oesophagus and can sometimes be appreciated on a plain chest film where there is a small or absent gastric fundal air bubble, the fluid-filled oesophagus widens the mediastinum and there is a mediastinal air–fluid level.

Recurrent episodes of *aspiration pneumonia* may complicate achalasia and lead to the development of bronchiectasis, lung abscesses or an empyema. Repeated aspiration may also cause basal pulmonary fibrosis. Prolonged food stasis may cause oesophagitis, with an

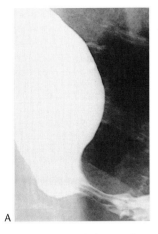
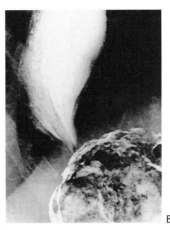

Fig. 18.45 Achalasia. The oesophagus is distended. (A) Intact oesophageal folds pass through the tapered narrowing, which corresponds to the site of the lower oesophageal sphincter. On fluoroscopy the impaired motility will be evident. (B) Sufficient barium has entered the stomach to coat the fundus and exclude an infiltrating gastric carcinoma as a cause.

increased risk of squamous cell carcinoma. This carcinoma usually develops in the midoesophagus and must be differentiated from food residue, which, if adherent, makes the walls of the oesophagus difficult to evaluate by barium swallow examination, and so it is important that all patients have an endoscopy. If the cricopharyngeus muscle prevents regurgitation, oesophageal distension may compress

and narrow the trachea to produce stridor. Massive oesophageal dilatation has resulted in sudden death from asphyxiation.

Treatment of achalasia consists of balloon dilatation of the gastro-oesophageal junction, local injection of botulinum toxin or a myotomy of the sphincter (*Heller's operation*). Oesophageal perforation and gastro-oesophageal reflux may complicate these procedures. After a myotomy a barium swallow may show a bulge of the oesophageal wall at the site where the muscle has been split.

Secondary achalasia or pseudoachalasia

When achalasia has developed rapidly, or after the age of 50, the possibility of an underlying neoplasm should be considered. Submucosal neoplastic infiltration of Auberach's plexus of the distal oesophagus may result from direct invasion from carcinoma of the stomach, extrinsic invasion from carcinoma of the tail of the pancreas or adjacent malignant lymph nodes, or metastatic invasion by carcinoma of the bronchus or breast. When investigating achalasia by barium meal it is not always possible to exclude gastric carcinoma as a cause (Fig. 18.45B). CT will demonstrate extrinsic malignant invasion, but endoscopic ultrasound is the only way of showing submucosal infiltration. In achalasia the muscularis propria of the lower oesophageal sphincter may appear thickened or thinned, but in pseudoachalasia the tumour infiltration can be seen.

Impaired relaxation of the lower oesophageal sphincter with slight dilatation of the oesophagus simulating achalasia may be seen as a transient phenomenon when vagal innervation to the lower oesophagus is disturbed, as may occur with bilateral truncal vago-

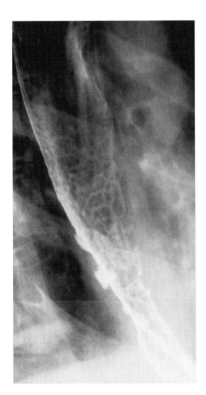

Fig. 18.46 Scleroderma. Incompetence of the gastro-oesophageal sphincter resulting in severe reflux oesophagitis with structuring, oedematous mucosa (mozaic pattern) and deep ulceration.

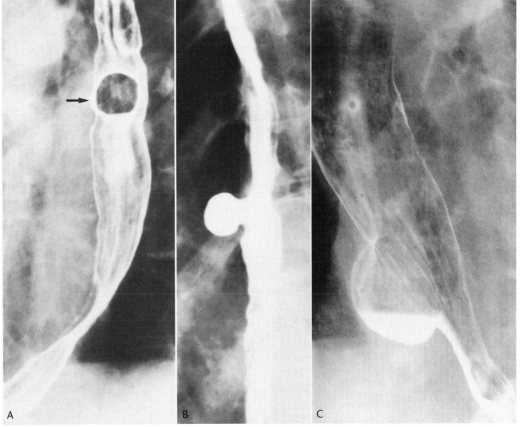

Fig. 18.47 Midoesophageal diverticulum seen (A) en face and (B) in profile. (C) Epiphrenic diverticulum.

tomy or a disease affecting the dorsal nucleus of the vagus, such as brainstem infarction.

The myenteric plexus is also damaged in chronic *Chagas's disease*, which is endemic to Central and South America. The protozoan *Trypanosoma cruzi* is transmitted as a result of the bite of the reduvid bug, which inhabits the walls and thatch of houses. A myocarditis leads to ventricular dilatation and often ventricular aneurysm formation. Bowel involvement results in achalasia and megacolon.

Oesophageal leiomyomatosis is a rare benign proliferation of smooth muscle, generally involving the distal oesophagus; it may resemble achalasia on a barium swallow. The condition generally presents in childhood with dysphagia and is sometimes associated with leiomyomas of the gastrointestinal tract and with hereditary nephritis (Alport's syndrome).

Scleroderma

In scleroderma a vasculitis damages the smooth muscle coat of the bowel. The lower two-thirds of the oesophagus are most frequently affected, although the proximal small bowel and, less frequently, the colon can be involved. Muscle damage results in a loss of primary and secondary motility and the development of tertiary contractions. As elsewhere in the bowel, it is mainly the circular muscle coat that is affected, and so the lower oesophagus dilates. Weakening of the lower oesophageal sphincter predisposes to reflux, which can lead to peptic ulceration (Fig. 18.46). Should a peptic stricture develop, the condition may have a similar appearance to achalasia. Up to a third of patients develop a Barrett's oesophagus, with the attendant risk of adenocarcinoma. Occasionally dermatomyositis, polymyositis and mixed connective tissue disease affect the oesophagus in a similar way to scleroderma.

Pulsion diverticula

Pulsion diverticula are rarely of clinical significance. They may develop when motility is abnormal, presumably as a consequence of high intraluminal pressures. They are wide necked and are mostly at the level of the carina (Fig. 18.47A,B) but may develop from the lower oesophagus (epiphrenic diverticula) (Fig. 18.47C). Sometimes, midoesophageal diverticula are produced by traction (*traction diverticula*) as a result of fibrosis from adjacent healing tuberculous lymph nodes.

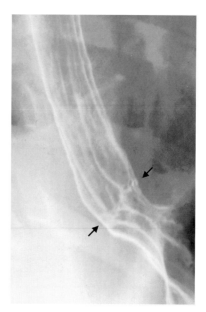

Fig. 18.49 Z-line (between the arrows) marks the junction of squamous (oesophageal) and columnar (gastric) epithelium. Gastric rugae are seen extending up to the line.

THE NORMAL OESOPHAGOGASTRIC JUNCTION

The diaphragmatic hiatus is the opening in the diaphragm which transmits the oesophagus and stomach. The phrenico-oesophageal membrane tethers the distal oesophagus to the diaphragm at the hiatus (Fig. 18.48) and stretches with the development of a hiatus hernia. The normal oesophagus shortens with swallowing, often, in adults, drawing the oesophagogastric junction above the diaphragmatic hiatus by as much as 2 cm. Movement beyond 2 cm results in the formation of a hiatus hernia and can only occur if the phrenico-oesophageal membrane stretches or ruptures.

The sling fibres are the innermost muscle fibres of the stomach wall and loop up around the notch between the oesophagus and the gastric fundus, forming the cardiac incisura. This is a useful landmark for the oesophagogastric junction, as the incisura can be seen above the diaphragmatic hiatus when there is a sliding hiatus hernia.

The change from squamous (oesophageal) to columnar (gastric) epithelium in the distal oesophagus is marked by an irregular line known as the Z-line, at which straight oesophageal folds abruptly give way to gastric rugae, or areae gastricae (Fig. 18.49). This line may lie some distance above the oesophagogastric junction if there is a columnar-lined oesophagus (Barrett's oesophagus).

The oesophagogastric junction (*cardia*) may also be identified on a barium swallow by a thin transverse mucosal fold known as the B-ring (*gastro-oesophageal ring*). Between 2 and 4 cm proximal to this ring is a thicker ring produced by active muscle contraction (Fig. 18.50), known as the A-ring (*inferior oesophageal sphincter*). The more distensible lower end of the oesophagus, between these two rings, is called the vestibule (or phrenic ampulla). The vestibule corresponds with the lower oesophageal sphincter, which, unlike the upper oesophageal sphincter, is not a distinct muscle but a high-pressure zone. The vestibule thus comprises the distal 2–4 cm of the oesophagus immediately above the oesophagogastric junction. If the patient breathes in during a prone barium swallow, the

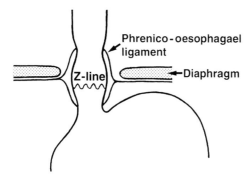

Fig. 18.48 The phrenico-oesophageal membrane tethers the distal oesophagus and stretches or ruptures with the development of a hiatus hernia. Normally the Z-line lies at the oesophagogastric junction.

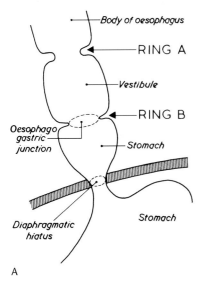

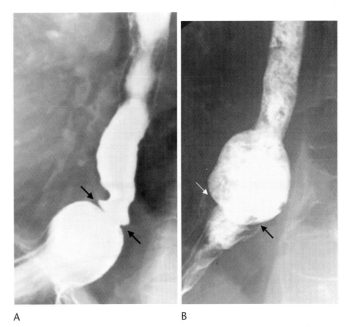

Fig. 18.51 (A) Schatski's ring (between arrows) demonstrated by barium swallow. (B) Bread soaked in barium has been swallowed and is lodged above the ring (between arrows).

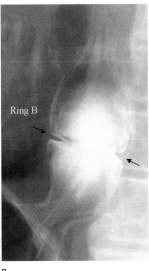

Fig. 18.50 The lower end of the oesophagus. (A) The B-ring may normally be within 2 cm above (as shown here) or below the hiatus. Thus the oesophageal vestibule may normally be above, or straddle, the diaphragmatic hiatus. (B) Small sliding hiatus hernia with normal B-ring (between arrows).

vestibule may bulge, as it is pinched at its lower end where it passes through the diaphragmatic hiatus.

Schatzki's ring

This is defined as a pathological annular narrowing at the oesophagogastric junction causing dysphagia, although some patients may present with bolus obstruction (Fig. 18.51A,B). Before dysphagia occurs, the lumen of the oesophagus has generally narrowed to less than 13 mm diameter. In some it may be congenital; in others there is inflammation and fibrosis, suggesting it is caused by reflux oesophagitis, and such cases may occasionally progress to a typical peptic stricture (Fig. 18.54A). It is always associated with a small sliding hiatus hernia, and is most consistently demonstrated when the oesophagus is distended during a prone barium swallow.

OESOPHAGEAL REFLUX AND REFLUX OESOPHAGITIS

Oesophageal reflux

Reflux can be a normal phenomenon, but oesophagitis results if reflux is excessive or particularly damaging to the mucosa. Excessive reflux results from an increase in the number or duration of episodes of relaxation of the lower oesophageal sphincter, as may be induced by fatty meals, drinking alcohol or coffee, or from cigarette smoking. Excessive reflux also results from weakening of the lower oesophageal sphincter from degeneration in elderly patients, or from diseases such as scleroderma. Reflux of acid and pepsin is the usual cause of oesophagitis, but the mucosa may be damaged by reflux of bile or pancreatic juice. Reflux is particularly damaging to the mucosa when the pH is unusually low, as may occur in Zollinger–Ellison syndrome or in patients with duodenal ulceration.

The lower oesophagus is normally protected by secondary peristalsis, which returns refluxed gastric juice rapidly back to the stomach. Failure of secondary peristalsis occurs when motility is disordered, a frequent finding in the elderly. Reflux oesophagitis itself may affect oesophageal motility and impair secondary peristalsis, thus further exposing the oesophagus to refluxed gastric juice.

A history of reflux is of more value than demonstrating reflux during a barium study, as reflux of barium may be observed in normal patients. Conversely, failure to demonstrate reflux may just reflect its intermittent nature. Hiatus hernias do not necessarily cause excessive reflux, as the function of the lower oesophageal sphincter may be maintained. However, an association between hiatus hernias and peptic oesophageal strictures exists, presumably because some hernias do predispose to reflux. Conversely in some patients reflux may be the initiating factor producing a stricture that shortens the oesophagus and draws the stomach into the chest.

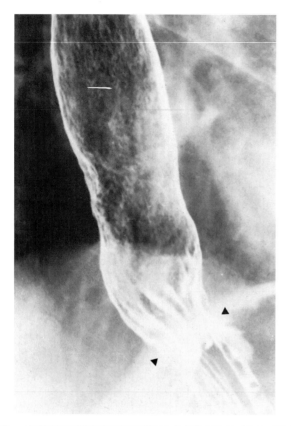

Fig. 18.52 Sliding hiatus hernia with peptic oesophagitis. The hiatus (between arrowheads) is wide (>3 cm) and at least three gastric folds are seen extending across it. The oesophageal mucosa is coarsely granular, indicating oesophagitis.

The association between peptic strictures and hiatus hernias is so strong that in the absence of a hernia an alternative cause for a stricture should be sought and biopsies performed to exclude neoplasia.

The definitive test for oesophageal reflux is 24 h pH recording, where a drop in pH below 4 defines a reflux event. Challenging the oesophageal mucosa with dilute hydrochloric acid is a useful test for acid sensitivity.

Reflux oesophagitis

The earliest changes of oesophagitis are seen at endoscopy: the mucosa becomes red and oedema results in loss of the vessel pattern and blurring of the squamocolumnar junction. It is only with more pronounced oedema that the earliest change of a fine mucosal nodularity is seen with a double-contrast barium swallow. The collapsed oesophagus shows thickened longitudinal folds (wider than 3 mm), which when nodular, give an appearance similar to that seen with varices. With further progression, multiple fine ulcers give the mucosa a punctate or granular appearance or larger discrete punched-out ulcers develop (Fig. 18.52). Ulceration is most pronounced immediately above the oesophagogastric junction and local circular muscle spasm may produce transverse folds. Scarring produces permanent folds that radiate from the margins of ulcers. When viewed in profile, outpouchings between folds can mimic ulceration (Fig. 18.53A), but unlike ulcers can be seen to change shape during the course of an examination. These coarse transverse folds are easily differentiated from the transient fine mucosal folds which are thought to result from contraction of the muscularis

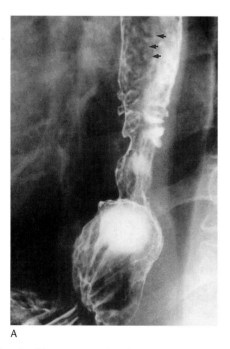
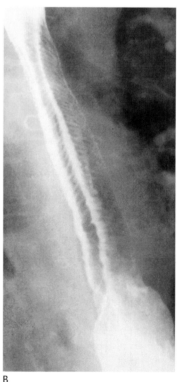

A   B

Fig. 18.53 (A) Hiatus hernia with an asymmetric stricture found to be benign on biopsy. Above the stricture are a number of ulcers together with transverse folds and pseudodiverticula produced by spasm and scarring. Mucosal erosions (arrows) are present in the oesophagus above this ulcerated segment. (B) Feline oesophagus. These fine mucosal folds are a transient finding produced by contraction of the muscularis mucosa. A similar appearance may be seen in cats. It is usually a normal variant but may be associated with gastro-oesophageal reflux.

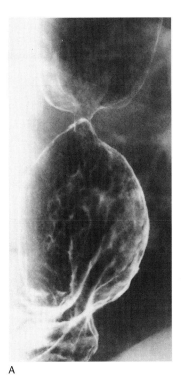
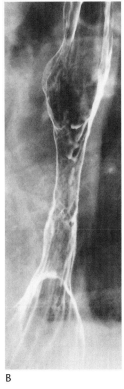
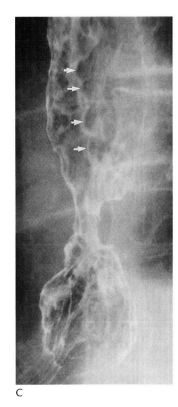
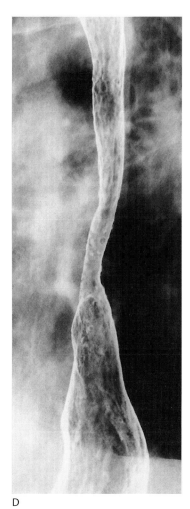

A   B   C   D

Fig. 18.54   (A) Annular peptic stricture at the oesophagogastric junction. Areae gastricae pattern is present below the stricture. (B) Benign peptic stricture above a hiatus hernia. The stricture has smooth tapered margins. (C) Benign peptic stricture. Asymmetric ulceration and scarring has produced a stricture with irregular and shouldered margins resembling a carcinoma. Erosions on oesophageal folds give them a lobular margin resembling varices (arrows). (D) Peptic oesophagitis with a long tapered stricture resulting from the presence of a nasogastric tube.

mucosa (*feline oesophagus*, Fig. 18.53B). These fine folds are prob-ably of no significance and relate to technique, as they are most often seen when the oesophagus is only partially distended.

Severe scarring results in stricture formation. Mild stricturing may be difficult to identify at endoscopy and is often better appre-ciated when the oesophagus is well-distended with barium. Should the patient be unable to take swallows of sufficient volume and rapidity to distend the oesophagus, the transit of bread or marshmallow soaked in barium is observed (Fig. 18.51). This is also worthwhile if there is a history of dysphagia for solids and the barium swallow has failed to find a cause. A peptic stricture above a hiatus hernia is typically short, and has a smooth lumen and tapered margins (Fig. 18.54A,B). However, asymmetric scarring and ulcer-ation may produce a stricture with irregular margins similar to that of a carcinoma (Fig. 18.54C). Long peptic strictures may be seen in Zollinger–Ellison syndrome or result from prolonged nasogastric intubation, as these tubes predispose to reflux (Fig. 18.54D).

Reflux oesophagitis may lead to columnar metaplasia develop-ing in the distal oesophagus (*Barrett's oesophagus*). Approximately 10% of patients with reflux oesophagitis have Barrett's oesophagus; of these, 15% develop adenocarcinoma. Endoscopic surveillance

and biopsy at yearly intervals have been recommended, although their efficacy has not been proven. At endoscopy the reddish-pink columnar mucosa extends circumferentially above the level of the gastro-oesophageal junction as finger-like projections or as multiple mucosal islands. Ulceration occurs at the junction of the columnar and the normal squamous oesophageal mucosa, so ulcers and stric-tures in Barrett's oesophagus often develop some distance above the gastro-oesophageal junction, and on occasions may even be seen in the midthoracic or cervical oesophagus. Islands of columnar mucosa give the oesophageal wall a fine reticular pattern (Fig. 18.55) and this is observed below the strictured or ulcerated segment.

OTHER TYPES OF OESOPHAGITIS

Candida oesophagitis

Candida oesophagitis most frequently develops in immunocompro-mised patients but occasionally it complicates food stasis in patients with achalasia or a peptic stricture. Patients present with odyno-phagia, dysphagia or haematemesis. Oral candidiasis, if present,

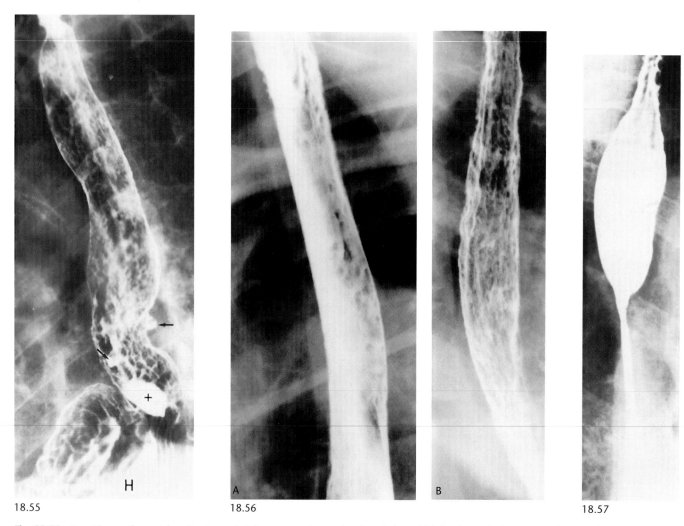

18.55   18.56   18.57

Fig. 18.55 Barrett's oesophagus. Ulceration (arrows) at the squamocolumnar junction, below which is a fine reticular pattern. This resembles the areae gastricae pattern of the stomach, and is produced by islands of columnar mucosa. + = Pool of barium; H = hiatus hernia.

Fig. 18.56 Candida oesophagitis. (A) Mucosal plaques. (B) Extensive mucosal nodularity.

Fig. 18.57 Corrosive stricture. Long stricture extending up to the midoesophagus resulting from swallowing lye as a child.

suggests the diagnosis. Double-contrast barium studies show mucosal plaques (Fig. 18.56A), which at endoscopy appear white on an erythematous background. The plaques run in the long axis of the oesophagus and on a barium swallow the background mucosa appears normal. Diffuse involvement may produce a granular or nodular mucosa (Fig. 18.56B), and in severe cases there is deep marginal ulceration. Rarely, barium may track beneath a sloughing pseudomembrane, or a fungal mass may form on the oesophageal wall and protrude into the lumen. Perforation, fistula and stricture formation are rare complications and are most frequently associated with AIDS-related candidiasis. A long oesophageal stricture is a rare complication of *chronic mucocutaneous candidiasis* in which an immunocompromised patient develops a persistent candidal infection of the mucous membranes, skin and nails.

Oesophagitis in the immunocompromised patient

Immunosuppression occurs in diabetics, debilitated patients and those with AIDS, and following chemotherapy, steroid treatment

and radiotherapy. The T-cell depression that results encourages infections with opportunistic organisms which are of low virulence and are normally present in mucosa and skin flora. In the oesophagus, candidal infection is the most frequent of these infections, and the oesophagitis may be severe, resulting in perforation, fistula and stricture formation. Cytomegalovirus (CMV), herpes simplex and tuberculous oesophagitis have all become more frequent with the current AIDS epidemic. In AIDS, candidal infection may coexist with herpes simplex or CMV oesophagitis. Actinomycosis may also involve the oesophagus in AIDS, producing deep ulcers and sinus tracts in the oesophageal wall. Acute and chronic HIV infection itself may produce giant oesophageal ulcers identical to those seen in CMV oesophagitis. If seen on barium studies, the patient should proceed to an endoscopic biopsy as HIV ulcers are treated with steroids, whereas CMV is treated with ganciclovir.

Herpes oesophagitis

Most patients with herpes oesophagitis are immunocompromised, but occasionally infection develops in an otherwise healthy individual. Oral herpetic lesions may suggest the diagnosis. Infection generally follows contact with herpetic lip lesions, and a prodromal flu-like illness precedes an acute onset of odynophagia. Vesicles in the upper and midoesophagus are shown as sessile filling defects on barium studies, and when they burst they leave punched out ulcers on a background of normal mucosa. In advanced disease the ulcers coalesce to produce diffuse ulceration. In most patients the disease resolves spontaneously in 2 weeks but with severe disease antiviral treatment is required.

Cytomegalovirus oesophagitis

This form of oesophagitis is rarely seen in the absence of AIDS. Discrete superficial ulcers develop, similar to those of herpes oesophagitis. Giant ulcers on a normal mucosal background are a feature of CMV oesophagitis. These ulcers must be differentiated from the identical appearing ulcers of HIV infection by performing an endoscopic biopsy, as treatment of HIV ulcers is with steroids, which causes CMV oesophagitis to progress.

Tuberculous oesophagitis

In *Mycobacterium tuberculosis* infection, caseating mediastinal nodes may compress or erode into the oesophagus to produce deep ulcers and fistulas. Infected sputum may be swallowed, producing mucosal plaques, ulcers and fistulas. Scarring and stricture formation may result. Similar features may be seen in *Crohn's disease*, although oesophageal involvement is rare in this disease and is invariably associated with severe disease of the ileum and colon.

M. tuberculosis and *M. avium-intracellulare* (MAI) both cause oesophagitis in AIDS. MAI produces discrete ulcers like those seen in herpes, CMV and HIV infection.

Drug-induced oesophagitis

Certain pills ulcerate the oesophagus if allowed to lie in contact with the mucosa for a prolonged period of time. Patients should therefore take tablets with a drink; particularly at bedtime. Tablets lodge at sites of oesophageal compression, and so ulceration occurs in the midoesophagus, above the aortic impression or that produced by the left main bronchus. The antibiotics tetracycline and doxycycline, which are acidic, are the most frequent causes of drug-induced oesophagitis. Potassium chloride and quinidine have been used in heart failure. They may lodge above the impression produced by an enlarged left atrium or left ventricle and cause deep ulceration which can lead to stricture formation. Non-steroidal anti-inflammatory drugs such as aspirin, phenylbutazone, indomethacin and ibuprofen cause contact oesophagitis or exacerbate reflux oesophagitis. Other causes include swallowing Clinitest tablets, ferrous sulphate, ascorbic acid and the antibiotics clindamycin and lincomycin. Most contact ulcers heal within a week of stopping the medication.

Radiation oesophagitis

If the oesophagus is included in the radiation field, doses in excess of 20 Gy will, after several weeks, produce a transient oesophagitis with odynophagia and dysphagia. A barium study shows mucosal granularity or discrete ulceration with narrowing of the lumen from mucosal oedema. The involved segment becomes aperistaltic or shows tertiary contractions. Doses in excess of 45 Gy, after an interval of about 6 months, cause an obliterative endarteritis resulting in severe oesophagitis, smooth tapered strictures, and sometimes deep ulceration which can fistulate to the trachea. Clinicians should be aware that acute and chronic radiation oesophagitis may be potentiated by doxorubicin or dactinomycin (actinomycin D).

Caustic oesophagitis

The ingestion of strong acids or alkalis causes a severe oesophagitis. Caustic household cleaning agents that may be swallowed include lye (sodium hydroxide), which is used as a drain cleaner, washing soda (sodium carbonate), iodine and bleaches. Initial mucosal necrosis is followed by ulceration and mucosal sloughing, and finally healing, often with fibrosis and stricture formation. Perforation may occur at any time within the first 2 weeks, and may result in fistulation to the pleural cavity or pericardium. Injury to the stomach generally involves the antrum, and is more frequent with acids, as alkalis are to some extent neutralised by gastric acid. Severe gastric damage may lead to perforation and peritonitis. A Gastrografin swallow will show if there is oesophageal or gastric perforation. The oesophagus may be narrowed from oedema and spasm and show ulceration, and sometimes Gastrografin is seen tracking underneath mucosa that is sloughing. The oesophagus may be atonic, show diffuse spasm or even achalasia if there is damage to the myenteric plexus. Long tapered strictures may develop as early as 2 weeks after the initial injury (Fig. 18.57), and these may involve the entire length of the oesophagus. Lye strictures are associated with an increased risk of squamous cell carcinoma, although there is a latent period of 20–40 years. Strictures may respond to balloon dilatation, but in severe cases colonic interposition surgery may be necessary.

Nasogastric tube oesophagitis

A nasogastric tube may render the lower oesophageal sphincter incompetent, and if the patient is being nursed supine a severe reflux oesophagitis may result. The condition has even been known to occur when the period of intubation has been as short as 3 days. A long tapered peptic stricture of the lower oesophagus may result (Fig. 18.54D).

Epidermolysis bullosa dystrophica and pemphigoid

Epidermolysis bullosa dystrophica is a hereditary skin disease affecting children, in whom minor trauma produces bulla formation. In some the oesophagus is also involved and may lead to stricture formation. Endoscopy can traumatise the mucosa, so a barium swallow is the preferred method of examining the oesophagus. Benign mucous membrane pemphigoid is a disease of middle age involving the conjunctiva and mucosa of the oral cavity and skin. Sometimes the upper oesophageal mucosa is also involved, with ulcers, webs and stricture formation.

Intramural pseudodiverticulosis

In this condition, oesophageal glands dilate and fill, and on barium studies are seen as multiple, flask-shaped outpouchings (Fig. 18.58A). There are normally about 300 oesophageal glands, and they are arranged longitudinally in rows with their ducts directed in

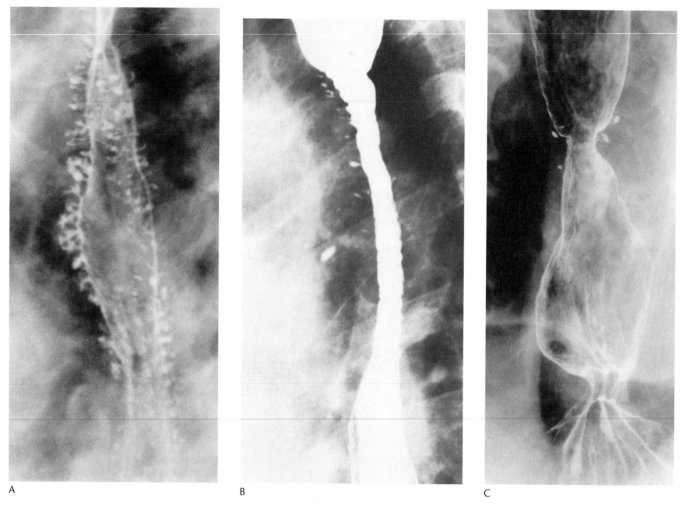

A   B   C

Fig. 18.58 Intramural pseudodiverticulosis. (A) Multiple flask-shaped projections produced by barium entering dilated oesophageal glands. (B) Midoesophageal stricture with small flask-shaped projections. (C) A few pseudodiverticula associated with a benign peptic stricture.

a slightly caudal direction. The duct orifices are small and the disorder is therefore difficult to diagnose by endoscopy. Gland dilatation is probably a consequence of oesophagitis, with reflux oesophagitis being the commonest cause. *Candida* spp may be grown from the oesophagus, but this is probably a secondary infection as a consequence of stasis of secretions within the glands. Fistulation may occur between the pseudodiverticula, and intramural abscesses may develop which can, rarely, perforate through the oesophageal wall. The oesophageal wall thickens and long tapered strictures develop, possibly as a result of inflammation and scarring (Fig. 18.58B). The disease often involves the entire length of the oesophagus but can be localised when pseudodiverticula are found in association with a peptic stricture (Fig. 18.58C). Pseudodiverticula may also be seen adjacent to an oesophageal carcinoma if it complicates a peptic stricture.

DIAPHRAGMATIC HERNIAS

Herniation of abdominal viscera into the thoracic cavity occurs through:

- The diaphragmatic hiatus (sliding and paraoesophageal hiatus hernias).

- A congenital defect (Bochdalek and Morgagni hernias). Failure of complete closure of the diaphragm during development produces a defect through which the thoracic and abdominal cavities are in direct communication.

- A diaphragmatic tear.

Sliding hiatus hernia

Sliding hiatus hernias are the most frequent type of diaphragmatic hernia. The presence of a sliding hiatus hernia is one of a number of factors that predisposes to gastro-oesophageal reflux, so not all patients with sliding hiatus hernias have excessive reflux and not all patients with reflux have a sliding hernia. They range in size from a small pouch to a hernia comprising most of the stomach. Phrenico-oesophageal ligaments extend from the margins of the diaphragmatic hiatus to the lower oesophagus and it is the stretching with age or the rupture of these ligaments that allows a hernia to develop. Small sliding hiatus hernias reduce in the standing or sitting posture, and appear in the recumbent or stooping positions. Large hiatus hernias often become 'fixed', with part of the stomach remaining permanently in the thorax. This is particularly liable to occur when the oesophagus shortens as a result of reflux peptic

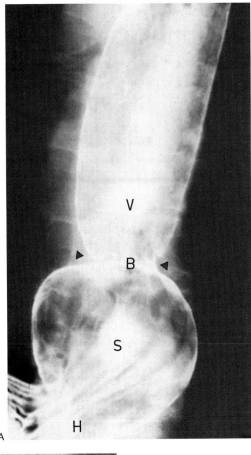

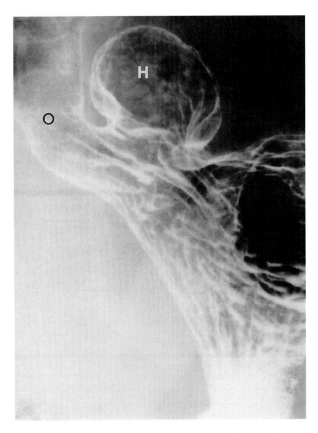

Fig. 18.60 Rolling (paraoesophageal) hiatus hernia. The gastric fundus (H) lies alongside the lower oesophagus (O).

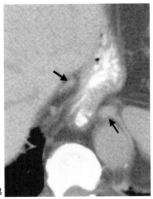

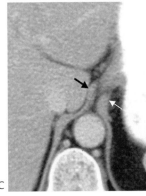

Fig. 18.59 (A) The radiographic features of a sliding hiatus hernia. H= hiatus, more than 3 cm wide with at least three gastric folds seen extending across the hiatus; S = stomach forming the hernia; B = B-ring, the oesophagogastric junction; V = vestibule. The A-ring is not visible. (B) CT scan showing the crura of the diaphragm (arrows) separated by 28 mm (normal is 15 mm or less). The fundus of the stomach is seen herniating through the diaphragmatic hiatus. (C) Normal CT of diaphragmatic hiatus for comparison. Crura of the diaphragm are arrowed.

oesophagitis. Such hernias can be seen behind the heart on a sufficiently penetrated plain chest radiograph.

The oesophagus normally shortens in length during swallowing and the elasticity of the phrenico-oesophageal ligaments allows the gastro-oesophageal junction to move up to 2 cm above the diaphragmatic hiatus. A sliding hiatus hernia is a pouch of stomach that protrudes more than 2 cm above the hiatus (Fig. 18.59A).

Three or more gastric folds may be identified passing from the stomach across the hiatus and the Z-line and areae gastricae are located above the hiatus. The hiatus is wide, measuring more than 3 cm in diameter. On CT the diaphragmatic crura are separated by more than 15 mm, and the hernia produces a mass of soft-tissue density that protrudes above the hiatus and which may be surrounded by mesenteric fat (Fig. 18.59B,C).

Large hernias may result in the entire stomach entering the chest. In such instances the gastro-oesophageal junction is normally sited but the stomach volves and comes to lie above the diaphragm with its greater curve uppermost, and the duodenum passes back through the hiatus. Such patients are often elderly and may be asymptomatic, but occasionally the volvulus causes oesophageal or duodenal obstruction or interferes with blood supply to the stomach, leading to gastric infarction.

Rolling hiatus hernia

The *paraoesophageal* or rolling hiatus hernia is a rare type of diaphragmatic hernia in which the cardia remains below the diaphragm while the fundus herniates through a weakness or tear in the phrenico-oesophageal membrane to lie alongside the lower oesophagus (Fig. 18.60). There is only a slight predisposition to reflux, the most frequent complication being anaemia from chronic bleeding. Most paraoesophageal hernias are not reducible.

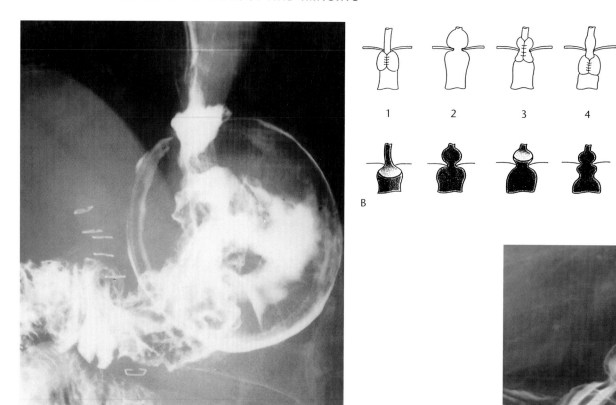

Fig. 18.61   (A) Angelchik prosthesis: a silicon ring that is placed around the intra-abdominal segment of the oesophagus to secure its position below the diaphragm. In this patient the ring has slipped down over the stomach and eroded into the stomach. Barium has leaked from the stomach around the prosthesis. (B) Radiological appearance of a failure of a fundoplication. Anatomical drawings top row, barium meal appearances bottom row. 1, Normal postoperative appearance; 2, complete disruption of wrap with recurrence of hiatus hernia; 3, wrap intact but herniates through diaphragmatic hiatus; 4, stomach slips up through wrap and bulges above diaphragm; 5, stomach slips up through wrap but remains below diaphragm. (C) Stomach slips up through wrap and bulges above diaphragm. Wrap is arrowed.

Occasionally a hiatus hernia with both a sliding and paraoe-sophageal component is demonstrated, giving rise to the term *mixed hiatus hernia*.

Hiatus hernia surgery

The Nissen fundoplication can be performed laparoscopically. The operation consists of pulling each side of the gastric fundus around the lower oesophagus and suturing the two sides together at the front to produce a 360° wrap. A barium swallow after fundoplication shows angulation and narrowing of the lower oesophagus, and there is a pseudotumour at the cardia. A similar but smaller pseudotumour is seen after a Belsey operation. This procedure requires a thoraco-tomy and consists of fixing the gastric fundus to 240° of the lower oesophagus. Knowledge of the nature of previous surgery avoids confusing a surgically fashioned fundal mass with a carcinoma. The Angelchik prosthesis is a split silicon ring that is tied around the intra-abdominal segment of the oesophagus to secure its position. The prosthesis contains a metallic marking ring which allows it to be recognised on plain films. Angelchik prostheses are no longer used, as complications were frequent and included migration of the ring so that it slipped over the stomach or oesophagus, or erosion of the ring into the stomach (Fig. 18.61A). Postoperative oedema is a common cause of dysphagia in the first few weeks after a fundoplication. Too tight a fundoplication may result in persisting dysphagia, a feeling of fullness and an inability to belch (the *gas bloat syndrome*). A pre-operative assessment with manometry or a barium swallow to ensure that motility is normal reduces the risk of these complications. Other complications include complete disruption of the fundoplication resulting in loss of the fundal pseudotumour, partial disruption resulting in loss of part of the pseudotumour and fundal outpouch-ing, herniation of the fundus through the diaphragmatic hiatus with an intact fundoplication, and telescoping of the cardia up through an intact wrap (Fig. 18.61B,C).

Congenital hernias

A hernia through the *foramen of Bochdalek* is a common diaphrag-matic hernia in infants, and may present as a respiratory emergency immediately after birth. There is associated malrotation of the bowel as the hernia interferes with the bowel's normal embryonic rotation. The radiographic findings depend upon the size of the defect and the contents of the hernia. The defect lies postero-laterally, and results from incomplete closure of the pleuroperi-toneal membrane. Closure occurs earlier on the right, which may explain why these hernias are much commoner on the left. The chest radiograph shows herniated bowel but the diagnosis is more difficult if the hernia only contains the spleen or kidney, or on early films when the bowel is still fluid filled.

The *foramen of Morgagni* hernia is rare and results from incomplete attachment of the diaphragm anteriorly to the sternum. These hernias are usually right sided and most are asymptomatic, so they may not be diagnosed until adult life. The contents of the hernia may include extraperitoneal fat, omentum, liver and transverse colon. Plain radiographs are usually sufficient for diagnosis.

Diaphragmatic tears

These may be small, from penetrating trauma, or large, from a sudden increase in abdominal pressure from blunt trauma. Penetrating trauma often necessitates surgery but the diagnosis of a tear following blunt trauma may be delayed. Tears of the diaphragm tend to occur at the musculotendinous junction. The diagnosis should be suspected if, in the appropriate clinical setting, there is paralysis, asymmetry or a change in diaphragmatic levels, abdomi-nal contents in the chest or an unexplained haemothorax. Helical CT with sagittal reformatting or MRI may show a waist around solid organs that have partially herniated through the tear. Obstruction of the herniated bowel is more likely with small tears, whereas large tears may cause respiratory problems.

BENIGN OESOPHAGEAL TUMOURS

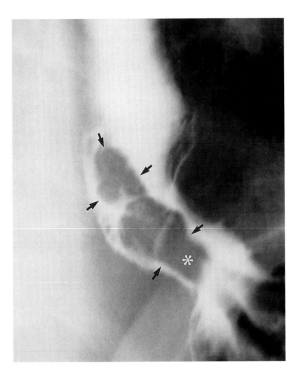

Fig. 18.62   Inflammatory polyp (arrows). The polyp lies at the end of a gastric fold (asterisk).

Squamous papilloma

These small 0.5–1.5 cm benign tumours consist of hyperplastic squamous epithelium with a fibrous core. They are generally an incidental finding on a barium study. They are ususaly single, sessile and have a smooth lobulated margin. Rarely, giant papillo-mas develop, which have a fronded surface that traps barium to produce a bubbly appearance, or a multitude of small papillomas cover the oesophageal mucosa, a condition known as *oesophageal papillomatosis*.

Adenoma

These rare benign tumours arise from Barrett's mucosa in the distal oesophagus. They are sessile or polypoid, and when found should be removed endoscopically, as, in common with colonic adenomas, they can be premalignant.

Inflammatory oesophagogastric polyp

Persistent gastro-oesophageal reflux may result in an inflammatory swelling developing at the top end of a lesser curve gastric fold. The distinctive feature of the polyp is that its lower margin merges with the gastric fold, and so the diagnosis is usually easily made (Fig. 18.62).

Glycogen acanthosis

In this benign degeneration of the oesophageal mucosa an accu-mulation of glycogen expands squamous mucosa cells; 1–2 mm white nodules are produced and can be readily appreciated at endoscopy. These nodules develop after the age of 50, increase in number with age, and are asymptomatic. They are usually mid-oesophageal but occasionally may be seen in the distal oesophagus. Rarely, plaques may form, which can be up to 1 cm size, and the radiological appearance may mimic candidal oesophagitis.

Leiomyoma

This well-encapsulated smooth muscle submucosal tumour is most often found in the lower two-thirds of the oesophagus because it is this part of the oesophagus that has a smooth muscle coat

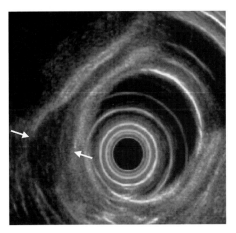

Fig. 18.63   Leiomyoma. An echopoor mass (between arrows) is continuous with the layer of the muscularis propria.

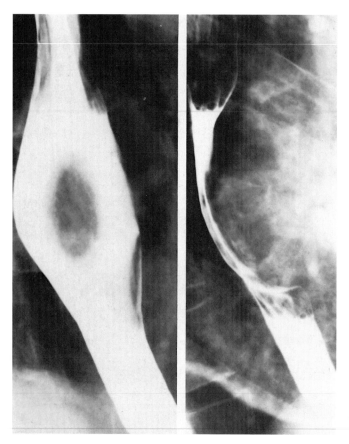

Fig. 18.64 Leiomyoma of the oesophagus. Two views showing features typical of an intramural or extrinsic lesion. There is a broad-based filling defect bulging into, and widening the lumen of the oesophagus.

(Fig. 18.63). Although generally solitary, rarely multiple tumours develop and are so numerous that they carpet the oesophagus. Leiomyomas are often large by the time of diagnosis, and if predominantly exophytic the chest film may show a mediastinal mass that sometimes contains punctate or amorphous calcification. The typical appearance on barium studies is of an intramural lesion with margins that make an obtuse angle with the normal oesophageal wall. Large tumours bulge into the oesophageal lumen, narrowing it in one plane but widening it in the other (Fig. 18.64). Typically leiomyomas appear as homogeneous ovoid masses of soft-tissue density eccentric to the lumen on CT. Rarely, a leiomyoma encircles and narrows the oesophagus, or a bulky tumour grows into the lumen and draws out a pedicle. The tumour may cause dysphagia, but bleeding is unusual, as, unlike their gastric counterparts, oesophageal leiomyomas rarely ulcerate. These tumours have no malignant potential, so if the patient is asymptomatic surgery may not be necessary. Oesophageal leiomyomas have been described in association with vulval leiomyomas and with hypertrophic osteoarthropathy.

Fibrovascular polyp

These tumours are covered by squamous epithelium and have a vascular core of fibrous and adipose tissue. They are usually solitary, arising from the upper cervical oesophagus, and may become pedunculated. Patients are generally male, elderly and asymptomatic but the tumours may become large and obstruct, ulcerate or bleed. Rarely, a tumour will prolapse up into the mouth or even into the larynx, causing asphyxia. On barium studies a bulky intraluminal mass is seen, which may move on swallowing. The fat content of the tumour can be recognized with CT and MRI. Surgery is performed if the tumour is large, as haemorrhage from the vascular core may complicate endoscopic removal.

Granular cell tumour

This is a rare benign tumour consisting of cells with an eosinophilic granular cytoplasm, which are thought to arise from Schwann cells. These tumours may be located anywhere in the body but most commonly arise in the oral cavity, subcutaneous tissues and breast. When they arise in the oesophagus they are generally found in the mid- or lower oesophagus, are submucosal and up to 2 cm in size. If diagnosed endoscopically, it is invariably an incidental finding and so can be left, as the tumour has no malignant potential.

Other rare submucosal tumours found in the oesophagus include lipomas, fibromas, neurofibromas, haemangiomas and hamartomas. Multiple oesophageal haemangiomas may develop in hereditary haemorrhagic telangiectasia (Osler–Rendu–Weber disease), producing a diffuse nodularity to the oesophageal mucosa. In Cowden's disease, multiple oesophageal hamartomas may produce a similar appearance.

Duplication cyst

These are round or tubular and occur in the lower posterior mediastinum. They often distort the distal oesophagus but only rarely communicate with the oesophageal lumen. A chest film may show a right-sided mediastinal mass, and if there is an associated vertebral abnormality this may also be seen. They can be shown to be fluid-containing by CT or MRI. Some have gastric mucosa in the cyst wall, in which case ulceration can cause bleeding into the cyst or perforation.

Retention cyst

Retention cysts result from obstruction to the ducts of oesophageal glands and produce one or more submucosal nodules that can be up to 2 cm in size. The cysts can be readily identified by EUS.

MALIGNANT OESOPHAGEAL TUMOURS
Oesophageal carcinoma
Squamous cell carcinoma

Sixty per cent of oesophageal carcinomas are of squamous cell type, although the incidence has been falling in the UK and USA for the last 20 years. They are evenly distributed throughout the length of the oesophagus. Cigarette smoking and alcohol consumption are risk factors which are thought to be synergistic for the development of squamous cell carcinomas, not only of the oesophagus but also of the larynx, pharynx and mouth. Different dietary contaminants are believed to account for the high prevalence in China, South Africa and parts of the Middle East. In China and South Africa infection with the human papilloma virus may be a contributory factor. Chronic mucosal injury as a result of food stasis may account for the increased risk in achalasia when carcinoma

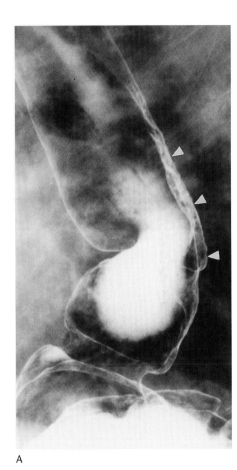

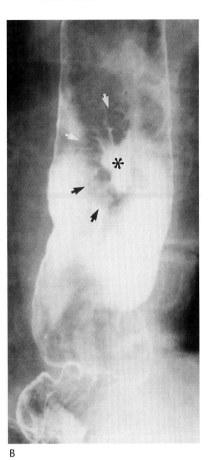

A   B

Fig. 18.65 Early oesophageal carcinoma. (A) A plaque lesion is seen in profile (arrowheads). (B) En face there is a central ulcer (asterisk) with a nodular margin (arrows).

develops after a latent interval of at least 20 years from the time of diagnosis. Other predisposing conditions with long latent intervals are chronic lye strictures, coeliac disease (despite adherence to a gluten-free diet), chronic radiation injury and asbestos exposure. Patients at risk from cigarette smoking and alcohol consumption who develop a squamous cell carcinoma of the oesophagus may also have synchronous squamous tumours in the pharynx, larynx or oral cavity. The mucosal changes in Plummer–Vinson syndrome predispose to the development of postcricoid oesophageal and pharyngeal carcinomas (Fig. 18.37). There is debate as to whether the increased risk in these conditions justifies periodic endoscopic surveillance, but in *tylosis palmaris et plantaris* the risk is so high that surveillance is certainly justified. In this hereditary autosomal dominant disorder there is hyperkeratosis of the palms of the hands and the soles of the feet, together with hyperkeratotic plaques in the oesophagus. It is from these plaques that foci of dysplasia and eventually carcinoma develop. Most of these patients will develop a carcinoma if they live long enough, and prophylactic oesophagectomy has been recommended.

Adenocarcinoma

Forty per cent of oesophageal carcinomas are adenocarcinomas arising in the lower oesophagus from dysplasia of metaplastic columnar epithelium that has developed as a result of longstanding reflux oesophagitis (Barrett's oesophagus). There is an increased risk of adenocarcinoma in scleroderma, as this disease predisposes to reflux and Barrett's oesophagus.

Early oesophageal carcinoma

Early oesophageal cancer is defined as a cancer limited to the mucosa and submucosa without lymph node involvement. The 5 year survival rate is 70%. These early cancers on barium radiology are depressed, polypoid or plaque-like (Fig. 18.65). In western countries the diagnosis of early oesophageal carcinoma is generally only made when growth is predominantly intraluminal, so that the patient presents early with dysphagia.

Advanced oesophageal carcinoma

Most patients with oesophageal carcinoma present with dysphagia and already have tumours that have spread to involve regional lymph nodes, so the prognosis is poor (5 year survival less than 10%). The tumour or enlarged regional lymph nodes occasionally produce a mediastinal mass on a plain chest film. Oesophageal dilatation and an air–fluid level may also be seen but these are more often features of achalasia and benign peptic strictures where dilatation is pronounced because of the slower onset of the obstruction. Barium radiology most frequently shows a stricture with an irregular lumen and rolled margins (Fig. 18.66A), unlike benign peptic strictures which have a smooth lumen and tapered margins. However, differentiation can be difficult, and so endoscopy and biopsy are always performed. Some tumours show pronounced ulceration (Fig. 18.66B), or are predominantly polypoid (Fig. 18.66C,D), or spread submucosally, producing thick and irregular oesophageal folds simulating varices (varicoid carcinoma, Fig. 18.66E).

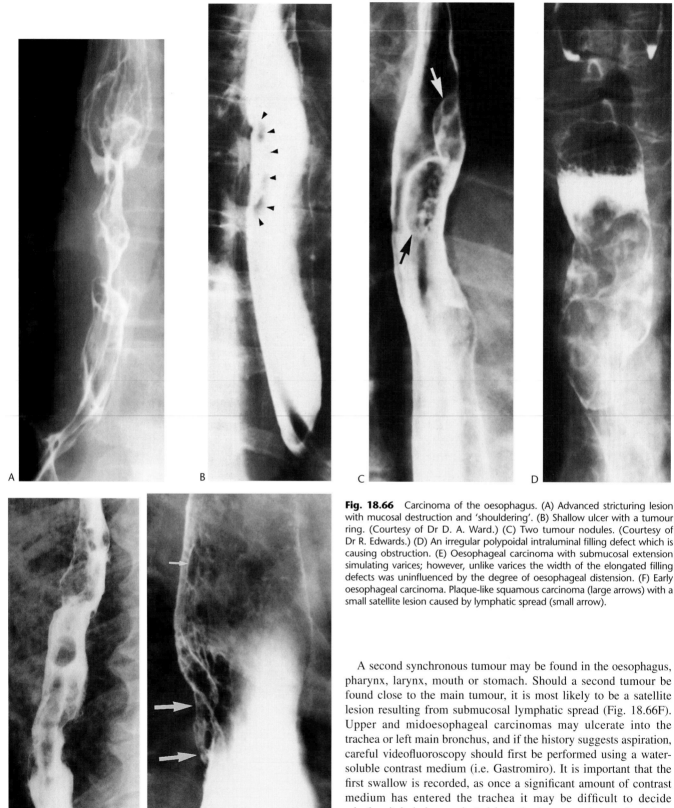

Fig. 18.66 Carcinoma of the oesophagus. (A) Advanced stricturing lesion with mucosal destruction and 'shouldering'. (B) Shallow ulcer with a tumour ring. (Courtesy of Dr D. A. Ward.) (C) Two tumour nodules. (Courtesy of Dr R. Edwards.) (D) An irregular polypoidal intraluminal filling defect which is causing obstruction. (E) Oesophageal carcinoma with submucosal extension simulating varices; however, unlike varices the width of the elongated filling defects was uninfluenced by the degree of oesophageal distension. (F) Early oesophageal carcinoma. Plaque-like squamous carcinoma (large arrows) with a small satellite lesion caused by lymphatic spread (small arrow).

A second synchronous tumour may be found in the oesophagus, pharynx, larynx, mouth or stomach. Should a second tumour be found close to the main tumour, it is most likely to be a satellite lesion resulting from submucosal lymphatic spread (Fig. 18.66F). Upper and midoesophageal carcinomas may ulcerate into the trachea or left main bronchus, and if the history suggests aspiration, careful videofluoroscopy should first be performed using a water-soluble contrast medium (i.e. Gastromiro). It is important that the first swallow is recorded, as once a significant amount of contrast medium has entered the trachea it may be difficult to decide whether it is being aspirated into the larynx or is entering via a fistula at a lower level.

Adenocarcinomas, unlike squamous carcinomas, frequently spread across the gastro-oesophageal junction to involve the gastric fundus, in which case there may be difficulty in deciding whether a

Box 18.1   TNM staging

Tis	Carcinoma in situ	N0	No nodal involvement
T1	Invading submucosa	N1	Regional nodes involved
T2	Invading muscularis propria		
T3	Invading adventitia	M0	No metastases
T4	Invading adjacent structures	M1a	Non-regional nodal involvement
		M1b	Other metastases

Table 18.3   Oesophageal tumours: non-regional nodal involvement

Tumour site	Non-regional nodes (M1a)
Upper third (thoracic inlet to carina)	Cervical, supraclavicular nodes
Mid third (Carina to halfway between carina and GOJ)	Not applicable
Lower third (halfway between carina and GOJ to GOJ)	Coeliac nodes

GOJ = gastro-oesophageal junction.
More distant node involvement is classified as distant metastases.

tumour has arisen in the stomach or the oesophagus. If the bulk of the tumour involves the fundus, it is generally classified as a gastric carcinoma, but if the majority of the tumour involves the oesophagus then it will be assumed to have arisen from the oesophagus.

Damage to the distal oesophageal mucosa from longstanding reflux oesophagitis may cause columnar metaplasia with the development of islands of gastric and intestinal epithelium (Barrett's oesophagus). Dysplasia of this epithelium may lead to the development of an adenocarcinoma. Adenomatous polyps are occasionally found arising from Barrett's mucosa and may also show dysplasia and lead to the development of an adenocarcinoma.

Cancer staging

The purpose of all staging systems is to give an indication as to the future behaviour of the disease process in question. The ultimate staging with cancers is histological, with outcome inversely proportional to the stage. The poor outcome of patients with advanced oesophageal tumours treated by surgery alone has led to therapeutic regimens using preoperative chemotherapy and radiotherapy. These treatments can lead to complete histological remissions in the resected specimens of some patients with T3 tumours. As treatment becomes more stage specific the demands on preoperative staging increase. EUS and CT have complementary roles to play in the staging of oesophageal carcinomas (Box 18.1, Table 18.3), and patients with tumours extending to the gastro-oesophageal junction may also be assessed with laparoscopy.

EUS shows layers of the oesophageal wall (Fig. 18.26) that cannot be resolved on CT and is therefore better for local tumour staging (T-staging, Fig. 18.67). Local lymph nodes not visible on CT can often be identified using EUS and criteria other than size can be applied to indicate involvement. Malignant nodes are round,

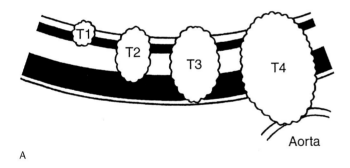

Aorta

A

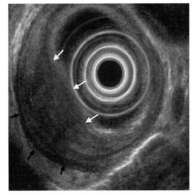

B

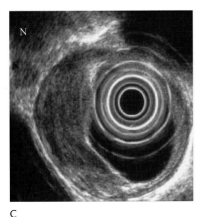

C

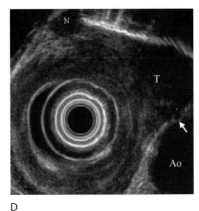

D

Fig. 18.67   Staging of oesophageal carcinoma by endoscopic ultrasound. (A) Diagram illustrating T staging. T1, Tumour limited to mucosa and submucosa. T2, Tumour infiltrates the muscularis propria. T3, Tumour involves adventitia. T4, Tumour invades adjacent structures, i.e. aorta, trachea, pericardium. (B) Stage T2. The muscularis propria has not been breached (black arrows). (C) Stage T2N1. The muscularis propria has not been breached. Adjacent involved malignant lymph nodes (N). Malignant nodes are round, hypoechoic and well defined with loss of internal structure. (D) Stage T4. Tumour has breached the muscularis propria and is invading the aortic wall (arrow). Ao = aorta; T = tumour; N = metastatic lymph node. (Courtesy of Dr K. Harris.)

hypoechoic and well defined, with loss of internal structure (Fig. 18.67C,D), whereas benign nodes are elongated, have echogenic centres and ill-defined margins. EUS is therefore more accurate in assessing lymph nodes that fall within the field of view. A drawback to EUS is that it is necessary to traverse the tumour with the endoscope, which may not be possible in up to 20% of cases. Nearly all adenocarcinomas and squamous cancers of the oesophagus are uniformly hypoechoic, with a homogeneous texture when small, becoming more disorganised as they outgrow their blood supply. EUS can also be of value in determining whether there is direct invasion of adjacent structures, as in the absence of invasion movement can be observed between the tumour and these structures. Staging accuracy with EUS is 80–90% for depth of tumour invasion and 85–95% for lymph node involvement.

The accuracy of CT in the staging of oesophageal tumours increases with more advanced disease. CT is of value in assessing locally advanced tumours, distant lymphadenopathy and other distant metastatic sites. The CT examination should extend from the lung apices to the bottom of the liver (extending to cover the cervical region for upper third tumours). This provides an overview of the tumour, its anatomical relationships and major metastatic sites. CT acquisitions with a collimation of 5 mm should be performed through the chest in an arterial dominated vascular phase and upper abdomen in the portal venous dominated phase. If possible the stomach should be distended so as to determine the extent of gastric involvement with lower third tumours. Water is ideal as a contrast agent, although patients with high-grade dysphagia may not be able to tolerate a sufficient volume to achieve adequate distension.

The normal wall of the oesophagus on CT has a maximal thickness of 3 mm but is often less than this, particularly when distended proximal to an obstruction; 5 mm is pathological and tumours usually appear as eccentric or circumferential mural thickening. Oesophageal distension proximal to an obstructing tumour helps to define its upper margin. The lower margin is more difficult to define: CT underestimates the length of oesophagus wall involvement by comparison with barium studies or histology. Local staging is largely confined to determining whether there is invasion of adjacent structures, and when deciding whether there is involvement of adjacent organs it is important to assess the integrity of intervening fat planes. In the posterior mediastinum fat is often absent between the oesophagus and the trachea, left main bronchus, aorta and pericardium, so absence of these fat planes, as a solitary finding, cannot be used as evidence of invasion. Tracheobronchial invasion is likely if the usual convex contour of the trachea or bronchus, at its interface with the oesophagus, is concave, and should be confirmed with bronchoscopy and biopsy (Fig. 18.68A). Posterior wall indentation, however, is a normal feature in the cervical oesophagus. Aortic involvement is relatively uncommon and is predicted on the basis of loss of the intervening fat plane. A circumferential interface with the tumour of >90° makes aortic invasion likely (Fig. 18.68B–D); with less than 45° of contact, invasion is unlikely; and between 45 and 90°, indeterminate. Using these criteria, accuracies of 80% have been reported. An alternative predictor of involvement is the obliteration of the triangle of fat between the spine, aorta and oesophagus, and this yields an accuracy of 84%. The presence of a pericardial effu-

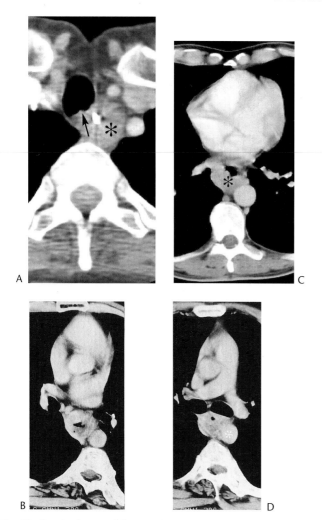

Fig. 18.68 Carcinoma of the oesophagus. (A) Carcinoma invading the trachea (arrow). A nasogastric tube is in situ, causing the high density artefact. (B) Thickened oesophageal wall but no aortic invasion as there is an intact fat plane between oesophagus and aorta. (C) Tumour (asterisk) surrounds the aorta over an arc of just under 90°, which is indeterminate for invasion. (D) Tumour surrounds the aorta over an arc of >90° and obliterates the triangle of fak between the spine aorta and oesophagus. Both of these features suggest aortic invasion.

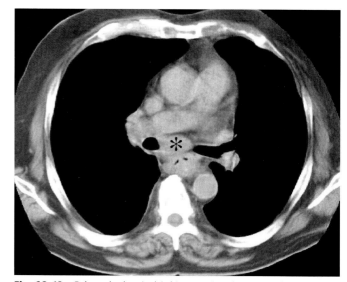

Fig. 18.69 Enlarged subcarinal (white arrow) and paraoesophageal (black arrows) lymph nodes in a patient with advanced oesophageal carcinoma. Note dilated oesophagus with air fluid level proximal to the tumour.

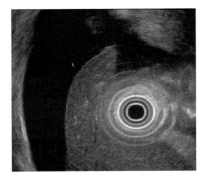

Fig. 18.70 Endoscopic ultrasound. A small amount of ascites at the margin of the left lobe of the liver.

sion, pericardial thickening or indentation of the left atrium suggests pericardial invasion. Direct contiguity of the tumour with the crus of the diaphragm over more than 1 cm suggests invasion, although this rarely precludes resection. CT performs relatively poorly in tumour staging, particularly with low stage tumours, with an accuracy of less than 40% for T1 and T2, 60–70% for T3 and 80–90% for T4 tumours. Overall there is a tendency for CT to underestimate involvement of adjacent structures, minimising the risk of patients being denied potentially curative surgery.

Lymphadenopathy (Fig. 18.69) is diagnosed on the basis of the short axis size criterion: 1 cm is usually taken as the threshold of significance for mediastinal and upper abdominal nodes, and 0.6 cm for retrocrural nodes, although clusters of smaller nodes are regarded as suspicious. As with all other cancers, lymphatic involvement can occur in normal size lymph nodes, and reactive lymph nodes can reach the dimensions of cancerous nodes. The accuracy of CT in predicting abdominal lymph node involvement is approximately 80%. CT is poorer at detecting perioesophageal lymph node involvement as this may be may be indistinguishable from the tumour mass. Management decisions based on the presence of lymphadenopathy need histological support. Unlike most cancers, distant lymphadenopathy of upper and lower third neoplasms contribute to the M stage of the tumour. At presentation the liver is the commonest extranodal site for metastases, being found in 35% of patients, followed by lungs 20%, bone 2%, adrenal 2% and brain 2%. CT provides a good means of surveying the majority of the sites, although the brain is not routinely imaged. Liver metastases are typically hypovascular and best demonstrated on portal venous images. Although the depth of penetration of EUS is limited, small metastases that are too small to detect with CT can be seen in the left lobe of the liver. A small peritoneal effusion resulting from peritoneal metastases may also be observed using EUS before it becomes apparent with CT (Fig. 18.70).

Positron emission tomography (PET) to detect oesophageal tumour spread relies on the tumour having an increased rate of glycolysis compared with normal tissues, and with ^{18}F-fluorodeoxyglucose (^{18}FDG) tumour involvement of normal sized nodes can be detected. Although only available in specialised centres, and offering relatively poor anatomical resolution, this technique is likely to be used with increasing frequency in tumour staging, as it allows metastases to be excluded with greater certainty.

Cancer management

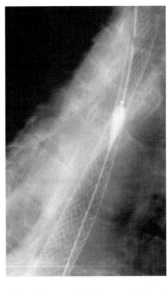

Fig. 18.71 Nitinol wallstent being deployed for an obstructing midoesophageal carcinoma. (Courtesy of Dr M. Sheridan.)

After chemoradiotherapy, CT and EUS are used to restage tumours before surgery; however, the tumour may appear identical to that of pretherapeutic scans despite histological regression, as necrosis, fibrosis and inflammation can have a similar appearance to that of the tumour mass. EUS and CT may also be of value for assessing tumour recurrence after resection, which predominantly arises deep to the mucosa or in contiguous nodes.

Stenting is now used to palliate malignant dysphagia, as surgical palliation is associated with a high operative mortality, radiotherapy improves dysphagia but only in about 50% of patients, and laser therapy, although effective, has to be repeated every 4–6 weeks. Nitinol metallic stents (Fig.18.71) have now replaced plastic stents. They are more expensive but are easier to place, less likely to result in perforation, provide a wider luminal diameter. Covered metallic stents are available for tumours associated with a tracheo-oesophageal fistula. They also reduce the problem of tumour ingrowth but have been unsuitable for deployment across the oesophagogastric junction where stent migration has been a problem. However, a conical shaped stent is now available with a polyurethane covering applied to the inside of the mesh (Flamingo Wallstent), which provides better fixation. Postprocedure pain is common and may last several days or even persist, requiring long-term analgesia. There is an increased risk of haemorrhage when stents are used after radiotherapy. Reflux and aspiration pneumonia can complicate stents placed across the gastro-oesophageal junction, although stents are now available that incorporate an antireflux valve.

Extrinsic malignant invasion

This is most frequently seen at the level of the carina, from malignant mediastinal nodes, usually secondary to carcinoma of the bronchus or breast. When direct invasion occurs, it is usually from an adjacent bronchial or thyroid carcinoma. There is initially a smooth indentation of the oesophagus and an adjacent soft-tissue mass, but eventually the mucosa is breached, and the tumour may spread circumferentially around the oesophagus to produce an appearance similar to that seen with a primary oesophageal carcinoma.

Haematogenous metastases to the oesophagus are rare and most are from breast carcinoma. Submucosal metastases to the distal

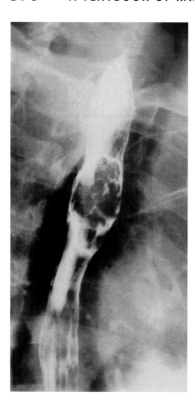

Fig. 18.72 Spindle cell sarcoma. A bulky polypoid tumour arising in the mid-oesophagus.

oesophagus from the breast, bronchus and pancreas may produce an achalasia-like picture. A metastasis may start as a smooth broad-based submucosal nodule and progress to a polypoid lesion or to a stricture, which can appear benign or malignant.

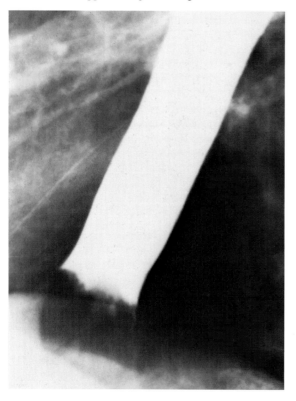

Fig. 18.73 Lower oesophageal obstruction produced by impaction of a large meat bolus.

Spindle cell carcinoma (carcinosarcoma, pseudosarcoma)

These rare tumours have both carcinomatous and spindle cell elements. They are generally bulky, polypoid tumours arising in the midoesophagus (Fig. 18.72). Occasionally the tumour mass has a pedicle, and torsion has been described. They generally develop in elderly men, and often there is a history of heavy smoking and excessive alcohol consumption.

Leiomyosarcoma

These tumours arise from smooth muscle and so are most frequently found in the lower two-thirds of the oesophagus because of its smooth muscle coat. They may be bulky and intraluminal or have a predominantly exophytic growth pattern. If a stricturing tumour develops, then it resembles a carcinoma. Like their benign counterparts, these tumours may produce a large posterior mediastinal mass which sometimes calcifies and may cavitate. A mass may be observed on a chest radiograph; CT often shows areas of low density from central necrosis; and on angiography the tumour is hypervascular.

Malignant melanoma

Malignant melanoma may metastasise to the oesophagus, but is also believed to develop as a primary tumour in the oesophagus, as a small percentage of the normal population have melanoblasts within the oesophageal mucosa. These also are often bulky, polypoid intraluminal tumours.

Lymphoma

Lymphoma of the oesophagus is rare, and when seen is usually non-Hodgkin's lymphoma in type. Primary lymphoma of the oesophagus generally resembles an oesophageal carcinoma, although rarely a diffuse nodularity is seen throughout the length of the oesophagus, which may suggest the diagnosis, or a submucosal nodule may develop, which ulcerates. Lymphomas may simulate achalasia if there is submucosal infiltration of the distal oesophagus. Gastric lymphomas may spread to involve the distal oesophagus, or lymphomatous mediastinal nodes may compress and invade the midoesophagus.

FOREIGN BODIES AND TRAUMA

Foreign body impaction

Most cases occur in children when a variety of foreign bodies may be swallowed. Most pass through the alimentary tract without lodging, but sharp objects such as open safety pins may arrest in the oesophagus. Metallic or dense foreign bodies are obvious on plain radiography.

The most common foreign body encountered in adults is an unchewed meat bolus arrested at a site of anatomical or pathological narrowing, such as a Schatzki's ring or peptic stricture (Fig. 18.73). Such non-opaque obstructing foreign bodies can be demonstrated by swallowing a small bolus of barium. An intraluminal filling defect such as a lump of meat may resemble a neoplasm, but the history of sudden onset of chest pain and dysphagia while eating is usually diagnostic. Following removal of this type of

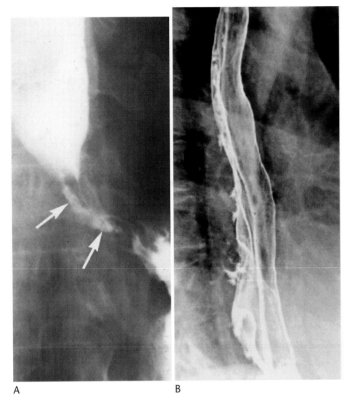

A   B

Fig. 18.74 (A) Mallory–Weiss syndrome. Tear in the oesophagus at its lower end caused by vomiting. Barium (arrows) has tracked through the defect to lie beneath the mucosa. (B) Mucosal tear and intramural haematoma spreading along the length of one side of the oesophagus. The patient had swallowed a meat bone.

foreign body, a barium swallow is necessary to exclude a pathological narrowing as the cause of hold-up.

Fish and meat bones are a particular problem as they tend to get caught above the bulge of the cricopharyngeus muscle, and if unrecognised may perforate the oesophagus and cause a retropharyngeal abscess. The bones may be of sufficient density to be seen with plain film radiography but care must be taken not to mistake normal laryngeal cartilage ossification for a foreign body. Meat and chicken bones are more likely than fish bones to be detected on plain radiographs. When plain radiography and barium swallow are unsuccessful in locating an impacted bone, the patient should be asked to swallow a piece of barium-soaked cottonwool in the hope that this will catch on the impacted object. Impacted foreign bodies are usually removed with an endoscope. A recently impacted meat bolus can sometimes be dislodged by the combination of swallowing an effervescent agent and using an antispasmodic. This should not be attempted if the diagnosis has been delayed, as, with time, the impacted bolus can cause pressure necrosis, increasing the risk of oesophageal perforation.

Mallory–Weiss tear

These tears result from a sudden increase in intraoesophageal pressure, as may occur from vomiting or retching. The tear causes a haematemesis which can be severe enough to necessitate blood transfusion, catheter embolisation or surgical repair. Endoscopically

the mucosal tear is above the gastro-oesophageal junction, and if a double-contrast barium study is performed the tear can sometimes be seen as a short vertical white line (Fig. 18.74A). Tears can also result from the ingestion of foreign bodies or from endoscopy. Haemorrhage may occasionally strip the mucosa from the underlying circular muscle coat to produce a smooth, broad-based filling defect which bulges into the lumen. *Oesophageal haematomas* that spread circumferentially produce an annular stricture, whereas those that spread longitudinally narrow the oesophageal lumen (Fig. 18.74B). On occasions barium may enter the tear and dissect under the mucosa.

Oesophageal perforation

Perforations of the cervical oesophagus are most frequently caused by endoscopic procedures. The endoscope perforates a pyriform sinus, or the posterior oesophageal wall immediately above the impression of the cricopharyngeus muscle or that produced by a cervical osteophyte, or it enters and perforates a posterior pharyngeal pouch. Untreated, a retropharyngeal or mediastinal abscess often develops, but such perforations can usually be managed conservatively with intravenous feeding and antibiotics.

The thoracic oesophagus may be perforated during stenting or dilatation procedures. Retching or vomiting can cause a lower oesophageal tear, which usually perforates at a point on the left posterolateral wall of the distal oesophagus (*Boerhaave's syndrome*). Patients present with severe lower chest pain, and subcutaneous emphysema may be felt in the neck. Untreated, a severe mediastinitis develops. The earliest chest X-ray feature is of extraluminal gas, which forms a radiolucent triangle behind the heart. Extraluminal gas is easier to recognise when it spreads and lifts the visceral pleura from the margins of the heart and aorta. Within a few hours of a perforation the gas has usually reached the neck. Mediastinitis causes sympathetic pleural effusions, or the mediastinal pleura may rupture to produce a hydropneumothorax. This is more common on the left where the mediastinal pleura is closely applied to the distal oesophagus.

Should the intra-abdominal segment of the oesophagus be perforated by an endoscope, then the perforation is usually into the lesser sac.

Providing there is no risk of aspiration, Gastrografin is used to demonstrate the site of perforation. Barium, as it is denser and more palatable, may show a small tear not evident with Gastrografin but Gastrografin should be given first, to exclude a sizeable leak, as significant amounts of barium in the mediastinum induce a fibrotic granulomatous reaction.

Thoracic oesophageal perforations are treated by immediate thoracotomy, closure of the perforation, and placement of mediastinal and pleural drains. However, perforation of malignant oesophageal tumours at endoscopy may be treated by placing a polyethylene- or polyurethane-covered self-expanding metal stent.

Varices

Oesophageal varices are dilated submucosal veins. In the lower oesophagus they occur chiefly as a consequence of portal hypertension in cirrhosis of the liver. These are uphill varices conveying portal venous blood to the azygos vein and are therefore seen in the lower two-thirds of the oesophagus. Downhill varices develop as a result of SVC obstruction; they are usually caused by tumour inva-

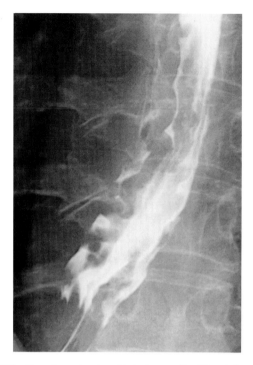

Fig. 18.75 Oesophageal varices. Typical worm-like filling defects.

sion or mediastinal fibrosis. If these varices bypass the SVC by conveying systemic venous blood from the upper half of the body to the portal vein and IVC, they will run the entire length of the oesophagus. However, if the obstruction is confined to the SVC above the entry point of the azygos vein, the varices will be confined to the upper thoracic oesophagus.

The demonstration of varices by barium swallow is best achieved by using an anticholinergic agent (Buscopan 20 mg i.v.) and a small amount of high-density barium. The administration of a gas-producing agent is optional. Multiple films of the oesophagus should be taken during a prone barium swallow, in different phases of respiration and during a Valsalva manoeuvre. Peristalsis temporarily obliterates varices, as does overdistension of the oesophagus.

Varices may be suspected on a chest radiograph by the presence of a posterior mediastinal mass behind the heart associated with a dilated azygos vein. On barium studies varices en face appear as beaded or serpiginous translucent filling defects (Fig. 18.75), and in profile as lines of nodular or scalloped filling defects. The demonstration of varices in a patient with haematemesis does not necessarily establish the origin of bleeding, as a third of such patients are bleeding from another cause, such as a peptic ulcer. Endoscopy or arteriography is preferable to barium examination for demonstrating the site of bleeding. Gastric varices can be difficult to demonstrate by endoscopy and barium studies but EUS will demonstrate varices within the gastric submucosa, together with the enlarged perigastric veins and collaterals. Contrast-enhanced CT shows varices as an enhancing thickening of the oesophageal wall.

Oesophagitis and carcinoma can simulate the barium swallow appearance of oesophageal varices. In oesophagitis there may be mucosal nodularity and thickened folds (Fig. 18.54C); and in the varicoid form of oesophageal carcinoma rigid thickened mucosal folds are seen, with loss of peristalsis of the affected area (Fig. 18.66E). Very rarely an isolated oesophageal varix develops in the absence of portal hypertension or venous obstruction and this may also cause variceal haemorrhage. Endoscopic sclerotherapy

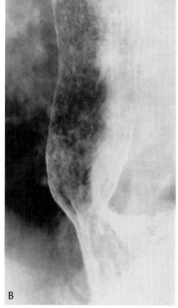

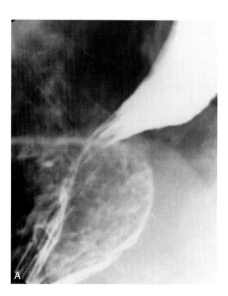

Fig. 18.76 Confluence of pulmonary veins behind the left atrium producing an extrinsic impression on the anterior oesophageal wall (arrows).

Fig. 18.77 Oesophageal displacement by a dilated aorta. (A) Lateral view shows narrowing at the gastro-oesophageal junction resembling achalasia but caused by displacement, as the oesophagus is of normal width in the frontal view (B).

can cause mucosal ulceration, oesophageal strictures and occasionally oesophageal perforation.

EXTRINSIC LESIONS AFFECTING THE OESOPHAGUS

The oesophagus traverses the posterior part of the middle mediastinum and is therefore closely related to the aorta and its branches, the tracheobronchial tree, the heart, the lungs and lymph nodes. Benign neoplasms of adjacent organs, lymph nodes and vascular anomalies tend to displace or press on the oesophagus, whereas malignant tumours and inflammatory conditions may spread to involve and invade the oesophagus.

The *aortic arch* and *left main bronchus* are two normal impressions on the left anterolateral aspect of the thoracic oesophagus which are seen best in the right anterior oblique view. Occasionally the confluence of pulmonary veins, as they enter the back of the left atrium, produces an extrinsic impression on the front of the oesophagus (Fig. 18.76).

A wide variety of *vascular anomalies of the aorta* and its *major branches*, and of the *pulmonary vessels*, cause extrinsic impressions on the barium-filled oesophagus. The most common aortic anomaly is a right-sided aortic arch and descending aorta. The oesophagus is indented on its right by the aortic knuckle, and the usual left aortic arch impression is absent. In coarctation of the aorta, a reversed-'3' impression may be produced on the left side of the oesophagus by the prestenotic and poststenotic dilatations. Aneurysms of the aortic arch and descending aorta frequently give rise to dysphagia by causing considerable localised displacement of the oesophagus.

As the aorta becomes atheromatous it assumes a tortuous course and displaces the lower end of the oesophagus anteriorly and to the side. Transient intermittent obstruction may occur, sufficient on rare occasions to produce dysphagia. Fluoroscopy of the barium-filled oesophagus shows transmitted pulsations. The distal oesophagus is narrowed in one plane by this extrinsic compression, and obstruction in the erect and supine positions may be relieved by turning the patient prone (Fig. 18.77).

An *aberrant right subclavian artery* arises from the aortic arch distal to the origin of the left subclavian artery, and passes upwards and to the right behind the oesophagus. This gives rise to a characteristic smooth, oblique indentation on the posterior wall of the barium-filled oesophagus (Fig. 18.78).

Enlargement of the *left atrium* produces an anterior impression on the barium-filled lower oesophagus which is displaced posteriorly and to the right. This can cause partial obstruction to a bolus of food or tablet, and certain tablets (usually containing potassium chloride) that lodge in the oesophagus at this point can ulcerate the mucosa and produce a stricture. Enlargement of the left ventricle produces a similar indentation to that of the left atrium but at a lower level.

Displacement of the middle third of the oesophagus is most often caused by mediastinal lymphadenopathy. Subcarinal nodal enlargement may be secondary to carcinoma of the bronchus, or result from lymphoma or infection. Although usually indenting the anterior margin of the midoesophagus, disease extension may produce a stricture resembling a primary carcinoma. Other masses in the middle or posterior mediastinum that indent the oesophagus include primary tumours and cysts of the mediastinum, abscess and hamartoma.

Enlargement of the thyroid gland frequently displaces and narrows the upper oesophagus and trachea. A large parathyroid tumour may also indent the lateral margin of the oesophagus.

Shift of the mediastinum, from whatever cause, displaces the oesophagus, so apical lung fibrosis will draw the mediastinum with the oesophagus to that side.

REFERENCES AND SUGGESTIONS FOR FURTHER READING

General
Caroline, D.F. (1987) Imaging of the oesophagus—update. *Current Opinion in Gastroenterology*, **3**, 812–819.
Eisenberg, R. L. (1996) *Gastrointestinal radiology: a pattern approach*, 3rd edn. Philadelphia: W.B. Saunders.
Federle, M. P., Megibow, A. J., Naidich, D. P. (1988) *Radiology of AIDS*. New York: Raven Press.
Gelfand, D. W., Ott, D. J. (1981) Anatomy and technique in evaluating the oesophagus. *Seminars in Roentgenology*, **16**, 168–182.
Gore, R. M., Levine, M. S. (2000) *Textbook of Gastrointestinal Radiology*, 2nd edn. Philadelphia: W.B. Saunders.
Levine, M. S. (1989) *Radiology of the Oesophagus*. Philadelphia: W. B. Saunders.
Margulis, A. R., Burhenne, H. J. (1989) *Alimentary Tract Radiology*, 4th edn. St Louis: Mosby.
Ott, D. J., Gelfand, D. W. (eds) (1994) Radiology of the upper gastrointestinal tract. *Radiological Clinics of North America*, **32**, 1167–1202.
Simpkins, K. C. (1988) *A Textbook of Radiological Diagnosis*, 5th edn, vol. 4. *The Salivary Glands and Hollow Organs*. London: Lewis.
Wegener, O. H. (1992) *Whole Body Computed Tomography*. Boston: Blackwell Scientific.

Salivary glands
Som, P. M. (1991) Salivary glands. In: Som, P. M., Bergerson, R. T. (eds) *Head & Neck Imaging*, 2nd edn, ch. 3. St Louis: Mosby Year Book.
Tabor, E. K., Curtin, H. D. (1989) MR of the salivary glands. *Radiologic Clinics of North America*, **27**, 379–392.

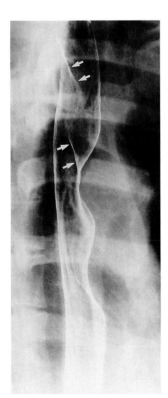

Fig. 18.78 Aberrant right subclavian artery producing characteristic extrinsic defect (arrows) of the oesophagus just above the level of the aortic arch. Left anterior oblique view.

Tegtmeyer, C. J., Keats, E. T. (1981) The salivary glands. In: Teplick, J. G., Haskin, M. D. (eds) *Surgical Radiology 3*, pp. 2582–2596. Philadelphia: W.B. Saunders.

Valvassori, G. E., Potter, G. D., Hanafee, W. N., Carter, B. L., Buckingham, R. A. (1982) *Radiology of the Ear, Nose and Throat*. Philadelphia: W. B. Saunders.

Pharynx and oesophagus

Dodds, W. J. (1997) Current concepts of esophageal motor function: clinical implications for radiology. *American Journal of Radiology*, **128**, 549–561.

Fishman, E. K., Urban, B. A., Hruban, R. H. (1996) CT of the stomach: spectrum of disease. *Radiographics*, **16**, 1035–1054.

Jones, B., Kramer, S. S., Donner, M. W. (1985) Dynamic imaging of the pharynx. *Gastrointestinal Radiology*, **10**, 213–224.

Laufer, I. (1982) Radiology of oesophagitis. *Radiological Clinics of North America*, **20**, 687–699.

Nuclear medicine

Bartlett, R. J. V., Parkin, A., Ware, F. W., Riley, A., Robinson, P. J. A. (1987) Reproducibility of oesophageal transit studies. *Nuclear Medicine Communications*, **8**, 317–326.

Harding, L. K., Donovan, I. A. (1988) Gastric emptying: gastro-oesophageal reflux. In: Davies, E. R., Thomas, W. E. G. (eds) *Nuclear Medicine: Applications to Surgery*, pp. 42–51. Tunbridge Wells: Castle House.

19

THE STOMACH AND DUODENUM

A. H. Chapman
with contributions from J. Ashley Guthrie and Philip J. A. Robinson

Endoscopy

Endoscopy is now usually used in preference to the barium meal for the investigation of upper gastrointestinal symptoms as it is more sensitive for detecting mucosal lesions and biopsies can be taken. In particular the barium meal is poor at detecting active ulceration when the mucosa is deformed from previous ulceration or gastric surgery. The barium meal is reserved for patients who are unable to tolerate endoscopy, when endoscopy is incomplete or confusing, or when morphological changes that are easier to appreciate with a barium meal are suspected, such as a modest lower oesophageal stricture or linitis plastica. CT of the stomach is used for tumour staging and to assess extraluminal tumour extension. Endoscopic ultrasound (EUS) is useful for local tumour staging and for determining the precise location of a tumour within the stomach wall.

Double-contrast barium meal

The barium meal examines the lower half of the oesophagus, the stomach and all of the duodenum. Patients fast for 6 h prior to the examination. They should also abstain from smoking as this increases gastric secretions, which impairs the barium coating of the mucosa. A history of previous gastric surgery is important as often this requires the radiologist to modify the examination.

A hypotonic agent, such as Buscopan (hyoscine butylbromide, 20 mg i.v.) or glucagon (0.1–0.2 mg i.v.) is administered; the patient then swallows an effervescent agent to distend the stomach with approximately 400 ml carbon dioxide. While standing in a right anterior oblique (RAO) position, 120 ml of high-density barium (250% w/v) is quickly swallowed to obtain well-distended double-contrast views of the lower oesophagus. The patient is turned to face the X-ray table and lowered to the horizontal, then turned onto the left side and finally to a supine position. Rolling the patient from side to side improves barium coating by washing mucus from the gastric wall. Films of the stomach are taken. When barium has entered the duodenum the patient is turned RAO to fill

Table 19.1 Typical filming sequence for a barium meal examination

Positioning		View
Erect	—RAO	Oesophagus (DC)
Supine	—RAO	Body and antrum with lesser curve in profile (DC)
	—AP	Body and antrum (DC)
	—LAO	Body with lesser curve en face (DC)
	—Right lateral	Fundus (DC)
Prone	—AP + pad under antrum	Duodenal loop (DC)
Supine	—RAO	Duodenal cap (DC)
Prone	—LPO	Oesophagus (SC)
Table to vertical		
Erect	—AP	Fundus (DC)
	—RAO	Antrum and cap (SC)

AP = anterior posterior; LAO = left anterior oblique; RAO = right anterior oblique; DC = double contrast; SC = single contrast.

the duodenum with gas, and double-contrast films of the duodenum are taken. A prone swallow with diluted barium (125% w/v) will distend the lower oesophagus and allow oesophageal peristalsis to be observed. Finally, the patient is brought back to a standing position and single-contrast films are obtained of the compressible parts of the stomach and duodenum (Table 19.1). The kilovolt range should be increased from 70–120 kV to 120–150 kV for single-contrast films.

Barium will quickly flood the jejunum if there has been a partial gastrectomy or a gastric drainage procedure such as a pyloroplasty or gastroenterostomy. It is then difficult to obtain satisfactory double-contrast images of the stomach, duodenum or anastomosis. To avoid early flooding, the examination sequence should be modified and the examination should start with a prone swallow using high-density barium. When barium reaches the duodenum or the gastroenterostomy, the patient is quickly turned supine for the double-contrast films of these structures. Double-contrast filming of the oesophagus and stomach can then follow.

The examination is also modified for the frail, immobile or elderly as the purpose of the examination is to detect a major lesion, so the study should be concluded as soon as the desired information is obtained. If a patient is unable to turn prone on the X-ray table, double-contrast barium coating cannot be achieved and a single-contrast examination will provide more information. For the single-contrast examination sufficient 100% w/v barium is swallowed to provide distended images of the oesophagus, stomach and duodenum. Compression is then applied to the accessible lower stomach and duodenum. This approximates the front and back walls of the stomach and duodenum so they are separated by a thin layer of barium and a protruding lesion is then seen as a radiolucent filling defect, whereas a depressed lesion, such as an ulcer, is seen as a focal extra density.

CT

The optimal demonstration of the gastric wall using CT is achieved when the stomach is enhanced with intravenous contrast and maximally distended with water. The gastric mucosa and most gastric tumours are vascular, with peak attenuation in the arterial dominated vascular phase. The low density of the water provides high contrast with the mucosa. There is considerable variation in precise CT technique employed. The technique is principally dependent on the objective of the examination, and, within the context of staging gastric tumours, the other investigations to be employed. CT should not be used as the primary diagnostic investigation because early gastric cancers may be occult and the principal finding of mural thickening is non-specific. If full CT staging is to be attempted then a biphasic technique should be performed, whereas if the patient is to undergo EUS a portal venous phase acquisition to detect lymphadenopathy and distant metastases is sufficient.

Prior to the examination the patient should be fasted for at least 6 h (longer with symptoms of gastric outlet obstruction). One litre of water is given in two equal aliquots, the first 15 min before the examination and the second once the patient is on the table; at this point a hypotonic agent, as described above, should be given. If, on a planning slice, the stomach is still poorly distended, more water should be given. For full staging, spiral acquisitions in arterial and portal venous phases should be obtained, typically using 150 ml iodinated contrast (300 g/l) delivered at 5 ml/s and starting acquisitions at 30 and 65 s with 5 mm collimation or less. Some prefer the patient to be scanned in the prone position to reduce artefacts from gas–fluid interfaces and to attempt to create a plane of separation between the stomach and the pancreas. There is an increasing tendency to make use of thinner slice techniques, with multislice scanners currently allowing a slice thickness of the order of 1 mm. This reduces partial volume effects and enables high-quality reformats, including virtual endoscopy, to be performed. It is yet to be seen whether there is any advantage of these newer techniques over EUS.

Endoscopic ultrasound

A forward-oblique viewing endoscope with an echoprobe mounted on its tip provides a 360° field of view. The frequency can be switched between 7.5 and 12 MHz. Higher frequency probes that can be passed through the forceps channel of the endoscope are available. As an alternative to using a water-filled balloon in the stomach and duodenum, deaerated water can be used as a coupling agent. Sometimes when using a balloon for contact the inner three layers of the stomach wall may merge, whereas with water immer-

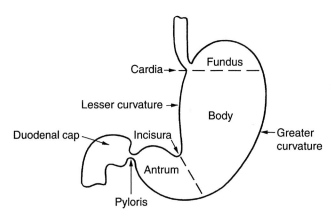

Fig. 19.1 Anatomy of the stomach.

sion all five layers are usually seen. Sometimes a thin hyperechoic layer can be seen at the interface between the two muscle layers of the gastric wall, and with higher frequency transducers even more layers of the gastric wall become apparent.

Radionuclide imaging

See pages 609–612.

ANATOMY OF THE STOMACH

The stomach communicates with the oesophagus by the cardia, and with the duodenal cap by the pyloric canal. The incisura angularis is a notch on the lesser curve that separates the body and antrum (Fig. 19.1).

Barium meal

The surface of the gastric mucosa has a reticular pattern produced by multiple interconnecting grooves. The grooves divide the surface into 2–4 mm polygonal islands known as *areae gastricae*. These

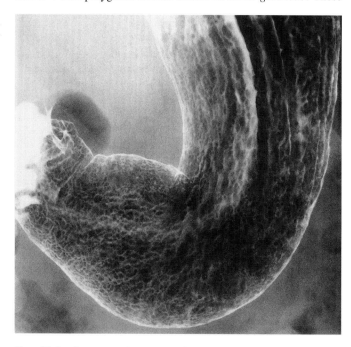

Fig. 19.2 Areae gastricae. Normal reticular pattern to the mucosa produced by areae gastricae.

can be seen in over half of good-quality double-contrast barium meals and produce a fine, medium or coarse reticular pattern that is most obvious in the distal two-thirds of the stomach (Fig. 19.2). The presence of this surface pattern makes diffuse atrophic gastritis unlikely, whereas enlargement of the areae gastricae (>4 mm) is a sign of gastritis. The mucosa of the fundus and body of the stomach is thrown into *longitudinal folds* or *rugae*. These are to some extent effaced when the stomach is distended, but where they are most prominent, along the greater curve, they are often still seen. When the stomach is distended, longitudinal folds may also be seen in the immediate prepyloric part of the antrum. Occasionally transient fine transverse folds are seen in the stomach, and are believed to be caused by contraction of the muscularis mucosa (Fig. 19.3). The *gastric cardia*, when viewed en face in the left anterior oblique position, shows a rosette of folds radiating from the oesophageal orifice, with a curved mucosal fold forming a hood over these emerging folds (Fig. 19.4).

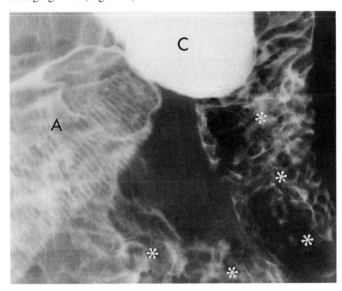

Fig. 19.3 Fine transverse mucosal folds. Prone view. A = antrum; C = duodenal cap. Asterisks mark the second and third parts of the duodenum.

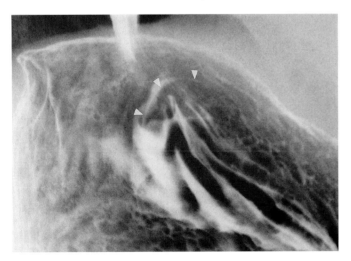

Fig. 19.4 The gastric cardia viewed en face in the left anterior oblique position. Lesser curve folds run to the oesophageal orifice, where a fold forms a hood (arrowheads) over the cardia.

CT

The maximal thickness of the stomach wall when adequately distended is 4 mm, with the antrum often a little thicker than the rest of the stomach. The thickness of the gastric folds should not exceed that of the adjacent gastric wall. During the arterial phase, with 5 mm collimation or less, the gastric wall appears as a two- or three-layered structure. The mucosa appears as a brightly enhancing inner layer with an intermediately enhancing outer layer and a variably demonstrated lower attenuation middle layer. The serosa usually has a sharp outer margin with the perigastric fat. Where the stomach wall traverses the scan plane at an oblique angle the wall may appear thickened and have a less discrete outer margin; this is most commonly observed at the gastro-oesophageal junction. This site is prone to thickening from 'pseudotumours' due to inadequate distension and compounded by hiatus hernias. A fat plane is often absent from the interfaces between the stomach and the crus of the diaphragm and the pancreas. In cachexic patients virtually all intra-abdominal fat may be absent.

Endoscopic ultrasound

The bowel wall when viewed with transducers in the 7.5–12 MHz range has five layers. Whereas in the oesophagus the fifth echogenic layer corresponds with the adventitia (see Fig. 18.17), in the stomach it corresponds with the serosa and subserosa. The wall of the distended stomach is approximately 3 mm in thickness.

Adjacent organs, such as the common hepatic and bile ducts, the pancreas and adjacent parts of the liver and spleen, can be seen through the wall of the stomach and duodenum (Fig. 19.5).

ANATOMY OF THE DUODENUM

The duodenum extends from the pylorus to the duodenojejunal flexure. Radiographically, the duodenum consists of a cap immediately beyond the pylorus, a second part (descending horizontal), third part (ascending) and fourth part.

Barium meal

The normal duodenal cap is symmetric and triangular (Fig. 19.6A). When distended and coated with barium a fine velvety reticular surface pattern may be seen due to the presence of villi (Fig. 19.6B). Sometimes barium gets caught in mucosal pits, giving the cap a spotted surface pattern—an appearance identical to that produced by incomplete erosive duodenitis (Fig. 19.26B). When the duodenal cap is undistended a fold pattern is seen and a prominent fold curves around the inferior bend between the first and second parts of the

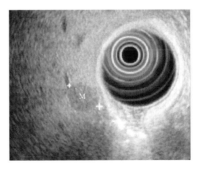

Fig. 19.5 Endoscopic ultrasound showing a metastasis (M) in the left lobe of liver. (Courtesy of Dr Keith Harris.)

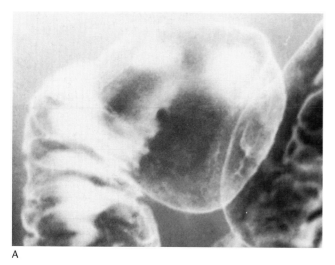

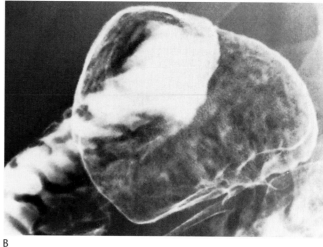

Fig. 19.6 The normal duodenal cap seen by double contrast. The mucosa has a velvety appearance due to the presence of villi. (A) Surface coating, almost homogeneous. (B) A fine velvety reticular pattern is produced by the villi.

duodenum. A small pool of barium may be caught under this fold, and should not be mistaken for an ulcer. Beyond the cap, mucosal folds are a normal feature and are seen as narrow bands that extend across the whole width of the duodenum (Fig. 19.7).

The *major papilla* (*of Vater*) projects into the lumen on the inner side of the second part of the duodenum (Fig. 19.7). Running down from the papilla are three folds: a central longitudinal fold with an oblique fold on either side. The two oblique folds join by forming an arch over the top of the papilla. Occasionally the *minor papilla* (*of Santorini*) is seen on the anterior wall, 2 cm proximal to the major papilla.

GASTRITIS, DUODENITIS AND PEPTIC ULCERATION

Helicobacter pylori

Helicobacter pylori is a spiral-shaped bacillus that lives in the mucus layer of the stomach. Infection affects approximately 50% of

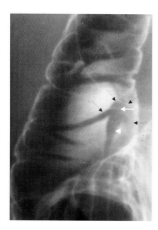

Fig. 19.7 The normal duodenal cap and loop. Routine double-contrast barium meal. Supine right anterior oblique view. The papilla of Vater (white arrow) has a longitudinal (arrowhead) and two oblique folds (black arrows) extending below it.

adults in developed countries and 100% in less developed countries. Infection is acquired in early childhood, probably as a result of poor hygiene, as it is particularly common in situations of domestic overcrowding and in people of poor socioeconomic status. Radiology department personnel who deal with instruments contaminated with gastric fluids are at risk of becoming infected with the organism: gloves and masks should therefore be worn when handling such equipment.

Adding the supernatant of a culture of a producing strain of cytotoxin *H. pylori* to a gastric cell line produces vacuolation within the cells. All strains of *H. pylori* cause chronic gastritis but it is patients with cytotoxin positive strains that are affected by ulceration and carcinoma. Chronic gastritis may involve the antrum, body or all of the stomach, the distribution being determined by the genetic make-up of the patient.

Approximately 65% of gastric ulcers develop in mucosa affected by chronic gastritis caused by *H. pylori* infection; most of the remainder are caused by aspirin and other non-steroidal anti-inflammatory drugs. These drugs inhibit the synthesis of *prostaglandins*, which maintain the integrity of the mucosal barrier. Damage to the mucosal barrier, predisposing to gastric ulceration, may also result from duodenogastric reflux of bile and pancreatic enzymes or from prolonged acid and pepsin contact as a result of impaired gastric emptying. Eradication of *H. pylori* may reduce gastric ulcer recurrence rates and is recommended for patients with gastric ulcers who are *H. pylori* positive.

Ninety-five per cent of patients with duodenal ulcers have stomachs infected with *H. pylori*. Patients with duodenal ulcers usually have an antral-predominant type of gastritis, which spares the body of the stomach so acid production is preserved. It is believed that the organism stimulates the release of *somatostatin* from the antral mucosa, and this affects the negative feedback mechanism controlling *gastrin*. The resulting increase in gastrin release causes parietal cell hyperplasia, increased basal gastric acid secretion and increased acid secretion in response to secretory stimuli. The increased gastric acid output is associated with gastric metaplasia of the duodenal mucosa and *H. pylori* colonisation such as omeprazole, clarithromycin and amoxycillin but alternatives are required for treatment failure due to antibiotic resistance. The colonised metaplastic mucosa is prone to erosion and ulceration. Eradication of the organism speeds ulcer healing and largely prevents relapse. Infection is eradicated by or triple therapy.

Gastric and duodenal ulcer treatment also involves reducing gastric acidity with a proton pump inhibitor. Gastric ulcers, when caused by non-steroidal anti-inflammatory drugs, can be treated with a synthetic prostaglandin analogue such as misoprostol, although usually a proton pump inhibitor is tried first. Surgery is reserved for the rare patients in whom medical treatment has failed or complications have developed. The most frequently performed operations are partial gastrectomy, vagotomy and pyloroplasty, and selective vagotomy.

The high gastric acid output associated with the Zollinger–Ellison syndrome causes severe duodenal ulceration. *Steroids* mask the symptoms of peptic ulceration and for this reason giant gastric ulcers and perforated gastric and duodenal ulcers are more frequent in patients being treated with steroids.

Approximately half the patients with chronic gastritis from *H. pylori* infection develop mucosal atrophy. Some will go on to intestinal metaplasia, a small proportion of these develop dysplasia, and over a 30 year period about 1% of those starting with chronic gastritis will have developed a carcinoma. *H. pylori* has also been incriminated in the development of a specific type of *gastric lymphoma*. This mucosa-associated lymphoid tissue (MALT) lymphoma is a low-grade B-cell lymphoma, and treatment to eradicate *H. pylori* may result in complete resolution of the tumour.

Acute erosive gastritis

Mucosal erosions are seen as small pools of barium en face, but are not seen in profile as they are too shallow, only reaching to the muscularis mucosae. The erosion may be surrounded by a translucent halo of oedema, but if the halo is absent they are referred to as 'incomplete erosions'. They often lie on rugal folds, giving the folds a scalloped margin. They are most frequently found in the antrum, and will be seen in up to 20% of good-quality double-contrast barium meals (Fig. 19.8). The causes of mucosal erosions are listed in Box 19.1.

Erosions associated with drug ingestion tend to occur at the site where the drugs dissolve and so are often found on the dependent part of the greater curve of the body of the stomach. Aspirin can produce erosions within 24 h but these heal rapidly when the drug is withdrawn.

Most patients are asymptomatic, but erosions may cause dyspeptic symptoms, and severe erosive gastritis is a cause of gastrointesti-

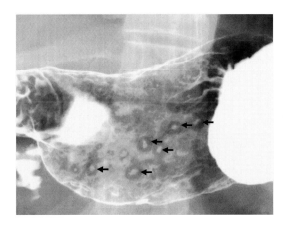

Fig. 19.8 Acute erosive gastritis. There are numerous erosions in the stomach (arrows). Each erosion consists of a small central collection of barium surrounded by a translucent ring (a small 'target' lesion).

Box 19.1 Causes of gastric mucosal erosions
Aspirin and other non-steroidal anti-inflammatory drugs, steroids or alcohol
Stress, trauma or burns
Bile reflux
Direct mucosal trauma i.e. from endoscopy
Crohn's disease
Viral and fungal infections

nal haemorrhage. Infusion of vasopressin or even embolisation of the left gastric artery can successfully control severe haemorrhage, but if such measures fail then a total gastrectomy may be necessary.

Chronic gastritis

H. pylori-associated gastritis

This is a histological diagnosis made by taking biopsies of the antrum and body of the stomach. It may be subdivided into antral predominant gastritis, pangastritis and corpus predominant gastritis.

Antral predominant gastritis is associated with duodenal ulceration; the body of the stomach and is mildly affected and so acid production is maintained. Folds of the upper two-thirds of the stomach may thicken (a condition sometimes referred to as *hypertrophic gastritis*), reflecting an increased parietal cell mass that is producing an increase in gastric acid output.

In *pangastritis* there is inflammation of both antral and corpus mucosa, which may progress to atrophy and intestinal metaplasia. Patients with gastric ulcers have severe pangastritis. Of patients with gastric ulcers, 75% are *H. pylori*-positive, and most of the remainder are taking non-steroidal anti-inflammatory drugs. It is believed that there is a sequence of gastritis to atrophy to intestinal metaplasia to dysplasia to neoplasia. Only about 50% of patients with gastric carcinoma are *H. pylori*-positive, probably because the number of organisms declines with mucosal atrophy. However, most will have antibodies to *H. pylori*, indicating past infection. Patients with *Helicobacter gastritis* develop lymphoid follicles in the gastric mucosa from which MALT-type gastric lymphoma may arise. Although a B cell lymphoma the proliferation is dependant on *H. pylori* reactive T-cells.

Corpus predominant gastritis progresses to mucosal atrophy of the body and fundus of the stomach. This may represent an end-stage of *H. pylori*-associated gastritis in patients with a genetic tendency to develop an autoimmune disease. There are circulating parietal cell antibodies and there is an association with Hashimoto's disease, Addison's disease and diabetes mellitus. Atrophic gastritis causes achlorhydria and a failure of intrinsic factor production. Intrinsic factor binds to vitamin B_{12}, enabling it to be absorbed by the terminal ileum, and so in severe cases pernicious anaemia may result. On barium studies the stomach is somewhat narrowed and shows a loss of fold pattern. Areae gastricae may be small or absent. Focal enlargement of areae gastricae may indicate intestinal metaplasia or early carcinoma, and is an indication for biopsy.

Other types of gastritis

Reactive gastritis

Bile and pancreatic reflux, alcohol and non-steroidal anti-inflammatory drugs may all cause mucosal injury. Antral folds are often thickened and the antrum may fail to distend (Fig. 19.9). Occasionally a thickened fold may be seen extending from the

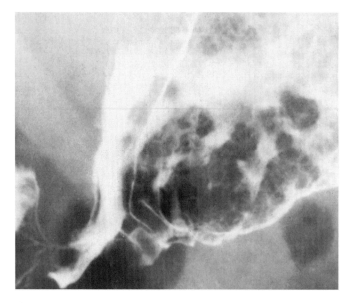

Fig. 19.9 Severe antral gastritis. Conical narrowing of the antrum with multiple thickened gastric folds.

pyloric canal a short distance along the horizontal part of the lesser curve. This needs to be differentiated from an early gastric carcinoma, and if there is uncertainty endoscopy and biopsy is advised.

Lymphocytic gastritis

An atypical response to *H. pylori* results in infiltration of the gastric surface epithelium by intraepithelial T cells. Endoscopy and barium radiology often show large 'varioliform' erosions in the body of the stomach. Treatment is with *H. pylori* eradication therapy.

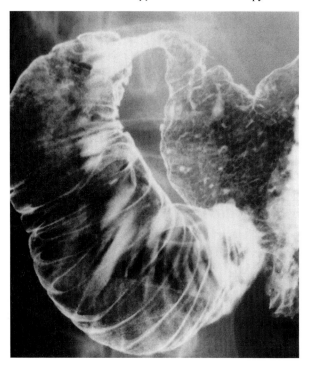

Fig. 19.10 Crohn's disease. Antral erosions and a tapered stricture involving the first part of the duodenum. The second part of the duodenum is dilated as a result of a further stricture of the third part.

Box 19.2 Causes of thick gastric folds	
Fundus and body	*Antrum*
Lymphoma, carcinoma	Lymphoma, carcinoma
Hypertrophic gastritis	Crohn's disease, tuberculosis
Ménétrier's disease	Amyloidosis, sarcoidosis
Zollinger–Ellison syndrome	Caustic ingestion, radiotherapy, 5-flurouracil
	Eosinophilic gastroenteropathy
	Watermelon stomach

Eosinophilic gastritis

This is a condition in which there is an eosinophilic infiltrate of the stomach. The small bowel may also be involved, and rarely the oesophagus. Fifty per cent of patients have a peripheral eosinophilia and a similar percentage have an allergic history. Patients frequently give a dyspeptic history, although if the small bowel is involved, malabsorption or a protein-losing enteropathy may result. In the stomach the antrum is most often involved, and is narrowed with rigid, thick nodular folds. The small bowel will also show thick nodular folds when involved.

Crohn's disease

Most patients with gastroduodenal Crohn's disease have ileocolic disease as well. The duodenum is more often involved than the stomach. When the stomach is involved it is usually the antrum and body that are affected (Fig. 19.10). Aphthous erosions, fold thickening, deep ulcers, skip lesions and scarring may all be observed. If severe, the gastric antrum or duodenum may obstruct.

The causes of thickened gastric folds are listed in Box 19.2.

Other gastric conditions

Watermelon stomach

This is a vascular ectasia of the antrum of the stomach which may be responsible for chronic blood loss. The condition is diagnosed at endoscopy when the ectatic submucosal vessels can be seen. Barium studies will show thickened folds similar to the submucosal varices that are sometimes seen in portal hypertension.

Ménétrier's disease

This is a rare disease of unknown aetiology that generally occurs in males over the age of 40. It is characterised by a pronounced hypertrophy of the glands of the body and fundus of the stomach. This results in large gastric folds, an increase in gastric mucus secretion and often a reduction in gastric acid output. A protein-losing enteropathy often develops, resulting in hypoproteinaemia and peripheral oedema. Gastric ulceration may occur and a hypercoagulation state with a tendency to venous thrombosis may develop. The excessive gastric mucus makes it difficult to coat the stomach when performing a barium meal. The stomach distends normally but there is gastric fold thickening which is most pronounced in the upper two-thirds of the stomach (Fig. 19.11), although occasionally it may extend throughout the stomach. The condition may remit spontaneously. Anticholinergics or even a vagotomy can be used to reduce the protein loss but if such measures fail a total gastrectomy may be necessary.

Amyloidosis, sarcoidosis and cystic fibrosis

When sarcoidosis involves the gastrointestinal tract it is usually the stomach that is affected. Amyloidosis and sarcoidosis may both produce gastric fold thickening and mucosal nodularity (Box 19.2).

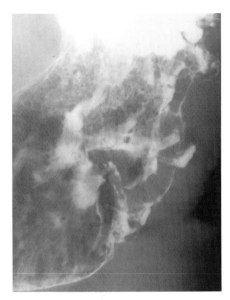

Fig. 19.11 Ménétrier's disease. Gross thickening of the folds of the upper two-thirds of the stomach. These patients often weep a protein-rich exudate from the stomach wall, and this excess of fluid in the stomach may impair barium coating.

The wall of the stomach may thicken and the lumen narrow; this may affect the antrum of the stomach or produce a general linitis plastica-type picture. Ulceration may be seen in sarcoidosis and chest X-ray changes may suggest the diagnosis.

Mucosal nodularity and fold thickening is often seen in the duodenum in patients with cystic fibrosis.

Peptic ulceration

In the West, duodenal ulceration is four times more common than gastric ulceration. In adults, duodenal ulceration has an even age distribution, whereas gastric ulcers tend to occur after the age of 40. Ulcers typically present with intermittent epigastric pain, which occurs shortly after meals if the ulcer is gastric or several hours after meals if the ulcer is duodenal. Many patients have no gastric symptoms and present with gastrointestinal blood loss.

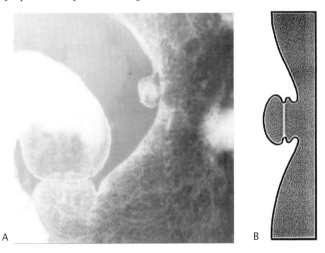

Fig. 19.12 Benign gastric ulcer. (A) Mid lesser curvature ulcer demonstrated in profile. The ulcer crater is projecting outside the wall of the stomach. (B) Diagram of benign ulcer with an oedematous collar. Beneath the collar, a thin lucent line may be seen across the mouth of the ulcer (Hampton's line).

Radiologically, gastric and duodenal ulcers are best demonstrated by performing a biphasic barium meal examination. Double-contrast views of the stomach are initially obtained and then the patient swallows dilute barium (100% w/v). This mixes with the 250% w/v barium in the stomach to produce a density that, in a thin layer, can be seen through. To produce this thin layer, compression is applied below the costal margin to the accessible lower two-

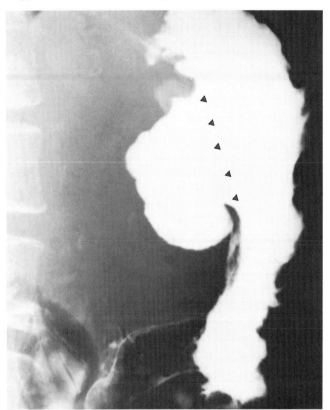

A

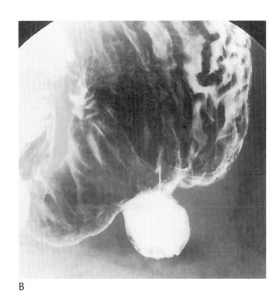

B

Fig. 19.13 Giant benign gastric ulcers. (A) Lesser curve gastric ulcer projecting from the posterior wall of the stomach (arrowheads) and penetrating into the pancreas. (B) Greater curve ('sump ulcer'). This ulcer is typical of those occurring in patients who are taking tablets which produce contact irritation and damage to the gastric mucosa (e.g. non-steroidal anti-inflammatory drugs, steroids, potassium chloride).

thirds of the stomach and the duodenum. The correct degree of compression results in an ulcer filling with barium and a tumour protruding into the barium and showing as a filling defect. This biphasic technique is particularly useful for demonstrating ulcers on the anterior wall of the stomach or duodenum, which otherwise can be missed if barium coating is poor.

Gastric ulcers

Benign gastric ulcers most frequently occur along the lesser curve of the stomach and the adjacent part of the posterior wall (Fig. 19.12). In older patients, ulcers are more often located high on the lesser curve (*geriatric ulcers*) and sometimes may be greater than 3 cm in diameter (giant ulcers (Fig. 19.13A)). Giant ulcers are also caused by aspirin and non-steroidal anti-inflammatory drugs, in which case they tend to develop on the dependent part of the greater curve because gravity deposits tablets at this site (Fig. 19.13B). Gastric ulcers associated with a hiatus hernia tend to develop high on the lesser curve where mucosa prolapses through the diaphragmatic hiatus and may result from ischaemic mucosal injury. Benign ulceration rarely involves the upper part of the greater curvature, so ulcers at this site should be suspected of being malignant.

When an ulcer is identified it should, where possible, be demonstrated en face and in profile. A benign ulcer in profile protrudes outside the expected line of the stomach wall, whereas a malignant ulcer at the apex of a protruding tumour mass will lie within the outline of the stomach (Fig. 19.14). Sometimes overhanging mucosa at the margins of a benign ulcer will be seen as a thin line separating a barium-filled ulcer from barium in the stomach (Hampton's line; Fig. 19.12B). Should the margins of the ulcer be oedematous, this line will be thick. When seen en face, an ulcer on the dependent wall of the stomach fills with barium, whereas an ulcer on the non-dependent wall is seen as a ring. Smooth folds radiate from the edge of a benign ulcer (Fig. 19.15A), or if the margin is oedematous the folds may stop some millimetres short of the margin. The fold pattern around posterior wall ulcers may be emphasised by turning the patient so that a thin layer of barium

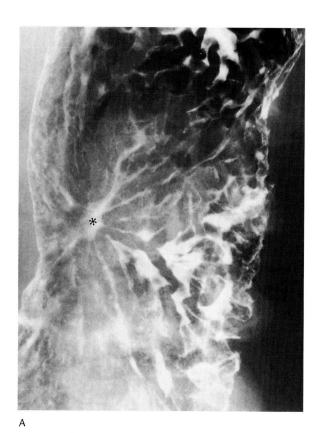

A

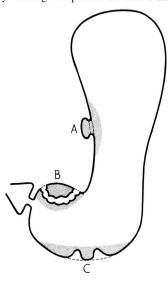

B

Fig. 19.15 (A) Benign gastric ulceration. Small posterior wall ulcer (asterisk) demonstrated en face. Radiating mucosal folds extend to the edge of the crater. (B) Healed benign gastric ulcer. Radiating folds from a central niche (arrow). In this patient the niche persists despite endoscopic evidence that the ulcer has healed.

runs across the surface of the ulcer. Single-contrast compression views are often best for demonstrating the fold pattern around anterior wall gastric ulcers. The areae gastricae pattern may be coarse and prominent at the margin of ulcers, possibly as a consequence of oedema.

With healing, ulcers decrease in size and change from being round to linear. Barium evaluation to assess healing is normally conducted after an interval of 8 weeks of medical treatment. Healing of the mucosa may be complete or there may be evidence of scarring. En face, scars are often seen as punctate or linear

Fig. 19.14 Three characteristic types of gastric ulcer; the shading represents barium. A = benign, projecting, lesser curvature ulcer with collar (broken lines); B = malignant, intraluminal ulcer with irregular nodular tumour rim; C = non-projecting benign greater curvature ulcer.

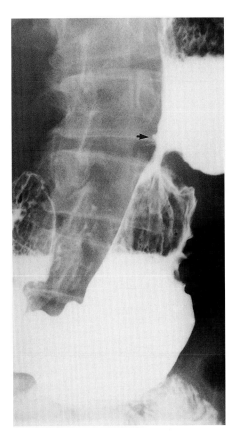

Fig. 19.16 Healing benign gastric ulcer. Incisura and 'hour-glass' stomach. A typical benign ulcer (arrow) on the mid lesser curvature of the stomach is associated with a prominent incisura which divides the stomach into two.

can be diagnosed as being benign with confidence, although it must be remembered that malignant ulcers may temporarily heal with medical treatment; a careful en face evaluation of the mucosa for nodularity or irregularity of the fold pattern is therefore essential. Benign ulcers may be misdiagnosed as malignant, especially if they are on the greater curve, where there is often associated spasm, which draws in the stomach wall (Fig. 19.14), and pronounced oedema thickens the adjacent mucosal folds. In practice most patients found to have gastric ulcers are assessed by endoscopy and biopsy. Benign gastric ulcers are multiple in 25% of patients but a benign ulcer can be associated with a malignant one, so each ulcer has to be assessed individually.

Duodenal ulcers

The majority of duodenal ulcers occur within the cap (Fig. 19.17). They involve the anterior and posterior walls with equal frequency. As in the stomach, an ulcer on the dependent wall fills with barium and shows radiating folds (Fig. 19.18A), which stop short of the margin if there is a rim of oedema. An ulcer on the non-dependent wall is etched by barium and appears as a ring (Fig. 19.18B). It can be difficult to coat the anterior wall of the duodenum and prone or erect compression views of the duodenal cap should therefore be obtained. Ulcers are generally round, but as with gastric ulcers may be linear (Fig. 19.19), especially when healing.

Spasm and scarring may draw in the margins of the duodenal cap, distorting its shape and often producing a characteristic clover-leaf appearance (Fig. 19.20). Healing duodenal ulcers have a similar range of appearances to healing gastric ulcers. The ulcer niche may persist, reduce in size, become linear or a depression may persist at the site of ulceration. If the duodenum has become scarred it can be difficult to diagnose recurrent ulceration; thus, if there is a history of past duodenal ulceration, endoscopy is the preferred investigation. Occasionally, postbulbar ulcers develop, and are usually on the medial wall of the duodenal loop above the papilla. They are often associated with oedema and pronounced spasm which pulls in the opposing duodenal wall (Fig. 19.21). Scarring from such ulceration may produce a permanent stricture of the postbulbar duodenum. When there are multiple ulcers or the ulceration extends beyond the papilla the possibility of the *Zollinger–Ellison syndrome* should be considered.

grooves from which smooth folds radiate evenly (Fig. 19.15B). In profile, scars cause a localised flattening of the mucosa. On occasions the mucosa heals over an ulcer crater but a depression persists, in which case the radiologist may believe the ulcer to be still active and it is only with endoscopy that healing is confirmed. If scarring has been pronounced, perhaps because of recurrent ulceration at the same site, gastric deformity may result and can lead to an hour-glass configuration to the stomach (Fig. 19.16). Gastric ulcers

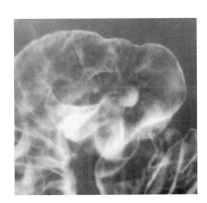

Fig. 19.17 Duodenal ulcer. Supine projection. Barium collects in an ulcer on the dependent (posterior) wall of the duodenal cap.

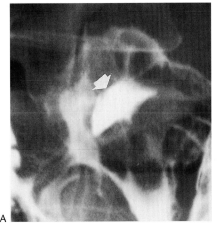

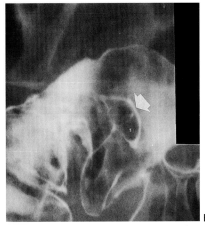

Fig. 19.18 Anterior wall duodenal ulcer. (A) Prone projection. The ulcer (arrow) is dependent, and so fills with barium. (B) Supine projection. The ulcer, which is now on the non-dependent wall of the cap, is outlined with a ring of barium (arrow).

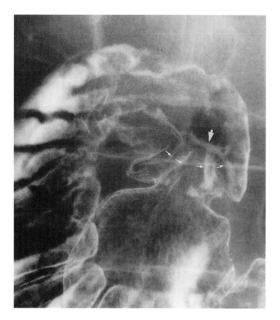

Fig. 19.19 Healing duodenal ulcer. The linear shape of the posterior wall ulcer is indicated (large arrow). Folds radiate to the ulcer (small arrows).

A giant ulcer may replace the whole of the duodenal cap, and, when smooth margined, such ulcers may be mistaken for a normal cap (Fig. 19.22). However, the giant ulcer will maintain its shape during a barium examination, whereas the normal cap can at times be seen to contract with peristalsis. Outpouchings or pseudodiverticula of a deformed cap can be mistaken for ulcers but will also change shape with peristalsis. Bleeding ulcers in the stomach or duodenum may contain a central filling defect produced by blood clot. Pyloric canal ulcers (Fig. 19.23) may simulate an annular carcinoma if surrounding oedema produces rolled margins at either end of the canal. Spasm, oedema and scarring from ulcers of the distal antrum, pyloric canal and base of the cap may produce gastric outflow obstruction. In such cases residual gastric content dilutes the barium so it is often best to empty the stomach with a nasogastric tube and then inject barium and air down the tube to complete the examination.

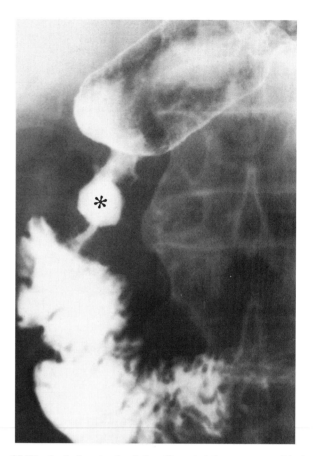

Fig. 19.21 Postbulbar duodenal ulcer. Characteristic appearance with ulcer crater (asterisk) in the middle of a stricture produced by spasm and oedema.

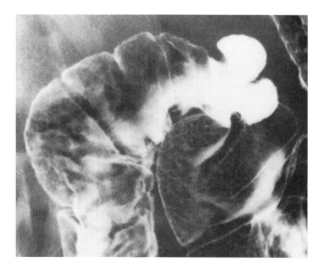

Fig. 19.20 Scarring of the duodenal cap resulting from a chronic duodenal ulcer which has now healed. The pouches produced by the scarring resemble the shape of a cloverleaf.

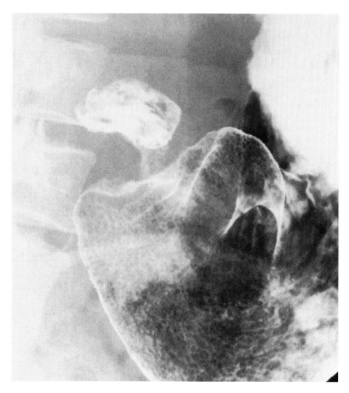

Fig. 19.22 Giant duodenal ulcer replacing the duodenal cap.

THE STOMACH AND DUODENUM

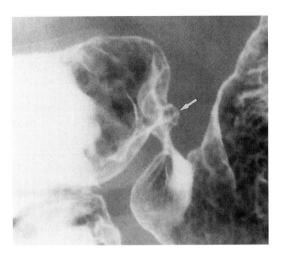

Fig. 19.23   Pyloric canal ulcer (arrow).

Perforated peptic ulcers

Ulcers on the anterior wall of the stomach or duodenum perforate into the peritoneal cavity, whereas those on the posterior wall perforate into the lesser sac or penetrate into the retroperitoneum and pancreas. The most frequent cause of a free peritoneal perforation is an anterior wall duodenal ulcer. Free peritoneal air, although readily recognised below the diaphragm on an erect chest film, is only seen in 60% of perforated duodenal ulcers. Insufficient time may be allowed for the gas to collect under the diaphragm, pre-existing adhesions may

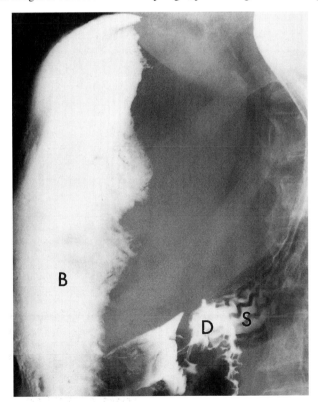

Fig. 19.24   Perforated duodenal ulcer. An unexpected, silent perforation which explains why barium has inadvertently been used as the contrast medium instead of Gastrografin. Fortunately the leak was localised to the right subphrenic and subhepatic space, otherwise a generalised barium peritonitis would have resulted. S = stomach; D = duodenum; B = leaked barium.

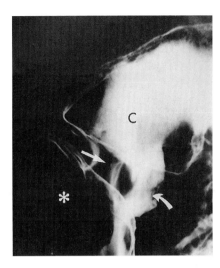

Fig. 19.25   Double pyloric canal. An antral ulcer has fistulated through to the base of the duodenal cap. Asterisk = antrum; C = duodenal cap; straight arrow = pyloric canal; curved arrow = fistula.

prevent gas reaching the subphrenic space, or the perforation may seal before a significant amount of gas has entered the peritoneal cavity. Gastrografin can be used to study patients with a perforation, and the right lateral decubitus position best demonstrates leakage from duodenal and lesser curve gastric ulcers (Fig. 19.24). Good mucosal detail is not obtained with Gastrografin, so it may be difficult to recognise a perforated ulcer that has sealed. When the perforation is into the lesser sac a gas shadow or air–fluid level develops behind the stomach. Small volumes of free intraperitoneal gas from perforations can be demonstrated using CT, which may be used in the context of diagnostic uncertainty in the acute abdomen. The site of the perforation itself is often not identified and has to be inferred.

An antral ulcer may fistulate to the duodenal cap to give the appearance of a 'double pyloric canal' (Fig. 19.25). Aspirin and non-steroidal anti-inflammatory drugs tend to produce ulcers on the greater curve, and these can fistulate to the colon or jejunum. Rarely, duodenal ulcers may fistulate into the common bile duct, causing cholangitis and air in the biliary tree.

Duodenitis

Duodenitis, like gastritis, may give rise to dyspepsia, and on rare occasions cause gastrointestinal haemorrhage. It predominantly affects the duodenal cap and may be associated with duodenal

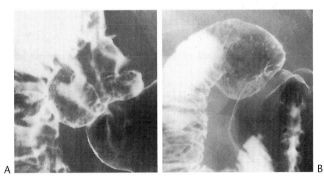

Fig. 19.26   Duodenitis. Typical appearances in the cap. (A) Thickened folds; several small ulcers are also present. (B) Multiple erosions.

Box 19.3   Causes of thickened duodenal mucosal folds

Duodenitis:	peptic including Zollinger-Ellison syndrome, Crohn's disease, AIDS, Crytosporidium, MAI and CMV
Pancreatitis	
Infestations:	Strongyloidiasis, Giardiasis
Neoplastic:	Pancreatic carcinoma
	Lymphoma
Varices	
Intramural haemorrhage	
Diffuse Infiltrative disease:	Whipple's disease, Amyloidosis
	Eosinophilic gastroenteritis
Intestinal lymphangiectasia	

ulceration. Most patients have *H. pylori*-associated antral gastritis and develop gastric metaplasia in the duodenal cap, which becomes colonised with *H. pylori*. Erosive duodenitis is considered to be part of the spectrum of duodenal ulceration and symptomatic patients are treated in the same way.

Barium radiology shows a coarsening of duodenal folds (Fig. 19.26A). Erosions, if present, are only seen en face when they show up as dots of barium, with or without a radiolucent halo (Fig. 19.26B). The combination of complete erosions and coarse folds gives the duodenal cap a 'cobblestone' appearance (Fig. 19.27A). Duodenitis may also be seen in patients with Crohn's disease and with the acquired immune deficiency syndrome (AIDS). In AIDS the organisms involved are *Cryptosporidium sp.*, *Mycobacterium avium-intracellulare* (MAI) and cytomegalovirus (CMV). The usual signs are thickening and nodularity of the folds, and often the small bowel is similarly affected. Other causes of thickening of the mucosal folds in the duodenum are listed in Box 19.3.

A cobblestone appearance to the duodenal cap is also seen in Brunner's gland hyperplasia (Fig. 19.27B), although there is not the irritability of the duodenal cap so often associated with duo-

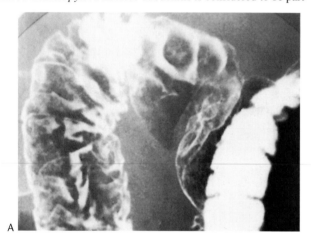

A

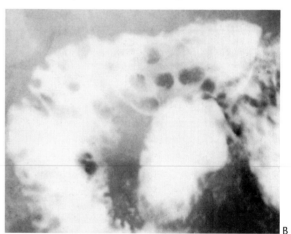

B

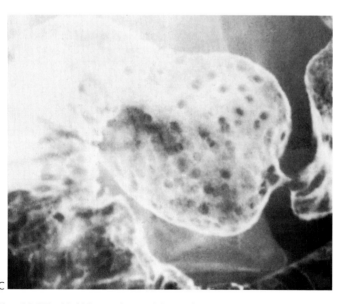

C

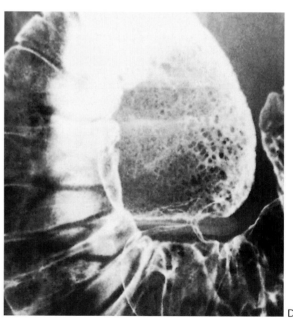

D

Fig. 19.27 'Cobblestone' caps (A) Duodenitis. Two large nodules are seen which are due to erosions on a single mucosal fold. (Courtesy of Dr J. Virjee.) (B) Hyperplasia of Brunner's glands. The nodules are clearly defined, discrete and randomly distributed in the duodenal cap and postbulbar region. (Courtesy of Dr A. Schulman.) (C) Nodular lymphoid hyperplasia is characterised by numerous small nodules all of the same size and evenly distributed. (Courtesy of Dr J. Virjee.) (D) Heterotopic gastric mucosa. The presence of gastric epithelium in the duodenal cap produces small nodules of various sizes and shapes extending from the pylorus toward the apex of the cap. (Courtesy of Dr J. Virjee.)

denitis. This is an uncommon condition, of uncertain aetiology and of no clinical significance, in which the submucosal duodenal glands (Brunner's glands) enlarge, causing the overlying mucosa to bulge.

A nodular appearance to the duodenum may result from *lymphoid hyperplasia*. This is a proliferation of submucosal lymphoid aggregates and is more often seen in the distal ileum and colon, although the duodenum is occasionally involved. There is an association with *Giardia* infection and hypogammaglobulinaemia. The double-contrast examination shows multiple round nodules, of uniform size (about 2 mm) and shape, evenly distributed throughout the duodenum (Fig. 19.27C).

Heterotopic gastric mucosa is a common finding on histological examination of the duodenal cap and is one that has a characteristic radiological appearance. Multiple small nodules of various shapes and sizes, ranging from 1 to 6 mm, are present, extending from the pylorus toward the apex of the cap (Fig. 19.27D).

Zollinger–Ellison syndrome

This syndrome is characterised by hypergastrinaemia, hypersecretion of gastric acid and severe peptic ulceration. The cause is *gastrinoma*, which is a non-islet cell tumour. Fifty per cent of gastrinomas are multiple and 50% are malignant, and 50% have metastasised to the liver by the time of diagnosis. The tumour is usually located within the pancreas but about 10% are found in the duodenal wall, and about 10% are found at ectopic sites such as the jejunum, stomach and ovary. A quarter of patients will have the hereditary syndrome of *multiple endocrine neoplasia type I*, with coexisting parathyroid, pituitary and adrenal tumours.

The large volume of gastric fluid impairs barium coating, thick folds in the stomach reflect an increased parietal cell mass, and mucosal oedema thickens duodenal and jejunal folds. There is gastric and duodenal ulceration. The ulcers are often multiple and in 25% ulceration extends beyond the duodenal cap and sometimes as far as the proximal jejunum. Reflux oesophagitis may lead to a peptic stricture and the high acid output inactivates pancreatic enzymes, causing steatorrhoea. Localisation of a gastrinoma may be difficult and involve endoscopic ultrasound, CT, abdominal angiography or selective portal venous sampling. Acid secretion can be controlled by the use of an H_2-receptor antagonist or a proton pump inhibitor. Tumours localised to the pancreas are usually resected.

A severe ulcer diathesis may also be seen in patients with hypergastrinaemia as a result of a G-cell hyperplasia of the antrum of the stomach (the Cowley syndrome).

BENIGN MUCOSAL TUMOURS

Gastric polyps are found in about 2% of double-contrast barium meals, and in common with colonic polyps, most are hyperplastic or adenomatous. Hyperplastic polyps are benign, whereas adenomatous polyps may undergo malignant change. The majority of gastric polyps are hyperplastic.

Hyperplastic polyps

These polyps consist of a local hyperplasia of the glandular tissue. They are small, smooth surfaced and generally sessile. They are usually no larger than a centimetre in size, and are often multiple, when they tend to all be of the same size. They are found predominantly in the fundus and body of the stomach (Fig. 19.28). The importance of these polyps is that, like carcinomas, they arise from mucosa affected by chronic atrophic gastritis, and so rarely a carcinoma will coexist.

A polyp on the dependent wall of the stomach is seen as a filling defect within the barium pool, whereas on the anterior wall a polyp is outlined by a thin rim of barium and shows as a ring. Rarely, giant polyps develop, and, if pedunculated, may prolapse through the pyloric canal to cause intermittent gastric outflow obstruction (Fig. 19.29). Small sessile polyps with a smooth surface can be confidently diagnosed as hyperplastic, so endoscopy is not required, whereas if the polyp's surface is irregular or the polyp measures more than a centimetre in size then endoscopy and biopsy is indicated.

Adenomatous polyps

The majority of these dysplastic polyps are tubular or tubulovillous and only a small percentage are villous. Adenomatous polyps are larger than hyperplastic polyps and generally measure over a centimetre in size. They are often solitary, are usually situated in the antrum of the stomach and frequently have a slightly nodular surface. They can be pedunculated, and may also prolapse into the

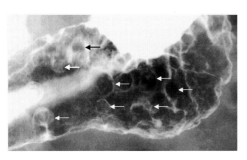

Fig. 19.28 Gastric polyps. Multiple benign hyperplastic polyps (arrows) evenly distributed throughout the stomach.

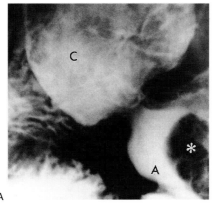
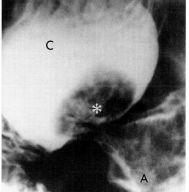

Fig. 19.29 Prolapsing giant hyperplastic polyp. (A) The polyp (asterisk) has a stalk and is seen as a filling defect arising from the antrum. (B) The polyp has prolapsed into the base of the duodenal cap. A = antrum, C= duodenal cap.

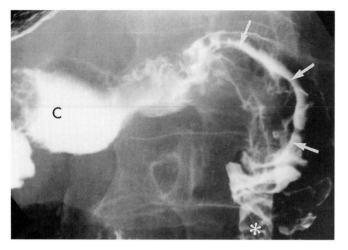

Fig. 19.30 Large villous tumour arising from the medial wall of the duodenum (arrows) close to the papilla (asterisk). Prone view. C = duodenal cap.

pyloric canal to cause gastric outflow obstruction. It is unusual for an adenomatous polyp to ulcerate, but when viewed en face, a droplet of barium hanging from the apex of the polyp may simulate ulceration. As with colonic polyps, the risk of malignant degeneration is related to size, with 50% of gastric polyps larger than 2 cm in diameter being neoplastic; adenomatous polyps greater than 1 cm in size should therefore be removed. These polyps also arise in areas of chronic atrophic gastritis, so carcinoma may coexist.

Duodenal polyps

Duodenal polyps are less common than gastric polyps and are usually adenomatous in type. Most are solitary and have a smooth surface, and, like their gastric counterparts, if larger than 1 cm in diameter should be removed because of their malignant potential.

Villous tumours

These generally present as polypoid masses, which by the time of diagnosis are invariably over 3 cm in size. They most frequently arise in the region of the papilla (Fig. 19.30). Barium caught

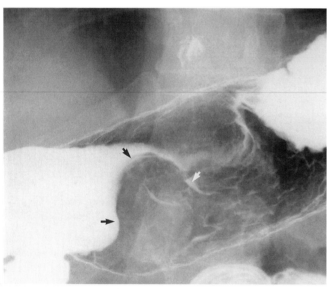

A

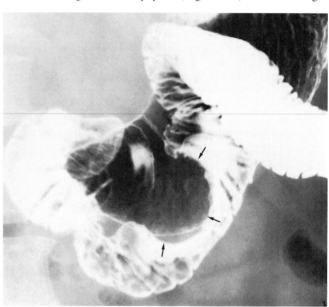

B

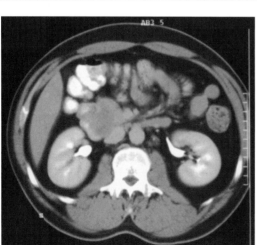

C

Fig. 19.31 (A) Benign gastric stromal tumour. The margins of this submucosal tumour make an obtuse angle with the adjacent normal mucosa. (B) Benign duodenal stromal tumour. Submucosal tumour of the third part of the duodenum. (Courtesy of Dr B. M. Carey.) (C) CT. Benign duodenal stromal tumour arising from the medial wall of the second part of the duodenum.

Box 19.4   Benign gastric submucosal tumours

Stromal tumour
Neurofibroma
Lipoma
Haemangioma
Lymphangioma
Glomus tumour
Neural tumour
Brunner's gland hamartoma
Duplication cyst
Ectopic pancreatic rest

between villi give the surface of the tumour a reticular appearance. Very large, bulky villous tumours may develop; they are soft and so rarely obstruct, and may be seen to change shape during the course of a barium study. In the fundus the tumour may prolapse up into the oesophagus or, if in the antrum, prolapse may occur into the duodenum. Antral or duodenal villous tumours may become the lead point for an intussusception. Fluid and electrolyte loss from the tumour is reabsorbed by the small bowel and colon, and so does not become a clinical problem.

Patients with *familial polyposis coli* and *Gardner's syndrome* frequently have gastric and duodenal polyps of both adenomatous and hyperplastic type. Periodic endoscopic surveillance is recommended because of the risk of developing gastric or duodenal carcinoma. Duodenal carcinomas are the more frequent and are generally periampullary.

In *Peutz–Jeghers syndrome*, hamartomatous polyps develop in the small bowel and tend to intussuscept. In 25%, hamartomatous polyps are also found in the stomach and duodenum, and, in 30%, polyps are found in the colon, but these are usually adenomas. In *Cowden's disease*, multiple hamartomatous polyps develop throughout the gastrointestinal tract. These patients have papillomatosis around the mouth and gingival hyperplasia, and are prone to develop breast and thyroid carcinomas.

BENIGN SUBMUCOSAL TUMOURS

The majority of benign submucosal tumours are stromal tumours. The other types of benign submucosal tumours are listed in Box 19.4. These tumours can be difficult to diagnose at endoscopy as the overlying gastric mucosa may be intact, although large submucosal tumours tend to ulcerate as a result of outgrowing their blood supply and causing pressure necrosis of the overlying mucosa. A submucosal lesion characteristically produces a smooth bulge into the bowel lumen, with margins that form a right angle or an obtuse angle with the normal bowel wall (Fig. 19.31B). Barium

will clearly define the margins, and if there is a central ulcer this will fill with barium to produce a 'target' or 'bull's-eye' appearance when viewed en face. On CT these are usually well-defined homogeneous tumours; larger tumours may show signs of necrosis or ulceration. Glomus tumours, carcinoid tumours and pancreatic rests can be relatively hypervascular masses, and stromal tumours, glomus tumours and haemangiomas may contain calcification visible on CT. Most are found incidentally, but large tumours may be symptomatic and ulceration is a cause of gastrointestinal bleeding. Occasionally a tumour protrudes into the lumen, becomes pedunculated, and, if near the pyloric canal, may cause gastric outflow obstruction or become the apex for an intussusception. Alternatively, most of the tumour growth may be extraluminal, so that the patient presents with a large abdominal mass. In such cases the tumour may drag on the gastric wall at its site of attachment, producing a characteristic niche (Fig. 19.32). Benign submucosal tumours are generally solitary and a more likely diagnosis for multiple submucosal tumours will be metastases, lymphoma or Kaposi's sarcoma. Submucosal tumours are rare in the duodenum (Fig. 19.31B).

Benign stromal tumours

It is often difficult for the radiologist and the histologist to distinguish benign from malignant gastric stromal tumours. Because of this difficulty and the tendency of these tumours, as they enlarge, to ulcerate and bleed, tumours larger than 3 cm are generally removed surgically. Malignant tumours grow faster, infiltrate into adjacent tissues, and metastasise by lymphatic and haematogenous spread. If the overlying mucosa remains intact, a normal areae gastricae pattern may be seen covering the protrusion caused by the tumour. Occasionally coarse calcification is present within these tumours. Endoscopic ultrasound shows a mass arising from the muscularis propria (Fig. 19.33) or muscularis mucosa, with benign tumours tending to be smaller, echo poor and better defined.

Lipomas

Lipomas are soft and may be seen to change shape with gastric peristalsis or palpation. Large tumours may ulcerate and, as in

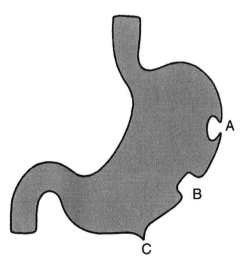

Fig. 19.32 Benign tumour growth. The margin of a mucosal tumour (A) forms a more acute angle with the normal mucosa than that of a submucosal tumour (B), which forms a right or obtuse angle with the mucosa. When growth is predominantly exophytic the tumour may drag on the gastric wall to produce a niche (C).

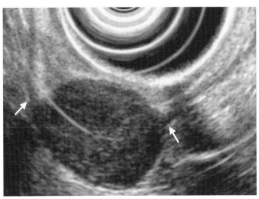

Fig. 19.33 Endoscopic ultrasound. Benign gastric stromal tumour. Echo-poor mass arising from the fourth hypoechoic layer, the muscularis propria. At the margins, the tumour can be seen to merge with the muscularis propria (arrows). Benign gastric stromal tumours can also arise from the second hypoechoic layer, the muscularis mucosa. (Courtesy of Dr Keith Harris.)

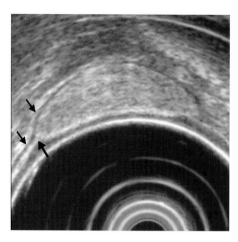

Fig. 19.34   Gastric lipoma. Echogenic well-defined tumour arising from and expanding the submucosal layer (black arrow). Muscularis propria is displaced but intact (smaller black arrows). (Courtesy of Dr Keith Harris.)

the small bowel and colon, may form the apex of an intussusception. Endoscopic ultrasound shows the tumour to be echogenic (Fig. 19.34). The diagnosis can be confirmed by demonstrating the fatty nature of the tumour with CT. *Liposarcomas* of the stomach and duodenum are very rare, and on CT show septation and an increased density to the fat.

Haemangiomas

These are capillary or cavernous in type. They have a characteristic endoscopic appearance, but on barium radiology look like any other submucosal tumour, although cavernous haemangiomas occasionally contain phleboliths which can be recognised radiologically. Haemangiomas may be solitary or multiple and may be distributed throughout the gastrointestinal tract. They are a cause of gastrointestinal bleeding.

Brunner's gland hyperplasia

Hyperplasia of these mucus-secreting duodenal glands may be caused by excessive gastric acid output and so be associated with enlarged gastric folds and duodenal ulceration. The glands lie deep to the muscularis mucosa, and enlargement produces submucosal nodules which predominantly involve the duodenal cap (Fig. 19.27B), but sometimes extend into the second part of the duodenum or the prepyloric region of the stomach. Rarely, a solitary gland enlarges (*Brunner's gland hamartoma*) to such an extent as to obstruct the duodenum or form the lead point for an intussusception (Fig. 19.35).

Duplication cysts

These are usually found on the greater curvature of the antrum or on the anteromedial aspect of the first or second part of the duodenum (Fig. 19.36). They result from a congenital failure of recanalisation of the bowel, and as such may be associated with other congenital abnormalities of the gastrointestinal tract, such as malrotation or biliary atresia. Gastric duplications generally present in early childhood but a proportion of duodenal duplications present in adult life. They are usually filled with a clear mucinous fluid, but, if there is gastric epithelium in the wall, ulceration may occur, and this can result in cyst perforation or bleeding into a cyst. They may enlarge and press on an adjacent structure, such as the bile or pancreatic duct, or obstruct the stomach or duodenum. They may be palpable and can become infected. Surgical resection is usually advised.

Ectopic pancreatic rest

These small 1–3 cm submucosal tumours are generally found toward the distal end of the greater curve of the antrum of the stomach or in the proximal duodenum between the cap and the papilla. If the tissue is well differentiated there will be a primitive ductal system, in which case a barium study may show a central

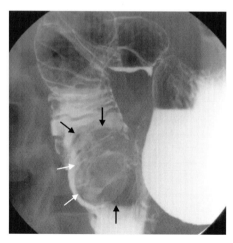

Fig. 19.35   Brunner's gland hamartoma (arrows) presenting as a large submucosal tumour arising from the medial wall of the second part of the duodenum. (Courtesy of Dr Keith Harris).

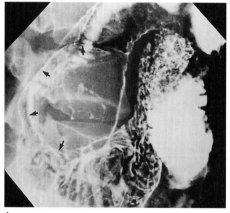

A

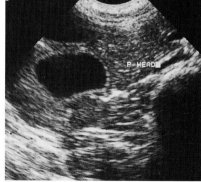

B

Fig. 19.36   Duodenal duplication cyst. (A) The cyst is impressing on the medial aspect of the second part of the duodenum (arrows) and did not communicate with the duodenal lumen. (B) Ultrasound shows fluid contents. (Courtesy of Dr R. Fowler.)

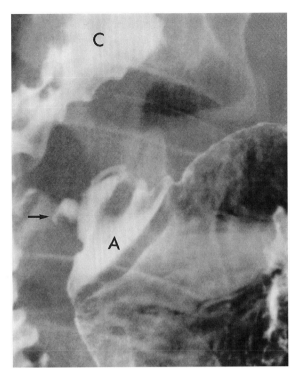

Fig. 19.37 Ectopic pancreatic rest. These are generally found in the distal antrum on the greater curve. The small diverticulum results from barium entering the primitive ductal system (arrow). Supine film. A = distal antrum; C = duodenal cap.

niche at the apex of the tumour (Fig. 19.37) or even fill a short branching ductal system. These rests are generally incidental findings, but occasionally they may be complicated by pancreatitis, pseudocyst formation or adenocarcinoma. On CT pancreatic rests have a variable appearance, ranging from homogeneous, strongly enhancing tumours of similar attenuation to normal pancreatic tissue through to avascular cystic lesions, depending on the acinar component of the rests and the formation of pseudocysts.

MALIGNANT TUMOURS

Gastric carcinoma

The prevalence of gastric adenocarcinoma is high in Japan, where successful screening programmes have been developed. Screening has not been established in western countries, as the disease prevalence is now four times lower than in Japan and has been declining for the last 20 years.

Atrophic gastritis predisposes to the development of gastric carcinoma. A sequence of events may follow atrophic gastritis, with the development of intestinal metaplasia, then dysplasia and finally neoplasia. A past infection with *H. pylori* is an important initiator of this sequence of events. Adenomatous polyps also develop from mucosa affected by chronic atrophic gastritis and so may coexist with carcino-

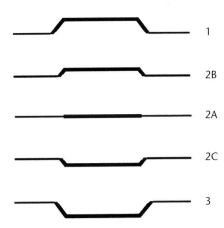

Fig. 19.38 The Japanese Endoscopic Society has classified early tumours into three types. Type 1, protrude more than 5 mm above the mucosal surface. Type 2, flat (2A), slightly elevated (<5 mm (2B)), or slightly depressed (2C). Type 3, ulcerating and penetrate the muscularis mucosa.

mas, although in a minority of cases these polyps undergo malignant change themselves. Patients with pernicious anaemia have an antiparietal cell antibody which produces atrophic gastritis involving the body and fundus of the stomach and so predisposes to gastric carcinoma. Partial gastrectomy also predisposes to gastric carcinoma, with the Billroth II operation being associated with a greater risk than the Billroth I operation; the majority of carcinomas develop close to the gastrojejunal anastomosis as a result of bile reflux. Bile reflux also accounts for the increased risk following a gastroenterostomy without gastric resection. Intake of *nitrates* may also be a risk factor as nitrates are converted to nitrosamines in the stomach; nitrosamines are known to be carcinogenic in animals. Conversely, diets rich in vitamin C prevent the formation of nitrosamines and are associated with a low risk of gastric carcinoma.

Unfortunately, symptoms do not usually develop until gastric carcinomas are advanced; they include loss of appetite, dyspepsia, weight loss and anaemia. Ulcerating tumours may haemorrhage, infiltrating tumours may cause early satiety, tumours obstructing the cardia cause dysphagia, whereas those obstructing the outflow to the stomach cause vomiting.

Early carcinomas

By definition these carcinomas are confined to the mucosa and submucosa, irrespective of whether or not regional lymph nodes are involved. Screening in Japan is aimed at detecting early carcinomas. These tumours have a 90% 5 year survival, as opposed to most gastric tumours, which present clinically at an advanced stage and have only a 10% 5 year survival. The Japanese Endoscopic Society has classified these early tumours into three types. Type 1 are elevated tumours protruding more than 5 mm above the mucosal surface. Type 2 are either flat (2A), slightly elevated (<5 mm (2B)), or slightly depressed but do not extend through the muscularis mucosa (2C) (Figs 19.38, 19.39A). Type 3 are ulcerating tumours which penetrate the muscularis mucosa. Some tumours may show a combination of appearances and are classified accordingly

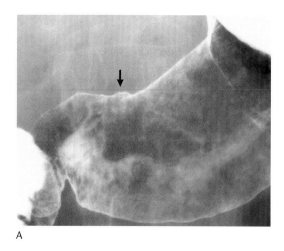

A

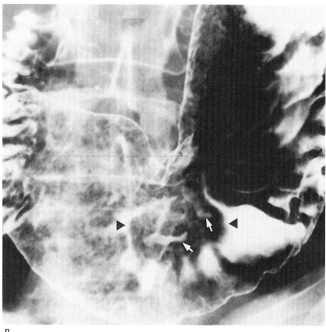

B

Fig. 19.39 Early gastric carcinoma. (A) Shallow ulcerating tumour, type 2C (arrow). (B) Mixed type (2B and C). An elevated tumour (between arrowheads) is outline by barium. Two small irregular ulcers are present (arrows).

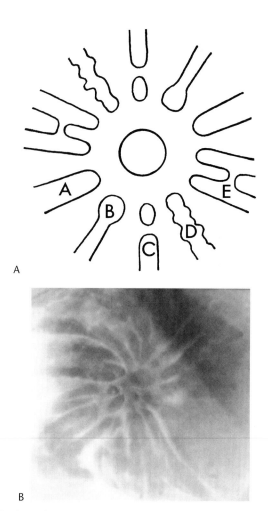

A

B

Fig. 19.40 Evaluating the folds around an ulcer. (A) The folds around an early or advanced gastric cancer may be thickened (A), clubbed (B), interrupted (C), nodular (D) or fused (E). Folds do not reach the margin of the ulcer, but this may be seen with benign ulcers if there is a rim of oedema around the ulcer. (B) Thickened, clubbed, interrupted, nodular and fused folds around a malignant ulcer.

(Fig. 19.39B). Recognition of flat lesions relies on the areae gastricae or fold pattern of the stomach being disturbed. Ulcerating lesions need to be differentiated from benign ulcers, so the adjacent mucosa must be carefully evaluated as malignant ulcers have folds radiating from their margins that are nodular, clubbed, interrupted or fused (Fig. 19.40). Rarely an ulcerating early carcinoma will temporarily heal with medical treatment, but the mucosal nodularity and the abnormal fold pattern persists.

Advanced carcinomas

By definition these tumours have invaded the muscularis propria. Carcinomas may protrude into the stomach lumen and be polypoid or fungating (Fig. 19.41A) or they may ulcerate (Fig. 19.41B) or infiltrate (Fig. 19.41C). When infiltration becomes extensive, the stomach develops a 'leather bottle' or 'linitis plastica' appearance (Fig. 19.41D). Often a combination of these appearances can be recognised.

Some adenocarcinomas produce an excess of extracellular mucin, and these mucin-producing carcinomas may show stippled calcification (Fig. 19.42). Large tumours protruding into the lumen of the stomach are unlikely to cause diagnostic problems. As with early gastric cancers, ulcerating tumours may resemble benign peptic ulcers, so the barium-coated adjacent mucosa needs to be carefully inspected for nodularity and fold changes (Fig. 19.40). In profile, malignant ulcers project into the lumen of the stomach, but benign greater-curve ulcers may do the same as a result of spasm and oedema. When viewed in profile and in single contrast, a meniscus sign, produced by the margin of an ulcerating tumour projecting into the barium-filled lumen of the stomach, may be observed (Fig. 19.4B).

Occasionally a gastric carcinoma will spread submucosally, leaving the mucosa intact, and in such cases an endoscopic biopsy usually returns negative. The desmoplastic reaction associated with

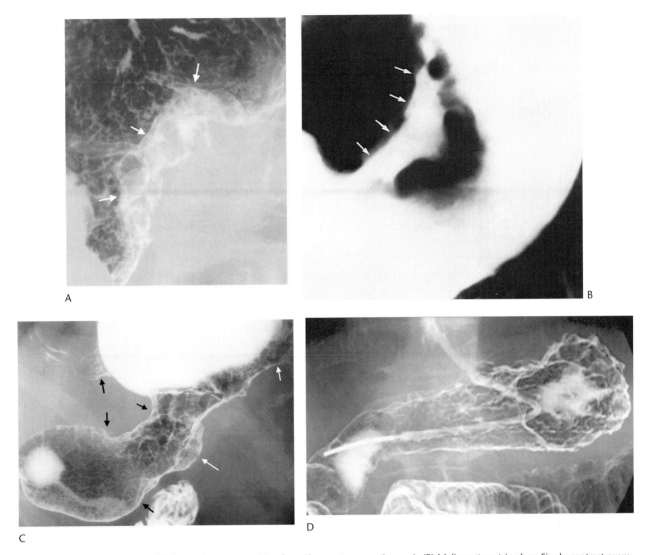

Fig. 19.41 Advanced gastric carcinoma. (A) Fungating cancer arising from the greater curve (arrows). (B) Malignant gastric ulcer. Single-contrast examination. The ulcer is situated close to the lesser curvature and near the incisura. The arrows indicate the base of the ulcer, which is in line with the lesser curvature, i.e. the crater is non-projecting. Tumour at the margin of the crater appears translucent and nodular creating a pool of barium, convex one side and concave the other (arrows) (meniscus sign). (C) Infiltrating and ulcerating gastric carcinoma. The proximal half of the stomach is involved with thickening of the wall, destruction of mucosa, and narrowing of the lumen (arrows). Ulceration is present on the greater curve (long arrow). (D) Small stomach as a result of diffuse submucosal infiltration (linitis plastica). Air has been injected down the nasogastric tube to distend the stomach.

such tumour infiltration makes the stomach wall rigid, with loss of peristalsis, and the gastric lumen narrows. If the whole of the stomach is involved, this is known as 'leather bottle' stomach or linitis plastica. In such cases the mucosa is nodular, and the fold pattern is lost or deformed (Fig. 19.41D). Other diseases narrowing the lumen of the stomach are listed in Box 19.5.

Cancers involving the distal antrum may have an 'apple core' shape which can be mistaken for the normal pyloric canal, particu-

Box 19.5   Diseases narrowing the lumen of the stomach

Entire stomach
Gastric cancer
Metastatic breast cancer
Hodgkin's disease
Kaposi's sarcoma

Antrum
Amyloidosis, sarcoidosis
Crohn's disease, tuberculosis, syphilis
Caustic ingestion, radiotherapy
Eosinophilic gastroenteropathy
CMV gastritis

Box 19.6   Tumour, node and metastases (TNM) staging

Primary tumour (T)
T1 Tumour limited to mucosa and submucosa
T2 Tumour infiltrates the muscularis propria or subserosa
T3 Tumour involves the visceral peritoneum without invasion of adjacent organs
T4 Tumour invades adjacent structures other than the duodenum and oesophagus, e.g. pancreas

Regional lymph nodes (N)
N0 Nodes not involved
N1 Involvement of 1–6 regional lymph nodes
N2 Involvement of 7–15 regional lymph nodes
N3 Involvement of >15 regional lymph nodes

Distant metastases (M)
M0 No metastases
M1 Distant metastases, e.g. liver, adrenal glands and distant lymph node groups

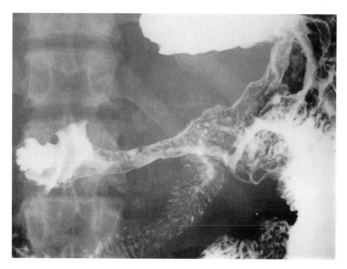

Fig. 19.42 Mucus-producing gastric adenocarcinoma. Faint calcification can be seen in the thickened wall of the antrum and distal body of the stomach.

larly if the tumour merges with the canal (Fig. 19.43). Carcinoma of the fundus may infiltrate submucosally into the distal oesophagus to produce an appearance that simulates achalasia.

Tumour staging (*Box 19.6*)

The role of staging procedures in gastric cancer is to stratify patients into those to be treated with primary surgery with curative intent, those who may benefit from chemotherapy and those in whom palliation is appropriate. The current staging procedures available are CT, EUS and laparoscopy, the deployment of each depending on the availability of local expertise and therapeutic philosophy. The main justification for the use of CT is to demonstrate distant metastases, principally in the liver, and distant lymphadenopathy. The use of CT for tumour staging (T-staging) of gastric carcinomas is more controversial, with EUS achieving a

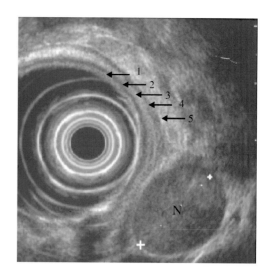

Fig. 19.44 Endoscopic ultrasound showing the five layers of the gastric wall and an enlarged, rounded, hypoechoic, metastatic lymph node (N). (Courtesy of Dr Keith Harris.)

higher accuracy. EUS has a high near-field spatial resolution and can demonstrate a greater number of layers in the gastric wall (Fig. 19.44). In addition, the real-time component to EUS can help to demonstrate relative movement or fixity between the stomach

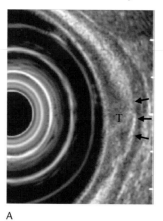

A

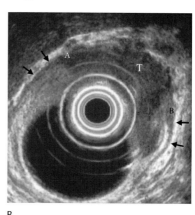

B

Fig. 19.45 Gastric carcinoma. (A) Tumour stage T1. The echogenic submucosal layer has not been breached (black arrows) by the tumour (T). (B) Tumour stage T3. Tumour (T) has breached muscularis propria between points A and B. Intact muscularis propria can be seen at the margins of the tumour (black arrows).

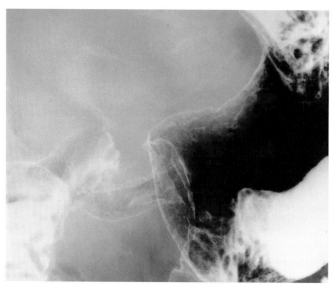

Fig. 19.43 Carcinoma of distal antrum. The rolled margins suggest the diagnosis. The differential diagnosis includes hypertrophic pyloric stenosis but in this condition the antrum tapers into the pyloric canal and the mucosa within the canal can be seen to be intact.

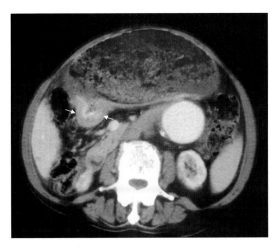

Fig. 19.46 Gastric carcinoma. The tumour is enhancing and thickening the wall of the antrum (arrows). The stomach is distended with food debris as a result of gastric outlet obstruction.

and adjacent organs. EUS is also of value in the assessment of local lymphadenopathy (Fig. 19.44). Laparoscopy is used to assess peritoneal disease and can be used to sample lymph node groups. CT is used to monitor the effects of chemotherapy.

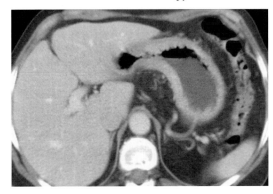

A

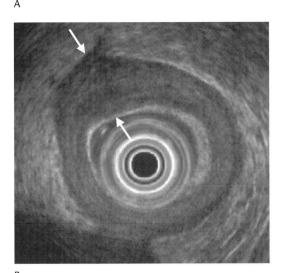

B

Fig. 19.47 Linitis plastica. (A) Diffuse thickening of the gastric wall demonstrated by CT. (B) Endoscopic ultrasound showing a narrowed gastric lumen and diffuse thickening of all layers of the gastric wall by tumour infiltration (between arrows).

EUS clearly shows the depth of cancer invasion (Fig. 19.45) through the gastric wall, enabling accurate T-staging (see Fig. 18.17). On CT, gastric cancers appear as focal wall thickening often associated with increased enhancement (Fig. 19.46). With early gastric cancers the low attenuation layer is preserved; with T2 lesions this layer is lost but the outer layer has a smooth margin and the adjacent fat is normal. Diffuse mural thickening with a small capacity stomach is found when there is extensive submucosal infiltration with linitis plastica (Fig. 19.47). Advanced tumours tend to be thicker, with greater mucosal irregularity due to the presence of ulceration, but size alone does not predict stage, as occasionally early tumours can be polypoid and several centimetres thick. Uncommonly, mucinous adenocarcinomas contain punctate calcifications. Strands of tumour extending into the perigastric fat indicate extension beyond the gastric wall. Direct tumour spread may involve the pancreas, diaphragm or liver, or spread may occur to the transverse colon and lead to fistula formation (Fig. 19.48C). Vascular encasement may also be seen (Fig. 19.48B).

Lymphatic spread

In the presence of gastric carcinoma, enlarged nodes are considered to indicate metastatic spread, but this is a crude index because normal-sized nodes may contain malignant deposits and enlarged nodes may just show reactive change. Generally, the larger the lymph node the greater the probability of metastatic involvement. Suggested thresholds for involvement are: gastrohepatic ligament and porta hepatis nodes 8 mm; coeliac axis to renal arteries 10 mm; and renal arteries to aortic bifurcation 12 mm. High attenuation (>100 HU) lymph nodes also more likely to be malignant, even if small. The accuracy of N-staging, using CT, ranges from 40 to 70%. EUS is more restricted in the nodal groups that can be visualised but has an accuracy of 65–80% for nodal involvement. A metastatic node is typically well defined, hypoechogenic and spherical. Enlarged lymph nodes often merge with the tumour mass, particularly in cachexic patients, but these nodes are removed at the time of surgery. Regional spread is to nodes that accompany the left gastric, splenic, coeliac and common hepatic arteries. Involvement of regional nodes is important, as this may change the extent of lymph node dissection at surgery. Enlarged retropancreatic and para-aortic lymph nodes are classified as distant metastases, and generally contraindicate surgery.

Peritoneal spread

Peritoneal spill results in fluid collections and tumour nodules developing at multiple sites throughout the peritoneal cavity. Gravity, the pattern of flow of peritoneal fluid and the pockets within the peritoneum make the pouch of Douglas, the superior aspect of the sigmoid mesocolon, the junction of the terminal ileum with the caecum, and the right paracolic gutter the commonest sites for peritoneal deposits. The mesentery may show stranding and soft-tissue thickening (Fig. 19.48C). Similar changes involve the omentum to produce an omental cake, although this is most frequently seen with carcinoma of the ovary. Peritoneal deposits may seed to the ovaries (*Krukenberg tumours*). They may involve one or both ovaries and have a cystic component but, unlike primary ovarian carcinomas, are rarely multicystic (Fig. 19.49). Other carcinomas (i.e. colon, breast and malignant melanoma) may metastasise to the ovaries, but carcinoma of the stomach is the most frequent.

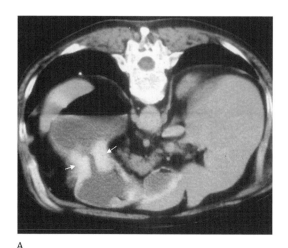

A

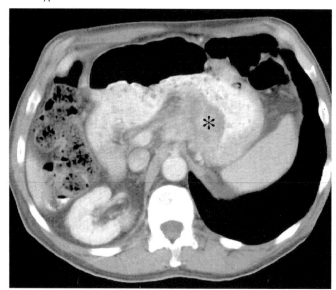

B

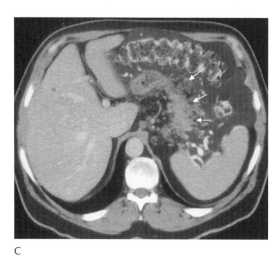

C

Fig. 19.48 (A) Gastric carcinoma constricting the body of the stomach (arrows). Stomach distended with water. Prone scan shows fat plane between tumour and pancreas, indicating that the pancreas is not invaded. (B) Gastric carcinoma (asterisk) extending beyond the serosa to encase the coeliac axis vessels. (Courtesy of Prof. R. W. Whitehouse.) (C) Extension into the transverse mesocolon (arrows) from a carcinoma of the antrum of the stomach.

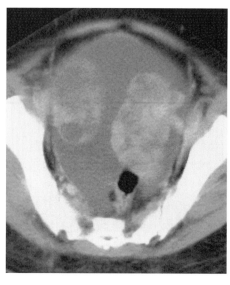

Fig. 19.49 Krukenberg tumours. Bilateral partly cystic ovarian tumours and malignant ascites. (Courtesy of Dr John Spencer.)

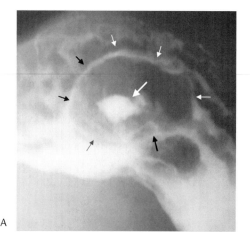

A

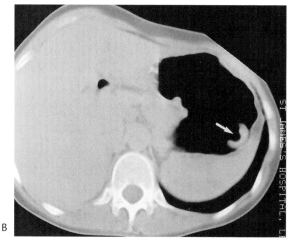

B

Fig. 19.50 Gastric 'target' lesion. (A) An ulcerating (large arrow) tumour in the fundus of the stomach (small arrows). This appearance is typical of an ulcerating submucosal metastasis from malignant melanoma. (B) CT scan shows the same tumour (arrow).

Haematogenous spread

This is primarily to the liver, but with modern chemotherapy metastases to the lungs, adrenals, kidneys and brain are now seen with increasing frequency.

Fundal adenocarcinomas involving the oesophagus have a similar appearance to oesophageal adenocarcinomas involving the fundus, but the tumour can be expected to have arisen from whichever structure shows the greater involvement. *Antral tumours* occasionally invade the duodenum, and although this pattern of spread is often associated with lymphoma it is more frequently observed with gastric carcinomas by virtue of their greater prevalence.

Metastatic disease

Malignant melanoma and *breast carcinoma* are the most frequent of the haematogenous metastases to involve the stomach. Prolonged survival with chemotherapy means that metastases to the gastrointestinal tract are now being seen more frequently with other carcinomas, such as those of the kidney, lung, thyroid and testes.

Melanoma metastases typically produce 'bull's eye' or target-type lesions as a result of ulceration of these submucosal deposits (Fig. 19.50). Breast carcinoma has a tendency to spread submucosally (Fig. 19.51), but the tumour produces less desmoplastic reaction than gastric carcinoma and so does not reduce the gastric volume to the same extent. Squamous carcinomas of the oesophagus may spread via the lymphatics in the oesophageal wall to produce satellite submucosal masses elsewhere in the oesophagus (see Fig. 18.17) or occasionally in the fundus of the stomach. Enlarged lymph nodes around the cardia may cause local extrinsic

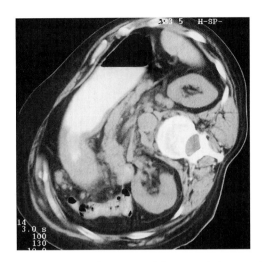

Fig. 19.51 Metastasis to the antrum of the stomach from carcinoma of the breast. The tumour has spread submucosally. CT scan. Lateral decubitus scan in an attempt to better distend the gastric antrum.

compression of the oesophagus and may sometimes invade the gastro-oesophageal junction to cause achalasia. Enlarged pancreatic lymph nodes may impress on the medial wall of the duodenum and widen the duodenal loop, giving an appearance more usually associated with enlargement of the head of the pancreas from pancreatitis or pancreatic carcinoma. Enlarged retroperitoneal nodes may compress the third part of the duodenum against the root of the superior mesenteric artery, and can even obstruct the duodenum at this site. Enlarged nodes around the coeliac axis may denervate the stomach to cause gastric dilatation.

Extrinsic infiltration of the stomach or duodenum by an adjacent tumour produces nodularity, spiculation and, finally, ulceration of the mucosa. Carcinoma of the head of the pancreas may infiltrate the inner wall of the second and third parts of the duodenum or occasionally the greater curve of the antrum of the stomach (Fig. 19.52). Tumours of the tail of the pancreas invade the fundus and upper posterior wall of the body of the stomach and the duodenojejunal flexure. Tumours of the transverse colon may spread by the gastrocolic ligament to involve the greater curve of the antrum and body of the stomach, whereas those of the right side of the transverse colon may involve the anterior wall of the second

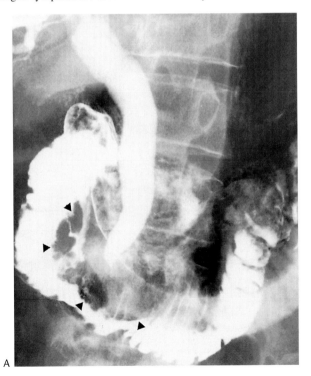

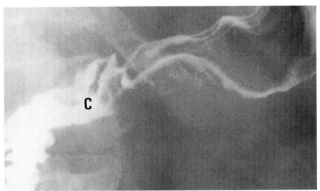

A   B

Fig. 19.52 Carcinoma of the pancreas. (A) Carcinoma of the head of the pancreas invading the medial wall of the duodenal loop. Note the reversed-'3' sign of Frostberg (arrowheads). A percutaneous transhepatic cholangiogram performed with the barium study shows the common bile duct to be obstructed at its lower end. (B) Pancreatic tumour producing an impression on and elevating the gastric antrum (the pad sign). C = duodenal cap.

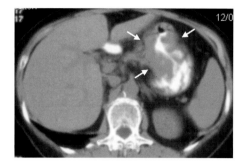

Fig. 19.53 MALT lymphoma. Multifocal tumour (arrows) thickening the gastric wall.

part of the duodenum where it is crossed by the attachment of the transverse mesocolon. Tumours of the gallbladder invade the adjacent first part of the duodenum, and those of the kidney the posterolateral aspect of the second part of the duodenum.

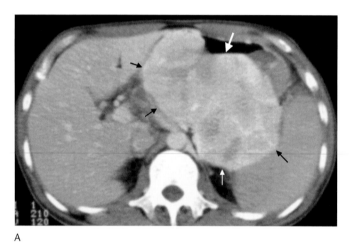

A

Lymphoma

The stomach is the commonest site for the development of gastrointestinal lymphoma. It may be the primary site or more rarely be secondarily involved as part of a generalised lymphoma. *H. pylori* gastritis is associated with the development of MALT in the lamina propria, which may progress to a MALT lymphoma, which is a low-grade B-cell lymphoma. High grade B cell lymphomas may arise de novo, or from low grade MALT lymphoma. Coeliac disease predisposes to small bowel lymphoma and rarely to lymphoma and carcinoma at other sites in the CI tract. These lymphomas are usually T cell presenting in patients with known or previously unrecognised coeliac disease.

Patients with gastric lymphoma are usually late middle-aged and there is a male predisposition. The presentation is generally with upper abdominal symptoms, weight loss or an epigastric mass. Low-grade MALT lymphomas produce gastric changes that are often focal and subtle (Fig. 19.53) compared with the more obvious changes of advanced tumours (Fig. 19.54A). The tumour may be polypoid, ulcerating or infiltrative, and so often has a radiological appearance identical to that of a gastric carcinoma, although sometimes an ulcerating lymphoma may resemble a benign gastric ulcer. The diagnosis of lymphoma may be suggested if there are giant cavitating lesions or multiple polypoid tumours, particularly if they show central ulceration giving them a 'bull's eye' appearance or if there is extensive infiltration producing pronounced thickening of the gastric folds (Fig. 19.54B). Diffuse submucosal infiltration thickens the gastric wall to produce an appearance that resembles linitis plastica. Most lymphomas produce little in the way of a desmoplastic reaction, and therefore distensibility of the stomach is generally preserved, with the exception of the occasional patient (about 10%) who has Hodgkin's disease. Antral tumours frequently spread to the duodenum (Fig. 19.54C). Less often, fundal tumours spread to involve the oesophagus. CT features which suggest lymphoma rather than gastric carcinoma include a bulky homogeneous

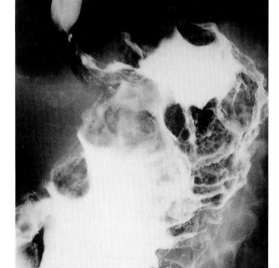

B

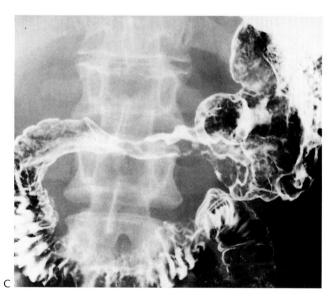

C

Fig. 19.54 Gastric lymphoma. (A) CT scan. A bulky tumour (small arrows) arising from the posterior wall of the stomach (large arrow). The tumour extends posteriorly to involve the pancreas and splenic hilum. (B) Gross thickening of folds in the fundus and body of this stomach infiltrated by lymphoma. (C) An irregular stricture is present in the distal stomach, also involving the duodenal cap. Adjacent nodal enlargement is producing an impression on the inside of the duodenal loop.

tumour with pronounced thickening of the gastric wall, preservation of the perigastric fat plane, transpyloric spread, multicentricity, widespread nodal disease and splenic enlargement. There is little lymphoid tissue in the duodenum, so duodenal involvement by lymphoma is generally from longitudinal gastric or jejunal spread or by extrinsic involvement from enlarged retroperitoneal lymph nodes.

Chest and abdominal CT is used for tumour staging (Box 19.7).

Some low grade tumours resolve following *H. pylori* eradication therapy. Gastric resection may be curative for intermediate- and high-grade stage 1 tumours but is combined with chemotherapy for stage 2 disease. Stage 3 and 4 disease may be treated with chemotherapy alone. Complete healing of ulcerating lesions may be seen with chemotherapy but in other cases the stomach may be left scarred. Occasionally tumour necrosis may result in haemorrhage or leave a large cavitating lesion that may perforate.

The mean 5 year survival for gastric lymphoma is 50%, although the prognosis for low grade MALT lymphomas approaches 90%.

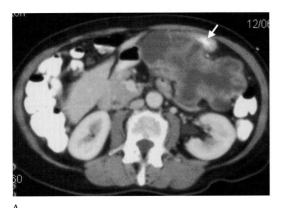

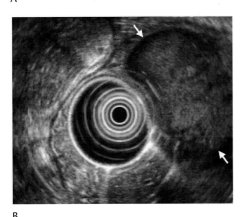

Fig. 19.55 Malignant gastric stromal tumour. (A) CT. This predominantly exophytic tumour is compressing the stomach (arrow). (B) Endoscopic ultrasound. These tumours tend to be less well defined and larger than their benign counterparts and to have a heterogonous echotexture, often with cystic spaces.

Malignant stromal tumours

These tumours comprise about 1% of gastric malignancies, and tend to develop in the fundus and body of the stomach. They only rarely arise from the duodenum. As with lymphoma, patients are usually middle-aged or elderly, and there is a male predisposition. They are often large intramural tumours that protrude into the stomach and have a tendency to central necrosis and ulceration. On occasions giant ulcers may result. These tumours may grow predominantly into the lumen of the stomach and become pedunculated, or they may grow beyond the stomach wall to invade the diaphragm, pancreas or colon. Exophytic growth is well shown by CT, and the tumour often has a low-density necrotic centre (Fig. 19.55). Occasionally, dystrophic calcification may be observed. An association with functional extra-adrenal paraganglioma and pulmonary chondromas has been described (*Carney's syndrome*).

Malignant stromal tumours metastasise to the peritoneal cavity, and haematogenous metastatic spread is to liver, lung and bone. Lymphatic spread is rare.

Differentiating benign from malignant stromal tumours can be difficult for the histologist even when the tumour has been resected. Benign stromal tumours are smaller (<10 cm) with a homogeneous consistency on CT and EUS. Liver metastases from malignant stromal tumours are vascular, although they often show central necrosis. In view of their vascularity, CT should include both arterial and portal venous phase scans of the liver.

Kaposi's sarcoma

This tumour of blood vessels develops in approximately a third of homosexual male patients infected with AIDS. Patients generally present as a result of an associated opportunistic infection, which will have its own radiological features. This sarcoma is generally multifocal, producing submucosal tumours throughout the gastrointestinal tract. The stomach, duodenum and small bowel are most frequently involved. Early diagnosis is by endoscopy, when haemorrhagic patches are recognised on the gastric mucosa. Barium radiology may show large polypoid masses, or submucosal nodules which later ulcerate to produce 'bull's eye' lesions. Submucosal infiltration thickens folds or produces a linitis plastica-type appearance. Retroperitoneal lymph nodes and splenomegaly are seen on CT.

Carcinoid tumour

Carcinoid tumours in the stomach or duodenum are rare. This slow-growing tumour tends to be found in the distal antrum and lesser curve of the stomach or the first and second parts of the duodenum (Fig. 19.56). It produces a submucosal nodule which can ulcerate or even become pedunculated. Occasionally a large tumour resembling a carcinoma develops. Unlike their small-bower counterparts, these tumours do not produce 5-hydroxytryptamine, and so the few that metastasise to the liver do not produce carcinoid syndrome. Both the primary tumour and the liver metastases are typically hypervascular, so arterial and portal venous phase CT should be performed.

Hypergastrinaemia predisposes to the formation of multiple benign gastric carcinoids, so in patients with chronic atrophic gastritis or Zollinger–Ellison syndrome a barium meal may show multiple small polyps in the fundus of the stomach. They have a similar appearance to hyperplastic and adenomatous gastric polyps.

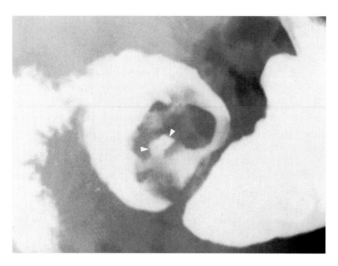

Fig. 19.56 Duodenal carcinoid tumour. There is an irregular, lobulated filling defect with central ulceration (arrowheads) in the duodenal cap. Stromal tumours, melanoma metastasis, and duodenal ulcer with oedema can also produce this appearance.

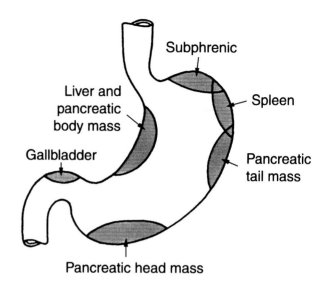

Fig. 19.57 Sites of extrinsic gastric compression.

MISCELLANEOUS CONDITIONS

GASTRIC DISPLACEMENT AND ROTATION

Extrinsic masses

Any intra-abdominal mass, if large enough, may impress on or displace the stomach. Frequent causes are hepatic and splenic enlargement, left subphrenic abscess and pancreatic tumours and cysts (Fig. 19.57). A splenic impression on the fundus may simulate a submucosal gastric tumour. Lesions of the head of the pancreas may displace the gastric antrum upwards and forwards and produce a smooth impression on the greater curve of the gastric antrum (the pad sign; Fig. 19.52B).

When an extrinsic impression or displacement is seen at endoscopy or during a barium meal an ultrasound or CT should be performed to determine the cause.

Gastric volvulus

Laxity of the gastrohepatic, gastrocolic and gastrolienal ligaments predisposes to gastric volvulus. Primary volvulus occurs in the absence of a diaphragmatic abnormality and in children may result from a congenital absence of some of the supporting ligaments of the stomach. Secondary volvulus is more common and occurs when the ligaments stretch as the stomach ascends to enter a diaphragmatic hernia or with diaphragmatic eventration. There are three types of gastric volvulus. The commonest is the *organoaxial volvulus*, in which the stomach rotates around an axis that runs between the relatively fixed duodenum and oesophagogastric junction. The greater curve rotates forwards and upwards (less often backwards and upwards) into the diaphragmatic defect or eventration (Fig. 19.58A,B). Rotation around an axis that runs between the midpoints of the greater and lesser curves is less common and is known as *mesenteroaxial volvulus* (Fig. 19.58C). The duodenum rotates anteriorly (less often posteriorly) from right to left so that the posterior surface of the stomach lies anteriorly and the greater

curve remains at the bottom. There is also a rare third type of chronic volvulus that is a combination of the other two.

Gastric volvulus is most often seen in elderly patients with a large diaphragmatic hernia. They are frequently asymptomatic, although some are troubled by dyspepsia and vomiting. Acute volvulus is rare and presents with retching and severe epigastric pain. The clinician is unable to pass a nasogastric tube from the oesophagus to the stomach and plain films show a gas- or fluid-distended viscus in the upper abdomen. A barium swallow confirms obstruction at the lower end of the oesophagus. Acute volvulus constitutes a surgical emergency, as, untreated, the stomach may infarct.

A '*cup and spill' stomach* is a normal variant that can simulate an organoaxial volvulus. The distinction is made by asking the patient to swallow barium while standing in a lateral position. The dependent part of the fundus fills and forms the 'cup', which is situated posteriorly. The barium then spills from this part of the fundus and 'cascades' down the posterior gastric wall.

DUODENAL DISPLACEMENT, OBSTRUCTION AND FISTULAS

Variations in peritoneal fixation produce either right or left paraduodenal fossae that predispose to internal herniation.

Paraduodenal hernias

These are the most frequent type of internal hernia. In the more common left-sided variety, loops of small bowel pass into a paraduodenal fossa behind the inferior mesenteric vein. The hernia extends into the transverse and descending mesocolon and here the incarcerated small bowel loops indent the back of the stomach or back of the left side of the transverse colon. CT will show the inferior mesenteric vein lying at the anterior border of the hernial opening. In the right-sided variety, small bowel passes into a paraduodenal fossa behind the superior mesenteric artery. This hernia protrudes below and lateral to the second part of the duodenum. Internal herniation, particularly of small bowel, may also occur through the foramen of Winslow.

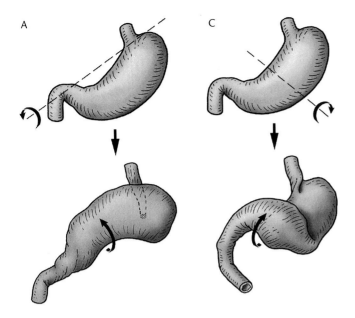

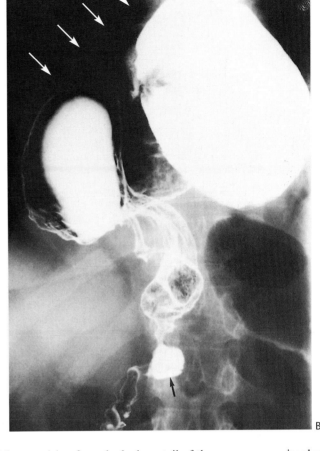

Fig. 19.58 Types of gastric volvulus. (A) Organoaxial. Rotation occurs around an axis connecting the pyloris to the oesophagogastric junction. (B) Organoaxial volvulus of an intrathoracic stomach. The greater curve is folded upward and to the right (small white arrows). There is a giant duodenal ulcer (arrow) which perforated 10 days later. (C) Mesenteroaxial. Rotation occurs around an axis connecting the middle of the greater curve to the middle of the lesser curve. Generally this type of volvulus is partial as a result of excess mobility of the antrum and duodenum and so the stomach often kinks and obstructs between the body and the antrum.

Extrinsic involvement

An abscess or tumour of the gallbladder may impress on or invade the duodenal cap. Tumours and abscesses of the right kidney may involve the posterolateral wall of the second part of the duodenum, whereas pancreatic tumours, cysts and abscesses affect the inner border of the duodenal loop or produce an impression on the inferior margin of the antrum of the stomach (pad sign) (Fig. 19.52B).

Masses arising from the body or tail of the pancreas may involve the third part of the duodenum and displace the stomach forward. When there is swelling of the pancreatic head from tumour or pancreatitis, the tethering influence of the papilla is responsible for a widened duodenal loop assuming a reversed-'3' configuration (*Frostberg's sign*) (Fig. 19.52A). The *transverse colon* crosses anterior to the second part of the duodenum, so a colonic carcinoma may invade at this site and a duodenocolic fistula may result.

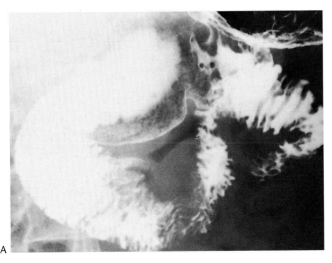

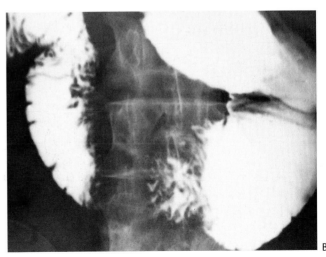

Fig. 19.59 Superior mesenteric artery syndrome caused by carcinoma of the pancreas involving the root of the mesentery. (A) Supine position. Compression of third part of duodenum. (B) Prone position. The compression persists and dilatation of the proximal duodenum is accentuated. (Courtesy of Drs J. R. Anderson, P. M. Earnshaw and G. M. Fraser, and the editor of *Clinical Radiology*.)

Extrinsic tumours initially indent the duodenal wall, then cause mucosal nodularity and spiculation and finally mucosal destruction and ulceration. Adjacent inflammation from pancreatitis or cholecystitis may cause spasm and oedema, which will narrow the duodenal lumen and thicken the folds.

Superior mesenteric artery syndrome

The third part of the duodenum lies in a fixed position and is bounded anteriorly by the root of the mesentery carrying the superior mesenteric artery, and posteriorly by the aorta and lumbar spine. When this compartment becomes narrowed, the third part of the duodenum may obstruct (Fig. 19.59); this is known as the superior mesenteric artery syndrome. Narrowing of the compartment may be caused by an aneurysm of the aorta or a retroperitoneal tumour. The condition is not entirely understood, as an association has also been reported with peptic ulceration, prolonged bedrest (often in a body plaster cast), severe weight loss and diminished duodenal peristalsis, as may be seen with scleroderma.

The duodenum dilates proximal to a broad, vertical band-like narrowing which crosses the third part of the duodenum as it passes over the spine. In most cases, with the exception of those with scleroderma, fluoroscopy shows vigorous to-and-fro peristalsis proximal to the site of obstruction. In some, the obstruction is related to posture, and by turning the patient prone or on to the left side the 'obstruction' is released. The attacks of abdominal pain and vomiting encountered in this condition tend to be intermittent, and radiological features are best demonstrated during an attack.

Aortoduodenal fistula

An aortic aneurysm may cause pressure necrosis of the posterior duodenal wall, or infection of the top end of a prosthetic graft may rupture into the duodenum (Fig. 19.60). Fistulation occurs at the site where the third part of the duodenum crosses the aorta.

Cholecystoduodenal fistula

In acute cholecystitis, a gallstone may erode from the gallbladder into the duodenum and, if large, the stone may obstruct the small bowel, causing *gallstone ileus*. A rarer cause of this type of fistula is a penetrating peptic ulcer that has eroded into the gallbladder. A

plain film will show air in the gallbladder, and in the biliary tree in cases where the cystic duct is patent.

VARICES, STRICTURES AND DIVERTICULA

Gastric varices

Possibly because of their subserosal location, gastric varices are a less frequent finding at endoscopy and barium meal than oesophageal varices, and less often cause gastrointestinal bleeding. They result from dilatation of the venous plexus of the fundus of the stomach, which normally communicates with the oesophageal venous plexus and drains into the coronary vein (left gastric) and short gastric veins. They are usually seen in association with oesophageal varices in patients with *portal hypertension*. Less often they are seen without oesophageal varices, when the splenic vein is occluded, as may result from pancreatitis or pancreatic carcinoma (Fig. 19.61). The varices produce a lobular contour to the fundus of the stomach (Fig. 19.62A). Occasionally, in severe portal hypertension, submucosal varices may develop elsewhere in the stomach and in the duodenum, producing multiple serpiginous folds. Rarely a solitary varix enlarges to produce a smooth submucosal tumour.

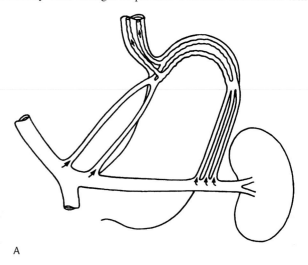

A

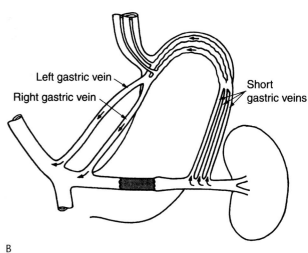

B

Fig. 19.61   Gastric varices associated with (A) portal hypertension, (B) splenic vein occlusion.

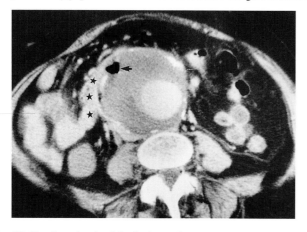

Fig. 19.60   Aortoduodenal fistula. Recent haematemesis. The third part of the duodenum (stars) is stretched over the aortic aneurysm, which contains thrombus. A fistula accounts for the gas in the aortic wall (arrow).

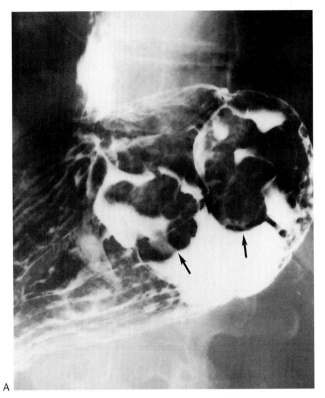

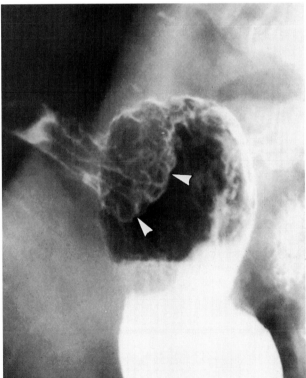

Fig. 19.62 Pseudotumours of the gastric fundus. (A) Gastric fundal varices. Filling defects (arrows) resembling a bunch of enlarged nodular mucosal folds. (Courtesy of Dr G. M. Fraser and the editor of *Clinical Radiology*.) (B) Intragastric prolapse of a sliding hiatus hernia. The mass (arrowheads) is composed of mucosal folds, and vanishes when the hernia expands above the diaphragm in the recumbent posture.

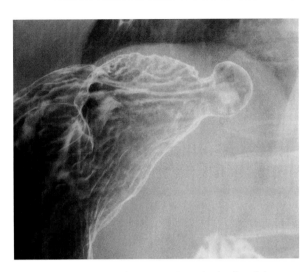

Fig. 19.63 Gastric diverticulum arising from the fundus of the stomach. Sometimes gastric folds can be seen entering the diverticulum, or areae gastricae can be seen within it.

CT or MR is useful for demonstrating portal venous and variceal anatomy and the underlying cause.

Gastric diverticulum

This is most frequently seen arising from the posterior wall of the fundus of the stomach (Fig. 19.63), but rarely may be prepyloric in location. Gastric diverticula tend to have a smooth outline and change shape during the course of a barium study, and the lining mucosa may show an areae gastricae pattern.

Gastric mural diverticulum

This is a localised invagination of gastric mucosa into the wall of the stomach. It is rare and usually found on the greater curve of the distal antrum. It needs to be differentiated from a small gastric ulcer or an ectopic pancreatic rest.

Antral diaphragm

This is a thin diaphragm with a small central opening that involves the antrum of the stomach (Fig. 19.64). It may be an inci-

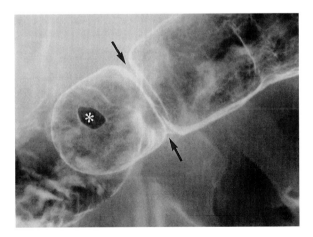

Fig. 19.64 An antral diaphragm (between the arrows). The pyloric canal is seen end on (asterisk).

dental finding or cause gastric outflow obstruction and, although congenital, may not present clinically until adult life.

Duodenal webs

Duodenal webs usually present in neonatal life with projectile vomiting, but less often present in adult life with obstruction. Rarely a congenital web in the second part of the duodenum causes partial duodenal obstruction and stretches to give a 'wind sock'-like appearance on barium studies (an *intraluminal diverticulum*).

Hypertrophic pyloric stenosis

There is an *infantile* and *adult* form of this congenital abnormality of the pyloric musculature. The adult form is probably a milder version of the infantile from. In the adult form stasis accounts for associated antral gastritis and gastric ulceration. The gastric antrum tapers into an elongated pyloric canal (>2 cm), which bulges into the base of the duodenal cap. Antral tapering and the absence of mucosal destruction, with intact mucosal folds passing through the pyloric canal, differentiate the condition from an annular carcinoma (Fig. 19.43).

Duodenal diverticulum

Duodenal diverticula are mucosal herniations through the muscle coat of the duodenum. They are often multiple, periampullary (Fig. 19.65) or arise from the third and fourth parts of the duodenum. They are usually asymptomatic but are a rare cause of haemorrhage, diverticulitis and perforation. Access to the papilla is difficult at ERCP if it opens into a diverticulum or if there is a periampullary diverticulum. Such diverticula may interfere with the drainage of the bile and predispose to a degree of biliary obstruction and the formation of bile duct stones.

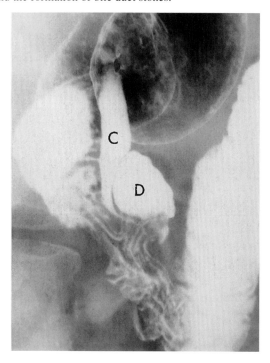

Fig. 19.65   Duodenal diverticulum into which the papilla is opening (D). Loss of continence has resulted in reflux of barium into the common bile duct (C).

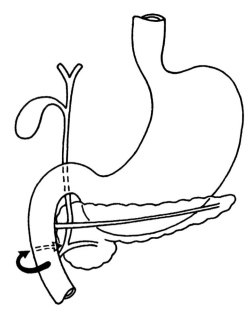

Fig. 19.66   Annular pancreas. The direction of rotation of the ventral pancreatic bud which joins the dorsal bud at the seventh week of embryonic life and finally comes to lie on the left side of the duodenum.

Duodenal ulceration with spasm or scarring may deform the duodenal cap to produce pseudodiverticula (Fig. 19.20). Unlike ulcers, pseudodiverticula change shape during the course of a barium meal examination.

Annular pancreas

In normal pancreatic development two ventral pancreatic buds and one dorsal pancreatic bud arise from the bile duct. One ventral pancreatic bud atrophies, whereas the other rotates around and behind the second part of the duodenum to join the dorsal pancreatic bud and eventually lie on the left side of the duodenum (Fig. 19.66). This ventral duct develops into the pancreatic head and uncinate process. In annular pancreas the other ventral bud fails to atrophy and both ventral buds contribute to a ring of tissue that surrounds the duodenum. Half present with obstruction as neonates, the rest present later when associated pancreatitis or periampullary peptic ulceration tips the patient into obstruction. On barium studies an annular narrowing of the second part of the duodenum with an intact mucosa suggests the diagnosis (Fig. 19.67A), and ERCP shows pancreatic duct branches encircling the duodenum. On ultrasound and CT the pancreatic head will look enlarged if the duodenum is not identified as it passes through the encircling pancreatic tissue (Fig. 19.67B).

GASTRIC SURGERY

Pyloroplasty and *gastroenterostomy* are operations used to drain the stomach (Fig. 19.68A,B) and are performed if there is outflow obstruction or poor motility. A pyloroplasty involves making a longitudinal incision in the line of the pyloric canal and then sewing the cut edges at right angles to the incision, which results in a widened channel. In the antecolic gastroenterostomy a proximal loop of

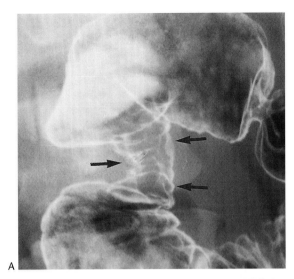

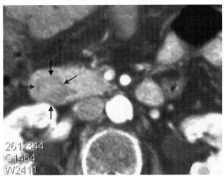

Fig. 19.67 Annular pancreas. (A) Producing a characteristic narrowing of the second part of the duodenum (arrows). (B) CT shows the gland encircling the duodenum (arrows).

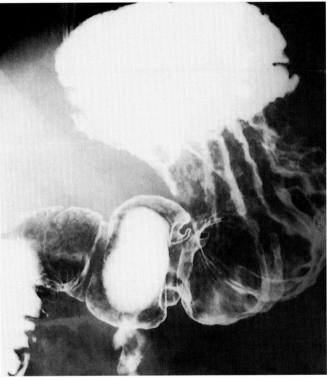

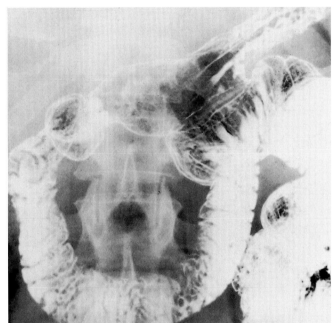

Fig. 19.68 (A) Pyloroplasty. A wide gastroduodenal channel has been produced. (B) Gastroenterostomy. (C) Normal postoperative barium examinations following Billroth I partial gastrectomy.

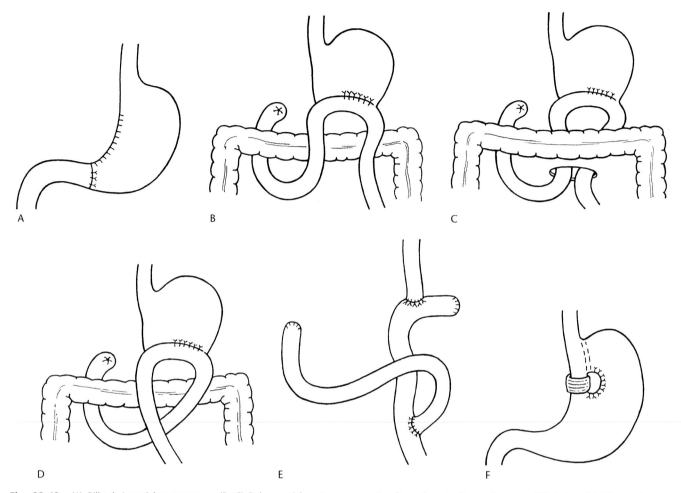

Fig. 19.69 (A) Billroth I partial gastrectomy. (B, C) Polya partial gastrectomy; antecolic and postcolic anastomoses. (D) Anteperistaltic anastomosis. (E) Postgastrectomy Roux-en-Y reconstruction. (F) Vertical banded gastroplasty.

jejunum is brought up in front of the omentum and transverse colon and anastomosed to the upper part of the anterior wall of the stomach. In the retrocolic operation an opening is made in the transverse mesocolon and a proximal loop of jejunum is anastomosed to the posterior wall of the stomach. The margins of the opening in the transverse mesocolon are sutured to the posterior gastric wall to prevent other loops of bowel herniating through the defect.

Partial gastrectomy is an operation in which the lower three-quarters of the stomach are resected. The Billroth I partial gastrectomy is performed for gastric ulcers and involves resecting the lower part of the stomach and suturing closed some of the end of the remnant, leaving enough open for the duodenal anastomosis (Figs 19.68C, 19.69A). The Billroth II or Polya operation is performed for duodenal ulceration. In this operation the duodenal stump is closed and a loop of jejunum is brought up, either in front of (Fig. 19.69B) or behind the colon (Fig. 19.69C), to drain the stomach. The anastomosis may be isoperistaltic or anteperistaltic. In the isoperistaltic operation the efferent loop runs away from the greater curve of the gastric remnant, whereas in the more common anteperistaltic operation the reverse applies (Fig. 19.69D). An alternative drainage procedure sometimes used with Billroth II operations is the Roux-en-Y anastomosis. Here the jejunum is transected, the distal end is drawn up to drain the stomach, and the proximal end is anastomosed to the side of this loop that has been brought up to the stomach.

A *total gastrectomy* usually involves an oesophagojejunostomy, for which a Roux-en-Y anastomosis may be constructed (Fig. 19.69E).

Increasingly, gastric surgery is being used as a weight-reducing procedure for morbid obesity. A variety of gastric operations have been devised to produce an early feeling of satiety when eating. The *vertical banded gastroplasty* involves stapling the stomach to produce a pouch along the upper part of the lesser curve and restricting the junction between this pouch and the body of the stomach to about 1 cm with a silastic band (Fig. 19.69F). Failure of the operation to control obesity may be caused by a breakdown of the staple line (Fig. 19.70), so when performing a barium study the staple line should be shown in profile. This is best achieved by examining the patient in an erect, steep oblique position, sometimes with the patient bent forward. Outlet obstruction may occur early in the postoperative period from oedema at the junction of the gastric pouch with the stomach. Late obstruction may be caused by too narrow a channel, and this can be managed by balloon dilatation. Benign ulceration may develop in the gastric pouch or in the distal stomach, and perforation has been described.

Early complications of gastric surgery

The commonest early complication to be encountered following gastroenterostomy is efferent loop obstruction from oedema or a

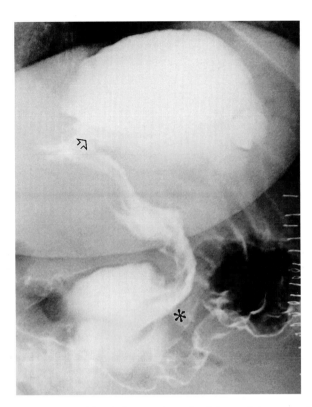

Fig. 19.70 Vertical banded gastroplasty. Breakdown of the top end of the staple line (arrow) with barium directly entering the fundus of the stomach. Site of banding marked with an asterisk.

haematoma at the stoma. If only the efferent loop side of the anastomosis is obstructed then an 'afferent loop circuit' movement may be observed, in which contrast medium passes through the pylorus and duodenum to the afferent loop and then passes back to the stomach via the anastomosis. Another cause of efferent loop obstruction following partial gastrectomy is entrapment of a jejunal loop within a postgastrectomy internal hernia.

Rupture of the duodenal stump is one of the gravest complications following gastric surgery, and occurs without warning any time during the first 3 weeks. Stump leakage may result in a right subphrenic abscess, whereas anastomotic leakage usually results in left subphrenic abscess. When stump rupture or an anastomotic leak is suspected, an urgent examination with a water-soluble contrast agent is indicated.

Late complications of gastric surgery

Following surgery for peptic disease, late problems include gastric obstruction and afferent loop obstruction, haemorrhage, post-operative ulcer disease, retained gastric antrum, fistula and post-gastrectomy syndromes.

Barium examination is useful in suspected stomal obstruction. The site and degree of obstruction are identified and often the cause can be determined. Prolapse of gastric mucosa through the stoma is usually symptomless, but can produce partial obstruction, and a polypoid mucosal filling defect in the stoma is shown with barium. A more serious complication is retrograde jejunogastric intussusception, which may be acute or chronic. Barium examination characteristically shows obstruction and a filling defect in the stomach

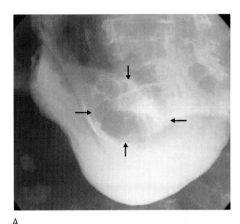

A

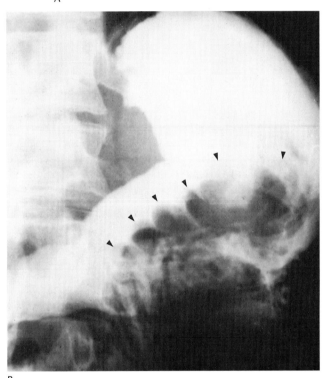

B

Fig. 19.71 Complications following gastric surgery. (A) Early post-operative oedema at a gastroenterostomy site (arrows). (B) Retrograde jejunogastric intussusception following gastrojejunostomy. The loops of jejunum within the stomach (arrowheads) have a characteristic 'coiled spring' appearance.

above the stoma, which can be identified as jejunum by the striated 'coiled spring' appearance of the oedematous valvulae conniventes (Fig. 19.71B). Strictures that develop at the site of an anastomosis or a pyloroplasty are amenable to endoscopic or fluoroscopically guided balloon dilatation. Phytobezoars occasionally develop in patients who have had gastric surgery, particularly partial gastrectomy with vagotomy, when the bezoar may obstruct the stomach.

Long afferent loops are best avoided when performing gastro-enterostomies as they can cause stasis of bile and pancreatic juice. This may cause epigastric discomfort and bile reflux. After a Polya gastrectomy, barium enters both afferent and efferent loops, although most goes down the efferent loop. Turning the patient on to the right side helps fill the afferent loop. In the *afferent loop syn-*

drome there is stasis in the afferent loop and this is characterised by postprandial epigastric fullness relieved by bilious vomiting. The usual cause is twisting or kinking near the gastric end of the loop. Stasis in the afferent loop may lead to bacterial overgrowth and anaemia. The distended afferent loop may be visible as a fluid-filled structure on plain radiography, ultrasound or CT. Barium examination may detect the point of obstruction, and sometimes in partial obstruction barium will enter the distended loop. Long afferent loops are also prone to internal herniation as they can slide behind the efferent loop and obstruct.

Following a Polya gastrectomy a portion of the gastric antrum may be unintentionally left behind so that it lies at the end of the afferent loop. In an alkaline environment this becomes a potent source of gastrin, so acid production continues and stomal ulceration results. The retained gastric antrum can be detected radiographically if there is sufficient barium filling of the afferent loop.

Suspected *anastomotic ulceration* (Fig. 19.72) is best investigated by endoscopy, as the distorted mucosa at the anastomosis site may be difficult to evaluate by barium studies.

Many patients develop diarrhoea after a gastrectomy. This may result from vagotomy, loss of pyloric hold-up, loss of coordination between the arrival of food and pancreatic and biliary secretions, and pancreatic insufficiency from lack of gastrin stimulation of the pancreas.

Vagotomy operations are performed to reduce gastric acid output in patients with duodenal ulcers, but unless the operation is highly selective there is a risk of gastric stasis, and so a gastroenterostomy or pyloroplasty should also be performed. Highly selective vagotomy involves cutting the branches of the vagus nerve that supply the fundus of the stomach and leaving the motor branches intact so that a drainage operation is not required.

Dumping syndrome is a complication of partial gastrectomy operations. About 15 min after a meal, patients suffer from epigastric discomfort, nausea, lightheadedness, flushing and sweating. It is thought that the rapid entry of food into the duodenum and jejunum draws fluid into the bowel lumen by osmosis, causing hypovolaemia. Rest after meals and dietary measures will control early dumping. Late dumping refers to a hypoglycaemic episode that occurs several hours after a meal. The rapid entry of food containing sugars into the duodenum and jejunum causes an early hyperglycaemia which is then followed by reflex hyperinsulinaemia and a reactive hypoglycaemia. This is a frequent symptom following gastric surgery, and usually adaptation occurs with time. It can be controlled by taking small, frequent meals and eating sugar a few hours after meals. Radionuclide imaging studies can be used to demonstrate gastric stasis and dumping (see p. 610).

Gastric acid is required for iron absorption, and following gastric surgery patients may develop a hypochromic anaemia. Loss of intrinsic factor may also cause a vitamin B_{12}-deficiency anaemia.

Bezoars

A bezoar is a mass of ingested material that has built up in the stomach. Patients may complain of a dragging sensation and a feeling of fullness. The word 'bezoar' is derived from Arabic and means 'antidote'; animal bezoars were treasured in the sixteenth century as an antidote to poisons. Most are masses of matted hair (trichobezoar) or vegetable or fruit pith (phytobezoar). The juice of unripe persimons coagulates with gastric acid, and this may form the basis of a phytobezoar. The edentulous are prone to develop phytobezoars, as are patients after gastric surgery, particularly partial gastrectomy with vagotomy, when the stoma may become obstructed. Young girls who chew the ends of their plaits and psychiatric patients who chew their hair or clothing may develop

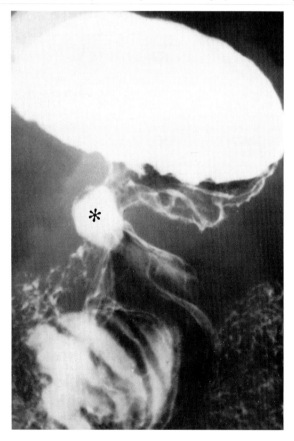

Fig. 19.72 Stomal (marginal) ulcer (asterisk) with scarring following Polya partial gastrectomy.

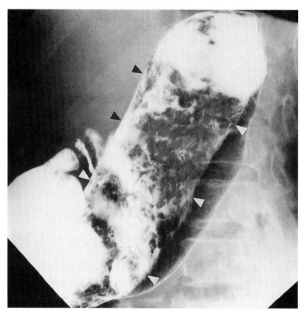

Fig. 19.73 Bezoar. There is a large filling defect (arrowheads) within the stomach; this proved to be a phytobezoar.

trichobezoars. Rapunzel's syndrome (named after the captive maiden in the Grimm's fairy tale) refers to severe cases of trichobezoar that extend from the stomach into the small bowel and may even reach the caecum. Gastric bezoars may obstruct the stomach and cause gastric ulceration. Barium outlines and often penetrates the mass, showing a filling defect in the stomach, which often has a mottled appearance (Fig. 19.73).

Percutaneous gastrostomy

This procedure is performed with increased frequency as an alternative to long-term parenteral or nasogastric tube feeding. The gastrostomy tube can be inserted using either a radiological or an endoscopic technique, so open surgical placement is now rarely necessary. The radiological technique involves passing a nasogastric tube and then inflating the stomach so that it can be punctured with a needle, a guide-wire introduced, a tract dilated and a gastrostomy tube placed (Fig. 19.74). The procedure may not be possible if the patient has had a partial gastrectomy, if an enlarged liver overlies the stomach, or if there is ascites or ulceration or tumour involving the anterior gastric wall. Coagulopathy may also contraindicate the procedure. Tube dislodgement is one of the commonest complications, and, if this occurs before a tract has formed between the stomach and the anterior abdominal wall, peritonitis may develop. Reflux and aspiration can be a problem, particularly for a patient being nursed flat. In such cases a longer catheter can be placed (percutaneous gastrojejunostomy) so that feeds can be introduced beyond the duodenojejunal flexure in order to prevent reflux. It is important that the gastrostomy site is kept clean, as abdominal wall infections can develop in these often debilitated patients. Tube blockage may necessitate tube replacement, which is simple once a mature tract has formed. A mature tract will also allow the gastrostomy tube to be replaced by a gastrostomy button which lies flush with the abdominal wall and is more comfortable for patients requiring long-term enteral feeding.

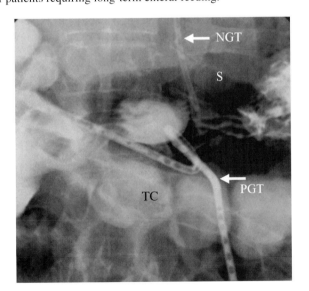

Fig. 19.74 Percutaneously placed gastrostomy catheter. Some oral barium had been given prior to the procedure to outline the colon. NGT = nasogastric tube; PGT = percutaneous gastrostomy tube; S = stomach; TC = transverse colon.

RADIONUCLIDE IMAGING OF GASTRIC MOTILITY

Numerous techniques have been used to investigate gastric function. A simple but crude approach requires the ingestion of a test meal including 10–20 *radio-opaque markers*. A single abdominal film 60 min later, or sequential films at 1–4 h, can then be obtained to check the progress of the opaque markers along the gastrointestinal tract. *Sonography* may be used to visualise gastric distension and peristalsis, and Doppler techniques have been described for estimation of flow through the pylorus. *Manometry* using an intragastric pressure monitoring device may help to differentiate mechanical obstruction (high pressure) from myopathies and neuropathies (low pressure) as causes for delayed emptying, while *electrogastrography* has been used to distinguish conduction deficits and dysrhythmias from muscular weakness or 'power failure'. *MRI* has been used to measure the frequency, amplitude and velocity of peristalsis in the stomach using a dynamic gradient-echo technique after a test meal, and gastric volume can also be measured using multislice fast spin-echo acquisition. Currently, however, *radionuclide imaging* is the preferred method, having the following advantages:

- Radionuclide methods are non-invasive and deliver only a very small radiation dose.

- The liquid and solid test meals used are 'physiological' in the sense that their constituents (apart from the radioactive label) can be chosen from normal dietary components.

- Continuous observation of the stomach after a test meal can be made over a prolonged period, commensurate with the normal timescale of gastric emptying.

- The results are quantifiable, so multiple studies can be compared within the same patient or between patients.

- The technique is simple for the patient, requires little cooperation and is suitable for all ages.

Indications

In patients suspected of gastric emptying problems, it is important that the presence of structural lesions is first excluded by endoscopy or barium meal. Gastric function can then be studied using a radiolabelled test meal. Conditions in which gastric emptying studies are helpful include the following:

- Patients with persistent nausea, vomiting, bloating or suspected dumping syndromes after gastric surgery.

- Patients with symptoms suggestive of outflow obstruction but normal endoscopy.

- Patients with suspected non-obstructive gastric stasis, e.g. autonomic neuropathy in diabetes, chronic renal failure, thyroid disorders, etc.

- Patients with severe or resistant reflux oesophagitis.

- Patients with biliary gastritis.

Normal gastric emptying

Solid phase

Solid food is retained in the stomach for a period of digestion, after which it is released gradually through the pylorus. Nutrients entering the small bowel provoke feedback mechanisms that subsequently maintain a constant rate of gastric emptying until all the food has left the stomach. This control mechanism produces a linear time–activity curve for normal emptying of solid food (Fig. 19.75A). However, in many patients there is an initial lag phase after ingestion of the meal, before emptying begins (Fig. 19.75B). The lag phase is partly explained by movement of the meal between the gastric fundus and the antrum, but may also be due to closure of the pylorus during the early stages of intragastric digestion.

Liquid phase

In contrast, the transit of non-nutrient fluids through the stomach is a passive process. The rate of emptying is proportional to the volume of fluid in the stomach, so it empties rather like a bucket with a hole in it—it approximates to a single exponential (Fig. 19.75). Because of this difference between active and passive emptying of solids and liquids, respectively, it is important to con-sider both phases when investigating gastric function. The preferred method uses separate radionuclides for labelling the liquid and solid elements of the meal, so that emptying curves for both phases can be obtained simultaneously.

Measurements

Because liquid phase emptying approximates to an exponential curve, a measurement of half-emptying time ($t\frac{1}{2}$) is an appropriate numerical description of the curve. The linear pattern of solid emptying can be described by the average gradient of the slope, but the length of the lag phase should also be taken into account. A simple but crude approach is to measure the proportion of the meal remaining in the stomach 1 h after ingestion, as well as $t\frac{1}{2}$.

Normal ranges

The normal ranges for liquid and solid emptying vary according to the details of the method used and also vary between different centres, so the following approach is suggested. Solid emptying is invariably slower than liquid emptying, so the diagnosis of dumping—accelerated transit of the nutritive meal into the small bowel—is made when the $t\frac{1}{2}$ of a solid meal is less than 30 min. Normal solid emptying requires that at least 50% of the meal remains in the stomach 30 min after ingestion, and at least 25% of the meal leaves the stomach by 60 min. Liquid-phase emptying normally takes place with $t\frac{1}{2}$ of 30 min or less, typically 10–20 min. A $t\frac{1}{2}$ of liquid phase longer than 30 min indicates gastric stasis.

Many factors affect the rate of gastric emptying, both in normal individuals and in disease. A summary of these is given in Box 19.8. Surprisingly, gastric emptying appears to be unaffected by *H. pylori* infection.

Postoperative gastric emptying

The most common cause of dumping syndromes is previous gastrectomy, particularly of the Billroth type, but any procedure

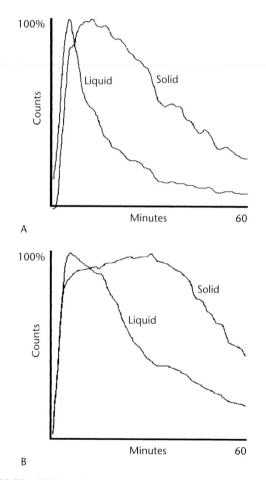

Fig. 19.75 (A) Normal gastric emptying curves showing approximately linear solid phase and exponential liquid phase. (B) Normal variant of gastric emptying pattern with lag period before onset of solid phase emptying.

Box 19.8 Factors affecting the rate of gastric emptying
Slower gastric emptying is associated with: Evenings Recumbent position Old age Ice cream or other cold foods Smoking Acute or chronic stress Acute or chronic alcoholism Strenuous exercise Drugs—morphine, buscopan, cimetidine, H_2 antagonists and L-dopa
Faster gastric emptying is associated with: Mornings Sitting or standing position Hot spicy foods Drugs—cisapride, metoclopramide, domperidone, erythromycin
Disorders that may cause delayed gastric emptying: Previous gastric surgery Diabetes mellitus and other causes of autonomic neuropathy Chronic renal failure Gastric ulcer Carcinoma of the stomach Systemic sclerosis and related conditions Thyroid disorders Electrolyte disturbances

which involves pyloroplasty or gastroenterostomy may lead to dumping. Vagotomy causes delayed emptying of solid meals, so procedures involving vagotomy and gastric drainage produce a characteristic pattern of rapid liquid-phase emptying with delayed solid emptying. Dyspeptic patients with gallstones often show delayed gastric emptying which reverts to normal after cholecystectomy, unless the dyspepsia persists, in which case the abnormality of emptying also remains. Not surprisingly, gastric emptying is often prolonged in patients who have undergone oesophageal resection with intrathoracic oesophagogastric anastomosis. If pyloroplasty is carried out at the same procedure, emptying of the intrathoracic stomach is less likely to be delayed, and is sometimes abnormally rapid.

Technique

The test meal

Either liquid or solid phases can be studied individually, but it is convenient to acquire both phases simultaneously using different radionuclides. Several different labels have been described; in the author's unit the liquid phase consists of 400 ml fruit juice labelled with ^{111}In-DTPA, while the solid phase comprises two slices of bread and a helping of scrambled egg labelled with ^{99m}Tc-colloid. Whatever label is chosen, it is important that the radionuclides are firmly bound to the components of the meal, are resistant to pH changes in the stomach and duodenum, and do not adhere to the mucosa. Dual multichannel analysers allow simultaneous acquisition of both phases, a correction being applied to take account of cross-talk between the two acquisition windows.

Data acquisition

After starving overnight to ensure that the stomach is as empty as possible, the patient is positioned sitting in front of the gamma camera and asked to eat the meal as quickly as possible. The acquisition is started as soon as the patient begins the meal, in order to avoid missing immediate emptying, which in some patients occurs with the first few mouthfuls of the meal. For basic gastric emptying studies, frames of 30–60 s duration are acquired for 60–90 min (Fig. 19.76). A comfortable chair is essential. If studies of antral peristalsis are to be made, a period of more rapid acquisition (10 s frames) can be included part way through the study.

Analysis

Results are analysed by producing time–activity curves for both liquid and solid phases. The breakthrough of each nuclide into the opposite channel is calculated and corrections are applied to the emptying curves. Interpretation requires visual inspection of the image frames and the curves. Calculation of $t\frac{1}{2}$ and the proportion of the meal remaining at 30 and 60 min after ingestion provide useful indices, as discussed above.

Interpretation

Four basic patterns may be observed:

- *Normal*. Liquid phase $t\frac{1}{2}$ is less than 30 min (typically 10–20 min); solid phase $t\frac{1}{2}$ is greater than 30 min but at least 25% of the meal leaves the stomach by 60 min (Fig. 19.75).

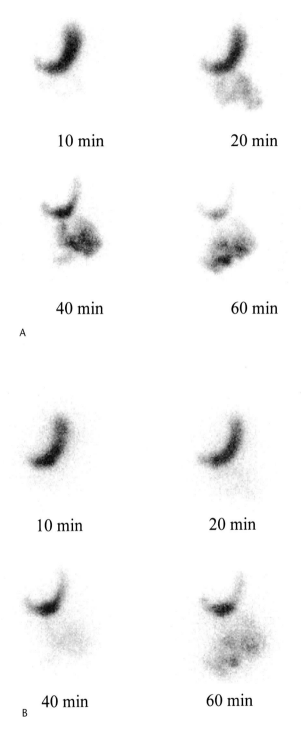

Fig. 19.76 Selected frames from a dual phase gastric study showing typical progression of liquid (A) and solid phase (B) emptying over 60 min after ingestion of the meal.

- *Vagotomy pattern*. Solid phase emptying is delayed, liquid phase is normal or rapid (Fig. 19.77).

- *Dumping pattern*. Both liquid and solid phases are abnormally rapid, with solid phase $t\frac{1}{2}$ less than 30 min (Fig. 19.78).

- *Gastric stasis*. Both liquid and solid phases are delayed (Fig. 19.79).

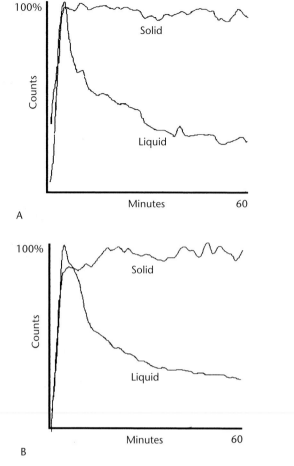

A

B

Fig. 19.77 (A, B) Typical gastric emptying curves after vagotomy in two patients, both showing rapid transit of liquid but delayed solid phase emptying.

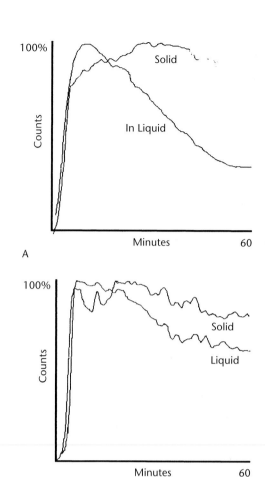

A

B

Fig. 19.79 (A, B) Delayed liquid and solid phase gastric emptying in two patients with gastroparesis.

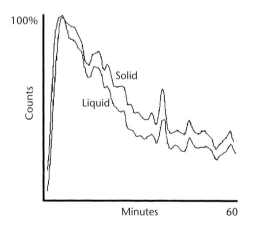

Fig. 19.78 Abnormally rapid solid phase gastric emptying in a patient with symptoms of dumping after gastric surgery.

REFERENCES AND SUGGESTIONS FOR FURTHER READING

General

Eisenberg, R. L. (1996) *Gastrointestinal Radiology: A Pattern Approach*, 3rd edn. Philadelphia: W. B. Saunders.

Federle, M. P., Megibow, A. J., Naidich, D. P. (1988) *Radiology of AIDS*. New York: Raven Press.

Gore, R. M. (1998) Stomach. In: Margulis, A. R. (ed). *Modern Imaging of the Alimentary Tube*. Berlin: Springer.

Gore, R. M., Levine, M. S. (2000) *Textbook of Gastrointestinal Radiology*, 2nd edn. Philadelphia: W. B. Saunders.

Gore, R. M., Smith, C. (1998) Postoperative findings. In: Margulis, A. R. (ed) *Modern Imaging of the Alimentary Tube*. Berlin: Springer.

Stomach and duodenum

Buck, J. L., Pantongrag-Brown, L. (1994) Gastritides, gastropathies and polyps unique to the stomach. *Radiologic Clinics of North America*, **32**, 1215–1231.

de Lange, E. E. (1987) Radiographic features of gastritis using the biphasic contrast technique. *Current Problems in Diagnostic Radiology*, **16**(6), 273–319.

Gohel, V. K., Laufer, I. (1978) Double-contrast examination of the postoperative stomach. *Radiology*, **129**, 601–607.

Lichtenstein, J. E. (1993) Inflammatory conditions of the stomach and duodenum. *Radiologic Clinics of North America*, **31**, 1315–1333.

Marshak, R. H., Lindner, A. E. (1971) Polypoid lesions of the stomach. *Seminars in Roentgenology*, **6**, 151–168.

Wyatt, J. I. (1995) Histopathology of gastroduodenal inflammation: the impact of *Helicobacter pylori*. *Histopathology*, **26**, 1–5.

Zomoza, J., Dodd, G. D. (1980) Lymphoma of the gastrointestinal tract. *Seminars in Roentgenology*, **15**, 272–287.

Computed tomography

Balthazar, E. J. (1991) CT of the gastrointestinal tract: principles and interpretation. *American Journal of Roentgenology*, **156**, 23–32.

Fishman, E. K., Urban, B. A., Hruban, R. H. (1996) CT of the stomach: spectrum of disease. *Radiographics*, **16**, 1035–1054.

Scatarige, J. C., DiSantis, D. J. (1989) CT of the stomach and duodenum. *Radiologic Clinics of North America*, **27**, 687–706.

Endoscopic ultrasound

Botel, J. F., Lighdale, C. J. (1991) Endoscopic sonography of the upper gastrointestinal tract. *American Journal of Roentgenology*, **156**, 63–68.

Chak, A., Cant, M. I., Rosch, T., et al (1997) Endosonographic differentiation of benign and malignant stromal cell tumours. *Gastrointestinal Endoscopy*, **45**, 468–473.

Harris, K. (1999) Endoscopic ultrasound of the upper gastrointestinal tract. *Accessing Reviews*, **5**, 14–17.

Nuclear medicine

Chatterton, B. E. (1994) Gastric motility. In: Murray, P. C., Ell, P. J. (eds) Nuclear Medicine in clinical diagnosis and treatment, pp. 393–405. Edinburgh: Churchill Livingstone.

Chaudari, T. K., Fink, S. (1991) Gastric emptying in human disease states. *American Journal of Gastroenterology*, **86**, 533–538.

Parkman, H. C., Miller, M. A., Fischer, R. S. (1995) Role of nuclear medicine in evaluating patients with suspected gastrointestinal motility disorders. *Seminars in Nuclear Medicine*, **25**, 289–305.

20

THE SMALL BOWEL AND PERITONEAL CAVITY

Steve Halligan

In contrast to large-bowel disease, small-bowel disease is relatively rare. Nevertheless, examination remains predominantly a radiological responsibility because of the relative inaccessibility of the small bowel. Although enteroscopy continues to develop, it is still principally confined to specialist centres, and modern push enteroscopes cannot examine the entire small bowel in most patients except during laparotomy. The small bowel is difficult to examine: there are multiple overlapping loops, which are highly mobile and, to make matters worse, are often furiously peristalsing!

ANATOMY

The small bowel is a convoluted tube, extending from the pylorus to the ileocaecal valve. It averages approximately 6–7 m in length and is divided into duodenum, jejunum and ileum. The duodenum is mostly retroperitoneal and lacks a mesentery. In contrast, the jejunum (literally 'empty'), which begins at the ligament of Treitz (duodenojejunal flexure) in the left upper abdomen, is suspended from a fan-like mesentery that runs obliquely along the posterior abdominal wall, which confers considerable mobility. The ileum (literally 'twisted') comprises the distal two-fifths of the small intestine and is also suspended from this mesentery. Arterial supply is predominantly from the superior mesenteric artery with venous drainage via the superior mesenteric vein. The jejunum tends to lie in the left upper quadrant and the ileum in the right lower quadrant, but it should be remembered that disease may alter this relationship, especially if obstruction is present. There is no reliable radiological demarcation between jejunum and ileum, although the valvulae conniventes, which are circumferential folds, are more prominent in the former. The most distal ileum is known as the terminal ileum and is important because many small-bowel diseases have a predilection for this site. Again there is no anatomical feature which distinguishes ileum from terminal ileum so it is convenient to define it as that length of small bowel that is generally available for ileoscopy once the ileocaecal valve has been intubated during colonoscopy—approximately 10–20 cm. Luminal calibre decreases along the length of the small bowel and maximum radio-

logical diameter will depend on the modality being used (for example, jejunal diameter should not exceed 3.5 cm on barium follow-through versus 4.5 cm for enteroclysis). The small-bowel wall comprises mucosa, submucosa, muscularis propria and serosa, and should not measure more than 1–2 mm thick when distended. Great care should be taken when assessing mural thickening or indeed any abnormal feature in underfilled, undistended loops. Normal undistended small bowel shows a 'feathery' pattern due to mucosal folds and the valvulae, although this may be absent in the distal ileum.

RADIOLOGICAL INVESTIGATION

Barium studies remain the cornerstone of small bowel imaging and still provide the best radiological assessment when subtle alterations of mucosal morphology are being sought. However, all cross-sectional modalities have made considerable inroads over the last decade, notably CT, and there are now several well-established indications for their use in luminal imaging.

Plain abdominal radiography

Plain films are widely available and are frequently requested to assess the small bowel, notably to diagnose obstruction (discussed below), and may also be used to visualise intestinal perforation. However, plain films can exclude neither and CT is more sensitive and specific in both.

Contrast studies
Barium follow-through

Historically, most small-bowel contrast examinations were performed as part of an upper gastrointestinal series: the 'barium meal and follow-through'. The small-bowel component of that examination was usually relegated to a series of overcouch films with little, if any, reliance on compression techniques; it is unsurprising the examination garnered a bad reputation among some radiologists. Now that there are site-specific barium suspensions available for each part of the gastrointestinal tract, it is no longer possible to combine a 'catch-all' type examination with state-of-the-art imaging and this latter approach should be rapidly abandoned.

There are several components to an adequate examination: patient preparation, the correct density and volume of barium suspension, spot filming combined with compression at frequent intervals and tailored to the clinical question being asked. The patient should be starved, preferably overnight, so that the small bowel and caecum are empty. Some investigators give a mild oral contact laxative the day before to aid this. It is also good practice to perform follow-through examinations during a morning session if possible because unsuspected slow intestinal transit may compromise examinations started later, due to difficulties obtaining room time and radiographic staff out of hours. A prokinetic agent such as metoclopramide 20 mg may be given orally as a tablet or syrup in order to accelerate transit (it mainly provokes gastric dumping); this is important so that an adequate continuous barium column is maintained and should ideally be administered at least 30 min before the study starts (Hare et al 2000). A lower density barium suspension than that used for the stomach is needed; about 50–100% w/v is ideal. An adequate volume must be administered; we have found that a single can (300 ml) of 100% w/v barium suspension diluted with an equal volume of water provides the best compromise of density and volume, giving 600 ml of 50% w/v suspension. Half of this solution is taken orally and a prone overcouch film taken at 10 and 30 min. However, modern digital fluoroscopic units allow overcouch films to be dispensed with altogether, so that the examination is completely radiologist based.

Visualisation of the villous pattern is a good guide to the technical adequacy of the radiographic technique employed (Gelfand & Ott 1981). If barium column progression is slow, or distension insufficient, the remaining suspension is administered. Spot filming continues until the terminal ileum has been completely opacified. The timing of compression and filming must be tailored to each individual request. For example, a history of vomiting should provoke close scrutiny of proximal small bowel, whereas known terminal ileal Crohn's disease will direct attention distally. Compression is mandatory to separate overlapping loops, assess mobility and define mucosal morphology, and each radiologist will have a preference for a particular device to achieve this; the author particularly likes a prone inflatable paddle (Fig. 20.1) (McClean and Bartram 1985). Tilting the patient head-down or angling the tube will help move loops out of the pelvis and visualise them. The study may be modified in several ways. Gas may be rectally insufflated in an attempt to distend the terminal ileum in order to better assess it—the 'peroral pneumocolon'. A double-contrast effect may be achieved by giving an oral effervescent agent (enough to produce 500–1000 ml gas) once contrast has reached the caecum, and allowing this to perfuse the small bowel. Alternatively, the agent may be given simultaneously with the barium suspension.

Enteroclysis (small-bowel enema)

Although described since the 1920s, intubation techniques for small-bowel contrast examinations did not become generally popular until the description by Sellink in the 1970s. Patients are prepared as for follow-through, with or without laxatives the previous day. Enteroclysis requires jejunal intubation with a purpose-designed catheter, usually via the nasal route (Fig. 20.2). Catheters are now generally 10 French diameter and can be smaller. The tip varies from type to type, some having a balloon, some a weighted tip, while others merely have infusion holes. A torqueable stiffening wire is common to each, and is used to direct the catheter tip, although it cannot be advanced out of the catheter. While the patient is sitting, the clearest nostril is identified (ask the patient to sniff) and lignocaine jelly syringed in with the head extended. After waiting a few moments for its effect, the catheter is then introduced and the patient asked to swallow, to aid passage. A few small sips of water may help. Once the catheter has entered the stomach, the patient lies supine on the fluoroscopy couch, the guide-wire is

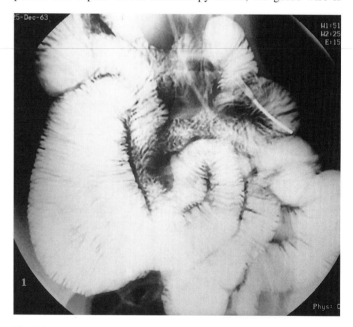

Fig. 20.2 Small bowel enema.

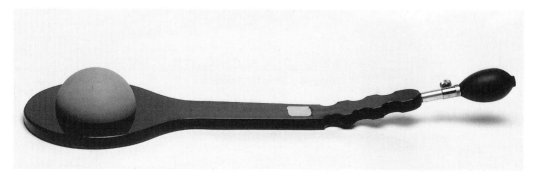

Fig. 20.1 Compression paddle. The patient lies prone on the paddle and the balloon is inflated to compress overlying small-bowel loops during fluoroscopy.

introduced into the catheter lumen, and its position checked fluoroscopically. The catheter tip is steered towards the gastric antrum by advancing it over the guide-wire; it is frequently necessary to partially withdraw the wire, and subsequently the catheter, in order to facilitate a directional change. The most technically demanding aspect of the procedure is usually crossing the pylorus. It may be helpful to form a slight bend on the guide-wire tip beforehand so that it can be directed more precisely, and a combination of positional change, manual compression and the introduction of some air to distend the stomach may also help. It also helps if the operator stands at the table top, beside the patient's head, as during endoscopy. Once the catheter tip is in the duodenum, advancement into the proximal jejunum is usually straightforward, with an ideal position a few centimetres distal to the ligament of Treitz. There are several good articles describing intubation technique in detail (Nolan and Cadman 1987), but there is no substitute for experience. The procedure is no more difficult than many interventional techniques, using essentially the same principles for catheter manipulation.

Once jejunal intubation has been achieved, contrast is optimally infused with an electric pump but cheaper handheld or gravity-assisted systems may be used. Flow is adjusted so that the barium column advances in an uninterrupted fashion with adequate but not excessive luminal distension; too fast, and undue distension with reflex hypotonia will result. About 75 ml per minute is ideal. A variety of regimens exist. Dilute barium (e.g. 18% w/v) may be used so as not to obscure overlapping loops (Nolan 1996). Alternatively, a barium suspension may be followed by 0.5% methylcellulose solution (1000–2000 ml), the purpose of which is to enable double-contrast views and also propel barium into the distal ileum: a biphasic examination. Air may also be used to achieve a double-contrast effect. As for the follow-through, spot filming and compression views are mandatory.

Which is better: follow-through or enteroclysis?

This debate has raged since enteroclysis was introduced, with passionate advocates for each technique. It is probably true to say that most specialised gastrointestinal radiologists favour enteroclysis, citing studies which apparently show its superiority. However, many of these studies are personal case series from expert gastrointestinal radiologists who have compared their enteroclysis in a tertiary referral setting to follow-through examinations performed by non-experts elsewhere. Furthermore, referral is often because of diagnostic uncertainty, perhaps due to an inadequate follow-through: a clear case of study spectrum bias. There are very few unbiased studies comparing the two techniques. In an attempt to prove the superiority of enteroclysis, Bernstein and coworkers performed a prospective, randomised, blind crossover study where patients with Crohn's disease had both studies performed by expert gastrointestinal radiologists (Bernstein et al 1997). The results surprised the authors: barium follow-through proved superior to enteroclysis, predominantly because of better mucosal detail. Furthermore, enteroclysis missed fistulas in two patients and duodenal disease in four patients. By way of explanation, advanced disease is easy to diagnose whatever the technique employed but small aphthous ulcers are probably best seen using a high-density barium and compression (Bartram 1996). It follows that, since Crohn's disease is the commonest primary small-bowel disease,

barium follow-through should be the preferred technique. Others have argued that the luminal distension produced by enteroclysis makes it easier to elicit morphological changes, just as it does for the stomach and colon (Nolan 1996). There seems to be little doubt that enteroclysis is superior for diagnosis of adhesions because of greater luminal distension. Technical preferences may also affect choice. Enteroclysis requires more room time per individual patient, and costs more because of this and the associated tubes and infusion equipment. It may also be associated with greater radiation burden. Whatever the choice, any technical difference is likely to be far outweighed by the interpretative skills of the observer (Robinson 1997). In any case, both must be carefully performed and supervised if radiologists are to retain prime responsibility for small-bowel imaging, one of the last bastions of barium radiology.

Ileostomy enema

Symptoms following ileostomy may be due to recurrent disease, for example Crohn's, adhesions related to the procedure, or a stomal hernia. Ileostomy enema is a simple method of assessing the neoterminal ileum while avoiding multiple overlapping loops of more proximal bowel. A Foley catheter is inserted into the stoma, its balloon inflated just deep to the anterior abdominal wall, and barium suspension injected via a syringe, followed by some air for a double-contrast effect (Fig. 20.3). Sometimes it is necessary to examine the distal limb of a loop stoma, usually to assess anastamotic integrity. The procedure is the same but water-soluble contrast is used. It is occasionally difficult to identify the distal limb stoma because of retraction; careful probing around the margins of the proximal spout will usually reveal it.

Water-soluble studies

Barium suspensions are contraindicated when intestinal perforation is possible, when surgery is highly likely (due to the risk of peritoneal spillage), or in rare cases of allergy. Furthermore, follow-

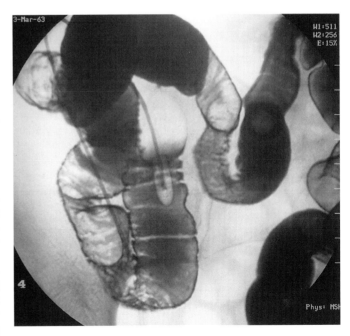

Fig. 20.3 Normal ileostomy enema.

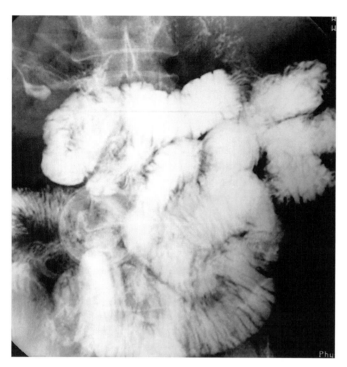

Fig. 20.4 Non-ionic, water-soluble follow-through performed using iohexol in a postoperative patient.

through examinations will seriously impair the quality of any subsequent CT because of barium related artefact. Water-soluble contrast is an alternative. There are essentially two choices, which will be determined by the clinical situation. Ionic agents such as Gastrografin are widely used and generally safe (unless there is a possibility of pulmonary aspiration). However, their hypertonicity draws water into the gut lumen so that radiographic density tends to get progressively worse, especially in the distal small bowel. This is exacerbated in obstruction because of slow transit. It should be borne in mind that these agents have therapeutic benefit in cases of obstruction and this consideration may outweigh radiographic disadvantages (discussed below). Non-ionic agents such as iohexol suffer less from dilution and provide better radiographic contrast (Jobling et al 1999) (Fig. 20.4).

CT and MRI

While resolution of fine mucosal detail only generally remains possible with contrast studies, CT has made very considerable inroads into small-bowel imaging over the last decade. CT is now equivalent to contrast studies in a variety of clinical scenarios, and superior in some, most notably obstruction. MRI has fared less well, usually because of poorer spatial resolution than CT. Also, longer acquisition times have seriously hampered small-bowel depiction, because of peristalsis. However, these problems are overcome by modern breath-hold sequences and MRI may eventually supplant CT, especially, for example, in Crohn's disease. These technique are pre-eminent for assessment of the peritoneal cavity and retroperitoneum.

Ultrasound

Like CT and MRI, technical advances over the last decade have pushed ultrasound evaluation of small-bowel disease to the fore-

front of modern gastrointestinal tract imaging. Bowel interrogation using ultrasound relies heavily on graded compression to assess mobility, and ultrasound is highly operator dependent. Nevertheless, in the right hands it is a formidable small-bowel imaging tool. Dedicated oral small-bowel contrast agents now exist and Doppler techniques raise the possibility of functional small-bowel assessment.

SMALL-BOWEL OBSTRUCTION

Mechanical intestinal obstruction accounts for approximately 20% of surgical admissions, approximately two-thirds of which are small bowel in origin. Causes may be generally divided into extrinsic and intrinsic groups. Extrinsic causes include *adhesions* (following surgery or peritoneal inflammation), *hernias* (inguinal, femoral or internal, particularly paraduodenal) and masses, most notably *disseminated peritoneal malignancy*. Congenital malrotation or peritoneal (Ladd's) bands are rarer extrinsic causes. Intrinsic *mural disease* may be due to inflammatory strictures, notably due to Crohn's disease or radiation enteritis, ischaemia, or rarely primary small-bowel tumours (which may also be accompanied by intussusception). *Intraluminal obstruction* may be due to gallstones or foreign bodies (often fruit pith). Non-steroidal tablets may cause *intestinal membranes*, resulting in obstruction. Adhesions, peritoneal malignancy and hernias account for about 80% of cases overall. In the west, most cases will be due to adhesions (up to 80% in some series), most of which will settle conservatively. Surgeons must decide between conservative management or laparotomy, which is life threatening if inappropriately delayed. Therefore, the relevant radiological questions are: Is there obstruction? If so, at what level? Is it partial or complete? What is the cause? Perhaps the most important question relates to *strangulation*. Strangulation is associated with a 30% mortality and occurs where there is irreversible ischaemia, usually precipitated by impaired venous outflow. Bowel becomes dilated and fluid filled, and arterial inflow is eventually compromised. Perforation follows, often with septicaemia and peritonitis. In *closed-loop obstruction* a segment of small bowel is obstructed at two points along its length by a single lesion, often a volvulus, perhaps associated with an adhesion. Unfortunately, preoperative clinical detection of strangulation is notoriously unreliable, and may miss 50–85% of cases, and it is this inability to differentiate ischaemic from simple obstruction that has driven most surgical controversy.

Plain abdominal films are usually the primary investigation in suspected obstruction. Diagnosis is by small-bowel distension down to the level of obstruction, with fluid levels and no distal gas (Fig. 20.5). However, it may take several hours for bowel to dilate and a similar time for distal gas to be resorbed. Also, problems occur when only a few loops are dilated in high obstruction (where there is also vomiting) or if loops are completely fluid filled (resulting in a 'grey' abdomen that is easily confused with ascites). A little residual gas may be trapped within adjacent valvulae; the 'string of beads' sign. The obstructive level is often difficult to define; it should be borne in mind that dilated jejunum may reach the right iliac fossa, and dilated distal ileum may reach the left upper quadrant. It is also occasionally difficult to distinguish distended small bowel from colon: small bowel tends to lie centrally and the valvulae conniventes are thinner than colonic haustra and also tend to

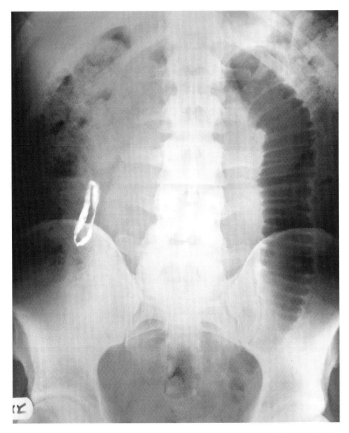

Fig. 20.5 Plain abdominal film reveals a dilated jejunal loop in this patient with obstruction secondary to an internal hernia (note residual contrast in the appendix from recent barium enema).

cross the bowel diameter completely. Erect films are now generally considered unnecessary, as they provide little information additional to supine films. Overall, plain films are diagnostic in 50–60%, equivocal in 20–30% and misleading in 10–20% (Maglinte et al 1997). A retrospective study comparing plain abdominal radiography, enteroclysis and CT found the overall accuracy of plain films to be 67%, compared with 67% for CT (Maglinte et al 1996). Plain films fared proportionately less well in patients with low-grade obstruction (56% sensitivity). However, the authors concluded that plain abdominal radiography should remain the initial method of imaging in these patients.

When plain film findings are unequivocal, further imaging, if any, will be determined by the clinical scenario. For example, if the patient is constitutionally unwell then early laparotomy for probable strangulation is indicated and further imaging will only serve to delay this. Where plain film findings are equivocal or normal but clinical features remain, the patient may undergo contrast studies or CT. If the plain film is entirely normal but intermittent adhesive subacute obstruction thought likely, then a contrast study is probably best, preferably during an attack of pain. If features are more developed, CT may be appropriate, and has assumed an increasingly prominent role over the last decade. In a landmark study of 84 patients believed to have small-bowel obstruction, Megibow and coworkers found CT had an overall accuracy of 95% (Megibow et al 1991). CT is attractive because the entire small and large bowel are rapidly assessed (as opposed to contrast studies) and dilatation is easily diagnosed (Fig. 20.6). Diagnosis of obstruction hinges on identification of dilated small bowel and a corresponding transition point where calibre

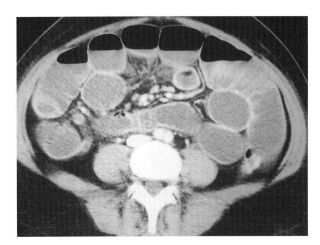

Fig. 20.6 CT shows unequivocal small bowel obstruction.

abruptly decreases; this will be the site of obstruction. Images are best viewed on a workstation in cine mode to facilitate this, and reformatted scans in orientations other than axial may also help. A *mass* should be identifiable at the transition point if obstruction is due to tumour (it is vital to elicit any history of previous laparotomy for malignancy). If no mass is visible then adhesions are the likely cause; the bands themselves are practically never visible (Fig. 20.7). It is important to include the hernial orifices on the study and to view the data on lung windows to facilitate visualisation of extraluminal air. CT will also make the diagnosis in the common scenario of small bowel obstruction due to a *caecal adenocarcinoma*. Whether oral contrast medium is necessary is debatable, as obstructed bowel is dilated and fluid filled. Oral contrast may also take hours to reach the site of obstruction, even if the patient is not vomiting, delaying intervention. The use

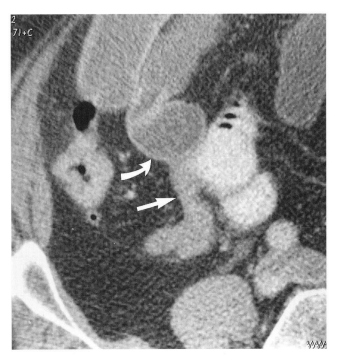

Fig. 20.7 Multislice CT with reconstruction shows no mass at the transition point between dilated (curve arrow) and undilated (straight arrow) small bowel. Diagnosis: adhesions, confirmed at subsequent laparotomy.

of intravenous contrast is also controversial but there is some evidence that mural enhancement, or lack of it, may help predict ischaemia (Frager et al 1996). CT is also useful to differentiate obstruction from paralytic ileus, again a common surgical problem.

Water-soluble studies are often requested by surgeons to diagnose acute obstruction. These are likely to be less useful than CT for diagnosis of the level and cause, predominantly because of slow transit coupled with distal contrast dilution. However, these studies may have valuable predictive value: a study of plain abdominal radiography 4 h after oral administration of 100 ml Gastrografin found that patients settled on conservative treatment if contrast had entered the colon but laparotomy was likely if it had not (Joyce et al 1992). Furthermore, surgeons have long believed that Gastrografin has a therapeutic effect in small bowel obstruction, a belief borne out in a randomised study of either 100 ml Gastrografin or conventional treatment, which found that the former significantly shortened obstructive episodes and hospital stay (Assalia et al 1994).

CT is probably less useful in the scenario of non-acute intermittent subacute obstruction. This is frequently due to adhesions, the diagnosis of which centres on demonstration of loop fixity and distensibility, especially when there is no actual obstruction at the time of examination. These features are best sought for using enteroclysis, although compression during follow-through techniques can be useful by demonstrating loop fixity and abrupt angulation (Bartram 1980) (Fig. 20.8).

ILEUS AND PSEUDO-OBSTRUCTION

There are many causes of *paralytic ileus*, which often needs to be differentiated from mechanical obstruction. In these patients there

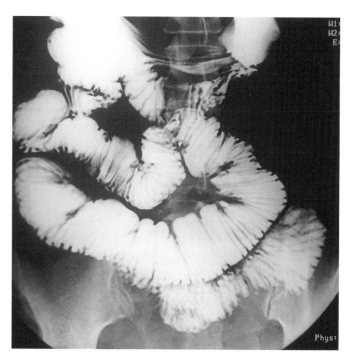

Fig. 20.9   Scleroderma.

is no focal obstructive lesion and both small and large bowel may be dilated. The commonest aetiologies are laparotomy and peritonitis but drugs, electrolyte imbalance and constitutional disease (e.g. heart failure, pneumonia, porphyria) may also be implicated. Some constitutional disease, for example *scleroderma* (systemic sclerosis) may be associated with a gut myopathy or neuropathy which gives rise to the clinical picture of intestinal pseudo-obstruction. The cardinal radiological feature of scleroderma is duodenal and jejunal dilatation associated with fold crowding and slow transit (Fig. 20.9), due to collagen replacement of intestinal smooth

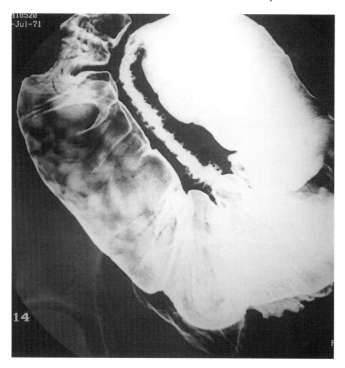

Fig. 20.8   Barium follow-through in a patient with adhesions. There is an abrupt transition point from dilated to undilated small bowel in this patient with obstruction to the afferent limb of an ileoanal pouch.

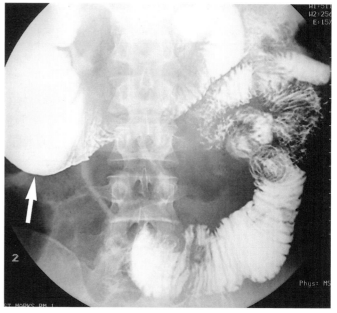

Fig. 20.10   Primary visceral myopathy. Note the characteristic, massively dilated duodenal loop (arrow).

muscle. Although commoner in the colon, small-bowel sacculation may occur and there may be associated distal oesophageal dilatation and aperistalsis. Pseudo-obstruction may also be primary, due to a visceral myopathy or neuropathy, usually of unknown cause (Fig. 20.10). Where this is a possibility, it is important to exclude an underlying paraneoplastic syndrome, notably due to small-cell lung carcinoma. Patients often present with intermittent obstructive attacks with accompanying abdominal pain and distension, which simulate a mechanical obstructive episode. Full-thickness intestinal biopsy is needed to reliably diagnose primary visceral myopathy/neuropathy, but this is unfortunately often overlooked when laparotomy, in the hope of finding mechanical obstruction, is performed. Diagnosis of ileus depends on demonstrating generalised atonic bowel dilatation. Ultrasound elegantly demonstrates atony, while CT or contrast studies will exclude an underlying obstructive lesion. Ileus may also be localised, classically afflicting loops adjacent to acute pancreatitis, appendicitis or cholecystitis: the 'sentinel loop'.

CROHN'S DISEASE

Crohn's disease is an idiopathic inflammatory disease which may afflict any part of the luminal gastrointestinal tract from mouth to anus. It is a disease of western civilisation and young adults, its prevalence is increasing, and its aetiology remains unknown. Characterised by discontinuous transmural ulceration, fistulation and spontaneous abscess formation, it is the commonest primary small-bowel disease in the west. Radiology is pivotal in the diagnosis and management of Crohn's disease for two reasons. First, because the small bowel (the commonest site affected) is only generally available to radiologists, and, second, because no single test suffices for primary diagnosis or assessment of disease activity, which is based on a combination of clinical, radiological, endoscopic and histological findings. The cardinal histological feature is the non-caseating granuloma, a collection of epitheliod histiocytes and giant cells. Most patients (60–80%) will have small bowel disease, with the terminal ileum most commonly affected (55% of all patients). About half of those with small-bowel disease also have colonic disease. Approximately 25% overall will have colonic disease only. It should be noted that disease distribution is different in children: approximately 20% of children with small-bowel disease have a normal terminal ileum, compared with only 6% of adults, so small-bowel disease cannot be excluded by normal ileoscopy (Halligan et al 1994).

Contrast studies remain the mainstay for diagnosis and assessment of both distribution and severity, predominantly because they are best able to demonstrate mucosal morphology. The radiological changes of Crohn's disease can be generally grouped into three categories; early, advanced and complicated. Although the earliest endoscopic manifestation is hyperaemia combined with an altered vascular pattern, this cannot be demonstrated on contrast studies because there is no change in epithelial surface contour. Villous oedema and blunting follow and are the earliest detectable radiological change, manifest as a granular pattern on high-quality contrast studies (Glick and Teplick 1985); the 'grains' are due to individual filling defects produced by the enlarged and inflamed vili and are best appreciated on compression views (Fig. 20.11). More generalised oedema, resulting in fold thickening may also occur

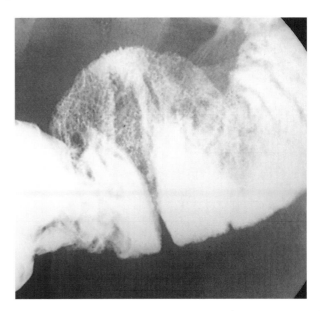

Fig. 20.11 Crohn's disease. Compression view reveals an intense mucosal granularity, caused by villous oedema.

(Fig. 20.12). Early ulceration is typically aphthoid, which describes small, shallow, circular, discrete ulcers surrounded by an oedematous halo. Again these are well demonstrated on high-quality contrast examinations, using compression techniques to reveal contrast within the central ulcer crater and its surrounding halo (Fig. 20.13). Granularity and aphthous ulceration represent the earliest detectable radiological changes and are the most challenging because they are subtle.

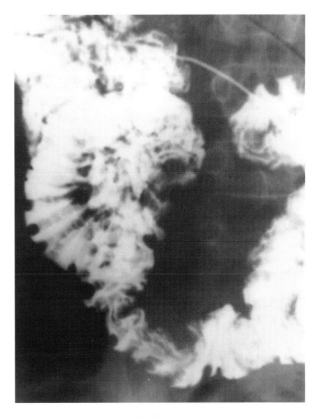

Fig. 20.12 Crohn's disease. Fold thickening.

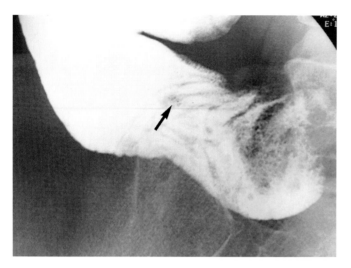

Fig. 20.13 Crohn's disease. Compression of an ileal loop reveals several aphthous ulcers (one of which is arrowed). Also note the background granularity caused by villous oedema.

Subsequent changes can be considered advanced and are generally easy to demonstrate whatever the radiological technique employed. As the features progress, ulceration becomes linear and deeper, with typical transmural penetration accompanied by mural thickening. Mucosal oedema and inflammation intervenes between these ulcers to cause the characteristic 'cobblestone' appearance (Fig. 20.14). Ulceration is frequently discontinuous and patchy and also asymmetrical along the bowel circumference; indrawing at the site of ulceration may be accompanied by ballooning of the contralateral wall, creating a characteristic pseudodiverticlar appearance (Fig. 20.15). Advanced disease may also be complicated by strictures, fistulation, abscess formation and, rarely, by tumour. Strictures are generally easy to demonstrate using contrast studies.

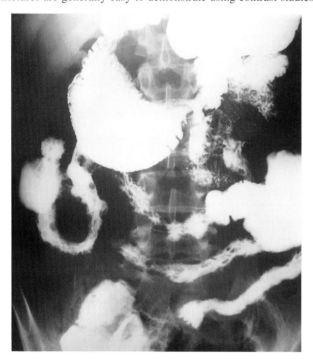

Fig. 20.14 Advanced Crohn's disease evidenced by several, long 'cobblestone' segments with intervening dilatation.

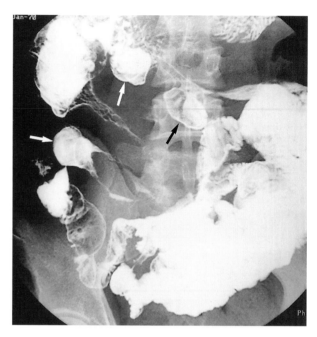

Fig. 20.15 Advanced Crohn's disease with several characteristic pseudodiverticulae (arrows).

Abdominal pain may be due to active disease, obstruction due to stricture, or a combination of the two, and differentiation between these possibilities is a common clinical scenario. It is important to remember that a considerable degree of spasm may accompany active disease, resulting in the impression of a tight stricture when the bowel is actually relatively distensible. Prestenotic dilatation suggests a degree of functional obstruction but the distensibility of a strictured segment is best assessed using enteroclysis due to infusion pressure. Massive small-bowel dilatation secondary to chronic strictures can occur and may be complicated by bacterial overgrowth. It is worth remembering that there may be little correlation between symptoms and the severity of disease as judged by contrast studies (Goldberg et al 1979).

Postoperative appearances

The likelihood of the necessity for surgery for Crohn's disease at some time is high and many patients examined will be postoperative. Right hemicolectomy is a common operation and anastamotic recurrence unfortunately frequent, tending to affect the neoterminal ileum; endoscopic surveillance of the neoterminal ileum following resection found recurrent disease in 73% of cases, although only 20% of these were symptomatic (Rutgeerts et al 1990).The radiological features are identical to those already described for the terminal ileum (Fig. 20.16). Anastamotic stricturing sometimes occurs and may be treated by endoscopic balloon dilatation (with or without steroid injection) if there is no endoscopic or radiological evidence of extensive active disease. Permanent ileostomy is a less frequent operation since the introduction of ileorectal anastamosis and the ileoanal pouch. Although the neoterminal ileal segment may be afflicted by recurrence, this is relatively uncommon, and the possibility of symptoms being due to a parastomal hernia or adhesional obstruction should be entertained. Demonstration of the presence and content of a parastomal hernia is particularly good using CT, which should be performed

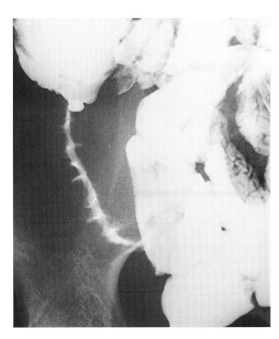

Fig. 20.16 Crohn's disease. Neoterminal ileal recurrence at right hemi-colectomy site.

with the patient lying in a position likely to precipitate the hernia (Fig. 20.17). Defunctioned loops may be assessed prior to restoration of intestinal continuity using a distal loop ileostomy enema. Strictureplasty may be performed in an attempt to conserve small bowel where further resection risks short-bowel syndrome and the need for total parenteral nutrition. The pseudotumour appearance of strictureplasty segments is well described (Kelly and Bartram 1993); it is helpful if the surgeon marks these sites with radio-opaque clips at the time of operation in order to avoid subsequent diagnostic confusion. The ileoanal pouch avoids a permanent stoma; a neorectum is fashioned from small bowel and anastamosed to the anus. Use of this procedure in Crohn's disease is controversial because of the possibility of recurrence within the

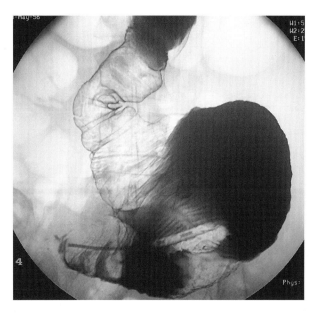

Fig. 20.18 Crohn's disease. Normal Kock pouch.

pouch (versus ulcerative colitis) but is becoming increasingly advocated as long as the patient understands the risks. Furthermore, because the aetiology of a colitis may be unknown at the time of pouch formation, subsequent disease within the pouch may alert clinicians to an underlying diagnosis of Crohn's disease. The Kock pouch is a similar procedure that involves anastamosing a small bowel pouch to the anterior abdominal wall (Fig. 20.18). A continent nipple is fashioned at the stoma site, allowing the patient to empty the pouch by self-catheterisation. Difficulty introducing the catheter or increasing incontinence raise the possibility that the continent nipple has failed, which can be revealed by infusing contrast directly into the pouch.

Ultrasound, CT and MRI

Although contrast studies are pre-eminent for assessment of endo-luminal disease, the cross-sectional capabilities of ultrasound, CT and MRI render these more suitable for diagnosis of extraluminal complications, namely fistula and abscess formation. All can readily assess mural thickening (Fig. 20.19). Concerning ultrasound, graded probe compression to displace bowel and assess mesenteric conpressibility is mandatory. Ultrasound assessment of fistula and abscess approaches the sensitivity of CT and MRI in

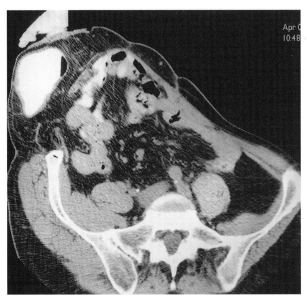

Fig. 20.17 Crohn's disease. CT reveals a parastomal hernia when the patient is in the right lateral position.

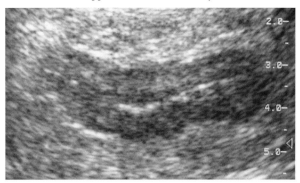

Fig. 20.19 Crohn's disease. Ultrasound reveals gross mural thickening in an ileal loop.

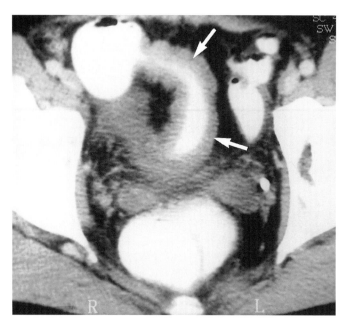

Fig. 20.20   Crohn's disease. CT shows the extent of terminal ileal thickening (arrows).

experienced hands (Gasche et al 1999), but is very operator dependent. Even in the best of hands, some sites remain poorly visualised, either due to overlying bowel gas, tenderness or because they are deep in the pelvis. Because of this, a negative ultrasound does not exclude an abdominopelvic collection or fistula. It should be noted that where the diagnosis is established in children, ultrasound is recommended for follow-up because children are technically easy to examine, avoiding exposing the patient to ionising radiation. In common with ultrasound, CT cannot diagnose early mucosal disease but bowel wall thickening is easily appreciated; surrounding fibrofatty proliferation is exquisitely demonstrated; and CT is superior for diagnosis of extramural complications, not least because it is less operator dependent and the whole abdominopelvic

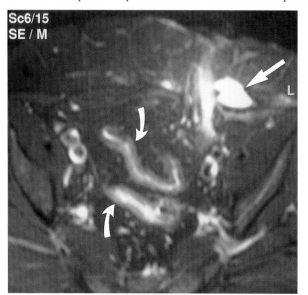

Fig. 20.21   Crohn's disease. Fat suppressed T$_2$-weighed MR scan shows thickened ileal loops (curved arrows) and also reveals a parastomal abscess (straight arrow).

cavity is easily imaged (Fig. 20.20). It is particularly suited to abscess detection, especially when a preliminary ultrasound has been negative but clinical suspicion remains high. CT may also detect extraintestinal complications, for example gallstones, pancreatitis, arthritis and nephrolithiasis. The role of MRI is similar to that of CT and there is increasing evidence that it may be superior. Fast breath-hold techniques in association with intravenous smooth muscle relaxants have eliminated problems with visceral movement during MRI. Furthermore, fat suppression techniques, combined with sequences which highlight fluid, emphasise abscesses and collections so that they may be better appreciated than with CT (Fig. 20.21). Moreover, because MR can image in any plane, the relationship between sepsis and adjacent anatomical structures is optimally demonstrated. This is especially relevant to perianal sepsis, where MR surpasses all other assessment techniques, including examination under anaesthetic. The choice between CT and MRI will largely depend on local availability and radiologist preference.

Assessment of disease activity is notoriously difficult because no one test is sensitive or specific enough to suffice. Assessment is therefore based on a combination of clinical, radiological, endoscopic and histological parameters. However, there is increasing evidence that functional radiological assessment may be at least as reliable as conventional tests, if not more so. *Superior mesenteric arterial flow*, measured by Doppler ultrasound, may indicate active small bowel disease when in excess of 500 ml per minute (van Oostayen et al 1994). Furthermore, the rate and degree of bowel wall enhancement after intravenous contrast during CT or MRI may reliably differentiate between active and inactive disease.

SMALL-BOWEL TUMOURS

Primary small-bowel tumours are rare and frequently difficult to diagnose because findings are non-specific and the diagnosis is often not considered, the latter often leading to late presentation and possibly poor prognosis. They account for less than 5% of all gastrointestinal tract tumours. It is likely that many benign tumours remain small and asymptomatic, so that patients presenting with symptoms tend to have malignant tumours. The possibility of a *polyposis syndrome* should be borne in mind.

Benign tumours

There are a variety of benign small intestinal tumours, of which adenomas and stromal tumours are the most common. Presentation usually occurs when they become large enough to cause intestinal obstruction. Otherwise occult bleeding and anaemia may cause symptoms. *Stromal tumour* is a term encompassing benign and malignant muscle tumours, as histopathological distinction between the two (e.g. leiomyoma versus leiomyosarcoma) is often very difficult and prognosis is more strongly associated with size and rate of growth than cellular features. Benign stromal tumours (leiomyomas), the commonest benign small-bowel tumour, arise from the smooth muscle of the muscularis propria. They are usually jejunal and may have endoluminal and exoluminal components. They are usually easy to demonstrate on contrast studies once large enough to cause obstruction or intussusception, and may also be

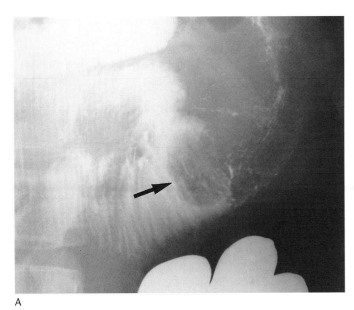

A

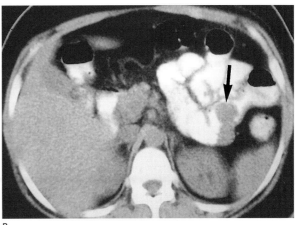

B

Fig. 20.22 Benign stromal tumour. (A) Barium follow-through reveals an intraluminal mass (arrow) on compression. (B) The tumour is also visible on CT (arrow).

seen on CT if large (Fig. 20.22). *Adenomas* are similar to their colonic counterparts both morphologically and histologically and are classified in a similar fashion: tubular, villous, tubulovillous. *Lipomas* may be recognised by their characteristic low attenuation on CT. Most are ileal and asymptomatic. When seen on contrast studies they are smooth and easily compressible. *Haemangiomas* may be capillary or cavernous. Most are too small to produce a filling defect but frequently present with anaema due to haemorrhage. *Neurogenic tumours* are rare and include neurofibromas (with or without systemic neurofibromatosis) and neurilemmomas.

Malignant tumours

Malignant small-bowel tumours have traditionally been associated with a dismal prognosis, not least because of their relatively late presentation. In contrast to the large bowel, *adenocarcinoma* is remarkably uncommon outside of a polyposis syndrome. There are well-documented associations with Crohn's and coeliac disease and

the morphology is essentially similar to that seen in the colon: an annular, shouldered, apple-core-type lesion (Fig. 20.23). *Lymphoma* is non-Hodgkin's in origin and is the commonest primary small-bowel malignant tumour in some series. Again, there is an association with coeliac and Crohn's disease (Greenstein et al 1992), and leukaemia. The association with AIDS is well recognised. Small-bowel lymphoma may also be secondary to lymphoma elsewhere. The morphology is highly variable, reflecting the protean nature of the disease, and it may be multifocal. At one end of the spectrum there may be diffuse, regular fold thickening without any obvious, localised tumour mass (Fig. 20.24). In contrast, other cases exhibit marked focal mural thickening with fistulation (often difficult to distinguish from Crohn's disease) and an obvious mass on CT or MRI (Fig. 20.25). Non-obstructing stricturing is common, as is

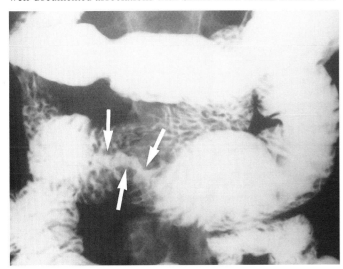

Fig. 20.23 Small bowel adenocarcinoma (between arrows) complicating Muir–Torre syndrome.

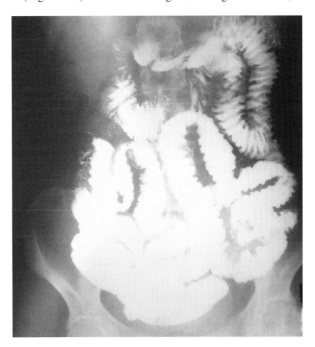

Fig. 20.24 Lymphoma. Diffuse fold thickening and nodularity.

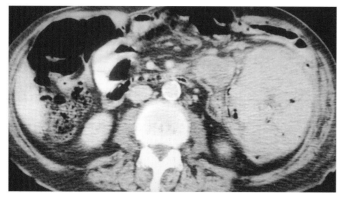

Fig. 20.25 Lymphoma. CT reveals a well-demarcated soft-tissue mass.

aneurismal dilatation, which is highly characteristic and due to cavitating necrosis, often following effective treatment. *Carcinoid* is a common finding at autopsy or incidentally during laparotomy, and the majority are in the distal ileum (although overall most occur in the appendix, where they are usually found incidentally).The primary tumour is usually small; tumours larger than 2 cm are frequently malignant, defined by metastasis. An intense desmoplastic response to the primary tumour is highly characteristic and is well demonstrated by CT (Fig. 20.26). The primary tumour rarely produces symptoms but the *carcinoid syndrome* may occur when significant liver metastasis prevents metabolism of secreted vasoactive serotonin and bradykinin, allowing them to reach the systemic circulation, and is characterised by episodic flushing and

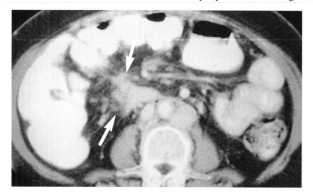

Fig. 20.26 CT reveals a desmoplastic reaction in a patient with carcinoid tumour.

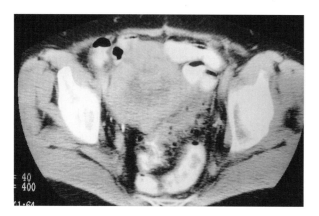

Fig. 20.27 CT reveals a large pelvic soft-tissue mass that proved to be recurrent stromal tumour.

diarrhoea. Prolonged survival, even in the presence of widely disseminated disease, is not uncommon. The difficulty differentiating benign and malignant *stromal tumours* on the basis of histological features has already been mentioned but large tumours are highly likely to behave in a malignant fashion. CT is especially well suited to their primary detection, as there is often a very large extraluminal component, and detection of local recurrence or metastatic spread (Fig. 20.27). The small bowel is frequently involved by *metastases* and may occasionally be the only site of dissemination. Intraperitoneal spread is the commonest route, whereby cells are deposited on the serosal bowel surface. Such seeded metastases are a frequent cause of malignant small-bowel obstruction and common primaries include stomach, colon, pancreas, ovary and breast. CT will demonstrate the presence of serosal deposits and the site and level of any associated obstruction. It is worth noting that *malignant melanoma* and *bronchial carcinoma* have a predisposition to small-bowel deposition via the haematogenous route, characteristically producing antimesenteric nodules. *Kaposi's sarcoma* afflicts almost 50% of homosexual men with AIDS and in approximately 50% of these the gastrointestinal tract is involved. Large submucosal nodules with central umbilication, small nodules, thickened folds and plaques are found, more commonly in the stomach than small bowel.

Polyposis syndromes

The small bowel may be afflicted by a number of polyposis syndromes, usually in association with large bowel polyposis as well. Adenomas in *familial adenomatous polyposis* (FAP) tend to cluster around the duodenal ampulla (Fig. 20.28) and may be innumerable. As with colonic adenomas, the larger the polyp, the greater the possibility of malignancy and there is also an association with *ampullary carcinoma*. FAP is also strongly associated with *desmoid disease* (Fig. 20.29), the origin of which is mesenteric rather than small bowel. *Peutz–Jeghers syndrome* is an autosomal dominant disease characterised by mucocutaneous pigmentation, often perioral, and gastrointestinal *hamartomas*. Polyps can be scattered throughout the

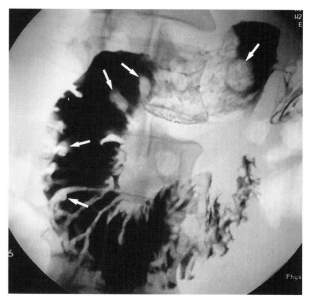

Fig. 20.28 Duodenal adenomas (some of which are arrowed) complicating familial adenomatous polyposis.

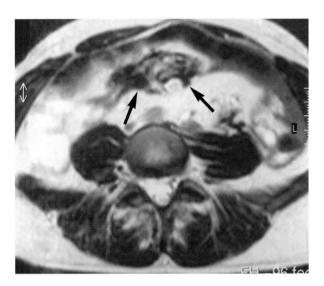

Fig. 20.29 Familial adenomatous polyposis. T_2-weighted MR image of a mesenteric desmoid tumour (arrows).

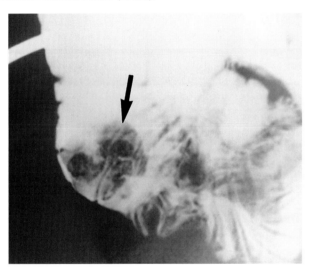

Fig. 20.30 Barium follow-through reveals an ileal hamartoma (arrow) in Peutz–Jeghers syndrome.

small bowel, with a duodenal and jejunal prediliction (Fig. 20.30). Intermittent obstruction is relatively common but small-bowel carcinoma is very rare, although these patients are at increased risk of stomach, duodenal and colonic carcinoma and, most notably, extraintestinal carcinoma, such as ovarian and breast. *Cowden's disease* also describes small intestinal hamartomas (and also adenomas, hyperplastic polyps and lymphomas), but the colon is more frequently involved. Diffuse inflammatory intestinal polyposis in *Cronkhite–Canada syndrome* is associated with neuroectodermal change, manifest as nail dystrophy and alopecia, and malabsorption.

INFECTIOUS ENTERITIS

Small-bowel enteritis (inflammation) may be due to a wide variety of causes. A convenient grouping is infectious and non-infectious. Small-bowel infection is extraordinarily common; all of use will have had *gastroenteritis* at some time, frequently due to food-poisoning because of enterotoxin ingestion. Indeed, it has been estimated that 20% of the UK population suffer at least one episode each year (Infectious Intestinal Disease Study 2000). A variety of organisms may be responsible, and symptoms of nausea, vomiting and diarrhoea are usually self-limiting. *Salmonella, Campylobacter* and *Staphylococcus* are all possible causative agents. Radiology has no role to play but appearances may be dramatic if patients are examined during an attack, with dilatation, ulceration and nodularity. *Chronic intestinal infection* is a different matter and, although uncommon, imaging may play an important role. However, although there may be obvious small-bowel abnormality, the radiological features are frequently non-specific: fold thickening and mild dilatation, for example. Consequently, although imaging may often raise the possibility of an underlying infection, identification of the causative organism is usually impossible on appearances alone.

Intestinal *tuberculosis* usually affects the ileocaecal area. Terminal ileal ulceration in association with a funnelled, contracted caecum are characteristic. Ulcers tend to be discrete and transverse or star-shaped, in contrast to Crohn's disease (the major differential), where they are usually longitudinal. Also, caecal disease tends to be more pronounced in tuberculosis, whereas the terminal ileum is usually the most afflicted in Crohn's disease. As in Crohn's disease, CT or ultrasound will show mural thickening and may reveal enlarged lymph nodes (possibly with central caseation and necrosis) and/or ascites. It is now uncommon to find associated respiratory disease and a normal chest X-ray should not discount the diagnosis, especially in an individual from a high-risk ethnic or social background. Chronic infection can result in fibrosis and obstruction. *Yersinia enterocolitica* also causes a terminal ileitis, the symptoms of which are frequently mistaken for appendicitis and the morphology of which is frequently mistaken for Crohn's disease. Fold thickening and aphthous ulceration are common but transmural ulceration is very rare, as is stricturing, both of which are common in Crohn's disease. Associated lymphadenopathy is also common and should raise the possibility when seen on ultrasound in a young person thought to have appendicitis.

A variety of parasites may inhabit the small bowel. *Ascaris lumbricoides* is a large roundworm which is extremely common worldwide, although uncommon in the west. Infestation is widespread, involving the liver, lungs and gut. Migration into the biliary tree, pharynx and even nasal cavity cause a variety of unpleasant symptoms, and they may be so numerous as to cause small-bowel obstruction. Their appearance on contrast studies is characteristic once the worms have swallowed contrast themselves; barium is seen within their intestinal tract. Hookworm (*Ancylostoma duodenale, Necator americanus*), tapeworm (e.g. *Taenia solium* and *saginata*) *Strongyloides* and *Anisakis* all parasitise the small bowel, eliciting non-specific findings of fold thickening, nodularity, mild dilatation and flocculation on contrast studies. Giardiasis, due to the protozoan *Giardia lamblia*, is increasingly seen in the west and chronic infection is an important cause of non-specific abdominal pain and diarrhoea. Again, radiological findings are non-specific, with mild fold thickening and dilatation. *Actinomycosis israelii* is a rare saphrophytic infection that may present as an ileocaecal mass, typically discharging yellow 'sulphur granule' pus through abdominal wall fistulas, which are frequently numerous. Schistosomiasis, South American blastomycosis and histoplasmosis are other infections that cause non-specific fold thickening, sometimes with stricturing.

Whipple's disease may also be considered an intestinal infection because of its association with the bacilli *Tropheryma whippelii*. It is a rare multisystem disease of middle-aged Northern European and North American men that presents with insidious systemic symptoms such as arthralgia and pyrexia. Intestinal biopsies reveal typical periodic acid–Schiff (PAS) macrophages. Diarrhoea, steatorrhoea and malabsorption are common and contrast studies typically reveal a micronodular mucosal pattern (which is also seen in *Mycobacterium avium-intracellulare* infection in AIDS). There may also be fold thickening and dilatation. Treatment is by antibiotics.

AIDS patients are prone to many of the infections already mentioned and others have a particular predilection for this group. *Cytomegalovirus* (CMV) is a herpes virus that frequently affects immunocompromised patients. Colitis is a common manifestation but the small bowel may also be involved, usually the terminal ileum, where there is deep ulceration and mural thickening. *Cryptosporidium parvum*, a cattle protozoan, is the commonest cause of an enteritis in AIDS but again the features are of non-specific duodenal and jejunal fold thickening and mild luminal dilatation. Although the incidence of tuberculosis is increased in AIDS, atypical mycobacteria are more common. *Mycobacterium avium* and *intracellulare* both cause a small bowel enteritis with diffuse fold thickening and mild dilatation. The typical micronodular mucosal pattern is due to villous distension. In AIDS, the possibility of multiple infections and/or an underlying malignancy should be considered.

NON-INFECTIOUS ENTERITIS

The small bowel is often unavoidably irradiated as a consequence of radiotherapy to abdominopelvic tumours. An acute radiation enteritis is followed by fibrotic healing which may precipitate an endarteritis obliterans. This causes ischaemia and the subsequent fibrosis and strictures that are characteristic of chronic *radiation*

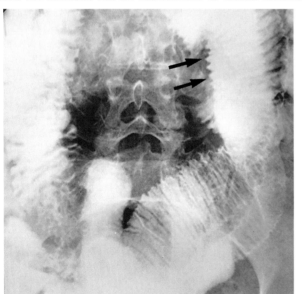

Fig. 20.31 Barium follow-through in a patient with extensive radiation enteritis reveals strictures, dilatation and a 'picket-fence' appearance (arrows).

enteritis. Inflammatory adhesions also develop and are widespread. Unfortunately it is difficult, if not impossible, to predict an individual's sensitivity to radiation but high-dose and closely spaced fractions increase the risk, as does extensive surgery prior to treatment. There is a characteristic temporal lag between therapy and symptom emergence, sometimes as much as 25 years. Radiology is rarely required during the acute phase as the diagnosis is obvious; the role of imaging is to examine those presenting later. There may be abrupt margination between affected bowel and normal adjacent bowel excluded from the radiation field. Initially the valvulae are thickened but may eventually become completely effaced. Extensive adhesions between the antimesenteric aspects of adjacent loops results in the phenomenon of 'mucosal tacking' and a 'picket-fence' appearance (Fig. 20.31). Superficial ulceration, stenosis and obstructive dilatation are common. CT is especially useful to demonstrate the extent of mural thickening and obstruction. Large bowel included in the field will also be affected, notably the rectosigmoid.

Eosinophillic gastroenteritis is a rare condition caused by widespread eosinophillic infiltration, which may be revealed on endoscopic biopsy. Peripheral blood eosinophillia may also be associated. The disease is usually self-limiting but characterised by remissions and relapses. The gastric antrum and small bowel are most frequently affected and nodular antral fold thickening is characteristic. Infiltration may be superficial or reach the serosa (resulting in normal superficial biopsies). Small-bowel folds are thickened and straightened. Nodular forms also exist.

Necrotising enteritis affects premature infants, especially those with additional problems such as respiratory distress. Cases sometimes occur in clusters, raising the possibility of an infective agent. Plain films reveal gastric and small-bowel dilatation. Intramural pneumatosis is a characteristic but late finding, as is portal vein gas and/or pneumoperitoneum, which indicates bowel perforation. Treatment is by bowel resection. Surviving children are prone to strictures, notably colonic, and often suffer from short-bowel syndrome as a consequence of bowel resection.

MALABSORPTION

Malabsorption describes impaired absorption of normal dietary constituents, namely protein, carbohydrates, fats, minerals and proteins. Steatorrhoea specifically describes fat malabsorption. The causes of malabsorption are legion but may be generally divided into several well-defined groups, for example those due to luminal disease, mucosal disease, bowel wall disease, and diseases outside the gastrointestinal tract, including drugs. It should be noted that any disease that either significantly destroys normal intestinal absorptive mucosa, or which grossly affects transit, may result in malabsorption. Therefore, many of the infective (Whipple's disease, parasitic infections) and non-infective (radiation enteritis, eosinophillic enteritis) enteritides may cause malabsorption, as can extensive tumours and endocrine disorders (diabetes, Zollinger–Ellison syndrome). Pseudo-obstructive syndromes are also associated, notably scleroderma. A major differential is between pancreatic and bile salt deficiency, and an enteropathy; the former tend to be selective for fat and protein malabsorption, whereas the latter affects all dietary constituents. Depending on the severity, patients present with diarrhoea, steatorrhoea, abdominal distension and weight loss. There may be some features specific to the deficient nutrient, for example glossitis. Malabsorption is confirmed by routine blood tests (albumin, folate, vitamins) and faecal fat estimation. Diagnosis of mucosal disease, such as tropical sprue and coeliac disease, is usually by endoscopic intestinal biopsy. The xylose breath test is specific for bacterial overgrowth, and the hydrogen breath test for lactase deficiency. Concerning imaging, many findings are non-specific and dilatation, oedematous fold thickening and impaired motility generally occur. Barium flocculation, once common, is now much reduced by newer, resistant suspensions. The role of imaging is therefore to reveal structural lesions that cause malabsorption, or gross motility abnormalities. A specific imaging diagnosis is then possible, for example with bacterial overgrowth due to blind loops or jejunal diverticulosis, Crohn's disease and extensive intestinal resection.

Coeliac disease

Coeliac disease (gluten-sensitive enteropathy) reflects hypersensitivity to the gliadin fractions of gluten (found in wheat, barley and rye). The histological hallmark is villous atrophy, which returns to normal after a gluten-free diet is instituted. The disease is especially prevalent in northern Europe, most notably Ireland, and there is some familial predisposition and linkage to HLA-DR3 leucocyte antigen. Classical presentation is with distension, steatorrhoea, skin pigmentation and glossitis but atypical features are common. The disease may not present until adulthood or even later in life. The classical radiological feature is ileal 'jejunisation'. Jejunal folds are either widely separated or absent altogether (five or more jejunal folds per 2.5 cm is normal) and this feature is accompanied by a paradoxical increase in ileal folds from the normal 2–4 per 2.5 cm to 4–6 (Herlinger & Maglinte 1986). Unfortunately, these classical features are often absent, and probably the commonest feature is luminal dilatation (La Seta et al 1992). Fold thickening may also occur, but usually because of oedema secondary to hypoalbuminaemia rather than as a primary feature. Transient painless intussusception is common and may be seen during follow-through and on CT or ultrasound. Positive infusion pressure during enteroclysis precludes this.

Coeliac disease has some notable associations that the radiologist should be aware of. Although it can occur as an isolated phenomenon, ulcerative jejunoileitis is most often seen in association with coeliac disease, which may be unsuspected. Ulceration may be acute or chronic and can be life-threatening. Another complication is enteropathy associated T-cell lymphoma, which may also occur where the underlying diagnosis of coeliac disease is unrecognised. Radiological features are similar to small-bowel lymphoma elsewhere. It is also worth remembering that carcinoma of the pharynx, oesophagus, duodenum and stomach are also increased in coeliac disease. Dermatitis herpetiformis is a well-recognised associated papulovesicular rash.

Tropical sprue

Tropical sprue is a postinfective malabsorption that also causes subtotal villous atrophy. It is due to small-bowel colonisation with a variety of organisms, and such infection is more common in the tropics, hence the nomenclature. Radiological findings are non-specific and symptomatic response to antibiotics and folate is dramatic.

Amyloidosis

Amyloidosis describes deposition of an insoluble glycoprotein in various organs. Gastrointestinal involvement is more common in primary amyloidosis and can diffusely involve the small bowel, producing non-specific dilatation, fold thickening and impaired motility, suggesting pseudo-obstruction. Ischaemia results from vascular deposition. Localised deposition is less common but results in filling defects, either macro- or micronodular (Tada et al 1991). Pain, diarrhoea and malabsorption may all result and the condition is frequently fatal.

Cystic fibrosis

Intestinal impaction and obstruction after childhood is termed 'meconium ileus equivalent' and small-bowel involvement later in life is increasingly well recognised. Indeed, 2% of patients are primarily diagnosed because of enteric or hepatobiliary symptoms in young adulthood. Malabsorption and steatorrhoea occur due to abnormal exocrine pancreatic secretion. In addition to non-specific small-bowel dilatation and fold thickening, duodenal sacculation is said to be characteristic and viscid secretions adhering to villi may produce a coarse reticular pattern. Although the corresponding colopathy is well described, it is increasingly well recognised that strictures also affect the small bowel.

Mastocytosis

Although abnormal mast cell infiltration usually involves the skin (resulting in urticaria pigmentosa), gastrointestinal infiltration may also occur. Mucosal and submucosal infiltration with consequent histamine release may cause pain, nausea, vomiting and diarrhoea. Small bowel findings are non-specific, with thickened, irregular folds, diffuse mucosal nodularity and occasionally larger urticarial-like lesions.

Intestinal lymphangiectasia
May be primary, due to congenital lymphatic dilatation, or secondary to occlusion of normal mesenteric lymph drainage channels, which raises pressure in peripheral lymphatics. The radiological hallmark is oedematous fold thickening with micronodules, representing villi distended by engorged lacteal channels.

Waldenström's macroglobulinaemia
Is a plasma cell neoplasm. The abnormal IgM proteins occasionally deposit in small-bowel lacteals, resulting in villous distension, oedema and malabsorption. Granularity on contrast examination reflects villous distension.

Abetalipoproteinemia
Is a recessively inherited disease characterised by fat malabsorption. Fat accumulates in enterocytes and the lymphatics are empty. Contrast studies may show a granular mucosa due to villous distension secondary to the lipid-laden enterocytes. Fold thickening and dilatation reflects malabsorption.

Zollinger–Ellison syndrome
Is characterised by gastric acid hypersecretion as a consequence of a gastrin-secreting neuroendocrine tumour (usually pancreatic). Hypersecretion results in diarrhoea and malabsorption. In addition to gastric fold thickening and widespread duodenal ulceration, contrast studies reveal thickened jejunal folds with increased luminal fluid.

VASCULAR DISEASE

Mesenteric ischaemia can be acute or chronic, arterial or venous. Arterial and venous bowel ischaemia due to obstruction has already been discussed. Acute superior mesenteric artery (SMA) occlusion, usually due to *atheromatous thrombus* or *embolus*, will result in small bowel and right colonic ischaemia. This can be intermittent or sustained and the consequences are related to the degree of ischaemia and its duration. Acute abdominal pain is common and peritonism occurs in severe cases. Like the colon, the mucosa is most sensitive, with early sloughing and ulceration. Small-bowel collaterals are more developed than in the colon and healing will ensue if these are adequate, sometimes with subsequent fibrotic stricture. Atherosclerosis commonly affects the origin of the SMA, with the result that most emboli are distal to this, resulting in segmental ischaemia. Abdominal films may reveal multiple, gas-filled, dilated small-bowel loops but diagnosis is often delayed because of failure to consider the diagnosis. Chronic arterial ischaemia ('intestinal angina') is likely to be more common than generally believed, given the prevalence of atherosclerotic disease. Pain is intermittent and classically follows eating.

Mesenteric vein thrombosis most often follows abdominal surgery but is associated with trauma, portal hypertension and hypercoagulative states. The superior mesenteric vein is involved in 95% of cases. There is bleeding into affected loops, with associated oedema, features which are more marked than in arterial occlusion. Again, plain films are non-specific, revealing distended, gas-filled loops with associated mural thickening (thumb-printing if marked), features that are elegantly revealed by CT, which may also reveal the intravascular embolus.

Intramural haemorrhage classically follows direct trauma or spontaneously occurs in individuals with a bleeding tendency, classically those taking anticoagulant therapy (Fig. 20.32), where it is said to affect 10–35% of patients. Diagnosis is now commonly initially by CT, which will reveal an isolated segment of mural thickening, with a clue to aetiology given by high attenuation. *Duodenal haematoma* typically follows blunt abdominal trauma, often in children, and may be sufficient to cause obstruction. Seat-belt injuries may be associated with small-bowel haematoma or rupture.

Vasculitides may also affect the small bowel. *Henoch–Schönlein purpura* typically affects children and young adults, who present

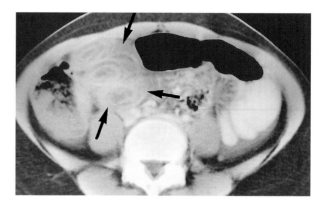

Fig. 20.33 Small-bowel thickening, causing a 'target' sign, in a young woman with Henoch–Schönlein purpura (arrows).

with a purpuric rash, abdominal pain and arthritis. There is small-bowel mucosal and submucosal haemorrhage in approximately 50% and perforation occurs rarely. Contrast examinations will reveal fold thickening in affected areas and CT will show the extent of mural haemorrhage (Fig. 20.33). *Behçet's disease*, the typical triad of orogenital ulceration, a rash and ocular inflammation, may affect the ileocaecal region, causing terminal ileal ulceration. *Rheumatoid arthritis, polyarteritis nodosa* and *systemic lupus erythematosus* may all cause a visceral vasculitis.

Vascular malformations are a relatively common cause of the *'obscure gastrointestinal bleeding syndrome'* and may occur in the small bowel, although colonic angiodysplasia is more likely. Small-bowel investigation usually follows when colonic and upper gastrointestinal tract causes have been excluded. Contrast studies are usually fruitless and the diagnosis is often reached using enteroscopy, which may need to be done during laparotomy via an enterotomy if the entire small bowel is to be examined. If lesions are large enough, angiography will suffice. Bleeding from the biliary tree should also be considered if the cause remains obscure. *Haemangiomas* may also occur in the small bowel and can be capillary or cavernous. Gastrointestinal haemangiomas are part of the blue rubber bleb naevus syndrome.

CONGENITAL LESIONS

Malrotation

In the normal course of fetal development the midgut herniates into the extraembryonic coelom and rotates around the superior mesenteric artery axis as it elongates. Completed rotation is approximately 270° anticlockwise and bowel retracts back into the abdomen towards the end of the first trimester, the mesenteries fusing with the posterior abdominal wall on their return. Rotation may be arrested at 90°, with the result that the caecum is the first part of the gut to return, settling on the left, with subsequent small bowel on the right—'non-rotation'. This may be complicated by volvulus because the mesentery is smaller and more centralised than usual. Clockwise 270° rotation results in true situs inversus, a mirror image of usual configuration, usually without detriment. A 90° clockwise rotation sites the transverse colon behind the duodenum and superior mesenteric artery—'reversed rotation'. Caecal descent on return to the abdomen may also be arrested and the resulting

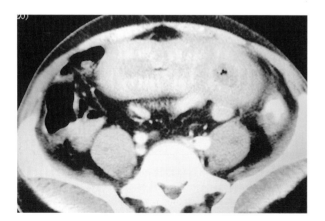

Fig. 20.32 Gross intramural jejunal haemorrhage revealed by CT in a young man taking oral anticoagulants.

peritoneal bands (Ladd's bands), which extend from the posterolateral abdominal wall to the caecum, may obstruct the duodenum. Congenital hernias may also occur when bowel loops become entangled in the colonic mesentery before they fuse to the posterior abdominal wall. The resulting paraduodenal (mesocolic) hernias may be right or left sided and cause intermittent obstruction. Paracaecal and lesser sac congenital hernias also occur. Many hernias encountered in clinical practice actually follow surgery.

Duplications

These may occur anywhere along the small bowel but are usually ileal. Size is highly variable and they may be cystic or tubular. Intramural duplications may cause obstruction, while others are usually mesenteric in origin. *Meckel's diverticulum* occurs in approximately 3% of the population, usually within the distal 100 cm of ileum. The diverticulum is a remnant of the vitelline duct and, while most are asymptomatic, the presence of ectopic gastric mucosa can result in bleeding. Fifty per cent of symptomatic cases present before the age of 2 years. The typical triradiate fold configuration of the diverticulum is infrequently visualised on contrast studies (Fig. 20.34), even when carefully sought, and scintigraphic techniques are more useful for diagnosis. Inverted Meckel's diverticulum is a rare but well-recognised cause of intestinal obstruction. Congenital stenoses and atresias also occur, usually because of incomplete vacuolisation, with the duodenum the most common site.

MISCELLANEOUS CONDITIONS

Nodular lymphoid hyperplasia is a common terminal ileal finding in children and is occasionally seen in young adults. Lymphoid follicles are aggregates of lymphocytes and enlarge in a wide variety of conditions in adults, including immunodeficiency, infection (often giardiasis), carcinoma and Crohn's disease. Nodular filling defects 2–3 mm in size are best seen on compression views

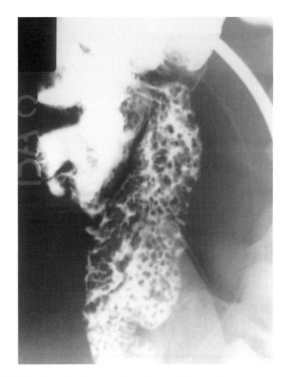

Fig. 20.35 Terminal ileum nodular lymphoid hyperplasia.

(Fig. 20.35) and in children are often mistaken for terminal ileal disease by less experienced operators, especially when the nodular morphology is less obvious.

Pneumatosis intestinalis describes gas in the bowel wall. This may be primary or secondary, due to infection, ischaemia or trauma, for example. It often occurs as an incidental finding in

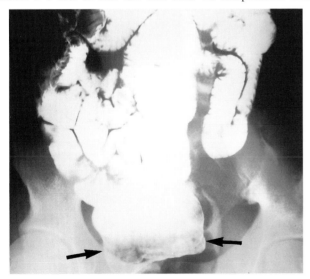

Fig. 20.34 Barium follow-through reveals a large Meckel's diverticulum (arrows).

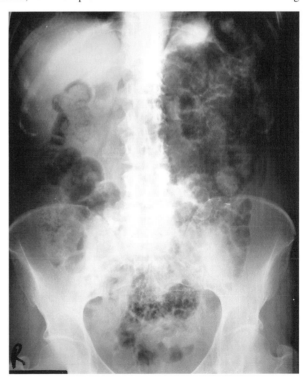

Fig. 20.36 Plain film showing pneumatosis intestinalis evidenced by innumerable air-filled cysts.

patients with chronic obstructive pulmonary disease or scleroderma. Hyperbaric oxygen therapy is used to treat patients in whom persistent cyst rupture is a cause of pneumoperitoneum. Plain film appearances of primary small-bowel pneumatosis are highly characteristic (Fig. 20.36) but CT is most sensitive for diagnosis, especially of secondary causes.

NSAID enteritis. Non-steroidal anti-inflammatory drugs may induce ileal diaphragms that can stenose the lumen to as little as 1 mm, causing intestinal obstruction (Lang et al 1988).

Graft-versus-host disease (GVHD) is seen after allogenic marrow transplantation and occurs when grafted tissue mounts an immunological response against the recipient. Acute gastrointestinal symptoms of abdominal pain and diarrhoea are accompanied by small-bowel fold oedema and occasionally total effacement, resulting in a 'toothpaste' or 'ribbon-bowel' appearance. Transit time is markedly reduced. Cross-sectional modalities reveal extensive jejunal and ileal mural thickening, and the colon is also often involved.

Typhilitis occurs in immunocompromised subjects, often those with leukaemia and lymphoma who are undergoing chemotherapy. It is characterised by terminal ileal and caecal inflammation and may be complicated by supra-added infection and ischaemia. Transmural inflammation can result in perforation.

THE PERITONEAL CAVITY

Anatomy

The peritoneum is a thin, translucent serous membrane that lines the abdominopelvic cavity (parietal layer) and either partially or completely invests the organs within (visceral layer). It consists of mesothelium and connective tissue, and the space between the

parietal and visceral layers (which are continuous with one another) is lubricated by serous peritoneal fluid. The space between the two layers is the peritoneal cavity and can be divided into the greater sac and smaller lesser sac, which lies behind the stomach (Fig. 20.37). It therefore follows that the peritoneum is thrown into a series of folds by the organs it suspends and these, along with its various attachments to the abdominopelvic cavity, form a series of spaces. These spaces can limit disease spread or, alternatively, the peritoneal folds themselves can act as direct conduits for contiguous disease spread. Similarly, the normal flow of peritoneal fluid occurs along these pathways, influenced by patient position and intraperitoneal pressure. Infected material and malignant cells within the peritoneal cavity will tend to follow the same routes and then collect in areas of relative stasis. For example, the peritoneal cavity is divided into supra- and inframesocolic spaces by the transverse mesocolon. The right and left inframesocolic compartments are separated by the root of the small-bowel mesentery. Whereas the left is open to the pelvis medially, the right is bounded by the ascending mesocolon, which is continuous with the small-bowel mesentery. This boundary means that pathology within this space tends to follow the superior aspect of the small-bowel mesentery as it attempts to reach the pelvis, finally reaching the medial aspect of the caecum. Similarly, pathology within the left infracolic space will involve the superior aspect of the sigmoid mesocolon before being liberated into the pelvis (to reach the lateral paravesical spaces and pouch of Douglas). Negative intrathoracic pressure tends to drive pelvic fluid up the paracolic gutters. However, although pelvic pathology may freely communicate with the right supracolic spaces (the right subphrenic and subhepatic spaces, and lesser sac) via the right paracolic gutter, the left gutter is partially bounded by the phrenicocolic ligament. This simple concept explains why metastases from ovarian carcinoma frequently involve the liver surface more often than the spleen

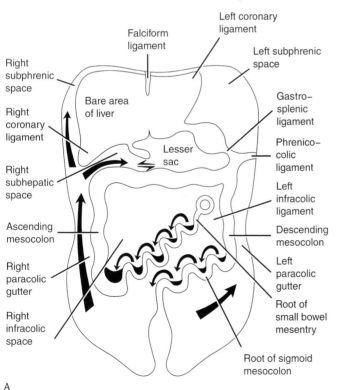

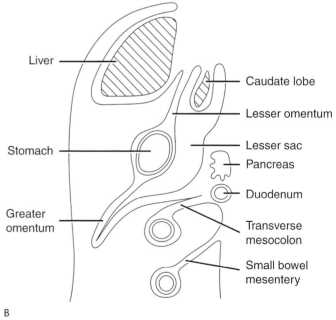

Fig. 20.37 Peritoneal attachments and potential spaces when viewed from the front (A) and side (B); (A) also demonstrates likely pathways for pathological spread.

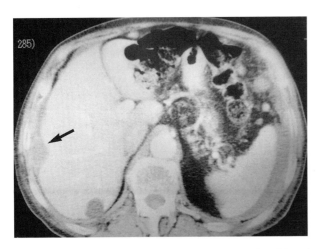

Fig. 20.38 CT reveals deposits on the liver surface (arrow) in this patient with ovarian carcinoma (note splenic ascites).

(Fig. 20.38). It follows that abscesses are most commonly found in the pelvis, right subhepatic space and right subphrenic space.

Intraperitoneal disease

The most commonly encountered peritoneal pathologies are abnormal *fluid collections*, either abscesses or ascites, and transcoelomic *metastatic disease* (typically ovary, colon, stomach, pancreas). Cross-sectional techniques are best suited to imaging because contrast studies usually only provide indirect evidence of intraperitoneal disease. Ultrasound is limited by its inability to visualise the central mesentry. Peritoneal seedings most commonly involve the pelvis (pouch of Douglas), the area bounded by the small-bowel mesentery root and adjacent ascending mesocolon, the superior aspect of the sigmoid mesocolon, and the right paracolic gutter (Meyers 1973). On CT these metastases appear as soft-tissue nodules or irregular plaques. Morphology is often bizarre and enhancement avid (Fig. 20.39). Ascites will often render very small nodules detectable. Sensitivity of CT for peritoneal metastasis is approximately 50% when compared directly with laparotomy or laparoscopy, but specificity approaches 90% (De Rosa et al 1995). Ascites, which describes non-loculated intraperitoneal fluid, may be a transudate (e.g. cirrhosis, heart failure) or exudate (e.g. carcinomatosis, pancreatitis) defined by its protein content. Loculated collections are usually abscesses following surgery, the prevalence

of which is almost certainly underestimated. Common primary causes include *appendicitis, diverticulitis* and *Crohn's disease*. Peritoneal infection also occurs in tuberculosis, which may be 'wet' with ascites or 'dry' when fibrosis predominates.

Primary peritoneal and mesenteric disease

Primary peritoneal and mesenteric malignancy is rare. *Malignant mesothelioma* is associated with asbestos exposure and is manifest as irregular serosal peritoneal thickening, sometimes with ascites. *Stromal tumours* also occur, notably fibrosarcoma. *Pseudomyxoma peritonei* follows rupture of an appendiceal mucocele and is manifest as multiple, lobulated low-attenuation fluid collections on CT, often with pronounced scalloping of the liver and spleen (Fig. 20.40). Prognosis is related to the underlying mucocele; if malignant, 5 year survival is less than 25%. Approximately 50% of patients with non-Hodgkin's *lymphoma* have mesenteric involvement. There are confluent central mesenteric messes; concomitant retroperitoneal lymphadenopathy will support the diagnosis. *Desmoid tumours* are benign but locally aggressive mesenchymal fibroblastic tumours that arise from the central mesentery and are a common cause of death in postcolectomy patients with familial ademomatous polyposis. There is a wide range of appearances, ranging from a precursor area of mesenteric scarring, often with a whorled appearance, to well-defined heterogenous mesenteric masses (Fig. 20.29) (Healy et al 1997). Mesenteric desmoplasia also classically occurs with small-bowel *carcinoid* tumours (Fig. 20.26). *Mesenteric cysts* may be enteric duplication cysts, pancreatic pseudocysts, lymphangiomas, teratomas and hamartomas. It should be noted that cystic ovarian disease may mimic primary mesenteric cystic disease. *Mesenteric panniculitis* (retractile mesenteritis, mesenteric lipodystrophy) is an idiopathic inflammatory process affecting mesenteric fat (Fig. 20.41). Fibrosis may predominate, resulting in a hard, fatty mass that may mimic a liposarcoma. Adjacent bowel is displaced and may be directly involved, producing dilatation or stenosis. *Sclerosing encapsulating peritonitis* most commonly occurs in patients on ambulatory peritoneal dialysis, who present with pain and a central abdominal mass, due to dense adhesions. Small-bowel obstruction may follow. Findings may be due to the dialysate or peritoneal infection, and a similar fibrotic peritonitis may follow some drugs, notably β-blockers. Primary idiopathic right-sided *segmental omental infarction* is a rare but well-recognised mimic of appendicitis in

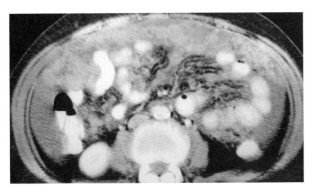

Fig. 20.39 Contrast-enhanced CT reveals plaques of high-attenuation peritoneal deposits in a patient with disseminated colorectal adenocarcinoma.

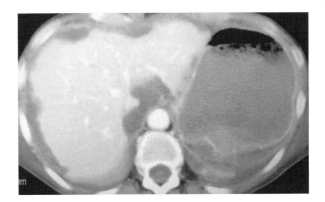

Fig. 20.40 CT reveals the liver scalloping typical of pseudomyxoma.

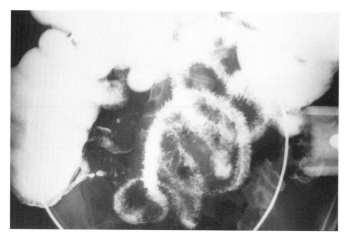

Fig. 20.41 Barium follow-through shows distal ileal encasement in mesenteric panniculitis.

men aged 20–40 years. CT reveals focally infiltrated right-sided omental fat (Puylaert 1992). The 'misty mesentery' is a well-recognised finding in patients where the normally low attenuation of mesenteric fat is increased. This can be focal or diffuse. The causes are legion but may be grouped into oedema (heart failure, cirrhosis), lymphoedema (malignancy, radiation), inflammation (diverticulitis, pancreatitis), haemorrhage (infarction, anticoagulation) and neoplasia (Mindelzun et al 1996).

REFERENCES AND SUGGESTIONS FOR FURTHER READING

Assalia, A., Schein, M., Kopelman, D., et al (1994) Therapeutic effect of Gastrografin in adhesive, partial small-bowel obstruction: a prospective randomised trial. *Surgery*, **115**, 433.

Bartram, C. I. (1980) The radiological demonstration of adhesions following surgery for inflammatory bowel disease. *British Journal of Radiology*, **53**, 650–653.

Bartram, C. I. (1996) Small bowel enteroclysis: cons. *Abdominal Imaging*, **21**, 245–246.

Bernstein, C. N., Boult, I. F., Greenberg, H. M., van der Putten, W., Duffy, G., Grahame, G. R. (1997) A prospective randomized comparison between small bowel enteroclysis and small bowel follow-through in Crohn's disease. *Gastroenterology*, **113**, 390–398.

De Rosa, V., Mangoni de Stefano, M. L., Brunetti, A., et al (1995) Computed tomography and second look surgery in ovarian cancer patients. Correlation, actual role and limitations of CT scan. *European Journal of Gynaecology and Oncology*, **16**, 123–129.

Frager, D., Baer, J. W., Medwid, S. W. (1996) Detection of intestinal ischaemia in patients with acute small-bowel obstruction due to adhesions or hernia: efficacy of CT. *American Journal of Roentgenology*, **166**, 67–71.

Gasche, C., Moser, G., Turetschek, K., Schober, E., Moeschi, P., Oberhuber, G. (1999) Transabdominal bowel sonography for the detection of intestinal complications in Crohn's disease. *Gut*, **44**, 112–117.

Gelfand, D. W., Ott, D. J. (1981) Radiographic demonstration of small intestinal villi on routine clinical studies. *Gastrointestinal Radiology*, **6**, 21–27.

Glick, S. N., Teplick, S. K. (1985) Crohn's disease of the small intestine: diffuse mucosal granularity. *Radiology*, **154**, 313–317.

Goldberg, H. I., Caruthers, S. B., Nelson, J. A., Singleton, J. W. (1979) Radiographic findings of the National Cooperative Crohn's Disease Study. *Gastroenterology*, **77**, 925–937.

Gore, R., Levine, M. (2000) *Textbook of Gastrointestinal Radiology*. London: W. B. Saunders.

Greenstein, A. J., Mullin, G. E., Strauchen, J. A., et al (1992) Lymphoma in inflammatory bowel disease. *Cancer*, **69**, 1119–1123.

Halligan, S., Nicholls, S., Bartram, C. I., Walker-Smith, J. A. (1994) The distribution of small-bowel Crohn's disease in children compared to adults. *Clinical Radiology*, **49**, 314–316.

Hare, C., Halligan, S., Bartram, C. I., Platt, K., Raleigh, G. (2000) Cisapride or metoclopramide to accelerate small-bowel transit during barium follow-through examination? *Abdominal Imaging*, **25**, 243–245.

Healy, J. C., Reznek, R. H., Clark, S. K., Phillips, R. K., Armstrong, P. (1997) MR appearances of desmoid tumors in familial adenomatous polyposis. *American Journal of Roentgenology*, **169**, 465–472.

Herlinger, H., Maglinte, D. D. T. (1986) Jejunal fold separation in adult celiac disease: relevance of enteroclysis. *Radiology*, **158**, 605–611.

Infectious Intestinal Disease Study Executive Committee (2000) *Report of the Infectious Intestinal Disease Study in England*. London: The Stationery Office.

Jobling, J. C., Halligan, S., Bartram, C. I. (1999) Non-ionic, water-soluble contrast agents for small-bowel follow-through examinations. *European Radiology*, **9**, 706–710.

Joyce, W. P., Delaney, P. V., Gorey, T. F., et al (1992) The value of water-soluble contrast radiology in the management of acute small-bowel obstruction. *Annals of the Royal College of Surgeons of England*, **74**, 422.

Kelly, I. M. G., Bartram, C. I. (1993) Pseudotumoral appearance of small bowel strictureplasty for Crohn's disease. *Abdominal Imaging*, **18**, 366–368.

Lang, J., Price, A. B., Levi, A. J., Burke, M., Gumpel, J. M., Bjarnson, I. (1988) Diaphragm disease: pathology of disease of the small intestine induced by non-steroidal anti-inflammatory drugs. *Journal of Clinical Pathology*, **41**, 516–526.

La Seta, F., Salerno, G., Brucellato, A., et al (1992) Radiological indicants of adult coeliac disease assessed by double contrast enteroclysis. *European Journal of Radiology*, **15**, 157–162.

McClean, A. M., Bartram, C. I. (1985) Prone compression with the pneumatic paddle during barium studies. *Clinical Radiology*, **36**, 213–215.

Maglinte, D. D. T., Balthazar, E. J., Kelvin, F. M., Megibow, A. J. (1997) The role of radiology in the diagnosis of small bowel obstruction. *American Journal of Roentgenology*, **168**, 1171–1180.

Maglinte, D. D. T., Reyes, B., Harmon, B. H., et al (1996) Reliability and role of plain film radiography and CT in the diagnosis of small-bowel obstruction. *American Journal of Roentgenology*, **167**, 1451–1455.

Megibow, A. J., Balthazar, E. J., Cho, K. C., et al (1991) Bowel obstruction; evaluation with CT. *Radiology*, **180**, 313–318.

Meyers, M. A. (1973) Distribution of intra-abdominal malignant seeding: dependency on dynamics of flow of ascitic fluid. *American Journal of Roentgenology*, **119**, 198–206.

Meyers, M. A. (1988) *Dynamic Radiology of the Abdomen: Normal and Pathologic Anatomy*. New York: Springer.

Mindelzun, R. E., Jeffrey, R. B., Lane, M. J., Silverman, P. M. (1996) The misty mesentery on CT: differential diagnosis. *American Journal of Roentgenology*, **167**, 61–65.

Nolan, D. (1996) Small bowel enteroclysis: pros. Abdominal Imaging, **21**, 243–244.

Nolan, D. J., Cadman, P. J. (1987) The small bowel enema made easy. *Clinical Radiology*, **38**, 295–301.

Puylaert, J. B. (1992) Right-sided segmental infarction of the omentum: clinical, US, and CT findings. *Radiology*, **185**, 169–172.

Robinson, P. J. A. (1997) Radiology's Achilles' heel: error and variation in the interpretation of the röntgen image. *British Journal of Radiology*, **70**, 1085–1098.

Rutgeerts, P., Geboes, K., Vantrappen, G. et al (1990) Predictability of the postoperative course of Crohn's disease. *Gastroenterology*, **99**, 956–963.

Tada, S., Iida, M., Matsui, T., et al (1991) Amyloidosis of the small-intestine: findings on double contrast radiographs. *American Journal of Roentgenology*, **156**, 741–744.

van Oostayen, J. A., Wasser, M. N., van Hogezand, R. A., Griffioen, G., de Roos, A. (1994) Activity of Crohn disease assessed by measurement of superior mesenteric artery flow with Doppler US. *Radiology*, **193**, 551–554.

21

THE LARGE BOWEL

Steve Halligan

with contributions by Philip J. A. Robinson

Imaging in coloproctology

Coloproctology is a well-defined surgical subspecialty, encompassing the entire range of large bowel pathology, from cancer to functional disorders. At the time of writing it is the most popular subspecialty choice among UK surgeons. The last decade has witnessed an explosion of investigative possibilities in coloproctology, largely due to imaging research. This has fuelled intense surgical demand for access to specialised imaging, such as anal endosonography, which has become pivotal in clinical decision-making. There has been a parallel demand for radiologists able to provide the full spectrum of coloproctological imaging; without such support, surgeons will cater for these examinations themselves.

ANATOMY AND FUNCTION

The colon is approximately 120–200 cm long and is distinguished from small bowel by three longitudinal muscular bands, the taenia coli (omentalis, mesocolica and libera), which form the haustral sacculations. Conventionally divided into caecum (including the appendix), ascending colon, hepatic flexure, transverse colon, splenic flexure, descending colon and sigmoid colon, these anatomical demarcations are difficult to define precisely in practice, not least because there is considerable individual variation in colonic configuration and calibre. Furthermore, although the transverse and sigmoid colons usually have a mesentery (mesocolon), its morphology is inconstant, resulting in further variation in colonic mobility and redundancy. This partially accounts for some of the technical difficulties occasionally encountered during barium enema and colonoscopy. Indeed, practically any segment of large bowel may have an associated mesocolon, although it is usual for the ascending and descending portions to be partly extraperitoneal. Rotational anomalies are uncommon. The most frequently seen is failure of caecal descent. In *situs inversus* the midgut loop fails to rotate so that the right colon is displaced to the left, with the caecum near the left iliac fossa. Lesser degrees of right colonic displacement are seen in *malrotation*. The caecum occasionally has its own mesentery and can be displaced superomedially. The rectum is the distal portion of the colon, defined by the third sacral segment, and generally begins where the sigmoid mesocolon ends. It is 15–18 cm long and expanded into an infraperitoneal ampulla. There are no haustra; instead the rectum is thrown into two or three full-thickness folds, the valves of Houston. The anal sphincter is the most complex sphincter in the human body and is closely integrated with pelvic floor function. Two sphincter muscles surround the anal canal: the striated external sphincter and the smooth muscle internal sphincter.

Colonic arterial supply is via ileocolic branches of the superior mesenteric artery (the right and middle colic arteries) and the inferior mesenteric artery (left colic artery). The sigmoid arteries are also branches of the inferior mesenteric artery. An anastamotic arch forms between the middle colic and ascending branch of the left colic, with a marginal artery running practically the entire medial colonic aspect. This creates a watershed region that is weakest at the junction of the mid- and hind-gut vessels at the splenic flexure, rendering this site vulnerable to ischaemia. The inferior mesenteric artery becomes the superior rectal artery on crossing the pelvic brim. The rectum is also supplied via branches from the internal iliac arteries and directly from the anal canal distally. Venous drainage of the right and left colon is essentially to the superior and inferior mesenteric veins, respectively.

Colonic mucosa is columnar, arranged in crypts. Deep to the epithelium are two muscular layers, the innermost muscularis mucosae (deep to which lies the submucosa) and the outermost muscularis propria. The latter essentially forms the muscular wall of the large intestine and is further divided into inner circular and outer longitudinal portions. The colon is not an essential organ (witness the success of total proctocolectomy) but is necessary for optimal absorption of nutrients, water and electrolytes, and the transit and storage of residue. Colonic innervation is extremely complex, with input from the autonomic central nervous system, extraintestinal autonomic ganglia, the enteric nervous system and local humoral factors. The colon forms a functional unit with the small bowel and the two are closely integrated physiologically. For example, caecal residue will slow small-bowel transit (the 'ileocaecal brake') and colonic transit varies in response to eating. Colonic contractions can be broadly subdivided into those that are *propagative* (e.g. 'mass' contractions) and those that merely mix intestinal content (*segmentation*). Again, individual colonic motility is highly variable, but generally accounts for at least 90% of intestinal total transit time. There are certain sites that are prone to *physiological narrowing*, notably at the ileocaecal valve, and spasm at these sites is easy to confuse with a malignant stricture. However, they are usually transient and may be abolished by smooth muscle relaxants combined with gas insufflation.

Lymphoid hyperplasia may be identified, particularly in children or young adults, and represents lymphoid follicle hypertrophy. In some instances this probably represents a normal anatomical variant but can occur secondary to inflammation or an abnormal immune response.

RADIOLOGICAL INVESTIGATION

Plain films

Intraluminal colonic gas is normal and the amount present varies considerably. There is usually enough to define the haustra and, in contrast to small bowel, several colonic fluid levels may be normal. The distribution of residue also varies considerably. The main role of abdominal films is to diagnose and monitor *obstruction* or *colitis*. Close temporal proximity to either sigmoidoscopy or colonoscopy may cause excess colonic gas, which should not be confused with pathology.

Barium enema

The barium enema remains the routine radiological technique for colonic examination, although CT has made considerable inroads in recent years. It remains the gold-standard technique for imaging fine mucosal detail and is also pre-eminent for best demonstration of general colonic configuration and calibre. Although single-contrast studies are widely practiced in the United States, the double-contrast technique has gained general acceptance elsewhere. Scrupulous colonic cleansing is mandatory for high-quality studies. The aim is for a clean but dry colon. A variety of purgative regimens have been described and local preference and availability will determine the choice. Modern regimens have rendered preliminary cleansing enemas redundant. Although useful for colonoscopy preparation where residual fluid is irrelevant, large volume irrigating electrolyte solutions (e.g. Klean-Prep and Golytely) tend to result in a wet colon with predictably poor mucosal coating (Bartram 1994). A better option is Picolax, which is a combination of magnesium citrate (an osmotic purgative) and sodium picosulphate. The latter is metabolised in the colon to the active metabolite of bisacodyl, a laxative that directly stimulates colonic contraction. This is usually combined with a low-residue diet the day before the examination, copious oral fluids to help purgation, followed by fluid restriction so that the colon is dry by the time of examination.

Because *barium peritonitis* is potentially fatal, barium suspensions are contraindicated if there is a risk of colonic perforation, for example in toxic megacolon. Unintentional full-thickness perforation is possible after mucosal biopsy using rigid forceps and sigmoidoscopes (or following snare polypectomy) but flexible biopsy via an endoscope channel is not usually a contraindication to immediate subsequent barium enema (biopsy or polypectomy often leaves a residual mucosal 'footprint' so close liaison with the endoscopist regarding the site of biopsy is necessary to avoid confusion). An intravenous smooth muscle relaxant is recommended (20 mg

hyoscine-*N*-butylbromide (Buscopan) or 1 mg glucagon) to aid distension. There has long been misconception relating to dangers of Buscopan in patients with glaucoma, as the only patients at risk are those who have undiagnosed disease, and will therefore not offer any suggestive history (Fink & Aylward 1995). Patients should, however, be told to seek urgent advice if they subsequently develop significant visual symptoms. It may be appropriate to substitute glucagon for Buscopan if the patient has a significant history of cardiac disease, as Buscopan can cause tachycardia. A rectal balloon catheter may be used in incontinent patients, with the proviso that perforation is more common using this device; the balloon should be inflated carefully and gently, after checking for rectal disease. A head-down position, muscle relaxant and controlled influx of barium will all help in this common scenario. If all fails, it may still be possible to perform a single-contrast study or convert to water-soluble contrast, which fills the colon more easily.

In general, the equipment available will determine the radiographic technique used. Traditionally the barium suspension was introduced to mid-transverse colon level using gravity, and the remainder of the colon is filled using a combination of gas insufflation and positional change. Carbon dioxide is preferable to air for insufflation because its rapid absorption decreases the incidence of subsequent abdominal pain (it is worth mentioning that barium enema immediately following failed colonoscopy is very difficult when air has been used by the colonoscopist, but carbon dioxide presents no problem). A series of overcouch films were then taken to image the entire colon in double contrast. A typical sequence would include prone straight and angled films, right and left 35° supine obliques, right and left lateral decubitus films, a left lateral rectal film and an erect 35 × 35 film to image the flexures. However, now that digital fluoroscopic equipment is widely available, many investigators prefer to image the colon using spot digital radiographs, progressively filming as the colon is filled (Rubesin et al 2000). In this scenario, the operator manipulates the barium pool in response to what he or she sees on the monitor. This technique allows the colon to be scrutinised during the examination, rather than on radiographs developed subsequently. Images can be taken during active gas insufflation and can also be immediately assessed for adequacy. Unlike conventional overcouch studies, the order in which various colonic segments are filmed is relatively unimportant and should be dictated by what appears well imaged on the monitor; most operators will have a set regimen, starting with the rectum and progressively imaging the sigmoid and descending colon, but being ready at all times to modify this when necessary. The flexures are best imaged in the upright position and a head-down position is needed to empty the caecum, usually the last segment imaged. Because it is impossible to obtain decubitus views unless there is a C-arm, cross-table decubitus films are required, especially if it has been difficult to fully drain the caecum.

Instant enema. This examination is useful in patients with known colitis, and is used to define the extent of disease during a relapse when the proximal extent cannot be seen sigmoidoscopically. Once toxic dilatation has been excluded by plain film, barium suspension is introduced to the mid-transverse colon or until residue is encountered, and gas then gently insufflated.

Gastrografin enema. A water-soluble enema, usually with dilute Gastrografin, may be used where there is a risk of colonic perforation, for example to check anastomotic patency, especially as Gastrografin will enter small tracks and fistulas more readily than barium. Water-soluble studies may also be suitable if a general

Table 21.1 Colorectal polyps and corresponding polyposis syndromes

Histology	Solitary	Multiple (polyposis syndrome)
Inflammatory	Inflammatory	Inflammatory, lymphoid
Hyperplastic (metaplastic)	Hyperplastic	Hyperplastic polyposis
	Serrated adenoma	Serrated adenomatous polyposis
Hamartoma	Juvenile	Juvenile polyposis, Peutz–Jeghers syndrome, Cronkhite–Canada syndrome, Cowden's disease, Ruvalcaba–Myhre–Smith syndrome
Adenoma (benign)	Adenoma	Familial adenomatous polyposis
Adenoma (malignant)	'Malignant polyp'	Familial adenomatous polyposis, Turcot's syndrome
Non-epithelial (benign)	Lipoma, connective tissue (neuroma, fibroma, myoma)	
Non-epithelial (malignant)	Lymphoma, metastasis, stromal	

assessment of colonic morphology is all that is required, for example when following up a known stricture or looking at rectal configuration in severe constipation, scenarios where bowel preparation is unnecessary.

Colostomy enema examines the large bowel proximal to a stoma. Full bowel preparation will be necessary if most of the colon remains and mucosal lesions are being sought. Barium is syringed into the colon via a large-gauge Foley catheter, preferably with its balloon inflated deep to the abdominal wall (this may be impossible with stomal prolapse or hernia). An inevitable mess can be avoided if the stoma bag is left in situ and the catheter is introduced via a small incision. Because of difficulties with lying the patient prone, it may be necessary to introduce large volumes of contrast to fill the transverse and right colon. Adequate filling and erect positioning should help achieve a complete study; Buscopan and air insufflation (via a balloon hand pump attached to the catheter) may be needed. Water-soluble contrast, without bowel preparation, may be all that is required if an assessment of colonic morphology, perhaps prior to further surgery, is all that is required.

Evacuation proctography (defecography) is a simple study that images rectal configuration during evacuation of a barium paste, while the subject is seated upright on a specially designed radio-opaque commode. It is used to investigate difficult rectal evacuation. It may be modified by the addition of bladder, vaginal and small-bowel contrast so that the entire pelvic floor is imaged.

Colonic transit studies are used to investigate severely constipated patients. The simplest studies involve measurement of whole-gut transit time using radio-opaque markers, which are ingested and followed by an abdominal film after an appropriate interval.

Rectal ultrasound for coloproctological practice normally uses a 360° rotating endoprobe that obtains high-resolution axial images of the rectal wall, and is primarily used to stage tumours.

Anal endosonography usually uses a modified rectal endoprobe to image the anal sphincters, providing information about sphincter integrity and morphology in patients who are anally incontinent.

CT and MRI have had very considerable impact on coloproctological imaging in recent years. While assessment of metastatic or recurrent tumour using CT probably remains the commonest indication, there are now several highly specific roles for these modalities. For example, MRI is pre-eminent for assessment of pelvic sepsis and is rapidly gaining ground in rectal tumour staging and anal sphincter imaging. The ability to characterise tissue and image in surgically relevant planes renders MR ever more suitable for

coloproctological imaging, especially as motion artefact is less relevant in the pelvis.

COLORECTAL TUMOURS

Polyps

A colorectal polyp may be defined as a mucosal elevation, the word deriving from the Greek 'polypos' for 'octopus'. Polyps are important because of their malignant potential, which depends on histology. There are several different types, with varying clinical implications, occurring both sporadically or as part of a polyposis syndrome (Table 21.1). Approximately 50–65% will be adenomatous and 10–30% metaplastic (hyperplastic). Inflammatory polyps comprise 10–30% of the remainder and other types such as hamartomas and lipomas are very uncommon.

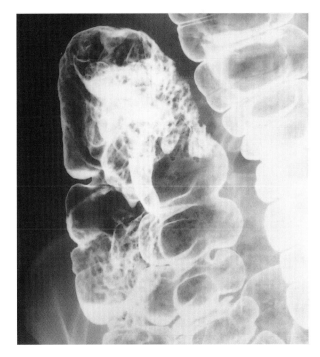

Fig. 21.1 Barium enema reveals two patches of filiform polyposis at the hepatic flexure in a patient with known Crohn's disease.

Re-epithelialisation of ulcerated colon may produce *inflammatory polyps*, which are dramatic in appearance but essentially only mucosal tags. They are classically filiform (Fig. 21.1) and may bleed. Inflammatory polyps carry no malignant risk, although rarely they can be so numerous as to cause colonic obstruction. They most commonly follow ulcerative colitis and Crohn's disease.

Metaplastic (hyperplastic) polyps are common, most notably in the rectum, where they appear as tiny pale, smooth nodules. They have a characteristic 'sawtoothed' epithelial lining but normal nuclei (cf. adenomas), and are generally not thought to carry any malignant risk. The term *serrated adenoma* describes the dysplastic hyperplastic polyp, up to 15% of which may contain a focus of adenocarcinoma.

Hamartomas may be either *juvenile* or associated with *Peutz–Jeghers syndrome* (see polyposis syndromes), and are developmental malformations composed of disorganised but otherwise normal intestinal tissue. Juvenile polyps show mucus retention cysts ('mucus retention polyps'), whereas hamartomas in Peutz–Jeghers syndrome show fibromuscular radiation between disorganised crypts. Solitary juvenile polyps are common in children and are frequently rectal, where they may present with bleeding. Isolated juvenile polyps are thought to carry no malignant risk.

Lipomas are submucosal, so that epithelial biopsy may be normal. They are easily deformable during compression, relatively radiolucent, and are typically right-sided (Fig. 21.2). Fatty infiltration of the ileocaecal valve may also occur and is difficult to distinguish from an adenoma afflicting the valve.

Adenomas are benign neoplasms of colorectal epithelium. By definition they are dysplastic and potentially premalignant, and their incidence increases with age. They may be tubular, tubulovillous or villous, the last being least common but with the greatest malignant potential and a propensity for rectosigmoid location. Villous adenomas have characteristic morphology, being broad based and relatively large, with a frond-like surface (Fig. 21.3). Most adenomas cause no symptoms but large polyps may bleed or cause electrolyte disturbance secondary to mucus secretion, especially if villous. The frequency of severe dysplasia increases with size, and size, villosity and dysplasia are the most important predictors of subsequent malignancy. The risk of malignancy in a 1 cm polyp is approximately 10% if villous. Malignancy is defined by invasive adenocarcinoma, i.e. cells penetrate the muscularis

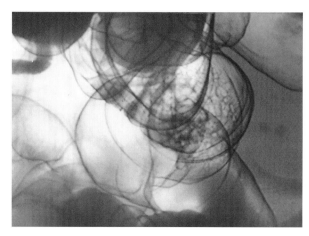

Fig. 21.3 A sigmoid villous adenoma, evidenced by a fine carpeting of frond-like projections.

mucosae to reach the submucosa. The term *malignant polyp* is used when a focus of invasive carcinoma is found within an excised adenoma. It is now generally appreciated that some adenomas are flat or depressed, and their morphology presents a considerable diagnostic challenge both for radiologists and endoscopists. Initially believed confined to oriental populations, there is increasing evidence that flat adenomas are found with equal frequency in the west if careful colonoscopy specifically aimed at their detection is performed (Rembacken et al 2000). Flat lesions may have greater malignant potential than elevated lesions.

Polyposis syndromes

Most histological types of polyp can be associated with a corresponding polyposis syndrome, all of which are relatively uncommon (Table 21.1). These syndromes are important because seemingly innocuous polyps that carry no risk of malignancy when single can convey increased risk when multiple. All patients whose risk of malignancy is significant require careful surveillance and consideration for prophylactic surgery.

Although metaplastic polyps are characterised by a lack of dysplasia, the polyps in *hyperplastic polyposis* may contain adenocarcinoma, raising the possibility of a separate syndrome, *serrated adenomatous polyposis*. Whereas isolated juvenile polyps are thought to carry no malignant risk, patients with the rarer *juvenile polyposis* (thought to be autosomal dominant and defined as five or more gastrointestinal polyps) are at risk of developing associated adenocarcinoma and require both upper and lower gastrointestinal surveillance. The role of prophylactic colectomy remains unclear.

Peutz–Jeghers syndrome is an autosomal dominant condition characterised by mucocutaneous pigmentation and intestinal hamartomatous polyps. As well as the large bowel, polyps occur in the stomach and small bowel and many patients suffer repeated episodes of intussusception. Epithelial displacement beneath the muscularis mucosae is commonly seen and has caused overdiagnosis of polyp malignancy. Nevertheless, these patients are at increased risk of malignancy, with approximately half of associated tumours occurring outside the gastrointestinal tract, including the breast, ovary, cervix and testis.

In *Cronkhite–Canada syndrome*, tiny hamartomatous polyps, usually in the stomach and colon, coexist with ectodermal changes, notably alopecia, nail loss and skin pigmentation. Diarrhoea may be

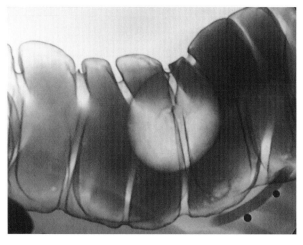

Fig. 21.2 Transverse colon lipoma. Note its exquisitely well-defined margins and compressibility under the compression paddle.

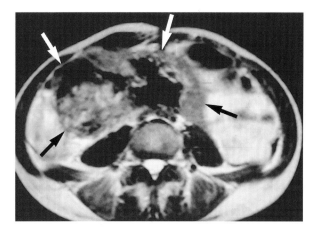

Fig. 21.5 Axial T$_2$-weighted MR image reveals a large central mesenteric desmoid tumour (arrows), with mixed signal.

is also evidence that high signal on T$_2$-weighted scans may indicate tumour activity (Fig. 21.5). Patients are also at risk of duodenal and periampullary carcinoma, and also liver, thyroid and brain neoplasms. Attenuated forms of FAP also exist, with patients presenting with fewer polyps later in life.

Gastrointestinal polyps can also occur in neurofibromatosis. Nodular lymphoid hyperplasia in children should not be mistaken for a polyposis syndrome, nor should pneumatosis coli. Barium enema in poorly prepared colons has also resulted in false-positive diagnoses of polyposis syndrome.

Radiographic appearance of polyps

Early lesions are usually sessile and, depending on size and location (dependent or non-dependent wall), appear on double-contrast barium enema as a barium-coated nodule projecting into the lumen (Fig. 21.6) or as a negative defect in the barium pool. Barium congregates in the angle where the polyp base meets normal colon, forming a 'meniscus', resulting in a ring shadow (Fig. 21.7). Because the polyp is a localised mass of soft tissue, its density is

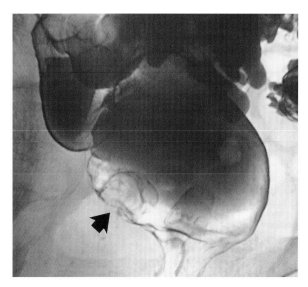

Fig. 21.6 A rectal adenoma visualised as a luminal nodule (arrow). This lesion was missed at sigmoidoscopy, presumably because of inadequate inspection during instrument insertion.

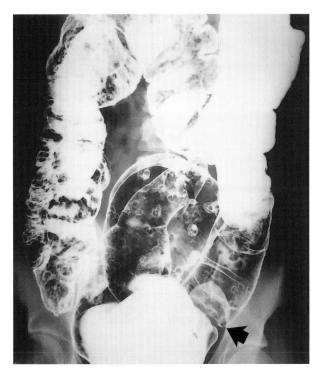

Fig. 21.4 Familial adenomatous polyposis (FAP). There are innumerable colonic adenomas. This adult woman refused colectomy, with the inevitable consequence of a cancer (arrow).

so severe as to cause death by malabsorption and protein loss. *Cowden's disease* is also an autosomal dominant multiple hamartoma syndrome, evidenced by skin and rectosigmoid polyps. Facial papillomas, extremity keratosis, pigmentation, lipomas, haemangiomas and neuromas also occur, as does colorectal, breast and thyroid cancer. *Ruvalcaba–Myhre–Smith syndrome* is possibly a variant of juvenile polyposis, characterised by ileal and colonic hamartomas, penile pigmentation and macrocephaly. *Turcot's syndrome* is an autosomal recessive association between colonic adenomas and carcinomas, and brain tumours.

Patients with *familial adenomatous polyposis (FAP)* comprise less than 0.5% of all those with colorectal cancers but are a clinically important group, not least because progression to cancer is inevitable if left untreated. FAP is an autosomal dominant syndrome due to mutations in the adenomatous poylposis coli (APC) gene and is characterised by innumerable colonic adenomas that develop with age (Fig. 21.4). Because the average patient will have developed colonic cancer by the age of 39 years, prophylactic colectomy with ileoanal pouch formation or ileorectal anastamosis (with subsequent surveillance of the rectal remnant) is advocated. In 1951, Gardner described a triad of skin, soft tissue and bony lesions (notably osteomas of the skull and mandible) but a growing list of associated features now precludes definition of a well-defined syndrome subset. Following colectomy, the commonest cause of death is from desmoid disease. Desmoids are benign but locally aggressive fibroproliferative tumours that are frequently mesenteric in FAP, resulting in intestinal obstruction. They are notoriously difficult to excise, not least because the belief that surgery may precipitate more aggressive tumours has resulted in a conservative approach and lesions are generally very large by the time laparotomy is attempted. CT and MR scanning are especially effective for monitoring desmoid disease and can detect precursor lesions. There

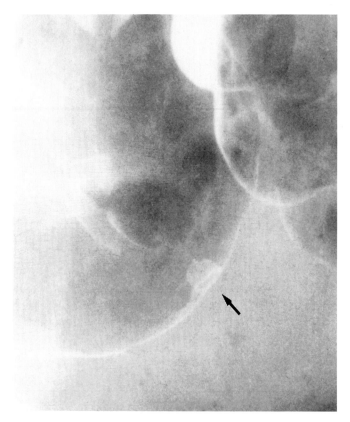

Fig. 21.7 A small polyp where the meniscal rim of barium between the polyp base and adjacent mucosa causes the 'bowler-hat' sign.

also increased in comparison to adjacent mucosa. Most difficulty arises when attempting to distinguish a possible polyp from a diverticulum or residue. In contrast to polyps, diverticulae have clearly defined outer margins, with gradual fading on the inside. Rotating

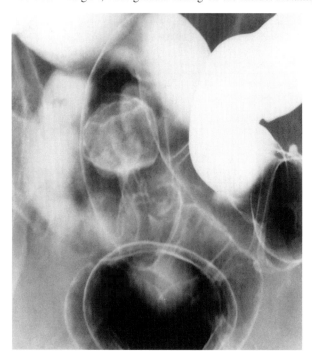

Fig. 21.8 A large, pedunculated sigmoid polyp.

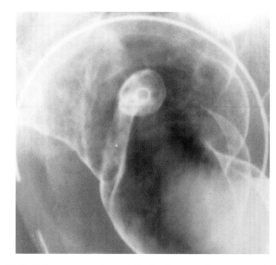

Fig. 21.9 When seen en face, stalked polyps produce a 'target' sign.

the patient so that the diverticulum is projected beyond the colonic lumen allows definitive distinction between the two. Residue can usually be persuaded to move by washing the barium pool over it or during compression.

As they grow, polyps become more elevated and surface nodularity becomes more pronounced. Some polyps, repeatedly exposed to the faecal stream, become pedunculated (Fig. 21.8). The stalk results in a 'target' sign when seen en face (Fig. 21.9). Although an attempt should be made to determine whether a polyp is benign or malignant on the basis of its morphology, this is frequently impossible. For example, large polyps tend to have irregular bases even when benign, and small polyps with smooth bases may be malignant. Radiologically, size alone is the best predictor of malignancy. Approximately 0.9% of adenomatous polyps 5–9 mm in size are malignant, compared with 5–10% measuring 10–20 mm and 10–50% measuring >20 mm (Morson 1974). Similarly, radiological morphology cannot reliably predict histology but on odd occasions this may be possible, for example with the typical fronds of a villous adenoma (Fig. 21.3) or deformability of a lipoma (Fig. 21.2). If one polyp is definitively demonstrated then a careful search for others should be made.

Colorectal cancer

Colorectal cancer is one of the commonest cancers in western Europe and the United States, with more than 300 000 cases a year. The cumulative lifetime risk is about 5%. Other types of malignant tumour comprise less than 1% of large bowel malignancies. Colorectal cancer occurs with roughly equal frequency in men and women and 5 year survival is approximately 50% overall. Most colorectal cancers are believed to arise from pre-existing adenomatous polyps via multistep accumulation of genetic faults: the 'adenoma–carcinoma sequence'. However, very few adenomatous polyps progress to cancer. Even then, an initiated polyp may grow for 10–15 years before becoming frankly malignant—'polyp dwell time'. It transpires that small adenomas are hardly ever malignant and a malignancy risk can be attributed according to polyp size, as described above. The whole issue of polyp measurement is fraught with difficulty whatever the modality used. Radiographic magnification of approximately 20% should be borne in mind when estimating polyp size from barium enema. Adenoma prevalence rises

Table 21.2 Distribution of adenomatous polyps and cancer

Site	Polyp frequency (%)	Cancer frequency (%)
Rectosigmoid	52	55
Descending colon	18	6
Transverse colon	11	11
Ascending colon	13	9
Caecum	7	13

with age, so that they occur in more than 50% of individuals over 70 years of age in most series. Paralleling this, colorectal cancer incidence also increases with age but mortality rates have fallen over recent years, probably due to polypectomy rather than any improvement in therapy. The distribution of adenomatous polyps also parallels the distribution of colorectal cancer, with most polyps and tumours being left sided (Table 21.2).

The risk of developing colorectal cancer is closely related to family history. Patients with an autosomal dominant condition such as FAP will inevitably develop colorectal cancer, and they account for approximately 1% of cases. In contrast, *hereditary non-polyposis colorectal cancer* (*HNPCC* or *Lynch syndrome*) accounts for approximately 5–10% of all colorectal cancers and is due to a dominantly inherited alteration within one of the DNA mismatch repair genes. To define the syndrome clinically, the patient should have colorectal cancer in at least three family members spanning two generations, with at least one case diagnosed before the age of 50 years—the 'Amsterdam' criteria (Lynch et al 1993). Tumours tend to be right sided and there may be associated urinary tract and gynaecological malignancy. The majority of colorectal cancers are believed to arise from sporadic adenomas ('adenoma–carcinoma sequence') but some cancers arise from non-polypoid dysplastic mucosa, for example occurring in inflammatory bowel disease.

Adenomas are defined by dysplasia, and cancer occurs when invasive adenocarcinoma crosses the muscularis mucosae to reach the submucosa. The prognosis of colorectal carcinoma is strongly related to this depth of penetration, or local stage. Working at St Mark's Hospital in London, Dukes devised the most simple and useful staging classification for rectal cancer, which combined bowel wall penetration (referring to the muscularis propria) with lymph node status (Table 21.3). Numerous other classifications exist, Dukes's original classification has been modified (e.g. B1/B2), and he has even been credited with stages (D) he never conceived!

The TNM classification for colorectal cancer is also widely used (Table 21.3). Radiological goals are the diagnosis of cancer and appropriate staging when this is necessary to direct appropriate therapy.

Typical presenting features include change in bowel habit, rectal bleeding and abdominal pain, although these symptoms are relatively common in older individuals without cancer. Radiological diagnosis of the primary tumour will usually be via barium enema. Any intraluminal shadow or line that cannot be confidently attributed to a normal feature must be viewed with suspicion. Frank carcinoma typically manifests as an annular, irregular, ulcerating lesion, giving rise to the classical 'apple-core' appearance (Fig. 21.10). In contrast to many benign or extrinsic strictures, carcinoma has abrupt, shouldered margins, and, as opposed to spasm, normal mucosal folds cannot be traced through the stricture lumen, indicating both a mucosal origin and destruction. Many cancers present as an eccentric tumour mass and some spread locally in a plaque-like infiltrative fashion where the lack of marked elevation makes detection difficult, especially when seen en face (Fig. 21.11). Overall, barium enema probably detects approximately 85% of colorectal cancers. Although technical factors such as poor distension, inadequate coating and overlapping loops all impair interpretation, most errors are perceptive in nature (Brady et al 1994). It is important to pay particular attention to those regions known to cause

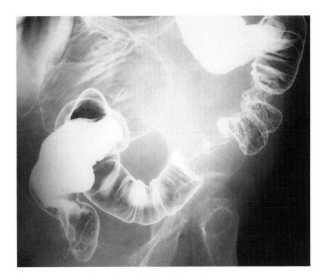

Fig. 21.10 Typical 'apple-core' sigmoid carcinoma.

Table 21.3 Comparison of Dukes's staging of rectal carcinoma and TNM classification for colorectal cancer

Dukes's stage		TNM classification	
A	Tumour confined to bowel wall	T1	Tumour involves submucosa
		T2	Tumour involves muscularis propria
B	Tumour penetrates bowel wall	T3	Tumour beyond muscularis propria
		N0	No involved nodes
C	Regional lymph nodes involved	N1	Up to three perirectal/colic nodes
		N2	Four or more perirectal/colic nodes
		N3	Apical node involved
		M0	No distant metastasis
(D)	Distant metastasis	M1	Distant metastasis

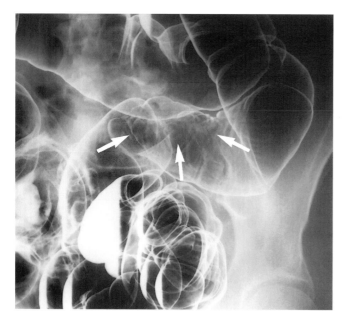

Fig. 21.11 Double-contrast barium enema reveals a diffuse, plaque-like sigmoid cancer (arrows).

problems, most notably the sigmoid colon (especially if there is diverticular disease), the ileocaecal valve and the rectum, where the enema tip may obscure pathology. The possibility of a synchronous cancer (5%) or polyp (25%) should be considered and sought if any lesion is detected.

Tumours disseminate via direct local extension, lymphatics (to local and distant nodes), veins (particularly to the liver and occasionally the lungs and bone) and peritoneum. In most instances the presence of disseminated disease will not prevent primary resection, so radiological detection of distant metastases before laparo-

tomy (during which time the surgeon takes time to directly inspect the abdomen and palpate the liver) is frequently unnecessary.

Although the features of colorectal cancer are usually typical, there is a differential diagnosis to be considered if radiological morphology is unusual. Secondary deposits (e.g. breast, gastric or pancreatic carcinoma) may exactly mimic a primary tumour, although long segments of bizarre stricturing and/or angulation should raise this possibility (Fig. 21.12). CT more elegantly demonstrates the nature and volume of extracolonic tumour and is useful in distinguishing between primary and secondary disease. Short segments of diverticular disease and ischaemic colitis may occasionally simulate a cancer, as may other primary large bowel tumours (discussed below). Inflammation due to Crohn's disease, amoebiasis and tuberculosis may also mimic a primary cancer, as may local segmental spasm. The apparent stricture produced by the latter may be persistent and appear remarkably like a carcinoma. The ileocaecal valve is a typical site. Further muscle relaxant and gas insufflation should help clarification.

Primary radiological diagnosis may also be achieved using other modalities, notably CT. In particular, CT is a viable alternative in frail elderly patients, in whom barium enema may be technically difficult and poorly tolerated. Bowel preparation is undesirable in the elderly but may not be necessary for CT because only large tumours are clinically relevant in this group. Furthermore, elderly patients have a high incidence of extracolonic disease, also detectable by CT. Several studies have found that minimal preparation CT does not miss significant colonic pathology in the elderly (Day et al 1993; Domjan et al 1998), suggesting it is a viable alternative to barium enema (Fig. 21.13). Ultrasound may also detect primary large bowel tumours, which are typically hypoechogenic.

It is worth mentioning that colorectal stenting may be used to overcome large bowel obstruction, either to palliate patients in whom surgery is not possible, or to avoid emergency surgery in those with acute obstruction, where morbidity and mortality are highest. Stent placement buys time for patient stabilisation and allows definitive surgery to be planned and performed at a later date. Stent placement is relatively straightforward: the colonic lumen is opacified with water-soluble contrast via a biliary manipulation or angiographic catheter, the catheter is advanced towards the distal edge of the stricture, and the stricture is crossed with a hydrophilic guide-wire. The catheter is then advanced through the tumour, the proximal colon opacified, and a metallic stent placed after exchange for a stiff guide-wire (Fig. 21.14).

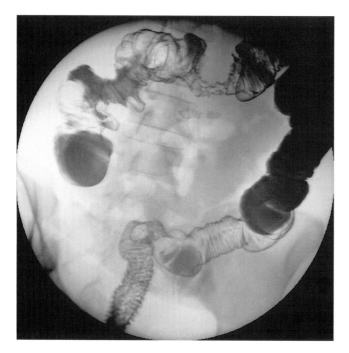

Fig. 21.12 Multiple bizarre strictures and mucosal pleating in a woman with extensive peritoneal carcinomatosis from an ovarian primary.

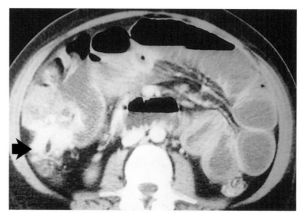

Fig. 21.13 CT reveals a strongly enhancing caecal carcinoma (arrow) in this elderly patient. Note associated small-bowel obstruction.

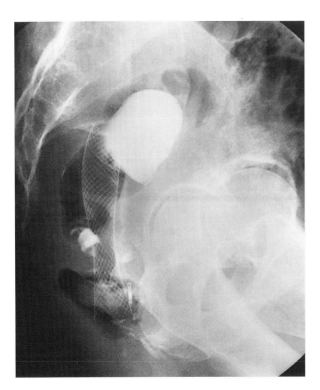

Fig. 21.14 Self-expanding metal stent crossing a low rectal tumour in a frail patient with extensive metastatic disease.

Rectal cancer

Approximately 40% of colorectal cancers occur in the rectum and may be considered a separate entity because the rectum is accessible and relatively immobile. Immobility permits accurate radiotherapy and accessibility allows transanal local excision if possible. Also, any tumour close to the anus raises the possibility of a permanent stoma, and adjuvant chemoradiotherapy may be able to 'downstage' these to avoid this. It therefore follows that rectal tumour staging is particularly useful. CT has been overtaken by MRI and transrectal ultrasound (TRUS) in this respect, with several studies confirming it lags behind because of an inability to visualise the muscularis propria (muscular rectal wall). However, it is unclear whether MRI or TRUS enjoy any advantage over one another. Both are able to demonstrate the muscularis propria (Fig. 21.15), and its relationship to any tumour. Local expertise and availability will most likely determine which is used.

Radiological assessment of recurrent disease

Surgery still offers the best chance of cure but approximately 20% of patients have disseminated disease at operation and a further 20% will harbor occult hepatic metastases. In the remainder, radical primary tumour clearance is the key to survival. Overall, approximately 50% will eventually die. Recurrence typically occurs within 2 years. *Local recurrence* (3–30%) is strongly related to operative experience and technique and carries a particularly poor prognosis; most patients die rapidly if symptomatic. Radiological diagnosis of local recurrence is frequently extremely difficult because of considerable overlap between the features of recurrence and those of postoperative fibrosis and radiotherapy change, both of which can be remarkably persistent. Generally tumour recurrence tends to form discrete masses, whereas fibrosis is more diffuse, but the degree of overlap is such that serial scans may be required and, even then, biopsy is often necessary. Both CT and MRI may be used, viable tumour returning high signal on T_2-weighted scans compared with fibrosis, which is low. It should be noted that oedema, inflamation and radiation change also return high signal. The multiplanar capabilities of MRI are particularly valuable when assessing the presacral space, using sagittal imaging, for recurrent rectal disease. Given the difficulties described, it may be worthwhile obtaining a baseline scan approximately 3 months after surgery, although there is considerable debate regarding the value of any type of structured follow-up because a definite survival advantage has not been demonstrated to date. Distant disease is predominantly hepatic and peritoneal and CT is generally satisfactory for detecting both of these.

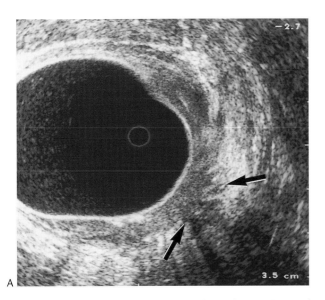

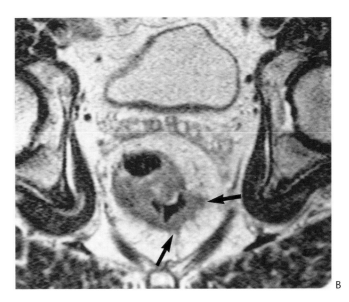

Fig. 21.15 (A) Transrectal ultrasound reveals a right posterior quadrant tumour that has penetrated the muscularis propria to reach surrounding tissue (arrows); stage uT3. (B) Axial T_2-weighted MR scan at the same level confirms the ultrasound finding of rectal wall penetration (arrows).

Screening for colorectal cancer

Mortality from colorectal cancer has remained relatively unchanged despite apparent advances in diagnosis and treatment. There is now considerable interest in screening for colorectal cancer because several studies have shown unequivocally reduced mortality. Screening aims to detect precancerous polyps or established cancer, but at an earlier stage, when 5 year survival is higher; 30% of screen detected cancer is Dukes's A, compared with 15% of symptomatic presentations. A variety of direct and indirect tests are advocated, including faecal occult blood testing (FOBT), barium enema, sigmoidoscopy and colonoscopy. The choice of screening modality is complex and controversial. FOBT is easy and cheap but detects less than half the prevalent cancers and large polyps. Colonoscopy is technically demanding, expensive and potentially dangerous. The barium enema is advocated on the basis of cost, safety and total colonic examination but may be insensitive for polyps in day-to-day practice (Rex et al 1997; Winawer et al 2000). Virtual colonoscopy is a CT-based technique that applies complex three-dimensional rendering algorithms to a helical CT of the gas-distended, cleansed colon (Fig. 21.16) (Halligan & Fenlon 1999). Initial assessment in pathology-enriched subgroups suggests that its accuracy for polyp and cancer detection exceeds that of barium enema and approaches colonoscopy (Fenlon et al 1999). If this proves to be true, then virtual colonoscopy will combine sensitivity and safety with total colonic examination, the 'holy grail' of colorectal cancer screening.

Other large bowel tumours

Over 99% of colorectal carcinomas are adenocarcinomas, 10% of the mucinous subtype. Other carcinomas, such as squamous and undifferentiated (oat), are described but very rare. Neuroendocrine *carcinoid tumours* may occur, notably in the caecum and rectum. *Stromal tumours* are composed of supportive tissues, for example neural and/or smooth muscle. Histological proof of malignancy

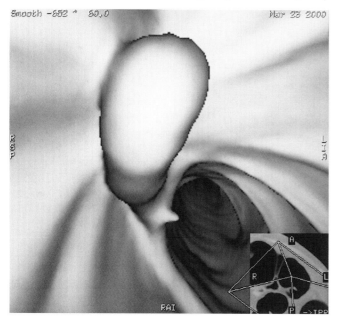

Fig. 21.16 Splenic flexure polyp revealed by virtual colonoscopy in a patient whose endoscopic colonoscopy had been normal.

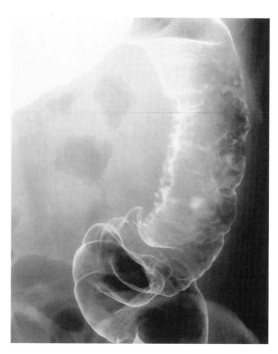

Fig. 21.17 Primary colonic non-Hodgkin's lymphoma. Note the irregular but intact mucosal line, suggesting the tumour has a submucosal origin.

may be difficult and size is often the best discriminator. Ulceration may indicate malignancy, although this also occurs in large, benign lesions. Most originate from the muscularis propria so that barium enema suggests a submucosal origin, with intact overlying mucosa. *Neural tumours* (neurilemmoma/fibroma) are rare, as are benign and malignant *haemangiomas*.

Colonic *lymphoma* usually arises from nodal disease and is rarely primary, accounting for only 0.5% of primary colorectal malignancy. Most lymphoid tissue occurs in the caecum and rectum and tumour distribution parallels this. The vast majority are non-Hodgkin's B-cell subtypes. Morphology is wide and varied, ranging from bulky polypoid lesions to diffuse, annular infiltrating forms (Fig. 21.17). The mucosa is usually intact, reflecting submucosal spread, and the lumen patent; obstruction is rare. CT findings of a bulky soft-tissue mass may suggest the underlying pathology. Colonic *Kaposi's sarcoma* is usually seen in association with AIDS or other causes of immunodeficiency.

Metastatic disease commonly involves the colon, either via intraperitoneal seeding (ovarian, gastric, pancreatic) or haematogenous routes (malignant melanoma, breast, lung). This diagnosis should be especially considered where there are multiple, bizarre, extrinsic lesions (Fig. 21.12). Particular sites also raise this possibility, most notably the pouch of Douglas. The colon may also be directly involved by contiguous spread from a primary tumour elsewhere, notably prostate, bladder and ovary, or by spread along an adjacent mesentery, for example pancreatic carcinoma via the transverse mesocolon to reach the transverse colon.

DIVERTICULAR DISEASE

Diverticular disease is ubiquitous in western civilisation, affecting approximately 30% over the age of 60 years and 60% over the age of 80 years. The disease was virtually unknown prior to 1900 and its subsequent incidence and geographic distribution suggest a direct relationship to industrialised methods of food processing. Inadequate dietary fibre as a consequence of carbohydrate refinement is believed to result in elevated colonic segmentation pressures. *Diverticulosis* describes the presence of acquired pulsion diverticula due to this pressure. These are mucosal herniations through vascular entry sites into pericolic fat, often between the mesenteric and antimesenteric taeniae. *Diverticulitis* implies superimposed inflammation, whereas the term *diverticular disease* encompasses both concepts. The sigmoid colon is typically affected, where there is muscular thickening due to elastosis, which results in luminal narrowing. This progressive elastosis, focused on the taeniae, also causes longitudinal foreshortening and accentuation of sigmoid corrugations. Furthermore, pericolic fibrosis and inflammation (due to micro- or macroperforation) also contribute. Muscle covering the diverticula tends to atrophy as they enlarge so that mucous membrane, connective tissue and peritoneum cover the mature diverticula. Less commonly, small protrusions of mucosa occur in the antimesenteric intertaenial area. These are frequently too small to reach the serosa (intramural diverticula), but sometimes do reach it to produce small transverse ridges.

Most patients are asymptomatic but many complain of vague left-sided abdominal pain and altered bowel habit, symptoms very similar to those of the irritable bowel syndrome. Approximately 10–25% of individuals with diverticulosis will experience bouts of diverticulitis that are evidenced by worsening left iliac fossa pain, constipation and/or diarrhoea, and possibly constitutional symptoms ('left-sided appendicitis'). The initial attack usually settles with bowel rest and antibiotics but more than 70% with symptoms will have recurrent episodes and 30% will eventually require surgery.

The distribution and severity of diverticular disease remains best demonstrated by barium enema. The diverticula themselves appear as flask-like or rounded outpouchings (Fig. 21.18). When seen en face they produce ring shadows. Differentiation from a polyp is a common problem (see above) but the definitive signs are projection beyond the bowel wall and the presence of a fluid level within it. Muscular change results in a concertina-like or serrated appearance (Fig. 21.18), frequently accentuated by pronounced and persistent spasm, which reflects abnormal motility.

Complications

Diverticulitis results in *pericolic abscess* and localised peritonitis. Barium enema is contraindicated acutely because of the risk of perforation; if the diagnosis needs confirmation, water-soluble contrast is preferred. Because of its ready availability, *ultrasound* is often the first imaging modality employed and can reveal mural thickening and pericolic inflammation, evidenced by altered fatty echogenicity, incompressibility and abscess. However, CT is of particular value in most hands, not only because it can also visualise mural thickening and attendant diverticula, but because it can precisely quantify diverticulitis, the hallmark of which is inflammatory change within pericolic fat (Fig. 21.19). CT-based staging systems have evolved which quantify the severity of pericolic disease and indicate prognosis:

Stage 0: Mural thickening and diverticula only
Stage 1: Abscess/phlegmon <3 cm in diameter
Stage 2: Abscess 5–15 cm in diameter
Stage 3: Abscess beyond the confines of the pelvis
Stage 4: Faecal peritonitis.

Stages 0 and 1 usually settle with conservative management, whereas stage 2 abscesses are ideal for percutaneous drainage under radiological guidance (Fig. 21.19). Stage 3 and 4 patients will need emergency surgery, although percutaneous drainage will temporise some stage 3 patients if clinically necessary. *Obstruction* may complicate an episode of diverticulitis, and spasm may be so severe as to obliterate the lumen. Occasionally small-bowel obstruction results from ileal adhesion to the inflammatory mass. Extension of inflammation to a neighbouring viscus or abdominopelvic wall may lead to the *fistulation*. The commonest is colovesical, between the sigmoid colon and the bladder, and occurs more often in males because of the interposition of the uterus between the colon and bladder in females. Symptoms include pneumaturia and recurrent urinary infection. CT is the most sensitive technique for demonstrating intravesical gas (Fig. 21.20). A water-soluble enema and/or cystogram will show the fistula in only approximately 30%; MRI may be more sensitive. Fistulas may also occur to the vagina, ileum or skin. Approximately 30% of patients with diverticular disease *haemorrhage*, typically from the vasa recta within a single uninflamed diverticulum. Although most cases are slight and occasional, diverticular disease is a well-recognised cause of torrential and life-threatening haemorrhage in the elderly and accounts for over 40% of major lower gastrointestinal bleeds in this age group.

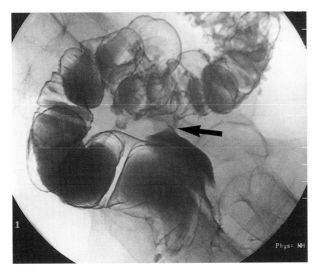

Fig. 21.18   Barium enema reveals severe sigmoid diverticular disease with a complicating fistula to the vagina (arrow).

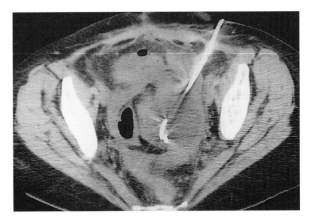

Fig. 21.19   CT was used to place a percutaneous drain into this large paracolic collection secondary to diverticular disease.

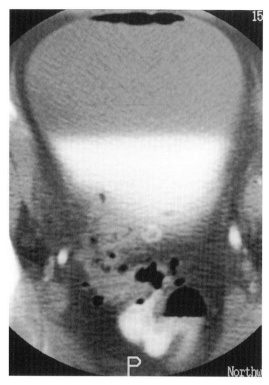

Fig. 21.20 CT reveals intravesical gas and the site of sigmoid fistulation on delayed scans.

Differential diagnosis

Differentiating between complicated diverticular disease and a perforated carcinoma is frequently difficult, even at laparotomy! A long segment of colonic thickening (>10 cm) in association with pericolic and mesenteric fluid suggests diverticulitis, whereas an abrupt mass with mesenteric lymph nodes favours carcinoma; however, there is considerable overlap in these appearances and liver metastasis found incidentally at CT is the only truly reliable differentiator. A water-soluble contrast enema is frequently helpful where the distinction remains in doubt but many individuals will have flexible endoscopy as the final arbiter once the acute episode has settled. Other differential diagnoses to consider include ischaemic colitis, inflammatory bowel disease (especially Crohn's colitis) and *primary epiploic appendagitis*, which refers to acute inflammation of an epiploic appendage, typified by a small pericolic mass which contains fat. There is no evidence that diverticular disease predisposes to malignancy but inevitably the two conditions sometimes coexist, as both are common, especially in older patients. The morphology of diverticular segments makes diagnosis of an underlying cancer difficult at the best of times but this should be considered in any patient where there is evidence of mucosal destruction or where a stricture is particularly irregular, shouldered, rigid, or contains no diverticula. It should be remembered that right-sided diverticulosis is a typically Asian phenomenon and diverticulitis in this instance will be difficult to distinguish from appendicitis, with CT again the most useful modality. Rectal diverticula are vanishingly rare.

The rarely encountered *giant sigmoid diverticulum* is believed to be secondary to a previous walled-off perforation following an acute attack of diverticulitis or due to a 'ball-valve' effect at the diverticular neck. *Giant caecal diverticulum* is equally rare but likely to be congenital.

COLITIS

Colitis describes colonic inflammation, which can be broadly subdivided into idiopathic, ischaemic and infectious aetiologies. The hallmarks of colitis are mucosal inflammation and ulceration, the nature of which is central to accurate radiological diagnosis. The morphology of mucosal ulceration remains best appreciated via contrast studies; indeed, many subtle forms can only be imaged this way. Because of this, contrast enemas remain the cornerstone of radiological differential diagnosis.

IDIOPATHIC INFLAMMATORY BOWEL DISEASE

Current theories of pathogenesis suggest that *Crohn's disease* and *ulcerative colitis* arise because of aberrant host responses to enteric environmental agents in genetically susceptible individuals. To date neither the genetic susceptibility nor the environmental agents have been elucidated so the term 'idiopathic inflammatory bowel disease' persists. There are idiopathic colitides other than Crohn's disease and ulcerative colitis, notably the *microscopic colitides*, but the former are by far the most prevalent. Histology is frequently unable to distinguish between the two, so diagnosis is often only possible by using a combination of clinical, radiological, endoscopic and histological features. The incidence of ulcerative colitis has remained static for several years but that of Crohn's disease continues to climb.

Ulcerative colitis

Ulcerative colitis is characterised by relapsing and remitting proctitis. The rectum is always affected but proximal spread occurs in a continuous fashion in approximately two-thirds of patients, half of whom will have total colitis at the time of presentation. The disease afflicts young adults (15–25 years), with a second smaller peak at approximately 60 years. It is a disease of developed countries, where patients are typically city-dwelling, white, non-smokers. Approximately 10–20% will have a similarly affected first-degree relative. Attacks are characterised by bloody diarrhoea, with or without constitutional symptoms. Although most patients will have a chronic low-grade illness, approximately 15% present with acute, fulminating colitis and are at risk of colonic perforation and death. Extraintestinal manifestations include arthralgia, erythema nodosum, pyoderma gangrenosum and sclerosing cholangitis. Because the rectum is always involved, proctoscopy and sigmoidoscopy with biopsy are essential. Loss of the normal mucosal vascular pattern is the earliest detectable change, and there may be contact bleeding. These changes progress through mucosal granularity and spontaneous haemorrhage to frank, continuous ulceration.

Plain films

The main role of plain films is the reliable and rapid assessment of disease extent and severity in *acute colitis*. A study of 97 patients in whom the extent of macroscopic colitis had been determined by colonoscopy or resection found that abdominal films could accu-

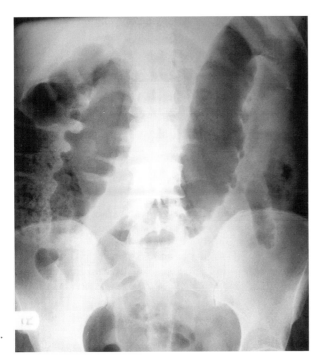

Fig. 21.21 Toxic megacolon. Luminal dilatation, abnormal haustration, mural thickening and mucosal islands.

rately diagnose extent in 78 (80%) (Prantera et al 1991). In total colitis the most reliable radiological features were 'irregularity of the mucosal edge' and 'increased thickness of the colon wall', which were present in 74% and 68%, respectively, of correctly classified patients. At least one of these features and/or 'loss of haustral clefts' and 'empty right colon' were present in 30 of 31 (97%) patients with total colitis (Prantera et al 1991). Since caecal residue is normally present, a totally empty colon in a patient with known disease suggests a total colitis. In the absence of enough spontaneous intraluminal air to assess the colonic wall, an informative gas shadow may be obtained by gentle insufflation of rectal air—the 'air enema'. Although colonoscopy is relatively safe in acute ulcerative colitis, the air enema can assess the entire colon more rapidly, and with less discomfort and probably with less risk (Almer et al 1996). There is excellent correlation between air enema and subsequent histopathology when severity and distribution of disease are assessed (Almer et al 1996).

Plain abdominal radiography is used to detect *acute toxic dilatation/megacolon* (diagnosed when transverse colonic diameter exceeds 5.5 cm) (Fig. 21.21). Toxic dilatation has a differential, including Crohn's disease, ischaemic colitis and amoebiasis, but is most common in ulcerative colitis and is accompanied by marked constitutional symptoms such as tachycardia and pyrexia. Diarrhoea is profuse. The transverse colon is the segment most often dilated on plain films, due to the patient's supine position. The haustra will be effaced or blunted, indicating that ulceration is transmural, causing neuromuscular degeneration. There will be no or little residue. The mucosal line is irregular, producing so-called 'mucosal islands' because of adjacent mucosal ulceration and sloughing. The colon has a consistency akin to wet blotting paper, so patients are at risk of perforation and ultimately death. Free air will be most apparent in either the erect or left lateral decubitus positions but CT remains the procedure of choice to exclude this; as little as 1 ml can be detected when scans are viewed on the appropriate imaging windows. Abdominal films should be performed daily where toxic dilatation is a possibility or established, or even more frequently if indicated, and are used to assess response to intensive medical therapy, and appropriately schedule emergency colectomy when necessary. Those patients whose plain films show excess small bowel gas are more likely to need surgery: a study of 75 patients with acute, severe disease found that all those whose abdominal film showed more than four loops of gas-filled small bowel failed medical therapy (Chew et al 1991).

Contrast studies

Double-contrast barium enema is more accurate than the single-contrast study in revealing early disease and is the radiological examination of choice to show disease extent and severity, with considerable value in the differential diagnosis of colitis. Double-contrast barium enema cannot visualise alterations in mucosal vascular pattern, with the result that proctosigmoidoscopy is approximately 15–20% more sensitive overall for primary diagnosis of early, distal ulcerative colitis. Barium enema also underestimates disease extent, and comparison with resection specimens suggests that the entire colon is involved histologically when changes on double-contrast barium enema extend as far proximally as the hepatic flexure (Bartram & Walmsley 1978). Contrast enema accurately assesses disease severity because depth of ulceration is readily appreciated. Contrast enema remains the most accurate technique for demonstrating overall colonic morphology and has a role in long-term management because of this, especially where the exact location and extent of any stricture needs to be defined, or

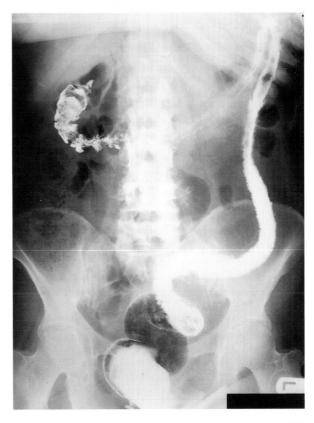

Fig. 21.22 Instant enema in a patient with ulcerative colitis reveals fine, continuous, symmetrical, left-sided ulceration.

where there is technical difficulty with colonoscopy. Faecal residue does not accumulate where there is active ulceration, so these patients do not require bowel preparation for an enema—the 'instant enema'. The instant enema provides a rapid assessment of the extent of colitis in those patients where its proximal extent cannot be seen sigmoidoscopically. Any barium examination is absolutely contraindicated if there is evidence of toxic dilatation or where a recent rectal biopsy increases the risk of perforation and subsequent barium peritonitis. A plain film should precede the contrast examination where there is doubt. The enema is conducted in the usual way except that the flow of barium is stopped if the patient complains of pain or when formed residue is encountered. The rectum is then drained and the colon insufflated, and prone, lateral and erect films obtained (Fig. 21.22).

The instant enema provides a rapid and accurate assessment of disease extent during an acute episode, where this cannot be determined sigmoidoscopically, and is used to guide treatment. In contrast, patients with longstanding disease in a quiescent phase require full bowel preparation and a conventional double-contrast study. The earliest radiological change is blurring of the mucosal line and a fine granularity when the mucosa is seen en face, due to oedema, abnormal barium adherence to altered colonic mucus and flecks of barium adhering to superficial erosions. As the disease progresses, this granularity becomes coarser and eventually frank ulceration develops, revealed by projections of barium outside the mucosal line and pools of barium in the en face view. Ulceration is continuous and tends to be superficial, although deeper ulceration does occur. It should be noted that, although ulcers may seem deep, this is an impresssion evinced by significant surrounding mucosal oedema. Ulceration always occurs against a background of a diffusely abnormal mucosa and, unlike Crohn's disease, discrete ulceration with intervening normal mucosa is never seen. Similarly, spontaneous transmural ulceration never occurs unless there is toxic dilatation (cf. Crohn's disease). Mucosal changes are accompanied by haustral blunting, luminal narrowing and colonic shortening due

to muscular abnormality rather than fibrosis, which is not a feature of this disease. A tubular, short, featureless colon is typical of longstanding total colitis. It should be noted that haustration may normally be absent from the mid-transverse colon distally.

The presacral space tends to widen owing to rectal narrowing and surrounding fatty proliferation. In those individuals with a total colitis, the ileocaecal valve becomes fixed and incompetent, resulting in terminal ileal granularity (back-wash ileitis), which should not be confused with the terminal ileitis of Crohn's disease (Fig. 21.23). The re-epithelialisation of ulcerated mucosa that follows a severe attack may result in *postinflammatory polyps*, which have a pathognomonic frond-like appearance (Fig. 21.1). These consist of granulation or fibrous tissue with an epithelial covering and form a 'road map' of previous severe disease. Although generally innocuous, they may be so numerous as to cause colonic obstruction. *Strictures* may also complicate longstanding disease and are usually smooth and symmetrical and will need to be differentiated from *carcinoma complicating ulcerative colitis*. These carcinomas arise from dysplastic mucosa rather than adenomatous polyps. Patients with longstanding (more than 10 years) total colitis are at most risk and frequently enter colonoscopic surveillance programmes, where they undergo multiple colonic biopsies at regular intervals to search for dysplasia. Although, when meticulously performed, double-contrast barium enema can detect approximately two-thirds of lesions associated with colonic dysplasia in ulcerative colitis (Matsumoto et al 1996), it is not recommended for primary diagnosis because it is likely that most dysplasia will be missed in the majority of hands. Furthermore, dysplasia cannot be reliably distinguished from inflammatory nodules. In some patients, double-contrast barium enema may direct the endoscopist to specific locations for biopsy.

Crohn's disease

In contrast to ulcerative colitis, Crohn's disease can involve any part of the gastrointestinal tract from mouth to anus. Like ulcerative colitis, it is a disease of young adults and extraintestinal features similarly occur. Over half will have *small-bowel disease*, with or without colonic disease, but approximately one-quarter will have disease limited to the large bowel and differential diagnosis from ulcerative colitis becomes relevant. Although the disease is also characterised by mucosal ulceration, this is typically transmural and discontinuous (cf. ulcerative colitis). The histopathological hallmark is the *non-caseating granuloma* but this is frequently absent. *Toxic megacolon* also complicates Crohn's disease and the comments above about the utility of plain films similarly apply.

Contrast studies

Contrast radiography plays a far greater role in the diagnosis and assessment of the distribution and severity of Crohn's disease, primarily because most patients will have small bowel disease, diagnosis of which remains mostly in the radiological domain. Concerning colonic disease, like ulcerative colitis, barium enema cannot demonstrate early vascular changes, so the first radiological features are granularity and *aphthous ulceration*. Aphthous ulcers are small and discrete, and are surrounded by slightly elevated oedematous mucosa. Barium collects in the central depression, with the surrounding elevation appearing as a radiolucent halo (Fig. 21.24).

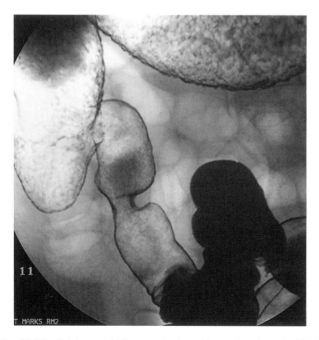

Fig. 21.23 Patulous, rigid ileocaecal valve with associated terminal ileal granularity ('back-wash ileitis') in a patient with total ulcerative colitis.

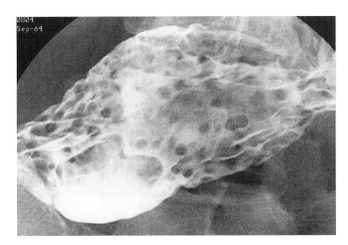

Fig. 21.24 Innumerable aphthoid ulcers in Crohn's disease.

Aphthous ulcers frequently occur on a background of otherwise normal mucosa. Although they are not specific to Crohn's disease (they also occur in tuberculosis, Behçet's disease, yersinia and amoebic colitis) they are not found in ulcerative colitis so their presence strongly suggests the former. As the disease progresses, ulceration becomes longitudinal and deeper; indeed, *transmural ulceration* is typical of Crohn's disease and results in deep, fissuring ulcers. Deep longitudinal ulcers combined with adjacent mucosal oedema results in a characteristic 'cobblestone' appearance (Fig. 21.25). Disease tends to be characteristically discontinuous, both longitudinally and circumferentially, i.e. one side of the bowel wall is affected while the other is spared. Contraction at the site of ulcer formation results in *pseudodiverticula*, which are characteristic of Crohn's disease (Fig. 21.26). Unlike ulcerative colitis, the rectum is histologically spared in approximately 50% of patients and, because of

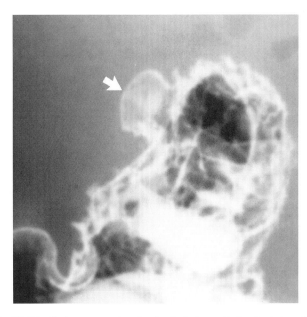

Fig. 21.26 Barium enema showing the typical pseudodiverticula found in Crohn's disease.

this, barium enema is superior to proctosigmoidoscopy for diagnosis. *Fistula-in-ano* is a characteristic complication, however, and an underlying diagnosis of Crohn's disease should be considered in any complex or recurrent fistula. The depth of ulceration predisposes to *pericolic abscess* formation and *fistulation*. Contrast studies may fill these but are frequently negative and cross-sectional imaging will be required for diagnosis (Fig. 21.27). Although the discontinuous nature of disease implies that the instant enema will be of limited use, in practical terms, this seems to make little difference. *Post-inflammatory polyposis* occurs as in ulcerative colitis, but in Crohn's disease this is more often patchy and segmental in distribution, reflecting the disease process. *Strictures* are very common and vary widely in their morphology. Although less than with ulcerative colitis, there remains an increased risk of *colonic carcinoma* (Connell et al 1994). The risk of *small-bowel carcinoma* is also increased, as is that of *lymphoma*. Additionally, long-standing anorectal disease may predispose to local carcinomatous change.

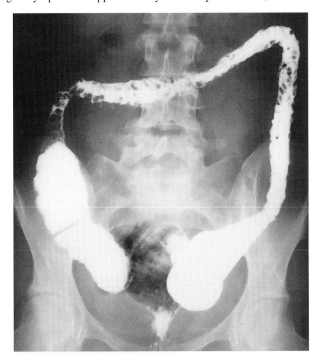

Fig. 21.25 Instant enema in Crohn's disease demonstrates extensive 'cobblestoning' due to linear ulceration and mucosal oedema. Note the rectum is relatively spared but contains aphthoid ulcers.

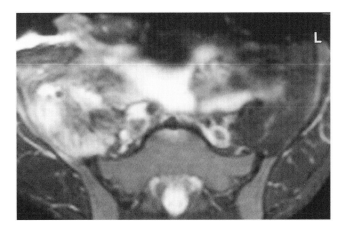

Fig. 21.27 T$_2$-weighted, fat-suppressed, axial MR scan demonstrates a right-sided psoas abscess (compare to the contralateral side).

Ultrasound, CT and MRI in inflammatory bowel disease

Ultrasound cannot diagnose early mucosal disease because its spatial resolution is inferior to double-contrast barium enema. However, ultrasound can readily diagnose bowel wall thickening. Graded probe compression to displace bowel and assess compressibility should be used. In experienced hands, ultrasound approaches the sensitivity of CT and MRI for assessment of complicated disease, notably fistulas and abscesses (Gasche et al 1999), and it is commonly requested to exclude these. However, ultrasound is highly operator dependent and, even in good hands, some sites remain poorly visualised, either due to overlying bowel gas, tenderness, or because they are deep in the pelvis; a normal ultrasound study does not exclude a pelvic collection. Ultrasound has a particular role in children where a diagnosis of Crohn's disease has been established because they are technically easy to examine, avoiding exposure to ionising radiation.

In common with ultrasound, CT cannot diagnose early mucosal disease but bowel wall thickening is easily appreciated and CT is superior to barium studies and endoscopy for the diagnosis of extramural complications. Because CT is less operator dependent and the whole abdominopelvic cavity is easily imaged, it remains superior to ultrasound for the diagnosis of extramural complications, notably abscesses, with a particularly relevant role when ultrasound has been negative but clinical suspicion remains high. CT may also detect extraintestinal complications, for example gallstones, pancreatitis, arthritis and nephrolithiasis.

The role of MRI is similar to that of CT, sharing many of its advantages. MRI is especially suited to the pelvis, and fat suppression techniques, combined with sequences that highlight fluid, emphasise collections more than is the case of CT (Fig. 21.27). MRI surpasses all other assessment techniques, including examination under anaesthetic, for the assessment of perianal sepsis in Crohn's disease (Halligan 1998). The choice between CT and MRI will largely depend on local availability and radiologist preference.

Table 21.4   Differential diagnosis between ulcerative colitis and Crohn's colitis on double-contrast barium enema

Abnormality	Ulcerative colitis	Crohn's disease
Mucosal change		
Granularity	++	+
Aphthoid ulcers	–	++
Deep ulceration	–	++
Discontinuous ulceration	–	++
Rectal sparing	–	+
Colonic configuration		
Colonic shortening	++	+
Haustral obliteration	++	+
Pseudodiverticula	–	++
Spontaneous enteric fistulas	–	++
Abscess formation	–	++
Small-bowel disease	–	++
Anal disease	–	++
Toxic megacolon	++	+

Distinguishing between ulcerative colitis and Crohn's disease

Radiologically, contrast studies remain the technique of choice to differentiate ulcerative colitis from Crohn's disease because they most elegantly demonstrate mucosal morphology (Table 21.4). An unequivocal diagnosis of Crohn's colitis is possible because of constellations of specific features: aphthoid ulceration, deep ulceration, discontinuous ulceration, asymmetric involvement and fistulas. A study of 53 patients with colitis found that barium enema was able to determine the underlying diagnosis in 28 of 29 (97%) with Crohn's disease and in 20 of 24 (83%) with ulcerative colitis (Kelvin et al 1978). It should be borne in mind that, although mucosal granularity and continuous distal involvement are more suggestive of ulcerative colitis, these may also be found in Crohn's disease. Because of this, an unequivocal barium enema diagnosis of ulcerative colitis is impossible. Where Crohn's colitis seems more likely, tuberculosis, yersinia and lymphoma should be considered if radiological or clinical features are atypical. Cross-sectional techniques are less helpful: although patients with Crohn's colitis generally have thicker colons than those with ulcerative colitis (mean thickness 13 mm versus 8 mm, normal maximal value 3 mm), CT is unable reliably to distinguish these on an individual basis unless there are associated features of small-bowel disease or extramural complications (Gore et al 1996). Ultrasound can distinguish individual bowel wall layers more reliably than either CT or MRI and it has been suggested that these layers remain visible in ulcerative colitis in contrast to Crohn's disease, despite mural thickening in both (Limberg & Osswald 1994). Stratification may also be apparent on CT, a phenomenon commonest in ulcerative colitis but again non-specific, also occurring in Crohn's disease, infectious enterocolitides, pseudomembranous colitis, irradiation and ischaemia. Because of this, CT cannot be recommended for primary diagnosis of colitis. Once toxic megacolon is established, even histology has very considerable difficulty establishing the underlying aetiology.

Surgery for ulcerative colitis and Crohn's disease

Because ulcerative colitis only affects the large bowel, colectomy will cure the disease, and is performed because of symptoms or where the risk of malignant transformation is unacceptably high. The simplest operation is *total proctocolectomy and ileostomy* but this leaves the patient with a stoma. *Colectomy and ileorectal anastamosis* leaves a rectal segment that remains susceptible to proctitis and which will need to be surveyed for dysplasia. Ileal reservoirs may be either the *Kock ileostomy*, which is a continent reservoir in place of a simple ileostomy (which the patient empties by self-catheterisation), or the *ileoanal pouch*, where an ileal reservoir is anastamosed directly to the anus, thereby avoiding a stoma. The Kock pouch remains continent because of a nipple valve, and pouchography to define this valve is performed if the pouch becomes incontinent or difficult to catheterise. Ileoanal pouches are usually created with a covering ileostomy; *water-soluble pouchography* is used to check anastamotic integrity before the ileostomy is taken down and continuity restored. Leaks usually occur from the posterior aspect of the ileoanal anastamosis, with tracking into the presacral space and abscess formation (Fig. 21.28). The choice of

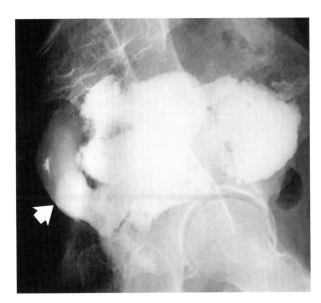

Fig. 21.28 Water-soluble pouchography reveals a presacral collection (arrow) originating from the posterior aspect of the pouch–anal anastamosis.

surgery is more complex in Crohn's disease because of its widespread and patchy nature. It is important to establish all sites of active disease; approximately 25% will have disease limited to the colorectum. Also, the possibility of postoperative complications, notably fistulation, has led to an understandable relative reluctance to operate. However, surgery is frequently performed for failed medical therapy and to treat complications. Ileoanal pouch formation, once relatively contraindicated, is now increasingly utilised.

ISCHAEMIC COLITIS

Mesenteric ischaemia can be acute or chronic, arterial or venous. The colon is particularly vulnerable to mesenteric ischaemia, notably the splenic flexure (see above, Anatomy and Function), and ischaemic colitis, once thought to be a rare condition, is actually very common. Most patients are elderly arteriopaths and ischaemia ranges from an imperceptible, transient assault to severe gangrene. Only those with significant symptoms usually come to hospital, so that the condition is probably underdiagnosed. Typical hospital presentation is with torrential rectal bleeding, with or without abdominal pain. The colonic mucosa is most susceptible to ischaemia, which causes oedema, haemorrhage and ulceration. The usual outcome is spontaneous healing but fibrosis following transmural ischaemia may eventually result in subsequent colonic stricturing. A proportion of cases with severe ischaemia will progress directly to gangrene and marked peritonism. There is also a well-described association with underlying carcinoma. Although there are a variety of well-established causes (for example, arterial thrombosis or embolism, venous thrombosis or embolism, diabetes, polyarteritis, slow-flow states, hypercoagulability), an underlying aetiology is rarely evinced.

Plain films are frequently taken and often reveal splenic flexure irregularity with mural thickening. The advent of colonoscopy has lessened the impact of barium enema for diagnosis, but where this has been performed, ulceration or the classical oedematous 'thumb-printing' may be seen acutely (Fig. 21.29). Haustration is lost. CT

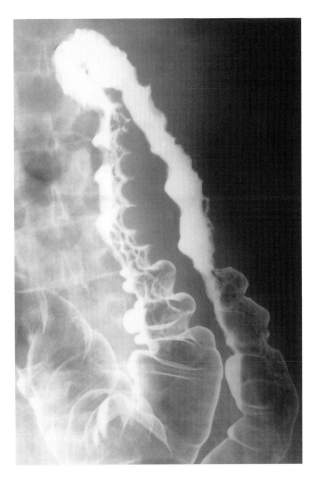

Fig. 21.29 Classical splenic flexure 'thumb-printing' diagnosing ischaemic colitis.

and ultrasound will demonstrate mural thickening but, because of overlap with other colitides, its distribution will be the only real imaging clue as to the underlying aetiology. Although routine subsequent barium enema to search for stricture formation is now no longer recommended, this remains the best study for demonstrating the presence and morphology of any stricture in those patients who develop symptoms. The stricture is often rather bizarre in configuration and large sacculations, rather redolent of Crohn's disease, are typical (Fig. 21.30).

INFECTIVE AND NON-INFECTIVE COLITIDES

A wide variety of organisms and their toxins may cause colitis, and differentiation between them, if necessary, is largely a microbiological or histopathological responsibility rather than radiological. Most cases are self-limiting and need no specific investigation. The presence or absence of concomitant *small-bowel disease* may give clues as to the organism responsible. Bacterial colitis is common and imaging usually reveals a non-specific segmental or pancolitis. Examples are infections caused by *Campylobacter, Salmonella, Shigella, Yersinia* spp and certain strains of *Escherichia coli*. Special mention must be given to *pseudomembranous colitis*, which is caused by overgrowth of *Clostridium difficile,* usually because broad-spectrum antibiotics administered in hospital have eradicated competing intestinal flora. Diagnosis is usually endoscopic, which reveals characteristic pseudomembranes, but occasionally patients

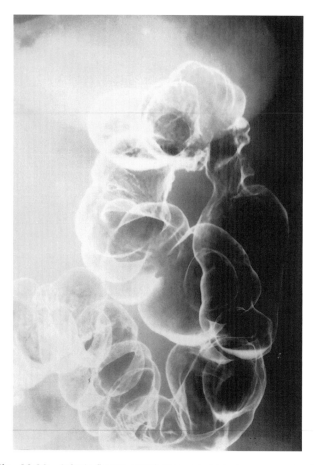

Fig. 21.30 Splenic flexure sacculation and stricturing as sequelae to ischaemic colitis.

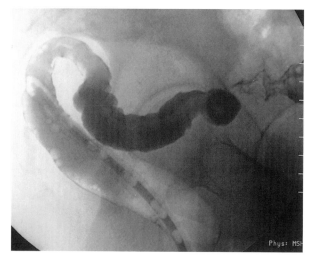

Fig. 21.31 Generally narrowed sigmoid and proximal rectum following radiotherapy.

non-specific colitis in susceptible patients. *Cystic fibrosis* is also associated with an inflammatory colitis and *fibrosing colonopathy*.

MISCELLANEOUS CONDITIONS

Appendicitis

Although historically a clinical diagnosis, a high negative laparotomy rate has driven the search for reliable preoperative imaging diagnosis. Currently ultrasound and CT both have their advocates. Ultrasound is highly operator dependent and relies heavily on graded compression, using the ultrasound probe to assess tissue compressibility. A thickened, dilated (more than 5 mm) appendix is highly suggestive of appendicitis (Puylaert et al 1987). In recent years CT has been suggested as a more reliable alternative (Rao et al 1997). The colon is filled with a large volume of dilute water-soluble contrast and scans limited to the right iliac fossa are taken. CT directly demonstrates periappendiceal inflammation, in contrast to ultrasound where it is revealed by periappendiceal incompressibility, and may be less operator dependent than ultrasound. However, ionising radiation may understandably limit its use in children.

Acquired immunodeficiency syndrome

Immunosuppression in AIDS predisposes to malignancy. Fifty per cent of patients with *Kaposi's sarcoma* of the skin and lymph nodes will also have a gastrointestinal tract tumour, which may be anywhere from pharynx to rectum. Tumours are often multiple and scattered throughout the gut. Lesions originate in the submucosa and may progress to large bulky masses. Patients may also develop other tumours, particularly *lymphoma*. Malignant melanoma and anal tumours are also described. Infective colitides are also common and AIDS may present with a non-specific proctitis. Cytomegalovirus may cause a local or diffuse colitis, and particularly affects the proximal colon. Initially the disease manifests as a diffuse nodular lymphoid hyperplasia, progressing to discrete multifocal ulceration. There may be progression to deeper ulceration and ultimately haemorrhage and perforation. *Tuberculous colitis is*

will come directly to imaging such as CT, often because the diagnosis remains unsuspected. *Tuberculosis* may cause colitis, the morphology of which is similar to Crohn's disease. A conical, contracted caecum is said to be characteristic and longitudinal and aphthoid ulcers may occur. Parasitic disease such as amoebiasis, strongyloidiasis, anisakiasis and schistosomiasis may also cause colitis, as can viruses such as CMV (especially in immunocompromised HIV patients), and fungal infection, such as histoplamosis and actinomycosis.

Radiation colitis may follow pelvic irradiation after a variable period, with a median of 2 years; 80% present within 5 years. Colitis is predominantly ischaemic, due to small vessel obliteration, with subsequent fibrosis. Diarrhoea with blood and mucus is frequent, as is stricture formation. Because of their relation to the irradiated field, strictures tend to be rather generalised and gradually segue into adjacent normal mucosa (Fig. 21.31). There may be accompanying ulceration or occasionally fistula formation. An appropriate history will clinch the diagnosis.

Microscopic colitis describes colitis where there is no radiological or endoscopic abnormality. Patients are grouped into those with either lymphocytic or collagenous forms, depending on the predominant histological infiltrate. *Eosinophilic colitis* may produce findings similar to ischaemia. *Neutropenic colitis (typhlitis)* occurs in immunocompromised patients, usually secondary to chemotherapy, and typically presents with right-sided inflammation. It was first described in leukaemic children but also occurs in adults, and is a diagnosis of exclusion. *Graft-versus-host disease* also causes a

relatively common but does not differ in its characteristics from non-AIDS-related disease. Colitis has also been described with *Mycobacterium avium* and *M. intracellulare*.

Colonic angiodysplasia

Angiodysplasia is a relatively common cause of lower gastrointestinal bleeding but is frequently difficult to diagnose because gross colonic morphology is unaltered; barium enema is normal. However, the lesions are readily visualised during colonoscopy. Unlike upper gastrointestinal bleeding, lower gastrointestinal bleeding rarely presents as an emergency, tending to be more indolent. When there is severe active bleeding, selective visceral angiography may demonstrate the site and cause (e.g. distinguishing between angiodysplasia and diverticular disease), thereby avoiding blind colonic resection and also raising the possibility of therapeutic embolisation. Other colonic vascular malformations also occur, for example hamartomas.

Volvulus

The colon may twist on its mesentery, resulting in intermittent obstruction. Prerequisites are a sufficiently redundant mesentery and associated loop to allow rotation around a fixed point. Sigmoid volvulus is commonest (60–75% of cases) and patients are usually elderly, suggesting that the condition is acquired. Caecal and transverse volvulus may also occur if the associated mesocolon is unusually long. Diagnosis is usually by plain film, although a water-soluble contrast enema may be needed for definitive diagnosis, especially where pseudo-obstruction is a possibility. An inverted 'U' without haustra suggests sigmoid volvulus and its apex frequently overlaps the transverse colon. There may be considerable proximal colonic gas and possibly small bowel gas but there is no rectal gas. The caecum is often ectopic in caecal volvulus (e.g. in the left upper quadrant), causing diagnostic confusion. Again there may be considerable small bowel gas but the remaining colon is usually deflated. CT will reveal a 'whorl' sign in all, due to the twisted mesentery and associated vessels.

Pseudo-obstruction

Intestinal pseudo-obstruction may predominantly affect the colon, causing gross dilatation that mimics mechanical obstruction on plain films. Contrast enemas will fail to reveal an obstruction. The underlying disorder is a visceral neuropathy or myopathy affecting gastrointestinal smooth muscle. Although often idiopathic, an association with underlying malignancy (e.g. oat cell lung carcinoma) is well described and this should be sought before a confident diagnosis is made.

Pneumatosis coli

Pneumatosis coli (pneumatosis cystoides intestinalis) is defined by multiple gas-filled cysts that lie submucosally or subserosally; overlying mucosa is normal. The idiopathic condition is rare but may be confused with life-threatening colonic disease. The small bowel is also affected. Pneumatosis may be secondary to bowel necrosis, for example necrotising enterocolitis or mesenteric thrombosis. It can also follow endoscopy or chronic obstructive pulmonary disease; it

is presumed that alveolar rupture allows air to track along the bronchi to reach the mediastinum and thence the retroperitoneum and mesentery. Cysts may be seen on plain film and produce multiple filling defects on barium enema if submucosal. Cysts are commonest in the sigmoid and descending colon, and symptoms, if they occur, are usually of pain, diarrhoea and occasionally bleeding. Treatment is by high-dose oxygen therapy, and response is monitored by plain films.

Endometriosis

Defined as ectopic endometrial tissue, endometriosis may involve the large bowel. The anterior rectosigmoid is the classic site because it closely approximates the pouch of Douglas. Implants are usually extrinsic or serosal but can rarely be intramural or intraluminal, and are a rare cause of a polyp. Contrast studies will show the extent of any stricture but MRI is most sensitive for diagnosis because of its ability to demonstrate blood.

Ileocaecal valve hyperplasia

Submucosal fat may congregate in the ileocaecal valve. Lack of a capsule differentiates this from a true lipoma. The normal upper limit of normal for ileocaecal valve diameter has been considered to be 4 cm, with no single lip exceeding 1.5 cm in thickness. The important differential is from a polyp arising on the valve. Crohn's disease may also thicken the valve.

Irritable bowel syndrome

Irritable bowel syndrome is the commonest condition seen by gastroenterologists in the west. Most patients are women and typical symptoms include abdominal pain and bloating, with alternating constipation and diarrhoea. Diagnosis is one of exclusion and radiology may be necessary to exclude an underlying organic cause: inflammatory bowel disease in the young and carcinoma in older patients. Excessive sigmoid spasm, haustral markings and pain precipitated by gas insufflation have been reported but their diagnostic relevance in individual subjects is unclear.

THE RECTUM AND PRESACRAL SPACE

Rectal neoplasia and inflammation have already been discussed. Although easily accessible to endoscopy, rectal lesions are not infrequently missed, often because the scope tip has already passed a low lesion by the time observation begins. For this reason, the entire rectum should always be examined during double-contrast barium enema. Haemorrhoids often produce distal ampullary filling defects but it should be remembered that the rectum is also a common site for cancer.

Constipation describes infrequent and/or difficult rectal evacuation. Although very common, constipation may be severe enough to cause considerable disability. The most severely afflicted are usually women. Many cases are functional in origin and may be conveniently divided into patients with slow colonic transit and those who have a specific problem with rectal evacuation, although there is considerable overlap. Impaired rectal evacuation may be predominantly structural in origin, perhaps due to a large rectocoele (Fig. 21.32), or functional, usually due to incoordination of pelvic

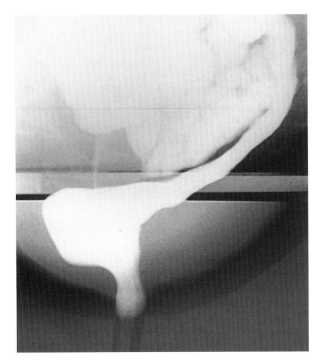

Fig. 21.32 Evacuation proctography demonstrates a moderate rectocoele.

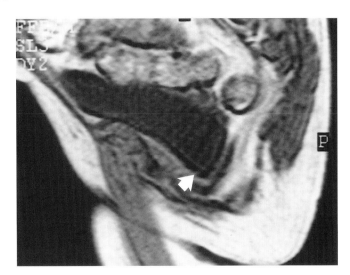

Fig. 21.33 Sagittal T$_1$-weighted MR during straining reveals a cystocoele (arrow), diagnosed by bladder descent below the symphysis pubis.

musculature. Evacuation proctography is frequently requested to distinguish between these possibilities and radio-opaque marker studies will determine colonic transit (Halligan & Bartram 1995). *Solitary rectal ulcer syndrome* is a specific diagnosis of an association between internal and external rectal prolapse, and functional impairment of rectal voiding. Repetitive straining leads to chronic rectal wall fibrosis, ulceration, cyst formation (colitis cystica profunda) and characteristic histological changes. It is increasingly recognised that prolapse syndromes may involve the pelvic floor generally, and there has been a trend towards global pelvic floor imaging because of this. Traditionally this has been achieved by combining bladder and vaginal opacification with evacuation proctography (Kelvin et al 1994) but there have been several reports advocating MRI as an alternative (Fig. 21.33) (Healy et al 1997).

The possibility of a congenital disorder should be considered in younger patients who are severely constipated and a water-soluble enema will rapidly determine rectal calibre and configuration, distinguishing between *Hirschprung's disease, congenital megarectum* and *congenital megacolon*. The rectum is massively dilated in each but only Hirschprung's disease shows *short-segment* narrowing, i.e. dilatation does not extend right down to pelvic floor level (Halligan & Bartram 1995). This segment arises as a result of congenitally absent myenteric ganglion cells and usually extends for 10–15 cm but ultrashort and ultralong segments can occur. In congenital megarectum the sigmoid colon is of normal calibre, unlike congenital megacolon.

In most individuals, the posterior rectal wall is closely applied to the anterior sacral hollow, so that the *presacral space* measures 1 cm or less. Pathological enlargement is usually due to inflammatory *proctitis,* especially ulcerative colitis but primary rectal and sacral tumours (e.g. *chordoma*) may both widen this space. Presacral pathology is historically notoriously difficult to diagnose but MRI is having a considerable impact in this rare group of disorders because of its ability both to tissue characterise and image in the

sagittal plane. Developmental cysts are relatively common at this site and include *dermoids, epidermoids, teratomas* and *tailgut cysts.* A neural origin is also possible and a presacral *meningocoele* should be borne in mind. *Pelvic lipomatosis* is a rare disorder characterised by excessive pelvic adipose tissue that can elongate, straighten and narrow both the rectum and bladder. Patients are at risk from renal failure secondary to ureteric obstruction, and sarcomatous transformation has been reported.

THE ANUS

The anus is the termination of the gastrointestinal tract and is surrounded by two sphincteric muscles, the internal and external anal sphincters. *Anal incontinence* is an extremely common and disabling complaint that may be due to either anal sphincter disruption or atrophy. Childbirth is the commonest cause of external sphincter disruption, which may occur in up to 30% of vaginal deliveries

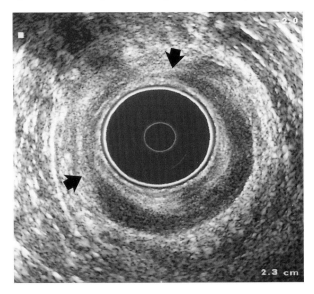

Fig. 21.34 Anal endosonography reveals an anterior external and internal sphincter tear due to obstetric injury (between the arrows).

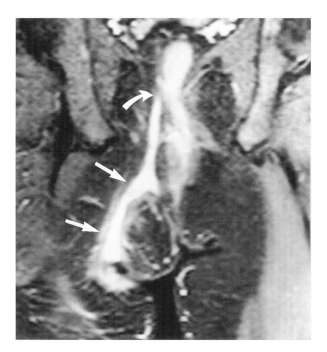

Fig. 21.35 Coronal MR STIR image reveals a right-sided extrasphincteric fistula (straight arrows) with its enteric communication in the rectum (curved arrow).

(Sultan et al 1993). Unintentional iatrogenic injury during anal surgery is the commonest cause of internal sphincter disruption. Anal endosonography directly visualises the sphincters in exquisite detail and is used to characterise sphincter morphology in anal incontinence so that treatment is guided appropriately; for example, patients shown to have external sphincter tears are candidates for surgical repair (Fig. 21.34), whereas those with sphincter atrophy are best treated medically initially.

Fistula-in-ano is a troublesome condition that is usually caused by chronic infection of the anal cryptoglandular glands. It has a tendency to recur, especially when there are remote septic extensions and abscesses from the primary fistula tract. The main role of radiology is preoperative identification of these extensions so that all areas of sepsis are adequately drained. Radiology should also determine the fistula course with respect to the anal sphincters so that any potential for subsequent incontinence secondary to sphincter division is fully appreciated, and sphincter-saving procedures employed when necessary. MRI has become pre-eminent in this field because it can both highlight sepsis and image in surgically relevant planes (Halligan 1998) (Fig. 21.35). Patients with recurrent fistula, apparently complex fistula on clinical examination, or underlying Crohn's disease are particularly suited to MR examination.

Primary *anal canal tumours* are relatively rare and most anal tumours are actually due to inferior extension of rectal carcinoma. Interestingly, the anal canal is one of the most pluripotential tumour sites in the human body and although primary tumours are usually squamous, a very wide variety of cell types can occur. For example, *malignant melanoma* accounts for 10–15% of primary anal tumours. Treatment is usually by chemoradiotherapy rather than surgery. Radiological staging of primary anal tumours will need to include the groins.

RADIONUCLIDE IMAGING OF THE SMALL AND LARGE BOWEL

Philip J. A. Robinson

Scintigraphic investigation of gastrointestinal bleeding

The clinical context of gastrointestinal (GI) bleeding has changed substantially over the last 2–3 decades. The incidence of peptic ulcer disease has fallen with the introduction of H_2 antagonists and there is an increase in proportion of patients in whom GI bleeding first presents as a complication or secondary phenomenon in patients with pre-existing illness. In one recent large series of cases more than half of the patients suffered their first episode of GI bleeding after being admitted to hospital with unrelated conditions.

The widespread introduction of early endoscopy not only allows increased accuracy of diagnosis for upper GI bleeding but also offers an opportunity for local treatment of the bleeding lesion, so the need for surgical exploration now occurs much less frequently. Currently about 80% of patients presenting with GI bleeding have a source in the oesophagus, stomach or duodenum, and about 20% are bleeding from an intestinal or rectal lesion. Early endoscopy has a very high success rate in showing the cause of upper GI bleeding, but the source of haemorrhage from the small bowel and colon is generally more difficult to establish. Even if colonoscopy or barium enema shows bowel pathology, evidence of recent bleeding is seen much less often than in upper GI examinations. Blood in the lumen of the colon may obscure the endoscopic view, and the time required for bowel preparation also reduces the opportunity to visualise a bleeding site. Intestinal haemorrhage is characteristically episodic, and in the majority of cases bleeding will stop spontaneously with supportive treatment.

The rationale for scintigraphic localisation of occult bleeding sites is based on the observation that patients in whom the source of bleeding is determined preoperatively have a better prognosis, whether or not they undergo surgery, than those in whom laparotomy is carried out without prior knowledge of the source of bleeding. The indications for scintigraphic investigation of occult GI bleeding may be summarised as follows:

1. Patients with recurrent episodes of bleeding.
2. Patients in whom endoscopy is inconclusive or negative.
3. Patients with comorbidities in whom surgical risks are likely to be high.
4. Patients with bleeding of sufficient severity to produce melaena.

TECHNIQUES AND INTERPRETATION

Two distinct approaches have been developed, both with specific advantages and drawbacks, but both are relatively simple non-invasive procedures.

Radiolabelled colloid

Colloidal particles in the size range 30–1000 nm are cleared rapidly from the circulation by the reticuloendothelial cells of the liver, spleen and bone marrow. In patients who are actively bleeding at the time of injection, leakage of the tracer into the lumen of the gut will produce a focus of activity that becomes increasingly conspicuous over the next few minutes as the background activity is cleared from the circulation (blood half-life about 2–3 min). Success with this technique depends on bleeding taking place during the first few minutes after the injection of the tracer. Subsequent uptake of the colloid in liver and spleen may obscure bleeding points in the stomach, duodenum and colonic flexures, but these can usually be deduced by the transit of the extravasated blood along the lumen of the bowel, shown on sequential images over the next 30 min or so.

Any technetium-labelled colloid of suitable particle size may be used, the choice depending upon availability and the speed of preparation. The activity administered is more than is conventionally used for liver/spleen scintigraphy, up to 400 mBq being used. Giving the labelled colloid as a fast bolus allows a rapid dynamic acquisition of sequential abdominal images in order to show aneurysms and other highly vascularised lesions. Subsequent images are obtained at intervals of up to 45 min, together with oblique views to improve visualisation of the colonic flexures.

^{99m}Tc-colloid – interpretation

Blood pool activity outlines the major vessels in the first 2 min but from 5 min onwards there is increasing localisation in the liver, spleen and bone marrow of the spine and pelvis. A small proportion of unbound pertechnetate may be excreted in the urine but bladder activity should not be a source of confusion because the timing of appearance of the tracer in the urine is quite different from the timing of GI extravasation. Intraluminal bleeding is usually seen within the first few minutes after injection. Extravasated blood from the small bowel tends to move along the lumen quite briskly so that sequential images show a change in the position of the abnormal focus (Fig. 21.36). Whilst small-bowel bleeding typically shows a central area of extravasation which moves relatively quickly around the centre of the abdomen, colonic activity tends to move fairly slowly around the periphery of the abdomen in a clockwise direction (Fig. 21.37). Extravasation first appearing in the jejunum after 15–20 min or so should be taken as an indication of a more proximal bleeding site initially obscured by activity in the liver and spleen.

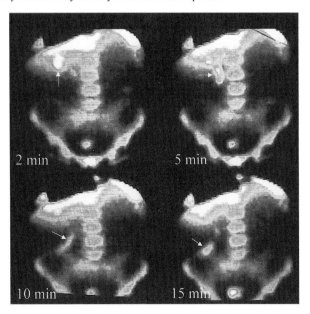

Fig. 21.36 Small-bowel bleeding. ^{99m}Tc-colloid study showing extravasated blood (arrows) moving along jejunal loops on consecutive images. Note normal uptake in bone marrow and in liver and spleen (partly excluded by lead screening placed on the patient).

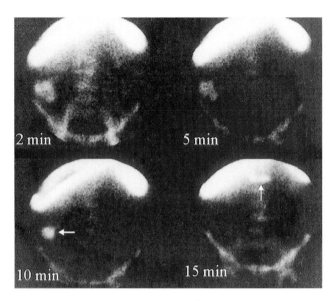

Fig. 21.37 Large-bowel bleeding. ^{99m}Tc-colloid study showing extravasation in caecum which remains static up to 10 min, but moves to the transverse colon at 15 min (arrows).

Radiolabelled red cells

Autologous red cells (RBCs) can be labelled either in vitro or in vivo with technetium. With effective labelling technique, the cells, which remain within the circulation, can be followed by gamma camera imaging for up to 24 h. The extravasation of labelled cells at a bleeding point produces a radioactive haematoma, which, if of sufficient volume, is detectable by external imaging. Because the blood background remains highly active, the volume of extravasated blood required to produce a visible abnormality is considerably greater than with the colloid method. About 50–70 ml of blood are required to identify an intraluminal bleed by this method, which is about the same volume as is required to produce a melaena stool. The success of this technique also depends on the rate at which extravasated blood moves along the bowel lumen and the vascularity of surrounding structures. The stability of the tracer within the vascular compartment allows sequential imaging for up to 24 h, which gives the opportunity of detecting bleeding which is episodic, or continuing at a slow rate.

In vivo red cell labelling is carried out by first tagging the cells with a reducing agent and subsequently injecting sodium pertechnetate. A more efficient binding can be achieved in vitro by labelling a 10 ml sample of autologous red cells by the same method, but washing the cells before reinjection. The in vitro method requires additional time and expertise but gives a higher binding efficiency, which reduces problems of interpretation arising from the urinary excretion of free pertechnetate.

A fast dynamic sequence of abdominal images can be obtained following a bolus injection of up to 400 mBq of ^{99m}Tc-RBCs. Subsequent images are obtained at 5 min intervals for about 1 h. If no abnormality has been found, further imaging may be continued at increasing intervals of up to 24 h.

^{99m}Tc-RBCs – interpretation

After the initial vascular phase, the blood pool activity within the liver, spleen and kidneys outlines these organs as well as the main vessels. The proximal small bowel often shows a persistent

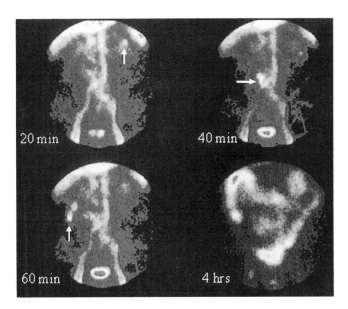

Fig. 21.38 Small-bowel bleeding. ⁹⁹ᵐTc-RBC study showing extravasation into small bowel loops at 20, 40 and 60 min (arrows), with the extravasation reaching the colon by 4 h.

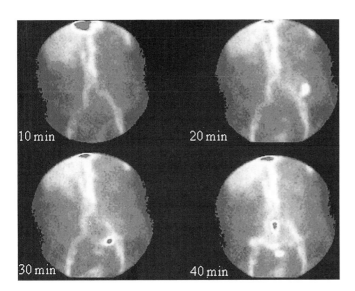

Fig. 21.39 Colonic bleeding. ⁹⁹ᵐTc-RBC study showing no bleeding up to 10 min, but a clear bleeding site at 20, 30 and 40 min following the line of the sigmoid colon.

vascular blush and in many cases the portal vein is visible. These appearances normally remain stable over the next few hours and extravasation is recognised as a focus of radioactivity outside the normal vascular landmarks which sequentially increases in activity compared with the background. Consecutive images showing the changing position of the extravasated focus help to locate the bleeding point, as described above with the colloid method (Figs 21.38, 21.39). Extravasation that is first seen on late images in the caecum may indicate a bleeding point in the right colon but can also result from slow or intermittent extravasation from a more proximal small-bowel site. However, in most cases of small-bowel bleeding the distal ileum is visualised as well as the caecum.

Choice of technique

Because of the rate at which labelled colloid is cleared from the circulation by the reticuloendothelial system. GI bleeding at the time of injection is detected within the first few minutes of the procedure. The rapid disappearance of background activity allows small volumes of extravasated blood to be visualised, and in positive cases the location of the bleeding site is usually clear. The major disadvantage of this method is that bleeding is episodic or intermittent in many cases, and if the patient has stopped bleeding at the time of injection a negative result will be obtained. The more widely used red cell method allows for the detection of intermittent bleeding but generally requires a longer period of observation, during which extravasated blood accumulates in the intestine. The combination of slow bleeding rates with movement of blood along the bowel lumen increases the difficulty of localising the site of origin. As a general rule, the sooner the bleeding point is recognised, the more accurate will be the localisation. Red cells studies which become positive only after 4 h or longer are less likely to correlate with subsequent angiographic or surgical finding than those which show an early positive result.

Results

In determining the accuracy of scintigraphic techniques, comparison has been made with angiography, endoscopy, barium studies and surgery. Initial studies with the colloid method showed that patients with negative scintigraphy never showed extravasation on subsequent arteriograms, suggesting the use of scintigraphy as a screening procedure before urgent angiography. However, other users had less success with labelled colloid and direct RBC/colloid comparisons in the same patients suggested that the red cell procedure would be positive in a higher proportion of patients. Numerous studies indicate a success rate of 75–90% in predicting the presence and approximate site of bleeding using labelled autologous red cells. Several surgical reports have confirmed a role for scintigraphic localisation of bleeding in those patients in whom endoscopy is negative or inconclusive. A positive scintigraphic result directs the subsequent surgery or angiography to the local pathology, and prior knowledge of the bleeding site reduces surgical morbidity and mortality. A negative scintigraphic result is also helpful in that it predicts better prognosis, reduced likelihood of surgical intervention being required, lesser transfusion requirements, and a shorter stay in hospital.

Meckel's diverticulum

Meckel's diverticulum, a remnant of the embryonic omphalomesenteric duct, persists into adult life in a small proportion of the population, probably about 2%. Only a minority of these produce clinical problems, usually arising from peptic ulceration within the diverticulum causing abdominal pain or occult bleeding. Chronic inflammatory reaction may result in scarring, which can lead to small bowel obstruction. Clinical presentation is most common in childhood but can occur at any age. Scintigraphic detection of Meckel's diverticulum depends upon the affinity of injected pertechnetate for the gastric mucosa contained in the diverticulum. The technique requires only a single intravenous injection and carries a low radiation burden compared with enteroclysis or angiography.

Technique

Intravenously injected pertechnetate distributes into the extracellular fluid space and is also cleared from the circulation by the thyroid, salivary glands and choroid plexus of the brain and also by the mucosa of the stomach and colon. The mechanism of uptake is not entirely clear but it is probably the mucus-secreting goblet cells which concentrate the pertechnetate. Uptake continues to accumulate for an hour or so after injection so serial images should be obtained during this period. Pertechnetate is also secreted into the lumen of the stomach by the gastric mucosa and is then free to move along the lumen. In order to avoid potentially confusing appearances from this effect, H_2-blocking agents are used to minimise the release of pertechnetate. The procedure visualises gastric mucosa in the stomach and also in ectopic sites, including Barrett's oesophagus and duplication cysts, as well as Meckel's diverticula.

Preparation

Adults should starve overnight to ensure the stomach is empty and to reduce the rate of gastric secretion. With infants and small children, it is sufficient to withhold one feed. H_2 blockade is prescribed in two doses, one the evening before the test and a second dose on the morning of the test.

Acquisition

After an intravenous injection of 200–400 mBq of sodium pertechnetate, images of the abdomen and pelvis are obtained with the patient supine. For infants and small children the dose is scaled down according to surface area and images may be obtained with the patient lying prone on the surface of the camera. Typically, images are obtained at 5 min intervals up to 45 min. Oblique or lateral views may be helpful and at the end of the procedure the bladder should be emptied and the postmicturition image obtained.

Interpretation

Pertechnetate is excreted by glomerular filtration so renal activity appears early and excreted pertechnetate gradually accumulates in the bladder. Abdominal lesions with an increased blood pool or extracellular fluid component (e.g. aneurysms, tumours, inflammatory masses) show maximum activity on early images, whereas gastric mucosa activity increases in intensity over 20–30 min (Fig. 21.40). If H_2 blockade is omitted, most patients will secrete activity into the lumen of the stomach; activity will then move on into small bowel (Fig. 21.41), and occasionally some small-bowel activity occurs even with the use of H_2 blockers.

Confusion should be avoided by reviewing the rate at which the activity appears in different sites. Areas of activity in the ureters may simulate Meckel's diverticulum but should be distinguishable on oblique or lateral views, and also by their transient nature.

Meckel's diverticulum appears as a focal area of uptake of pertechnetate which is remote from but synchronous with the normal gastric mucosa. Although other intra-abdominal sites have been described, the majority of Meckel's diverticula lie in the right iliac fossa or in the right side of the true pelvis (Fig. 21.42).

Results

The reliability and accuracy of the tests vary in different reports, but in a large multicentre series over 10 years scintigraphy correctly established the presence or absence of a Meckel's diverticulum in about 75% of patients who subsequently underwent surgery, with a sensitivity of about 85%. The procedure is less likely to be successful in adults, but in another multicentre study of patients of all ages presenting over 13 years with a variety of complications of Meckel's diverticulum, the detection rate for scintigraphy was 83%.

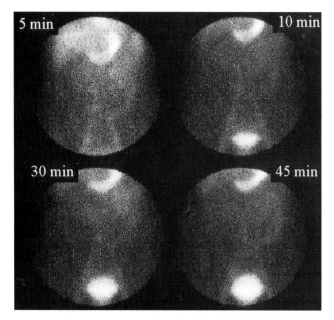

Fig. 21.40 Meckel's study. Normal appearance after injection of ^{99m}Tc-pertechnetate showing concentration in the normal gastric mucosa, and also renal excretion outlining the bladder.

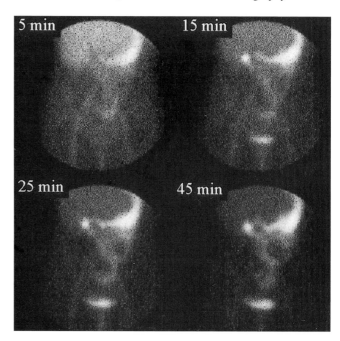

Fig. 21.41 Meckel's study. The patient did not take H_2 blockade as requested, and the later images show pertechnetate in the lumen of the small bowel, resulting from gastric secretion of the tracer.

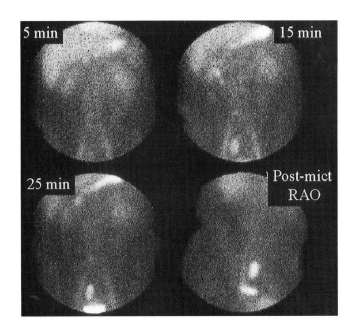

Fig. 21.42 Meckel's study. Typical appearance of Meckel's diverticulum in the right side of the pelvis (surgically confirmed).

Radionuclide imaging of inflammatory bowel disease

Numerous different radiotracers have been tried in the search for a reliable marker of infection and inflammation. Labelled colloids and human immunoglobulin have been disappointing; gallium citrate retains niche applications in selected clinical cases; while labelled antibody fragments (e.g. sulesomab) and [99mTc]-labelled ciprofloxacin appear promising for some applications. The most widely used and successful current technique uses autologous white cells labelled either with technetium-99m or with indium-111. In outline, a sample of white cells is harvested from the patient, labelled in vitro with a radiotracer, and reinjected into the patient. Images obtained over the next few hours demonstrate the localisation of white cells and, in particular, will show abnormal foci of infection or inflammation.

Choice of technique

Early development work used indium-111 combined with one of several chelating agents, of which tropolone is now usually chosen. The white cells from 30–50 ml of the patient's blood are labelled in vitro with ^{111}In-tropolone under sterile conditions, and the cells are resuspended and injected back into the patient. Meticulous technique is needed to avoid damaging the cells and to achieve a high level of labelling efficiency. Images of the abdomen and pelvis (or of other areas if they are of clinical interest) are obtained at 4 and 24 h after injection.

The original validation work for the use of labelled white cells in infection, and particularly in inflammatory bowel disease, showed high degrees of correlation with histological criteria and clinical indices. For acute infection, there are some advantages to using labelled granulocytes rather than mixed white cell populations, but the technical difficulty of fractionating the white cells may outweigh the marginal advantage in sensitivity which it achieves.

The introduction of technetium-labelled hexamethyl-propyl-amine-oxime ([99mTc]-HMPAO), which also binds to white cells in vitro, offered an alternative method with a number of advantages. The radiation dose from technetium-99m is relatively less than from indium-111, so more activity and a higher count rate can be achieved with less radiation hazard to the patient. Localisation with technetium-99m appears to be more rapid and images can be diagnostic at 1 h, with delayed views being obtained at 4 h. HMPAO can be kept on the shelf, whereas indium-111 with its $t_{1/2}$ of 68 h has a relatively short shelf life. The labelling procedure itself is also a little quicker with [99mTc]-HMPAO. Disadvantages of the technetium-99m technique include a greater proportion of renal excretion, more bone marrow uptake of the agent, generally slightly less labelling efficiency, and also the phenomenon of migration of the agent into the lumen of the bowel, particularly in the colon, within a few hours of injection.

In general, [99mTc]-HMPAO is preferred because of its relative technical simplicity, reduced radiation dose and faster turnaround of result. However, some centres still prefer to use ^{111}In-labelling, particularly as there is a more extensive literature validating its results in comparison to histology, to other imaging, and to clinical indices of disease. With [99mTc]-HMPAO, images of the abdomen are obtained 1 and 4 h after injection.

Interpretation

Labelled white cells normally accumulate in liver, spleen and bone marrow, with the most intense uptake being seen in the spleen. With [99mTc]-HMPAO, low-grade activity in the colon or terminal ileum is a normal feature at 4 h, although not at 1 h after injection. Bowel activity identified at 1 h may be taken as evidence of inflammatory disease. Most lesions are more apparent on the delayed images than on the initial images. With ^{111}In-labelling, inflammatory disease should be recognisable at 4 h, and abscesses are best seen at 24 h. Patients undergoing immunosuppression, or those on prolonged steroid therapy, may show negative results in the face of active infection. These patients will usually have a depressed white count in the peripheral blood, and this also adds to the difficulty of labelling the cells.

Bowel uptake is seen not only in Crohn's disease and ulcerative colitis but also in other active inflammatory colitides, including infections. It has also been described in patients with GI bleeding or

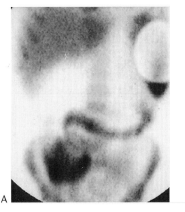 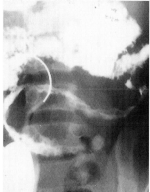

Fig. 21.43 Crohn's disease. Labelled white cell study shows a single long loop of abnormal small bowel (A). Barium study (B) shows diffuse narrowing and mucosal irregularity affecting the same segment.

bowel infarction, and in rare cases of tumours in which there is an inflammatory component. Taken overall however, there is a high level of correlation between positive white cell scintigraphy and active inflammatory disease shown by endoscopy, barium examination and histology (Fig. 21.43), and also a good correlation with clinical indices of disease activity.

Applications

Detecting inflammatory bowel disease

In the early stages of disease, WBC scintigraphy may be the only positive test, particularly in early small bowel Crohn's disease (Fig. 21.44) and in 'minimal change' colitis with normal barium enema or colonoscopy. Particularly in children, WBC scintigraphy is a simpler procedure than small bowel barium examination, and probably more sensitive.

Assessing the extent and location of abnormal bowel

In patients in whom the presence of disease has been established, scintigraphy can show which areas of the small bowel and colon are involved, and also assess the intensity of inflammatory change in each area (Figs 21.45–21.47). This may be particularly useful in monitoring the effects of treatment and in patients with recurrent episodes of abdominal symptoms. The distribution of abnormalities may also indicate the type of inflammatory colitis. The presence of skip lesions, predominant right-sided disease, perianal infection, and sparing of the rectum all favour Crohn's rather than ulcerative colitis.

Follow-up

In assessing the progress of disease, WBC scintigraphy offers a relatively non-invasive method that is well tolerated by patients.

Assessing complications

Abscess detection may be problematic in patients with extensive small-bowel disease and previous surgery. WBC scintigraphy will differentiate between infected collections and pockets of sterile fluid or localised loops of dilated small bowel, which may be confusing on ultrasound or CT. In assessing strictures, those which

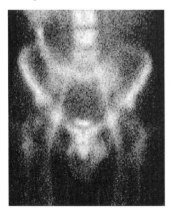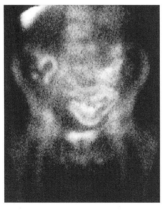

Fig. 21.44   Early Crohn's disease. Labelled WBC study shows low-grade disease localised to distal ileum 1 h after injection of ⁹⁹ᵐTc-HMPAO-WBC. Note normal uptake in bone marrow. Concurrent barium examination was negative, but the patient later developed overt signs of disease.

Fig. 21.45   Extensive small-bowel Crohn's disease. ⁹⁹ᵐTc-HMPAO-WBC study at 1 h after injection showing multiple loops of abnormal small bowel.

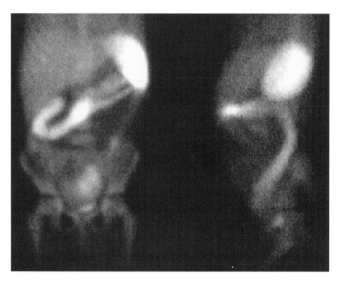

Fig. 21.46   Ulcerative colitis. ⁹⁹ᵐTc-HMPAO-WBC study (left, anterior view; right, left lateral view) showing extensive involvement of transverse and descending colon, but no small-bowel disease.

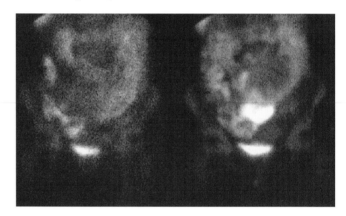

Fig. 21.47   Crohn's disease. ⁹⁹ᵐTc-HMPAO-WBC study (left, 1 h; right 4 h) showing patchy abnormality in both large and small bowel.

show inflammatory change may be amenable to medical treatment, whereas strictures which are inactive on WBC scintigraphy are more likely to need surgical intervention.

Somatostatin receptor scintigraphy (SRS)

Somatostatin is a peptide of 14 amino acids which is unstable in blood, with a half-life of only a few minutes, and relatively short acting in vivo. Octreotide is a synthetic analogue with eight amino acids which is more stable (blood half-life 2–3 h), has a more prolonged activity, and also binds to somatostatin membrane receptors which occur in cells of neuroendocrine origin and also in some other tissues containing activated lymphocytes. When labelled with ¹¹¹In-DTPA, octreotide is used to localise tumours of neuroendocrine origin, both primary and secondary, and also several other types of tumour which exhibit somatostatin receptors.

Applications   Neoplasms of neuroendocrine origin include pancreatic islet cell tumours, carcinoids, vipomas and apudomas, some pituitary adenomas, medullary thyroid cancers, phaeochromocytomas, neuroblastomas and paragangliomas. Other tumour types showing positive results with SRS include small-cell lung cancer, malignant lymphomas, particularly Hodgkin's disease, and breast cancer. Octreotide uptake is also seen with some chronic granulomatous diseases, including rheumatoid arthritis and sarcoidosis. The value of SRS in these latter conditions still needs to be explored, and for the localisation of adrenal medullary tumours and paraganglioma, scintigraphy with metaiodobenzyl-guanadine (mIBG) is usually preferable (see Ch. 27). The major applications for SRS are in the localisation of pancreatic islet cell tumours and their metastases (see Chs 25, 36) and in the investigation of gastrointestinal carcinoids, apudomas and related tumours, and their metastases.

Technique Theoretically, treatment with unlabelled octreotide may reduce tracer uptake by the tumour, so it is arguably desirable to stop such treatment for 2–3 days before the test, if it is possible to do so without endangering the patient. If long-acting depot preparations of octreotide are being used, interruption of treatment would take months, so is inappropriate in most circumstances. About 110 MBq of indium-111 chelated with DTPA, which is itself bound to 10–20 μg of carrier octreotide, is given intravenously (220 MBq is given if single photon emission CT (SPECT) is planned). Whole body images are obtained at about 4 and 24 h. SPECT acquisition at the second visit is often helpful, particularly if seeking deep-seated lesions in the upper abdomen which could be obscured by normal activity in the overlying liver and spleen. With the usual activity given, radiation dose to the patient is approximately 14 mSv (compared with 5–10 mSv for CT of the abdomen). Since much of the activity is excreted in the urine, the bladder should be emptied immediately before acquiring the images.

Interpretation In the normal subject, about 90% of the injected activity is excreted in the urine by 24 h, so images typically show fairly intense uptake in the kidneys and also some bladder accumulation. A high level of uptake is typical in the spleen, and rather lower grade activity throughout the liver parenchyma. A small proportion of the injected dose is excreted via the biliary tract, so low-grade activity in the colon is normal at 24 h. There is also fairly intense activity in the normal thyroid and the pituitary takes up enough to be just visible on planar views of the head.

Results Compared with other imaging techniques, SRS is highly accurate (probably more sensitive than CT or MRI) in detecting primary bowel carcinoids (Fig. 21.48) and their metastases in mesenteric lymph nodes. SRS is particularly useful in patients presenting with liver metastases when the primary site is not known (Fig. 21.49). In differentiating carcinoids from non-functioning tumours, SRS may eliminate the need for biopsy. SRS is also useful for staging of carcinoid tumours, particularly detecting extrahepatic and extra-abdominal disease (Fig. 21.50). The intensity of uptake on SRS can also be used as an indication of disease activity after treatment.

Functioning tumours which show marked uptake of octreotide on SRS usually also respond well to unlabelled octreotide for the relief of symptoms. Further, the feasibility of delivering a therapeutic dose of indium-111 for local radiotherapy of malignant lesions can also be predicted from the intensity of uptake on SRS.

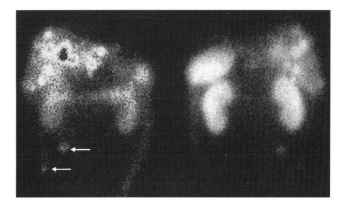

Fig. 21.49 Primary and metastatic carcinoid. SRS (left, anterior view; right, posterior view) shows a small active lesion in the right iliac fossa and an adjacent lymph node deposit (arrows) together with multiple liver metastases.

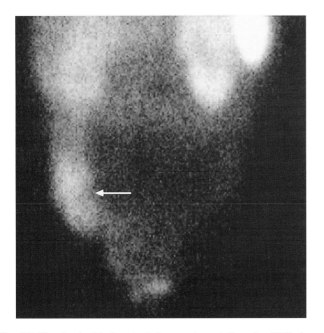

Fig. 21.48 Carcinoid. Somatostatin receptor scintigraphy (SRS) shows functioning tumour in the right iliac fossa (arrow).

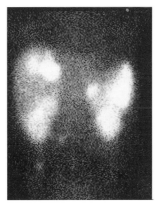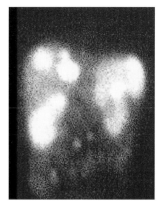

Fig. 21.50 Primary and metastatic carcinoid. SRS (left, 4 h; right, 24 h) shows multiple functioning liver tumours, but also shows nodal disease in midabdomen and primary focus in the right iliac fossa, best seen on delayed images at 24 h.

REFERENCES AND SUGGESTIONS FOR FURTHER READING

Almer, S., Bodemar, G., Franzen, L., Lindstrom, E., Nystrom, P., Strom, M. (1996) Use of air enema radiography to assess depth of ulceration during acute attacks of ulcerative colitis. *Lancet*, **47**, 1731–1735.

Bartram, C. I. (1983) *Radiology in Inflammatory Bowel Disease*. New York: Marcel Dekker.

Bartram, C. I. (1994) Bowel preparation—principles and practice. *Clinical Radiology*, **49**, 365–367.

Bartram, C. I., Walmsley, K. (1978) A radiological and pathological correlation of the mucosal changes in ulcerative colitis. *Clinical Radiology*, **29**, 323–328.

Brady, A. P., Stevenson, G. W., Stevenson, I. (1994) Colorectal cancer overlooked at barium enema examination and colonoscopy: a continuing perceptual problem. *Radiology*, **192**, 373–378.

Chew, C. N., Nolan, D. J., Jewell, D. P. (1991) Small bowel gas in severe ulcerative colitis. *Gut*, **32**, 1535–1537.

Connell, W. R., Sheffield, J. P., Kamm, M. A., Hawley, P. R., Lennard-Jones, J.E. (1994) Lower gastrointestinal malignancy in Crohn's disease. *Gut*, **35**, 347–352.

Day, J.T., Freeman, A.H., Coni, N.K., et al (1993) Barium enema or computed tomography for the frail elderly patient. *Clinical Radiology*, **48**, 48–51.

Domjan, J., Blaquiere, R., Odurney, A. (1998) Is minimal preparation computed tomography comparable with barium enema in elderly patients with colonic symptoms? *Clinical Radiology*, **53**, 894–898.

Fenlon, H. M., Nunes, D. P., Schroy, P. C. III, Barish, M. A., Clarke, P. D. Ferrucci, J.T. (1999) A comparison of virtual and conventional colonoscopy for the detection of colorectal polyps. *New England Journal of Medicine*, **341**, 1496–1503.

Fink, A. M., Aylward, G. W. (1995) Buscopan and glaucoma: a survey of current practice. *Clinical Radiology*, **50**, 160–164.

Gasche, C., Moser, G., Turetschek, K., Schober, E., Moeschi, P., Oberhuber, G. (1999) Transabdominal bowel sonography for the detection of intestinal complications in Crohn's disease. *Gut*, **44**, 112–117.

Gore, R., Levine, M. (2000) *Textbook of Gastrointestinal Radiology*. London: W. B. Saunders.

Gore, R. M., Balthazar, E. J., Ghahremani, G. G., Miller, F. H. (1996) CT features of ulcerative colitis and Crohn's disease. *American Journal of Roentgenology*, **167**, 3–15.

Halligan, S. (1996) Imaging anorectal function. *British Journal of Radiology*, **69**, 985–988.

Halligan, S. (1998) Imaging fistula-in-ano. *Clinical Radiology*, **53**, 85–95.

Halligan, S., Bartram, C. I. (1995) The radiological investigation of constipation. *Clinical Radiology*, **50**, 429–435.

Halligan, S., Fenlon, H. M. (1999) Virtual colonoscopy. *BMJ*, **319**, 1249–1252.

Healy, J. C., Halligan, S., Reznek, R. H., Watson, S., Phillips, R. K. S., Armstrong, P. (1997) Patterns of prolapse in women with symptoms of pelvic floor weakness: assessment with MR imaging. *Radiology*, **203**, 77–81.

Henry, M. M., Swash, M. (1992) *Coloproctology and the Pelvic Floor*. Oxford: Butterworth-Heinemann.

Kelvin, F. M., Maglinte, D. D. T., Benson, J. T., Brubaker, L. P., Smith, C. (1994) Dynamic cystoproctography: a technique for assessing disorders of the pelvic floor in women. *American Journal of Roentgenology*, **163**, 368–370.

Kelvin, F. M., Oddson, T. A., Rice, R. P., Garbutt, J. T., Bradenham, B. P. (1978) Double contrast barium enema in Crohn's disease and ulcerative colitis. *American Journal of Roentgenology*, **131**, 207–213.

Limberg, B., Osswald, B. (1994) Diagnosis and differential diagnosis of ulcerative colitis and Crohn's disease by hydrocolonic sonography. *American Journal of Gastroenterology*, **89**, 1051–1057.

Lynch, H. T., Smyrk, T. C., Watson, P., et al (1993) Genetics, natural history, tumour spectrum and pathology of hereditary non-polyposis colorectal cancer: an updated review. *Gastroenterology*, **104**, 1535–1549.

Matsumoto, T., Iida, M., Kuroki, F., et al (1996) Dysplasia in ulcerative colitis: is radiography adequate for diagnosis? *Radiology*, **199**, 85–90.

Meyers, M. A. (1988) *Dynamic Radiology of the Abdomen: Normal and Pathologic Anatomy*. New York: Springer-Verlag.

Morson, B. C. (1974) The polyp–cancer sequence in the large bowel. *Proceedings of the Royal Society of Medicine, 67*, 451.

Nicholls, R. J., Dozois, R. (1997) *Surgery of the Colon and Rectum*. London: Churchill Livingstone.

Phillips, R. K. S., Spigelman, A. D., Thomson, J. P. S. (1994) *Familial Adenomatous Polyposis and Other Polyposis Syndromes*. London: Edward Arnold.

Prantera, C., Lorenzetti, R., Cerro, P., Davoli, M., Brancato, G., Fanucci, A. (1991) The plain abdominal film accurately estimates extent of active ulcerative colitis. *Journal of Clinical Gastroenterology*, **13**, 231–234.

Puylaert, J. B, Rutgers, P. H., Lalisang, R. I., et al (1987) A prospective study of ultrasonography in the diagnosis of appendicitis. *New England Journal of Medicine*, **317**, 666–669.

Rao, P. M., Rhea, J.T., Novelline, R. A., et al (1997) Helical CT technique for the diagnosis of appendicitis: prospective evaluation of a focused appendix CT examination. *Radiology*, **202**, 139–144.

Rembacken, B. J., Fujii, T., Cairns, A., et al (2000) Flat and depressed colonic neoplasms: a prospective study of 1000 consecutive colonoscopies in the UK. *Lancet*, **355**, 1211–1214.

Rex, D., Rahmani, E., Haseman, J., et al (1997) Relative sensitivity of colonoscopy and barium enema for detection of colorectal cancer in clinical practice. *Gastroenterology*, **112**, 17–23.

Rubesin, S. E., Levine, M. S., Laufer, I., Herlinger, H. (2000) Double contrast barium enema technique. *Radiology*, **215**, 642–650.

Sultan, A. H., Kamm, M. A., Hudson, C. N., Thomas, J., Bartram, C. I. (1993) Anal sphincter disruption during vaginal delivery. *New England Journal of Medicine*, **329**, 1905–1911.

Winawer, S. J., Stewart, E. T., Zauber, A. G., et al (2000) A comparison of colonoscopy and double contrast barium enema for surveillance after polypectomy. *New England Journal of Medicine*, **342**, 1766–1772.

Radionuclides

Alavi, A. (1982) Detection of gastrointestinal bleeding with Tc99m sulphur colloid. *Seminars in Nuclear Medicine, 12*, 126–138.

Charron, M. (1999) Technetium-leukocyte imaging in inflammatory bowel disease. *Current Gastroenterology, 1*, 245–252.

Chiti, A., Briganti, V., Fanti, S. et al (2000) Results and potential of somatostatin receptor imaging in gastroenteropancreatic tumour imaging. *Quarterly Journal of Nuclear Medicine, 44*, 42–49.

Conway, J. J. (1980) Radionuclide diagnosis of Meckel's diverticulum. *Gastrointestinal Radiology, 5*, 209–213.

Gostout, C. J., Wang, K. K., Alqist, D. A. et al (1992) Acute gastrointestinal bleeding—experience of a specialised management team. *Journal of Clinical Gastroenterology, 14*, 260–267.

Kusumoto, H., Yoshida, M., Tachahashi, I. et al (1992) Complications and diagnosis of Mecekl's diverticulum in 776 patients. *American Journal of Surgery, 164*, 382–383.

Kwekkeboom, D. J., Krenning, E. P. (1997) Radiolabelled somatostatin analog scintigraphy in oncology and immune diseases: an overview. *European Radiology, 7*, 1103–1109.

Robinson, P. (1993) The role of nuclear medicine studies in acute gastrointestinal bleeding. *Nuclear Medicine Communications, 14*, 849–855.

Weldon, M. J. (1994) Tc99m-HMPAO planar white cell scanning. *Scandinavian Journal of Gastroenterology. Supplement, 203*, 36–42.

Winzelburg, G. G., McKusick, K. A., Froelich, J. W. et al (1982) Detection of gastrointestinal bleeding with ^{99m}Tc labelled red blood cells. *Seminars in Nuclear Medicine, 12*, 139–146.

22

THE ACUTE ABDOMEN

Stuart Field, Iain Morrison

Patients with an acute abdomen comprise the largest group of people presenting as a general surgical emergency. Following the history and clinical examination, plain film radiographs have traditionally been one of the first and most useful methods of further investigation. In spite of the recent increased use of other imaging techniques, plain films still retain this position as one of the most useful initial investigations.

In most acute abdominal conditions, the radiological diagnosis depends on gas patterns, for example the distribution of gas in dilated and non-dilated bowel and the presence of gas inside or outside the bowel lumen. Plain films are likely to remain the best method of imaging these gas shadows for many years to come, and radionuclide studies, computed tomography and magnetic resonance imaging are unlikely to play any major role in the initial investigation of the acute abdomen. In certain specific conditions, however, where gas shadows play a relatively minor role, e.g. acute cholecystitis, ultrasound has become the initial imaging technique of choice. However, the presence of moderate or large amounts of intraabdominal gas, which acts as a barrier to ultrasound waves, can make the ultrasound examination of an acute abdomen difficult or sometimes impossible.

Interpretation of plain films in the acute abdomen may present a formidable challenge to the radiologist, for, while in many cases a specific diagnosis can be made, not infrequently the appearances are non-specific or even positively misleading and further investigations using contrast media, ultrasound, radionuclides or CT may be required. When the radiological diagnosis is specific or supports the clinical finding, surgery is often indicated without further investigation. However, if there are clinical signs to indicate that surgery should be performed, negative or equivocal radiology should be ignored.

The radiologist has one major role, to help the surgeon decide whether or not a patient with acute abdominal pain needs to have an operation. He or she should then try and indicate to the surgeon whether the operation should be performed immediately or whether time can be spent in resuscitating the patient or carrying out further investigations.

It is often of value to view the radiographs initially in the absence of any clinical information. An objective evaluation of the radiological signs can then be made and a full differential diagnosis considered without being biased by the clinical findings. It is absolutely essential, however, that before a final opinion is given, the radiologist should be aware of the full clinical history so that minor abnormalities are not overlooked or the wrong interpretation placed on certain signs.

Radiographic technique

A supine abdomen and an erect chest can be regarded as the basic standard radiographs. A horizontal-ray abdominal radiograph, either erect or left lateral decubitus, is frequently taken to add more information and to demonstrate fluid levels.

The clinical condition of the patient will determine whether he or she can sit or stand for the erect radiograph. Sometimes it is possible to obtain a lateral decubitus or even a supine radiograph with a horizontal ray in patients who are too ill to be moved. It is essential that patients should be in position for 10 min prior to the horizontal-ray radiograph to allow free gas time to rise to the highest point. Wherever possible, the bladder should be emptied before the supine radiograph is taken, and this should always include the area from the diaphragm to the hernial orifices.

CHEST X-RAY

A chest radiograph can be regarded as an essential examination for any patient presenting with an acute abdomen. The reasons are as follows:

1. The erect chest film is the best radiograph for showing the presence of a small pneumoperitoneum, particularly on the right side between the liver and the diaphragm. It is superior to the erect abdominal film for this purpose because in the latter the divergent X-ray beam penetrates the gas at the top of the diaphragm obliquely and this area is also relatively dark due to overexposure; in the erect chest film, however, the top of the diaphragm and the gas beneath are penetrated almost tangentially by the X-ray beam, and the exposure of the diaphragm is optimal to show small amounts of gas.

2. A number of chest conditions may present as acute abdominal pain and mimic an acute abdomen exactly (Box 22.1). They may be suspected on the chest radiograph.

3. Acute abdominal conditions may be complicated by chest pathology. For example, pleural effusions frequently complicate acute pancreatitis, elderly patients may have heart failure, or aspiration pneumonia may follow prolonged vomiting in intestinal obstruction. Up to 10% of patients with an acute abdomen may have acute unsuspected chest conditions, which will be diagnosed on the chest radiograph.

4. Even when the chest radiograph is normal it acts as a most valuable baseline. Postoperative chest complications and subphrenic abscesses are relatively common following emergency surgery for an acute abdomen. Comparison with a previously normal film may allow subtle new changes to be detected, and so enable an early diagnosis of complications to be made.

ABDOMINAL RADIOGRAPHS

The supine abdominal radiograph is probably the single most useful film. It allows the distribution of gas and the calibre of bowel to be determined and may show displacement of bowel by soft-tissue masses. Furthermore, obliteration of fat lines normally visualised, for example psoas outlines, may indicate fluid or inflammatory exudate in these regions.

Traditionally an erect abdominal radiograph is taken 'to show fluid levels and free gas'. As discussed already, the erect chest radiograph is superior to the erect abdominal film for the demonstration of a pneumoperitoneum. Furthermore, the presence of fluid levels in bowel rarely contributes to the overall diagnosis in an acute abdomen. This is because there are numerous causes of small-bowel fluid levels and the number, distribution and length will not usually help to distinguish between the two commonest causes, obstruction and paralytic ileus, or any of the others (Box 22.2). A small number of short fluid levels are frequently present, and sometimes as many as 26 fluid levels up to 10 cm long may be seen in normal patients. Although most of these

fluid levels lie within the colon, they may be difficult to differentiate from small-bowel fluid levels. However, three or more small-bowel fluid levels longer than 2.5 cm are abnormal, and indicate dilated small bowel, usually with stasis.

Horizontal-ray films, either erect or lateral decubitus, by allowing redistribution of gas within distended bowel, may enable its exact location and identity to be determined. If gas shadows are demonstrated which are suspected as lying outside the bowel, then horizontal-ray films are often particularly helpful by demonstrating that air–fluid levels lie within a confined space and are thus likely to represent an abscess cavity.

A left lateral decubitus abdominal radiograph is one taken with the patient lying on the left side but with the X-ray beam horizontal. In patients who are unfit to sit or stand for an erect film, it is the projection of choice to show a small pneumoperitoneum. Some have suggested that it should be the first film taken when searching for a pneumoperitoneum. In this projection, free gas may be trapped between the edge of the liver and the lateral abdominal wall, or sometimes over the pelvis when this is the highest point, which is more likely to occur in females. In the left lateral decubitus position, air will preferentially leave a perforated duodenal or antral ulcer, while fluid is more likely to leak when the patient is erect. Furthermore, if air is present in the lesser sac of the peritoneum following a perforated posterior gastric ulcer, it will enter the main abdominal cavity and be more readily identified. A gas-filled dilated duodenal loop, one of the commonest signs of acute pancreatitis, is best shown in this projection.

A lateral abdominal view may demonstrate calcification in an aortic aneurysm which has not been detected on the supine view.

It has been suggested that as many as six standard films are the minimum requirement for an acute abdomen. However, there is considerable merit and saving in time and film costs in taking an erect chest and a supine abdominal radiograph and only proceeding if these films do not confirm the clinical diagnosis or if abnormalities are detected which need further elucidation.

To obtain good radiographic contrast between the water density of the soft tissues and the relative transradiancy of fat, the kilovoltage used should be kept low, ideally in the range 60–65 kV, and the output of the set must be sufficient to keep the exposure time short. Blurring, due to even slight respiratory movement, may obscure details of fat line, small gas bubbles and calcification.

Normal appearances

Organ identification on plain radiographs depends on anatomical position, helped by the tissue–fat interface, and the presence of gas, fluid or food residue within the bowel.

Relatively large amounts of gas are usually present in the stomach, which can be identified by its position and the gastric rugae on supine radiographs, and it is common to see a long air–fluid level in the fundus of the stomach when erect. The duodenal cap is often gas-filled and frequently contains a fluid level on erect films.

Small-bowel gas is extremely variable: usually, relatively small amounts of gas are present and are insufficient for more than a short length of fluid level to be demonstrated. Sometimes, however, with air swallowing, such as in breathless patients or those with abdominal pain, there may be enough air for longer lengths of small bowel to be outlined and the valvulae conniventes identified (Fig. 22.1). In the non-obstructed patient it is, however, rare to see the thin bands of valvulae conniventes stretching over more than a short segment of

Most of the gas in the bowel has been swallowed and it normally reaches the colon within 30 min. In severe pain, or when respiration is laboured, as in pneumonia or asthma, people increase the amount of air they swallow, often resulting in a dramatic plain abdominal radiograph. The gas-filled, slightly dilated loops of bowel so produced contain relatively little fluid; the term 'meteorism' is applied to this appearance. It is sometimes difficult to distinguish meteorism produced, for example, by renal colic, from intestinal obstruction. A clinical history and examination frequently enable the radiological findings to be correctly interpreted.

The posterior extraperitoneal fat pad, which completely surrounds the kidneys, psoas muscles and the posterior borders of the liver and spleen, extends anteriorly and laterally to surround the parietal peritoneum and so is also intimately related to intraperitoneal organs. The fat lines produced are responsible for the visualisation of most of these intra-abdominal organs. These fat lines can be displaced if the organs are enlarged and may be blurred or effaced by inflammation or fluid. However, visualisation of these structures by fat lines is not universal. In 19% of normal people the right psoas outline is blurred, and the lower border of the spleen can only be visualised in 58%. This is particularly important in children, where the psoas outlines are lost in 52% and the properitoneal fat line is lost in 18% of normals. These factors must therefore be considered carefully before undue emphasis is placed on these signs in the abnormal patient.

Pneumoperitoneum

The demonstration of a small pneumoperitoneum in a patient presenting with acute abdominal pain is one of the most significant

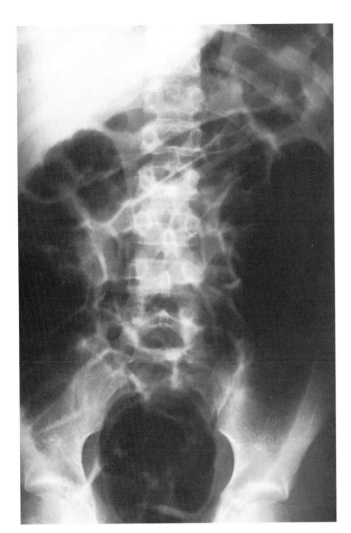

Fig. 22.1 Air swallowing. There is slight gaseous distension of both small and large bowel, but this extends down to the rectum. A 7-year-old girl admitted to hospital with abdominal pain and distension following a single episode of vomiting. At the time of admission she was distressed and crying. Shortly after admission her bowels were opened normally and the abdominal distension and pain disappeared.

small bowel. Fluid is a normal constituent of small bowel, and short fluid levels are not abnormal. A small-bowel calibre exceeding 2.5 cm is abnormal and indicates dilated small bowel.

Enough gas is usually present in the colon for it to be readily identified by its position and haustra. However, the calibre of the colon varies more than that of any other viscus, and no satisfactory measurement of the upper limit of normal diameter is possible. Old, mentally subnormal, psychiatric or institutionalised patients may have enormous colons measuring 10–15 cm in diameter and yet apparently be without symptoms. Their colonic diameters frequently exceed those of younger patients with clear-cut large-bowel obstruction. In inflammatory bowel disease, however, a transverse colonic diameter exceeding 5.5 cm has been suggested as the upper limit of normal, and above this megacolon should be diagnosed. In patients with large-bowel obstruction, a transverse caecal diameter exceeding 9 cm is the level above which a state of 'impending perforation' exists.

Colonic fluid levels are a normal finding, and some which are several centimetres long may be seen. Eighteen per cent of normal people also have a caecal fluid level.

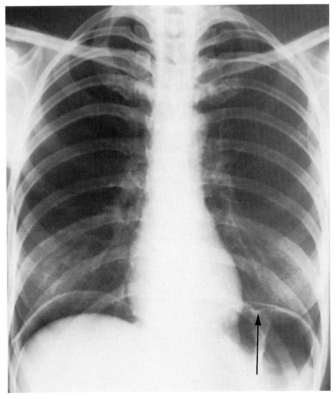

Fig. 22.2 Pneumoperitoneum. Erect chest film. Free intra-abdominal gas is clearly demonstrated under the right hemidiaphragm. Under the left hemidiaphragm a small triangular collection of free gas can be identified between loops of gas-filled bowel (arrow).

signs in medicine. In over 90% of cases the cause of the pneumoperitoneum will require emergency surgery.

It is possible, by careful radiographic technique, to demonstrate as little as 1 ml of free gas on erect chest or left lateral decubitus abdominal films. However, radiographic technique and positioning are important and a patient should be in position for 10 min before the film is taken, for it takes this time for free gas to rise to the highest point in the abdomen (Fig. 22.2).

The demonstration of a pneumoperitoneum on plain film following a perforated viscus is, however, not invariable, and most series show that in only 75–80% of perforations is free gas demonstrable. A number of reasons for this have been suggested, including sealing of the perforation, lack of gas at the site of perforation, or adhesions around the site of the perforation. However, radiographic technique is also important: a pneumoperitoneum can be detected in 76% of cases using an erect film only, but when a left lateral decubitus projection is included, a pneumoperitoneum can be demonstrated in nearly 90% of cases.

If a perforated viscus is suspected, then a horizontal-ray radiograph, either an erect chest or decubitus abdomen, is mandatory. However, in many patients—particularly following trauma, the elderly or critically ill, and those who are unconscious—perforation may be clinically silent or is overshadowed by another serious medical or surgical condition. A supine abdominal radiograph, frequently taken using a mobile unit, may be the only radiograph that has been obtained. It is therefore important to recognise the signs of pneumoperitoneum on these.

About 56% of patients with a pneumoperitoneum may have free gas detectable on a supine radiograph. Almost half the patients will have a collection in the right upper quadrant adjacent to the liver and lying mainly in the subhepatic space and the hepatorenal fossa (Morison's pouch), and visible as an oval or linear collection of gas (Fig. 22.3). Visualisation of the outer as well as the inner wall of a loop of bowel (Rigler's sign) is a valuable indication of a pneumoperitoneum (Fig. 22.4). However, this sign may be misleading if gas-distended loops of bowel are in contact, with apparent visualisation of outer and inner walls, when in fact the inner walls of two loops of bowel are seen. Small triangular collections of gas between loops of bowel may sometimes be identified and are a valuable sign of pneumoperitoneum in supine radiographs.

Reflections of the peritoneum normally present on the inner surface of the anterior abdominal wall are not usually identified, but may be visualised by large amounts of free gas when it lies on either side. Thus the falciform ligament (Fig. 22.3), medial and lateral umbilical ligaments and the urachus can occasionally be identified when relatively large amounts of gas are present.

Relatively large amounts of gas may accumulate beneath the diaphragm (the 'cupola' sign) or in the centre of the abdomen over a fluid collection (the 'football' sign). Free gas may also be identified in the fissure for the ligamentum teres.

CT is, however, the most sensitive method for the detection of peritoneal free gas, with even tiny bubbles of gas being visible. The radiologist should review the images on wide window settings in order to appreciate small volumes of gas, as the gas adja-

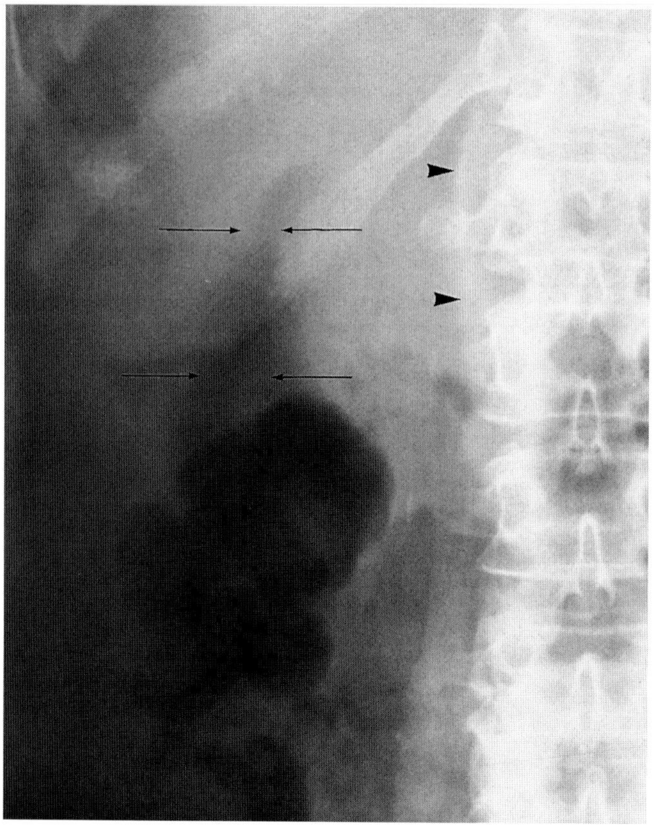

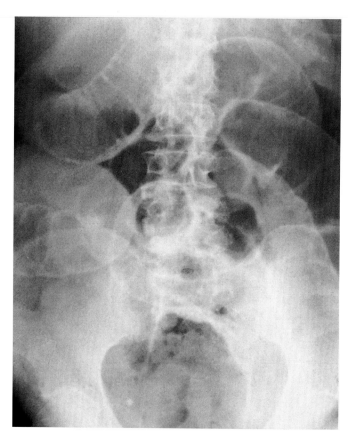

Fig. 22.3 Pneumoperitoneum. Abdomen, supine. A triangular collection of free gas is demonstrated in the subhepatic region (arrows). The falciform ligament is also outlined (arrowheads).

Fig. 22.4 Pneumoperitoneum. Abdomen, supine. Visualisation of both sides of the bowel wall (Rigler's sign). Both the inside and outside wall of multiple loops of small bowel can be clearly identified.

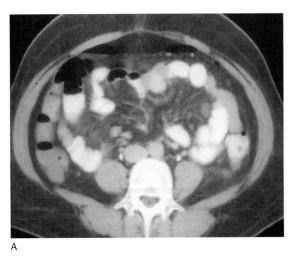

A

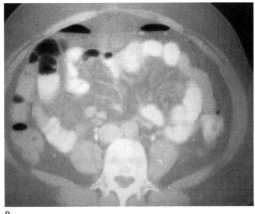

B

Fig. 22.5 Free intraperitoneal gas. (A) On abdominal windows the free gas is not well seen anteriorly. (B) On wide window settings, the free gas is much more obvious.

cent to neighbouring fat and bowel loops is otherwise easy to miss. Free gas tends to collect over the liver, anteriorly in the mid abdomen, and in the peritoneal recesses (Fig. 22.5).

Pseudopneumoperitoneum

A number of conditions have been described which simulate free air in the peritoneal cavity on plain film (pseudopneumoperitoneum) (Box 22.3). These are important because failure to

---

Box 22.3   Causes of pseudopneumoperitoneum

Chilaiditi syndrome
Subdiaphragmatic fat
Curvilinear pulmonary collapse
Uneven diaphragm
Distended viscus
Omental fat
Subphrenic abscess
Subpulmonary pneumothorax
Intramural gas in pneumatosis intestinalis
Apposition of gas-distended loops mimicking the double wall sign

---

Box 22.4   Causes of a pneumoperitoneum without peritonitis

Silent perforation of a viscus, which has sealed, related to steroid therapy, in the elderly, in coma, in the presence of other serious medical conditions
Postoperative
Peritoneal dialysis
Perforated jejunal diverticulosis
Intra-abdominal therapeutic embolisation
Air from pneumatosis intestinalis
Leakage through distended bowel (e.g. stomach at endoscopy)
Laparoscopy
Entry through the female genital tract
Associated chest conditions
　Pneumonia
　Emphysema
　Carcinoma of the lung
　Pneumomediastinum
　Intermittent positive-pressure ventilation
　Pulmonary peritoneal fistula

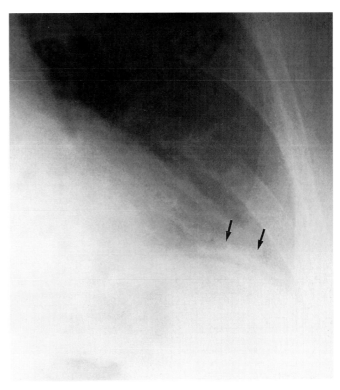

Fig. 22.6 Pseudopneumoperitoneum. A band of curvilinear pulmonary collapse (arrows) with a crescent of normal lung beneath it simulates a pneumoperitoneum almost exactly.

recognise them may lead to an unnecessary laparotomy in search of a perforated viscus. One of the commonest of these conditions is distended bowel, usually hepatic flexure of the colon, interposed between the liver and the diaphragm (the Chilaiditi syndrome). Subdiaphragmatic fat, an extension from the posterior pararenal fat, is a common normal finding and frequently can be identified as a lucent crescent under the diaphragm; this may simulate a pneumoperitoneum. Its constant position in decubitus views will enable the correct diagnosis to be made. Sometimes curvilinear pulmonary collapse parallel to and just above the diaphragm may simulate a pneumoperitoneum exactly (Fig. 22.6). An

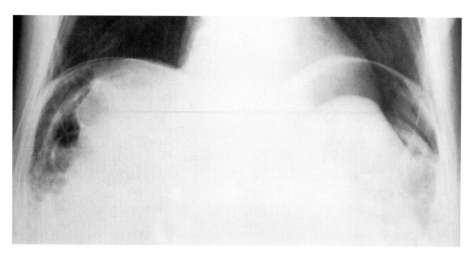

Fig. 22.7 Pneumoperitoneum without peritonitis. Small-bowel pneumatosis. Free gas is readily identified under the left hemidiaphragm and there is a thin crescent of gas under the right hemidiaphragm. The typical cysts of pneumatosis can be identified in the small bowel under the right hemidiaphragm. A 69-year-old man admitted with haematemesis. (Courtesy of Dr A. R. Carter.)

uneven diaphragm, distended bowel and omental fat between the liver and the diaphragm may also simulate free gas on occasions.

Pneumoperitoneum without peritonitis

Occasionally, asymptomatic patients or those with very minimal signs and symptoms are found to have a pneumoperitoneum. Many of these patients will subsequently be found to have perforated an ulcer which has sealed itself, or to have not yet developed the signs of peritonitis. Numerous other conditions that may produce a spontaneous pneumoperitoneum without peritonitis have been described (Box 22.4; Fig. 22.7).

Postoperative pneumoperitoneum

About 60% of all postlaparotomy patients will have evidence of a pneumoperitoneum. Although, in most patients, the air will have been absorbed within a few days, a delay of up to 24 days before all the air has disappeared has been reported. A pneumoperitoneum occurs in the postoperative period more commonly in thin patients than in obese ones, and the rate of absorption is faster in the obese—in these, the air has usually all been absorbed by the third postoperative day. Provided that identical radiographic technique is used, and adequate time is spent in positioning the horizontal-ray radiograph, any increase in the volume of gas postoperatively indicates an anastomotic leak or a further perforation.

Use of contrast media in suspected perforation

If a patient with severe upper abdominal pain has equivocal clinical signs and no free gas is seen on plain films, further investigations may be needed to exclude a perforation. A nasogastric tube is normally in position and 100 ml of air can be injected down the tube and a further film taken after the patient has been lying in the left lateral decubitus position for 10 min. More than 80% of perforations occur in the duodenum or pyloric antrum, and this technique will facilitate the passage of air into the peritoneal cavity. Alternatively, 50 ml of non-ionic contrast medium can be given orally, the patient placed on the right side and a further abdominal film taken after 5 min. A leak of contrast medium may occur in ulcers which have perforated but which do not show free gas. Furthermore, an oedematous stretched duodenal loop may be seen

in patients with acute pancreatitis. A CT scan will usually be valuable where there is doubt.

INTESTINAL OBSTRUCTION

Dilatation of bowel occurs in mechanical intestinal obstruction, pseudo-obstruction, paralytic ileus, air swallowing and several other conditions. The radiological differentiation depends mainly on the size, mucosal appearance, and the distribution of the loops of bowel. The diagnosis of intestinal obstruction depends on the demonstration of dilated loops of bowel proximally with non-dilated or collapsed bowel distal to the presumed point of obstruction.

GASTRIC DILATATION

Dilatation of the stomach can be caused by four main groups of conditions: mechanical gastric outlet obstruction, paralytic ileus, gastric volvulus and air swallowing. These are summarised in Box 22.5.

The 'paralytic ileus' group of conditions is frequently referred to as 'acute gastric dilatation', often occurs in old people and is associated with considerable fluid and electrolyte disturbance; as a result it carries a high mortality (Fig. 22.8).

Box 22.5   Causes of a massivelly dilated stomach
Paralytic ileus
Postoperative
Trauma
Peritonitis
Pancreatitis
Cholecystitis
Diabetic coma
Hepatic coma
Mechanical gastric outlet obstruction
Duodenal ulceration
Antral carcinoma
Extrinsic duodenal compression
Gastric volvulus
Air swallowing
Intubation
Secondary to intestinal obstruction
Drugs

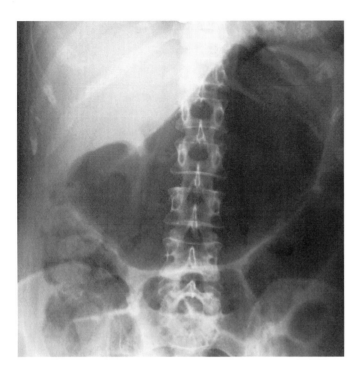

Fig. 22.8 Acute gastric dilatation. Abdomen, supine. A 38-year-old woman admitted in diabetic precoma.

Mechanical gastric outlet obstruction, caused by peptic ulceration or a carcinoma of the pyloric antrum, often leads to a massive fluid-filled stomach which occupies most of the upper abdomen and is demonstrable as a large soft-tissue mass with little or no bowel gas beyond. Fortunately, a little gas is usually present within the stomach and this can be identified on horizontal-ray films, which allow the organ to be identified.

Volvulus of the stomach is a relatively uncommon condition and may result from the stomach twisting around the longitudinal or mesenteric axis. In a gastric volvulus the dilated stomach usually contains both air and fluid, is identified as a spherical viscus, displaced upward and to the left, and is associated with elevation of the hemidiaphragm. It is usual for the small bowel to be collapsed and it is uncommon to see any gas shadows beyond the stomach. It is important to differentiate a volvulus of the stomach from a caecal volvulus; both may produce a distended viscus containing fluid and air lying beneath the left hemidiaphragm. If contrast medium is given in a case of suspected gastric volvulus there may be complete obstruction at the lower end of the oesophagus, or if contrast medium does enter the stomach it may not pass beyond the obstructed pylorus.

Frequently after resuscitation and intubation large amounts of gas enter the stomach and may lead to massive dilatation. This may sometimes occur after air swallowing alone, for example in hysteria or in near-drowning.

When supine, the gas-filled stomach can usually be identified, with the wall of the greater curvature convex caudally and the pyloric antrum pointing cranially. It is very important to differentiate a distended stomach from a caecal volvulus, which may also be positioned beneath an elevated left hemidiaphragm, as noted above. However, with caecal volvulus, one or two haustra can frequently be identified and the inferior part of the caecum usually points caudally, in contrast to the pyloric antrum which points cranially.

THE DISTINCTION BETWEEN SMALL- AND LARGE-BOWEL DILATATION

When a radiograph shows dilated bowel it is important to try to determine whether it is small or large bowel, or both. Useful differentiating features depend on the size, distribution and marking of the loops and are summarised in Table 22.1.

Although the features listed in Table 22.1 are useful, there is often considerable overlap of these signs. For example, problems in distinguishing the lower ileum from the sigmoid colon are relatively frequent as both may be smooth in outline and occupy a similar position low in the midline in the abdomen. Haustra usually form thick, incomplete bands across the colonic gas shadow; however, sometimes they may form complete transverse bands. Usually these can still be distinguished from valvulae conniventes because they are thicker and further apart than the small-bowel folds. Haustra may be completely absent from the descending and sigmoid colon, although they can usually still be identified in other parts of the colon even when it is massively distended.

The small-bowel folds, or valvulae conniventes, usually form thin complete lines across the dilated small bowel. They are prominent in the jejunum but become less marked as the ileum is reached. The valvulae conniventes are situated much closer together than colonic haustra and become thinner when stretched, but still remain relatively close to each other even as the calibre of the small bowel increases. However, if the small bowel blood supply becomes compromised and the bowel becomes oedematous or gangrenous, the valvulae conniventes may become greatly thickened and may then be extremely difficult to distinguish from colonic haustra.

When numerous loops of dilated bowel are present, this almost invariably indicates that the small bowel is dilated. However, in large-bowel obstruction, both the large and the small bowel may be dilated.

Although the diameter of the bowel may be extremely variable in intestinal obstruction, in small-bowel obstruction it is unusual for it to greatly exceed 5 cm except in cases of longstanding obstruction. Equally, in large-bowel obstruction it is unusual for the calibre of the large bowel to be less than 5 cm; indeed it usually greatly exceeds this.

The causes and management of small-bowel obstruction are very different from those of large-bowel obstruction and so it is essential to differentiate between them wherever possible. In most patients, this is relatively easy but some can present a major diagnostic problem, and further investigation may be needed.

Table 22.1 The distinction between small- and large-bowel dilatation

	Small bowel	Large bowel
Valvulae conniventes	Present in jejunum	Absent
Number of loops	Many	Few
Distribution of loops	Central	Peripheral
Haustra	Absent	Present
Diameter	3–5 cm	5 cm+
Radius of curvature	Small	Large
Solid faeces	Absent	Present

SMALL-BOWEL OBSTRUCTION

Due to the high incidence of elective surgery the commonest cause of small-bowel obstruction in the developed world is adhesions due to previous surgery, comprising 75–80% of all cases. Strangulated hernias, which were once the commonest cause, now comprise only 8%, although in underdeveloped parts of the world they still remain the commonest cause. Complete obstruction of the small bowel usually causes small-bowel dilatation with accumulation of both gas and fluid and a reduction in calibre of the large bowel. The amount of gas present in the large bowel depends on the duration and completeness or otherwise of the small-bowel obstruction. It frequently takes several bowel movements to empty the large bowel entirely of gas and faeces. Plain film changes in small-bowel obstruction may appear after 3–5 hrs if there is complete small-bowel obstruction, and such changes are usually marked after 12 h. With incomplete obstruction, or if films are taken very shortly after the onset of symptoms, plain films may be normal and barium studies or ultrasound may have to be done to establish a diagnosis.

In most cases of small-bowel obstruction, however, dilated gas-filled loops of small bowel are readily identified on the supine radiograph, multiple fluid levels are present on erect films, and in most cases there is little diagnostic difficulty (Fig. 22.9). However, one must resist the temptation to diagnose obstruction by the pres-ence of fluid levels alone, as there are many other causes of these. Dilated fluid-filled loops of small bowel may be identified as sausage shaped, oval or round soft-tissue densities that change in position in different views. In dilated small bowel which is almost completely filled with fluid, small bubbles of gas may be trapped in rows between the valvulae conniventes on horizontal-ray films; this is known as the 'string of beads' sign (Fig. 22.10). This sign, if present, is virtually diagnostic of small-bowel obstruction and does not occur in normal people.

In about 6% of small-bowel obstruction, small-bowel loops may be predominantly fluid filled, with little or no gas visible. Fluid-filled loops should be carefully searched for in patients who are clinically suspected of having intestinal obstruction, otherwise diagnosis may be delayed and, as a result, the seriousness of the condition increased. The normal tinkling obstructive bowel sounds, which are so characteristic of small-bowel obstruction, are caused by fluid moving in a predominantly gas-filled dilated bowel. When little or no gas is present and the dilated loops are predominantly fluid filled, the classic obstructive bowel sounds may be absent, and so it is even more important for the radiologist to consider fluid-filled loops in small-bowel obstruction.

If the initial radiographs are considered normal, there is frequently a delay in making the diagnosis of small-bowel obstruction. If there is persistent diagnostic difficulty, repeat films taken within a

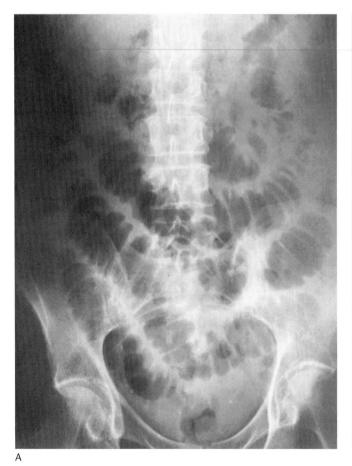

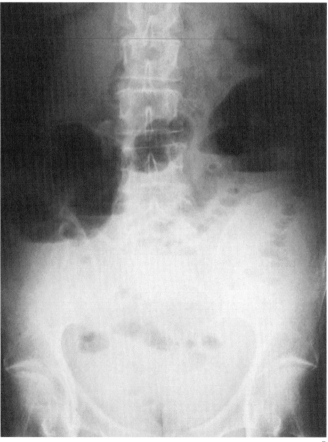

A   B

Fig. 22.9 Small-bowel obstruction: (A) supine; (B) erect. Multiple dilated loops of both gas-filled and fluid-filled small bowel are readily identified. There is little or no gas in the large bowel. Multiple fluid levels are noted on erect film. A 77-year-old woman with a past history of several abdominal operations. The small-bowel obstruction was presumed to be due to adhesions and resolved with conservative management.

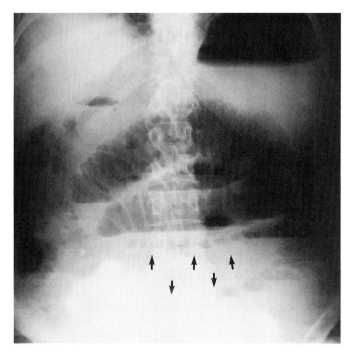

Fig. 22.10 Small-bowel obstruction, 'string of beads' sign. Erect film. The dilated proximal small bowel is predominantly gas filled with a few long fluid levels. More distally, the small bowel is fluid filled and bubbles of gas are trapped between the valvulae conniventes, producing a chain of bubbles.

few hours of the first will often solve the problem—if not, oral barium should be given. Giving barium in suspected small-bowel obstruction is not harmful, due to the large amounts of fluid present, and it will not complete an otherwise incomplete obstruction.

Some authors advocate giving an oral dose of 100 ml of non-ionic contrast medium and taking a plain film of the abdomen at 4 h. In those patients where the contrast has not reached the caecum at 4 h, there is a high likelihood of surgery being required for small bowel obstruction during that admission.

Ultrasound can be used to demonstrate the dilated fluid-filled loops of small bowel obstruction, and an assessment of the peristaltic activity can be made at the same time. The cause of obstruction is unlikely to be evident, and if there is an excessive quantity of gas the examination becomes difficult.

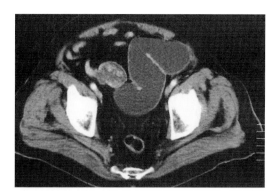

Fig. 22.11 Small-bowel obstruction due to a metastatic deposit. Very dilated small bowel leads into the mass at the point of transition to collapsed small bowel.

If a confident clinical and radiological diagnosis of small bowel obstruction has been made, and the patient has not had previous abdominal operations, he or she is likely to proceed to laparotomy. Increasingly, CT scanning is used for diagnosis because it demonstrates the presence of bowel calibre change, and the level. Fluid-filled loops are difficult to visualise on plain film, but are clearly visible on CT. In order to establish the level of obstruction one may need to follow the dilated bowel loops with the eye forwards from the duodenojejunal flexure, or backwards from the ileocaecal valve (Fig. 22.11). 'Paging' through the images on the CT console may assist in this assessment.

The cause of obstruction is occasionally evident on plain film, for instance when there is a groin hernia, volvulus or gallstone ileus, but obstructing lesions are identified much more frequently by CT (Fig. 22.12). CT should be performed whenever there is a history of previous abdominal malignancy, as extraluminal disease in the peritoneum, nodes and liver will be demonstrated, and may change the management of the patient.

Although peritoneal adhesions are usually a diagnosis of exclusion in the presence of obstruction, adhesions can be suspected on CT when bowel loops are seen to converge to a point where there is no mass, sometimes appearing beaked or triangulated. The CT sensitivity for adhesions is around 73%.

The initial management of a patient who has small-bowel obstruction which is presumed to be due to adhesions is usually conservative, using a 'drip and suck' regimen. Prolonged conserva-

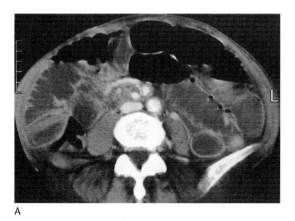

A

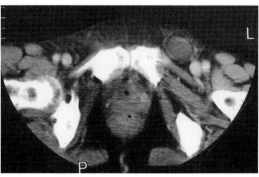

B

Fig. 22.12 Small-bowel obstruction due to left femoral hernia. (A) Dilated small-bowel loops in the midabdomen. (B) There is a left femoral hernia containing a bowel loop.

tive management warrants repeat supine radiographs, to assess the bowel diameter, thickness of the bowel wall and valvulae conniventes, so that radiological progress can also be monitored. Radiological evidence of failure to respond, or evidence of increasing obstruction or of bowel necrosis, are indications for surgery.

If there is clinical doubt about the diagnosis, or when non-operative management is being planned, CT scanning is valuable in furthering the diagnosis and helping to exclude complications of obstruction. Plain films are generally poor at detecting bowel strangulation and ischaemia. Mortality from small-bowel obstruction rises dramatically if strangulation is present.

Strangulating obstruction

'Strangulating obstruction' means mechanical small-bowel obstruction caused when two limbs of a loop are incarcerated by a band or in a hernia, frequently compromising the blood supply due to compression of the mesenteric vessels. The closed loop may fill with fluid and be palpable, or it may be visible on the radiograph as a soft-tissue mass or 'pseudotumour'. The strangulated loop uncommonly contains gas; the limbs of the loop, separated only by the thickened intestinal walls, may resemble a large coffee bean. If gangrene occurs, lines of gas may be seen in the wall of the small bowel. However, the appearance in strangulating obstruction, with all its lethal potential, may be indistinguishable from that of simple small-bowel obstruction.

CT is much more sensitive for bowel loop strangulation than plain films. A closed loop is usually fluid-filled, and V-shaped or radial, with mesenteric vessels converging towards the point of obstruction. The loop may be triangular, and show a whorl or beak. If the loop is strangulated it becomes thickened with venous congestion of the mesentery locally (Fig. 22.13). If there is haemorrhage the bowel wall may be of increased attenuation, but this sign is masked if bowel and intravenous contrast have been given. If necrosis is present, gas may be seen in the bowel wall. Viewing on wide or 'lung' windows will make bowel wall gas more conspicuous. CT is also very sensitive for peritoneal fluid, but this cannot be relied upon as a sign of strangulation.

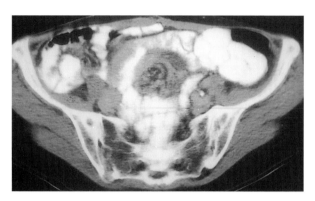

Fig. 22.13 Strangulated small bowel loop. There is whorled mesenteric thickening with an adjacent loop of small bowel with a thickened wall.

Volvulus of the small intestine

Volvulus of the small bowel may occur as an isolated lesion or be combined with obstruction due to adhesive bands. It is often associated with congenital abnormalities of the mesentery and there is frequently malrotation. In children, incomplete rotation, malrotation or non-rotation of the gut may be associated with a massive small-bowel volvulus which may occur in the neonatal period, or months or even years after birth. There is frequently an impaired blood supply in the small bowel so that intramural gas or thumbprinting may be seen. However, it is not usually possible to distinguish simple obstruction, strangulating obstruction or small-bowel volvulus on plain radiographs alone.

When a **strangulated external hernia** is the cause of obstruction, it is usually detected clinically. However, sometimes this is overlooked due to obesity, and so it is important to search the radiograph for evidence of a hernia. Many strangulated hernias will be fluid filled and not visible on a plain film; furthermore, the mere presence of a hernia does not mean this is the cause of obstruction. However, if dilated bowel is identified ending at a hernial orifice, then the hernia is probably the cause of obstruction.

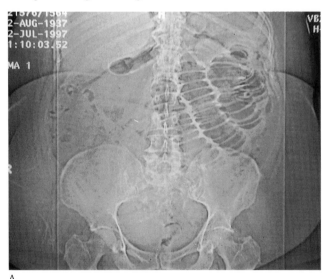

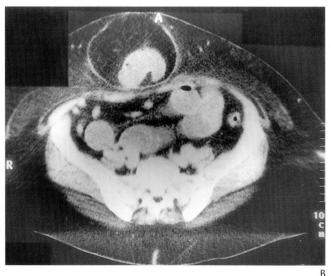

Fig. 22.14 Small-bowel obstruction due to an incisional hernia in an obese patient. (A) CT scout image showing dilated small bowel, and illustrating the degree of obesity. (B) CT demonstrating the midline incisional hernia containing a bowel loop.

CT is very effective at detecting hernias, not only at the groin, but also elsewhere in the abdominal wall (Fig. 22.14), and within the peritoneum. It will also help establish if the hernia is the cause of the obstruction.

An **appendix abscess** may present as small-bowel obstruction due to small bowel becoming adherent to the wall of the abscess. The appendix abscess may be identified as a soft-tissue mass which may contain gas and indent the caecum (Fig. 22.15).

Crohn's disease sometimes presents as small-bowel obstruction. When this occurs the abnormal segment of small bowel causing the obstruction is never identified as plain film and the appearances are those of non-specific small-bowel obstruction.

The presence of a distended caecum in someone with small-bowel obstruction suggests a carcinoma of the ascending colon or caecal volvulus.

The majority of patients who present with small-bowel obstruction have adhesions and the cause cannot be identified on plain films. The main value of plain films is in assessing the degree and severity of the obstruction.

Gallstone ileus

Gallstone ileus is mechanical intestinal obstruction caused by the impaction of one or more gallstones in the intestine, usually in the terminal ileum, but rarely in the duodenum or colon. The patient, most commonly a middle-aged or elderly woman, will often have had recurrent episodes of right hypochondrial pain characteristic of cholecystitis. The most recent attack may have been more severe and associated with prolonged vomiting. The gallstones pass into

the duodenum or rarely into the colon by eroding through the inflamed gallbladder wall.

Gallstone ileus comprises about 2% of all small-bowel obstruction, but in elderly women who have not had a previous laparotomy it is much more common. Gallstone ileus is an important condition because the operative mortality is high and the diagnosis is frequently delayed or missed, even though specific radiological signs may be present in nearly 40% of cases. Over half the patients will have evidence of intestinal obstruction and about one-third will have gas present in the biliary tree (Fig. 22.16).

Gas in the biliary tree can be recognised by its branching pattern, with the gas more prominent centrally; gas in the portal vein, from which it must be distinguished, tends to be more peripherally located, in small veins around the edge of the liver. The obstructing gallstone, which is frequently located in the pelvic loops of ileum overlying the sacrum, will be identified in about one-third of patients either on plain radiographs or barium examinations. However, visualisation of the obstructing gallstone on plain films is frequently difficult, because it is often composed almost entirely of cholesterol with only a thin rim of calcium within it. Furthermore,

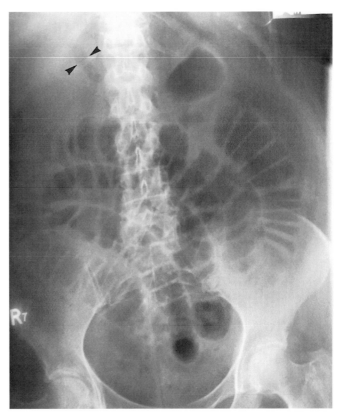

Fig. 22.16 Gallstone ileus. Supine film. Multiple dilated loops of small bowel are seen. A band of gas in the right hypochondrium (arrowheads) lies within the common bile duct. The obstructing gallstone cannot be identified.

Box 22.6 Signs of gallstone ileus
Gas within the bile ducts and/or the gallbladder   Complete or incomplete small-bowel obstruction   Abnormal location of gallstone   Change in position of gallstone

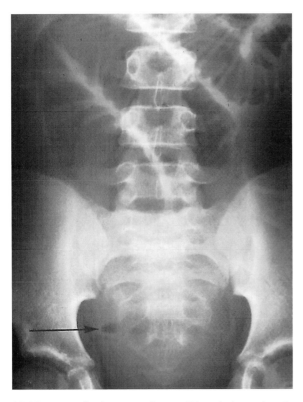

Fig. 22.15 Appendix abscess causing small-bowel obstruction. A small gas bubble which lies within the abscess (arrow) is seen in the right iliac fossa. Age 11 years, vomiting with some diarrhoea for 1 week.

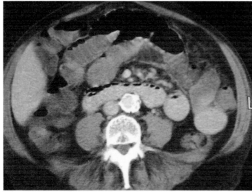

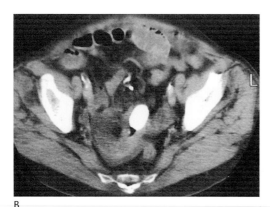

A

B

Fig. 22.17 Small-bowel obstruction due to an ileal faecolith. (A) Dilated small bowel loops. The gallbladder appeared normal. (B) Image through the pelvis. At the transition from dilated to collapsed bowel is a large densely calcified intraluminal faecolith.

the gallstone is often located over the sacrum and is further obscured by dilated small bowel. Change in position of a previously observed gallstone is uncommon and only occurs in 6% of cases. Signs of gallstone ileus are summarised in Box 22.6.

The small bowel dilatation, gas within the biliary tree and the gallstone at the point of obstruction may all be demonstrated elegantly on CT. Occasionally small bowel obstruction may be caused by a bezoar or enterolith (Fig. 22.17).

Gas in the biliary tree

Gas in the biliary tree is most commonly seen following sphincterotomy biliary surgery or interventional procedures. Anastomoses between the gallbladder or bile duct and the duodenum or jejunum will almost invariably result in gas in the biliary tree, and it is therefore essential to know of any such interventions before interpreting plain films. On occasions, malignant disease of the duodenum or colon may involve the gallbladder or bile ducts, resulting in a

---

Box 22.7 Causes of gas in the biliary tree
Following biliary surgery Gallstone fistula—gallbladder usually small Emphysematous cholecystitis—gallbladder usually enlarged Malignant fistula Perforated peptic ulcer into bile duct Physiological—due to lax sphincter

---

fistula. A posterior perforation of a peptic ulcer into the bile duct is a further means of communication between the bowel and a bile duct. Emphysematous cholecystitis or cholangitis may result in gas filling the gallbladder and bile ducts, but in this situation the gallbladder is usually enlarged. Sometimes gas in the biliary tree may be identified in small-bowel obstruction which is not due to gallstone ileus. In these cases the gas is presumed to have entered through a physiologically lax sphincter. Causes of gas in the biliary tree are summarised in Box 22.7.

Intussusception

The incidence of intussusception varies considerably in different countries, but in general it is most frequently seen in children under 2 years of age. In children it usually commences in the ileum as the result of inflammation of the lymphoid tissue and tends to be associated with mesenteric adenitis. The enlarged lymphatic patches are forced into the ileum by peristaltic movement and, acting as a tumour, one part of the ileum is pulled into the other and finally pulled into the colon. Although the condition is usually recognised clinically by pain, vomiting, blood in the stool and a palpable tumour, the diagnosis may not be apparent initially and further investigations may be needed.

Plain films may show evidence of small-bowel obstruction, or the intussusception itself may be identified as a soft-tissue mass some-

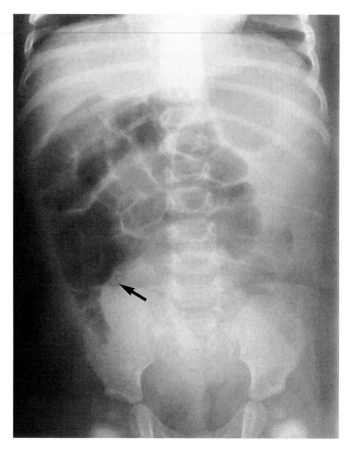

Fig. 22.18 Intussusception. Supine film. There are multiple gas-filled loops of slightly dilated small bowel. In addition, there is a soft-tissue mass in the right iliac fossa (arrow). A 5-month-old child with mesenteric adenitis.

times surrounded by a crescent of gas and most frequently identified in the right hypochondrium (Fig. 22.18). More recently the 'target sign' has been described, comprising two concentric circles of fat density lying to the right of the spine—often superimposed on the kidney. It is probably due to the layers of peritoneal fat surrounding and within the intussusceptum alternating with the layers of mucosa and muscle but seen 'end on' as it passes forward from the right paraspinal gutter in the transverse colon. However, a barium enema is frequently required to establish a definite diagnosis and, providing certain precautions are taken, can also be used to reduce it. In adults, an intussusception is invariably caused by a tumour of the bowel, which may be large or small, benign or malignant. Any part of the small bowel may be involved, although the terminal ileum is still the most common site for the underlying pathology. Classical pathologies include lipoma of the terminal ileum, lymphoma, and metastases from melanoma; abnormalities that are found in the submucosa. Symptoms may be severe and sudden, or chronic with recurrent episodes of colicky abdominal pain.

CT readily demonstrates intussusception, often with a characteristic feature of fat centrally due to mesenteric fat being brought up the lumen of the intussuscipiens behind the intussusceptum. The intussusception appears as a sausage-shaped mass or a target mass, depending on its orientation in relation to the CT plane (Fig. 22.19).

Mesenteric thrombosis—small intestinal infarction

Necrosis of the small bowel is the most serious abdominal condition caused by thrombosis or embolism of the superior mesenteric artery. The clinical diagnosis is often uncertain until laparotomy, but the sudden onset of abdominal pain, often associated with bloody diarrhoea, in an elderly person is very suggestive of this condition. Gas-filled, slightly dilated loops of small bowel with multiple fluid levels, or fluid-filled loops of small bowel, are frequent plain film findings. The walls of the small bowel may be thickened due to submucosal haemorrhage and oedema. Linear gas streaks in the bowel wall may be seen if there is gangrene, and free

gas may be present if perforation has occurred. Colonic distension may also be present if there is a generalised paralytic ileus. Gas in the portal vein may occur secondary to bowel necrosis and is a grave prognostic sign in adults. In small bowel infarction, bowel wall thickening is the most common feature on CT. This is due to oedema and haemorrhage in the submucosa, and may be diffuse or forming submucosal nodules. The density may be low if predominantly oedematous, or of increased attenuation if due to the presence of haemorrhage. There may be engorgement of the mesenteric veins, and increased attenuation of the mesenteric fat. All of these signs are non-specific, but gas within the bowel wall is far more suggestive of the diagnosis, although a less commonly seen sign. Even less common is gas in the mesenteric veins and portal venous system. This is a bad prognostic sign, as is bowel perforation in ischaemia. It may be possible to identify non-enhancement of the superior mesenteric artery and vein after intravenous contrast.

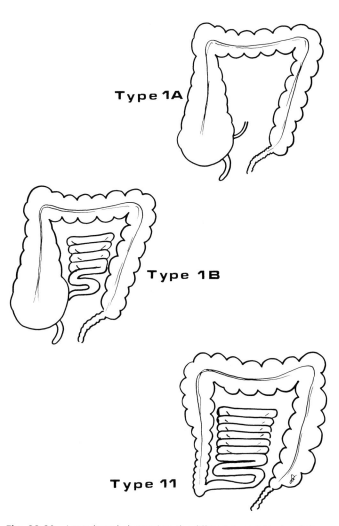

Fig. 22.20 Large-bowel obstruction: the different types (after Love). Type IA: Competent ileocaecal valve. Distended large bowel, particularly ascending colon and caecum. No distension of small bowel. Type IB: Competent ileocaecal valve. Caecal distension and small-bowel distension. Type II: Incompetent ileocaecal valve. No distension of caecum and ascending colon but distension of small bowel. Caecal perforation is much more likely to occur in type I large-bowel obstruction.

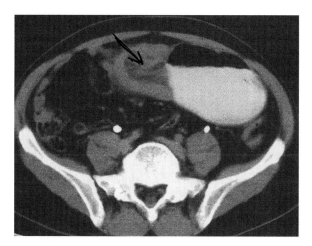

Fig. 22.19 Small-bowel obstruction due to a small-bowel melanoma metastasis which has caused jejunal intussusception. The grossly dilated loop of jejunum contains oral contrast medium, and leads into the intussusception, which contains the characteristic central mesenteric fat (arrow).

LARGE-BOWEL OBSTRUCTION

The commonest cause of large-bowel obstruction is carcinoma, of which about 60% are situated in the sigmoid colon. Diverticular disease as a cause of obstruction has decreased in frequency since the introduction of high-fibre diets. Volvulus of the colon comprises about 10% of large-bowel obstruction in the USA and Europe, but in less developed parts of the world volvulus accounts for 85%.

The key to the radiological appearances of large-bowel obstruction depends on the state of competence of the ileocaecal valve. Three patterns (Fig. 22.20) of obstruction have been described. In type IA the ileocaecal valve is competent and the radiological appearance is one of dilated colon with a distended thin-walled caecum but no distension of small bowel (Fig. 22.21). As this type progresses, small-bowel distension occurs (type IB), probably secondary to the tightly closed ileocaecal valve. Both type I obstructions can lead to massive caecal distension, which is then at risk of perforation secondary to ischaemia. A transverse caecal diameter of 9 cm has been suggested as the critical point above which the danger of perforation exists. In type II obstruction the ileocaecal valve is incompetent and the caecum and ascending colon are not distended, but the back-pressure from the colon extends into the small bowel and there are numerous dilated loops of small bowel which may simulate small-bowel obstruction.

The obstructed colon almost invariably contains large amounts of air and can usually be identified by its haustral margin around the periphery of the abdomen. However, on occasions the right half

of the colon may be filled with fluid and massive caecal distension may be overlooked. Even more rarely, the whole colon up to the point of obstruction may be filled with fluid and so the diagnosis may be overlooked initially.

When both small- and large-bowel dilatation are present in large-bowel obstruction, the radiographic appearances may be identical to those of a paralytic ileus. However, the clinical signs will usually help to differentiate. If problems in interpretation still occur, however, a left lateral radiograph, by demonstrating air in the rectum, may differentiate paralytic ileus from low large-bowel obstruction.

There are numerous causes of colonic distension without obstruction. These include all forms of paralytic ileus and pseudo-obstruction. It is extremely important, therefore, that prior to surgery for 'obstruction' a single-contrast diluted barium enema examination is performed as an emergency to confirm mechanical obstruction and to exclude pseudo-obstruction or colonic ileus. If the patient appears to be unfit for an enema, the same information can be obtained from a CT.

The cause of simple large-bowel obstruction cannot usually be determined from plain radiographs alone, although sometimes a pericolic abscess secondary to diverticular disease may be identified.

Pseudo-obstruction

Pseudo-obstruction is a disorder of bowel which symptomatically, clinically and radiologically may mimic intestinal obstruction. It may be acute and self-limiting and associated with pneumonia, septicaemia or certain drugs, or chronic with acute flare-ups, as seen in diabetes mellitus, collagen disorders, neurological disorders and amyloid disease.

A large proportion of patients, however, have no associated medical condition and these cases are called 'idiopathic intestinal pseudo-obstruction' (Fig. 22.22). A large quantity of bowel gas is usually present and there may be gastric, small- or large-bowel distension with associated fluid levels just as great as in true obstruction. If an unnecessary operation is to be avoided it is essential that barium studies are performed to exclude true organic obstruction.

Large-bowel volvulus

A prerequisite for the formation of a volvulus is that a long and freely mobile mesentery must be present. This occurs normally in the sigmoid, which is the commonest organ involved. Occasionally the caecum and ascending colon are on a mesentery, which is often associated with a degree of malrotation, and they comprise the second most common organs involved. Volvuli of the transverse colon or flexures do occur, but they are exceedingly rare in developed countries. A compound volvulus involving the intertwining of two loops of bowel, such as an ileosigmoid knot, is very rare in developed countries, but not uncommon in Africa. Large-bowel volvulus is the commonest cause of large-bowel obstruction in certain less-developed parts of the world.

Caecal volvulus (right-colon volvulus)

Caecal or right-colon volvulus can only occur when the caecum and ascending colon are on a mesentery, and this is often associated with a degree of malrotation (it has been estimated that this occurs in about 11% of the population). Caecal volvulus accounts for less than

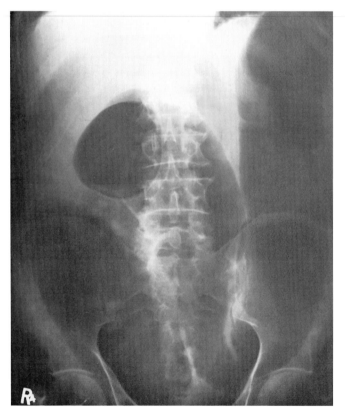

Fig. 22.21 Large-bowel obstruction type IA (competent ileocaecal valve). Supine film. There is gaseous distension of the large bowel from the sigmoid backward, including the ascending colon and caecum. The dilated caecum lies in the pelvis. There is no visible small-bowel distension. (Carcinoma of the sigmoid.)

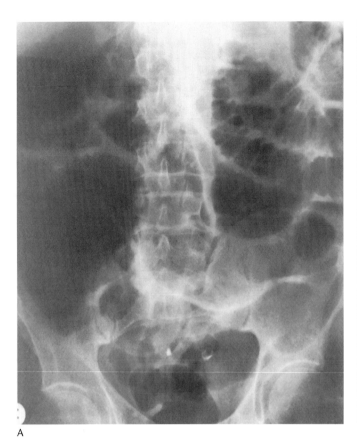 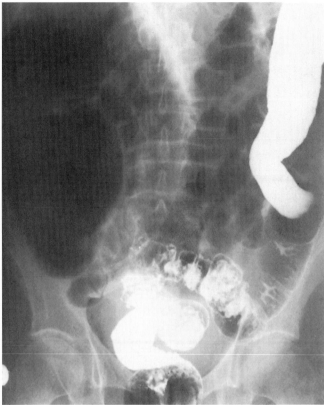

A   B

Fig. 22.22 Pseudo-obstruction: (A) supine abdomen; (B) barium enema. On the plain film, gas-filled loops of both small and large bowel can be identified, with gas extending down to the rectum. The barium examination demonstrates diverticular disease in the sigmoid but this is not obstructing, and barium flows freely into the dilated descending colon. Conservative management, using a flatus tube, failed and a laparotomy had to be undertaken. Dilated small and large bowel were found but there was no obstructing lesion. A caecostomy was performed.

2% of all cases of adult intestinal obstruction. It is usually found in a relatively young age group—30–60 years. Gangrene may occur early in the course of the condition, and it is therefore vital that an accurate diagnosis be made promptly. The diagnosis of acute caecal volvulus is rarely made on clinical grounds alone, so the radiological diagnosis becomes much more important. In about half the patients the caecum twists and inverts so that the pole of the caecum and appendix occupy the left upper quadrant. In the other half it twists in an axial plane without inversion, and then the caecum still occupies the right half or the central part of the abdomen. Even though there is considerable distension of the volved caecum, one or two haustral markings can usually be identified, unlike sigmoid volvulus where haustral markings are usually absent. The distended caecum can frequently be identified as a large gas- and fluid-filled viscus situated almost anywhere in the abdomen. Identification of an attached gas-filled appendix confirms the diagnosis. Moderate or severe small-bowel distension is present in about half the cases, but the remainder only show minimal small-bowel distension. The left half of the colon is usually collapsed (Fig. 22.23).

Sigmoid volvulus

This is the classic volvulus, occurring in old, mentally subnormal or institutionalised people. The usual mechanism is twisting of the sigmoid loop around the mesenteric axis; only rarely does one limb twist in an axial torsion. Sigmoid volvulus is usually chronic, with intermittent acute attacks; less commonly, a true acute torsion occurs. Although plain film diagnosis is often easy, up to one-third of cases can present diagnostic difficulty, the main problem being to differentiate the sigmoid volvulus from distended but non-twisted sigmoid, or distended transverse colon looping down into the pelvis (pseudovolvulus). Signs are summarised in Box 22.8. The essential feature for diagnosis is to identify the wall of the twisted sigmoid loop separate from the remaining distended colon. When a sigmoid volvulus occurs, the inverted U-shaped loop is usually massively distended and it is commonly devoid of haustra (ahaustral). This is a most important diagnostic point. The ahaustral margin can often be identified overlapping the lower border of the liver shadow—the 'liver overlap' sign. Where the ahaustral margin of the volvulus overlies the haustrated and dilated descending colon, the term 'left flank overlap sign' has been used. The apex of the sigmoid volvulus usually lies high in the abdomen, under the left hemidiaphragm, with its apex at or above the level of T10.

Inferiorly, where the two limbs of the loop converge, three white lines, representing the outer walls and the two adjacent inner walls of the volved loop, meet. This is called the inferior convergence; it is usually on the left side of the pelvis at the level of the upper sacral segments. Frequently a huge amount of air is present in sigmoid volvulus and an air–fluid ratio greater than 2:1 is usual (Fig. 22.24). The 'left flank overlap', apex above T10 and inferior convergence on the left are highly specific and sensitive signs.

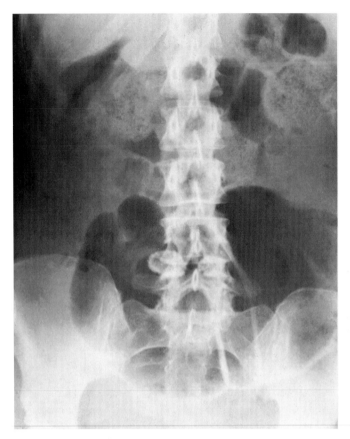

Fig. 22.23 Caecal volvulus. Supine. The considerably distended caecum with its haustral markings is readily identified lying low in the central abdomen. There is no significant small-bowel distension.

The initial treatment of a sigmoid volvulus frequently involves the insertion of a flatus tube per rectum. However, if there is a doubt about the diagnosis on the plain films, a barium enema should be performed. Features seen at the point of torsion include a smooth tapered narrowing—the 'bird of prey' sign—and the mucosal folds often show a screw pattern at the point of twist. In chronic sigmoid volvulus, shouldering may be seen at the point of torsion, and this corresponds to the localised thickening which is frequently found in the wall of the sigmoid at the site of the chronic volvulus.

Ileosigmoid knot

An ileosigmoid knot is a compound volvulus involving the small bowel and the pelvic colon. It is not uncommon in developing countries, but rare elsewhere. An abnormally mobile loop of small bowel passes round the base of the pelvic colon below the attach-

Box 22.8 Identification of the loop in sigmoid volvulus
Ahaustral margin
Left flank overlap sign
Apex above T10
Apex under the left hemidiaphragm
Inferior convergence on the left
Liver overlap sign
Air–fluid ratio greater than 2:1

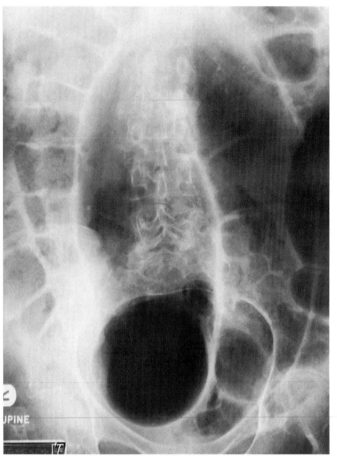

Fig. 22.24 Sigmoid volvulus. Supine film. The hugely dilated ahaustral loop of sigmoid can be seen rising out of the pelvis in the shape of an inverted U. Haustrated ascending and descending colon can be identified separate from the volved sigmoid loop.

ment of the pelvic mesocolon and forms a knot. The clinical onset is frequently abrupt, with a fulminating course and intense pain in the abdomen and back. The key radiological features are a dilated loop of pelvic colon, evidence of small bowel obstruction, and retained faeces in an undistended proximal colon. The dilated loop usually lies in the right side of the abdomen.

PARALYTIC ILEUS

Paralytic ileus occurs when intestinal peristalsis ceases and, as a result, fluid and gas accumulate in the dilated bowel. It is very common but most frequently occurs in peritonitis and in the postoperative period. When it is generalised, it results in both small- and large-bowel dilatation and, on horizontal-ray films, multiple fluid levels will be seen. Sometimes it can be very difficult to distinguish paralytic ileus from some types of large-bowel obstruction (Fig. 22.25). There are numerous causes of a generalised paralytic ileus and these are summarised in Box 22.9.

Sometimes local inflammatory processes such as pancreatitis, cholecystitis or appendicitis may result in a localised ileus leading to dilatation of one or two adjacent loops of bowel only. These appearances are not specific and they sometimes mimic small- or

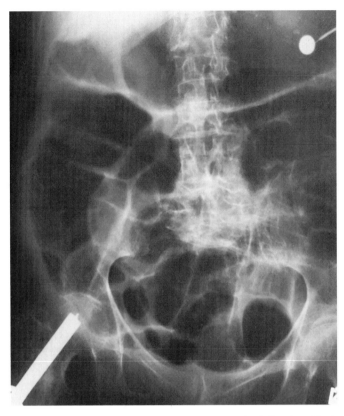

Fig. 22.25 Paralytic ileus. Supine film. There is generalised dilatation of both small and large bowel. An 84-year-old woman with generalised peritonitis following perforation of a gastric ulcer.

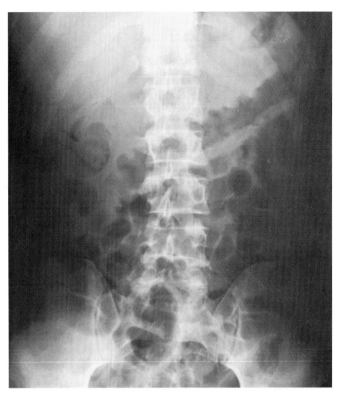

Fig. 22.26 Acute inflammatory bowel disease. Supine film. Loss of haustration and irregular mucosa, with mucosal island formation, are most readily identified in the transverse colon. A 35-year-old man with progressive severe bloody diarrhoea, subsequently proven to have ulcerative colitis.

Box 22.9	**Some of the causes of a paralytic ileus**
Postoperative	Pneumonia
Peritonitis	Renal failure
Inflammation	Renal colic
Appendicitis	Leaking abdominal aortic aneurysm
Pancreatitis	Hypokalaemia
Cholecystitis	Drugs, e.g. morphine
Salpingitis	General debility or infection
Trauma	Vascular occlusion
Spine	
Ribs	
Hip	
Retroperitoneum	
Congestive cardiac failure	

even large-bowel obstruction. Clinically a paralytic ileus is characterised by a 'silent abdomen' with absence of bowel sounds.

Postoperative abdomen

The same general principles of interpretation which apply to preoperative radiographs apply to the postoperative films. However, the features are frequently complicated by paralytic ileus and a postoperative pneumoperitoneum. Sometimes abdominal films are requested in the postoperative period in patients who remain distended and who continue to vomit. If both large and small bowel are filled with gas, it is usually impossible to distinguish incomplete small-bowel obstruction from paralytic ileus.

ACUTE COLITIS

Acute inflammatory colitis

The plain abdominal radiograph can usually predict the extent of mucosal lesions in acute inflammatory disease of the colon. An assessment of the extent of the colitis, the state of the mucosa, the depth of the ulceration and the presence or absence of megacolon and/or perforation can be made. The state of the colonic mucosa can be assessed from the faecal residue, the width of the bowel lumen, the mucosal edge and the haustral pattern. In left-sided disease the proximal limit of faecal residue will usually indicate the extent of active mucosal lesions, and where the mucosal edge is smooth and the haustral clefts are sharp, there is unlikely to be any mucosal change. Fuzzy mucosal edges, widened clefts or absent haustrations indicate active disease. Coarse irregularity of the mucosal edge and absence of haustrations are associated with marked ulceration (Fig. 22.26). Where extensive mucosal destruction has taken place, 'mucosal islands' or 'pseudopolyps' may be seen, which may precede 'toxic dilatation' and have themselves been suggested as an indication for surgery. When there are signs of left-sided disease, the presence of large amounts of faeces in the caecum and ascending colon is always associated with a severe disease process.

When intracolonic air is present, the mucosal state can be accurately assessed. However, severe mucosal changes can be missed on the plain radiograph if there is no air to outline the mucosa. A 'gasless colon' in someone with known inflammatory bowel disease is strongly suggestive of severe disease.

The absence of ulceration or dilatation means that a patient is not in any immediate danger and may be managed medically. Ulceration is responsible for the major complications and so places the patient at risk. When the bowel becomes dilated to above 5.5 cm diameter, the ulceration has penetrated the muscle layer, and the patient moves into a higher-risk group where urgent surgery must be considered. The patient must then be monitored by daily plain abdominal radiographs to detect any changes in colonic diameter, detect early megacolon or identify a perforation which may be masked clinically if the patient is taking steroids. Radiological evidence of failing medical treatment is a strong indication for surgery.

Toxic megacolon

Toxic megacolon is a fulminating form of colitis with transmural inflammation, extensive and deep ulceration and neuromuscular degeneration. Perforation and peritonitis are common complications, with a mortality as high as 30%. The most important radiological signs are mucosal islands and dilatation; both are usually seen together. In severe cases, the mean dilatation may be as much as 8 cm (Fig. 22.27). Changes are most frequently seen in the transverse colon, as gas collects here because it is the highest part in the supine position.

Perforation of the colon may occur during an acute attack of ulcerative colitis; the sigmoid is the most common site. Perforation

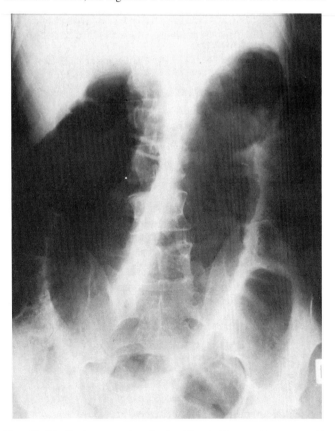

Fig. 22.27 Toxic megacolon. Supine film. A 37-year-old woman with progressively severe diarrhoea over a period of 3 weeks, which failed to respond to medical treatment, subsequently requiring a total colectomy. Final diagnosis: Crohn's disease.

results from deep ulceration, which may be localised or associated with a toxic megacolon. Perforations may be free, when a pneumoperitoneum will usually be detected, but sealed perforations also occur which cannot be detected reliably on plain radiographs.

Pseudomembranous colitis (*Clostridium difficile*-associated colitis)

Pseudomembranous colitis may follow the administration of antibiotics, particularly the clindamycin and lincomycin groups, and *Clostridium difficile* is frequently cultured in the stools. Thumb-printing, thickened haustra, abnormal mucosa and dilated bowel may be identified on plain films in about one-third of cases, and involvement of the whole of the colon differentiates the condition from ischaemic colitis. Dilated colon is more commonly seen in the right half and nodular haustral thickening in the left half. Associated small-bowel dilatation is frequently seen and the presence of ascites is a further pointer to the diagnosis. Appearances may mimic acute inflammatory bowel disease.

Ischaemic colitis

Ischaemic colitis is a disorder caused by vascular insufficiency and bleeding into the wall of the colon. It is characterised by the sudden onset of severe abdominal pain, often occurring in the early hours of the morning, followed by bloody diarrhoea. It most commonly occurs in middle-aged and elderly patients, and affects the splenic flexure and descending colon preferentially. The affected wall of the colon is greatly thickened due to submucosal haemorrhage and oedema. This may be identified as thumb-printing on plain films although barium studies are frequently required to demonstrate this. The involved area of the colon usually acts as an area of functional obstruction, so that the right side of the colon is frequently distended.

INTRAPERITONEAL FLUID

Fluid within the peritoneal cavity is commonly present in acute abdominal conditions, but even moderate amounts can be quite difficult to diagnose from plain films alone. The pelvis is the most dependent part of the peritoneal cavity in both the erect and supine positions, and fluid preferentially accumulates here. As more fluid collects it passes into the paracolic gutters and on the right side reaches the subhepatic and subphrenic spaces. The earliest signs are fluid densities within the pelvis, visualised superiorly and laterally to the bladder or rectal gas shadows. As more fluid accumulates it displaces the bowel out of the pelvis and, as the fluid enters the paracolic gutters, it displaces colon medially from the flank fat stripes. Fluid in Morison's pouch can obscure the fat interface with the posterior inferior border of the liver and results in failure to visualise its lower border.

Ascitic fluid between the liver and the lateral abdominal wall may result in the visualisation of a lucent band, the fluid being slightly less dense than liver tissue (Hellmer's sign). Blood has a similar density to liver, and a haemoperitoneum does not demonstrate this sign.

When huge amounts of fluid are present within the abdomen, it causes separation of bowel loops, and the general distension of the abdomen causes thinning of the flank stripes laterally. Large amounts of fluid cause a generalised haze over the abdomen and the scattered radiation produced results in poor visualisation of normal structures, such as psoas and renal outlines.

In the pelvis, tumours, particularly when bilateral and of gynaecological origin, can simulate free fluid. In addition, fluid-filled loops of small bowel in the pelvis and in the flanks can also mimic free fluid exactly.

Ultrasound and CT are very sensitive for small amounts of peritoneal fluid.

INFLAMMATORY CONDITIONS

Intra-abdominal abscesses

Abscesses are mass lesions, usually of soft-tissue density, which may be identified by displacement of adjacent structures or by loss of visualisation of normal fat lines following their involvement by the inflammatory process. Many abscesses contain gas which can be identified as one or several tiny bubble-like lucencies, which on first appearance may look like faeces. Others may contain much larger quantities of gas, exhibit long air–fluid levels on horizontal-ray films, and mimic gas in normal or dilated bowel. Others may fill anatomical spaces.

Most subphrenic abscesses appear in the postoperative period, following elective or emergency surgery, and many are related to anastomotic leaks. Most of the remainder are caused by perforated peptic ulcers, appendicitis and diverticulitis, or follow other perforations of the gastrointestinal tract or penetrating abdominal injuries.

Knowledge of the basic anatomy of the peritoneum and its reflections, together with an understanding of the spread of intraperitoneal infections, is a prerequisite for radiological diagnosis and localization. Meyers (1994) has made a comprehensive study of this topic.

The spread and location of infection within the peritoneal cavity are governed by a number of factors. The site, nature and rapidity of outflow of the escaping visceral contents, together with the nature of the disease processes which lead to the escape, are clearly of major importance.

The pelvis, being the most dependent part of the peritoneal cavity, is the most common site of residual abscess formation following generalised peritonitis. Furthermore, spreading infection from two common inflammatory conditions, appendicitis and diverticulitis, will readily enter the pelvis. Displacement and compression of the bladder and pelvic colon frequently occur and can be observed on plain films. However, ultrasound and CT will provide greater sensitivity and specificity in diagnosis and are usually of considerable help in further evaluation. They can also help plan and guide percutaneous drainage.

Subphrenic and subhepatic abscesses

Upper abdominal abscesses continue to have a bad prognosis and, in spite of modern antibiotics and surgical techniques, the mortality remains at nearly 30%. A negative upper abdominal pressure in both erect and supine positions, secondary to diaphragmatic movement, favours the passage of fluid out of the pelvis into the right paracolic gutter. Here it drains into the most dependent part, which is Morison's pouch. Once in the subhepatic space, fluid can readily enter the right subphrenic space, but is usually prevented from passing to the left side by the falciform ligament. Left subphrenic abscesses do not often follow pelvic disease, but more commonly arise locally from anterior perforation of the stomach or duodenum or, more frequently, following gastric or colonic surgery or splenectomy.

In addition to the primary signs of an abscess, secondary manifestations of subphrenic and suphepatic abscesses frequently occur. A chest X-ray of a patient who has a postoperative pyrexia often provides vital clues to the presence of a subphrenic or subhepatic abscess. Over 80% of subphrenic abscesses will show a raised hemidiaphragm, 70% evidence of a basal consolidation, and 60% a pleural effusion. In a postlaparotomy patient, a subphrenic abscess is the commonest cause of a unilateral pleural effusion (Fig. 22.28). Other signs are decreased diaphragmatic movement, generalised or localised paralytic ileus, scoliosis toward the lesion and decreased

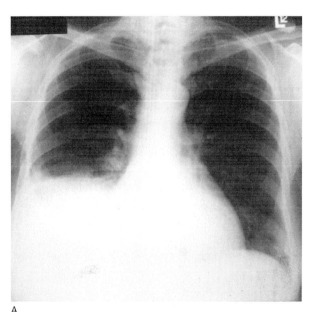

A

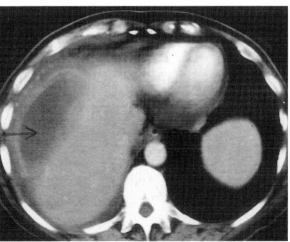

B

Fig. 22.28 Postoperative right subphrenic abscess. (A) Chest X-ray showing a raised right hemidiaphragm and small pleural effusion. (B) CT demonstrates the subphrenic collection (arrow).

organ mobility. Ultrasound is the investigation of choice for diagnosing these collections.

Right paracolic abscess

Abscesses in the right paracolic gutter are most likely to originate from appendicitis, although they may be secondary to a subphrenic abscess tracking down toward the pelvis. The ascending colon would be displaced medially on plain films.

Left paracolic abscess

The left paracolic gutter is limited superiorly by the phrenicocolic ligament, but it communicates freely with the pelvis inferiorly. Abscesses here are most commonly caused by perforated diverticular disease, although they may be caused by ascending infection from the pelvis.

Diagnosis of intra-abdominal sepsis

Plain film diagnosis of abscesses requires a high degree of suspicion combined with meticulous perusal of the radiographs in search of small gas bubbles, which are usually unchanged in position on consecutive films, displacement of organs and bowel from their usual anatomical position and effacement of fat lines normally present. Although plain film changes may be present in nearly 70% of subphrenic abscesses, less than 50% of abscesses elsewhere in the abdomen will show plain film changes. Frequently ultrasound, radionuclide studies or CT are required to make a definite diagnosis.

Plain radiography combined with ultrasound is diagnostic in about 90% of cases and is the initial preferred method of investigation if there are localising signs.

CT scanning is a highly accurate method of detecting intra-abdominal abscesses and is diagnostic in over 90% of cases. A pathological mass with an attenuation value of 15–35 HU is common, and when gas is present it is always seen on CT. Ring enhancement after intravenous contrast medium is characteristic. CT is excellent for therapeutic planning, particularly when percutaneous abscess drainage is being considered. This technique has revolutionised the treatment of intra-abdominal abscesses, and provides a safer and simpler alternative to laparotomy in seriously ill patients (Fig. 22.29).

Leucocyte scanning

The development of in vitro cell labelling procedures has allowed leucocyte scanning to be used to locate intra-abdominal sepsis. The most commonly used radionuclide is indium-111, chelated to leucocytes with either oxine or tropolone.

[111]In-labelled leucocyte scans have been shown to have a sensitivity and specificity greater than 90% in the localisation of intra-abdominal sepsis (Fig. 22.30). The technique is particularly useful within the abdomen, as it can identify sepsis at any site, including in prosthetic grafts and pre-existing cysts. The technique demon-

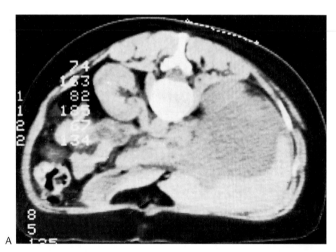

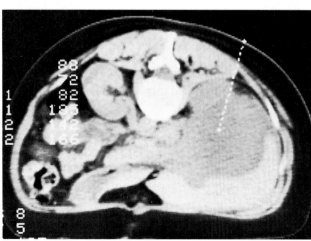

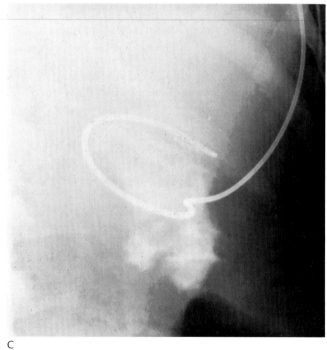

Fig. 22.29 (A,B) CT scans of prone patient showing a large right subhepatic abscess secondary to gallbladder surgery. Electronic cursors are used to measure (A) distance from midline to avoid kidney, and (B) distance to centre of abscess. (C) Prone X-ray, showing catheter in situ after insertion from posterior approach. A small amount of contrast medium has been injected. (Courtesy of Dr David Sutton.)

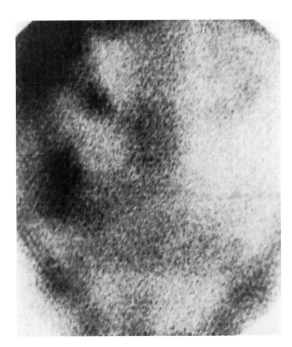

Fig. 22.30 Intra-abdominal abscess. ^{111}In-leucocyte scan, 24 h film. Postoperative repair of aortic aneurysm. No localising clinical signs. Accumulation of isotope in the right iliac fossa, with isotope in the right side of the colon indicating enteric communication. (Courtesy of Dr A. J. Coakley.)

strates when abscesses have enteric communication. The main causes of false-positive examinations are other inflammation (e.g. inflammatory bowel disease) and non-infected thrombus. False negatives are rare but can occur with chronic abscesses with a low inflammatory response.

If localising signs are absent, ^{111}In scanning is the technique of first choice. Ultrasound or CT may sometimes be needed in addition if the result is equivocal, or to help plan drainage. When localising signs are present, ultrasound or CT is likely to be the first investigation, the choice depending on the site. Leucocyte scanning will be needed in some cases, particularly when it is unclear whether a fluid collection is purulent.

More recently, in vitro cell labelling with technetium-99m HMPAO (hexamethylpropylene amine oxine) has been described, but this technique is of limited value within the abdomen as there is physiological activity in the gastrointestinal and genitourinary tracts. Other techniques not requiring an in vitro labelling procedure (e.g. using non-specific immunoglobulins or monoclonal antibodies to granulocytes) are still under evaluation, but generally appear less satisfactory than labelled leucocyte techniques.

Appendicitis

Acute appendicitis is the commonest acute surgical condition in the developed world and it carries an overall mortality of about 1%. When clinical findings are typical, a prompt diagnosis is usually made and there is no indication for taking abdominal radiographs. In older patients who present with atypical findings, a chest X-ray should be taken, predominantly to act as a baseline in case of postoperative complications.

In a significant minority of patients, particularly the young and the old, clinical features of appendicitis are obscure and the diagno-

sis is difficult; plain films are frequently taken to elucidate the cause of abdominal pain and may subsequently play a significant role in making the diagnosis. The radiological signs result from the localised inflammatory change, which may then progress to perforation and abscess formation with an associated paralytic ileus.

Abscess formation results in indentation of the caecum on its medial border; when inflammation permeates into the adjacent fat, the lower part of the properitoneal fat line and the right psoas muscle shadow will disappear. Intestinal obstruction may occur as several loops of small bowel become matted together or stuck to the inflamed appendix (Fig. 22.15). There is a high correlation between the presence of a calcified appendicolith and appendicitis, and these can be identified in about 13% of cases. About 90% of patients with right lower quadrant pain and ring-shaped calcification in the same area are found to have acute appendicitis, and a gangrenous appendix is found in about three-quarters of these.

Ileal and caecal fluid levels can be seen in nearly 50% of cases. It should be remembered, however, that a number of the signs of appendicitis are non-specific, and caecal fluid levels and loss of the right psoas outline may occur in about one-fifth of normal people. Air in the appendix may be seen in acute appendicitis, but this is also found in normals and in cases of large-bowel obstruction and paralytic ileus, particularly if the appendix is high and retrocaecal. The signs of acute appendicitis are summarised in Box 22.10.

Ultrasound in acute appendicitis

The graded compression technique for ultrasound examination of the appendix was described by Julien Puylaert in 1986. Using a probe of at least 7 MHz over the point of maximum tenderness in the right iliac fossa, pressure is gradually increased over the area in order to displace the bowel loops. The appendix may then be seen overlying the psoas muscle. The ultrasound features of appendicitis are listed in Box 22.11. The most sensitive sign is a non-compressible appendix with a diameter of 7 mm or greater. The surrounding echogenic non-compressible fat represents the mesentery and omentum (Figs 22.31, 22.32). An appendicolith is obstructing the lumen in up to 30% of cases. An accompanying

---

Box 22.10   Signs of acute appendicitis

Appendix calculus (0.5–6 cm)
Sentinel loop—dilated atonic ileum containing a fluid level
Dilated caecum
Widening of the properitoneal fat line
Blurring of the properitoneal fat line
Right lower quadrant haze due to fluid and oedema
Scoliosis concave to the right
Right lower quadrant mass indenting the caecum
Blurring of the right psoas outline—unreliable
Gas in the appendix—rare, unreliable

Box 22.11   Acute appendicitis: ultrasound signs

Blind-ending tubular structure at the point of tenderness
    Non-compressible
    Diameter 7 mm or greater
    No peristalsis
Appendicolith casting acoustic shadow
High echogenicity non-compressible surrounding fat
Surrounding fluid or abscess
Oedema of caecal pole

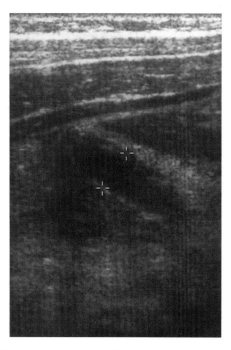

Fig. 22.31 Acute appendicitis. Ultrasound in the right iliac fossa demonstrating a hypoechoic non-compressible tubular structure measuring more than 6 cm in diameter, with surrounding hyperechoic fat.

ileus and/or free peritoneal fluid may be seen. A sensitivity of around 90% has been claimed. It should be remembered that there are pitfalls in the ultrasound diagnosis of appendicitis. Scenarios

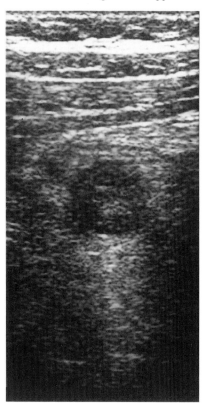

Fig. 22.32 Acute appendicitis. Ultrasound in the right iliac fossa demonstrating a non-compressible thickened appendix in transverse section, with surrounding hyperechoic fat.

Box 22.12 Diseases mimicking appendicitis diagnosed at ultrasound
Ectopic pregnancy
Ovarian cyst +/− torsion
Salpingitis
Endometriosis
Diverticulitis
Infectious ileocaecitis
Crohn's disease
Malignancy
Intussusception
Meckel's diverticulitis
Cholecystitis
Urolithiasis
Mesenteric adenitis

leading to false-negative examinations include appendicitis of the appendiceal tip, retrocaecal appendicitis, gangrenous or perforated appendicitis, or gas-filled appendix. If the appendix has perforated, it may become compressible, and if there is generalised peritonitis it may be difficult to perform the technique. Pitfalls leading to a false-positive examination include resolving appendicitis, dilated fallopian tube, inflammatory bowel disease and inspissated stool mimicking an appendicolith.

Some experienced operators claim to find the normal appendix in the majority of cases using this technique, but in most hands the normal appendix is not visualised, and this is the major drawback of the investigation. Although a positive diagnosis can be made when an abnormal appendix is seen, appendicitis cannot be excluded when an appendix has not been found. Ultrasound or CT examination should not be a substitute for a good clinical history and examination, and where the surgeon is confident of the diagnosis there should not be a need for further investigations. However, there are many conditions which mimic appendicitis clinically and may be diagnosed at ultrasound of the abdomen and pelvis (Box 22.12). Since the more common of these are gynaecological conditions, it is reasonable to perform an ultrasound in young women with suspected appendicitis in order to exclude some of these conditions. Many would also recommend scanning children and pregnant women in this situation. Ultrasound and CT is usually performed if there is significant clinical doubt in other patients, but practices vary locally, and depend on the availability of ultrasound expertise. Ultrasound has not been shown to be of proven clinical benefit in some studies, and a delay in treatment while scans are being organised may have an adverse effect on the clinical outcome.

CT in acute appendicitis

CT signs of appendicitis include an appendix measuring greater than 6 mm in diameter, failure of the appendix to fill with oral contrast or air up to its tip, an appendicolith, and enhancement of its wall with intravenous contrast (Fig. 22.33). Surrounding inflammatory changes include increased fat attenuation, fluid, inflammatory phlegmon, caecal thickening, abscess, extraluminal gas and lymphadenopathy (Fig. 22.34). Sometimes the lumen of the caecum can be seen pointing towards the obstructed opening to the appendix (the 'arrow-head' sign). Prospective trials have demonstrated that CT is a highly accurate test for confirming or excluding appendicitis; however, there is no consensus regarding the best scanning technique in this situation. Spiral scanning is more accurate than conventional axial scanning, and scanning with oral contrast and/or

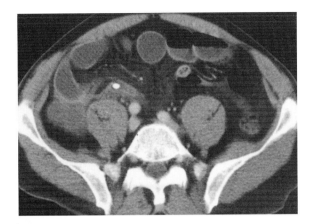

Fig. 22.33 Acute appendicitis. CT showing an appendix which contains a dense appendicolith, with surrounding inflammatory changes.

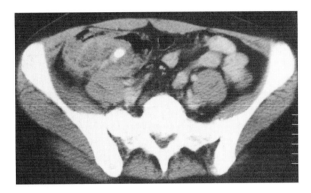

Fig. 22.34 Appendix inflammatory mass. CT shows soft-tissue density in the right iliac fossa containing an appendicolith. Abscess formation was seen on adjacent images.

colonic contrast is more accurate than without. Intravenous contrast is not considered to be essential. A focused technique examining the abdominopelvic junction exposes the patient to approximately one-third of the radiation dose of a full abdomen and pelvis scan (~3 mSv versus 10 mSv). Some studies indicate that the normal appendix can be identified in the majority of cases, and others do not, but there is no doubt that the normal appendix is more frequently seen on CT than at ultrasound. This is a major advantage that CT has in this situation.

Proponents for spiral CT in suspected appendicitis have published sensitivities and specificities approaching 100%, but these are interpreted by radiologists with a particular interest in this field, and it cannot be assumed that all radiologists will be able to reproduce these results. These series also include cases where the diagnosis of acute appendicitis is deemed highly likely on clinical assessment, and in many centres CT will not be considered necessary in such cases. Imaging should not be a substitute for good clinical assessment, and it is reasonable that imaging should only be requested where there is real clinical doubt.

Acute cholecystitis

Almost all cases of acute cholecystitis are associated with gallstones, and most are caused by obstruction of the cystic duct. However, only about 20% of gallstones contain sufficient calcium to be visible on plain radiographs, and only rarely does the wall of

Box 22.13   Signs of acute cholecystitis

Gallstones seen in 20%
Duodenal ileus
Ileus of hepatic flexure of colon
Right hypochondrial mass due to enlarged gallbladder
Gas within the biliary system

the gallbladder itself calcify. It is uncommon to identify a normal-sized gallbladder on plain films because it is not surrounded by fat. However, in cholecystitis the gallbladder may enlarge due to obstruction, and a mass may be visualised by displacement of adjacent gas-filled structures. The duodenum and hepatic flexure of the colon may show an ileus secondary to the inflamed gallbladder, and rarely gas may be seen in the lumen and wall of the gallbladder itself. However, in two-thirds of cases, the plain radiographs will be completely normal or show only borderline dilatation of small or large bowel. Signs of acute cholecystitis are summarised in Box 22.13 but many of these are noted to be non-specific.

Ultrasound is widely used for the diagnosis of acute cholecystitis. A thickened echogenic gallbladder wall with a hypoechoic margin can be identified in about 50–70% of cases (Fig. 22.35). Other signs include an indistinct contour to the gallbladder wall and fluid around the fundus of the gallbladder. Gallstones are readily identified and cast acoustic shadows. A stone obstructing the cystic duct may produce a grossly distended gallbladder. Echogenic sediment may be seen in the lumen, caused by inspissated bile or pus.

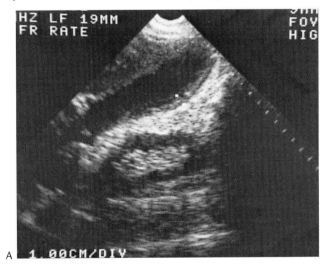
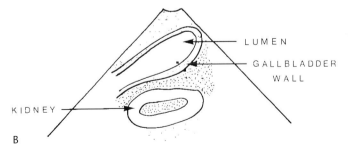

Fig. 22.35 Acute cholecystitis. (A) Ultrasound examination. (B) Diagram. A distended gallbladder has been identified, with a considerably thickened gallbladder wall. Markers placed across the gallbladder wall indicate a thickness of 9 mm. No gallstones have been identified. (Courtesy of Dr M. O. Downes.)

Tenderness of the gallbladder as it lies immediately beneath the ultrasound transducer is also a very reliable sign that the gallbladder is inflamed (positive sonographic Murphy sign). The reader is referred to Chapter 24.

Scintigraphy, using ^{99m}Tc-labelled derivatives of aminodiacetic acid (HIDA), is a simple and highly accurate method of diagnosing acute cholecystitis. The technique depends on the fact that acute cholecystitis occurs in association with a blocked cystic duct.

The scan is considered positive when, in the fasted patient, the gallbladder is not visualised but the bile duct and duodenum are visualised promptly. Although the method is highly accurate, not everyone is enthusiastic about radionuclides. False-positive scans occur in chronic malnutrition (e.g. in alcoholics) and in patients receiving parenteral nutrition.

Obstruction of the common bile duct, producing biliary colic, may present as an acute abdomen and is usually indistinguishable clinically from cholecystitis. Plain film findings in acute bile duct obstruction are usually absent, although occasionally the obstructing stone may be seen on the right, adjacent to the transverse process of L1 or L2.

An *empyema of the gallbladder* may be identified on plain films or ultrasound, when a distended gallbladder is seen as a large soft-tissue mass. Sometimes the obstructing stone may be identified in the cystic duct or Hartmann's pouch.

Emphysematous cholecystitis

Emphysematous cholecystitis is characterised by gas in either the wall or the lumen of the gallbladder, and in 20% of cases gas will also be present in the bile ducts. The cystic duct is usually obstructed, followed by ischaemia and proliferation of gas-forming organisms. *Clostridium welchii* is the most common infecting organism. About 30% of cases are diabetic and, unlike ordinary cholecystitis, the condition is much more common in men. A substantial number of patients will have no evidence of stones in the gallbladder.

Clinically, patients present with cholecystitis, but plain films will usually reveal a gas collection whose position is constant in the right hypochondrium: either lines of gas bubbles parallel to the wall, or an oval collection of gas within the gallbladder lumen. Air in the gallbladder from a gallstone ileus or enteric fistula may simulate emphysematous cholecystitis but will usually demonstrate a small or normal-sized gallbladder, while in emphysematous cholecystitis the gallbladder is usually enlarged. Small-bowel fluid levels may be seen in both conditions.

Patients frequently undergo ultrasound examination, and air within the gallbladder wall and in the lumen of the gallbladder has a characteristic appearance.

Although the condition is rare, diagnosis is important because gangrene of the gallbladder is common and the mortality is higher than in conventional cholecystitis. Most authorities, therefore, advise early surgery for this condition.

Acute pancreatitis

The clinical diagnosis of acute pancreatitis can be extremely difficult and, in the initial stages, other acute abdominal conditions such as perforated peptic ulcer or acute cholecystitis have to be included in the differential diagnosis. Morbidity is on the increase and most cases are related to gallstones or alcohol abuse. Plain abdominal radiographs are frequently taken as part of the initial investigation and a great many plain film signs have been described. The pathological changes of acute pancreatitis include oedema, haemorrhage, fat necrosis and infarction, which is sometimes followed by acute suppuration. The inflammatory process may extend into the gastrocolic ligament or the duodenal area, and follow the root of the mesentery or extend out of the peritoneum into the pararenal space. The clinical diagnosis is usually confirmed by a markedly elevated serum amylase level. However, this test has a number of well-recognised limitations, and the amylase levels may also be raised in perforated peptic ulcers, acute cholecystitis and intestinal obstruction.

A large number of radiological signs have been described in acute pancreatitis; many of these are uncommon, most are non-specific, and in two-thirds of cases plain films may be normal or show only borderline dilatation of bowel. As a result, most of the signs are of little or no value in the diagnosis of acute pancreatitis in individual cases. Gas in a dilated duodenal loop is optimally demonstrated in the left lateral decubitus position and this view should be included in all patients with suspected pancreatitis. Demonstration of gas within the pancreas, usually as multiple small bubbles giving a mottled appearance, is diagnostic of a pancreatic abscess, and the prognosis is grave. Other signs frequently seen are dilated loops of bowel (small bowel, terminal ileum, ascending and transverse colon) and a generalised paralytic ileus. Loss of the left psoas outline may also occur. Other signs which may occur relatively frequently are, however, non-specific and so are unlikely to be of any use in distinguishing between pancreatitis and other acute abdominal conditions. These include opaque gallstones, pancreatic calcification, pancreatic enlargement, gastrocolic separation, absent right psoas shadow, elevated left hemidiaphragm and the 'renal halo' sign.

Four different types of colon 'cut-off' sign have been described; this can lead to great confusion and so this term is best avoided and a description of the colonic dilatation used instead. A very rare but diagnostic sign is faint mottling over the pancreas due to fat necrosis.

Plain films will occasionally enable an indirect diagnosis of acute pancreatitis to be made. Their main value is to exclude other acute abdominal conditions.

Ultrasound or CT can be used to make a specific diagnosis of pancreatitis; however, some cases may yield negative results on both ultrasound and CT.

The pancreas can be directly imaged with ultrasound but the full length of the organ cannot be visualised in all patients, often due to obesity or overlying air. In acute oedematous pancreatitis, ultrasound may show organ enlargement, indistinct boundaries, diminished echogenicity due to oedema, duodenal atony and wall thickening. With necrotising pancreatitis, liquid or semiliquid tissue may be identified spreading beyond organ boundaries to the retroperitoneal and pararenal spaces and into the lesser sac of the peritoneum. Pleural effusions and ascites may be detected. The view of the pancreas at ultrasound may be poor in some patients, but ultrasound will provide valuable information regarding the biliary tree where common bile duct obstruction must be excluded.

CT may demonstrate necrosis, haemorrhage and solid parenchyma that enhances with intravenous contrast medium. The localisation of extrapancreatic fluid collections can be established without the administration of contrast media. Differentiation from necrotic tissue is accomplished by means of a bolus injection.

A pancreatic pseudocyst may complicate the later stages of acute pancreatitis. This may be identified on plain films as a large soft-

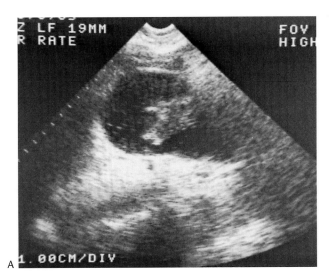

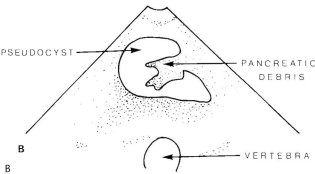

Fig. 22.36 Acute pancreatitis—pancreatic pseudocyst. (A) Ultrasound. (B) Diagram. A large transonic area is demonstrated in the region of the head of the pancreas, and, within it, irregular echoes represent pancreatic debris. Ten days following an attack of acute pancreatitis. (Courtesy of Dr M. O. Downes.)

tissue mass, or on ultrasound examination as a transonic mass (Fig. 22.36). CT is useful for assessing patients with complications of acute pancreatitis, because pseudocysts, abscess, haemorrhage, necrosis and ascites are all readily detected. A patient with acute pancreatitis who is not improving clinically should undergo regular ultrasound or CT examinations in order to detect pseudocyst formation and other complications as early as possible.

INTRAMURAL GAS

Sometimes gas is found within the walls of a hollow viscus. This can be easily recognised radiologically and different patterns distinguished. Cystic pneumatosis is in most cases a relatively benign condition, but the identification of linear gas shadows in the bowel wall is usually a sign of bowel necrosis.

Cystic pneumatosis (pneumatosis cystoides intestinalis)

This is an uncommon condition comprising cyst-like collections of gas in the walls of hollow viscera, and is most frequently seen in the gastrointestinal tract, where it is called pneumatosis cystoides

intestinalis. Although it may occur anywhere in the gastrointestinal tract, the left half of the colon is the site most commonly affected, and the condition is then termed pneumatosis coli. Most patients are past middle age and the symptoms include vague abdominal pain, diarrhoea and mucous discharge. However, in some patients air cysts are discovered by chance during the investigation of other symptoms. The cysts vary in size from 0.5 to 3 cm in diameter and they lie both subserosally and submucosally. Plain film findings are typical, with the gas-containing cysts producing a characteristic appearance easily distinguishable from normal bowel gas shadows. Occasionally these cysts rupture, producing a pneumoperitoneum without evidence of peritonitis, but it is extremely important to recognise that pneumatosis is the cause of the pneumoperitoneum and so avoid an unnecessary laparotomy (Fig. 22.7). The condition is also discussed in Chapter 21.

Interstitial emphysema

This is a rare condition where linear gas, in single or double streaks, is found in the bowel wall and is not associated with infection. The commonest sites are the stomach and the colon. A breach in the mucosa, with an increase in the intraluminal pressure, would seem to be important aetiologically. In the stomach, gastroscopy and pyloric stenosis have been implicated as a cause. In the colon it is associated with toxic megacolon and is a sign of impending perforation.

Gas-forming infections

Numerous bacteria are capable of producing gas, but those most commonly involved in humans are *Escherichia coli*, *Clostridium welchii* and *Klebsiella aerogenes*. Such infections usually give rise to severe constitutional disturbance and toxaemia with a high mortality. However, over half of all gas-forming infections occur in diabetics; the infecting organism is frequently *Escherichia coli* and in this group the constitutional disturbance is usually much less.

Emphysematous gastritis
This results from a severe infection in the wall of the stomach, producing a contracted stomach, with a frothy or mottled radiolucency visible in the left upper abdomen due to gas within the stomach wall. It has a high mortality.

Emphysematous cholecystitis
This occurs most frequently in elderly male diabetics and is often associated with an absence of gallstone. The clinical findings are suggestive of acute cholecystitis and this has been previously discussed.

Emphysematous enterocolitis
This occurs predominantly in premature babies and is discussed in Chapter 28. In adults it is associated with profound constitutional disturbance and usually indicates necrotic bowel. It may be associated with gas in the portal vein, a sign which, in an adult, has a grave prognosis.

Emphysematous cystitis
Emphysematous cystitis causes linear gas streaks and gas cysts within the wall of the urinary bladder and is frequently associated

with gas within the lumen of the bladder itself, *E. coli* and *K. aerogenes* are the usual infecting organisms and the condition is much more common in diabetics. Emphysematous cystitis must be distinguished from gas within the lumen of the bladder due to a vesicocolic fistula. The latter is not usually associated with gas within the wall of the bladder.

RENAL COLIC

A large number of patients with acute ureteric obstruction due to a stone present with an acute abdomen. Although most ureteric calculi are opaque, they are frequently small and difficult to identify on plain films alone, or, if identified, are impossible to place within the ureter with certainty. Phleboliths within the pelvis are a frequent source of potential confusion, but their appearance, with smooth outline and radiolucent centre, is quite different from that of stones, which are frequently less calcified, oval and with no radiolucent centre.

The severe pain which accompanies renal colic frequently leads to air swallowing and this, together with an associated paralytic ileus, which is common, frequently results in gas-filled small and large bowel, which is often slightly distended and may contain fluid levels. Sometimes colonic distension may be so great as to mimic large-bowel obstruction. An intravenous urogram is required to confirm the diagnosis and to identify the degree and site of obstruction. It is important to confirm the diagnosis, for many patients who are initially thought to have ureteric colic have a normal emergency IVU and are eventually found to have another abnormality. A normal intravenous urogram, done while the pain is still present, excludes the diagnosis of renal colic; a normal urogram done once the pain has ceased is much less helpful. The author believes that the IVU should be done as an emergency and as soon as possible.

Sometimes ureteric colic is complicated by the spontaneous rupture of the renal pelvis or the calyces. This can lead to a retroperitoneal collection of urine—a urinoma. A urinoma may be identified on plain films as a soft-tissue mass causing loss of the renal and psoas outlines. It is frequently associated with a marked paralytic ileus. Diagnosis is confirmed by emergency urography.

Emphysematous pyelonephritis may be recognised by gas bubbles within the kidney or linear gas beneath the renal capsule. It occurs most commonly with uncontrolled diabetics or is associated with obstructive uropathy.

LEAKING ABDOMINAL AORTIC ANEURYSM

A leaking aortic aneurysm frequently presents as an acute abdomen and sometimes may simulate renal colic. Although clinical diagnosis may be obvious and urgent surgery indicated without any further investigations, the diagnosis is often missed on admission to hospital. If confirmation is required, ultrasound will establish the diagnosis of an aortic aneurysm but a leak or a retroperitoneal haematoma may be difficult to diagnose except by CT. Frequently, however, a leaking aneurysm is not suspected clinically, and plain films are

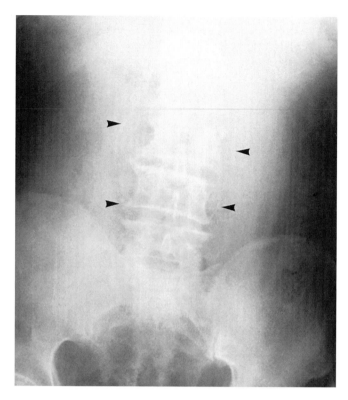

Fig. 22.37 Leaking aortic aneurysm. Supine film. The faintly calcified rim of an aortic aneurysm is identified (arrowheads). In addition, there is a large soft-tissue mass outside the aneurysm, indicating a retroperitoneal haematoma. The outlines of the psoas and renal margins on the left are lost.

taken to investigate the cause of the abdominal pain. An aneurysm may be detected as a central soft-tissue mass which may obscure the psoas outline on the left. Frequently curvilinear calcification may be seen on the anteroposterior view, but if confirmation is required it is usually better demonstrated on a lateral film. The mere demonstration of an aortic aneurysm does not necessarily indicate that leaking has occurred. If, however, a soft-tissue mass can be identified outside the calcified wall of the aneurysm, or bowel gas is displaced anteriorly, or the psoas or renal outlines are obscured by a soft-tissue mass, this is usually strong confirmation of a leak (Fig. 22.37). These signs may be detected on plain films in up to 90% of cases.

ACUTE GYNAECOLOGICAL DISORDERS

The primary disorder may produce specific signs within the pelvis, while secondary signs within the peritoneal cavity may result from free fluid or a paralytic ileus. Torsion of an ovarian cyst may produce a pelvic mass, and an ovarian dermoid can be diagnosed if it contains calcification, teeth or fat. Salpingitis often produces a localised paralytic ileus but it cannot usually be distinguished from appendicitis or diverticulitis on plain films. A ruptured ectopic pregnancy may produce a pelvic mass, free fluid and a paralytic ileus, but ultrasound is usually of particular value in these patients.

CALCIFICATION ASSOCIATED WITH ACUTE ABDOMINAL CONDITIONS

There are numerous causes of calcification within the abdomen. However, only a very few of these are associated with conditions which may give rise to an acute abdomen. These are summarised in Table 22.2.

Table 22.2 Abdominal calcification associated with an acute abdomen

Calcification	Acute condition
Appendix calculus	Appendicitis
Gallstone	Acute cholecystitis
	Acute pancreatitis
	Biliary colic
	Empyema of gallbladder
	Gallstone ileus
Calcified gallbladder wall	Cholecystitis
Limy bile	Cholecystitis
Calculus in Meckel's, sigmoid or jejunal diverticulum	Acute inflammation or perforation
Pancreatic calculi	Pancreatitis—chronic and acute
Calcified aneurysms: aortic, iliac, splenic, hepatic	Rupture
Teeth or bone in ovarian dermoid	Torsion
Ureteric, renal calculus	Ureteric, renal colic

REFERENCES AND SUGGESTIONS FOR FURTHER READING

The acute abdomen

Baker, S. R., Cho, K. D. (1999) *The Abdominal Plain Film with Correlative Imaging.* Stamford: Appleton & Lange.

Balthazar, E. J., Birnbaum, B. A., Megibow, A. J., Gordon, R. B., Whelanm, C. A., Hulnick, D. H. (1992) Closed-loop and strangulating intestinal obstruction: CT signs. *Radiology,* **185**, 769–775.

Bartnicke, B. J., Balfe, D. M. (1994) CT appearance of intestinal ischemia and intramural hemorrhage. *Radiologic Clinics of North America, * **32**, 845–860.

Birnbaum, B. A., Jeffrey, R. B. (1998) CT and sonographic evaluation of acute right lower quadrant abdominal pain. *American Journal of Roentgenology,* **170**, 361–371.

Hahn, H. B., Hoepner, F. U., Kalle, T. V, et al (1998) Sonography of acute appendicitis in children: 7 years experience. *Pediatric Radiology,* **28**, 147–151.

Jeffrey, R. B., Jain, K. A., Nghiem, H. V. (1994) CT Sonographic diagnosis of acute appendicitis: interpretive pitfalls. *American Journal of Roentgenology,* **162**, 55–59.

Maglinte, D. D. T., Balthazar, E. J., Kelvin, F. M., Megibow, A. J. (1997) The role of radiology in the diagnosis of small bowel obstruction. *American Journal of Roentgenology,* **168**, 1171–1180.

Meyers, M. A. (1994) *Dynamic Radiology of the Abdomen.* New York: Springer.

Puylaert, J. B. C. M., Rious, M., van Oostayen, J. A. (1999) The appendix and the small bowel. In Meire, H, Cosgrove, D, Dewbury, K, Farrant, P (eds) *Clinical Ultrasound: A Comprehensive Text, * pp. 841–864. Edinburgh: Churchill Livingstone.

Rao, P. M. (1998) Technical and interpretive pitfalls of appendiceal CT imaging. *American Journal of Roentgenology,* **171**, 419–425.

Rao, P. M., Boland, G. W. L. (1998) Imaging of acute right lower abdominal quadrant pain. *Clinical Radiology,* **53**, 639–649.

Rao, P. M., Rhea, J. T., Novelline, R. A., et al (1997) Helical CT technique for the diagnosis of appendicitis: prospective evaluation of a focussed appendix CT examination. *Radiology,* **202**, 139–144.

23

THE ABDOMEN AND MAJOR TRAUMA

Otto Chan and Ioannis Vlahos

Epidemiology of trauma

Trauma causes an estimated 10% of worldwide deaths and is the third commonest cause of death after malignancy and vascular disease. Trauma is the leading cause of death in the first four decades of life (1–44 years) and potentially the leading cause of loss of life years. There are over 150 000 deaths annually in the USA and for each death 2–3 people are permanently disabled, at an estimated cost of $400 billion. There has been a significant reduction in trauma-related deaths in the past two decades.

Causes of trauma deaths (*Table 23.1*) Road traffic accidents (RTAs) are the commonest cause and account for up to 50% of trauma-related deaths. There has been a significant reduction in RTAs, due predominantly to legislation, e.g. seat belts, speed limits. The percentages of deaths from all other causes have remained relatively stable.

Imaging

Abdominal trauma contributes 10% of overall trauma mortality and considerably more in terms of morbidity. The underappreciation of abdominal injuries represents a significant cause of preventable trauma deaths. Following the initial primary survey of the trauma patient, and the acquired routine plain films, a more detailed secondary appraisal of the trauma patient can begin. The role of further imaging is central to this evaluation. Several diagnostic modalities are available, all of which exhibit different advantages and disadvantages.

Ultrasound Ultrasound is a fast technique, which can be brought to the patient's bedside and can give rapid information on even quite

Table 23.1 Causes of trauma-related deaths

Cause	%
RTAs	<50
Suicides	15–20
Homicides	15
Falls	10
Burns	5
Other	<5

haemodynamically unstable patients. The value of ultrasound in detecting haemoperitoneum in these patients is well established, with a sensitivity of between 80 and 100% and a specificity nearing 100% (Fig. 23.1). In a haemodynamically unstable patient, the presence of a haemoperitoneum on ultrasonography mandates a laparotomy. However, ultrasonographic assessment can often be hampered by limited access to the patient due to a combination of factors, including bandages and dressings, surgical emphysema, other working trauma team members and the acute time constraints. In addition, the inability of ultrasound to accurately detect parenchymal injuries (sensitivity 40–80%), and injuries of the retroperitoneum in general, further limits its value. Due to these limitations, when positive for haemoperitoneum, ultrasound alerts to the presence of significant injuries, but the absence of detected haemoperitoneum does not exclude injury. Nonetheless, the use of a FAST protocol examination (*Focused Assessment for the Sonographic examination of the Trauma patient*) reviewing abdominal quadrants for free fluid is an invaluable tool in the initial evaluation of the acutely injured patient.

Computed tomography Contrast-enhanced CT, and in particular the use of faster helical CT, has revolutionised the management of haemodynamically stable trauma patients. Its advent has practically eliminated the need for invasive diagnostic peritoneal lavage (DPL). DPL is at least as sensitive as CT in the detection of haemoperitoneum, with sensitivities of both techniques above 90%; however,

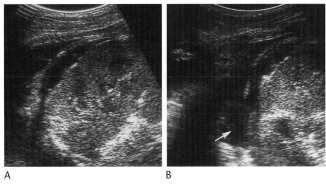

A   B

Fig. 23.1 (A, B) Ultrasound of the left hypochondrium showing the presence of haemoperitoneum, pleural fluid and a defect in the left hemidiaphragm more posteriorly, consistent with diaphragmatic rupture (arrow).

the lack of specific organ information and of retroperitoneal assessment is a major limiting factor of DPL. In addition, DPL is invasive, with a significant false-positive rate that in one series resulted in non-therapeutic laparotomies in 29% of patients. The higher accuracy (approximately 98%) of CT in solid viscera assessment, including contained intraparenchymal organ injuries, and assessment of the retroperitoneum has defined its role in trauma. The superior organ-specific trauma staging capabilities of CT have prompted a reduction of exploratory surgery and have been largely responsible for the trend to monitored non-operative management of solid intra-abdominal trauma.

Further benefits are offered by the new multislice spiral CT machines, which can visualise the whole abdomen within 20 s (see Ch. 59).

Other modalities *Magnetic resonance imaging (MRI)* has been demonstrated to be a near-equivalent technique to CT in the accurate appraisal of individual organ injuries. However, the use of MRI at present confers no additional advantages in the initial trauma evaluation. Moreover, the limited access to patients for monitoring and resuscitation and the need for MR-compatible equipment pose major disadvantages. In addition, while individual organs can be relatively quickly assessed, an assessment of the entire abdomen and pelvis requires numerous sequences increasing the total imaging time. At present MRI is reserved for problem solving after the acute phase of trauma has passed.

Angiography remains a useful adjunct in the management of trauma, although the emergence of CT and ultrasound have all but eliminated the need for primary diagnostic examinations. The investigation of persistent haemorrhage and the use of embolisation have an increasing role in the non-operative management of abdominal trauma.

Spleen

The spleen is the most commonly injured organ in blunt abdominal trauma, accounting for approximately 40% of all solid organ injuries. Splenic injuries are present in 25% of patients with left renal trauma and 45% of patients with hepatic trauma. Contributory factors include its potential for injury from fractured ribs, intra-abdominal compression and its rich vascular supply. As many as 20% of patients with left lower rib fractures have associated splenic trauma, although approximately 60% of splenic injuries have no associated fractures. The presence of splenomegaly or of splenic disease, e.g. infectious mononucleosis, increases this susceptibility to trauma. The incidence of penetrating trauma of the spleen is relatively low, as this relates roughly to the surface area of the spleen (approximately 7% of the abdominal surface). On the whole, management protocols relate to the treatment of blunt injury, as penetrating injury is usually treated far more aggressively due to the increased incidence of vascular injuries.

Choice of investigation Contrast-enhanced CT is the definitive radiological investigation for the detection of splenic injuries. The utility of CT in the detection of splenic trauma was established with non-spiral CT. In haemodynamically stable patients, CT studies have repeatedly demonstrated a very high sensitivity, specificity and accuracy in the detection of splenic injuries (all in excess of 95%). Undoubtedly, these figures are somewhat biased by the use of successful non-operative management as the gold standard of absence of injury, particularly as splenic injuries may often heal

with conservative measures. A more significant analysis of the effect of CT has been the demonstration that it has reduced the total number of trauma laparotomies and the number of negative and non-therapeutic laparotomies.

A manifestation of the potential inaccuracy of CT is the entity of delayed splenic rupture. This is defined as bleeding due to splenic injury occurring more than 48 h after blunt trauma *following an apparently normal CT examination* and must be differentiated from delayed presentation of splenic rupture due to an injury initially thought minor, or from cases of delayed or insufficient initial imaging. Most of these latter cases are due to ruptures of sub-capsular splenic haematomas. The mechanism of rupture of these haematomas may relate to clot lysis with subsequent osmotic shift of fluid due to oncotic pressure or initial tamponade of the haematoma by surrounding organs. Due to the delay in diagnosis, the mortality rate in these patients may be as high as 5–15%, compared with 1% in patients with acutely detected injuries. It is notable that all cases of false-negative CT with subsequent delayed rupture were recorded on non-spiral CT equipment and the validity of this entity with newer generation equipment has yet to be confirmed.

CT imaging findings On contrast-enhanced CT, splenic lacerations appear as linear low-attenuation defects that contrast well with the high-attenuation vascular spleen (Fig. 23.2). Complex interconnecting lacerations may combine, resulting in a shattered spleen. Intrasplenic haematomas appear as more diffuse hypo-attenuating regions (Fig. 23.3). Although initially postulated that the use of postcontrast images alone could miss haematomas that might appear hyperdense on unenhanced CT but become isodense with respect to the enhancing splenic parenchyma following contrast administration, it has subsequently been demonstrated that parenchymal haematomas always appear far more conspicuous after contrast administration. Splenic haematomas must be distinguished from the more triangular peripheral non-enhancing regions

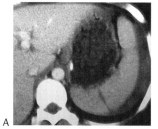
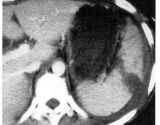
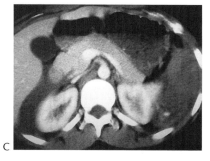

Fig. 23.2 Multiple splenic injuries in the same patient. (A) Splenic low-attenuation linear defect due to a splenic laceration. (B) More inferiorly a splenic fracture with separation of fragments is present. Haemoperitoneum is localised to the left upper quadrant. (C) In the splenic bed active extravasation of contrast is identified.

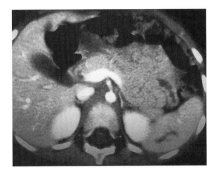

Fig. 23.3 Intrasplenic haematomas are characterised by irregular margins and swelling of the spleen, altering the normal crescentic contour.

that are characteristic of splenic infarcts. Subcapsular haematomas may occur alone or in combination with other injuries and result in low-attenuation collections that indent the splenic margin (Fig. 23.4). As in the interpretation of CT of the injured liver, the routine use of liver windows has not been demonstrated to increase significantly the conspicuity nor alter the staging of splenic injuries.

Imaging pitfalls Uniform enhancement of the spleen occurs approximately 50–60 s after contrast administration and is the optimal timing for the detection of intrasplenic injuries. Imaging during the earlier arterial phase may be useful in the detection of active extravasation and of traumatic pseudoaneurysms. These vascular injuries appear as ill-defined and well-defined regions of early arterial enhancement, respectively. However, during this earlier phase of enhancement the cord-like geographical enhancement of the splenic pulp may mimic intrasplenic lacerations, and delayed supplementary confirmatory images should therefore be obtained whenever there is doubt. Normal splenic enhancement should exceed that of the liver; however, two studies have reported reduced splenic enhancement in trauma even when the spleen itself is not injured. This phenomenon is thought to relate to adrenergic stimulation reducing arterial perfusion to the spleen during hypotension. Another manifestation of this adrenergic stimulation is the increase in splenic size by more than 10% that occurs in over half (57%) of patients with splenic trauma during the first post-traumatic week. This is believed to reflect a return to normal splenic size following reversal of adrenergic contraction in the acute period coupled with increased fluid replacement and does not signify clinical deterioration (Fig. 23.18). Congenital splenic clefts may be distinguished from lacerations by their superior location and slightly lobulate contour. Further confirmation of a normal variant may be offered by the absence of adjacent perisplenic haematoma and the clarity of the surrounding perisplenic fat (Fig. 23.5).

Haemoperitoneum Splenic injuries are almost invariably associated with haemoperitoneum. This is initially localised to the left upper quadrant and as the volume increases may extend to other peritoneal compartments. The higher density of blood around the

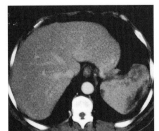

Fig.23.4 Resolving splenic lacerations and haematomas. A peripheral crescentic low-attenuation collection is due to a subcapsular haematoma and, although small, poses a risk of delayed rupture.

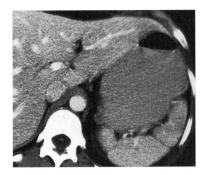

Fig. 23.5 Normal splenic clefts. These can be distinguished from lacerations by their relatively superior location, lobulate contour and the absence of perisplenic haemoperitoneum. Note the preservation of the fat planes around the spleen.

spleen may often indicate the source of haemoperitoneum. This sentinel clot sign may be also utilised to identify other solid-organ origins of intraperitoneal bleeding. On occasion, haemoperitoneum may be identified only within the dependent pelvis and, therefore, justifies the extension of the CT examination to include the pelvis. Even in isolated splenic injury blood can track into the anterior pararenal space via the potential space of the splenorenal ligament, which connects the splenic hilum to the left anterior pararenal space. In a study of 96 children with isolated splenic injuries, 8% demonstrated such extension, with two patients demonstrating fluid dissecting the splenic vein and pancreas—a feature considered specific for pancreatic injury.

Staging and management The knowledge of the risk of overwhelming sepsis and of susceptibility to coccal infections has led to a desire to preserve splenic function whenever possible. Non-operative management of even quite severe splenic trauma has been successfully demonstrated in children following the observation that splenic bleeding has often ceased by the time of laparotomy. In fact it is considered that the haemodynamic state of the child, rather than the CT appearance of splenic injuries, dictates the need for surgery. The extension of this approach to adults has met with quite variable success. Postulated reasons for the difference in outcome following non-operative management in children and adults include: a relatively thicker capsule in comparison to adults; a vascular supply more sensitive to adrenergic stimulation; and the reduced risk of fractured rib impalement due to greater rib elasticity.

Due to the higher failure rate of non-operative management in adults with the consequence of increased morbidity and mortality of delayed surgery, several attempts at classifying splenic injury have been proposed. These include the Buntain and subsequent Mirvis classifications (Box 23.1). The objective of these classifications has been to attempt to segregate successfully those patients in whom surgical management should be operative or non-operative. The majority of these studies are retrospective and inherent problems in such classification systems are that a decision to operate may not

Box 23.1	**CT grading (blunt splenic trauma)**
Grade 1	Capsular avulsion, superficial laceration(s) or subcapsular haematoma <1 cm
Grade 2	Parenchymal laceration(s) 1–3 cm deep, central/subcapsular haematoma(s) <3 cm
Grade 3	Laceration(s) >3 cm deep, central/subcapsular haematoma(s) >3 cm
Grade 4	Fragmentation (>3 segments), devascularised (non-enhancing) spleen

From Mirvis et al (1994).

have necessarily been correct and that patients with isolated splenic injuries will behave differently to those patients with multiple intra-abdominal injuries. Unsurprisingly, all the classification systems demonstrate that, in general, higher grades or scores of injury (rupture, complex lacerations) correlate with the need for surgery. However, significantly, several patients with low grades of injury (simple small lacerations, subcapsular collections) subsequently required surgery. In addition, retrospective reviews of patient records using such analyses demonstrate that several patients with high-grade injuries have been successfully treated non-operatively.

In the adult population, despite the use of CT grading systems, the choice of expectant management in selected patients is contentious, due to the varied reported rates in the need for subsequent delayed surgery. Depending on the stringency of the applied criteria, these may vary from as low as 3% to as high as 70%. For most sizeable studies (greater than 100 subjects), the use of criteria of low CT grade, haemodynamic stability following initial resuscitation and absence of associated intra-abdominal injuries results in approximately 15–30% of patients with splenic injury being appropriate for conservative management. Within this subset, approximately 10–30% will fail conservative treatment.

Apart from the potential for increased mortality, one of the main concerns regarding delayed surgical intervention appears to be the reduced rate of splenic salvage. In one retrospective review the rate of reparative splenorrhaphy reduced from 67% in the operative group to 21% in the non-operative limb. Other groups have expressed similar results.

The observation that a significant proportion of splenic injuries may require delayed surgery has led to investigations for further factors to guide management in individual patients more reliably. In one study of expectant management, patients older than 55 years had only a 9% successful non-operative course, compared with a 66% success rate in patients under 55 years of age with similar CT grades of injury and overall injury severity scores. Caution is therefore advised in this subgroup of patients.

Angiography and embolisation Angiography may be performed in haemodynamically stable patients with splenic injuries diagnosed on CT to determine whether active extravasation is present (Fig. 23.6). Using an algorithm in which splenic injuries are treated with bed-rest alone, and splenic extravasation is treated with embolisation of the splenic artery distal to the dorsal pan-

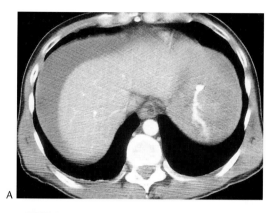

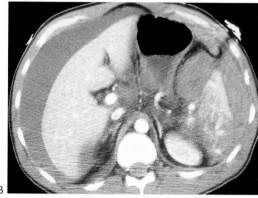

Fig. 23.7 (A, B) Contrast-enhanced CT: there is frank arterial bleeding from the splenic artery associated with a fragmented spleen. Extensive haemoperitoneum is also present.

creatic artery, the success of non-operative management can be significantly improved. By the use of such an approach even higher CT grade injuries have been successfully managed non-operatively. This approach may result in non-operative management in up to 90% of patients, with a successful non-operative outcome in over 90%. Although such high non-operative rates are desirable, there is animal evidence to suggest that antigenic clearance is better in models with partial splenectomies than in those with interrupted blood supply to whole spleens. The long-term results of splenic hypoperfusion in humans are not yet known.

In view of the significant impact of angiographically detected active extravasation, it is not surprising that on contrast-enhanced CT examinations active extravasation or the presence of pseudoaneurysms or arteriovenous malformations of the splenic vasculature have been demonstrated as important indicators of the need for operative care independently of CT grade (Fig. 23.7). Limiting diagnostic angiography to those patients with these CT abnormalities has been suggested as a means of reducing the number of unnecessary angiograms. Such an approach would have an 83% accuracy in predicting the need for splenic injury treatment.

Recovery CT can be utilised to monitor the recovery from splenic injury, although the value of such a practice is contentious. In a study of 37 children with splenic injuries treated conservatively, grade 1 and 2 injuries (modified Mirvis) showed CT evidence of healing within 4 months, grade 3 injuries tended to heal within 6 months, and grade 4 injuries could take as long as 11 months. A similar grade-related time course to splenic healing has been recorded by use of ultrasound. It is not, however, known whether

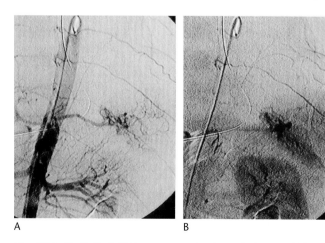

Fig. 23.6 (A, B) Flush DSA aortogram showing splenic arterial bleeding with a persistent blush in the spleen on the delayed image.

resolution of sonographic or CT appearances correlates with structural splenic healing. On ultrasound, the spleen may not revert to an entirely normal appearance, with a residual echogenic band thought to represent a fibrous band. Occasionally small cysts may form, thought to represent resolving haematoma. Rarely foci of calcification may also develop. Moreover, the importance of follow-up imaging is questionable, as nearly all splenic lesions heal with no significant sequelae, particularly in children.

At present the high accuracy of CT in excluding injury and in documenting the degree of splenic injury and associated other intra-abdominal injuries is undoubted. This information must be coupled with a clinical haemodynamic assessment of the patient's fluid/blood requirements, age and associated injuries to provide information towards an individual patient's care. In the future the constant evolution of CT technology and the use of angiographic signs on CT or fluoroscopy combined with interventional therapy may further improve the management of splenic injuries.

Liver and biliary tract

The liver is the second most frequently injured organ in the abdomen, damage occurring in 20–30% of blunt trauma overall. In patients haemodynamically stable enough to be examined by CT, splenic and hepatic injuries are almost equal in incidence. The relatively large surface area of the liver also makes penetrating trauma a relatively frequent occurrence. The discrepancy in size between the two lobes dictates that right lobe injuries are four times more frequent than those of the left lobe. Injuries to the liver are, in over 50% of cases, accompanied by other injuries. Left lobe injuries are frequently accompanied by splenic (45%) or pancreatic trauma, while those of the right lobe are frequently accompanied by rib (33%) (Fig. 23.8) or adrenal injuries.

The assessment and management of hepatic trauma draws many corollaries with the evaluation of splenic trauma. As in the case of splenic trauma, it has been noted that many hepatic injuries had ceased to bleed by the time of laparotomy and that a large proportion of such operative interventions were non-therapeutic. Stimulated by the successful expectant management of hepatic injuries in children, the approach was rapidly extended to adults.

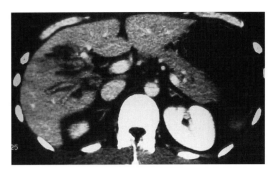

Fig. 23.9 Multiple right lobe lacerations. This configuration has been described as a 'bear claw' appearance.

Imaging findings Contrast-enhanced CT remains the best investigative modality for the accurate detection and characterisation of hepatic injuries in haemodynamically stable patients. The commonest types of injury are low-attenuation defects in linear or stellate patterns that correspond with hepatic lacerations. When these extend to involve the capsule, the volume of haemoperitoneum increases. Multiple radiating lacerations have been described as a 'bear claw' appearance (Fig. 23.9). Haematomas are often seen in association with lacerations as more ill-defined areas of low attenuation. Subcapsular haematomas indent the liver margin and are frequently identified in the anterolateral aspect of the right lobe (Fig. 23.10). These injuries do not appear to have the same potential for delayed rupture as in trauma of the spleen, and in part the relative infrequency of delayed severe haemorrhage has led to increased confidence in non-operative management. The dual blood supply of the liver protects the liver from traumatic regional infarction unless there has been gross disruption of parenchyma (Figs 23.11, 23.12).

Periportal low-attenuation tracking along the distribution of the portal veins is a common finding in trauma, particularly in children (Fig. 23.13). The condition has also been noted to occur in a variety of other hepatic (malignancy, inflammation and hepatic transplantation) and systemic (leukaemia, right heart failure) conditions. It is postulated that the visualised low-attenuation within Glisson's capsule represents either blood or obstructed lymphatics secondary to hilar obstruction by haematoma or tense haemoperitoneum. However, in the context of trauma one of the likeliest causes for this appearance is probably overtransfusion during resuscitation, a fact reflected by the often isolated presence of this finding and its rapid resolution on follow-up imaging. The available evidence at

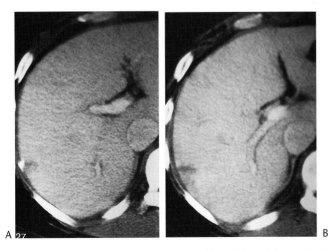

Fig. 23.8 (A,B) Motorcyclist after a road traffic accident. A fractured rib has caused a direct small peripheral laceration to the right lobe of the liver.

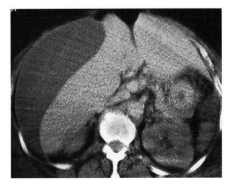

Fig. 23.10 Subacute subcapsular haematoma of the liver. The low-attenuation collection indents the liver margin. Unlike splenic subcapsular collections, these collections are not thought to predispose to delayed rupture.

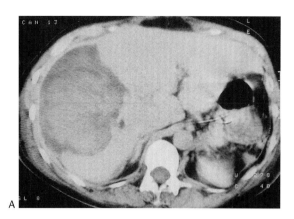
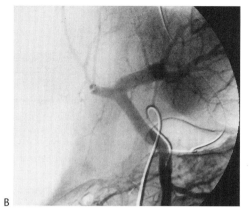

Fig. 23.11 (A) Contrast-enhanced CT: a large right hepatic lobe contusion with acute haematoma extending into the right portal vein. (B) The venous phase of the superior mesenteric angiogram demonstrates an acute cut-off to the right portal vein.

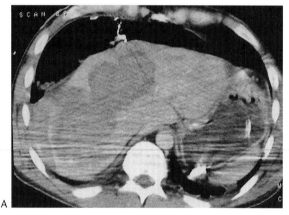
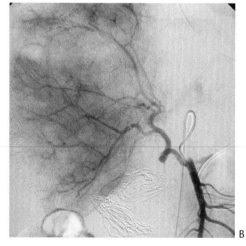
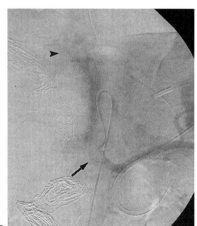

Fig. 23.12 (A) Massive central haematoma (grade 4) with laceration extending through the liver capsule in a patient with a ruptured liver. (B) The right hepatic artery arises from the superior mesenteric artery. The angiogram demonstrates areas of devascularisation and separation by the extrahepatic haematoma seen on CT. No arterial bleed is seen. (C) The venous phase of the angiogram shows complete disruption of the portal vein (arrow) and contrast extravasation (arrowhead).

present suggests that the finding of its own accord in hepatic trauma is not a cause for concern, although lobar or segmental distributions of the appearance should prompt scrutiny of the local region for associated lacerations.

Limited studies with MRI have demonstrated that at least an equivalent imaging assessment can be performed as that achievable with contrast-enhanced CT; however, currently MRI presents no clear advantage to justify the additional time requirement of the examination and the limited access to the patient during this period.

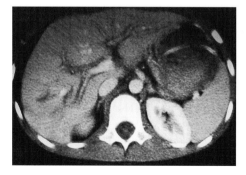

Fig. 23.13 Periportal low attenuation. Extensive periportal low attenuation is identified in a central and peripheral distribution in an 11 year old. As is frequently the case, no hepatic laceration was identified.

Pitfalls in imaging Several pitfalls may cause diagnostic error in the correct interpretation of hepatic trauma on CT. Streak artefacts from nasogastric tubes, dense oral contrast or poor breath-holding may cause false-positive interpretations of lacerations. A similar misinterpretation may occur with diaphragmatic slip insertions. Small areas of hepatic low attenuation, due to beam hardening, just deep to ribs must not be misconstrued as hepatic haematomas. It has been reported that low-attenuation lacerations may be missed in very fatty livers due to little difference in attenuation. The use of liver-specific windowing has been advocated as a means of avoiding this possibility, although overall there appears to be no significant advantage in the routine use of such windows. Superficially, multiple radiating lacerations may sometimes mimic dilated intrahepatic ducts, although the true nature of the injury should be appreciated by analysis of contiguous images and by the detection of associated haemoperitoneum (Fig. 23.9).

Staging and management The critical determination of the feasibility of non-operative management of hepatic trauma is the haemodynamic stability of the patient and the absence of other associated injuries. The patient must be appropriately resuscitated and in an environment that permits constant physiological monitoring and ready access to surgery should there be clinical deterioration. The role of CT, therefore, is to identify liver injuries, determine the quantity of haemoperitoneum and exclude the presence of other organ involvement. While the classification of liver

---

Box 23.2   CT grading (blunt hepatic trauma)

Grade 1	Capsular avulsion, superficial laceration(s) (<1 cm deep), subcapsular haematoma (<1 cm thick), isolated periportal blood tracking
Grade 2	Parenchymal laceration(s) 1–3 cm deep, central/subcapsular haematoma(s) 1–3 cm
Grade 3	Laceration(s) >3 cm deep, central/subcapsular haematoma(s) >3 cm
Grade 4	Massive central/subcapsular haematoma (>10 cm), lobar tissue destruction (maceration) or devascularisation
Grade 5	Bilobar tissue destruction (maceration) or devascularisation

From Mirvis et al (1994).

---

injuries may in general terms predict the outcome of patient groups, the fact that 50–80% of adults with hepatic trauma are currently managed conservatively has reduced the relevance of specific staging. The AAST (American Association for the Surgery of Trauma) has proffered a staging system that is of use in comparing trials of different patients. Mirvis has adapted this classification to a more practical CT grading (Box 23.2).

Vascular complications and angiography It has become clear that non-operative management can be potentially successful in up to 90% of patients with isolated injuries; however, the propor-

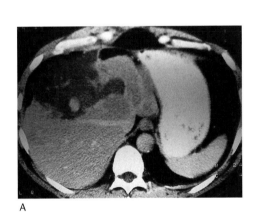

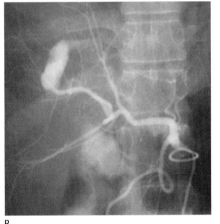

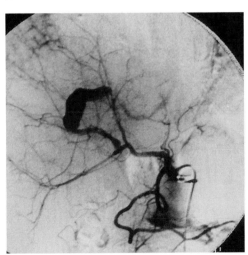

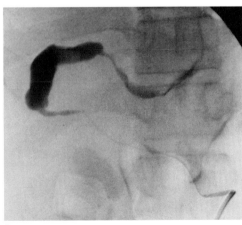

Fig. 23.14 Embolisation of a traumatic false aneurysm in a patient with liver laceration. (A) Dynamic CT scan showing an area of liver laceration. There is abnormal tubular enhancement in the lacerated area. (B) Hepatic artery angiogram demonstrates a traumatic false aneurysm. (C) Embolisation: hepatic arteriogram, again showing the aneurysm with abnormal vascular blush in the lacerated liver. (D) A supraselective coaxial catheterisation of the right hepatic artery leading to the false aneurysm, which was successfully embolised.

tion of haemodynamically stable patients in which such therapy is attempted varies from as low as 16% to as high as 72%. There is generalised consensus that isolated grade 1–2 injuries will have an excellent non-operative course. Although overwhelmingly higher grade injuries will have a successful non-operative course, the CT grading system alone is not accurate in predicting which patients will fail conservative management or suffer complications. At least two groups have demonstrated non-operative success of up to 100% in all haemodynamically stable patients with liver injuries, by using diagnostic angiography, and where appropriate selective embolisation, in all patients with grade 3–5 injuries. In order to reduce the requirement for angiography and the rate of non-therapeutic angiographic intervention, other CT parameters have been evaluated. The presence of active contrast extravasation or pooling, or of traumatic vascular malformations, are warnings that conservative management alone may fail and should at least prompt angiographic assessment (Fig. 23.14). Complex or perihilar injuries involving large branches of the portal veins, or injuries that extend into the hepatic veins or IVC, should be more aggressively managed (Fig. 23.15). In one recent retrospective series such injuries were associated with an approximately three times greater incidence of hepatic arterial injury at angiography and almost seven times greater rate of surgical management. Nevertheless, 56% of haemodynamically stable patients with a grade 4 injury and laceration extending into the hepatic veins were successfully treated non-operatively. This data reflect the potential of conservative management even in the severest of injuries. However, there is limited experience with grade 5 injuries, which are usually not isolated injuries and rarely haemodynamically stable.

Gallbladder and biliary tree Injuries to the gallbladder and biliary tree in blunt abdominal trauma are rare and rarely occur without concomitant hepatic injury. Such injuries are more common with penetrating injury or iatrogenic procedures, and in particular following laparoscopic gallbladder surgery. Gallbladder or biliary tree disruption is particularly difficult to diagnose. Such injuries will usually be accompanied by biliary leakage or a more discrete biloma; however, there are no discriminating features on CT between such collections and other serous or blood collections (Fig. 23.16). The presence of hyperdense blood in the gallbladder may be mimicked by gallbladder debris. The gallbladder wall thickening or collapsed lumen appearances of trauma may resemble a normally collapsed gallbladder or the features of chronic cholecystitis. Haematoma in the gallbladder fossa may be another

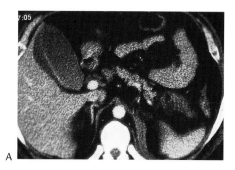
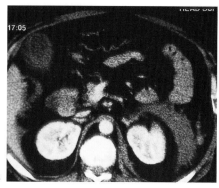

Fig. 23.16 Non-specific findings in an adult male following a fall. (A). Pericholecystic free fluid. This finding may be due to gallbladder injury but is more frequently due to other injuries. (B) Anterior pararenal haemorrhage. This is a frequent site of haematoma secondary to renal injuries but also pancreatic tail injuries. The visceral injury is often not visible.

indicator of gallbladder injury; however, the specific sign of gallbladder wall interruption is infrequently identified (Fig. 23.17). Traditionally, suspected biliary leakage has been investigated by radionuclide imaging, which, however, lacks spatial resolution. More recently helical CT following intravenous biliary contrast material administration has proved a valuable alternative that both detects and localises biliary disruption and may reduce the need for the more invasive ERCP, with its inherent risks of superadded pancreatitis. Magnetic resonance cholangiopancreatography (MRCP) has a well-defined role in the assessment of iatrogenic trauma to the biliary tree following laparoscopic surgery. MRCP is in these cases frequently accompanied by magnetic resonance angiography (MRA) of the hepatic arterial system, which may be concomitantly injured.

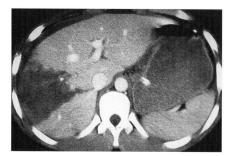

Fig. 23.15 Large irregularly marginated segmental right lobe contusion. The contusion extends to the IVC and is associated with only minimal haemoperitoneum anterior to the liver. Such injuries may be significantly underestimated by ultrasound, particularly if the haemoperitoneum is not detected.

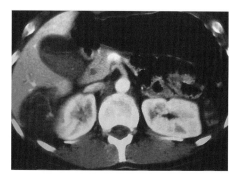

Fig. 23.17 Layered high-attenuation haematoma is present in the injured gallbladder. Additional active extravasation in the hepatorenal angle is noted within a hepatic haematoma.

Complications and injury resolution Following hepatic trauma, delayed complications occur in a fifth of patients overall, although these are more common in surgically treated patients. The main liver complications are delayed haemorrhage and infective collections. Involvement of the biliary system may result in bilomas, haemobilia, bile peritonitis and delayed strictures of the extrahepatic biliary tree. Unless there are clinical signs or parameters suggesting such complications, there is little value in the routine follow-up of hepatic injuries to monitor resolution. Serial CT following injury to the liver demonstrates that, unless there is persistent haemorrhage, there should be significant reduction of haemoperitoneum within 3–7 days. Intraparenchymal lacerations or haematomas initially expand and become more sharply defined as the damaged peripheral parenchyma is resorbed. The attenuation of the focal abnormality often falls owing to clot lysis and water osmosis. The time course of resolution of injuries over weeks or months often exceeds that of comparable splenic injuries, due to the inhibitory effect of stasis of bile products at the injury margins (Fig. 23.18). Injuries may heal completely, or result in small cysts or serous collections. Focal intraparenchymal collections developing following hepatic trauma may relate to resolving haematomas, abscesses or bilomas. Distinguishing one from the other can be difficult, relying largely on the clinical context but often ultimately on diagnostic aspiration. Infective abscesses may develop thick enhancing walls and on occasion contain gas bubbles. The latter finding has, however, been described in sterile resolving lacerations (Fig. 23.19). Extension of the infection may result in subcapsular empyemas, which may demonstrate enhancement along their margin. Bilomas tend to occur following deep injuries to the central periportal biliary tree. They usually present weeks to months after injury as simple thin-walled cysts with low-attenuation contents. Occasionally, how-

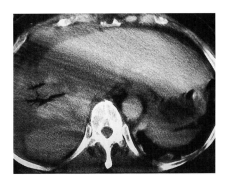

Fig. 23.19 Air within a hepatic laceration. This CT was performed a week after a therapeutic selective embolisation. This finding is well described in resolving lacerations and does not necessarily indicate infection. Associated peritoneal and pleural collections are present.

ever, septations may develop due to secondary infection or haemorrhage. Their communication with the biliary tree can be confirmed by hepatobiliary-specific isotope studies. MRI may help distinguish bilomas from haematomas.

Haemobilia, due to the communication of the vascular tree with the biliary tree, also usually presents in a delayed fashion with pain, jaundice and gastrointestinal bleeding. CT may demonstrate the presence of high-attenuation blood in a dilated biliary tree. The use of interventional assessment and selective embolisation has reduced the morbidity and mortality of operative intervention. Biliary peritoneal leaks may result in biliary peritonitis following secondary infection. The suspicion of such a leak may be raised by the low attenuation of the peritoneal fluid (0–20 HU compared with >50 HU in haemoperitoneum), although this is usually confirmed by diagnostic aspiration.

Kidney and ureters

Renal injury occurs in 8–10% of all blunt and penetrating abdominal trauma. Blunt injury accounts for 85–90% of all injuries, while the remaining penetrating injuries are attributable predominantly to stabbings and iatrogenic procedures. This latter contribution is often underestimated. A recent study demonstrated a 90% incidence of CT-detected retroperitoneal haemorrhage 24–72 h after renal biopsy (Fig. 23.20).

Certain anatomical variants predispose to renal injury. These include horseshoe, cross-fused and pelvic or transplanted kidneys. This susceptibility is due to their relatively anterior location and the potential for compression against the spine. The presence of con-

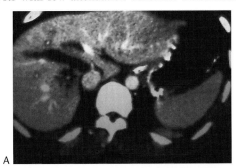
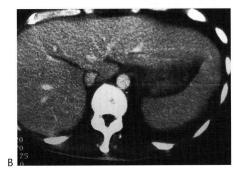

Fig. 23.18 Laceration recovery. (A) Acute phase imaging demonstrates a complex laceration extending to the IVC. Despite this extension the patient was successfully treated conservatively. (B) One month after injury the laceration has almost healed. The splenic size had significantly increased from the initial scan, presumably due to reversal of adrenergic stimulation.

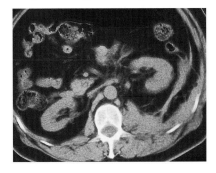

Fig. 23.20 After a renal biopsy extensive haemorrhage is present, splitting the renal fascia (interfascial). In addition, haematoma has spread to the psoas and left flank soft tissues.

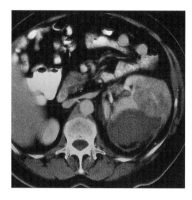

Fig. 23.21 Renal cell carcinoma detected incidentally following minimal trauma. A large anterolateral renal cell carcinoma is present. A posterolateral subcapsular haematoma indents the renal contour and displaces the kidney anteriorly.

genital or acquired cystic disease, hydronephrosis and solid vascular lesions (e.g. angiomyolipomas, renal cell carcinomas) also predisposes to injury (Fig. 23.21).

Choice of imaging modality The advent of rapid CT imaging has revolutionised the management of renal trauma. Intravenous urography can be negative in 21–34% of significant injuries and, even when positive, the findings are often non-specific and correlate poorly with renal injury severity. Intravenous urography is now limited to the occasional need for a peroperative 'one-shot' IVU examination. This full-length film following intravenous contrast administration is often useful to trauma surgeons if the patient has been too haemodynamically unstable for CT. The examination is used to confirm the presence of a functioning kidney on the contralateral side of a suspected renal injury, prior to a retroperitoneal exploration. Ultrasound fares little better in the analysis of the retroperitoneal kidney. In one series only 35% of isolated renal injuries demonstrated associated free fluid, and only 8 of 37 parenchymal injuries were identified. Acute retroperitoneal or renal haematoma appears hypoechoic, becoming more hyperechoic with time. Unfortunately the acoustic architecture is often so minimally disrupted that even the most severe of injuries may be missed or seriously underappreciated.

The accuracy of CT in the diagnosis of blunt abdominal trauma has been reported to be as high as 98%. Equally importantly, CT allows accurate staging of injury and also demonstrates the associated injuries that occur in 20% of blunt and 80% of penetrative injuries. Normality of renal appearances on CT effectively excludes any significant renal injury.

CT imaging findings High accuracy in detecting renal injuries can be obtained with 10 mm sections through the abdomen and pelvis in the nephrographic phase (60–70 s). However, if the examination is performed primarily for the kidneys then thinner collimation images (5–8 mm) are advised, with additional early scans in the corti-

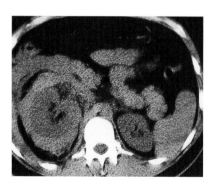

Fig. 23.22 Unenhanced CT. Extensive hyperdense perirenal haematoma is present. Unenhanced CT is not essential in the analysis of renal trauma as most significant haematomas are sufficiently conspicuous on postcontrast imaging alone.

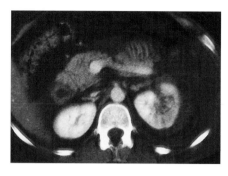

Fig. 23.23 Central irregular low attenuation of the left kidney due to a traumatic contusion. There is associated perirenal haematoma surrounding the renal margin. Further pararenal haemorrhage is separated from this haematoma by perirenal fat bounded by Gerota's fascia. Intraperitoneal haemorrhage is present in both flanks.

comedullary phase (30 s). These images help determine the extent of renal laceration, detect traumatic vascular lesions and active vascular extravasation. Later phase excretory images (3–6 min) should be used when urinary extravasation or ureteropelvic disruption is suspected. In this latter case a supplementary plain film may be of use to demonstrate ureteropelvic integrity and ureteric filling. Precontrast images are not essential but may assist for localisation and to identify hyperdense acute haematoma (Fig. 23.22).

Renal parenchymal injuries may be accurately depicted on CT. Contusions appear as ill-defined areas of low attenuation with irregular margins and are often associated with focal or diffuse swelling (Fig. 23.23). In contrast, traumatic segmental infarcts are well defined and wedge-shaped (Figs 23.24, 23.25). Peripherally, a thin

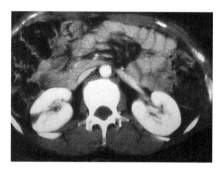

Fig. 23.24 A segmental peripheral low-attenuation wedge is noted in the right kidney consistent with a peripheral infarct. These injuries are seen relatively frequently post-traumatically but may also predate the injury in older patients with concomitant vascular disease.

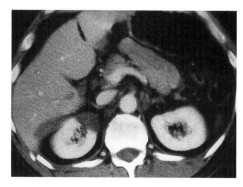

Fig. 23.25 Well-demarcated area of hypoperfusion secondary to traumatic infarction. Haemoperitoneum is present in the hepatorenal angle.

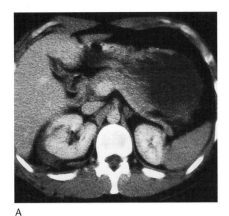

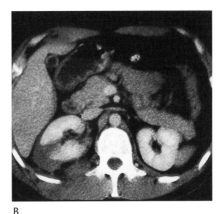

Fig. 23.26 Renal lacerations. Two stabbing injuries are identified in the same patient. (A) Superficial laceration limited to the cortex. (B). Deep laceration extending to the medulla. Such injuries are more frequently associated with urinary leakage. Associated perirenal haematoma is present.

rim of perfusion may persist due to an intact capsular blood supply. Lacerations appear as linear disruptions that may extend into the medulla, causing urinary extravasation (Fig. 23.26). Lacerations are often associated with intrarenal or extrarenal haematomas. Intrarenal haematomas tend to expand the kidney, whereas subcapsular haematomas distort the renal contour owing to the tight fascial con-

straint. Large perirenal haematomas are circumferential and usually bounded by Gerota's fascia. Most frequently these are predominantly posterior and displace the kidney anteriorly. If a large medial perirenal collection is present, ureteropelvic disruption should be excluded by delayed scanning. Perirenal haemorrhage can occasionally be due to adrenal haemorrhage alone.

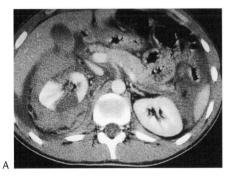

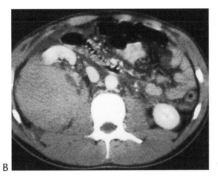

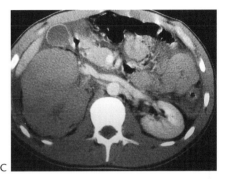

Fig. 23.27 (A–C) Major renal trauma with multiple devascularised segments. Such injuries are traditionally treated surgically, although in haemodynamically stable patients angiography and embolisation may obviate the need for nephrectomy.

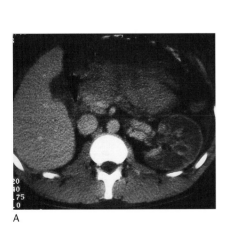

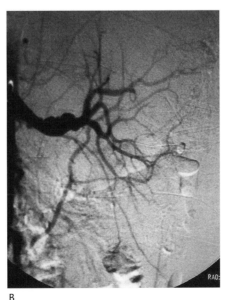

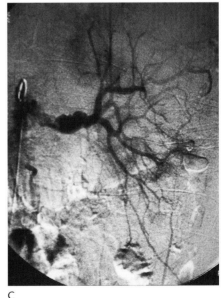

Fig. 23.28 (A) Contrast-enhanced CT following blunt trauma demonstrates a largely absent left nephrogram except for preserved rim cortical perfusion. The left renal artery is dilated. The right kidney is congenitally absent. (B) Selective arteriography demonstrates a dissection of the renal artery with poor distal perfusion. (C) Delayed phase: poor and patchy nephrogram appearances (Images (A) and (B) reproduced with kind permission from McAlinden et al 2001.)

More severe renal injuries are well delineated by CT and this has resulted in a reduction of exploratory staging surgery. Fractured and shattered kidneys are accurately defined, as well as the extent of the devascularised fragments (Fig. 23.27). CT may often determine the presence of pedicular injuries, reducing the need for angiography. This results in expedited surgery, increasing the success rate of revascularisation. Renal arterial injury is characterised by absent renal perfusion or a rim nephrogram, abrupt cut-off of the renal artery with periarterial haematoma and retrograde filling of the renal vein (Fig. 23.28). Renal vein injuries are often underdetected and are suggested when the kidney is enlarged with an, often thick, rim nephrogram. An expanded renal vein with thrombus is diagnostic.

Ureteropelvic junction injuries are uncommon and in the past were erroneously considered to be restricted to children. Uretero-pelvic junction disruptions are characterised by medial perirenal collections, good renal excretion, an intact calyceal system and focal extravasation.

Indications for imaging While it has become clear that CT is an excellent tool for the detection and characterisation of renal injuries, more debate has centred on the indications for imaging in suspected renal trauma. Clearly CT is inappropriate for haemo-dynamically unstable patients. In adults with blunt trauma the presence of gross haematuria or the combination of microscopic haematuria and shock (<90 mmHg systolic) are indications for imaging to exclude renal injury and other associated intra-abdominal injuries. Twenty-five per cent of patients with gross haematuria will have significant renal injuries. In a meta-analysis of 2873 patients with blunt trauma, microscopic haematuria and no shock, only 10 significant injuries were identified. Of these, only one did not have other associated injuries that would have necessitated abdominal imaging or surgery that would have identified the renal injury. Thus, the restriction of imaging to those patients with microscopic haematuria and shock is justified, with a failed detection rate of only 0.03%. While it has been stated that renal pedicle

abruption can rarely occur without haematuria, a review of the literature reveals all such injuries have been associated with other significant injuries that necessitated imaging.

Unlike blunt trauma, the indications for renal imaging in penetrative trauma are based solely on the site of injury and are irrespective of the presence of haematuria. This approach is justified because the rate of significant renal injuries can be as high as 67% in penetrating trauma, as opposed to 4% in blunt trauma. Moreover, penetrating injuries are more likely to result in renal loss. In a large series of proven stab injuries to the kidney 9% had no haematuria. Other studies have demonstrated no relationship between the degree of haematuria and the severity of renal injury.

In children a lower threshold for imaging must be applied as hypotension may be absent or delayed in significant injuries. Many centres recommend investigation for any degree of haematuria in children, while others argue that, as most of these injuries will heal spontaneously, imaging is only indicated when microscopic haematuria greater than 3+ on dipstick is present.

Box 23.3   CT grading (blunt renal injury)*

Grade I	Contusion or non-expanding subcapsular haematoma without laceration
Grade II	Non-expanding perirenal haematoma or cortical laceration (<1 cm) without urinary extravasation
Grade III	Laceration (>1 cm) without urinary extravasation, larger perinephric haematomas
Grade IV	Laceration through the corticomedullary junction and into collecting system or segmental renal artery or vein with contained haemorrhage
Grade V	Shattered kidney or avulsion of the renal pedicle

*Grade based on most accurate assessment of radiology, surgery or autopsy. Advance one grade for multiple injuries.
From Moore, E. E., et al (1989) *Journal of Trauma-Injury Infection and Critical Care,* **29**, 1664–1666.

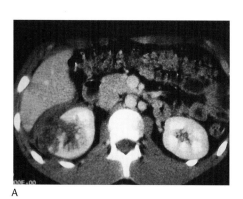
A

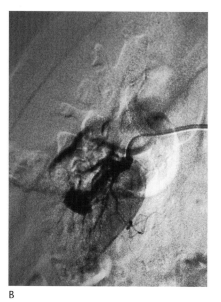
B

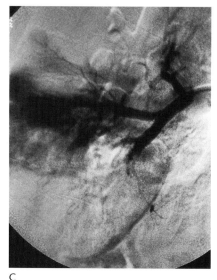
C

Fig. 23.29   (A) CT following blunt trauma demonstrates a right renal contusion with perirenal haemorrhage. The patient was haemodynamically stable and treated conservatively. (B) Angiography performed for persistent haematuria demonstrates a traumatic false aneurysm. (C) Successful embolisation of the supplying branch artery. (Courtesy of Dr C. Blakeney, Royal London Hospital.)

Staging and management The retroperitoneum represents a relatively closed compartment that can contain and to a degree tamponade haemorrhage from a renal injury. Several staging systems have been postulated to segregate renal injuries into different management protocols. The most widely used is the AAST classification (Box 23.3).

Consensus has been established that, providing the patient is haemodynamically stable and there are no associated injuries requiring treatment, grade I–III injuries can be successfully treated non-operatively. These injuries are considered minor and constitute the vast majority of renal injuries (85–90%). Higher grade injuries are considered significant and their treatment is more variable and in constant evolution, with many centres now advocating that even the most severe of injuries can be conservatively managed. Devitalised segments were once considered an absolute contraindication to non-operative management; however, if there are no associated bowel or pancreatic injuries, these have been demonstrated to be treated with similar success non-operatively. Complete ureteropelvic disruptions are an indication for surgery, although partial tears can be treated by antegrade stenting. Renal pedicle injuries have the worst overall prognosis, with poor operative revascularisation rates. Early experience suggests that endovascular stenting may prove a viable alternative.

Angiography and embolisation The indications for angiography in renal tract injuries remain predominantly the investigation of delayed or protracted bleeding and the treatment of CT-detected traumatic vascular malformations (Figs 23.29, 23.30). Angiography and selective embolisation have increased the success of non-operative management of higher grade injuries, with haemostasis successfully achieved in approximately 90%. Angiographic techniques result in a greater preservation of renal parenchyma and are, therefore, the first line of treatment in transplant kidneys. Diagnostic angiography may also assist when CT imaging suggests that there may be an underlying renal anomaly that predisposed to injury (Fig. 23.31).

Bladder

Bladder injuries may be the result of blunt or penetrative injuries. The propensity to injury depends largely on the degree of bladder distension at the time of injury. Haematuria is almost invariably present in bladder injuries and is usually gross in nature. Injuries may be classified as contusions or lacerations that may result in rupture. Intraperitoneal ruptures are usually the result of blunt trauma to a distended bladder. By contrast, extraperitoneal ruptures

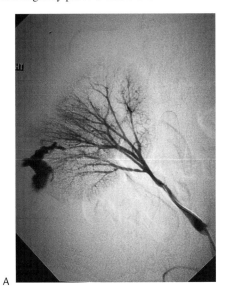

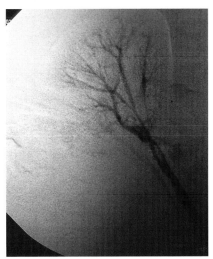

Fig. 23.30   Persistent haemorrhage (same patient as Fig. 23.26). (A) Diagnostic angiography demonstrates active extravasation. (B) Following embolisation haemorrhage has ceased, although perfusion to the lower pole of the left kidney was sacrificed. (Reproduced with kind permission from McAlinden et al 2001.)

A   B

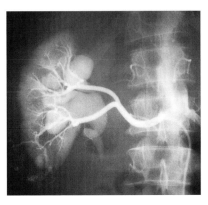

Fig. 23.31   Angiography for persistent haemorrhage demonstrates abnormal vasculature due to a renal angiomyolipoma. (Reproduced with kind permission from McAlinden et al 2001.)

are associated with pelvic fractures in over 95% of cases. Although traditionally these are believed to be due to direct bony penetration, many injuries probably also occur due to shearing injuries of the bladder base. Isolated extraperitoneal injuries are more common (50–85%) than isolated intraperitoneal ruptures (15–45%) or combined injuries (0–12%).

The relevance in determining whether a rupture is intraperitoneal or extraperitoneal lies in the different treatment for these two injuries. Intraperitoneal injuries require surgery, whereas extraperitoneal injuries may be treated by catheterisation alone. Traditionally the gold standard for evaluation has been conventional cystography (Fig. 23.32). Cystography must always be preceded by ascending urethrography in male patients in order to exclude a urethral injury as the cause of haematuria.

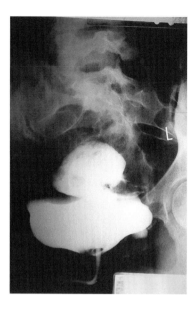

Fig. 23.32 Contrast cystography. Following trauma there is an intraperitoneal rupture of the bladder dome. Contrast is starting to line the small bowel in the left iliac fossa. (Courtesy of Dr T. Fotheringham, Royal London Hospital.)

Choice of imaging and findings Conventional CT with intravenous contrast may detect contusions of the bladder wall appearing as wall thickening or hyperdense intravesical haematoma. However, CT is poor at depicting bladder lacerations, due to inadequate distension and the absence of intravesical contrast at the time of pelvic scanning. Delayed scanning at 5 min is still insensitive due to inadequate vesical distension. More recently thin-collimation pelvic CT has been performed following contrast instillation into the bladder as a supplement to normal abdomino-pelvic scanning. Contrast should not be instilled into the bladder before the routine abdominopelvic scan for trauma because extravasation from disrupted pelvic vasculature or bowel contrast leaks may be misinterpreted as an intraperitoneal bladder rupture. Results suggest at least comparable performance to conventional cystography, eliminating the need for multiple plain films. Intraperitoneal rupture is characterised by free spill of contrast around pelvic small-bowel loops and in the paracolic gutters. Extraperitoneal rupture results in localised collections of contrast in the prevesical space of Retzius and around the bladder base (Fig. 23.33). These latter collections must be distinguished from extravasations due to urethral disruption. If the urogenital diaphragm is disrupted, these collections can extend into the perineum and the upper thigh.

Pancreas

Blunt pancreatic injuries are relatively uncommon, occurring in 3–12% of abdominal trauma. Such injuries are mainly the result of compression of the neck and body of the pancreas against the vertebral column by steering wheels or seat belts in adults and bicycle handlebars in children. These mechanisms of injury result in associated injuries to the duodenum, spleen, kidneys or lumbar spine in over 90% of cases. It is these associated injuries that are largely responsible for the increased mortality levels of 10–25% in combined injuries, compared with 3–10% for isolated injuries.

The initial clinical and biochemical parameters may be non-specific, with epigastric pain and mild leucocytosis. Serum amylase measurements are elevated in 60% of cases, although these changes may be delayed, and the serum amylase level does not correlate with the level of injury. In addition, in blunt abdominal trauma only 10% of patients with elevated serum amylase have a pancreatic injury; however, persistently normal amylase levels have a 95% negative predictive value for pancreatic injury.

CT imaging findings CT is the most accurate available modality for the detection and gradation of pancreatic injury; however, even using optimal CT techniques pancreatic injury is often missed on initial appraisal. Up to 40% of pancreatic injuries may not be visible on CT obtained within 12 h of trauma. Injuries may be very subtle, and frequently unopacified bowel loops or streak artefacts may cause false-positive interpretations. Acute assessment of the pancreas by ultrasound is often hampered by the presence of air in the stomach and small bowel secondary to aerophagy caused by pain. Even when visualisation is not impeded, the retroperitoneum is poorly assessed. Hence pancreatic injuries may often go undetected and, unless they are associated with other injuries or pancreatic duct disruption, may well resolve spontaneously. Often these injuries are identified incidentally at laparotomy for other injuries.

As with lacerations and contusions in other solid organs on contrast-enhanced CT, these usually appear as areas of lower attenuation on the background of a well-enhancing pancreas. More severe injuries usually occur in the neck or proximal body just anterior to the vertebral body and include transection and disruption (Fig. 23.34). Unfortunately the direct injury to the pancreas itself is not easily visible and ancillary secondary signs must be used to alert to pancreatic injury. These include presence of localised oedema, retroperitoneal haematoma or fat infiltration, localised collections of fluid in the lesser sac, or anterior pararenal fascia thickening (Fig. 23.16). Tracking of fluid between the splenic vein and the pancreatic body is considered a relatively specific sign of pancreatic injury.

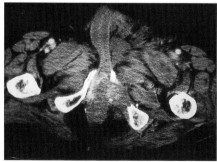

A

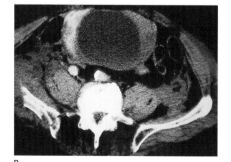

B

Fig. 23.33 (A) Extraperitoneal bladder base rupture. Following an ascending urethrogram, contrast surrounds the bladder base within the perineum. (B) Contrast has tracked around the bladder, which still contains urine. There are associated fractures of the right iliac blade and of the left pubic rami.

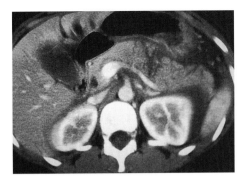

Fig. 23.34 Pancreatic laceration following a go-karting car accident. Complete transection of the junction of the body and tail with fragmentation. The pancreatic duct would almost certainly be disrupted in such an injury. Associated extensive peritoneal and retroperitoneal haematoma is present. Note that despite the significant injury the splenic vein is not separated from the pancreas, demonstrating the low sensitivity of this sign.

Box 23.4   CT grading (blunt pancreatic injury)*

Grade I	Minor contusion or laceration without duct injury
Grade II	Major contusion or laceration without duct injury or tissue loss
Grade III	Distal transection or parenchymal injury with duct injury
Grade IV	Proximal transection (to the right of mesenteric vein) or parenchymal injury involving ampulla
Grade V	Massive disruption of pancreatic head

*Grade based on most accurate assessment of radiology, surgery or autopsy. Advance one grade for multiple injuries.
From Moore, E. E., et al (1990) *Journal of Trauma-Injury Infection and Critical Care*, **30**, 1427–1429.

Staging and management Pancreatic injuries may be graded according to the OIS (Organ Injury Scale) classification (Box 23.4), which recommends that grade I and II injuries can be conservatively managed. Although pancreatic duct trauma cannot be directly visualised on CT, the deeper the laceration the more likely it is that there will be ductal disruption; 80% of major lacerations (>50% thickness) are associated with ductal injury, whereas superficial lacerations (<50% thickness) are rarely associated with duct damage. The presence of pancreatic duct disruption (grade III–V) is associated with a higher morbidity and mortality due to the development of pancreatic pseudocysts, fistulas and abscesses. A surgical approach is, therefore, mandated, and with deeper lacerations attempts must be made to exclude ductal injury by endoscopic retrograde or peroperative pancreatography. MRCP may offer a future potential role in stable patients, although experience is still limited. In severe injuries of the pancreas particular attention must also be paid to the integrity of the splenic, mesenteric and portal veins.

Delayed imaging After an initial delay in diagnosis pancreatic injuries may often become more apparent owing to the development of localised oedema and autodigestion due to pancreatic enzyme leakage. Vigilance is therefore required when there is persistent epigastric pain or an elevated amylase level, and a repeat scan may be rewarding within the first 24 h. The release of pancreatic enzymes may trigger a post-traumatic pancreatitis with the sequelae of pseudocyst formation or vascular complications.

As pancreatic injuries are difficult to detect in the acute phase, even with optimal technique, diagnosis is based on careful scrutiny of secondary signs and may require supplementary repeat imaging. The identification or suspicion of ductal disruption and of associated injuries is paramount, as these significantly increase the morbidity and mortality of the injuries.

Bowel and mesentery

Bowel and mesenteric injuries occur in approximately 5% of blunt abdominal trauma cases and are, therefore, relatively unusual injuries. These injuries often demonstrate subtle or minimal signs on CT imaging and can hence cause interpretative problems. Even when the diagnosis is suspected, several of the described signs of injury have a low diagnostic specificity. Detection of these injuries is of importance as, in contradistinction to the trend to non-operative management of solid intra-abdominal organ injuries, the optimal treatment for bowel and mesenteric injuries remains early surgical repair. A delay in diagnosis, and hence treatment, increases morbidity and mortality.

Deceleration injuries tend to cause shearing forces at the points of fixation of the bowel, such as the retroperitoneal duodenum, the ligament of Treitz, the ileocaecal valve and any incidental hernias. These forces may precipitate mesenteric tears or bowel wall injuries. Compressive forces tend to cause an increase in intraluminal bowel pressure resulting in direct rupture. Lap seat belts, in particular in children, have been associated with such injuries. Penetrating injuries tend to the affect the colon more due to its relative size and fixation. Blunt trauma injury to the colon is rare.

CT technique Although CT is far superior to other modalities such as ultrasound in the detection of bowel and mesenteric injuries, the technique employed must be appropriate and observers need to have a high index of suspicion. In particular, oral contrast must be administered in addition to intravenous contrast in order to maximise sensitivity. Although the visualisation of direct contrast leakage is a relatively rare but specific finding, bowel contrast also allows the detection of bowel wall thickening and of small collections between bowel loops. Previously many centres avoided oral contrast, fearful of aspiration pneumonitis. In a series of studies seeking evidence of contrast-related aspiration pneumonitis no documented adverse effects have been found in over 1000 adult and 50 paediatric patients. For suspected rectal and colonic injuries rectal contrast is an essential adjunct.

CT imaging findings The most specific signs of bowel injury include oral contrast extravasation, direct visualisation of disrupted bowel and extraluminal mesenteric gas or pneumoperitoneum. The detection of this last finding is facilitated by the use of lung window settings but it may be present in fewer than 50% of cases. These relatively infrequent specific findings constitute indications for early laparotomy (Fig. 23.35). The presence of peritoneal fluid in the absence of an identifiable solid organ injury should also cause suspicion, except in the case of small amounts of free fluid in the pelvis of women of reproductive age, which may be normal. Bowel related peritoneal fluid is often of lower attenuation than haemoperitoneum and if aspirated often has a high amylase content.

Other signs of bowel injury include focal bowel thickening due to intramural haematoma (commonest in the second part of the duodenum) (Fig. 23.36) and abnormal bowel wall enhancement (Figs 23.37–23.39). However, the low specificity for significant

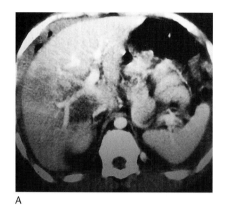

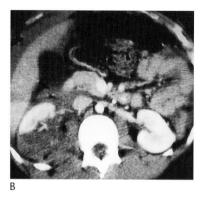

Fig. 23.35 Gunshot injury to the abdomen. (A) There is an intrahepatic contusion with haemoperitoneum. Within the haemoperitoneum air bubbles are identified due to an associated large bowel injury. (B) There is a further large devascularising injury of the posterior right kidney but no other bowel injury localising signs were identified.

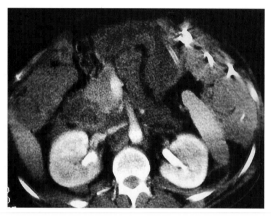

Fig. 23.36 Duodenal rupture with leakage into the right anterior pararenal space.

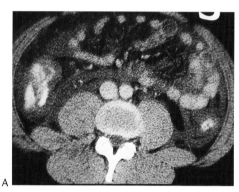

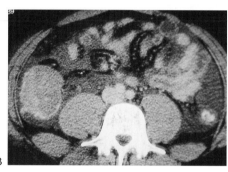

Fig. 23.38 Bowel trauma. There is extensive intraperitoneal free fluid with no evidence on other images of a solid visceral injury. (A) The ascending colon demonstrates intense staining of the wall and lumen consistent with haemorrhage. (B) More inferiorly a large haematoma compresses the colonic lumen.

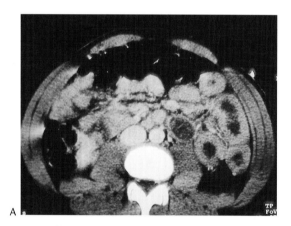

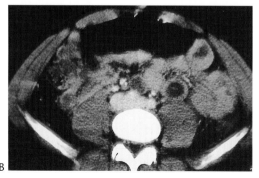

Fig. 23.37 (A,B) Localised bowel wall thickening due to small bowel haematoma following blunt abdominal trauma.

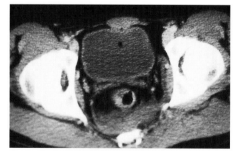

Fig. 23.39 Haematoma is present in the perirectal space secondary to a 20 metre fall resulting in blunt injury to the rectum.

bowel injury in these signs does not justify immediate surgical intervention. The presence of bowel wall thickening and intense enhancement without peritoneal fluid may simply be part of the hypoperfusion–reperfusion complex, commonly known as 'shock bowel' and does not necessarily imply bowel rupture (Fig. 23.40).

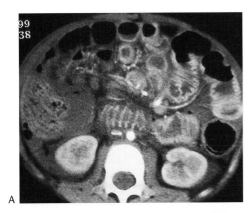

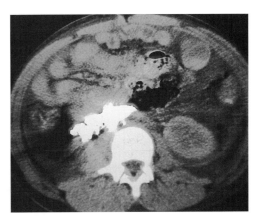

Fig. 23.41 Laceration of the IVC in a child after a 15 metre fall. Contrast has been instilled via a femoral line. Active contrast extravasation into the retroperitoneum is noted. There is almost no contrast in the systemic circulation and hence the kidneys.

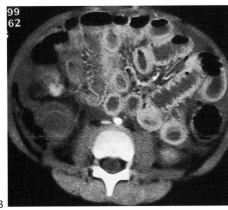

Fig. 23.40 Bowel findings in a 7 year old following a road traffic accident. (A) The diffuse fluid dilatation of the small bowel with brightly enhancing walls suggest 'shock bowel'. This is supported by the collapsed IVC and the small calibre aorta. (B) The focal dilatation and thickening of the terminal ileum with extraluminal air lateral to the colon suggests bowel trauma with perforation. The findings of trauma and 'shock bowel' may coexist and be difficult to differentiate.

Mesenteric injuries may occur in isolation or in combination with bowel perforation. The presence of active vascular contrast extravasation with a large haematoma reflects a patient at high risk for subsequent bowel ischaemia and rupture and is an indication for surgery. However, lesser degrees of haematoma or 'misting' of the mesentery do not necessarily indicate a need for surgery and may require follow-up examinations coupled with clinical observation.

In the detection of bowel and mesenteric injuries careful review of the images is paramount because the signs, if present, may often be minimal. When there is clinical suspicion of such injuries, delayed repeated imaging may be of assistance.

Major blood vessels

Blunt injuries to the inferior vena cava and the aorta are unusual except at the junction of the hepatic veins with the IVC. At this point hepatic lacerations may extend directly into the IVC, which is relatively fixated by its opening into the diaphragm. Injuries to the retroperitoneal infrarenal course of these vessels in the abdomen is unusual, and even less frequently imaged, as these patients are usually very haemodynamically unstable and have significant associated injuries. Injuries due to penetrating causes are relatively more common but still very rare unless they are due to gunshot wounds. Iatrogenic manipulations during angiography, or interven-

tional procedures such as inferior vena caval filter insertions, represent a small subset of these injuries.

The mortality of patients surviving initial transfer to hospital with major caval or aortic injuries is very high and even for isolated injuries has been reported as 9% and 20% for caval and aortic injuries, respectively, and up to 75% for combined injuries.

CT imaging findings Contrast-enhanced CT represents an excellent tool for the detection of these injuries and often obviates the need for diagnostic angiography. In caval injuries the lumen of the IVC is often irregular or compressed by haematoma and active vascular contrast extravasation may be observed (Fig. 23.41). Injuries of the infrarenal IVC have a better prognosis than those of the retrohepatic IVC, due to the tamponading effect of the retroperitoneum. These injuries may initially respond to fluid resuscitation and, therefore, delay presentation. A collapsed IVC, particularly in the absence of pericaval haemorrhage, should alert the careful observer to the possibility of extreme hypovolaemia. This finding is useful in children and young adults, who can initially maintain their blood pressure despite significant volume loss.

Abdominal aortic injuries are also well detected by contrast-enhanced CT. These injuries are usually infrarenal and in blunt trauma associated with significant lumbar spine injuries. Patients are usually in shock with poor peripheral pulses, or paraplegic due to associated spinal cord injuries. The presence of an underlying aneurysm is an associated risk factor for blunt injury. CT may demonstrate contrast extravasation, large psoas or mesenteric haemorrhages or, in cases of contained intimal rupture, an enhancing pseudoaneurysm. Traumatic thrombosis is a rare but appreciated complication.

Pelvic vasculature Injuries to the iliac vessels and their subdivisions are relatively common. Significant injuries occur almost exclusively in association with associated pelvic fractures. The superior gluteal vessels are particularly prone to injury in their close proximity to the bony pelvis. As with other vascular injuries, helical contrast-enhanced CT is a very useful non-invasive modality at detecting active bleeding sites or vascular abnormalities, with a sensitivity and specificity of approximately 85%. Associated pelvic injuries and haematomas are also simultaneously depicted.

Angiography and embolisation Angiographic evaluation remains the gold standard for the diagnosis of traumatic vascular injuries. Although CT often provides sufficient information to proceed to surgery, angiographic techniques offer the possibility of minimally invasive therapy. This is particularly important in the pelvis, where a surgical approach is associated with significant morbidity and mortality.

Embolisation of pelvic arterial injuries is a well-established technique that can be life saving. An approach is recommended from the contralateral side to the suspected injury. This allows easier access to the internal iliac vessel on the traumatised side, which is the most frequent source of injury. Embolisation should be performed as selectively as possible with a combination of gelfoam and coils, and may result in immediate haemodynamic response. It is noted that a collaborative approach with orthopaedic colleagues is mandatory, as an unstable pelvis can cause further haemorrhage following a successful embolisation. Emergency external fixation is, therefore, an essential adjunct to vascular control.

The utilisation of angiographic techniques and treatments depends largely on the preplanning for such events. Angiographic suites must be in close proximity to emergency rooms, with 24 h availability of staff. Although there are ever-expanding possibilities for endovascular stenting and the treatment of vascular injuries, the decision to use these techniques relies as much on these factors as on the local expertise and knowledge of trauma surgeons and radiologists.

REFERENCES AND SUGGESTIONS FOR FURTHER READING

Becker, C. D., Spring, P., Glattli, A., Schweizer, W. (1994) Blunt splenic trauma in adults: can CT findings be used to determine the need for surgery? *American Journal of Roentgenology,* **162**, 343–347.

Benya, E. C., Bulas, D. I., Eichelberger, M. R., Sivit, C. J. (1995) Splenic injury from blunt abdominal trauma in children: follow-up evaluation with CT. *Radiology,* **195**, 685–688.

Bodner, D. R., Selzman, A. A., Spirnak, J. P. (1995) Evaluation and treatment of bladder rupture. [Review.] *Seminars in Urology,* **13**, 62–65.

Brown, M., Casola, G., Sirlin, C., Patel, N., Hoyt, D. (2001) Blunt abdominal trauma: screening US in 2693 patients. *Radiology,* **218**, 352–358.

Butela, S. T., Federle, M. P., Chang, P. J., et al. (2001) Performance of CT in detection of bowel injury. *American Journal of Roentgenology,* **176**, 129–135.

Cerva, D. S., Mirvis, S. E., Shanmuganathan, K., Kelly, I. M., Pais, S. O. (1996) Detection of bleeding in patients with major pelvic fractures: value of contrast-enhanced CT. *American Journal of Roentgenology,* **166**, 131–135.

Dinkel, H. P., Moll, R., Gassel, H. J., et al (1999) Helical CT cholangiography for the detection and localization of bile duct leakage. *American Journal of Roentgenology,* **173**, 613–617.

Dowe, M. F., Shanmuganathan, K., Mirvis, S. E., Steiner, R. C., Cooper, C. (1997) CT findings of mesenteric injury after blunt trauma: implications for surgical intervention. *American Journal of Roentgenology,* **168**, 425–428.

Erb, R. E., Mirvis, S. E., Shanmuganathan, K. (1994) Gallbladder injury secondary to blunt trauma: CT findings. *Journal of Computer Assisted Tomography,* **18**, 778–784.

Federle, M. P., Yagan, N., Peitzman, A. B., Krugh, J. (1997) Abdominal trauma: use of oral contrast material for CT is safe. *Radiology,* **205**, 91–93.

Gavant, M. L., Schurr, M., Flick, P. A., Croce, M. A., Fabian, T. C., Gold, R. E. (1997) Predicting clinical outcome of nonsurgical management of blunt splenic injury: using CT to reveal abnormalities of splenic vasculature. *American Journal of Roentgenology,* **168**, 207–212.

Glancy, K. E. (1989) Review of pancreatic trauma. [Review.] *Western Journal of Medicine,* **151**, 45–51.

Godley, C. D., Warren, R. L., Sheridan, R. L., McCabe, C. J. (1996) Nonoperative management of blunt splenic injury in adults: age over 55 years as a powerful indicator for failure. *Journal of the American College of Surgeons,* **183**, 133–139.

Hagiwara, A., Yukioka, T., Ohta, S., Nitatori, T., Matsuda, H., Shimazaki, S. (1996) Nonsurgical management of patients with blunt splenic injury: efficacy of transcatheter arterial embolization. *American Journal of Roentgenology,* **167**, 159–166.

Hagiwara, A., Yukioka, T., Ohta, S., et al (1997) Nonsurgical management of patients with blunt hepatic injury: efficacy of transcatheter arterial embolization. *American Journal of Roentgenology,* **169**, 1151–1156.

Jurkovich, G. J. (2001) Injuries to the duodenum and pancreas. In: Feliciano, D. V., Moore, E. E., Mattox, K. L., (eds) *Trauma,* pp. 573–594. Stamford: Appleton & Lange.

Klein, S. R., Baumgartner, F. J., Bongard, F. S. (1994) Contemporary management strategy for major inferior vena caval injuries. *Journal of Trauma-Injury Infection and Critical Care,* **37**, 35–41.

Kluger, Y., Paul, D.B., Raves, J. J., et al. (1994) Delayed rupture of the spleen—myths, facts, and their importance: case reports and literature review. *Journal of Trauma,* **36**, 568–571.

Lane, M. J., Mindelzun, R. E., Sandhu, J. S., McCormick, V. D., Jeffrey, R. B. (1994) CT diagnosis of blunt pancreatic trauma: importance of detecting fluid between the pancreas and the splenic vein. *American Journal of Roentgenology,* **163**, 833–835.

McAlinden, P., Vlahos, I., Matson, M., Chan, O. (2001) Imaging of renal trauma. *Imaging,* **13**, 44–58.

McGahan, J. P., Richards, J. R., Jones, C. D., Gerscovich, E. O. (1999) Use of ultrasonography in the patient with acute renal trauma. *Journal of Ultrasound in Medicine,* **18**, 207–213.

Meredith, J. W., Young, J. S. Bowling, J., Roboussin, D. (1994) Nonoperative management of blunt hepatic trauma: the exception or the rule? *Journal of Trauma,* **36**, 529–534.

Miller, K. S., McAninch, J. W. (1995) Radiographic assessment of renal trauma: our 15-year experience. *Journal of Urology,* **154**, 352–355.

Mirvis, S. E. (1996) Trauma. *Radiologic Clinics of North America,* **34**, 1225–1257.

Mirvis, S. E., Shanmuganathan, K., Erb, R. (1994) Diffuse small-bowel ischemia in hypotensive adults after blunt trauma (shock bowel): CT findings and clinical significance. *American Journal of Roentgenology,* **163**,1375–1379.

Novelline, R. A., Rhea, J.T., Bell, T. (1999) Helical CT of abdominal trauma. *Radiologic Clinics of North America,* **37**, 591–vii.

Patel, S. V., Spencer, J. A., el Hasani, S., Sheridan, M. B. (1998) Imaging of pancreatic trauma. *British Journal of Radiology,* **71**, 985–990.

Patten, R. M., Gunberg, S. R., Brandenburger, D. K., Richardson, M. L. (2000) CT detection of hepatic and splenic injuries: usefulness of liver window settings. *American Journal of Roentgenology,* **175**, 1107–1110.

Peng, M. Y., Parisky, Y. R., Cornwell, E. E., Radin, R., Bragin, S. (1999) CT cystography versus conventional cystography in evaluation of bladder injury. *American Journal of Roentgenology,* **173**, 1269–1272.

Poletti, P. A., Mirvis, S. E., Shanmuganathan, K., Killeen, K. L., Coldwell, D. (2000) CT criteria for management of blunt liver trauma: correlation with angiographic and surgical findings. *Radiology,* **216**, 418–427.

Ruess, L., Sivit, C. J., Eichelberger, M. R., Gotschall, C. S., Taylor, G. A. (1997) Blunt abdominal trauma in children: impact of CT on operative and nonoperative management. *American Journal of Roentgenology,* **169**, 1011–1014.

Schurr, M. J., Fabian, T. C., Gavant, M., et al (1995) Management of blunt splenic trauma: computed tomographic contrast blush predicts failure of nonoperative management. *Journal of Trauma,* **39**, 507–512.

Sclafani, S. J., Shaftan, G. W., Scalea, T. M., et al (1995) Nonoperative salvage of computed tomography-diagnosed splenic injuries: utilization of angiography for triage and embolization for hemostasis. *Journal of Trauma,* **39**, 818–825.

Shanmuganathan, K., Mirvis, S. E. (1998) CT scan evaluation of blunt hepatic trauma. *Radiologic Clinics of North America,* **36**, 399–411.

Shanmuganathan, K., Mirvis, S. E., Sover, E. R. (1993) Value of contrast-enhanced CT in detecting active hemorrhage in patients with blunt abdominal or pelvic trauma. *American Journal of Roentgenology,* **161**, 65–69.

Shanmuganathan, K., Mirvis, S. E., Boyd-Kranis, R., Takada, T., Scalea, T. M. (2000) Nonsurgical management of blunt splenic injury: use of CT criteria to select patients for splenic arteriography and potential endovascular therapy. *Radiology,* **217**, 75–82.

Sivit, C. J., Frazier, A. A., Eichelberger, M. R. (1999) Prevalence and distribution of extraperitoneal hemorrhage associated with splenic injury in infants and children. *American Journal of Roentgenology,* **172**, 1015–1017.

Wong, Y. C., Wang, L. J., Lin, B. C., Chen, C. J., Lim, K. E., Chen, R. J. (1997) CT grading of blunt pancreatic injuries: prediction of ductal disruption and surgical correlation. *Journal of Computer Assisted Tomography,* **21**, 246–250.

Yoshii, H., Sato, M., Yamamoto, S., et al (1998) Usefulness and limitations of ultrasonography in the initial evaluation of blunt abdominal trauma. *Journal of Trauma,* **45**, 45–50.

Abdominal trauma—general

Cornelius, R. S., Leach, J. L. (1995) Imaging evaluation of cervical spine trauma. *Neuroimaging Clinics of North America,* **5(3)**, 451–463.

Cowley, R. A. (1977) Trauma center: a new concept for the delivery of critical care. *Journal of the Medical Society of New Jersey,* **4**, 979–986.

Dalal, S. A., Burgess, A. R., et al (1989) Pelvic fractures in multiple trauma: classification by mechanism is key to pattern of organ injury, resuscitative requirements and outcome. *Journal of Trauma,* **28(7)**, 981–1002.

Enderson, B. L., Maull, K. I. (1991) Missed injuries: the trauma surgeon's nemesis. *Surgical Clinics of North America,* **71**, 399.

Gavant, M. I., Flick, P., Menke, P., Gold, P. E. (1996) CT aortography of thoracic aortic rupture. *American Journal of Roentgenology,* **166(4)**, 955–961.

Gens, D. R., (1992) Imaging priorities in the admitting area. In: Mirvis, S. E., Young, W. R. (eds) *Imaging in Trauma and Critical Care,* pp. 1–22. Baltimore: Williams & Wilkins.

Samuels, L. E., Kerstein, M. D. (1993) 'Routine' radiologic evaluation of the thoracolumbar spine in blunt trauma patients: a reappraisal. *Journal of Trauma,* **34(I)**, 85–89.

Abdominal trauma—imaging strategies

Baron, B. J., Scalea, T. M., Sclafani, S. J., et al (1993) Nonoperative management of blunt abdominal trauma: the role of sequential diagnostic peritoneal lavage, computed tomography, and angiography. *Annals of Emergency Medicine,* **22(10)**, 1556–1562.

Boulanger, B. R., Brenneman, F. D., McLellan, B. A., et al (1995) A prospective study of emergent abdominal sonography after blunt abdominal trauma. *Journal of Trauma,* **39(2)**, 325–330.

Grieshop, N. A., Jacobson, L.E., Gomez, G. A., et al (1995) Selective use of computed tomography and diagnostic peritoneal lavage in blunt abdominal trauma. *Journal of Trauma, Infection and Critical Care,* **38(5)**, 727–731.

Kinnumen, J., Kivioja, A., Poussa, K., et al (1994) Emergency CT in blunt abdominal trauma of multiple injury patients. *Acta Radiologica,* **35**, 319–322.

Mirvis, S. E., Dunham, C. M. (1992) Abdominal/pelvic trauma. In: Mirvis, S. E., Young, W. R. (eds) *Imaging in Trauma and Critical Care,* pp. 148–242. Baltimore: Williams & Wilkins.

Myers, D. M., Thal, E. R., Coln, D., et al (1993) Computed tomography in the evaluation of children with blunt abdominal trauma. *Annals of Surgery,* **217(3)**, 272–276.

Rozycki, G. S. (1995) Abdominal ultrasonography in trauma. *Surgical Clinics of North America,* **75(2)**, 175–191.

Splenic trauma

Benya, E. C., Bulas, D. I., Eichellberger, M. R., et al (1995) Splenic injury from blunt abdominal trauma in children: followup evaluation with CT. *Radiology,* **195**, 685–688.

Kohn, J. S., Clark, D. E., Isler, R. J., Pope, C. F. (1994) Is computed tomographic grading of splenic injury useful in the non surgical management of blunt trauma? *Journal of Trauma,* **36(3)**, 385–389.

Mirvis, S. E., Whitely, N. O., Gens, D. R. (1989) Blunt splenic trauma in adults: CT-based classification and correlation with prognosis and treatment. *Radiology,* **171**, 33.

Hepatobiliary injury

Boone, D. C., Federle, M., Billiar, T. R., Udekwu, A. O., Peitzman, A. B. (1995) Evolution of management of major hepatic trauma: identification of patterns of injury. *Journal of Trauma,* **39(2)**, 344–350.

Croce, M. A., Fabian, T. C., Menke, P. G., et al (1995) Nonoperative management of blunt hepatic trauma is the treatment of choice for haemodynamically stable patients. Results of a prospective trial. *Annals of Surgery,* **221(6)**, 744–753.

Erb, R. E., Mirvis, S. E., Shanmuganathan, K. (1994) Gallbladder injury secondary to blunt trauma: CT findings. *Journal of Computer Assisted Tomography,* **18(5)**, 778–784.

Shanmuganathan, K., Mirvis, S. E. (1995) CT evaluation of the liver with acute blunt trauma. *Critical Review of Diagnostic Imaging,* **36(2)**, 73–113.

Renal, adrenal and bladder injury

Gomez, R. G., McAninch, J. W., Carroll, P. R. (1993) Adrenal gland trauma: diagnosis and management. *Journal of Trauma,* **35(6)**, 870–874.

Guerriero, W. G. (1988) Etiology, classification and management of renal trauma. *Surgical Clinics of North America,* **68**, 1071–1084.

Herschorn, S., Radomski, B., Shoskes, D. A., et al (1991) Evaluation and treatment of blunt renal trauma. *Journal of Urology,* **146**, 274–277.

Matthews, L. A., Spirnak, J. P. (1995) The nonoperative approach to major blunt renal trauma. (Review.) *Seminars in Urology,* **13(1)**, 77–82.

Miller, K. S., McAninch, J. W. (1995) Radiographic assessment of renal trauma: our 15-year experience. *Journal of Urology,* **154(2 Pt 1)**, 352–355.

Moore, E. E., Shackford, S. R., Pachter, H. L., et al (1989) Organ injury scaling: spleen, liver, and kidney. *Journal of Trauma,* **29**, 1664–1666.

Nguyen, H. T., Carroll, P. R. (1995) Blunt renal trauma: renal preservation through careful staging and selective surgery. (Review.) *Seminars in Urology,* **13(1)**, 83–89.

Pancreatic injuries

Carr, N. D., Cairns, S. J., Lees, W. R., Russell, R. C. (1989) Late complications of pancreatic trauma. *British Journal of Surgery,* **76(12)**, 1244–1246.

Jeffrey, R. B., Laing, E. C., Wing, V. W. (1986) Ultrasound in acute pancreatic trauma. *Gastrointestinal Radiology,* **11**, 44–46.

Lane, M. J., Mindelzun, R. E., Sandhu, J. S., et al (1994) CT diagnosis of blunt pancreatic trauma: importance of detecting fluid between the pancreas and the splenic vein. *American Journal of Roentgenology,* **163(4)**, 833–835.

Injury to the bowel and mesentery

Hamilton, P., Rizoli, S., McLellan, B., et al (1995) Significance of intra-abdominal extraluminal air detected by CT scan in blunt abdominal trauma. *Journal of Trauma,* **39(2)**, 331–333.

Levine, C. D., Patel, J. J., Wachsberg, R. H., et al (1995) CT in patients with blunt abdominal trauma: clinical significance of intraperitoneal fluid detected on a scan with otherwise normal findings. *American Journal of Roentgenology,* **164(6)**, 1381–1385.

Rizzo, M. J., Federle, M. P., Griffiths, B. G. (1989) Bowel and mesenteric injury following blunt abdominal trauma: evaluation with CT. *Radiology,* **173**, 143.

24

THE BILIARY TRACT

John Karani

ANATOMY OF THE BILIARY TREE

Correct interpretation of biliary pathology requires a thorough understanding of biliary anatomy, the common developmental anomalies, and their relevance to surgical techniques of biliary exposure and drainage. Consequently radiological anatomy parallels that of surgery. The currently accepted descriptions are those of Couinaud, and Healey and Schroy, and it is these that follow.

Intrahepatic bile duct anatomy

Bile drains from the ductular and canalicular network of the acini. These ducts run with branches of the portal vein and hepatic artery in the portal triad. The smallest interlobular ducts join to form septal bile ducts, and these finally unite to form the left and right hepatic ducts. The liver is divided into two major parts and a caudate lobe. The left (segments 2, 3, 4) and right (segments 5, 6, 7, 8) halves are divided by the principal plane which passes from the middle of the gallbladder bed anteriorly to the left side of the inferior vena cava posteriorly. Each of these halves is then divided into two sectors by the right and left fissures, corresponding to the line of the left and right hepatic veins. The caudate lobe, termed segment 1, is best considered an autonomous part of the liver with separate vascular and biliary apparatus.

The left hepatic duct drains the three segments of the left liver, and the right hepatic duct the four segments of the right liver. The right hepatic duct arises from the union of two main sectorial ducts: an anterior division draining segments 5 and 8 and a posterior division draining 6 and 7. The caudate lobe (segment 1) has a variable drainage pattern but in the majority (78%) drainage is into both main ducts.

Extrahepatic bile duct anatomy

The right and left main hepatic ducts fuse at the hilum, anterior to the bifurcation of the portal vein, to form the common hepatic duct, which runs caudally in the free edge of the omentum. The extrahepatic segment of the right duct is short but the left duct has a much longer extrahepatic course and hence, when exposed surgically at the level of the hilar plate, can facilitate a wide biliary–enteric anastomosis.

The main bile duct is divided into two segments: the common hepatic duct and common bile duct, divided by the cystic duct insertion. While the cystic duct joins the common hepatic duct in its supraduodenal segment in 80%, it may extend downward to a retroduodenal or retropancreatic site. The common bile duct passes inferiorly posterior to the first part of the duodenum and pancreatic head. In the majority it then forms a short common channel with the main pancreatic duct within the wall of the duodenum, termed the ampulla of Vater. Variance in this anatomical path may have pathological sequelae; for example, the association of a long common channel proximal to the duodenal wall and choledochal cysts is well documented.

The gallbladder, acting as a reservoir, lies in the cystic fossa. Rarely, it may be embedded in liver parenchyma or alternatively may be on a long mesenteric attachment, which may then render it liable to volvulus.

Arterial supply

A knowledge of the blood supply is important because of the contribution of ischaemia to the development of biliary strictures, now increasingly recognised following laparoscopic cholecystectomy and transplantation. Three segments of supply are described: hilar, supraduodenal and retropancreatic. The supply to the supraduodenal part is essentially axial from the retroduodenal artery, right hepatic artery, cystic artery and gastroduodenal artery. The majority of this supply (60%) runs upward from the major vessels, with 38% descending from the intrahepatic divisions of the right hepatic artery, while 2% is non-axial from the main trunk of the hepatic artery. Hilar ducts recruit their supply from a network in continuity with the supraduodenal supply, while the retropancreatic common bile duct supply is derived from the retroduodenal artery.

Developmental anomalies of biliary anatomy

Intrahepatic anomalies

The normal biliary confluence of left and right hepatic ducts as described is reported in between 57 and 72% of individuals. Variations described are:

1. Triple confluence of the right posterior sectoral, right anterior sectoral and main left hepatic duct (12%)
2. Direct insertion of the right sectoral duct into main bile duct (20%)
3. Insertion of right sectoral duct into left hepatic duct (6%)
4. Absence of main hepatic confluence (3%)
5. Insertion of right posterior sectoral duct into the cystic duct or gallbladder.

Failure to recognise these anatomical variations at cholangiography or surgery, either laparoscopic or open, may result in biliary leaks or impaired biliary drainage, with its clinical sequelae of cholangitis and secondary biliary cirrhosis.

Extrahepatic anomalies

A number of anomalies with important radiological implications have been described:

1. Agenesis of the gallbladder. This is rare, with an incidence of less than 0.1% of the population. Hindgut malformations of imperforate anus and rectovaginal fistula are documented associated anomalies.
2. Bilobar gallbladder with a single cystic duct but two fundi.
3. Folded gallbladder. This may be retroserosal between the body and fundus, commonly termed the Phrygian cap deformity and present in up to 18% of individuals. Alternatively, it may be serosal between the body and infundibulum.
4. Congenital diverticulum.
5. Duplication of the cystic duct with a unilocular gallbladder.
6. Septum of the gallbladder.

The importance of the above anomalies lies in their association with calculus formation.

7. Anomalies of gallbladder position. Left-sided gallbladder arises as part of complete transposition of the abdominal viscera in situs inversus or as a result of abnormal migration with the gallbladder developing to the left of the falciform ligament. The gallbladder may also lie in an intrahepatic, suprahepatic or retrohepatic site or herniate through the epiploic foramen. Uncomplicated by disease, these anomalies represent interesting entities, but if pathology develops they carry a high morbidity and present a major challenge to the surgeon and interventional radiologist.

8. Anomalies of cystic duct insertion into either the left or right hepatic ducts or into the retroduodenal or retropancreatic segment of the common bile duct. These anomalies contribute to the complication of laparoscopic bile duct injury as they may be inadvertently divided, resulting in postoperative biliary leak. They also are a factor in the development of Mirrizzi syndrome where a distended cystic duct and gallbladder, often with stone impaction, compress the common duct, resulting in biliary obstruction.

METHODS OF INVESTIGATION

With a careful clinical history and examination coupled with standard biochemical tests of liver function, biliary disease can be reliably diagnosed. For instance an elevated alkaline phosphatase, even in the presence of otherwise normal liver function, should prompt investigation of the biliary tract. Although the last 10 years have

seen a revolution and evolution of techniques which shows no sign of abating, it should be recognised that no imaging technique stands alone and it remains important to use the appropriate method for rational investigation. Imaging protocols are of value but should be tailored to the individual patient. Errors of diagnosis generally occur not because of lack of availability of techniques and images but through failure to collate all the clinical and radiological data, whether it be plain films, ultrasound, magnetic resonance or sophisticated cholangiography, to a single diagnosis.

The plain radiograph

The plain abdominal radiograph has been superseded by ultrasound as the first-line investigation of the biliary tract. Often it is performed in the clinical context not of questionable biliary disease but as part of the sequence of investigation of abdominal pain. However, specific radiological signs may be present and biliary disease reliably diagnosed.

Calcified gallstones It is estimated that approximately 20–30% of gallstones are radiopaque. Gallstones are a mixture of cholesterol, pigment and calcium bile salts. They are precipitates of an abnormal balance of the normal constituents of bile.

The densest stones are almost pure calcium carbonate and are often described as 'mulberry' stones (Figs 24.1–24.3). However, the majority of stones have mixed constituents. The characteristic

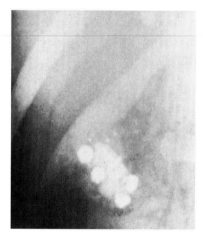

Fig. 24.1 Calcium carbonate ('mulberry') stones.

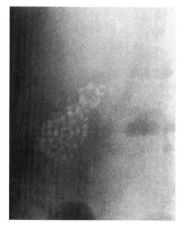

Fig. 24.2 Small, very dense stones, probably calcium carbonate.

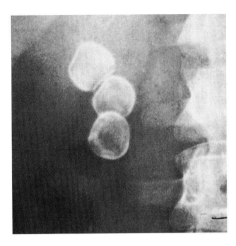

Fig. 24.3 'Mixed stones' showing lamination and facets.

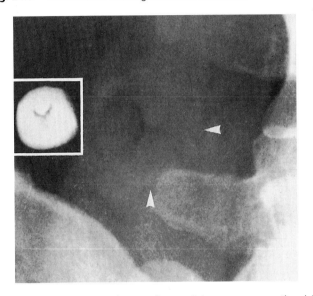

Fig. 24.4 'Mercedes Benz' stone; characteristic appearance on the plain radiograph (arrowheads) and after removal (insert).

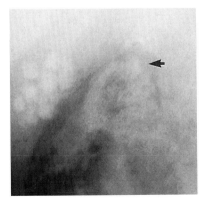

Fig. 24.5 'Mulberry stones' in gallbladder and bile duct (arrow).

feature of these, if radiopaque, is a stellate faceted appearance with gas-containing fissures (Mercedes Benz sign) (Fig. 24.4). In older patients, common duct stones producing choledocholithiasis may coexist and significantly increase the morbidity of stone disease. However, calcification within these is less common (Fig. 24.5).

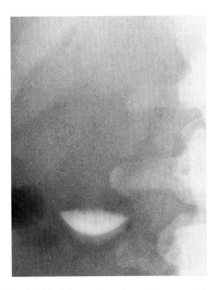

Fig. 24.6 'Limy bile' (calcium carbonate sand) on erect film.

Limy bile This appearance represents bile with a high calcium content. A layering effect is seen on a horizontal-ray projection. Calculi and chronic cholecystitis may be coexistent features (Fig. 24.6). This entity should not be confused with the often misused ultrasound diagnosis of 'biliary sludge', which may only represent hyperconcentrated bile. This is often seen in patients in intensive care on prolonged parenteral nutrition and is not of pathological significance.

Mural calcification Rarely the gallbladder wall may undergo calcification consequent to chronic inflammatory change, producing a 'porcelain gallbladder' with its predisposition to malignant change (Fig. 24.7).

Mural gas Emphysematous cholecystitis develops from severe cholecystitis, often with gas-forming organisms. It is recognised particularly in diabetics and as a complication of hepatic artery embolisation (Fig. 24.8).

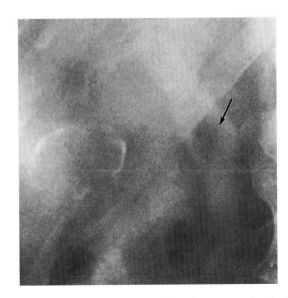

Fig. 24.7 Calcified ('porcelain') gallbladder; the common duct is dilated and contains a large stone (arrow).

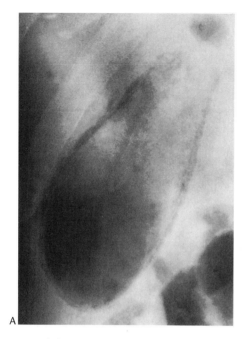
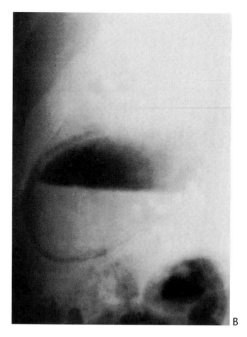

Fig. 24.8 Emphysematous cholecystitis showing (A) gas in the lumen and wall of the gallbladder and (B) a gas–fluid level in the erect posture.

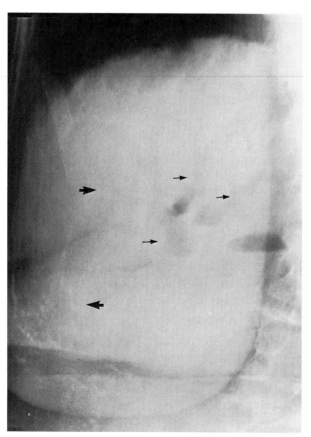

Fig. 24.9 Gas in biliary tree following endoscopic sphincterotomy (→). Note overlying benign calcifying breast disease (←).

Gas in the biliary tree The distribution of gas centrally and anteriorly in the distribution of the left and anterior sectoral right duct system is indicative of aerobilia (Fig. 24.9). It can be distinguished from portal venous gas, which is characteristically peripheral in distribution. A number of causes are recognised but the history of previous surgical or endoscopic intervention coupled with other secondary radiological signs often prompts a definitive diagnosis.

Important causes are:

- Reflux of duodenal gas through an incompetent sphincter of Oddi consequent to a previous endoscopic sphincterotomy, operative sphincteroplasty or passage of a stone. Alternatively there may be no pre-existing intervention in elderly patients, reflux being due to failure of closure of the smooth muscle of the sphincter.
- Reflux of enteric gas; this is recognised as a result of previous surgery with disconnection of the bile duct and construction of a biliary bypass with a biliary–enteric anastomosis, now almost exclusively to the jejunum through a Roux loop. Alternatively an abnormal communication between the biliary tree and either the duodenum, small bowel or colon may develop from fistulation of a calculus, local invasion of a malignant enteric or biliary tumour, duodenal ulceration, or as a complication of surgery or other trauma.

Supportive radiological features of fistulation from calculous cholecystitis are abnormal small bowel with signs of obstruction and radiopaque intraluminal gallstones. This is the classic radiological triad of 'gallstone ileus'.

Review of the abdominal radiograph may also reveal signs supportive of but not specific to biliary disease, such as calcification of chronic pancreatitis and intrahepatic gas within abscesses communicating with the biliary tree (Fig. 24.10).

Ultrasound

Ultrasound is the technique which answers most of the clinical questions posed in patients with suspected biliary tract pathology. Specifically, in the investigation of the jaundiced patient, differentiation of a hepatocellular 'medical' from an obstructive 'surgical'

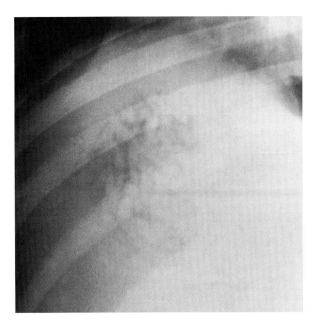

Fig. 24.10 Chronic *Ascaris* abscess of liver. The worms are seen in contrast against gas in the cavity.

cause lies at the fulcrum of the diagnostic algorithm. Failure to recognise dilated ducts of biliary obstruction or parenchymal tumour infiltration will direct the patient along a potentially fruitless diagnostic path. Equally, ultrasound is often the only investigation necessary in confirming calculous disease. Its sensitivity in detection of such pathologies means that careful correlation between the clinical presentation and ultrasound findings has to be made to ensure that unnecessary treatment is not carried out, particularly cholecystectomy in patients with gallstones as an incidental finding.

The normal gallbladder Fasting for a minimum of 6 h should ensure distension of the gallbladder for visualisation of the lumen. Scanning in two positions, supine and left lateral, ensures optimal visualisation with a 3.5 or 5 MHz probe. The normal gallbladder contains anechoic bile and has a mural thickness of 3 mm or less. High-frequency scanning is able to define the three layers of the mucosa, muscularis and serosa. Contraction is demonstrable following a fatty meal but this feature rarely aids in diagnosis. The spiral valves of Heister appear echogenic with acoustic shadowing and have to be differentiated from calculi.

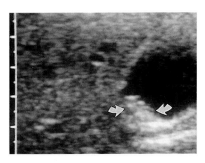

Fig. 24.12 Multiple small stones (arrows) in the dependent part of the gallbladder. No acoustic shadow.

Gallstones The accuracy of ultrasound in detection of gallstones is over 98%; false negatives are usually due to observer error or technical limitations such as patient obesity. Gallstones are characteristically echogenic, with posterior acoustic shadowing consequent to their crystalline matrix, and often lie within the dependent portion of the gallbladder. They may be freely mobile as the patient's position changes but this is an inconsistent feature (Figs 24.11, 24.12).

Cholecystitis In acute cholecystitis, recognised features are a circumferential halo of low echogenicity with mural thickening of greater than 3 mm in the fasting state (Fig. 24.13). Calculi may be present but acalculous cholecystitis is a recognised although uncommon entity. Local tenderness on scanning is a key feature as there are conditions which result in 'mural thickening' in the absence of active biliary disease; these are portal hypertension with or without cirrhosis, acute hepatitis, ascites of any cause and chronic renal failure.

Echogenic bile, which occurs as a result of stasis and hyperconcentration of bile, may be present, but obstruction and not inflammation is the aetiological factor—hence its occurrence in prolonged fasting, parenteral nutrition and extrahepatic biliary obstruction.

Chronic cholecystitis results in a contracted gallbladder, sometimes with obliteration of the lumen, so that acoustic shadowing at the porta may be all that is visible (Fig. 24.14).

Gallbladder polyps and cholesterol deposits These are an important differential in the demonstration of echogenic foci. However, they do not cast acoustic shadowing or exhibit postural movement (Fig. 24.15).

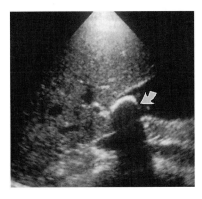

Fig. 24.11   Large stone (arrow) impacted in the neck of the gallbladder. Note the dense acoustic shadow.

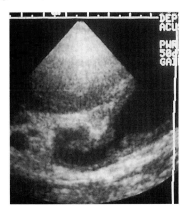

Fig. 24.13 Acalculous cholecystitis. The gallbladder wall is thickened and reduced in echogenicity.

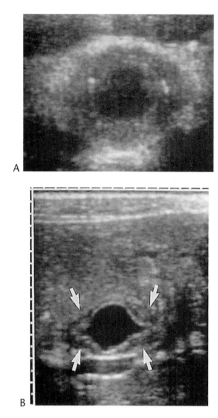

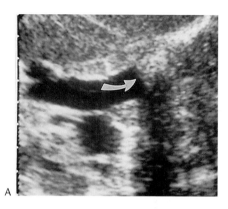

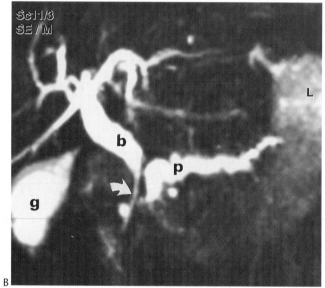

Fig. 24.14 (A) Chronic cholecystitis (see text). (B) Inflammatory thickening of the wall of the bile duct seen in transverse section at the level of the bifurcation (arrows).

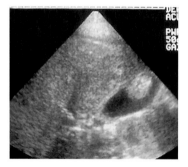

Fig. 24.15 Gallbladder polyp fixed to the ventral wall of the gallbladder.

Intra- and extrahepatic biliary tree The normal common bile duct measures up to 8 mm in adults. However, in asymptomatic patients with normal liver function and no evidence of biliary dyskinesia, a duct of up to 12 mm may be observed. This may occur following cholecystectomy, with the duct fulfilling a reservoir function, or in patients with a previous episode of obstruction. Equally, it should be emphasised that the presence of normal calibre ducts does not definitively exclude obstruction—dilatation can only occur if the adjacent parenchyma is compliant. Cirrhotic or infiltrated parenchyma may prevent duct dilatation, producing a low-volume but high-pressure duct system. For example, if a patient with established cirrhosis develops obstructive liver function tests, it is mandatory to exclude choledocholithiasis as a cause even if ultrasound demonstrates undilated ducts.

In the presence of biliary obstruction, ultrasound is reported to define the level in 95% and cause in up to 88% of patients, with a

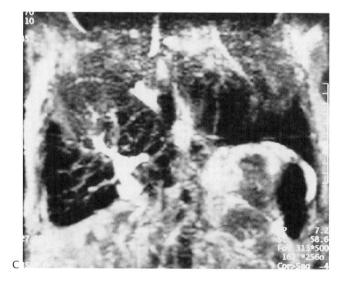

Fig. 24.16 (A) Calculus obstruction. Note acoustic shadow and the thin rim of bile around the front edge of the stone (arrow). (B) Coronal MIP image of an MR cholangiopancreatogram (MRCP) (TSE 2320/380) showing proximal stenoses (arrow) of the common bile (b) and pancreatic (p) ducts from a cholangiocarcinoma. There is a plastic F5 catheter in situ within the common bile duct which is not producing any signal artefact. g = gallbladder; L = left. (Courtesy of Dr J. P. R. Jenkins.) (C) MR cholangiography showing biliary dilatation due to anastomotic bile duct stricture following liver transplant.

diagnostic accuracy of up to 79% for common duct stones (Fig. 24.16).

The ultrasound appearances of certain biliary disorders may be characteristic; in cases of choledochal cysts the fusiform dilatation and long common pancreaticobiliary channel may be demonstrable. The cholangiopathies may demonstrate areas of segmental duct dilatation with or without increased periductal echogenicity, but such appearances are not pathognomonic and serve only to direct investigation toward biliary disorders with direct cholangiography.

Endoscopic ultrasound

This is now an established technique for investigation of biliary disorders. It has a developing role in the evaluation of bile duct tumours at the ampulla or liver hilum to determine operability. Experienced operators can also survey the common duct for bile duct stones before or after cholecystectomy and evaluate choledochal varices or other submucosal pathologies invisible to conventional endoscopy and radiology.

Computed tomography

The sensitivity of CT in differentiating hepatocellular from obstructive jaundice and in determining the level and cause of obstruction parallels that of ultrasound. The density of gallstones is an indicator of their constituent matrix. For instance, pure cholesterol stones have a density approximating to that of fat. This finding, coupled with absence of calcification, defines those patients who may benefit from dissolution therapy. However, ultrasound has the advantage in cost, availability and the lack of irradiation.

CT is reserved for those patients in whom there is doubt as to the cause of obstruction and in staging of biliary tumours, particularly cholangiocarcinoma. Lobar atrophy, vascular encasement or occlusion, and the presence of lymphadenopathy are CT criteria which adversely affect outcome.

Magnetic resonance imaging

Magnetic resonance cholangiography (MRC) is becoming established as a non-invasive alternative for evaluating the biliary tree (Fig. 24.16B,C). This technique uses either a body coil or multicoil in magnets of greater than 0.5 T field strength. The high-signal ('bright bile') techniques are commonly preferred and can be performed using either contrast-enhanced Fourier-acquired steady-state (CE-FAST) or fast spin-echo (FSE) pulse sequences in the coronal plane without intravenous contrast media. The former is a variant of gradient-echo imaging and utilises a heavily T_2-weighted breath-hold sequence. This sequence is extremely motion sensitive and to date the published series have been limited to using a body coil only, resulting in reduced resolution. The FSE method is a variant of spin-echo imaging with long echo and repetition times. Although repeated acquisitions are required, the use of multicoil or flexible surface coils allows higher signal to noise ratio and a smaller field of view, resulting in improved resolution. Fat suppression further enhances image quality. Both techniques require image processing with a maximum intensity projection (MIP) algorithm, allowing rotation of the summed image and display of the cholangiogram to best advantage.

Currently, visualisation of the common bile duct, common hepatic duct and main right and left ducts is achievable in the normal subject. The diagnostic sensitivity of the techniques varies according to the pathology. Preliminary experience indicates that the FSE technique is more successful in diagnosing the cause of obstruction in malignant biliary or pancreatic disease, with sensitivities up to 89%, whereas CE-FAST appears more accurate in demonstrating choledocholithiasis. There is evidence that MRC may be diagnostic in non-dilating biliary disorders.

MRC is rapidly evolving, and as the stronger gradients of echo planar imaging become more widely available a combination of these two techniques will emerge, allowing improved accuracy with rapid breath-hold sequences without compromise of signal intensity. The combination of conventional axial MRI scanning with MR angiography (MRA) of the hepatic vasculature and MRC has the potential to produce a complete morphological view of the liver by a single non-invasive means.

Radionuclide imaging

[131]I rose Bengal has now been superseded by derivatives of ^{99m}Tc-labelled N-substituted iminodiacetic acid, e.g. ^{99m}Tc-HIDA, as the agents to study the action of the biliary tree (Figs 24.17, 24.18).

Technique Between 2 and 10 mCi of ^{99m}Tc-HIDA is administered intravenously after a 2 h fast. Images are acquired over the next hour at 1 min intervals. Subsequent images may be required at various intervals over 24 h to evaluate excretion.

The normal ^{99m}Tc-HIDA scan provides functional and morphological information about the hepatic parenchyma in the first 10 min, the extrahepatic biliary tree by 20 min and excretion into the bowel by 1 h.

Falsely abnormal results may occur in a normal subject following an inadequate period of starvation. Physiological gallbladder con-

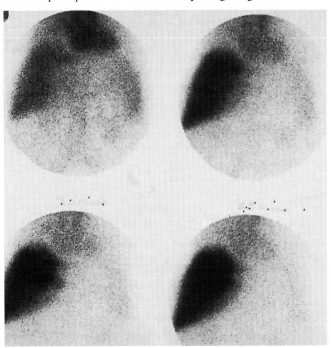

Fig. 24.17 ^{99m}Tc-HIDA scan. Biliary obstruction. Activity on the serial images is concentrated in the liver and none has traversed the biliary tree into the gut. Cardiac activity is shown to decrease as more and more of the active agent is extracted by and concentrated in the liver. (Courtesy of Professor E. Rhys Davies.)

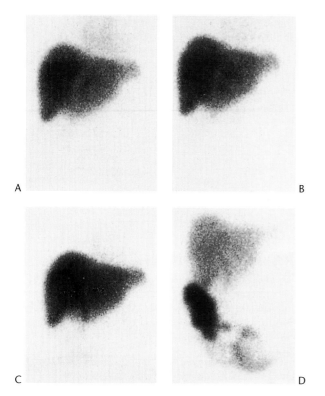

Fig. 24.18 (A–D) ^{99m}Tc-dimethyl-IDA. Serial images at 7 min, 15 min, 80 min and 270 min, showing transit of radioactivity through the liver into the small gut and ascending colon. The gallbladder is not shown, indicating cystic duct obstruction. (Courtesy of Professor E. Rhys Davies.)

traction may occur up to 6 h after enteric stimulation and biliary scintigraphy should not be carried out during this period. Conversely, prolonged starvation may be equally misleading, as the tracer may not enter an abnormally distended gallbladder. These patients should be pretreated with cholecystokinin analogues prior to the study.

Specific indications for imaging are the following.

Neonatal and childhood jaundice Excretion scintigraphy has an important role in neonatal jaundice in defining surgically correctable disorders such as biliary atresia. This condition can be excluded if tracer enters the small intestine. Secondly, any biliary connection to a hepatic 'cyst' can be confirmed by the demonstration of tracer within it.

Cholecystitis Biliary scintigraphy has a high sensitivity in the diagnosis of acute cholecystitis. Persistent non-visualisation of the gallbladder is an indicator of cystic duct obstruction. Chronic cholecystitis may be excluded when stimulation with cholecystokinin analogue allows passage of bile with delayed visualisation of the gallbladder. Other positive findings for acute cholecystitis include the 'rim sign' and 'cystic duct sign' where increased tracer uptake is present within the adjacent liver and cystic duct proximal to the obstructing calculus.

Biliary obstruction The cause and level of obstruction is best determined by other methods. If there has been a previous surgical biliary–enteric anastomosis, cholangitis may result from obstruction of the Roux loop or more distal small bowel. Scintigraphy will confirm non-obstructed bile ducts but stasis within a proximal segment of bowel with delayed transit through

the small bowel. Scintigraphy may thus be indicated in children who have undergone a previous portoenterostomy for biliary atresia presenting with cholangitis, where a distinction has to be made between the diagnoses of progressive intrahepatic disease and Roux loop obstruction, where surgery may be necessary.

Biliary leaks Bile leaks may occur following surgery or trauma. Loculated or free tracer may then be demonstrable in the peritoneal cavity.

Indirect cholangiography

Oral cholecystography

Now superseded by ultrasound as the primary investigation for suspected cholelithiasis, oral cholecystography still has a limited role in anatomical and functional assessment of the gallbladder.

The media in common use are sodium ipodate (Biloptin) and calcium ipodate (Solubiloptin). These are tri-iodinated benzene ring compounds whose concentration in the gallbladder is dependent upon ingestion and adequate absorption in the gut, take-up in the liver, excretion in the bile, enterohepatic recirculation and a patent cystic duct. Any factor influencing this pathway will result in failure of opacification and a 'non-functioning gallbladder'.

Therefore, non-biliary causes of failure of opacification that need to be considered are:

1. Failure of transfer, e.g. non-compliant patient, oesophageal achalasia, pyloric stenosis
2. Failure of absorption, e.g. diarrhoea, small-bowel bypass or resection
3. Parenchymal liver disease, in particular intra- or extrahepatic cholestasis
4. Biliary–enteric fistulas or surgical anastomosis
5. Acute pancreatitis.

Optimum technique includes a preliminary plain radiograph, followed by coned (low kV) films, either screened or with standardised prone oblique, supine oblique and a horizontal-ray projection at an interval of 12–15 h following ingestion of 3 g of contrast medium. Anomalies of gallbladder position should be excluded with an abdominal radiograph if these standardised coned views fail

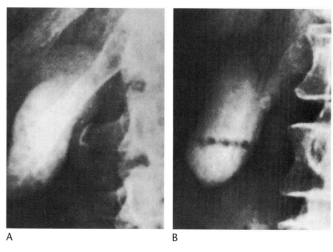

Fig. 24.19 Small cholesterol calculi which float in the erect posture. (A) Prone. (B) Erect.

to visualise the gallbladder. Ingestion of contrast can also be confirmed, with the radiopaque medium demonstrated within bowel.

The diagnostic accuracy of oral cholecystography in demonstrating gallstones in a functioning gallbladder is of the order of 85–90% (Fig. 24.19).

Intravenous cholangiography

Endoscopic retrograde cholangiography (ERCP) has virtually replaced intravenous cholangiography in the assessment of the extrahepatic biliary tree, although it enjoyed a brief resurgence in some surgical circles with the advent of laparoscopic cholecystectomy and the inherent limitation for operative cholangiography.

The contrast media in use are ioglycamide (Biligram) and iotroximate (Biliscopin). They differ from the oral compounds in that they are highly soluble, become rapidly bound to albumin, and do not undergo significant enterohepatic circulation.

Its relatively poor resolution compared with ERCP, technical limitations in up to 40% of studies, and hypersensitivity reactions, with a mortality quoted at up to 1 in 5000, are further factors which limit the acceptability of intravenous cholangiography.

Percutaneous cholangiography (PTC)

Direct puncture of the intrahepatic ducts using a fine-gauge Chiba needle allows demonstration of the biliary tree with relative safety. Expert operators can opacify the duct system in over 98% of cases in both adults and children. Technical success is reduced with undilated duct systems and in less experienced hands. There are specific indications:

1. To define the level and cause of obstruction in patients with dilated bile ducts on ultrasound in the presence of jaundice.

2. In patients with clinical and biochemical indicators of obstruction but undilated ducts on ultrasound. Although in the majority of cases, endoscopic cholangiography fulfils this role, if there has been previous surgery with disconnection of the bile duct with drainage through a Roux loop, access to the bile ducts can only be by a transhepatic route. For example, in children who develop cholestasis following a previous portoenterostomy for biliary atresia or following construction of a hepaticojejunostomy for a choledochal cyst or orthotopic segmental liver graft, percutaneous cholangiography is used to evaluate the biliary anastomosis and Roux loop drainage.

3. In defining biliary–enteric or biliary–cutaneous fistulas.

4. In defining the level of a bile leak.

5. To map the biliary tree as a preliminary to establishing external or internal biliary drainage with stent placement.

Technique Under antibiotic cover and following correction of any pre-existing coagulopathy, the liver is punctured using a fine-gauge Chiba needle under fluoroscopic and, if necessary, ultrasound guidance. On slow withdrawal of the needle and injection of contrast, the ducts are identified as contrast flows away from the needle tip centrally toward the hilum of the liver. Ducts can be distinguished from hepatic vasculature by the pattern of contrast flow. Contrast injected into hepatic veins flows in a cephalad direction toward the retrohepatic inferior vena cava and right atrium, while contrast injected into portal vein divisions flows to the periphery of the liver. Errors in diagnosis are generally due to

failure to identify all intrahepatic segmental ducts, particularly of the left liver, and inadequate demonstration of the level and length of the obstruction through suboptimal filling.

Complications In a comprehensive multi-institutional review, serious complications occurred in 3.4% of over 2000 studies. Sepsis (1.4%), biliary peritonitis (1.45%) and haemorrhage (0.35%) were the most common. Less common were pneumothorax and puncture of viscera. These complications can be reduced by ensuring fastidious technique, with a single puncture of the liver capsule, avoiding overdistension of ducts which may allow reflux of infected bile into the circulation through hepatic sinusoids, and ensuring that manoeuvres are carried out in suspended respiration.

Endoscopic retrograde cholangiopancreatography (ERCP)

ERCP and PTC should not be seen as competitors but as allies in the evaluation of the biliary tract. Advantages of ERCP are that both the biliary and pancreatic ducts are studied, and that it allows direct inspection and biopsy of the papilla and duodenum and therapeutic procedures of sphincterotomy and stone extraction. As with PTC, a diagnostic procedure can become a therapeutic one with stent placement and relief of jaundice. In patients with obliterative cholangiopathies, such as sclerosing cholangitis, or with biliary hypoplasia, opacification of the biliary tree may be technically easier by a retrograde approach. Conversely, if there has been previous surgery with a hepaticojejunostomy or if there is duodenal obstruction from a pancreatic carcinoma, then there is no access for an endoscopic examination. This illustrates the importance of a biliary team—radiologist, endoscopist and hepatobiliary surgeon—matching the needs of the patient to local expertise and availability.

This technique carries a low morbidity (less than 3%) and mortality (0.2%) pancreatitis, and duodenal perforation or bleeding following sphincterotomy for impacted ductal stones are significant contributors to these figures.

Operative cholangiography

Specific indications for operative cholangiography prior to further surgery are well defined. Of these the most common is determining the need for exploration of the common bile duct at the time of cholecystectomy. Ten per cent of patients presenting with gallstones necessitating cholecystectomy will have common duct stones; it is estimated that worldwide about 15 000 patients per year will present with stones following cholecystectomy, a significant proportion of these stones having been missed at the time of the original surgery. This second group of patients can be treated endoscopically. Operative cholangiography with demonstration of stones, together with clinical criteria of cholangitis with duct dilatation, pancreatitis or palpable stones at surgery, are the indications for exploration of the bile duct with a high positive predictive value.

Other indications for cholangiography at the time of surgery include demonstration of anomalous duct anatomy, and defining developmental disorders of the biliary tree such as biliary hypoplasia and biliary atresia prior to surgical drainage if the preoperative investigations are equivocal.

Postoperative cholangiography through a T-tube is indicated to ensure that all stones have been removed following exploration of the bile duct. Further indications are evaluation of the anastomosis and intrahepatic biliary tree of a liver transplant. Although T-tubes may not be routinely used, a specific operative indication is when there is disparity in calibre between the donor and recipient bile duct.

DISORDERS OF CHILDHOOD

Development disorders of the biliary tree

The majority of newborn infants develop a serum hyperbilirubinaemia, predominantly unconjugated, but this physiological jaundice generally resolves spontaneously within 2 weeks. Persistent jaundice beyond this period is pathological. Medical causes such as the neonatal hepatitis syndrome, a_1-antitrypsin deficiency, intrauterine acquired infection and metabolic disorders such as the glycogen storage diseases constitute the prevalent aetiologies. However, prompt investigation is mandatory to identify those with a structural obstructive component who would benefit from surgery. The accepted principles of investigation of jaundice with ultrasound, direct cholangiography, biliary excretion scintigraphy and liver biopsy are applicable to this age group and diagnostic in most cases.

Biliary atresia

Atresia of the extrahepatic bile ducts in newborn infants is the end-result of a destructive inflammatory process of unknown aetiology. It occurs with a similar incidence of 0.8–1.0 per 10 000 live births throughout the world. The association of biliary atresia with other anomalies, such as polysplenia, situs inversus, malrotation and absent inferior vena cava, is recognised in up to 30% of cases. Three anatomical types are recognised, reflecting the degree of bile duct obliteration. Atresia of the whole duct system with no normal intrahepatic ducts carries the highest morbidity and is by far the most common.

Presentation is with prolonged conjugated hyperbilirubinaemia accompanied by non-pigmented stools. Although babies may thrive

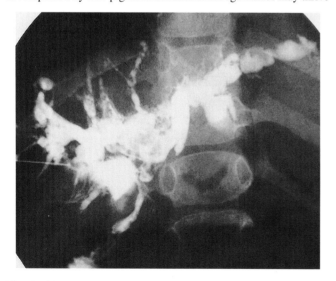

Fig. 24.20 Percutaneous cholangiography demonstrating an intrahepatic cholangiopathy of biliary atresia following portoenterostomy. There is some preservation of normal duct morphology but intrahepatic strictures and calculi are features.

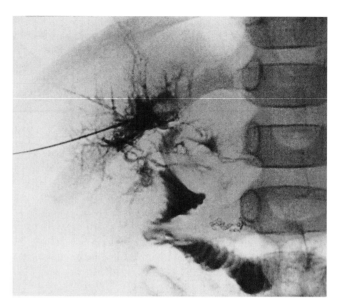

Fig. 24.21 Severe biliary atresia with obliteration of intrahepatic bile ducts. Hyperplastic lymphatics allow some drainage of bile into the constructed portoenterostomy (Kasai procedure). This is the most common type and carries the worst prognosis.

for up to 3 months, irreversible liver damage will by then have occurred. Early surgery with a portoenterostomy (Kasai operation) should be carried out if cirrhosis and its sequelae are to be deferred.

In the majority of cases the diagnosis is made with the combination of liver biopsy and excretion scintigraphy. Visualisation of small bowel using the isotope ^{99m}Tc-DISIDA (di-isopropyliminodiacetic acid) excludes biliary atresia with characteristic histological features seen in over 80% of liver biopsies. Supportive ultrasound features are a hypoplastic gallbladder, a cystic cavity at the porta, the features of established cirrhosis early in life, and recognition of the aforementioned accompanying anomalies as part of the biliary atresia–splenic malformation syndrome.

Percutaneous or endoscopic cholangiography is generally reserved for cases where doubt remains following these investigations. Hypoplastic or atretic ducts, often with hyperplastic lymphatics, are pathognomonic signs (Figs 24.20, 24.21). Equally, demonstration of an anatomically and functionally normal biliary system differentiates biliary atresia from the medical disorders which may exhibit parallel clinical and pathological pathways.

Biliary hypoplasia This condition may present with conjugated hyperbilirubinaemia in infancy. It may be seen as part of Alagille's syndrome (arteriohepatic dysplasia) with accompanying syndromic features of abnormal facies, pulmonary stenosis and segmental vertebral anomalies. Biliary cirrhosis and its complications develop but their onset is dependent upon the severity of biliary obstruction and may not become significant until adolescence or adulthood.

A characteristic pattern of attenuated ducts is present on cholangiography and this affords the only accurate method of diagnosis.

Choledochal cyst

Cystic dilatation of the extrahepatic bile ducts is a rare abnormality with a female preponderance of 4:1. The majority are now diagnosed in childhood, with jaundice from obstruction and cholangitis

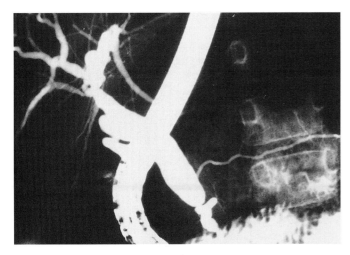

Fig. 24.22 Fusiform choledochal cyst with a long common channel and associated stricture at the pancreaticobiliary junction.

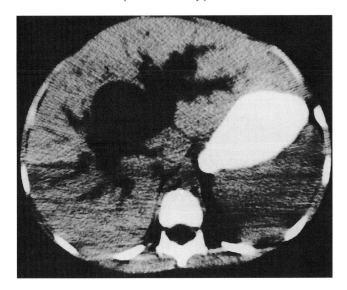

Fig. 24.23 CT of a large choledochal cyst with biliary obstruction.

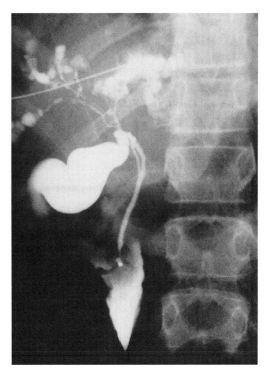

Fig. 24.24 Caroli's disease with characteristic strictures and segmental intrahepatic dilated ducts.

(80%) and abdominal pain (55%), often from pancreatitis, the most common clinical presentations. The association of a long common pancreaticobiliary channel, demonstrable on cholangiography in up to 75% of cases, would seem to be an important factor in the development of pancreatitis (Figs 24.22, 24.23). However, up to 10% of cases may present with-established cirrhosis, and intraductal carcinoma is a recognised primary presentation.

Five types are described in the most commonly used classification (Todani):

Type I—cystic (51%) or fusiform (10.6%)
Type II—diverticulum
Type III—choledochocele of intraduodenal common bile duct
Type IV—extra- and intrahepatic cysts (28.5%)
Type V—intrahepatic dilatation (4.6%)

This classification relates to the cholangiographic appearances and allows preoperative surgical planning, with radical excision of the cyst and hepaticojejunostomy being the most common operative treatment. The increasing recognition of this disorder is in part due to the high diagnostic yield of ultrasound in demonstrating fusiform duct dilatation, often in patients with non-specific abdominal symptoms. Rarely, such cysts are so large that their relationship to the biliary tree can only be determined non-invasively by pooling of isotope within them on excretion biliary scintigraphy (HIDA scan).

Caroli's disease

The relationship between Caroli's disease and the more common type of intrahepatic choledochal cysts is unclear, but probably represents a spectrum of disease. Typical cholangiographic features are those of an irregular intrahepatic duct system, which may be total, lobar or segmental in distribution (Fig. 24.24). Stone formation and cholangitis develop. It is usually associated with congenital hepatic fibrosis and cystic disease of the kidneys. This condition is now usually termed autosomal recessive fibropolystic disease, with varying representation within the liver and kidneys, ranging from chronic renal failure to minor urographic abnormality of renal duct ectasia in the renal tract and from minor bile duct dilatation to severe cirrhosis and portal hypertension necessitating transplantation in the liver.

Acquired disorders of the biliary tree

Inspissated bile plug syndrome Infants may present with jaundice secondary to plugs of thickened bile or more rarely calculi obstructing the biliary tree. Prematurity and prolonged parenteral nutrition, haemolysis, developmental choledochal anomalies and cystic fibrosis are recognised aetiological factors. Jaundice and acholic stool are presenting features.

Ultrasound demonstrates proximal bile duct obstruction, often with echogenic bile plugs within the common bile duct and gallbladder. Percutaneous cholangiography is diagnostic, confirming

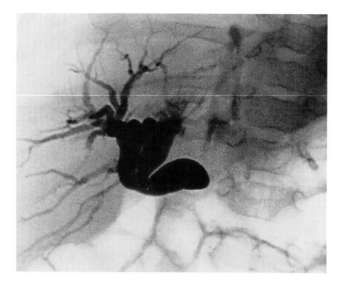

Fig. 24.25 Biliary obstruction secondary to an acquired 'atresia' in a neonate following a perforated bile duct.

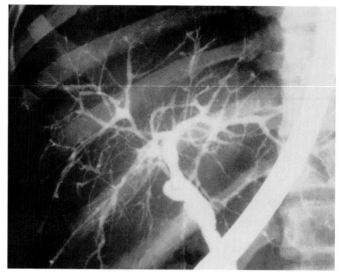

Fig. 24.26 Characteristic intrahepatic strictures of sclerosing cholangitis.

intraluminal obstruction and defining any associated anatomical anomaly. Saline irrigation of the bile duct at percutaneous cholangiography may result in clearance of the plugs but surgical exploration is often necessary.

Spontaneous perforation of the bile duct This rare condition of infancy presents within the first 2 months of life with jaundice and biliary ascites. The site of perforation is invariably at the junction of the cystic and common hepatic duct. Biliary obstruction, rarely with an atretic segment of bile duct, may ensue (Fig. 24.25).

The radiological diagnosis is based on the ultrasound demonstration of ascites associated with a complex periduodenal mass. Excretion biliary scintigraphy may demonstrate accumulation of isotope within the peritoneum or in a fibrinous periduodenal mass.

Bile duct tumours Although the malignant hepatocellular tumours, namely hepatoma and hepatoblastoma, may be associated with jaundice by compression or direct invasion, primary bile duct tumours are a potential cause. Of these, rhabdomyosarcoma is the most reported. However, it remains a rarity, comprising only 0.8% of all rhabdomyosarcomas. The tumour arises from mesenchymal cell rests beneath the biliary epithelium. Consequently the radiological appearances reflect both the intraductal invasion, with grape-like projections on cholangiography, and periductal, parenchymal and vascular involvement, best demonstrated on ultrasound and axial imaging. Generally, by the time of presentation (often with a long history of fluctuating jaundice), all these features are present, thus limiting curative surgical treatment. The prognosis is therefore poor.

Cholelithiasis Cholelithiasis is being increasingly diagnosed in childhood. Prolonged parenteral nutrition, phototherapy, infection and ileal resection contribute to this rising incidence. However, haemolytic diseases with formation of pigment stones remain the most significant factor. The incidence in hereditary spherocytosis may be as high as 60%. It is lower in sickle-cell disease, occurring in between 10 and 20% of homozygotes.

The complications of cholecystitis, empyema, perforation and the Mirrizzi syndrome have all been reported in childhood.

Radiological diagnosis does not differ from that used in adults. However, spontaneous resolution is reported in infancy; conservative management is therefore advisable if the condition is asymptomatic.

Biliary strictures Trauma, pyogenic or parasitic cholangitis, and sclerosing cholangitis in association with inflammatory bowel disease are the most common causes of biliary strictures. The spectrum of ductal involvement in sclerosing cholangitis presenting in childhood is wide, varying from a single hilar stricture to involvement of all duct orders resembling the adult pattern (Fig. 24.26). As with adults the degree of histological liver damage and severity of radiological change are not necessarily in accord but the cholangiographic appearances are an important diagnostic criterion.

Cholangiopathies of childhood Rarer causes of a generalised intrahepatic cholangiopathy with stricturing and segmental dilatation include cystic fibrosis, Langerhans' cell histiocytosis, α_1-antitrypsin deficiency and the opportunistic infections of HIV disease. There are no pathognomonic cholangiographic features by which these can be reliably distinguished, so correlation with clinical presentation and other imaging is the key to diagnosis.

DISORDERS OF THE GALLBLADDER

Gallstones

Prevalence and aetiological factors It is estimated that up to 17% of the adult population have gallstones but a significant proportion of these are silent with no clinical sequelae. Studies have shown that up to 50% of detected calculi remain asymptomatic over a 10 year period.

There is an increasing incidence with age, with a preponderance in females and in patients with chronic liver disease, haemolytic disorders and diabetes. Cholelithiasis is rare in prepubescent children unless associated with a haemolytic disease, congenital anomaly of the biliary tree or rare conditions such as immunoglobulin A deficiency. Recognition in infancy, although an uncommon occurrence, is now increasing. Total parenteral nutrition in preterm infants with lack of enteral stimulation of the biliary tree, phototherapy, ileal resection and sepsis are contributory factors.

Types of stones Three main types of stones are recognised according to their constituent matrix. Mixed stones form the majority, with cholesterol and pure pigment stones being less common. Predicting the type of stone has historically been based on recognition of important aetiologic factors coupled with the radiological findings. For instance, pigment stones are preponderant in patients with haemolytic disorders and in patients with chronic liver disease and recurrent cholangitis, particularly if secondary to parasitic infection. Equally, up to 30% of cirrhotic patients may have silent cholesterol stones, so predictive factors on clinical criteria may be misleading. A role for imaging has been defined in dissolution therapy with the bile salt derivatives chenodeoxycholic and ursodeoxycholic acid where the number of, and presence of calcification within, stones is important. Well-defined criteria have been established for this therapy: radiolucent stones of less than 15 mm within a functioning gallbladder. Even with such prescriptive criteria a recurrence rate of up to 30% is reported.

However, in practice, such distinctions of type are of little importance but there is a clear role for radiology in confirming the presence of stones and their complications.

Calculous cholecystitis

In the vast majority of cases this results from a stone obstructing the cystic duct with resultant infection of static bile and the gallbladder mucosa. Transmural infection may result in a gangrenous gallbladder that may perforate and give rise to either a localised abscess or biliary peritonitis. An empyema or mucocele may result if there is continuing cystic duct obstruction. Infection with specific coliform organisms or *Clostridium welchii* may result in emphysematous cholecystitis, particularly in patients with diabetes or those who are immunosuppressed, with mural air visible on a plain radiograph.

Fistulation of stones may occur to the small or large bowel, with associated enteric obstruction, termed gallstone ileus.

Ultrasound is the pre-eminent diagnostic technique; the following key features may be established in the acute phase:

1. Presence of calculi as echogenic intraluminal foci
2. Mural thickening greater than 3 mm with a halo of low reflectivity and associated local tenderness
3. Pericholecystic abscess formation
4. Development of an empyema or mucocele with a thickened gallbladder assuming a spherical shape and containing highly reflective bile and stones (Fig. 24.27).

The features differ in chronic calculous cholecystitis where the gallbladder may be contracted around the stones. Oral cholecystography to determine non-function, although historically important, has now been virtually replaced by ultrasound; the features listed above and an appropriate clinical history are indications for cholecystectomy.

Supportive evidence may be obtained with an excretion HIDA scan. Failure of demonstration of the gallbladder confirms cystic duct obstruction with a reported sensitivity of 95%. However, this finding is not pathognomonic of acute cholecystitis, occurring in any cause of cystic duct obstruction. It is of value in the patient

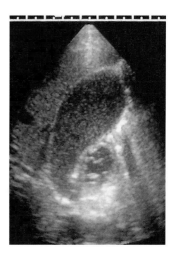

Fig. 24.27 Empyema of the gallbladder. The true nature of the fine internal echoes can only be determined by aspiration.

with gallstones on ultrasound who presents with abdominal pain and there is doubt as to whether presentation is due to cholecystitis or to another cause.

Mirrizzi syndrome This syndrome occurs when an impacted calculus within the cystic duct causes acute cholecystitis. Extension of the local inflammatory process involves the common hepatic or common bile duct. This compressive effect may result in biliary obstruction and jaundice. Cholecystectomy alone often results in the re-establishing of biliary drainage and relief of jaundice.

Acalculous cholecystitis The aforementioned radiological findings, excluding the presence of stones, are applicable to this relatively uncommon condition (Fig. 24.13). Recognised causes are:

1. Septicaemia, often in patients with multiorgan failure or severe burns
2. Typhoid or actinomycotic infection
3. As part of an acute cholangitis secondary to common duct stones or a choledochal abnormality, e.g. choledochal cysts
4. Secondary to cystic duct obstruction from indwelling stents or infiltrating tumour
5. Secondary to ischaemia from torsion of the gallbladder.

Cholesterosis In this condition there is diffuse deposition of cholesterol on the gallbladder mucosa. Deposits are of the order of 1–2 mm, multiple and fixed on scanning. Differentiation from a

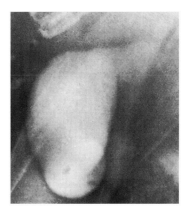

Fig. 24.28 Cholesterosis, showing fixed mural defects.

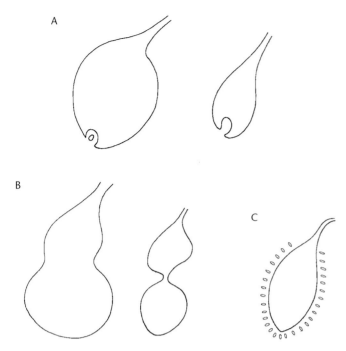

Fig. 24.29 Types of adenomyomatosis. (A) A fundal nodule before and after contraction. (B) Stricture before and after contraction. (C) Rokitansky–Aschoff sinuses.

polyp is not possible. The condition is generally asymptomatic; the majority of patients develop cholesterol stones (Fig. 24.28).

Adenomyomatosis (cholecystitis glandularis proliferans) This condition of unknown aetiology has distinct has pathological features, with round-cell infiltration, muscle hypertrophy and formation of epithelial mucosal sinuses (Rokitansky–Aschoff sinuses), and occurs in three distinct types with well-documented features on oral cholecystography (Figs 24.29–24.32):

1. A fundal nodular filling defect
2. Strictures which occur at any site within the gallbladder and which become accentuated after gallbladder contraction
3. Epithelial sinuses, which may only become apparent following contraction with contrast within small mural diverticula.

Xanthogranulomatous cholecystitis This condition is characterised histologically by a destructive inflammatory process with varying proportions of fibrous tissue, inflammatory cells and lipid-laden macrophages. The presence of gallstones is variable. Its locally invasive nature may result in biliary structuring at intra- or extrahepatic level, masquerading as a neoplastic process.

Gallbladder carcinoma Adenocarcinoma of the gallbladder is associated with stones in over 90% of patients. There is a female to male ratio of 3:1. Porcelain gallbladder and sclerosing cholangitis are predisposing factors. Characteristically the tumours are scirrhous and locally infiltrative, involving the intrahepatic biliary tree and common duct, with resulting obstruction and jaundice as a common presenting feature. Involvement of the hepatic artery and portal vein at the porta are the main reasons why curative surgery is often not possible and treatment is palliative.

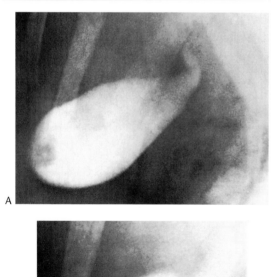

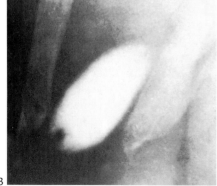

Fig. 24.30 (A,B) Fundal nodule of adenomyomatosis before and after gallbladder contraction. Note long cystic duct medial to common bile duct, a congenital anomaly.

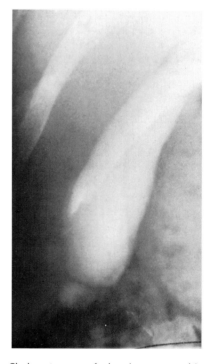

Fig. 24.31 Cholecystogram of phrygian cap resulting from partial septum across the fundus of an otherwise normal gallbladder. This is a normal variant.

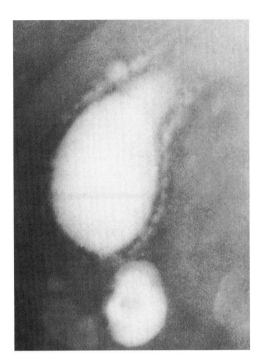

Fig. 24.32 Rokitansky–Aschoff sinuses shown on the after fatty meal film at cholecystography. Stricture is also present.

Ultrasound and CT may demonstrate a soft-tissue mass within and adjacent to the gallbladder, often with direct extension into the parenchyma of the related liver segments. Cholangiographic features are biliary stricturing, often with intrahepatic duct dilatation. These features are similar to those of a cholangiocarcinoma, which, although histologically different, often has the same clinical presentation and outcome. However, the differential diagnosis includes benign sequelae of a complicated cholecystitis with development of the Mirrizzi syndrome or xanthogranulomatous cholecystitis, which obviously carry differing therapeutic and prognostic implications, hence the need for a histological diagnosis by guided biopsy.

Gallbladder intervention

Many techniques of minimally invasive management of benign gallbladder disease have been superseded by the rapid development and acceptability of laparoscopic cholecystectomy. Many of the therapies designed to treat gallstones independent of cholecystectomy, namely extracorporeal shock-wave lithotripsy (ESWL), percutaneous cholecystolithotomy and percutaneous cholecystectomy with contact lithotripsy and dissolution with agents such as methyl-tertiary-butyl-ether (MTBE), have significantly high rates of recurrent gallstones, estimated at 10% each year, equivalent to 50% at 5 years. In addition, entry criteria for ESWL exclude 85% of patients with gallstones. Treatment with MTBE requires an average treatment time of 5 h/day for up to 3 days; residual debris >5 mm is present in the majority of patients, although this is silent in the short term. More than 90% of patients with gallbladder carcinoma have stones. Prospective studies have shown that the risk of developing a gallbladder carcinoma in patients with asymptomatic stones is less than 1%. All these data are regarded as compelling evidence for cholecystectomy as the best treatment for symptomatic gallstones.

Percutaneous cholecystotomy

This technique, in selective circumstances, has withstood the evidence displacing the aforementioned radiological techniques. It remains important because, although cholecystectomy is a successful operation with a mortality rate of 0.5–1.8%, both mortality and morbidity rise in parallel with increasing age, patients over 65 accounting for 70% of deaths. The mortality rate from emergency cholecystectomy (13.3%) is 10 times that of elective surgery (1.3%) in this age group and rises to 25% if an empyema of the gallbladder has developed. The surgical option in these circumstances is a two-stage procedure of open cholecystotomy and subsequent cholecystectomy.

Percutaneous cholecystotomy, with placement of a drainage tube into the gallbladder under imaging control, is now considered an alternative to the first stage, carrying a lower morbidity and equal technical success and patient outcome. In elderly patients with cardiovascular or respiratory disease that precludes general anaesthesia it may be the only alternative. Subsequent cholecystectomy may be deferred or avoided if the stone can be extracted along the tube track.

This technique can also be used to establish external biliary drainage, provided that the obstruction is distal to a patent cystic duct. This is often reserved for the intensive care situation where the patient cannot be moved to a screening unit and the procedure can be carried out solely under ultrasound control.

DISORDERS OF THE BILE DUCTS

Common bile duct and intrahepatic stones

The spectrum of presentation of common duct stones (choledocholithiasis) is wide, ranging from septicaemia resulting from untreated biliary obstruction and cholangitis to an incidental finding on ultrasound. Coexistent stones within the gallbladder are present in the majority of patients. It is estimated that 10% of patients will have common duct stones at the time of cholecystectomy. However, a number of predisposing factors are recognised in the development of common duct and intrahepatic stones, bile stasis and infection being common denominators (Fig. 24.33). These are:

1. Postcholecystectomy; about 5% of patients will have persistent symptoms following surgery, with choledocholithiasis or biliary dyskinesia requiring exclusion with direct cholangiography and functional studies such as excretion HIDA scans or a morphine stimulation test.
2. Choledochal anomalies, e.g. choledochal cysts, Caroli's disease.
3. Acquired disorders of the bile duct, e.g. sclerosing cholangitis, parasitic cholangiopathy.
4. Ampullary obstruction, e.g. periampullary diverticulum, common channel anomalies.
5. Hyperconcentration of bile and lack of enteral stimulation, e.g. total parenteral nutrition in infants.
6. Following surgery when stricturing of a surgical anastomosis or obstruction of a fashioned Roux loop develops.
7. Chronic liver disease and haemolytic disorders.
8. Pancreatic abnormalities; it has been well documented that common duct stones are significant in the development and morbidity of pancreatic inflammatory disease, but in addition

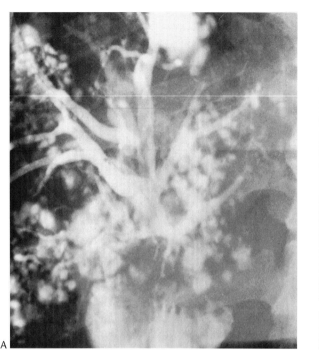

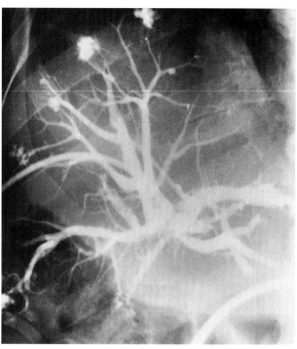

A

B

Fig. 24.33   Acute suppurative cholangitis. (A) Abscess cavities communicating with dilated ducts following stricture of choledochoenterostomy for malignant disease. (B) After 5 days external drainage via transhepatic tubes, most of the abscess cavities have healed and the ducts are less distended. Biliary sepsis rarely occurs in association with malignant obstruction unless there has been previous intervention.

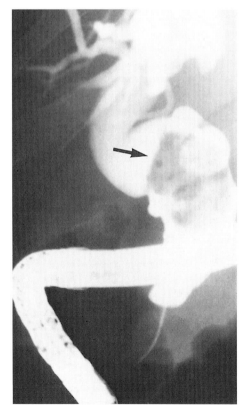

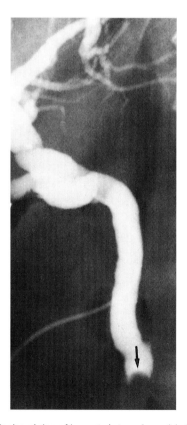

Fig. 24.34   Very large gallstone (arrow) in dilated bile duct shown at ERC.   **Fig. 24.35**   'Meniscus' sign of impacted stone (arrow) in bile duct.

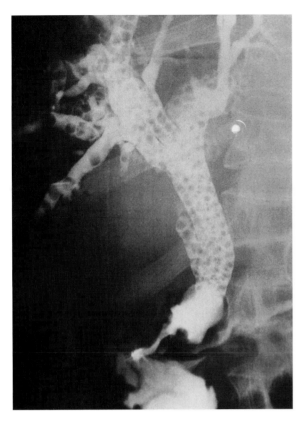

Fig. 24.36 Multiple calculi forming within the common duct following a distal bile duct trauma.

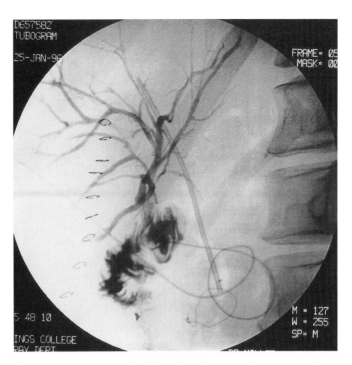

Fig. 24.37 Correction of a bile leak with surgical drainage via a Roux loop of a sectorial right duct transected at cholecystectomy. The stent demarcates the line of the common bile duct, into which the transected duct had an anomalous insertion which was not recognised at laparoscopic cholecystectomy.

anomalies of pancreatic duct development or acquired stricturing of the common bile duct result in biliary stasis and stone formation independent of the aetiology of the pancreatitis (Figs 24.34–24.36).

Benign biliary strictures

Postsurgical strictures

The variable anomalous anatomy and vascular supply of the bile duct contribute to postsurgical stricturing. This is often compounded by the difficulty of exposure of an undilated duct in the presence of inflammation or invasive tumour. Accurate preoperative radiology will help to reduce this potential sequel. Four main groups of operation carry the risk of stricture formation:

1. Cholecystectomy (open or laparoscopic). Bile duct injury, with transection or devascularisation of the bile duct, may result in a postoperative bile leak or stricture formation. The common hepatic duct at the cystic duct insertion is at highest risk. Failure to recognise the normal anatomy or anomalous duct insertions, and diathermy injury are factors which contribute to the morbidity of laparoscopic cholecystectomy, particularly if the surgeon is inexperienced (Figs 24.37, 24.38).

2. Biliary disconnection and drainage of the bile ducts. Roux loop anastomosis to the common hepatic duct or segment 3 duct and portoenterostomy (Kasai operation) carry a risk of anastomotic stricturing. This occurs particularly if the primary operation was carried out for a complex biliary injury (Figs 24.39, 24.52).

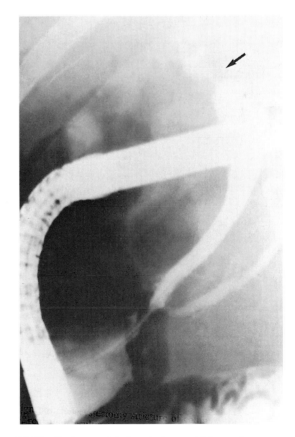

Fig. 24.38 Benign postcholecystectomy stricture of common duct (arrow). Typical site at level of ligation of cystic duct.

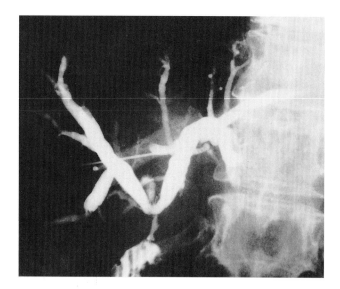

Fig. 24.39 Stricture of a hepaticojejunostomy.

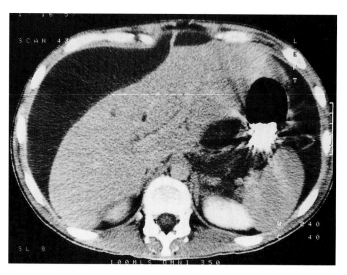

Fig. 24.41 Subcapsular bile leak following blunt liver trauma.

3. Hepatic resection. Although major resection leaving single liver segments is possible, these operations carry a risk of arterial devascularisation of the bile duct (Fig. 24.40).

4. Transplantation. An anastomotic stricture will occur in 5–14% of liver transplants, prompted by ischaemia, harvesting injury and surgical trauma. An increased incidence is seen in end-to-end anastomoses. Non-anastomotic strictures carry a significantly poorer prognosis because of the association of hepatic artery thrombosis in 50%.

Blunt or penetrating liver trauma

Injury to the bile duct or gallbladder occurs in approximately 5% of liver trauma cases with segmental or lobar devascularisation or transection leading to biliary leaks and stricture formation. Rarely, in the most serious liver injury there is avulsion of the portal vasculature and the bile duct. Such an injury carries an extremely high mortality and transplantation may be the only surgical option (Figs 24.41, 24.42).

Primary sclerosing cholangitis (PSC)

This is a disease of unknown aetiology, characterised by an inflammatory process affecting the intra- and extrahepatic ducts. The presentation and course is highly variable. Although the condition commonly presents in early childhood with features of cholestasis, it may begin in infancy or in old age. There is a wide range in the interval between presentation and death or transplantation, varying from 2 to 20 years. Biliary cirrhosis and hepatic failure ensue, with up to 20% of patients requiring transplantation.

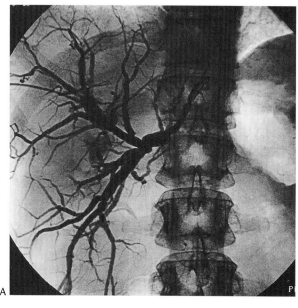

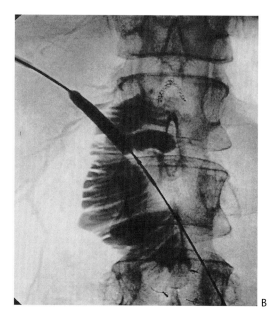

Fig. 24.40 Bile duct stricture developing following hepatic resection (A). Recurrent stricturing following biliary reconstruction which was successfully treated by balloon dilatation (B).

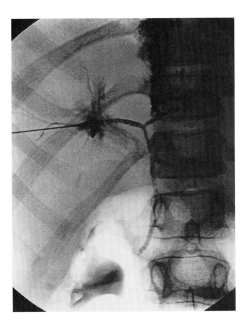

Fig. 24.42 Percutaneous cholangiography demonstrating a leak from the bile duct following blunt abdominal trauma.

Recognised associations are:

1. Inflammatory bowel disease (30%)
2. Retroperitoneal and mediastinal fibrosis
3. Riedl's thyroiditis
4. Orbital pseudotumour.

There is a predisposition to development of bile duct cancer. In the patient who develops decompensating disease, it becomes important to exclude the development of a cholangiocarcinoma. Transplantation in the presence of a cholangiocarcinoma carries a poor prognosis with a 1 year survival of less than 15%, compared with over 85% in those patients with PSC transplanted without tumour.

Cholangiography demonstrates multifocal stricturing of the bile ducts. Up to 86% of patients will have both intra- and extrahepatic involvement. Strictures of the extrahepatic bile duct may be long or short and multiple; if long (>5 mm) and associated with proximal dilatation and a short history of increasing jaundice, then stenting of these 'dominant' strictures may improve liver function. Outside these criteria, there is no evidence that dilatation or stenting alters the natural history of the disease. Equally, the 'severity' of intrahepatic cholangiopathy does not predict the severity of histological liver damage or act as a prognostic indicator. Severity of extrahepatic involvement may carry a worse prognosis but this varies between series (Fig. 24.43).

Ultrasound and CT may demonstrate segmental duct dilatation and there is increased periductal reflectivity on ultrasound, with regional lymphadenopathy recognised in up to 15% of cases. This may be associated with features of established cirrhosis and portal hypertension.

Cholangiopathy of acquired immune deficiency syndrome

Opportunistic infection of the bile duct, with cryptosporidium, cytomegalovirus or *Pneumocystis carinii*, results in an obliterative cholangiopathy with a picture similar to PSC. Abdominal pain and cholangitis are the predominant presentations and endoscopic sphincterotomy may result in symptomatic and biochemical improvement.

Chronic pancreatitis

Any cause of pancreatitis may result in a low bile duct stricture with biliary obstruction (Figs 24.44, 24.45). Associated factors are common duct stones or anomalaous anatomy of the pancreatic and bile ducts, e.g. pancreas divisum and the long common channel.

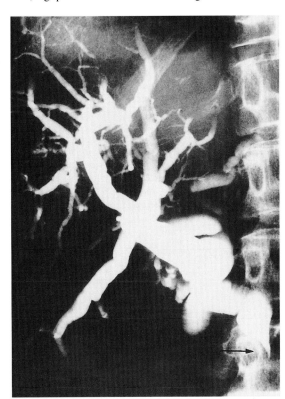

Fig. 24.44 Low common bile duct stricture, with characteristic features of extrinsic compression from a pancreatic mass (arrow).

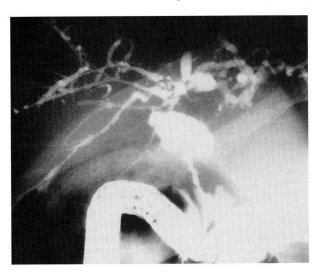

Fig. 24.43 Characteristic stricturing of sclerosing cholangitis involving the intra- and extrahepatic biliary system.

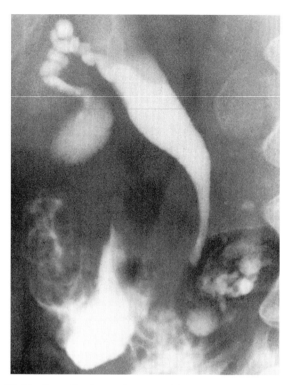

Fig. 24.45   'Rat-tail' stricture of common bile duct due to chronic pancreatitis. Note calcification in pancreatic head.

Parasitic infection

The common parasites which infest the biliary system are:

1. *Clonorchis sinensis* This is endemic in South-East Asia and enters the human host from undercooked and contaminated fish. Live worms within the biliary tree cause periductal fibrosis and stone formation. Although up to 75% of patients are asymptomatic, a minority develop recurrent cholangitis and biliary cirrhosis. Adenocarcinoma is a recognised development but the relative risk is unknown.

2. *Ascaris lumbricoides* Endemic in Asia, Africa and South America, this worm infests the small bowel; up to 10% of patients will have biliary infestation. Of these, 40% will have significant complications. Septic cholangitis with biliary abscess formation, cholecystitis with empyema formation and biliary stricture are the sequelae which carry the highest morbidity (Fig. 24.46).

3. *Echinococcus granulosus* Hydatid disease of the liver classically produces a complex intrahepatic cyst characterised by loculation and mural calcification, diagnosed by its CT and ultrasound features. Biliary manifestations of cholangitis and jaundice result from rupture of the cyst into a bile duct, causing occlusion by daughter cysts and hydatid sand. In such patients preoperative endoscopic cholangiography is essential, as when the cyst is opened surgically it is swabbed with a scolicide. These agents—formalin,

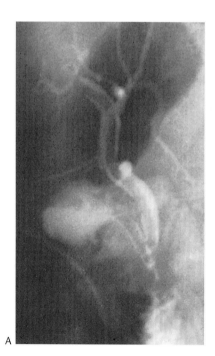

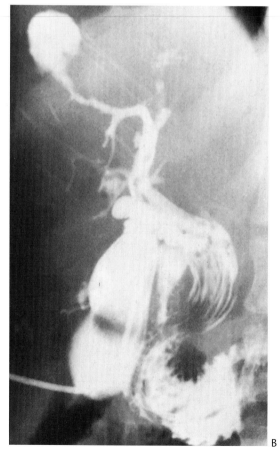

Fig. 24.46   *Ascaris lumbricoides.* (A) *Ascaris* worm in the biliary ducts. (B) Cholecystostomy tube study showing multiple worms extending from common bile duct into duodenum. Note associated abscess in right lobe of liver.

hypertonic saline and silver nitrate—are all potentially toxic to biliary epithelium, producing an obliterative cholangiopathy. Any biliary communication must therefore be identified and closed prior to their instillation.

4. *Entamoeba histolytica* Amoebiasis may produce liver abscesses which communicate with segmental bile ducts, producing cholangitis.

Choledochal varices

The choledochal veins of Petren and Saint form a lattice around the bile duct. In portal vein thrombosis with cavernous transformation these veins hypertrophy and may compress the bile duct, producing a smooth stricture (Fig. 24.47). Stones may then form above the stricture with development of jaundice. Regression occurs following operative portosystemic shunting with decompression of this variceal bed.

Tumours of the bile duct

Cholangiocarcinoma

First described by Klatskin, this tumour develops at a relatively young age, with one-third of patients presenting under the age of 50 years. There is a male preponderance. Sclerosing cholangitis and choledochal cysts have been recognised as predisposing diseases. It has also been described in association with inflammatory bowel disease in the absence of pre-existing cholangiopathy.

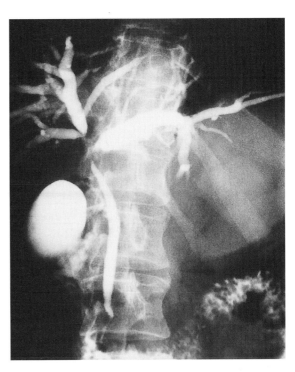

Fig. 24.48 Cholangiocarcinoma of the hilum with a characteristic stricture involving the confluence of the main left and right hepatic ducts.

Histologically the tumours are characterised by a marked scirrhous reaction, with clumps of carcinoma cells surrounded by fibrous tissue resulting in a malignant stricture (Fig. 24.48). The tumours

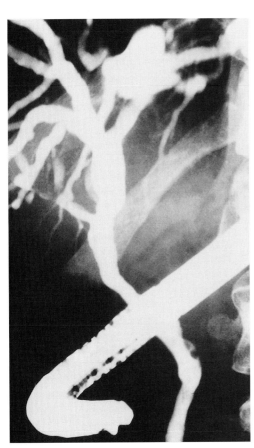

Fig. 24.47 Extrinsic compression along the line of the common duct from choledochal varices secondary to portal vein thrombosis.

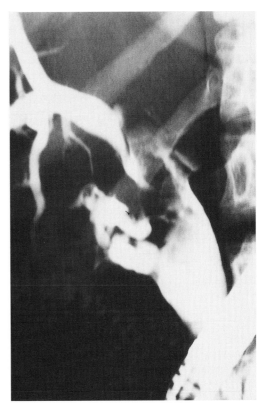

Fig. 24.49 Papilliferous tumour infiltrating and expanding the common bile duct.

are slow growing but are locally invasive with involvement of the hepatic artery and portal venous system. The tumour has to be distinguished from peripheral cholangiocarcinoma arising from peripheral bile ducts. These tumours are distinct in their clinical presentation and course, with the peripheral type only complicated by jaundice at a later stage, whereas, in hilar or extrahepatic tumours, biliary obstruction is an early manifestation. Rarely a papilliferous tumour may occur, expanding the bile duct (Fig. 24.49). Distant metastatic spread is not a major feature, occurring in only 12% of patients at presentation.

Despite the low biological activity of the tumour and accurate radiological assessment, the prognosis is poor, with a survival of only 2 months if untreated. Even with an aggressive surgical approach and staging by cholangiography, CT and indirect portography, resection is contraindicated in up to 68% of patients. Exclusion criteria include bilateral extension beyond the second-order intrahepatic ducts, and involvement of the main portal vein or hepatic artery by tumour. Further vascular exclusion criteria are involvement of both the left and right first-order portal venous divisions or involvement of the portal vein to one lobe and hepatic artery of the other. A further 10–12% of patients will either be unfit for radical surgery or the tumour will be irresectable at laparotomy when preoperative staging has underestimated the volume of disease. Thus the respectability rate falls to approximately 10%, and one-third of these will die from recurrent disease within 2 years.

Biliary decompression, either surgical, percutaneous or endoscopic, significantly improves survival. Adjunctive chemotherapy with internal and external irradiation may further improve survival.

Biliary cystadenoma and cystadenocarcinoma

These rare tumours of the biliary epithelium present as complex, often cystic masses within liver parenchyma which may infiltrate segmental bile ducts (Fig. 24.50). Histological categories include a better prognostic group containing ovarian stroma but there is no radiological criterion by which these may be distinguished.

Radiological assessment is based on determining respectability on the segmental distribution and vascular relationships rather than on cholangiographic criteria.

Ampullary and pancreatic carcinoma

These are the most common causes of a malignant bile duct stricture (Fig. 24.51). Pancreatic pathologies are covered elsewhere but, in summary, specific indications for radiological assessment are to:

1. Define the site and size of the tumour.
2. Confirm a tissue diagnosis by guided biopsy.
3. Determine operability by excluding: (i) local involvement of the coeliac trunk, superior mesenteric and splenic arteries and (ii) the portal venous system, particularly at the junction of the superiorior mesenteric and splenic veins; (iii) regional pathological lymphadenopathy; (iv) ascites; (v) distant metastatic spread to the lungs and mediastinum. All these are exclusion criteria for curative surgery.
4. Determine suitability for palliative biliary drainage, either percutaneous, endoscopic or surgical.

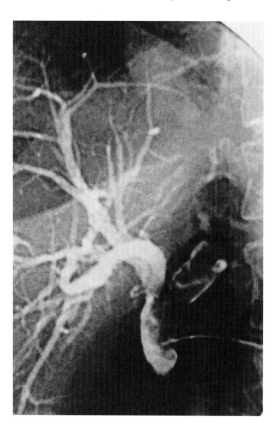

Fig. 24.50 Direct cholangiography defining the intraductal extension of a biliary cystadenoma of the left liver.

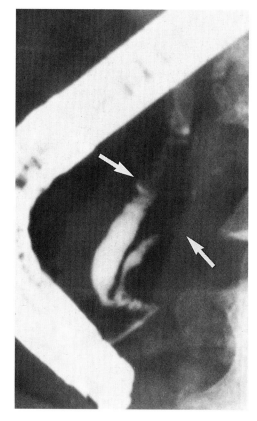

Fig. 24.51 'Double duct' sign. Concomitant strictures of pancreatic duct and bile duct (arrows) diagnostic of carcinoma of head of pancreas.

Bile duct intervention

Endoscopic techniques

Endoscopic management of benign and malignant disease of the bile duct is now widely practised, particularly in the investigation of jaundice. In a series of over 2500 patients choledocholithiasis (55%) and malignant bile duct strictures (26%) were the most common indications for intervention. Endoscopic sphincterotomy using a diathermy sphincterotome was the first interventional technique, and now has well-defined indications:

1. Common duct stones with or without gallbladder stones
2. Common duct stones following cholecystectomy with or without a T-tube in place
3. Ampullary carcinoma
4. Malignant bile duct strictures prior to stent insertion
5. Benign papillary stenosis
6. Postsurgical strictures before dilatation or stent placement
7. Choledochal fistula
8. Choledochocele (type III choledochal cyst).

Stone extraction Stone extraction with a Dormia basket may follow sphincterotomy. Used in conjunction with contact lithotripsy and stone crushers, over 95% of common duct stones may be successfully removed.

Cholangioscopy Tumours of the bile duct may be directly inspected following coaxial introduction of a fine-gauge endoscope into the bile duct percutaneously or endoscopically. This may facilitate guided biopsy or assessment of intraductal lesions, differentiating stones from tumour. Although various types of cholangioscope have been available since 1981, their role and impact on biliary disease remain limited.

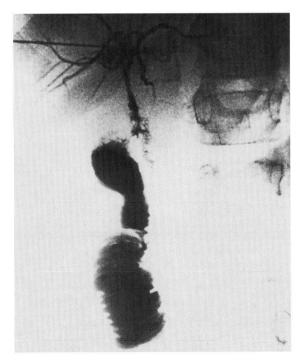

Fig. 24.52 Percutaneous cholangiography demonstrating obstruction of the Roux loop following hepaticojejunostomy.

Percutaneous techniques Biopsy This is now well established in hepatobiliary disease, with a high diagnostic yield (up to 90% in malignant disease) and low morbidity (<4%). Under CT or ultrasound guidance lesions of under 1 cm can be targeted. Histological as opposed to cytological specimens allow characterisation of malignant tumours but cytological assessment may suffice in confirming malignancy. For instance, fine-needle aspiration may be diagnostic in 50% of hilar cholangiocarcinomas. Coagulopathy remains a relative contraindication but often the benefit of obtaining a tissue diagnosis outweighs the risk. With careful technique and image guidance and with administration of corrective clotting factors, complications can be kept to a minimum.

Percutaneous stone extraction T-tube track Residual gallstones in the main bile duct occur in up to 4% of patients. These may be extracted along a mature T-tube track, which generally forms at least 4–5 weeks following surgery. Using a steerable catheter and Dormia basket, up to 90% of stones can be cleared, either using the track or advancing the fragments through the papilla following stone crushing. A morbidity of 4% is reported from cholangitis, pancreatitis and perforation of the sinus track with development of biliary peritonitis. Endoscopic extraction is a favourable alternative.

Access loop Similar instrumentation can be used for clearance and irrigation of the bile ducts following hepaticojejunostomy if an access loop has been fashioned at the original biliary disconnection. In this operation the afferent segment of the Roux loop is sutured on to the posterior surface of the anterolateral abdominal wall and tagged with a metal marker. Under fluoroscopic guidance the segment can be identified and entered using a Seldinger technique, facilitating catheter entry into the bile ducts for stone extraction, stricture dilatation or stent placement (Fig. 24.52).

Biliary dilatation Radiologically guided balloon dilatation of benign strictures provides an alternative to surgical intervention. All types of benign strictures—anastomotic, post-traumatic and sclerosing cholangitis—are theoretically amenable to balloon dilatation once the bile ducts have been entered either percutaneously, endoscopically or via an access loop. The best results are seen in patients with a dominant single anastomotic stricture. Conversely there is no evidence that the natural history of PSC is altered by dilatation.

There is little consensus as to the appropriate number of dilatations, length of inflations, balloon inflation pressures or the best predictor of success. However, in a multicentre review, there was no discernible difference between different methodologies of technique. Obliterating the waisting effect with a high-pressure balloon would seem to be an early predictor of success but how this relates to long-term outcome is unknown.

The complication rate is related to the morbidity of establishing biliary drainage rather than the dilatation itself, sepsis and haemorrhage being the most significant complications.

Biliary drainage and stenting Establishing internal biliary drainage to relieve jaundice is achievable in over 90% of patients with malignant biliary obstruction and this forms the main indication for endoscopic or percutaneous stenting (Figs 24.53, 24.54).

Tumours suitable for stenting include:

1. Pancreatic carcinoma
2. Cholangiocarcinoma

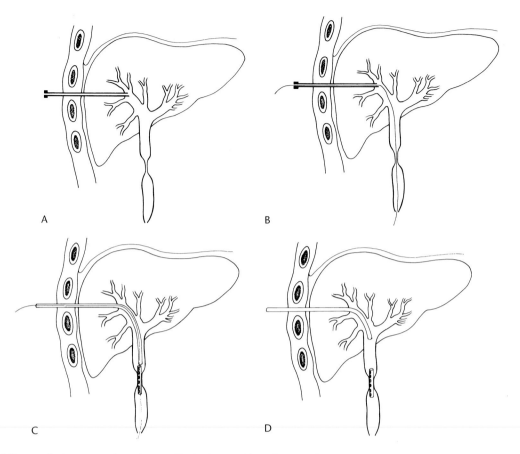

Fig. 24.53 (A) A fine-needle duct system is used to opacify the ducts and introduce a catheter. (B) An appropriate guide-wire is manipulated through the stricture. (C) A sheath introduction system is then placed into the ducts to allow delivery of the plastic or metallic stent. (D) The sheath is removed and external drainage may be used for the first 24 h if necessary. This will allow subsequent cholangiography to confirm optimum stent deployment and internal drainage.

3. Metastatic disease to the liver and portal nodes with biliary obstruction
4. Hepatocellular carcinoma with intraductal invasion or compression.

Specific indications for benign bile duct disorders include:

1. As a prelude to definitive surgery in iatrogenic transection of the bile duct with biliary leak
2. Early structuring or anastomotic leak following liver transplantation
3. Failed stone extraction or a large impacting stone associated with biliary obstruction
4. Benign strictures such as Mirrizzi syndrome in patients unfit for surgical exploration
5. Recurrent anastomotic stricturing following surgery where refashioning would be technically difficult; for instance in the presence of portal hypertension
6. Dominant extrahepatic stricture in patients with sclerosing cholangitis presenting with a short history of progressive jaundice.

Types of stent There has been considerable debate about the 'ideal' stent. Any discussion of the material characteristics must evaluate three major properties. First, biocompatibility with surrounding tissue and bile. Second, stability in maintaining the original surface property. This is the major factor in stent failure and occlusion, affecting both plastic and metallic stents. Finally, handling properties of length, gauge, surface friction and elasticity which ensure ease of deployment. This has led to two major debates: whether to use metallic or plastic stents, and whether endoscopic or percutaneous placement is the optimum. With regard to the latter, both techniques in experienced hands carry approximately the same success rate (89–95%), the same morbidity (10–15%) and an equivalent mortality (5–8%). Choice of technique should be guided by the local expertise within the biliary team of radiologist, endoscopist and surgeon.

Plastic stents are usually made of Teflon; a variety of methods of deployment are used.

Metallic stents can be divided into self-expanding and balloon-expandable designs. Self-expanding stents are held in a constrained position in the delivery system and expand to their preset diameter on deployment (Wallstent & Gianturco—Rosch Z stent). Balloon-expandable stents are dilated to their final size with balloon catheters at the time of deployment (Palmaz stent).

Metallic endoprostheses were developed because studies had shown that plastic stents were prone to occlusion and migration in 6–23% of cases. Recent studies have shown a lower occlusion rate with metallic stents of 7–15%. However, the potential advantages and disadvantages should be assessed in each individual patient.

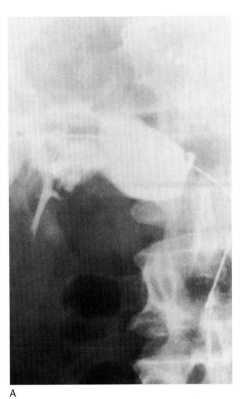
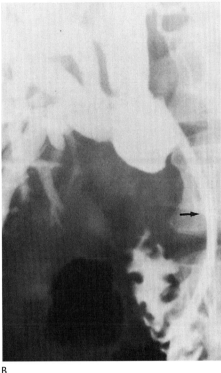
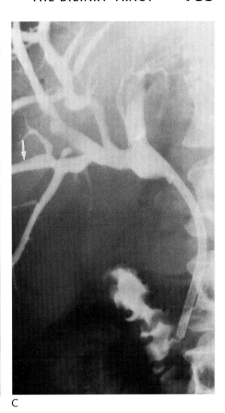

A B C

Fig. 24.54 Transhepatic endoprosthesis. (A) A guide-wire has been manipulated through the completely obstructing lesion of the common hepatic duct. (B) An endoprosthesis (arrow) has been positioned through the stricture. (C) Two days later, cholangiography through the external drain (arrow) shows that the prosthesis is functioning (contrast in duodenum) and that the intrahepatic ducts have been decompressed. The external drain is now removed.

Advantages of metallic stents

1. They can be introduced through small introduction systems, reducing morbidity and increasing patient acceptance.

2. They have a large internal diameter of 10–12 mm compared with a functional lumen of 4–5 mm for plastic stents and result in higher long-term patency rates.

3. They have a low mass and surface area. Experimental studies have shown that bacterial colonisation of the stent surface and subsequent fibrous deposition and occlusion is directly proportional to the surface area of the stent.

Disadvantages of metallic stents

1. They become incorporated into the bile duct mucosa and cannot be easily removed, even at open surgery. Placement in benign disease therefore requires careful consideration of the natural history of the disease and potential future surgical options. If the stent is infected, there will be continuing cholangitis even if drainage can be re-established by balloon recanalisation or further stent placement.

2. Shortening of up to 40% may occur following deployment, therefore multiple stents may be required in long-segment obstructions to ensure coverage of the length of the stricture.

3. The cost of a metallic stent is up to 10 times that of a plastic stent. The need for multiple stents and dilatation with a balloon catheter postdeployment further enhances this differential cost. It should be remembered that the vast majority of patients requiring stenting are elderly and have inoperable pancreatic carcinomas. The majority will succumb from a non-biliary cause with continued

patency of a plastic stent effectively decompressing their biliary tree.

Angiographic intervention

The main indication for angiographic intervention is embolisation in the presence of haemobilia. Jaundice and gastrointestinal bleeding with melaena are the presenting features.

Recognised causes are:

1. Iatrogenic trauma, either surgical or following percutaneous liver biopsy
2. Blunt or penetrating liver trauma
3. Liver tumours; malignant tumours of either hepatocellular or cholangiocellular origin are recognised causes.
4. Vascular malformations
5. Multiorgan failure with disseminated intravascular coagulation.

Ultrasound shows characteristic features of reflective material within a dilated gallbladder and bile duct. Endoscopic cholangiography may not only demonstrate clot within the bile duct but active bleeding may be visible at the papilla. Angiography or cholangiography defines any arteriobiliary communication and embolisation is curative in the majority of cases.

REFERENCES AND SUGGESTIONS FOR FURTHER READING

Anatomy
Couinaud, C. (1957) *Le Foie. Etudes Anatomiques et Chirurgicales.* Paris: Masson.

Healey, J., Schroy, P. (1953) Anatomy of the biliary ducts within the human liver. Analysis of the prevailing pattern of branchings and the major variations of the biliary ducts. *American Medical Association Archives of Surgery*, **66**, 599–616.

Smadja, C., Blumgart, L. (1944) *The Biliary Tract and the Anatomy of Exposure. Surgery of the Liver and Biliary Tract*. Edinburgh: Churchill Livingstone.

Methods of investigation and intervention

Burhenne, H. J. (1990) Interventional radiology of the biliary tract. *Radiologic Clinics of North America*. Philadelphia: W. B. Saunders.

Cosgrove, D., Meire, H., Dewbury, K. (1993) *Clinical Ultrasound—A Comprehensive Text*, Vol. 1. Abdominal and General Ultrasound. Edinburgh: Churchill Livingstone.

Haaga, J., Lanzieri, C. (1994) Computed tomography and magnetic resonance imaging of the whole body. St Louis: Mosby-Year Book.

Mitchell, D., Stark, D. (1992) *Hepatobiliary MRI*. St Louis: Mosby-Year Book.

Mujahed, Z., Evans, J., Whalen, J. (1974) The non-opacified gall bladder on cholecystography. *Radiology*, **112**, 1–4.

Biliary strictures and tumours

Blumgart, L. (1994) *Surgery of the Liver and Biliary Tract*. Edinburgh: Churchill Livingstone.

Farrant, M., Hayllar, K., Wilkinson, M., Karani, J. (1991) Natural history and prognostic variables in primary sclerosing cholangitis. *Gastroenterology*, **100**, 1710–1717.

Paediatric biliary disorders

Howard, E. R. (1991) *Surgery of Liver Disease in Children*. London: Butterworth-Heinemann.

Liver transplantation

Kane, P., Karani, J. (1995) The radiology of liver transplantation. *Imaging*, **7**, 195–203.

Williams, R., Portmann, B., Tan, K. C. (1995) *The Practice of Liver Transplantation*. Edinburgh: Churchill Livingstone.

25

THE LIVER AND SPLEEN

Robert Dick and Anthony Watkinson
with contributions from Richard W. Whitehouse, Philip J. Robinson and Julie F. C. Olliff

THE LIVER

Liver imaging fulfils four purposes. First, it assesses the causes of hepatomegaly or of a localised liver mass. Second, it diagnoses a suspected neoplasm, either primary or metastatic. Third, it confirms or excludes hepatic inflammatory or parasitic disease. Finally, it aids planning of therapy—medical, interventional radiological, or surgical.

Imaging techniques

Many different techniques are available for imaging the liver. They include the long-established traditional simple X-rays, the second generation tools of arteriography, radionuclide scanning and ultrasound and, since the 1970s, computed tomography (CT) and magnetic resonance imaging (MRI). Fast scanning spiral (helical) CT, recently introduced, is a superb investigative technique for all liver pathologies. Angiography, once widely used in diagnosis, is now more applicable (as digital subtraction angiography or DSA) to interventional techniques and therapy. MRI also provides multidisplay information in a great range of liver diseases, and may make a successful diagnosis when other modalities fail. It provides details of vessels and bile ducts with ever-increasing resolution, MR angiography (MRA) being particularly helpful to a surgeon contemplating liver resection.

Hepatomegaly is a common clinical finding with numerous and varied causes (Box 25.1).

Abdominal X-ray

Being the bulkiest body organ, the liver casts an appreciable shadow on a radiograph, although modified by individual variations of shape and orientation. Its outline is deduced from contrast differences between the right lobe and adjacent tissues, namely the right lung and hemidiaphragm above, the properitoneal fat line along its lateral border, and the right kidney and extraperitoneal fat below the sloping posterior border. The anterior edge of liver, the surface palpated clinically, is not directly seen on a plain film, although gas in the hepatic flexure of colon may indicate its position.

Box 25.1   Causes of generalised liver enlargement

Vascular
Congestive heart failure
Congestive pericarditis
Budd–Chiari syndrome

Cirrhosis
Hypertrophic nodular
Congenital cystic disease with hepatic fibrosis

Infiltrative
Fatty infiltration
Reticulosis
Storage disease (histiocytosis, amyloid)

Biliary
Obstructive jaundice

Blood disorders
Myelofibrosis
Thalassaemia

Infection and infestation
Portal pyaemia
Pyogenic and amoebic abscess
Hydatid disease, actinomycosis
Hepatitis, infectious mononucleosis
AIDS

Neoplasm
Adenoma
Hepatoma, fibrolamellar carcinoma
Cholangiocarcinoma
Metastases

The left lobe of the liver is less easily seen radiographically due to its smaller size and central position over the spine. However, it may be indirectly outlined by air in the stomach (Fig. 25.1). Reidel's lobe is an inferior tongue-like extension from the lateral margin of the right lobe of liver, and is found more often in women (Fig. 25.2).

Plain radiographs to assess hepatomegaly should ideally include the diaphragm and the pubic symphysis on the same film. Gross enlargement is usually obvious (Fig. 25.3). Nevertheless, clinical and radiological assessment of liver size may not tally. Early enlargement may be palpable, yet a supine radiograph appear normal. Should the liver enlarge in a purely upwards direction then it may be clinically impalpable, yet sequential chest films may demonstrate changes in either the height or contour of the diaphragm (Fig. 25.4). On the other hand, an enlarging left lobe may usually be palpated anteriorly, even though not yet apparent on film, while a large caudate lobe, which occurs in many cirrhoses and in the Budd–Chiari syndrome, can be suspected from anterior displacement of gas or barium in the duodenal cap.

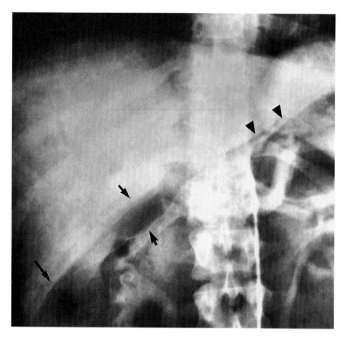

Fig. 25.1 Liver of normal size and shape. Hepatogram following coeliac angiogram. Lower right lobe related to hepatic flexure (single arrow). Caudate lobe to duodenum (facing arrows), left lobe to gastric fundus (arrowheads).

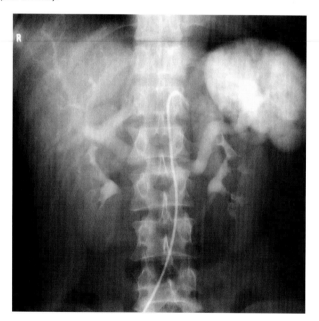

Fig. 25.2 Indirect portal venogram. Note large Reidel's lobe (segment VI) projecting downwards on right.

Radiological signs of liver enlargement are;

1. *Right lobe*
   a. elevated right hemidiaphragm
   b. depressed hepatic flexure and duodenum
   c. depressed right kidney (occasionally it remains high)
   d. bulging of the right properitoneal fat line
   e. occasionally, splaying of the lower right ribs.
2. *Left lobe*
   a. gastric fundus displaced downwards and laterally

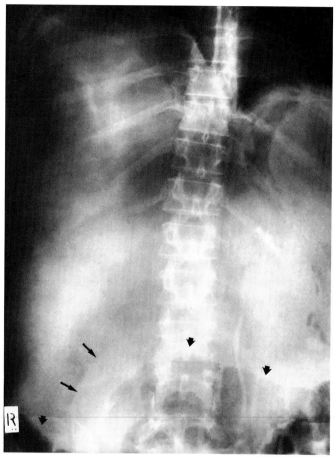

Fig. 25.3 Multiple large-bowel metastases causing gross hepatomegaly. Elevated right hemidiaphragm, depressed right kidney (thin arrows) and transverse colon (thick arrows).

   b. intra-abdominal oesophagus elongated
   c. extrinsic pressure on lesser curvature of stomach
   d. sometimes, posterior stomach displacement on lateral film.

Other imaging modalities, such as ultrasound, radionuclide scanning, CT or angiography, will readily reveal enlargement of one or both lobes and may characterise the pathology in some (Figs 25.5, 25.6). Only CT and MRI can fully assess the contours of the liver surface (Fig. 25.7).

Before hepatomegaly is diagnosed clinically or radiologically, it is essential to check on the position of the diaphragm. If low, as in patients with obstructive airways disease or an asthenic body habitus, the liver may be readily palpable. Similarly, spinal abnormalities such as severe kyphoscoliosis may cause pseudohepatomegaly.

Localised masses

In the liver such masses are detectable on plain X-ray if they lie adjacent to, or deform, one of the visible borders, or cause a change in an adjacent structure such as the diaphragm (Fig. 25.8). Masses invisible on simple X-ray may be readily shown by ultrasound, radionuclide scanning or CT.

Subphrenic abscess

The affected hemidiaphragm will show diminished excursion during fluoroscopy, and later it will be become raised or immobile,

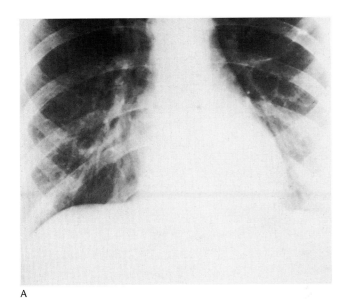

A

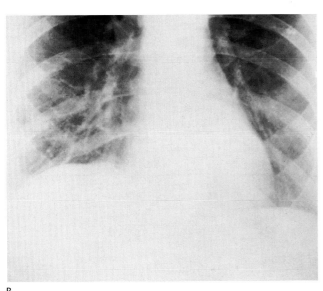

B

Fig. 25.4 (A) Patient with carcinoma of the stomach. Right hemidiaphragm normal preoperatively. (B) The same patient 3 months later. Elevation of right hemidiaphragm with slight humping medially is a highly significant abnormality. Liver biopsy: metastatic adenocarcinoma.

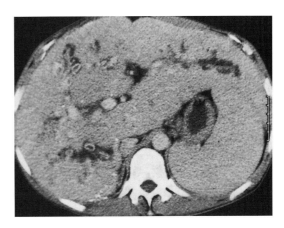

Fig. 25.5 Contrast enhanced CT. Hepatosplenomegaly. Dilated bile ducts containing many stones. Congenital hepatic fibrosis with secondary portal hypertension.

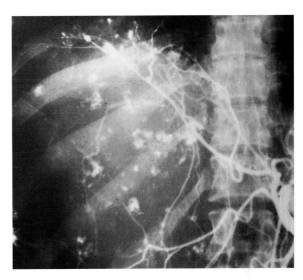

Fig. 25.6 Selective hepatic arteriogram. Multiple small, dense, well-defined stains arise from normal-sized hepatic arteries, and persist over 26 s. Haemangiomas.

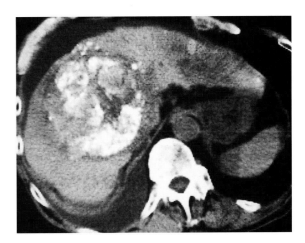

Fig. 25.7 Unenhanced CT. Irregular anterior liver border indicates cirrhosis. Overall increased density is due to haemochromatosis. Intra-arterial Lipiodol has been taken up by hepatomas. Note ascites.

or show paradoxical movement with sniffing. The important differential diagnosis is postoperative gas, which may persist under the diaphragm for 10 days after a laparotomy or laparoscopy. Hence the value of repeated screening, since any increase in gas, or the formation of a fluid level, indicates a subphrenic abscess. A sympathetic pleural effusion is common, and results from irritation of the parietal pleura by the inflammatory process. On the left the abscess lies between the gastric fundus, spleen and diaphragm (Fig. 25.9). Postoperative pulmonary collapse with effusion and pulmonary infarction may mimic the diaphragmatic signs of subphrenic abscess. Collapse usually occurs in the early postoperative period and infarction in the first week, when it may be accompanied by haemoptysis.

Ultrasound is the most cost-effective investigation for subphrenic, hepatic and subhepatic abscesses, and may be performed at

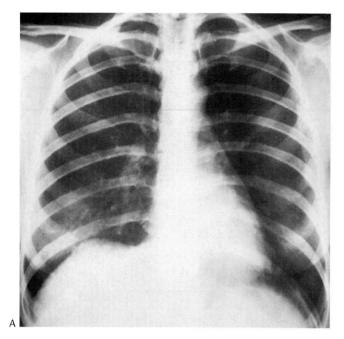

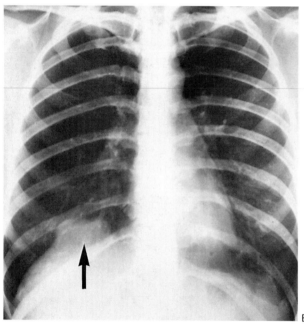

Fig. 25.8 (A) Chest film of 28-year-old woman with fever, reported as normal. (B) Repeat film after 1 week shows marked localised hump of diaphragm (arrow). Aspiration: amoebic abscess. The shape of the abnormal diaphragm contour does not help in distinguishing an inflammatory from a neoplastic cause. However, a change over days favours an abscess, and over months a slower-growing lesion such as a hepatic cyst or tumour.

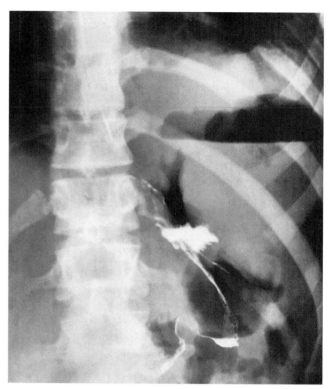

Fig. 25.9 Left subphrenic abscess 12 days after perforated gastric ulcer. Barium has shown the stomach to be compressed and displaced medially by the abscess, with fluid level. High hemidiaphragm with fluid above.

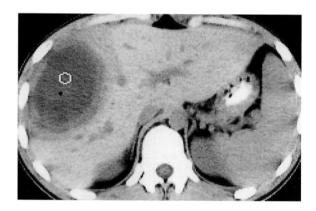

Fig. 25.10 CT in patient with high fever after a foreign holiday. The semiliquid mass in the right lobe of the liver has concentric walls (compressed liver tissue) and a central speck of gas. An abscess can be diagnosed with certainty (aspirate: amoebae).

the patient's bedside. Radionuclide scanning and CT may also prove useful (Fig. 25.10).

Calcification

Whether it is localised or diffuse, calcification can often be detected on plain radiographs. Its pattern may characterise the pathology (Fig. 25.11). Most but not all echinococcal (hydatid) cysts calcify in part, the appearance resembling a crumpled eggshell. In a live growing cyst, the ectocyst itself may be faintly radiopaque. Even dense compact calcification does not exclude live scolices in the cyst centre.

Primary hepatocellular carcinoma (HCC or hepatoma) may rarely exhibit either faint stippled calcification (Fig. 25.12) or very rarely 'sunburst' type. *Mucus-secreting adenocarcinoma* deposits from large bowel may contain multiple areas of faint fluffy calcification, as may *calcitonin-secreting metastases* from medullary carcinoma of thyroid (Fig. 25.13). Sometimes the nature of the tissue *adjacent* to the calcium gives a clue to the pathology, and to assess this, plain X-ray may be complemented by CT (Fig. 25.14).

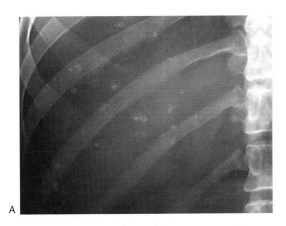

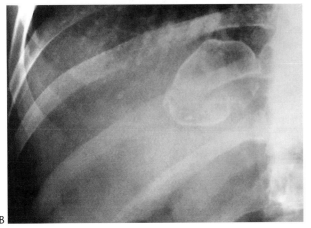

Fig. 25.11 (A) Multiple hepatic calcifications are typical of phleboliths: haemangiomas. (B) Typical egg-shell calcification: echinococcal cyst.

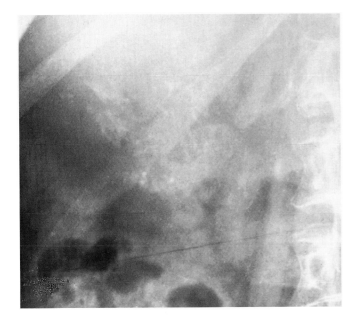

Fig. 25.12 Faint amorphous calcification within liver. Biopsy: primary liver cancer.

Generalised increased radiodensity of the liver

This occurs in haemochromatosis, or following previous Thorotrast or Lipiodol injection. It may not be readily seen on simple X-ray

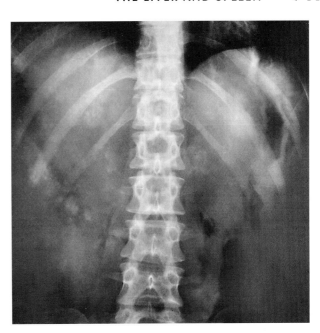

Fig. 25.13 Multiple areas of fluffy calcification in a patient with metastases from carcinoma of the thyroid. All the signs of hepatomegaly are present.

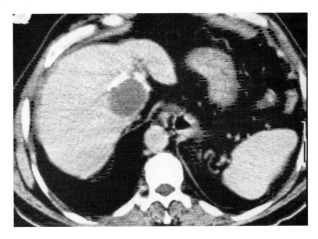

Fig. 25.14 CT scan of high right lobe of liver. A small rim of calcification lies adjacent to a cyst, suggesting that it is hydatid. Strongly positive hydatid serology.

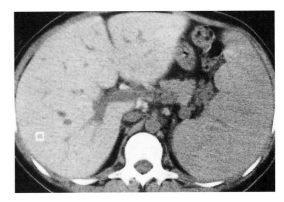

Fig. 25.15 Non-enhanced CT scan of liver in haemochromatosis. Portal vessels appear as strikingly low-density channels within the denser iron-loaded liver (liver density 90 HU). Splenomegaly.

but is reliably shown by MRI or CT, which also quantify liver iron with accuracy (Fig. 25.15). Selective hepatic arterial embolisation of primary or metastatic liver tumours using an emulsion of Lipiodol and cytotoxic drugs or radioactive isotopes is commonly employed and results in a striking increase in liver density at tumour sites; non-tumorous liver usually clears Lipiodol within 14 days (Fig. 25.7).

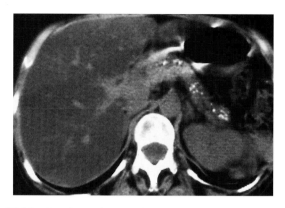

Fig. 25.18 Unenhanced CT in alcoholic. Low-density liver is due to excess fat, although segment 1 around the inferior vena cava is spared. Note calcific pancreatitis.

Increased transradiancy of the liver

This may be due to gas localised within an abscess (Fig. 25.10). It may occur in necrotic tumour after hepatic embolisation. If present in a vascular or ductal structure, gas is linear in distribution. Gas in the biliary tree generally accumulates in the common hepatic or major bile ducts (see Ch. 24). It is often seen after endoscopic sphincterotomy and surgical biliary-enteric bypasses. Gas in portal vessels is rare, but is clinically ominous, the gas exhibiting a branching pattern extending to the liver periphery (Fig. 25.16). A degree of hepatodiaphragmatic interposition of the colon is a not unusual finding (Fig. 25.17), although gross forms of Chilaiditi syndrome are most frequent in elderly patients. To the unwary this may resemble free gas under the diaphragm or a gas-forming right subphrenic abscess; fortunately, a haustral pattern of bowel can usually be discerned. Diagnosis of a *fatty liver* is only rarely suspected on plain radiographs, although the condition is strikingly obvious on ultrasound or CT (Fig. 25.18).

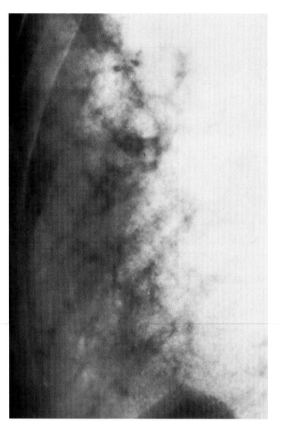

Fig. 25.16 Portal pyaemia following mesenteric artery infarction. Gas is present in peripheral branches of the portal vein.

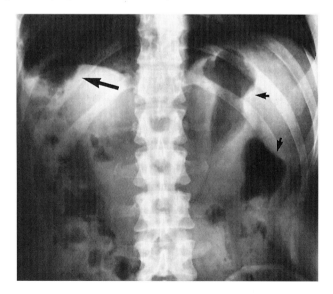

Fig. 25.17 46-year-old man. There is partial interposition of colon between the liver and the right hemidiaphragm (large arrow). Note normal spleen size and its relationships to stomach and colon (small arrows).

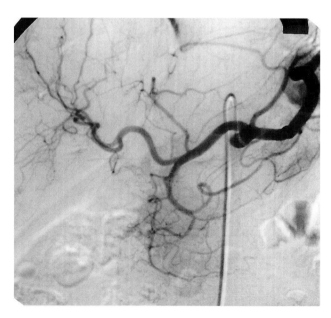

Fig. 25.19 DSA. Normal coeliac angiogram. The hepatic arteries are regular.

Angiography

Hepatic angiography was originally used mainly for the assessment and differential diagnosis of liver masses. Its diagnostic role has rightly diminished with the ascent of ultrasound, CT and MRI. Notwithstanding this, its use in interventional procedures such as embolisation and transhepatic portosystemic shunts (TIPS) has expanded greatly. Whether angiography is being undertaken as a diagnostic or therapeutic procedure, it is important to demonstrate fully both the arterial and venous (portal and hepatic) vascular supply to the liver. Arteriography requires selective catheterisation of the coeliac axis followed by the superior mesenteric artery, ensuring that the total hepatic arterial supply has been accounted for, as there are many variations in anatomy. Occasionally a free-flush aortogram will be necessary to search for additional arteries. DSA allows the procedure to be undertaken safely on a daycare

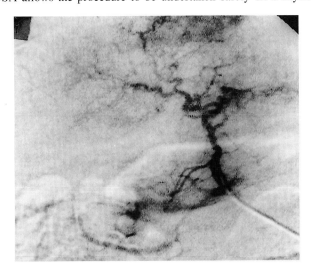

Fig. 25.20 DSA. Selective hepatic arteriogram in cirrhosis. Note corkscrewed arteries in a small liver.

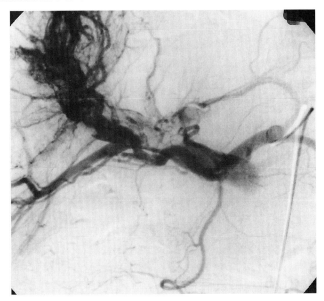

Fig. 25.21 Selective hepatic angiogram (DSA). Arteries feeding a vascular liver tumour communicate in this early frame with the portal vein, which fills retrogradely and contains tumour thrombus. This appearance is diagnostic of hepatocellular cancer (HCC).

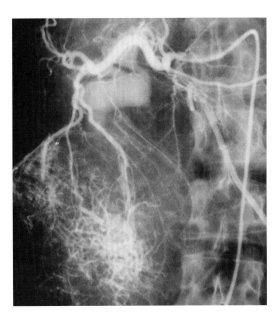

Fig. 25.22 Hepatic arteriogram performed because of palpable right lobe of liver. A large localised vascular tumour mass is seen in Reidel's lobe. Both liver adenoma and well-defined HCC (hepatoma) could have this appearance. A vascular metastasis does not usually have such large feeding arteries.

basis using 5F preshaped catheters, some of which are hydrophilic and able to take 0.038 inch guide-wires. In the adult, 35–30 ml of non-ionic contrast injected into each artery over a 7–10 s period, image acquisition continuing for 30 s to ensure a rich portogram when the contrast returns from either the spleen or bowel. Figure 25.19 shows the ordered division and distribution of hepatic arterial branches within the normal liver. Compare this with the irregular pattern in cirrhosis (Fig. 25.20), a tumour circulation with or without venous shunts (Figs 25.21, 25.22), the typical appearance of benign haemangiomas (Fig. 25.6) and the grossly abnormal angiogram in hereditary haemorrhagic telangiectasia (Fig. 25.23).

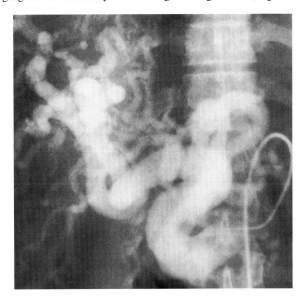

Fig. 25.23 Osler–Rendu–Weber syndrome (hereditary haemorrhagic telangiectasia). Selective hepatic arteriogram. Grossly dilated hepatic arteries, which shunted early to hepatic veins. No tumour circulation.

Pharmacoangiography (20 μg adrenaline (epinephrine) injected into the hepatic artery before contrast) has been used in the past to highlight poorly vascularised neoplasms by redirecting flow from vasoconstricted normal vessels, although the main requirement for any satisfactory angiogram is an adequate volume of contrast medium delivered by an appropriate rate selectively into the liver, coupled with high-quality digital radiography. Portal and hepatic phlebography are discussed below.

Interventional angiography

Procedures in the liver, as in other body regions, aim to deliver therapeutic alternatives to surgery, or sometimes provide an adjunct to it. *Embolisation* has been performed both for vascular lesions and for tumours. Embolisation of a bleeding site following liver biopsy, or of a traumatic blood–bile fistula or false aneurysm, is usually successful at a single session and prevents a major operation (Fig. 25.24). Advances in technology have resulted in easier access for

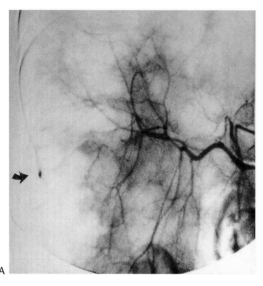
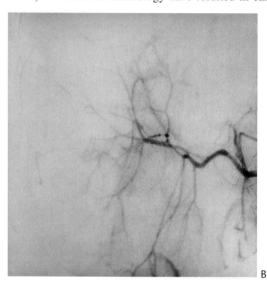

Fig. 25.24   DSA in a patient with multiple metastases who developed haemoperitoneum after liver biopsy. (A) Hepatic arteries stretched around avascular masses. A bead of contrast laterally (arrow)—bleeding site. (B) Bleed has ceased after selective embolisation with polyvinyl alcohol particles.

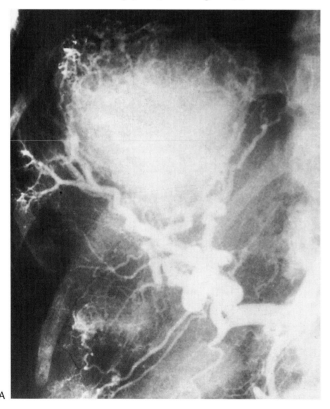
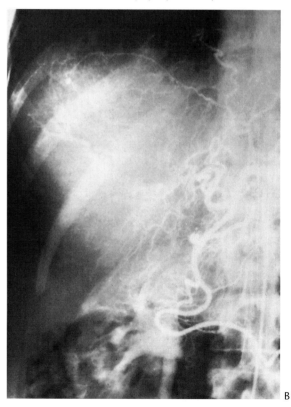

Fig. 25.25   (A) 45-year-old woman who had taken the contraceptive pill for 16 years. Vascular adenomas in the liver (biopsy proof). (B) Angiogram postembolisation with dextrose, Gelfoam and absolute alcohol. No tumour circulation. No further therapy. Asymptomatic 14 months later. This is an example of embolisation as an alternative to surgery.

guide-wires and catheters in the hepatic artery. Although a 'tracker' system introducing a fine wire or catheter through an outer 8F catheter is available (but expensive), success is usually achieved using a standard or hydrophilic 5F Simmonds or 'sidewinder' shaped catheter, which may be sufficiently pliable to enter the hepatic artery origin form the coeliac. A variety of floppy 'J' wires or hydrophilic (glide) wires will travel along the length of the hepatic artery and allow a curved catheter to straighten and advance well into the liver towards the desired site.

Embolisation with small metal coils or particulate matter such as polyvinyl alcohol (PVA) may be a definitive treatment for benign liver tumours (adenoma), or tumour-like conditions (focal nodular hyperplasia), both of which may follow use of the contraceptive pill or be seen in older patients on hormone replacement therapy (Fig. 25.25). For very vascular tumours preoperative embolisation may both devascularise and reduce tumour bulk (Fig. 25.26). Particulate embolic material should be mixed with contrast medium and be injected carefully during fluoroscopy, ensuring that no reflux

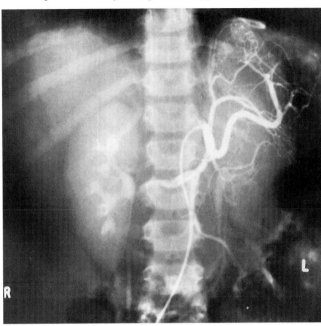

Fig. 25.26 (A) Boy aged 5 with a rapidly enlarging liver and highly vascular unusual 'tumour' in the left lobe of the liver. Embolised prior to surgery. (B) Postembolisation angiogram. Note wire coil in mouth of the left hepatic artery (right hepatic originated from superior mesenteric). This is an example of embolisation as an aid to surgery.

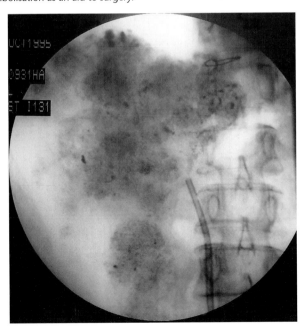

Fig. 25.27 DSA after Lipiodol has outlined multiple vascular malignant tumours. Radioactive Iodine-131 has been incorporated in the injection. Note the presence of a biliary stent.

occurs into the coeliac trunk, splenic artery or gastroduodenal artery. Applying pressure over the gastroduodenal artery with a lead-gloved hand is recommended by Japanese radiologists to prevent undesirable flow to the duodenum should the catheter position become precarious.

Embolisation in primary liver cancer can be used for reducing tumour size as well as for pain control. For the procedure to be successful, the patient must have a patent portal vein and no liver decompensation. An emulsion of Lipiodol, contrast agent and a chemotherapeutic agent such as deoxyrubicin or cisplatinum is injected into the right and left hepatic arteries to label hepatomas for later CT, and for therapy. Radioactive iodine is an alternative to the cytotoxic drug (Fig. 25.27). Patients usually tolerate this, and indeed all liver embolisations, very well, although a 24 h period of nausea, fever and abdominal pain is not uncommon.

As the great majority of hepatic metastases are avascular, angiography has a diminishing role. Delivery of chemotherapeutic drugs via arterial catheter is not clearly superior to systemic therapy. To detect the number and distribution of liver metastases, CT portography performed as a dynamic study during a slow (2 ml/s) injection of a large volume (120 ml) of contrast into the superior mesenteric artery will provide dramatic visualisation of tumours as a negative defect within the very dense portogram (Fig. 25.28). In some patients, increasingly aggressive surgery can improve survival rates

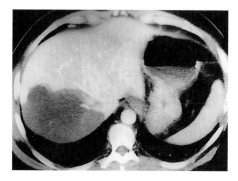

Fig. 25.28   CT portogram. The avascular filling defect high in the right lobe posteriorly abuts the inferior vena cava and compressed right hepatic veins, while the remainder of the (normal) liver enhances. Diagnosis: solitary large-bowel metastasis, predicted as suitable for resection.

to 40% at 5 years, even with extensive metastatic disease. If the left lobe residual (non-tumour) volume is less than 30%, embolisation of the right portal vein branch preoperatively will allow swift left lobe hypertrophy, followed by a subsequent extended right hemi-hepatectomy.

Perhaps the most generally agreed indication for liver tumour embolisation is the presence of neuroendocrine metastases such as *carcinoid*. Patients undoubtedly tolerate this well and obtain both pain relief from reduction in volume of the very large liver and loss of systemic symptoms following embolic blockage of hormone release. With multiple deposits, embolisation is best performed in stages (Fig. 25.29).

Biopsy

Obtaining tissue under image control is now a frequent interventional procedure. A common indication is the small liver 'missed'

on a ward biopsy (Fig. 25.42), although the more usual indication is accurate biopsy of a localised region of pathology (Fig. 25.30). Should even a small tumour have taken up Lipiodol, confidence in entering it should be high. In patients with coagulopathy, the biopsy track requires plugging with embolic material or wire coils. The technique of transjugular biopsy is discussed later.

THE SPLEEN

Images of the spleen may be obtained by simple X-rays, radionuclide scanning and CT. Non-invasive techniques such as ultrasound and MRI (including MR angiography) have a useful role. Since the diagnosis of significant splenic enlargement is confidently made by clinical examination, plain X-ray and more expensive imaging techniques are rarely used, although ultrasound is an inexpensive and

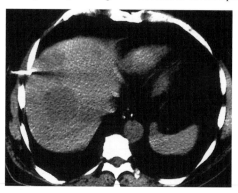

Fig. 25.30   Multiple liver metastases high right lobe. Biopsy site carefully selected, and tissue obtained from viable periphery of lesion: metastases from haemangiopericytoma.

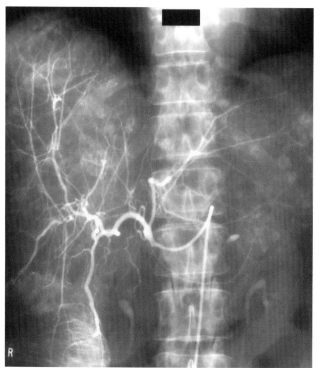

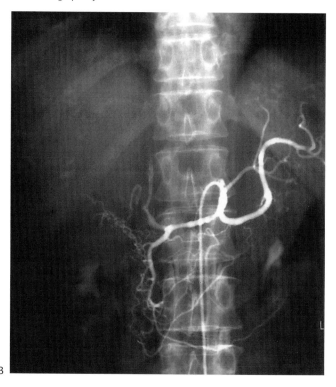

Fig. 25.29   (A) Hepatic arterial study. Both lobes are large and contain numerous vascular carcinoid tumour metastases. Patient highly symptomatic. (B) Study after embolisation with polyvinyl alcohol, dextrose and Gelfoam. Patient alive 10 years later.

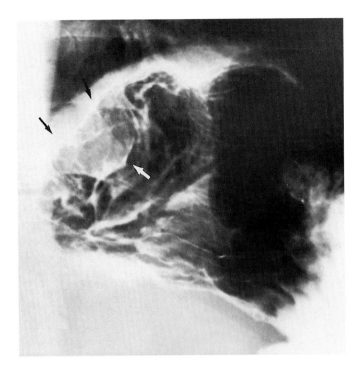

Fig. 25.31 Barium meal. Indentation on gastric mucosa (arrows) was due to a splenunculus.

accurate means of assessing splenomegaly in doubtful cases, and in assessing serial enlargement.

Simple X-ray

Although the spleen must be moderately enlarged in order to be clinically palpable, even a normal-sized organ is usually visible on good quality radiographs. A small spleen can also be detected, especially if calcified as a result of infarction, such as may occur in sickle-cell anaemia.

Good-quality abdominal films show the spleen to lie posteriorly in the cavity of the left ninth, tenth and eleventh ribs with the left hemidiaphragm above, the stomach medially and the colonic splenic flexure inferiorly (Fig. 25.17). On CT, it can always be identified and measured (Fig. 25.28). In adults, the long axis of the spleen should not exceed 11 cm, and over 15 cm is regarded as certain splenomegaly.

Accessory spleens are not uncommon, lying along the splenic artery, near the hilum, or in the omental ligaments around the spleen. Such 'splenunculi' occur in normal people and sometimes enlarge following splenectomy. Although rarely diagnosed on plain X-rays, an accessory spleen may appear as an extrinsic mass indenting the stomach (Fig. 25.31) and may have been previously misdiagnosed as a pancreatic or adrenal mass. Splenunculi can be readily identified by isotope scanning or CT and should not be mistaken for tumours such as a gastric leiomyoma or a large gastric varix.

Splenomegaly

The aetiology is broad ranging and is classified in Box 25.2. *Plain films* will sometimes provide a clue as to the cause of a large spleen. For example, small pigment stones in the gallbladder and abnormal bony trabeculation affecting all bones suggests thalassaemia; an overlying rib fracture may occur with traumatic splenic haematoma; a miliary lung pattern is seen with miliary tuberculosis; with

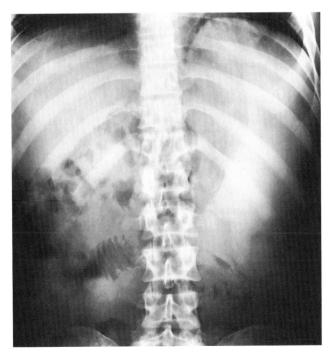

Fig. 25.32 Gross splenomegaly in the Banti syndrome. Note elevation of left hemidiaphragm.

myelosclerosis all of the bones may be dense and the liver prominent due to extramedullary haemopoiesis within it.

An enlarged spleen extends downwards, anteriorly and to the right. The stomach is displaced forward and medially and the left diaphragm may rise. Loss of the left psoas margin and depression of the left kidney are variable signs, the kidney perhaps staying high (Fig. 25.32). Although a depressed splenic flexure is a seminal sign of splenomegaly, the large spleen occasionally grows to lie

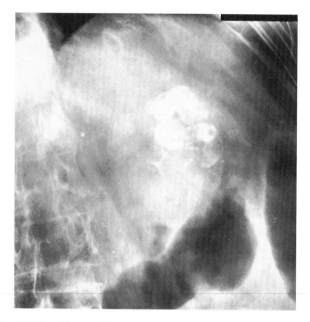

Fig. 25.33 89-year-old woman, plain X-ray of abdomen. Tortuous parallel-line calcification in splenic artery.

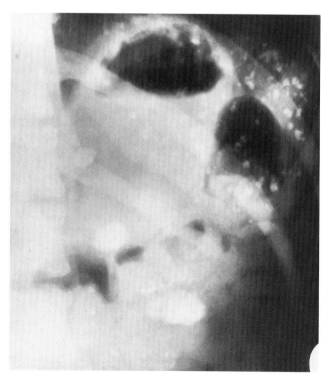

Fig. 25.34 31-year-old Arab man. Known previous tuberculosis affecting spleen and left kidney; both shows areas of calcification.

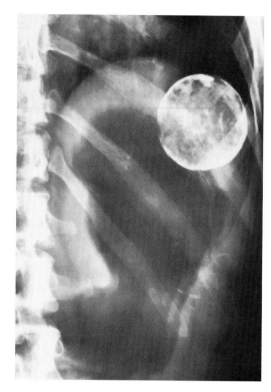

Fig. 25.35 39-year-old woman. Calcified non-parasitic cyst in spleen.

totally *below* the flexure. CT demonstrates fully the extent of splenomegaly (Fig. 25.15).

Calcification

Calcification in or adjacent to the spleen is common, especially after the age of 50. Calcific plaques in the splenic artery (or aneurysms of it) are frequent chance findings on abdominal X-rays (Fig. 25.33). Splenic vein calcification is uncommon but may follow portal pyaemia or splenectomy, while phleboliths, although rare, have the typical appearance of those seen in the pelvis. Granulomas such as tuberculosis produce single or multiple well-defined calcifications in the parenchyma (Fig. 25.34). Rarely, old splenic abscesses and haematomas calcify. Splenic cysts show typical curvilinear or oval calcification (Fig. 25.35). A completely infarcted spleen, such as occurs in sickle-cell anaemia, may occur late in the course of the disease, appearing as a small curved calcified structure below the left hemidiaphragm.

Thorotrast spleen

Although long obsolete and rarely seen now, it should not be mistaken for multiple calcifications. Thorium dioxide was widely used for angiography up to 1950; thus, some patients are still harbouring the medium, which was finally deposited in the spleen and other organs of the reticuloendothelial system such as coeliac lymph nodes and liver. In the spleen it is seen as multiple closely aggregated dense punctate opacities.

Gas transradiancy

This is seen within the spleen in splenic abscess. Although very rare, it is important to diagnose, as the patient is gravely ill. The condition may follow embolisation of the splenic artery, and is usually associated with restricted left diaphragm movement and a

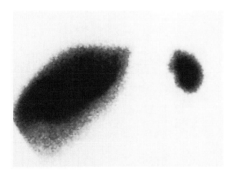

Fig. 25.36 ⁹⁹ᵐTc-colloid scan in patient with severe left hypochondrial pain. Small infarcting spleen.

left basal pleural effusion. It must not be confused with the mottled appearance of gas or faeces in the colonic splenic flexure. A fluid level in the erect radiograph may clinch the diagnosis. If no gas is present, an abscess may be suggested by isotope scanning, although the area of reduced uptake is non-specific. Ultrasound or CT may be definitive, and guide a needle aspiration to diagnose and treat the condition.

Splenic infarcts

Infarcts, such as occur in sickle-cell disease, can be shown as localised defects on radionuclide studies, as well as wedge-shaped defects on CT (Fig. 25.36).

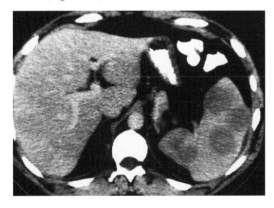

Fig. 25.37 CT. Multiple metastases in spleen from carcinoma of thyroid.

Splenic tumours and cysts

The latter are commonly pseudocysts following old haematoma or infarcts. Less comon cysts are epidermoid, presumably congenital, and usually presenting in children, or hydatids, which are seen in adults. All three types, but especially the last two, may show marginal calcification on simple X-rays. If they do not, as with most pseudocysts, ultrasound or CT will be required to confirm the diagnosis. Isotope scanning will show the cyst as a photopenic defect with sharp margins, but a similar defect is present with abscess and haematoma, and the clinical setting is all important. With state-of-the-art ultrasound or fast CT, solid or cystic neoplastic masses as small as 0.5–1 cm may be shown, allowing accurate and safe diagnostic aspiration with a needle (Fig. 25.37).

Splenic rupture

This may follow either a direct penetrating wound or closed abdominal trauma. Simple X-ray may show a mass in the left hypochondrium with indistinct margins to the spleen, left kidney or psoas. One or more lower left ribs may be fractured, although this is not invariable. Isotope scanning shows a defect due to the haematoma, as should ultrasound, but CT usually proves diagnostic as it is able to show increased density at the site of recent haemorrhage. Dynamic enhanced CT is important to show the extent of the tear and the remaining viable splenic tissue, which is much help to surgical management, as splenectomy is normally indicated if there is significant splenic haemorrhage (Fig. 25.38). CT is advantageous in showing damage to the other major organs, seen within continuous cuts through the abdomen, including liver, left kidney and aorta.

Following splenectomy for whatever cause, the radiologist must be aware of two common complications: early sepsis (particularly in children), and splenic or portal vein thrombosis (a late complication).

Asplenia, polysplenia

These rare congenital abnormalities have been described in association with congenital heart and gut lesions, in particular 'situs ambiguus'.

PORTAL HYPERTENSION

Liver cirrhosis is by far the commonest cause of portal hypertension. Ultrasound remains the simplest first-line test in detecting

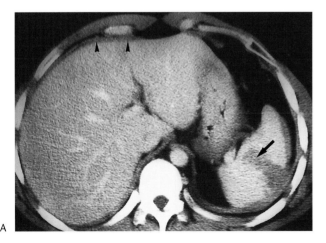

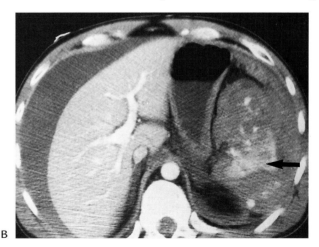

Fig. 25.38 (A) Enhanced CT. Triangular non-enhancing defect in spleen after trauma (arrow). Subcapsular hepatic fluid (arrowheads). (B) Another patient. Spleen pulped from major trauma. Enhanced CT. Arrow indicates only viable tissue. Note dense fluid in peritoneum (blood).

HAEMATEMESIS
↓
Endoscopy
↓
Varices   No varices
(= portal hypertension)

Varices (= portal hypertension):
↓
Visualise portal vein
(Doppler/CT)
↓
Measure portal pressure
(wedge hepatic phlebogram)
↓
Therapeutic endoscopy ⟶ STOP
(sclerotherapy, banding)
↓
Rebleed
↓
TIPS

No varices:
↓
Continued bleeding
↓
Arteriography
(+/– embolisation)
↓
STOP

Fig. 25.39 Investigation of bleeding in suspected portal hypertension.

diffuse liver disease. Radionuclide scanning, although a functional technique, is now used rarely. Many patients with bleeding oesophageal varices will require angiography. The type of imaging used in the management varies between the acute bleeder and the patient with intermittent bleeding, and is listed in a simple algorithm (Fig. 25.39).

Due to the risk of haemorrhage associated with coagulopathy in these patients, diagnostic venography is performed rarely by the direct trans-splenic or transhepatic routes, but more often indirectly, by arterioportography, where the portal venous system and oesophageal collaterals (varices) are visualised from the return of contrast after it is injected selectively into the splenic or superior mesenteric arteries (technique previously described).

The appearance of a normal splenic artery, spleen, splenic and portal veins is shown in Fig. 25.40. In portal hypertension the splenic artery dilates, and aneurysms may develop in its extra- or

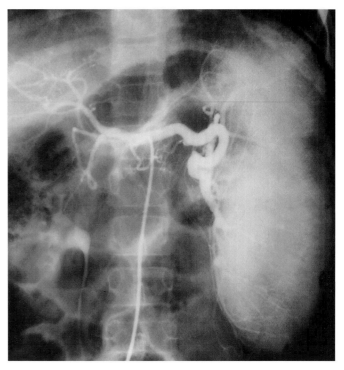

Fig. 25.41 Coeliac angiogram in portal hypertension. Sparse liver arteries. Enlarged tortuous splenic artery with aneurysms on main trunk and divisions. Intrasplenic branches stretched within grossly enlarged spleen which has vertical axis (cf. Fig. 25.40A).

intrahepatic portions (Fig. 25.41). Due to dilution of contrast in the enlarged spleen, the best indirect portograms in patients with raised portal pressure (above 12 mmHg) often follow superior mesenteric rather than coelic or splenic arterial injection. A small catheter (4F or 5F) should be used in view of the underlying coagulopathy. DSA is recommended to show the full extent of varices in the addition to the major veins (Fig. 25.42A). Angiograms are useful as a 'road map' for planning surgical portosystemic shunts (or showing them to be contraindicated). They are now only an occasional requirement in patients being considered for liver transplantation, being replaced by MR angiography. *Direct transplenic portography* is now rarely performed, as ultrasound will show the state of portal circulation, and both perisplenic varices and ascites, both of which

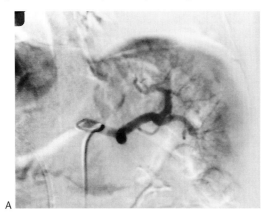
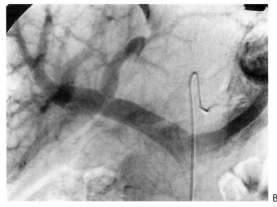

Fig. 25.40   (A) Splenic arteriogram (digital subtraction). Normal arteries and non-enlarged spleen. (B) Venous phase. Normal splenic and portal veins, with no filling of tributaries or collaterals.

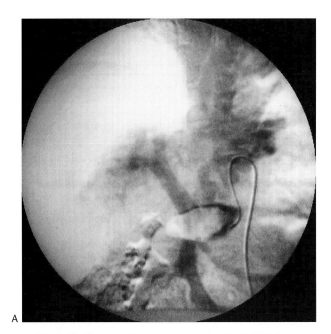

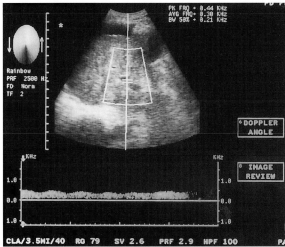

Fig. 25.42 (A) DSA. Venous phase superior mesenteric artery injection. Portal vein widely patent. Liver tiny in size—ascites suspected. Note filling of left gastric (coronary) vein thence gastric and oesophageal varices. (B) Duplex Dopper ultrasound. Ascites is confirmed. Portal vein flow is 24 cm/s.

would contraindicate a transperitoneal approach to the spleen (Fig. 25.42B). *Helical CT scanning* in portal hypertension is of special value in showing the position and extent of varices, especially if reformatting is carried out (Fig. 25.43). It will show the patency or thrombosis of a surgical shunt.

Hepatic vein catheterisation

Using an occlusion balloon catheter, this is a useful and safe procedure, simple to perform, which will provide hepatic phlebograms and sinusoidograms as well as pressure measurements. The small vessel pattern varies between normal (Fig. 25.44) and grossly pathological (Fig. 25.45), while corrected pressure measurements can pinpoint the level of portal hypertension as well as indicating its progress. Changes in portal pressure in response to drug therapy and diet may also be assessed and influence patient management.

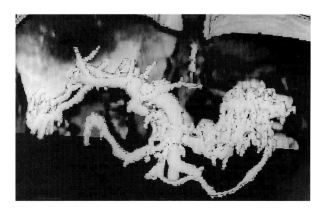

Fig. 25.43 Reformat of spiral CT axial image to show portal vein and gastric varices in coronal projection.

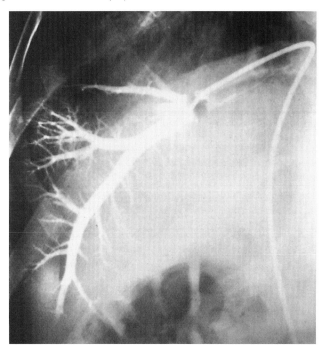

Fig. 25.44 Hepatic phlebogram. Occlusal balloon method. Normal major and minor veins. Occlusion pressure normal at 6 mmHg.

Interventional procedures in portal hypertension

As cirrhosis is the most frequent aetiology, **liver biopsy** is usually required. It is common to ask the radiologist to perform this under ultrasound or CT control, particularly if the liver is small. Embolising the percutaneous needle track with polyvinyl alcohol or steel coils is advisable. Biopsy may also be undertaken using a needle–catheter assembly introduced by the transfemoral or transjugular routes (usually the latter), both transvenous approaches being safe (Fig. 25.46).

Should portal hypertension be due to a posthepatic cause, such as hepatic vein thrombosis or web, **balloon dilatation** to re-establish hepatic vein patency is a therapeutic option, while in prehepatic portal hypertension due to portal vein thrombosis, **clot thrombolysis** via a transhepatic approach is feasible. Thrombolysis has also been used in the hepatic artery in patients with thrombosis of small

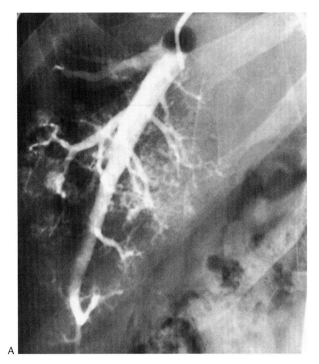

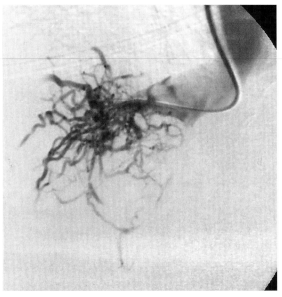

Fig. 25.45 (A) Hepatic phlebogram. Occlusal balloon method. Irregular hepatic vein radicles and bizarre sinusoidogram. Corrected pressure 16 mmHg: cirrhosis. (B) DSA hepatic venogram. The right vein occludes close to site of its caval entry. Contrast outlines 'spider's web' of new venous collaterals. Budd–Chiari syndrome.

hepatic veins. **Dilatation of stenosing portocaval or other shunts** after introducing a balloon catheter from the inferior vena cava may re-establish the surgical shunt in appropriate patients.

Increased interest in the medical control of portal hypertension has led to investigating splanchnic blood flow and its response to various drugs. A Doppler probe can be placed through a catheter in the superior mesenteric artery. Information gained has been shown to be more accurate than Doppler studies performed through the anterior abdominal wall (Fig. 25.47).

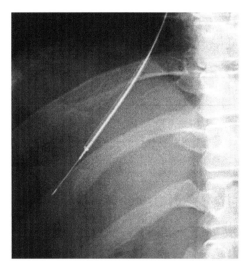

Fig. 25.46 Transjugular liver biopsy. Cutting needle introduced via right hepatic vein.

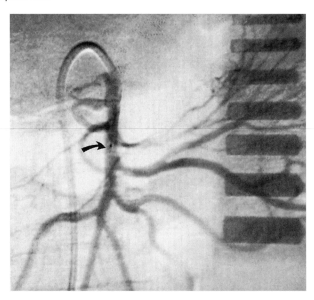

Fig. 25.47 DSA of superior mesenteric artery, assessing effect on flow of various drugs. Fr 8 catheter houses Fr 3 microtip disposable Doppler catheter (arrow). Note graduated markers on right (4–10 mm).

Embolisation of the splenic artery

This has largely been superseded as a treatment for hypersplenism but is sometimes performed for left-sided portal hypertension (secondary to splenic vein thrombosis). It is not without hazard and has resulted in splenic infection and abscess formation, particularly if not performed in stages. Timely one-stage embolisation immediately prior to laparoscopic splenectomy may reduce blood loss and splenic volume, and so help both patient and surgeon.

Transjugular intrahepatic portosystemic shunt (TIPS)

TIPS is the creation of an image-guided connection between a major hepatic vein (usually right-sided) and a major intrahepatic branch of the portal vein. Since 1987 TIPS has replaced surgical shunting in many centres worldwide as effective treatment of acutely bleeding oesophageal or gastric varices. A catheter–needle

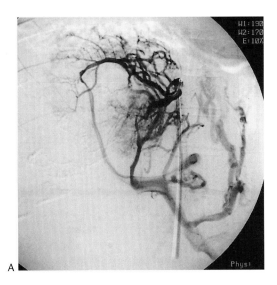

A

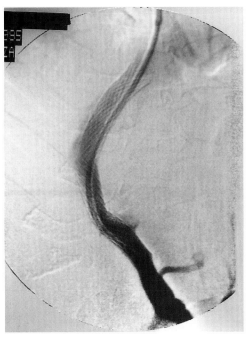

B

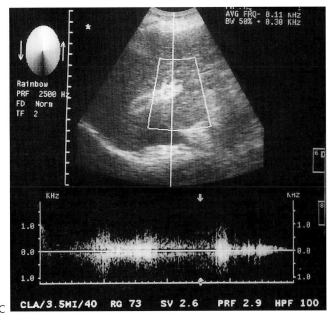

C

Fig. 25.48 TIPS procedure (DSA). (A) Phlebogram shows right hepatic vein occlusion near its caval junction. Note reflux via spider's web network into portal vein, thence into left gastric vein (patient had acutely bleeding varices). (B) TIPS completed. A 12 mm diameter metal stent has relieved the portal hypertension. (C) Follow-up Doppler ultrasound. Turbulent flow enters the stent.

assembly, guide-wires and balloon catheters contribute to the formation of a transhepatic tract, which is then maintained by an expanding metal stent of at least 10 mm diameter and of appropriate length. Carbon dioxide is a useful 'negative' contrast agent to use in these compromised patients to show reliably the portal vein from a wedge hepatic vein injection of the gas, and fluoroscopy and ultrasound help guide the needle and catheter. TIPS succeeds in over 90% of patients (Fig. 25.48). Cessation of bleeding following the predictable drop in portal blood pressure is invariable, however encephalopathy can ensue. TIPS is therefore lifesaving, though to guarantee technical success the radiologist needs to undertake it other than infrequently.

COMPUTED TOMOGRAPHY OF THE LIVER AND SPLEEN

Robert Dick, Anthony Watkinson and Richard W. Whitehouse

Normal appearances

Both radiologists and surgeons need familiarity with liver anatomy so clearly displayed on CT. In unenhanced scans liver veins are seen as tubes of lower density than the parenchyma, which reads 50–60 HU due to its high glycogen content. The three major hepatic veins are visible in the higher cuts as convergent on the intrahepatic vena cava, while the horizontally orientated main portal vein is seen in lower cuts (Fig. 25.49). The porta hepatis is a cleft containing hepatic artery, portal vein and bile duct, and lying on the medial liver surface. Normal hepatic artery and biliary ducts are too small to be shown on conventional scanners, but multislice multidetector scanners may show them. The caudate lobe (segment I) lies behind the porta hepatis, between it and the inferior vena cava. If enlarged, it is readily identified (Fig. 25.50).

The segments of the liver are shown in Fig. 25.51. The physiological left lobe lies to the left of a line joining the inferior vena cava to the gallbladder fossa, and is divided into lateral and medial parts by the falciform ligament. The medial part consists of segment II superiorly and III inferiorly, the lateral part being segment IV, known as the quadrate lobe. The right lobe of liver has segment V anteroinferiorly, VI posteroinferiorly, VII posterosuperiorly, and VIII anterosuperiorly.

Splenic parenchyma is homogeneous in attenuation on unenhanced scans, with a similar density to blood in nearby aorta. On dynamic enhanced scans, the spleen may show swirls of contrast prior to homogeneity, this being a normal appearance, especially with spiral CT. Normal-sized liver and spleen do not extend below the costal margins. Reformatted images from contrast-enhanced helical CT can strikingly demonstrate the configuration and patency of the splenic and portal veins (Fig. 25.52).

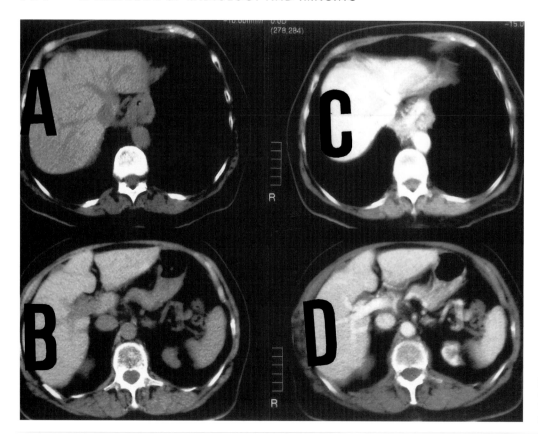

Fig. 25.49 (A, B) Unenhanced CT showing hepatic and portal veins. (C, D) Enhanced study of these veins.

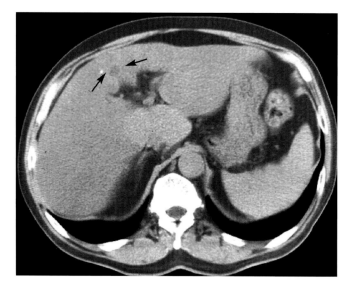

Fig. 25.50 Non-enhanced CT. Fatty infiltration of liver, with focal sparing and mild hypertrophy of caudate lobe in cirrhosis. The small arrowed defect is a hepatoma.

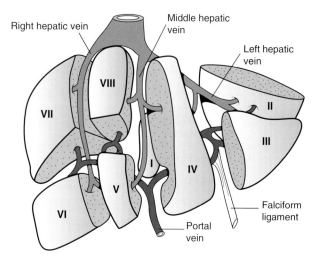

Fig. 25.51 Surgical segments of the liver.

Technical considerations

Whereas conventional CT allows two or three contiguous scans before a pause for another breath, resulting in breathing artefacts and misregistrations, helical (spiral) scanning (now widely available) allows the entire liver to be scanned in a single breath-hold, with overlapping 8–10 mm thick sections reconstructed from the data. After a control scan, intravenous contrast is given by an injec-

tor at 3 ml/s for a total of 100 ml. The hepatic arterial phase scan is done 25 s after the start of injection, and the portal venous phase at 70 s, when the parenchyma enhances by around 40 HU. In first-generation scanners the postcontrast scan was obtained very late and many lesions were missed. With helical CT, the triple phase will show many more tumours, and often characterise their nature (Fig. 25.53).

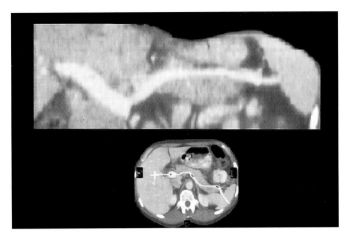

Fig. 25.52 Normal study. Curved plane reformation from a contrast-enhanced spiral scan of the upper abdomen, demonstrating the splenic and portal veins.

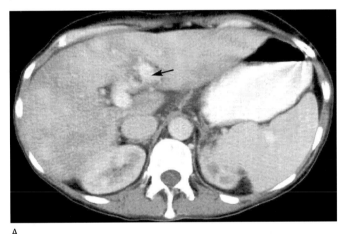

A

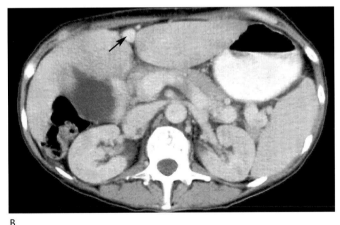

B

Fig. 25.54 (A, B) Patchy irregular enhancement of the hepatic parenchyma due to altered portal blood flow in cirrhosis with portal hypertension. Recanalisation of the umbilical vein in the falciform ligament is arrowed.

Cirrhosis and diffuse liver disease

The early stages of hepatitis, regeneration and fibrosis are not detectable on CT, although in established cirrhosis focal regenerative nodules may distort liver outline and liver volume may be

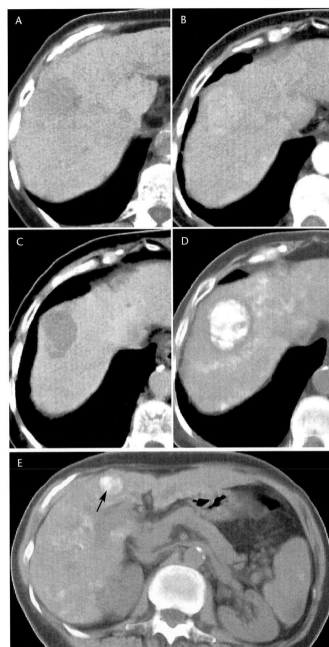

Fig. 25.53 (A) Non-enhanced scan shows poorly defined low-density mass—hepatoma. (B) Dynamic enhanced scan. Arterial phase shows greater enhancement in the defect than in surrounding liver: vascular hepatoma. (C) Delayed postcontrast venous phase scan shows persistent parenchymal density but loss of enhancement in the hepatoma, increasing its conspicuousness. (D) 10 days post-Lipiodol angiogram shows strong Lipiodol staining of the tumour. (E) CT at another level (post-Lipiodol) shows a satellite lesion in the left lobe of the liver (segment IV) (arrow) not seen on earlier scans.

reduced, sparing or even hypertrophy of the caudate or left lobes being noted. Liver parenchyma enhances irregularly (Fig. 25.54) and ascites may be seen (Fig. 25.57). Splenic enlargement and widening of splenic and portal veins with attendant varices and collaterals secondary to portal hypertension are common. Underlying fat in the liver may confuse the enhancement pattern and small

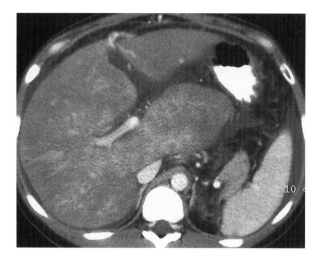

Fig. 25.55 CT in Budd–Chiari syndrome. Large oedematous liver, with huge caudate lobe. No hepatic vein radicles. Collateral veins in falciform ligament. Ascites.

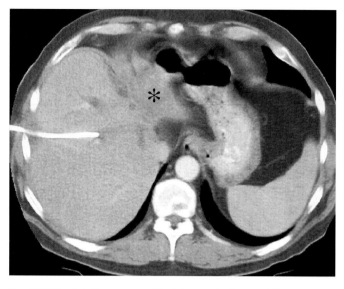

Fig. 25.56 Klatskin tumour of the left hepatic duct resulting in marked atrophy of the left lobe of the liver (asterisk). Some dilated right lobe ducts are evident, a percutaneous biliary drain is in situ.

hepatomas can be missed (Fig. 25.50). Note that a 'normal' parenchymal appearance on CT may sometimes be seen in the presence of a widespread infiltrate.

Iron deposition in *haemochromatosis* increases the CT number (Figs 25.7, 25.17) and can be quantified by use of a calibrated dual energy CT scan. Hepatic parenchymal density may also increase with iodine deposition in patients treated with *amiodarone* and by increased glycogen content in those with *glycogen storage disease*.

Reduced liver density occurs in *fatty infiltration*, which may be diffuse or regional (Fig. 25.18). Circular areas of parenchyma spared by fat must not be mistaken for neoplasms. Fat infiltrating liver may be seen in diabetes mellitus, alcoholism, patients with obesity or hypertriglyceridaemia, in those on intravenous alimentation, steroids or chemotherapy. It may be reversible. Infiltration by *sarcoid* or *amyloid* does not affect the parenchymal CT number.

With hepatic venous thrombosis (*Budd–Chiari syndrome*), CT shows typical hypertrophy and bright enhancement of the caudate lobe, the remainder of the liver being of low density due to congestive oedema, and the hepatic veins failing to obtain contrast (Fig. 25.55).

Primary malignancy

Hepatoma (primary hepatocellular cancer) is increasing in incidence worldwide, especially in those with hepatitis B, hepatitis C, cirrhosis and alcoholic liver disease. It may also complicate haemochromatosis and glycogen storage disease. If cirrhosis is present, small 1 cm tumours can be missed on CT in up to 50% of patients but are being increasingly seen with newer scanners. Hepatomas appear as solitary or multiple masses, or as a diffusely infiltrating lesion of liver. Striking but transient early enhancement is common as lesions are vascular (Fig. 25.53). Areas of necrosis within tumour may be seen as low-density non-enhancing areas. Tumour invasion of the portal vein, and less often the hepatic vein or the hepatic cava, occur, and show as distension of the vein with a filling defect on contrast-enhanced CT.

Hepatic arterial catheterisation and injection of 10 ml emulsified Lipiodol is used to highlight focal hepatic tumours. Hepatomas retain the Lipiodol for months, allowing small satellite cancers to

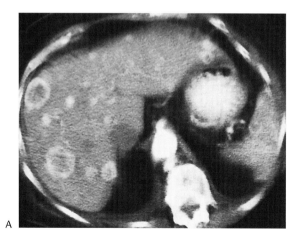

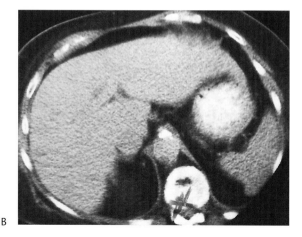

Fig. 25.57 (A) Arterial phase CT. Numerous metastases with ring enhancement. (B) Scan in equilibrium phase shows lesions are isodense with normal liver. They would be missed with slow scanning techniques. Biopsy: adenocarcinoma.

be identified (Figs 25.7, 25.53). Serial CT scans will follow tumour growth or regression.

Fibrolamellar hepatoma is a rare tumour, usually in a younger age group, and not associated with any predisposing cause. On CT the tumour is often well circumscribed and may be hard to detect due to uniform contrast enhancement. Between 30 and 40% may have a central scar or calcification. The tumour may recur, or metastasise after surgery.

Cholangiocarcinoma arises from the bile ducts, commonly close to the bifurcation of right and left main ducts (Klatskin's tumour). The primary lesion is often invisible on CT as it infiltrates the duct; however, proximal duct dilatation is produced. If slowly growing, atrophy of the obstructed duct and lobe can occur (Fig. 25.56).

Metastatic lesions

In the adult, hepatic metastases are 20 times more frequent than primary malignancy. They are usually similar to, or slightly lower in attenuation than the adjacent liver on unenhanced scans, but become of much lower attenuation if they contain areas of necrosis or cyst formation. Mucin-producing metastases (from *colon*, *stomach*, *ovary*) are low in attenuation, and may contain faint cumulous areas of calcification, allowing a confident diagnosis to be made on the unenhanced CT. Even small lesions close to normal liver density should be made visible on good triple-phase CT. Hypervascular metastases such as those from *endocrine* or *renal* primary tumours are readily visible (Fig. 25.57).

Greater degrees of normal parenchymal enhancement can be achieved by performing *arterioportography* combined with helical CT. The superior mesenteric artery is catheterised and 150 ml contrast injected at 2–3 ml/s with the patient on the CT table. The liver is scanned after 30–40 s. As the portal vein supplies 80% of liver blood input, the contrast results in normal liver enhancing by 150–190 HU. Liver malignancies receive virtually all their blood supply from the hepatic artery and will thus show as negative defects, as at the time of the scan contrast has not yet reached the aorta and hepatic artery (Figs 25.28, 25.58). The technique is used especially to plan surgical resection in patients with colorectal metastases.

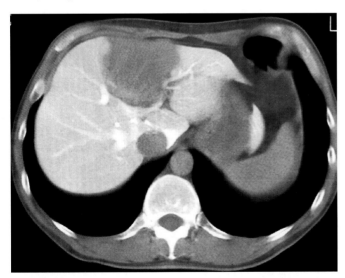

Fig. 25.58 Spiral scan through the liver during contrast injection into the superior mesenteric artery. Large solitary non-enhancing metastatic lesion demonstrated in the left lobe of the liver (segment IV). (Courtesy of Dr N. Chalmers.)

Benign hepatic masses

Haemangioma

This common capillary lesion occurs in up to 10% of the population. It may be single or multiple, varying in size between 5 mm and 15 cm. Over 50% have a characteristic sequence of contrast enhancement with a precontrast density less than normal liver, peripheral and nodular clumps of contrast appearing during dynamic scanning, followed by centripetal 'diffusion' of contrast into the centre of the lesion on sequential CT scans over the next 10–60 min (Fig. 25.59). Giant 'cavernous' haemangiomas have even less internal circulation, and may not fill so fully due to central areas of cystic change or haemorrhage. They may replace an entire lobe. Haemangiomas rarely if ever rupture and remain benign.

Adenoma and focal nodular hyperplasia (FNH)

Both are more common in females, particularly with the use of oral contraceptives. They are vascular on CT, and may be multiple. FNH

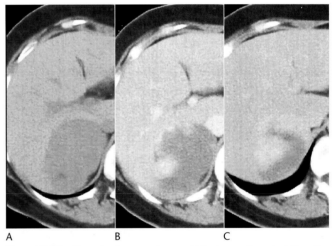

A   B   C

Fig. 25.59 Hepatic haemangioma. This is a characteristic site. (A) Unenhanced scan shows a mass of identical attenuation to that of the IVC. (B) During dynamic contrast enhancement, the periphery of the lesion takes up pools of contrast. (C) On delayed postcontrast scans the enhancement travels centripetally into the lesion.

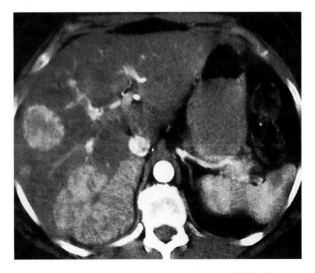

Fig. 25.60 Enhanced CT. Large vascular lesion in right lobe has a central scar: focal nodular hyperplasia. Other lesions. Note fatty liver.

has a central scar, whereas adenoma can have a central haematoma or may rupture externally. Patients on hormone therapy, such as occurs in gender reorientation, may develop adenomas. Fresh blood within them is of high density; old blood within the mass sometimes forms a low-density fluid level containing basal sediment. Adenoma and FNH may mimic each other on CT, and may even be difficult to distinguish from hepatoma if small (Fig. 25.60).

Cysts and abscesses

Between 10 and 13% of the population have congenital hepatic cysts, either single or multiple. On CT the cysts have well-defined margins and are of uniform water density. Larger cysts may be multilocular with thin internal septa. Multiple liver cysts are seen in 45% of patients with polycystic renal disease (Fig. 25.61). Small (1 cm diameter) hepatic cysts may be hard to characterise on CT (Fig. 25.62). Repeat scanning may be necessary to prove stability. Cystic hepatic lesions may also be postinflammatory, posttraumatic or parasitic (hydatid disease). Some cysts show curvilinear calcification in their wall.

Hepatic abscesses are usually low-density lesions with rim enhancement (Fig. 25.63). The high right lobe is the commonest position. Gas may be present within them (Fig. 25.10). Very large

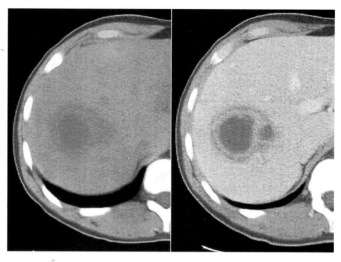

Fig. 25.63 CT. Hepatic abscess. The thick peripheral onion ring in the postcontrast scan (right) is typical.

abscesses can be seen in amoebiasis. Others from haematogenous or biliary origins may be confluent.

SPLENIC MASSES

Splenic abscesses

Splenic abscesses are rare and have similar appearances to infarcts and haematomas, appearing as a rounded area of low density within splenic tissue. Cysts and haemangiomas are the commonest benign splenic neoplasms, with similar appearances to cysts and haemangiomas in the liver, although splenic haemangiomas may not exhibit central contrast enhancement on delayed scans.

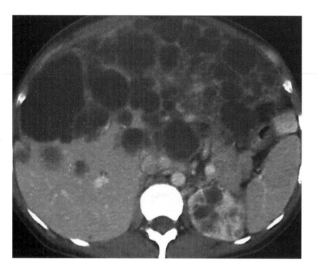

Fig. 25.61 Unenhanced CT. Hepatomegaly. Polycystic hepatic and renal disease.

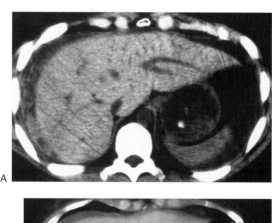

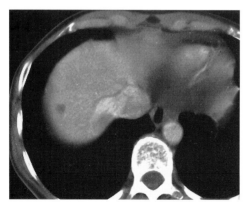

Fig. 25.62 CT. Small peripheral 'cyst' in right lobe is indeterminate. The nature is sometimes only clarified on follow-up.

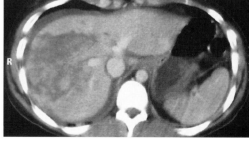

Fig. 25.64 (A) CT after blunt liver trauma: subcapsular haemorrhage. (B) Major trauma. Non-enhancing cleavage area in right lobe is nonviable. Right hepatic vein intact.

Splenic primary malignancy

Splenic primary malignancy is very rare; angiosarcoma can occur as multiple focal lesions. *Splenic metastases* generally occur in the presence of widespread metastases elsewhere, and are usually necrotic, low-density focal lesions on CT (Fig. 25.37). *Lymphomatous* involvement of spleen is relatively common. Multiple focal low-attenuating lesions are seen, but the usual CT finding is splenic enlargement per se, without an identifiable focal abnormality.

Hepatic and splenic trauma

CT is the procedure of choice to demonstrate lacerations, subcapsular and parenchymal haematomas, and areas of devitalised (and hence non-enhancing) parenchyma in both liver and spleen following major upper abdominal trauma (Figs 25.38, 25.64). Trauma is not often managed conservatively, thus sequential CT scans may be needed to show the development of *bilomas* (water-density bile collections at the site of hepatic injury), and the progression of subcapsular haematomas, which are typically lentiform collections with relatively high heterogeneous density initially due to the presence of blood clot. These subsequently enlarge and reduce in density due to osmotic effects (see Ch. 24).

RADIONUCLIDE IMAGING OF THE LIVER AND SPLEEN

Philip J. Robinson

The liver parenchyma is made up of hepatocytes, which perform the excretory and synthetic functions of the liver, and a smaller proportion of Kupffer cells, which have a reticuloendothelial function. Both of these cell populations can be investigated with ^{99m}Tc-labelled tracers, and further techniques are available for investigating the vascular compartment: blood pool studies using labelled red cells, and blood flow studies using a first-pass technique. The resolution of radionuclide imaging of the liver is such that lesions of 1–2 cm should be detectable if they are close to the liver surface, but deep-seated lesions of this size will usually not be detected. Single photon emission CT (SPECT) imaging improves the resolution at depth, but still does not approach the detail available with ultrasound, CT and MRI. For this reason the use of liver scintigraphy as a screening procedure for detecting liver lesions is now obsolete, and, while scintigraphy is of primary value in biliary tract disease, its use for investigation of liver lesions is now limited to a few specific applications.

Radiopharmaceuticals based on imidodiacetic acid (IDA) are taken up by functioning hepatocytes, excreted unchanged in the bile, and not reabsorbed from the gut. Studies with IDA compounds allow imaging of functioning liver parenchyma and also trace the flow of the bile in the ducts, gallbladder and bowel.

Labelled colloids demonstrate the distribution of functioning tissue by targeting the reticuloendothelial (RE) cells of the liver, spleen and bone marrow. Mass lesions which contain no functioning RE cells (the vast majority of pathologies) are shown as non-functioning areas. Blood pool imaging using radiolabelled autologous red blood cells (RBCs) has been used to differentiate haemangiomas from other liver tumours, as a result of their characteristically increased blood volume, but these applications have been largely overtaken by improved ultrasound, CT and MR techniques. Other obsolete nuclear techniques for the liver include tumour imaging with selenomethionine or gallium.

Somatostatin receptor scintigraphy (SRS) is used to demonstrate the presence and the functional activity of carcinoids, pancreatic islet cell tumours, and similar tumours of argentaffin cell type, including both abdominal primaries and metastatic deposits in liver or lymph nodes.

First-pass blood flow studies using ^{99m}Tc-colloid have been used to detect the subtle changes of increased arterial and reduced portal inflow fraction, which may be the first manifestation of early metastatic disease. Other techniques which look promising but have not yet reached routine clinical application include tumour imaging using positron emission tomography (PET) and single-photon techniques using labelled monoclonals or antibody fragments.

Techniques

Hepatocyte-based imaging

If the biliary tree is the primary area for investigation, the patient should be starved for 12 h before the study to encourage filling of the gallbladder; 150 MBq (scaled down for children) of di-isopropyl IDA or other IDA compound is given intravenously. Images are obtained sequentially up to about 45 min. Anterior or right anterior oblique projections may be used. Further oblique views or a right lateral view of the upper abdomen may be helpful to identify the gallbladder separately from overlapping bowel loops. In the normal subject, peak liver uptake occurs 15–30 min after injection, depending on the particular pharmaceutical used. If liver tumours are suspected, a SPECT acquisition obtained around the time of peak liver activity may be helpful.

If the gallbladder and bile ducts are demonstrated by 45 min but no tracer has passed into the bowel, a fatty meal or cholecystokinin (CCK) infusion may be used to provoke biliary drainage. If the gallbladder is not demonstrated by 60 min and acute cholecystitis is suspected, imaging should be continued up to 4 h, as some patients with chronic gallbladder disease show delayed filling. Absence of filling at 4 h is a good indication of acute cholecystitis with mechanical or functional obstruction of the cystic duct. Gallbladder function may be further investigated by recording the effect of CCK infusion on the contractility of the full gallbladder—normal gallbladders will react briskly, so that at least 35% of their contents will be evacuated 20 min after starting CCK. Most normal gallbladders show a 20 min ejection fraction of 70–80%.

Colloid scintigraphy

No preparation is required; 80 MBq of a ^{99m}Tc-labelled colloid (particle size 30–1000 nm) are given intravenously. With normal liver function, the blood clearance half-life of labelled colloids is 2–3 min, so uptake in the liver, spleen and bone marrow is virtually complete by 15 min after injection. The label remains in the cells, so multiple spot views can be obtained starting 15 min after injection. Anterior, posterior and oblique views are obtained, and SPECT acquisition is used if seeking small or deep-seated intrahepatic lesions.

Interpretation

Hepatocyte-based imaging

With normal liver function, liver uptake is homogeneous and peaks 15–30 min after injection. The left and right hepatic ducts and common duct are visualised about the same time, and gallbladder filling begins from 10 min onwards. High-quality images may also show segmental ducts but a particular prominence or beading of the secondary and tertiary ducts suggests obstructive or fibrotic duct disease. Delayed uptake with increased renal excretion is seen in patients with impaired liver function, and delayed clearance following normal uptake indicates a degree of biliary tract obstruction. Non-filling of the gallbladder by 60 min indicates either acute or chronic cholecystitis, and if images up to 4 h still show no filling the cystic duct is obstructed.

Colloid scintigraphy

With normal liver function about 80% of the injected dose is trapped in the liver, 15% in the spleen and about 5% in bone marrow. Liver uptake is homogeneous in relation to the distribution of liver tissue. Mass lesions within the liver, except those with functioning RE cells (see below) appear as photon-deficient areas within the parenchyma.

Diffuse liver disease results in impaired liver uptake with correspondingly increased splenic and bone marrow activity. Cirrhosis produces a characteristic appearance with reduced activity in the liver, which is usually small, increased activity in the enlarged spleen, and increased bone marrow uptake, which highlights separation of the liver from the costal margin by ascites. In Budd–Chiari syndrome, about half of all affected patients show a characteristic

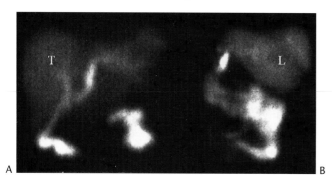

Fig. 25.65 Regional liver function shown by ⁹⁹ᵐTc-IDA: shortly after auxiliary liver transplantation (A), the transplant liver (T) occupying the normal position of the right lobe provides virtually the whole of the patient's liver function. Nine months later (B) the patient's own left lobe (L) has regenerated and the transplant has been allowed to undergo rejection and atrophy.

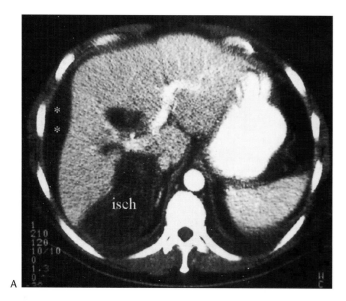

scintigraphic appearance, with hypertrophy of the actively functioning caudate lobe and atrophy of the remainder of the liver, which shows diminished function.

Applications

Applications of hepatobiliary scintigraphy in liver disease include the assessment of regional liver function (e.g. where the left or right hepatic duct has been damaged at surgery), demonstration of bile leaks in liver trauma, and the differential diagnosis of hepatocellular liver tumours. Applications in biliary tract disease include the investigation of biliary obstruction, bile leaks, suspected biliary atresia, choledochal cyst or other anomalies of the biliary tree, detection of abnormalities of bile flow in the gut, including duodenogastric reflux and afferent loop obstruction, and the demonstration of gallbladder function, including cystic duct obstruction as a marker of acute cholecystitis, biliary dyskinesia, and sphincter of Oddi dysfunction in patients with atypical or postcholecystectomy right upper quadrant pain. These latter applications are discussed in Chapter 24.

In liver *trauma*, or after surgical *resection* or liver *transplantation*, IDA imaging may be used to demonstrate the functional integrity of the liver parenchyma, including differential function of individual lobes or segments (Fig. 25.65). The pathway of biliary drainage is also shown so that leaks, obstructions and collections can be identified (Fig. 25.66).

In differentiating benign *hepatocellular tumours* from metastases or primary malignancies, radionuclide imaging using IDA or labelled colloid is sufficiently specific to allow biopsy to be avoided in the majority of cases. Focal nodular hyperplasia (FNH) is relatively common and most often presents as an incidental finding in patients with no related symptoms. Biopsy may be avoided if a convincing demonstration of functioning liver tissue within the lesion can be achieved by targeted imaging. FNH is the only liver tumour which consistently contains functioning RE cells and so shows uptake of labelled colloids. The degree of uptake may be a little less than in adjacent normal liver tissue, but occasionally appears more intense than adjacent liver (Fig. 25.67A). FNH also contains functioning hepatocytes, and takes up IDA compounds (Fig. 25.67B). Histology typically shows the presence of bile duc-

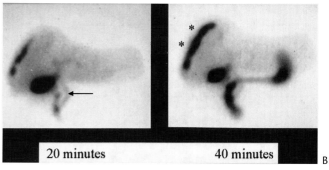

Fig. 25.66 Bile leak following liver trauma. Contrast-enhanced CT (A) showed a subcapsular fluid collection (asterisks) with segmental ischaemia (isch) but surgical exploration found no injury to the extrahepatic ducts. ⁹⁹ᵐTc-IDA scintigraphy (B) showed normal extrahepatic bile ducts (arrow) but leakage of bile from damaged intrahepatic ducts forming a subcapsular collection (asterisks).

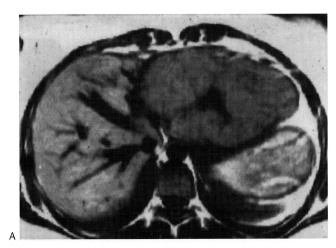

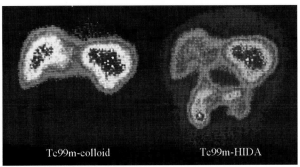

Fig. 25.67 Focal nodular hyperplasia. T₁-weighted MRI (A) shows a large mass in the left lobe with typical morphology for FNH. (B) Scintigraphy with ⁹⁹ᵐTc-colloid (left) shows that the mass exhibits at least as much reticuloendothelial cell activity as the normal liver in the right lobe, while ⁹⁹ᵐTc-IDA scintigraphy (right) shows active hepatocyte function with prolonged retention of tracer in the area of FNH.

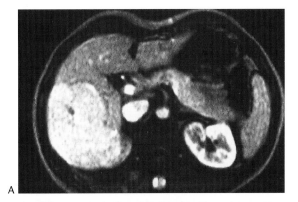

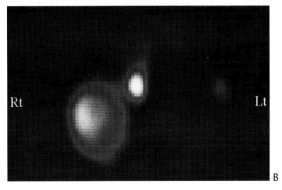

Fig. 25.68 Focal nodular hyperplasia. Gadolinium-enhanced T₁-weighted MRI (A) shows a highly vascularised lesion in the right lobe. SPECT imaging after ⁹⁹ᵐTc-IDA (B) shows prolonged retention of the tracer in the abnormal area. The focus of activity anteromedial to the mass in (B) represents the confluence of the hepatic ducts and common duct.

tules within FNH, but the ducts do not communicate with the biliary tree so there is no excretory pathway. This explains why FNH lesions characteristically show prolonged retention of IDA on delayed images when the tracer has cleared from the normal liver parenchyma (Fig. 25.68).

Hepatocellular adenoma has less consistent functional characteristics, but is also much less common than FNH. Probably a minority of adenomas contain functioning RE cells and, although most contain hepatocytes, the degree of IDA uptake is less predictable than with FNH. However, the demonstration of significant uptake of either colloid or IDA by a suspected adenoma is useful confirmatory evidence of its benign nature.

Hepatocellular carcinoma (HCC) contains little or no functioning liver tissue. Cases of colloid uptake in HCC are exceptionally rare, and although well-differentiated HCC may take up a small amount of IDA, the degree of uptake is much less than with FNH, although it may overlap with that of adenoma. Regenerative nodules in the cirrhotic liver show preservation of colloid uptake in contrast to the diminished activity shown in areas of fibrosis.

Somatostatin receptor scintigraphy (SRS)

The technique of SRS is described in Chapter 21 in relation to primary carcinoid lesions in the bowel, and their lymph node metastases. This technique is also the most sensitive non-invasive method currently available for detecting pancreatic islet-cell

tumours (see Ch. 26). The tracer used, ¹¹¹I-DTPA linked to octreotide, accumulates at all sites where there are sufficient somatostatin receptors, and this includes normal liver tissue. Even so, the presence of functioning liver metastases from pancreatic islet cell tumours, carcinoids, intestinal vipomas and other tumours of neuroendocrine origin can be shown (Fig. 25.69). Optimum images for liver lesions are those obtained at 24 hours since at this time the activity in normal liver parenchyma has diminished, while uptake in tumours remains high, and even small lesions may be

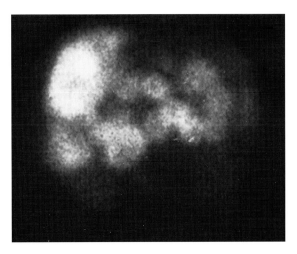

Fig. 25.69 Somatostatin receptor scintigraphy (SRS) in a patient with multiple liver metastases from pancreatic gastrinoma.

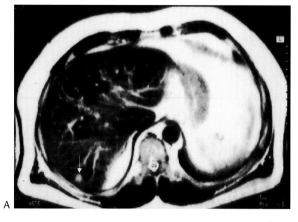

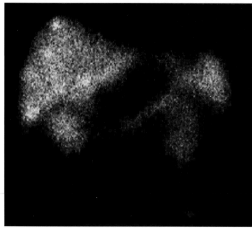

Fig. 25.70 Small liver lesions shown by SRS in a patient with metastatic carcinoid. SPIO-enhanced MRI (A) shows a 1 cm lesion in the periphery of the right lobe (arrow). SRS (B) shows multiple small lesions against a background of normal activity in adjacent liver.

identified (Fig. 25.70). Scintigraphy may be used to identify the presence of these lesions in the liver, to differentiate them from other types of liver tumour (Fig. 25.71), and to assess whether targeted radiotherapy is likely to be useful, using a much larger dose of a somatostatin analogue labelled with an appropriate therapy nuclide.

SPLEEN SCINTIGRAPHY

Imaging splenic disorders is achievable in the great majority of cases using ultrasound, CT or MRI, so scintigraphic examination of the spleen, which has been widespread in the past, is now rarely needed. However, there are still a few clinical problems in which splenic scintigraphy can be a very useful second-line technique.

Reticuloendothelial cells in the spleen take up intravenously-injected colloids. The particle size usually used for liver imaging with colloid, as described above, also demonstrates functioning splenic tissue. In the normal subject about 15% of the injected activity reaches the spleen, but in patients with cirrhosis or hypersplenism, a much greater proportion of the injected particles will be trapped in the spleen, as a result of its increased blood flow and the relative reduction in blood flow to the liver. More specific splenic imaging is obtained by injecting autologous red cells which have been incubated at about 50 °C and labelled with technetium ('heat-

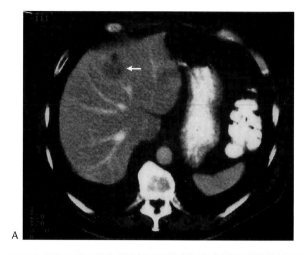

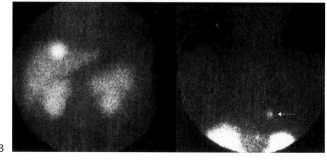

Fig. 25.71 Carcinoid metastases presenting as a solitary liver lesion (arrow) on CT (A), with neuroendocrine activity shown by positive SRS (B). Note also an unsuspected lung metastasis shown on SRS (arrow).

damaged RBCs'). With this agent, a much higher proportion of the injected activity is trapped in the spleen, so there is less interference in the images from overlying liver.

Splenic imaging in trauma and the investigation of mass lesions in the left upper quadrant is usually achieved with ultrasound or CT, but if there is difficulty in identifying the presence of splenic tissue, colloid scintigraphy is helpful. It is also used to differentiate splenunculi from other solid nodules found in the upper abdomen and is the first-choice technique when what is required is to localise sites of functioning splenic tissue in the absence of a normal spleen. This

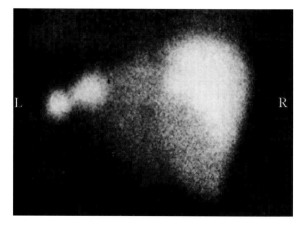

Fig. 25.72 ⁹⁹ᵐTc-colloid imaging in a patient with two unidentified rounded nodules in the left upper quadrant several years after splenectomy: focal uptake confirms the presence of splenunculi.

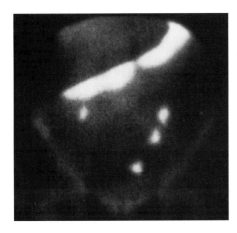

Fig. 25.73 ⁹⁹ᵐTc-colloid study following splenectomy for trauma. Fragments of splenic tissue entering into the omentum at surgery are now shown to be viable and functioning (liver uptake shielded on this image).

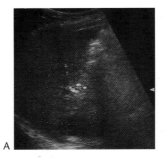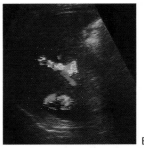

Fig. 25.74 (A) Interrogation of the porta hepatis, using a 2.5 MHz probe, failed to reveal normal flow within the portal vein. (B) Following intravenous administration of ultrasound contrast medium (Levovist), reverse flow is now readily seen in the portal vein using the same settings as in (A).

includes patients with the polysplenia/asplenia syndromes, those with haematological evidence of splenic function persisting after splenectomy (Fig. 25.72), and those with splenic implants deliberately or accidentally placed at the time of surgery (Fig. 25.73).

⁹⁹ᵐTc-colloid should be used as the first-choice technique for these applications, but if the liver obscures the area of interest (e.g. in polysplenia) heat-damaged red cells may be used. The latter technique is also helpful in searching for residual splenic tissue in patients with functional or congenital asplenia.

Splenic scintigraphy is also used in a few specific haematological applications. Autologous platelets, labelled with indium-111, may be used to demonstrate the increased rate of clearance of circulating platelets in patients with idiopathic thrombocytopenic purpura who may benefit from splenectomy. Similarly, in some patients with haemolytic anaemia, demonstrating abnormally rapid clearance of undamaged red cells from the circulation into the spleen may be used as an indicator of likely improvement with splenectomy.

ULTRASOUND OF THE LIVER AND SPLEEN

Julie F. C. Olliff

Ultrasound is the initial examination performed in most patients with suspected hepatic or splenic abnormality. Interrogation with ultrasound is best performed using a 5 MHz curvilinear probe but in large patients a lower frequency probe may be necessary. Complete examination usually requires both subcostal and intercostal scanning. Near and far gain settings should be adjusted to give a uniform reflectivity. Tissue harmonic imaging, which is available on many new ultrasound machines, improves the image resolution from a greater depth and decreases artefacts. This technique uses the phenomenon that a tissue insonated by the ultrasound wave resonates at twice the frequency of the beam, and the transmitted signal is free of background noise. The technique is helpful in the difficult patient and is particularly useful when scanning the obese patient with suspected hepatic metastatic disease. It can also be useful in the distinction of hypoechoic solid liver masses from cystic lesions. The normal liver parenchyma has a solid homogeneous echotexture. The parenchyma echoes appear as moderately short dots or lines. Discontinuities are produced by cross-section of

vessels. In the normal adult the liver is of higher reflectivity than the kidney and of lower reflectivity than the pancreas.

Ultrasound contrast media

Media which survive passage through the pulmonary bed may be useful in the Doppler assessment of liver vessels. These contrast media usually consist of microbubbles and have only relatively recently been released for clinical use. They are of potential use in patients in whom an inadequate Doppler examination has been performed (Fig. 25.74). They may also be of use in the assessment of tumour vascularity and in the investigation of hepatic metastatic disease. They produce an increase in the backscatter of blood. At higher acoustic pressures, resonant signals at second and other harmonic frequencies start to appear. As sound pressures increase, microbubble destruction causes transient ultrasonic signals. This effect is called stimulated acoustic emission (SAE). After the contrast agent clears the blood pool phase, transient wide-frequency Doppler signals may be seen from normal hepatic and splenic parenchyma which are destroyed by the act of scanning and are thought to be due to SAE.

Normal anatomy

The liver is divided into right and left lobes by the middle hepatic vein. Further division into segmental anatomy is achieved by the course of the right and left hepatic veins and the right and left portal vein branches. Segment I is the caudate lobe, which lies anterior to the intrahepatic IVC. Segment II lies medial to the left hepatic vein and superior to the left portal vein. Segment III lies lateral to the left hepatic vein and inferior to the left portal vein. Segment IV lies between the middle and left hepatic veins and may be further divided by the portal vein into segments IVA and IVB. Segment VIII lies between the middle and right hepatic veins superior to the right portal vein branch. Segment VII lies lateral to the right hepatic vein and superior to the right portal vein. Segment VI lies lateral to the right hepatic vein inferior to the right portal vein branch, and segment V lies between the right and middle hepatic veins inferior to the right portal vein branch.

Portal vein

Approximately 25% of the flow into the liver is supplied by the hepatic artery, the remainder by the portal vein. The portal vein walls are seen as well-defined parallel reflective thin lines. Normal portal venous flow is hepatopetal and is usually monophasic with

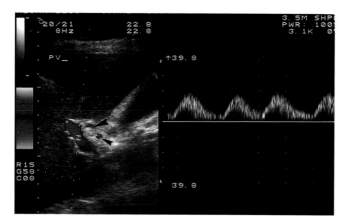

Fig. 25.75 Oblique intercostal scan in the right upper quadrant of the liver demonstrates forward flow (encoded red) in the portal vein. The hepatic artery is seen as a small focus of colour flow (small arrowhead) lying between the portal vein and bile duct (large arrowhead).

some fluctuation due to respiration and cardiac activity (Fig. 25.75). Thus, when colour flow is being used to assess the portal vein, flow into the liver will conventionally appear red. Portal vein pulsatility may be seen in thin healthy subjects, in patients with congestive heart failure and in a very few patients with liver disease. The pulse repetition rate (PRF) may need to be reduced to detect flow in patients with portal hypertension (Fig. 25.76).

Hepatic artery

The hepatic artery can be identified in most patients at the porta hepatis lying between the portal vein and common bile duct (Fig. 25.75). In a small percentage of patients this anatomy may be altered and the hepatic artery may lie anterior to the bile duct. Colour flow imaging allows rapid differentiation of bile duct from hepatic artery. In older patients with an ectatic hepatic artery or in patients with a dilated hepatic artery, which can occur in alcoholic hepatitis and cirrhosis, this may prevent misinterpretation of a dilated common duct. The hepatic arterial wave form characteristically has a high diastolic phase due to the low resistance of the hepatic vascular bed.

Hepatic veins

There are usually three hepatic veins—the right, the middle and the left—which drain into the IVC. These may be differentiated from portal vein radicles not only by their anatomical position and pattern of drainage but also by the lack of reflectivity of the hepatic vein wall (Fig. 25.77). They are best interrogated either by scanning transversely in the epigastrium or by scanning transversely using

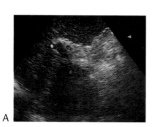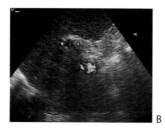

Fig. 25.76 (A) Oblique intercostal scan demonstrates flow in the hepatic artery but no flow within the portal vein. (B) Scanning in the same position but with a lower PRF flow is now demonstrated within the portal vein.

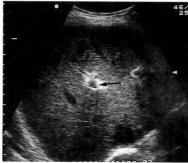

Fig. 25.77 Portal vein radicals have reflective walls (arrow) in contrast to the poorly reflective walls of hepatic vein branches.

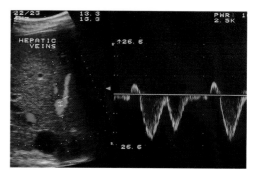

Fig. 25.78 This scan, obtained by scanning transversely in an intercostal space, shows the three hepatic veins. The left hepatic vein has been sampled with duplex Doppler and shows a triphasic wave form which reflects right atrial and inferior vena caval pressures.

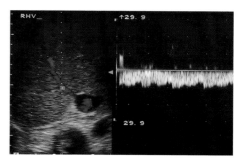

Fig. 25.79 The right hepatic vein has been sampled in a patient with portal hypertension and ascites due to cirrhosis. This scan shows flattening of the normal triphasic wave form.

an intercostal approach. The hepatic veins characteristically have a triphasic wave form which reflects right atrial and inferior vena caval pressures (Fig. 25.78). This results in flow in the hepatic veins being predominately coded blue, i.e. away from the probe on the colour Doppler, but with some phases being coded red. Loss of the triphasic wave form of the hepatic vein (Fig. 25.79) is seen in patients whose livers have lost compliance, for example in cirrhosis, acute hepatitis and liver transplant rejection.

Diffuse liver changes

Liver enlargement

The objective ultrasound assessment of liver enlargement can be quite difficult. The liver is a large organ with a very variable shape. The most commonly used measurement is an increased length of the right

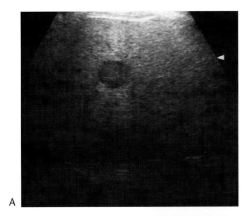
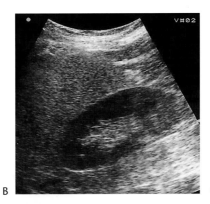
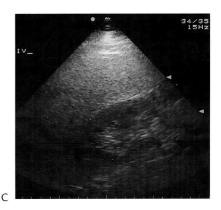

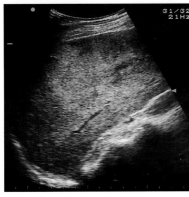

Fig. 25.80 (A) Colorectal cancer metastasis in a patient with a fatty liver following chemotherapy. Note the apparent posterior acoustic enhancement caused by the relative lack of attenuation of the ultrasound beam by the metastasis. (B) Longitudinal scan of the right lobe of the liver and right kidney in a patient with fatty change demonstrating attenuation of the ultrasound beam with the upper pole of the right kidney appearing less reflective than the lower pole. Note the bright liver and loss of vascular detail. (C) Longitudinal ultrasound scan of a patient with an enlarged liver demonstrates an attenuating liver with the beam failing to penetrate posteriorly even using a 2.5 MHz probe. The right kidney appears of relatively low reflectivity. (D) An area of geographical fatty change is seen with a vessel running through this irregular area of increased reflectivity.

lobe measured from the dome of the diaphragm to the inferior edge of the right lobe of the liver in the midclavicular line. Several authors have found a measurement of 15.5 cm to be a reliable indicator of enlargement, with the liver being enlarged in 85% of cases. If the liver measures 13 cm or less in length it is normal in 93% of cases. Another commonly used sign of liver enlargement is extension of the right lobe of the liver inferior to the lower pole of the right kidney, but thin patients may have long narrow livers. Thus some authors have suggested including an anteroposterior measurement of the right lobe of the liver. Loss of the normal concavity of the inferior margin of the left lobe of the liver is another indicator of hepatic enlargement.

Hepatomegaly may be due to cardiac failure. In this case the liver parenchyma may be less attenuating. In right heart failure the IVC and hepatic veins are dilated and there will be loss of the respiratory variation in the calibre of the IVC. A diameter of the hepatic vein exceeding 1 cm at a distance of 2 cm from the confluence of the hepatic veins and IVC should be considered abnormal. It has been found that hepatic vein dilatation, Doppler waveform alteration and portal vein pulsatility changes correlate well with New York Heart Association functional classes of heart failure in a selected group of patients.

Fatty infiltration or steatosis

This is the metabolic complication of various insults to the liver. It is commonly seen in patients with diabetes mellitus and in alcoholics. Other causes include obesity, hyperlipidaemia, parenteral nutrition, glycogen storage disease, severe hepatitis and chemotherapy (Fig. 25.80A). The normal liver parenchyma reflectivity should be midway between renal cortex and pancreas. Fatty infiltration will cause an increase in reflectivity. The liver will be more attenuating (Fig. 25.80B,C), resulting in poor definition of the posterior liver,

and the hepatic veins will be less well seen. The reflectivity of the portal vein walls will be lost and the parenchyma will become featureless. The degree of increased echogenicity is roughly proportional to the level of steatosis. The liver will be enlarged in 75–80%. The involvement of the liver may be diffuse or focal. Four patterns of focal fatty infiltration have been described: (1) hyperechoic nodule, (2) multiple confluent hyperechogenic lesions (Fig. 25.80D), (3) hypoechoic skip nodules, (4) irregular hyperechoic and hypoechoic areas. The commonest areas of focal fatty sparing (hypoechoic skip nodules) are in segment IV anterior to the portal vein bifurcation next to the gallbladder bed (Fig. 25.81) and in subcapsular regions. Areas of focal fatty change and fatty sparing may simulate mass lesions and may give rise to difficulty in the treated oncology patient. These areas do not have mass effect and colour Doppler may be useful to demonstrate vessels running through the areas of altered echogenicity. An angular or interdigitating geometric margin is also characteristic of focal fat. There may be rapid changes with time, depending on the clinical condition. Ultrasound has an 85% accuracy in the diagnosis of this condition, with a sensitivity of 100% and specificity of 56%.

Hepatitis

This is the term used to describe acute or chronic inflammation of the liver. This can result from infection: viral, bacterial, fungal and rickettsial. It can also be caused by a large number of toxins, including alcohol, halothane, isoniazid, chlorpromazine, oral contraceptives, methotrexate, etc.

Viral hepatitis

Although liver is almost always involved in haematogenous viral infection, the term 'viral hepatitis' is used clinically to denote liver

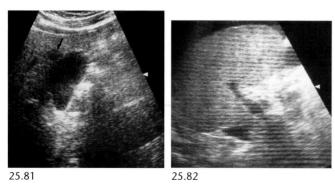

25.81   25.82

Fig. 25.81 A small area of focal fatty sparing (arrow) in a typical position close to the gallbladder in a patient with an otherwise bright fatty liver which is very attenuating. Note how ill-defined the vessels seem.

Fig. 25.82 Diffusely echobright liver in a patient with alcoholic hepatitis and cirrhosis.

involvement by a small group of viruses. *Hepatitis A* usually has a benign self-limiting course. It rarely causes fulminant hepatitis and does not cause chronic liver disease. *Hepatitis B*, however, can cause an asymptomatic carrier state, acute hepatitis, chronic hepatitis, fulminant hepatic failure and hepatocellular carcinoma.

Hepatitis C (non-A, non-B) can cause either acute or chronic hepatitis, with at least 50% of acute cases progressing to chronic hepatitis; 10–20% of these patients go on to develop cirrhosis.

In acute viral hepatitis the liver is enlarged in 70% of patients and there is splenic enlargement in 20%. The liver parenchyma is of decreased echogenicity in severe cases and the portal vessel walls are more echogenic than is usual. This has been observed in up to 60% of patients. This pattern is not specific for viral hepatitis and has been seen in other conditions such as toxic shock syndrome, leukaemia and cytomegalovirus infection. Gallbladder wall thickening may also be observed. Severe chronic hepatitis increases the echogenicity of the liver, with loss of the portal vein wall echogenicity. Lymphadenopathy may be seen in the gastrohepatic ligament in patients with chronic active hepatitis, which may help differentiate this condition from fatty infiltration. The major role of ultrasound in patients with acute hepatitis is to exclude biliary obstruction as a cause of jaundice.

Alcoholic hepatitis This is part of the spectrum of alcoholic liver disease which also consists of fatty liver and cirrhosis. It is due to acute liver cell necrosis following an alcoholic binge. In acute alcoholic hepatitis the liver is echogenic because of underlying fatty change (Fig. 25.82). The liver may be enlarged, but as the disease progresses to cirrhosis it will become atrophic.

Toxin and drug-induced liver disease cause fairly non-specific findings of hepatomegaly, fatty infiltration and cirrhosis.

Cirrhosis

This is a term used to describe chronic liver disease with diffuse parenchymal necrosis, active formation of fibrous tissue leading to fibrosis of the liver, and nodular regeneration. Regenerating nodules have been classified as siderotic or non-siderotic, with the siderotic nodules having a greater tendency to undergo malignant transformation. Micronodular cirrhosis, which is common in alcohol-related liver disease has diffuse nodules measuring less than 3 mm in size with thin fibrous septa. Viral hepatitis results in macronodular cirrhosis which is characterised by nodules greater than 3 mm in

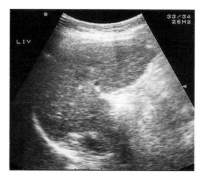

Fig. 25.83 Ultrasound of a cirrhotic liver. There are coarse echoes and vessels are difficult to identify.

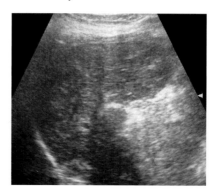

Fig. 25.84 An irregular liver margin with coarse echoes in a patient with hepatitis C cirrhosis.

size and thick fibrous septa. Both types lead to progressive hepatic fibrosis, liver failure and portal hypertension. Cross-sectional imaging cannot reliably differentiate the types of cirrhosis. When large nodules are appreciated they are likely to be associated with macronodular cirrhosis.

There is significant overlap between the ultrasound appearances of fatty infiltration and cirrhosis, with both causing an increase in liver reflectivity, decreased beam penetration and poor depiction of intrahepatic vessels (Fig. 25.83). The two often also coexist. While ultrasound has up to a 98% positive predictive value for the presence of diffuse hepatic parenchymal disease, it cannot reliably differentiate between the two. Cirrhosis should be suspected if a reduction of liver size, nodularity of the liver surface (Fig. 25.84),

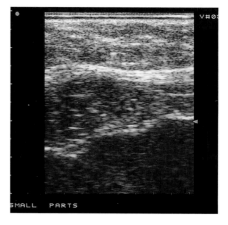

Fig. 25.85 Ultrasound using a linear probe demonstrates an irregular liver margin (arrow) in a patient with cirrhosis and no ascites.

accentuation of the fissures, marked coarsening of the liver texture, regenerating nodules, ascites or signs of portal hypertension are seen. Irregularity of the liver surface has a reported sensitivity of 88% for the presence of cirrhosis. This is best detected using a high-frequency linear probe (Fig. 25.85). Enlargement of the caudate lobe and lateral segment of the left lobe may occur, as may atrophy of the right and medial segments of the left lobe. There are various measurements that may be made to determine whether cirrhosis is likely to be present based upon these findings but measurement of the transverse diameter of segment IV (left wall of the gallbladder to ascending portion of left portal vein where it gives off the branch to segment IV) has been found to have a sensitivity of 74% and specificity of 100% if a lower limit of normal of 30 mm is used. Regenerating nodules may be seen and be difficult to differentiate from a hepatocellular carcinoma. Some studies have reported a sensitivity of approximately 50% of ultrasound screening of cirrhotic patients for hepatocellular cancer but a specificity of 98% for any discrete lesion. The incidence of gallstones is increased in patients with cirrhosis.

Portal hypertension

Portal hypertension is due to increased resistance to portal flow and/or to increased portal blood flow. It is defined as an increase in portal pressure above the normal range of 6–10 mmHg or a gradient of more than 5 mmHg between the hepatic veins and the portal vein. Development of this condition may cause enlargement of the extrahepatic portal vessels and development of spontaneous portosystemic collaterals (Fig. 25.87). Causes of portal hypertension may be divided into: prehepatic, due to obstruction of the portal, superior mesenteric or splenic vein (portal vein thrombosis, aplasia or hypoplasia, infection, trauma and malignancy); intrahepatic, including cirrhosis, congenital hepatic fibrosis, hepatitis, myeloproliferative disorders and schistosomiasis; and suprahepatic, due to obstruction of the blood flow out of the liver—Budd–Chiari syndrome. Cirrhosis is the commonest cause of portal hypertension in Europe and North America.

Doppler examination may be used to determine the presence and direction of flow within the portal vein. It must be remembered that flow velocity may be slow and appropriate Doppler settings used to prevent the inappropriate diagnosis of portal vein thrombosis (Fig. 25.76). The normal oscillations tend to disappear in portal hypertension as the flow becomes slow and turbulent. Some authors have identified that a portal vein with a diameter over 17 mm is 100% predictive for large varices. Many other factors, such as respiration, postural changes and food intake, will influence the diameter of the portal vein. A normal diameter portal vein will not, however, exclude portal hypertension. Reversed portal vein flow

may occur in up to 8% of patients with cirrhosis (Fig. 25.86) and is generally associated with a reduction in the diameter of the portal vein. Patients with hepatofugal flow have a decreased incidence of bleeding. Reversed flow in intrahepatic vessels only may be observed occurring in advanced cirrhosis more frequently than complete reverse flow. Intrahepatic flow reversal can also be seen in hepatocellular cancer, Budd–Chiari syndrome when there is a differential pressure in differing parts of the liver, and in a patent umbilical vein when the left portal vein branches will flow towards the patent umbilical vein and the right portal vein branches may demonstrate reversed flow. Flow can become alternating when pressures are similar in the intrahepatic and collateral bed. Flow in the balanced state may be difficult to detect and may lead to the erroneous diagnosis of portal vein thrombosis. Ultrasound may be used to detect the presence of spontaneous portosystemic collaterals. Collateral vessels may be seen sonographically in up to 88% of patients with portal hypertension. The *umbilical vein* running within the ligamentum teres can become recanalised in patients with portal hypertension, and collateral vessels may be readily identifiable with colour flow Doppler (Fig. 25.87). This is a highly specific sign of portal hypertension. This vein may also be detected outside the liver with blood flowing away from the liver. Other collaterals, such as the *coronary vein* which branches from the portal vein (Fig. 25.88) or splenic vein, may again be readily identifiable using colour flow Doppler. The presence of oesophageal varices may be difficult to assess directly with ultrasound but can be inferred by thickening of the oesophageal wall, irregularity of the oesophageal lumen and variation of the oesophageal wall thickness with respiration. Collateral vessels may also be seen in relation to the spleen, with splenorenal collaterals originating from the splenic hilum and running toward the left kidney (Fig. 25.89), and short gastric veins appearing as vessels near the upper pole of the spleen. Less commonly, collaterals can be seen within the gallbladder wall

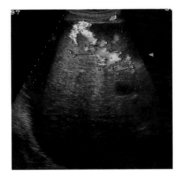

Fig. 25.87 This scan shows recanalisation of the ligamentum teres with blood flowing in the ligamentum teres toward the Doppler probe, i.e. away from the liver.

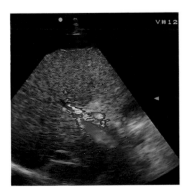

Fig. 25.86 Oblique coronal scan through the porta hepatis of a patient with cirrhosis. Note the irregular liver margin, ascites and coarse liver reflectivity showing normal forward flow (encoded red) within the hepatic artery and reversed flow within the portal vein (encoded blue).

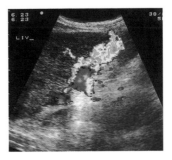

Fig. 25.88 Colour Doppler study demonstrating flow within enlarged collaterals in the position of the coronary vein running along the inferomedial aspect of the left lobe of the liver.

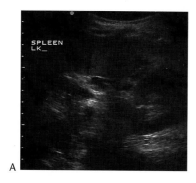

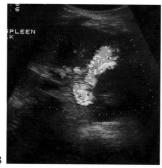

Fig. 25.89 (A) This scan has been performed without colour Doppler, showing the spleen and left kidney. (B) When colour Doppler is used, abnormal large collateral vessels can be appreciated running between the spleen and left kidney—splenorenal collaterals.

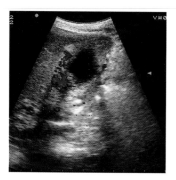

Fig. 25.90 Colour Doppler study reveals a thickened gallbladder wall containing abnormal vessels with colour flow within them.

(Fig. 25.90). This is often seen in association with portal vein thrombosis.

Liver cirrhosis is the commonest underlying condition for the development of *portal vein thrombosis* but this may be caused by haematological disorders or by gastrointestinal disorders, including pancreatitis and pancreatic tumours. Recent thrombosis may be anechoic and thus undetectable with ultrasound imaging. As the

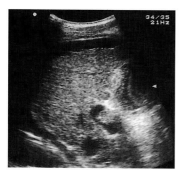

Fig. 25.91 Ultrasound of echogenic bland thrombus partially occluding the portal vein.

thrombus becomes established, it becomes visible as echogenic material within the lumen of the vessel (Fig. 25.91). In chronic thrombosis highly echogenic fibrous tissue replaces the portal vein. *Cavernous transformation of the portal vein* may develop in patients with complete occlusion. On colour Doppler ultrasound this appears as a rounded mass of small collateral vessels with variable direction low-velocity flow at the porta hepatis (Fig. 25.92). Portal vein thrombosis may also be due to tumour thrombus from, most commonly hepatocellular carcinoma (Fig. 25.93). In these patients it may be possible with colour and duplex Doppler to identify neovascularity within the tumour tissue invading the portal vein. Because the hepatic artery takes over the entire hepatic blood supply in patients with portal thrombosis, high-frequency arterial signals are seen at the porta hepatis and within the hepatic parenchyma with no demonstration of portal vein flow.

Hepatic vein thrombosis

This most often occurs in patients with haematological disorders or with other coagulopathy. This results in the *Budd–Chiari syndrome*. Other causes of the Budd–Chiari syndrome include hepatic vein obstruction by inferior vena caval web, stenosis, clot or tumour. Hepatic vein thrombosis may be investigated using colour flow Doppler and duplex Doppler. In this situation, thrombus may be identified within these hepatic veins with lack of colour flow within the normal veins, but abnormal collateral vessels may be seen heading toward the surface of the liver (Fig. 25.94). High-velocity jets may be seen on interrogation of the IVC in patients with significant IVC stenosis when colour Doppler is used. Flow reversal is commonly seen in the portal vein but is not pathognomonic of Budd–Chiari syndrome. Power Doppler has the advantage that it is

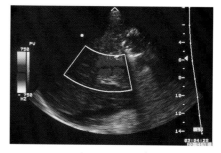

Fig. 25.92 This scan, obtained using an intercostal approach and with colour Doppler, shows a mass of collateral vessels at the porta hepatis, a cavernoma. No normal portal vein can be seen.

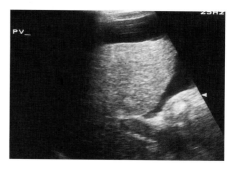

Fig. 25.93 There is tumour thrombus in the portal vein in this patient with multifocal hepatoma in a cirrhotic liver and ascites.

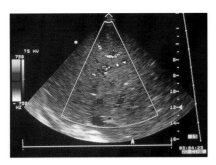

Fig. 25.94 A transverse intercostal scan. No normal hepatic veins are seen. Some thrombus is seen in a middle hepatic vein. Some abnormal flow away from the probe is seen, with other abnormal collateral vessels close to the surface of the liver with blood flowing out of the liver and coded red.

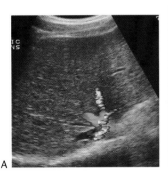
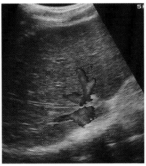

Fig. 25.95 (A) Transverse intercostal scan showing the three hepatic veins with colour flow Doppler. Note that because of the poor angle of interrogation of the right hepatic vein, colour flow is not seen within this vessel. (B) In the same position, power flow Doppler has now been used to interrogate the three hepatic veins and flow is readily seen within the right hepatic vein despite the poor angle of interrogation.

not angle dependent. This is useful, most often, when assessing *patency of the IVC*, when on coronal scanning and transverse scanning the angle of interrogation is often unfavourable (Fig. 25.95).

Duplex Doppler and colour Doppler may also be used to evaluate *portosystemic surgical shunts* (Fig. 25.96). The patency of the shunt may be assessed in 75% of cases. Splenorenal shunts are more easily demonstrated than portocaval shunts. An indirect sign of shunt patency is the presence of flow reversal in the portal vein when, prior to shunt surgery, flow had been demonstrated in a hepatopetal direction. This finding will not apply to distal spleno-renal shunts.

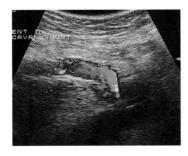

Fig. 25.96 A stent has been placed within a mesocaval shunt and its patency is readily demonstrated with colour flow Doppler.

Focal liver lesions

Simple hepatic cysts

Simple hepatic cysts are developmental, with their incidence increasing with age. They are found in 3–7% of patients over the age of 60 but in less than 1% of patients younger than this. Cysts may occur in younger patients with polycystic liver disease, auto-somal dominant polycystic kidney disease (25–33% of patients) and von Hippel–Lindau disease. Symptoms are uncommon. The cyst is usually single with a thin well-defined wall and anechoic contents (Fig. 25.97) with posterior acoustic enhancement. Size is variable. Thin septations are common. Simple cysts may be simulated by cystic metastases, particularly from ovarian cancer, treated liver abscesses and hydatid cysts, and may be acquired following trauma. Simple cysts are usually solitary. One of the associated polycystic diseases should be considered if more than 10 cysts are present.

Congenital hepatic fibrosis and polycystic liver disease

The majority of patients present in childhood with portal hypertension. Multiple cysts are seen within the liver with occasional wall calcification. The cysts may contain haemorrhage and fluid levels.

Biliary cystadenoma

Biliary cystadenoma is a premalignant cystic tumour of the liver which is usually solitary. It is generally multiloculated and mural nodules may be seen in both the cystadenoma and cystadeno-carcinoma. Calcification may be seen within the wall (Fig. 25.98).

Cavernous haemangiomas

Cavernous haemangiomas are the most common benign neoplasm, occurring in 1–4% of individuals. They are rarely seen in young children. Most are small and asymptomatic but, if large, may present with symptoms related to mass effect. Very rarely they may haemorrhage. They can enlarge during pregnancy. They are often peripheral or subcapsular in position in the posterior part of the

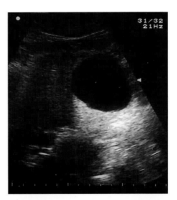

Fig. 25.97 There is a small well-defined lesion with a very thin wall; anechoic contents consistent with a cyst.

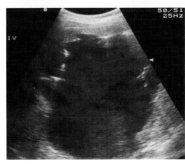

Fig. 25.98 A large intra-hepatic cystic mass with calcification within its wall proved to be a biliary cyst-adenoma.

right lobe of liver. They are multiple in 10% of patients. Small lesions are generally well-defined spherical or ovoid in shape, of increased reflectivity compared with normal liver (Fig. 25.99), with or without small central regions of decreased reflectivity, and between one- and two-thirds show posterior acoustic enhancement. Although these appearances are highly suggestive of a cavernous haemangioma, a number of other hepatic lesions, such as hepatocellular carcinoma and metastases, may occasionally have these appearances. Most persist unchanged on follow-up. Colour Doppler rarely reveals flow within the lesion. Power Doppler may reveal such flow. This is non-specific and may also be seen in metastases and hepatocellular cancer. Larger lesions may well be more heterogeneous in texture, with solid and cystic areas within the mass (Fig. 25.100). Confirmatory imaging with dynamic contrast-enhanced CT or MRI is recommended in patients with known malignancy or at high risk, e.g. in patients with cirrhosis. Some authors, however, have found that follow-up imaging is not necessary in patients at low risk.

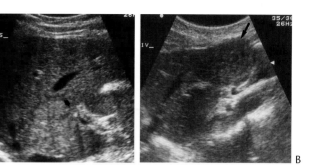

Fig. 25.101 Two lesions in the same patient proved to be due to focal nodular hyperplasia. One deep within liver parenchyma (arrow) is slightly hyper-reflective (A). The other, causing a focal hump on the left lobe (arrow) of the liver, is of similar reflectivity to normal liver parenchyma (B).

Focal nodular hyperplasia

Focal nodular hyperplasia is a tumour-like condition with a central fibrous scar surrounded by nodules of hyperplastic hepatocytes and small bile ductules. Vessels course through the tumour and are most abundant in the central scar. On ultrasound it appears as a well-defined mass of hypo-, iso- or hyper-reflectivity relative to normal liver (Fig. 25.101). A central scar may be visible. High-velocity flow may be detectable within the lesion.

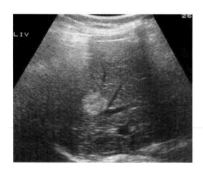

Fig. 25.99 Cavernous haemangioma measuring less than 2 cm in diameter demonstrates the typical features of a well-defined hyper-reflective mass with some posterior acoustic enhancement.

Hepatic adenomas

Hepatic adenomas are composed of hepatocytes but lack portal tracts. They may be of similar reflectivity to normal liver (Fig. 25.102A). They are of variable size, with a propensity to haemorrhage and necrosis. These produce areas of decreased reflectivity within a hyper-reflective tumour (Fig. 25.102B). Fresh haemorrhage will cause fluid areas (Fig. 25.102C). Colour Doppler US demonstrates peripheral arteries and veins. Intratumoural veins may also be seen. This finding is absent in FNH and may be used to discriminate between the two. Rarely hepatic adenomas may be multiple (Fig. 25.102).

Nodular regenerative hyperplasia

Nodular regenerative hyperplasia is rare. Many small nodules are seen and may be confused with metastatic disease and cirrhosis. It is associated with myeloproliferative and lymphoproliferative syndromes, chronic vascular disorders, rheumatological disorders, systemic lupus erythematosus, steroids and following chemotherapy. It may lead to portal hypertension.

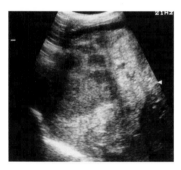

Fig. 25.100 There is a heterogeneous mass with some free fluid around the liver. This was subsequently shown to be a large haemangioma which had bled.

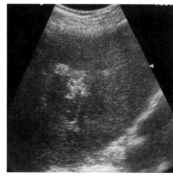

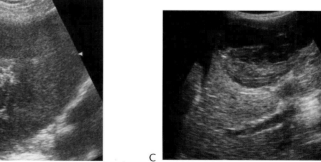

Fig. 25.102 Ultrasound examination of a patient presenting with right upper quadrant pain and shock due to haemorrhage within an adenoma. Multiple lesions are seen. (A) demonstrates a lesion of similar reflectivity to normal liver with a further area of mixed reflectivity (B). Bleeding had occurred in a superficial lesion (C). The patient later underwent resection of this lesion.

Hepatic **lipomas and angiomyolipomas** are seen in 10% of patients with tuberose sclerosis. They are highly reflective lesions resembling haemangiomas.

Infantile haemangioendothelioma

Infantile haemangioendothelioma is a relatively common tumour in childhood that may produce cardiac failure but slowly involutes with time. Single or multiple lesions may be seen with variable reflectivity. There may be large draining veins.

Abscess

Bacterial hepatic abscess

Bacterial hepatic abscess can develop via five major routes: biliary, portal vein, hepatic artery, direct extension from contiguous organs, and traumatic. Necrotic hepatic metastases may also become infected. Pyogenic abscesses have a variable contour on ultrasound. The abscess wall is typically hyporeflective and irregular. Early lesions tend to be hyperreflective and may be difficult to see. The contents of an abscess may be anechoic (50%), hyper-reflective (25%) or hyporeflective (25%). The internal contents may show debris, fluid levels and septations. Posterior acoustic enhancement may be present (Figs 25.103, 25.104). Gas, if present, will appear as brightly reflective areas with posterior reverberation.

Approximately 10% of the world's population is infected by *Entamoeba histolytica*. Of these, 3–7% will develop hepatic **amoebic abscess**, which is the commonest extraintestinal manifestation of this parasite. It is usually seen as a well-defined round or ovoid mass lying peripherally, containing homogeneous fine low-level echoes seen at high gain settings with some distal acoustic enhancement (Fig. 25.105). More than 90% of hepatic amoebic abscesses respond to antimicrobial therapy. Guided ultrasound intervention may be required to establish the diagnosis, for a large

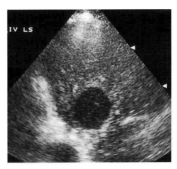

Fig. 25.105 A well-defined area close to the diaphragm containing fine low-level echoes and some posterior acoustic enhancement in a pyrexial patient with a recent history of foreign travel proved to be due to an amoebic abscess.

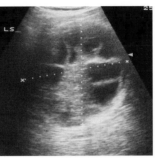

Fig. 25.106 The spokewheel appearance of a hydatid cyst.

symptomatic abscess, for patients who fail to respond to treatment, suspected superadded bacterial infection, in pregnancy, and as an alternative to surgery when an abscess ruptures. Amoebic abscess is more likely to have a round or ovoid shape than a pyogenic abscess (82 versus 60%) and a hypoechoic appearance with fine low-level echoes (58 versus 36%).

Hydatid

Most patients acquire **hydatid** (*Echinococcus granulosus* and *E. multilocularis*) disease in childhood but the are not diagnosed until the third or fourth decade, when they slowly enlarging echinococcal cysts become symptomatic. On ultrasound a cyst may appear as a well-defined anechoic cyst, an anechoic cyst with debris, a multiseptate cyst with daughter cysts (Fig. 25.106) and echogenic material between the cysts, a cyst with an undulating membrane (the waterlily sign) or a densely calcified mass. Response to medical therapy includes reduction in cyst size, membrane detachment, progressive increase in cyst reflectivity and wall calcification. *E. multilocularis* is the less common but more aggressive form: irregular necrotic regions may be seen, microcalcification and biliary obstruction are common, with spread to the hepatic hilum.

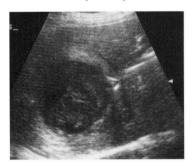

Fig. 25.103 Thick-walled abscess containing mixed reflectivity material with a little through transmission. *Enterococcus* and *Streptococcus* species were grown from the pus aspirated under ultrasound guidance.

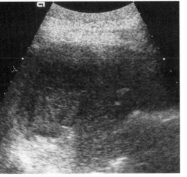

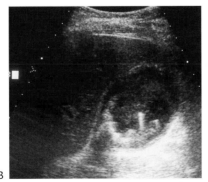

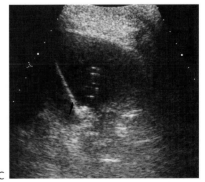

Fig. 25.104 An ill-defined area of decreased reflectivy in a pyrexial patient demonstrates some posterior acoustic enhancement (A). The adjacent gallbladder was also abnormal (B). The abscess was successfully drained by inserting a pigtail catheter (arrow) which can be seen within the abscess (C).

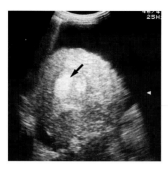

Fig. 25.107 A predominantly hyper-reflective mass (arrow) within a cirrhotic liver due to a hepatoma.

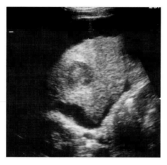

Fig. 25.108 A mixed reflectivity mass within a cirrhotic liver due to a hepatoma.

Hepatic candidiasis is becoming more common with increasing chemotherapy and AIDS. Blood cultures are positive in only 50% of patients. Four different patterns may be seen on ultrasound: a central necrotic hyporeflective nidus with a reflective rim surrounded by a peripheral zone (the wheel within a wheel); a bull's eye lesion, a small 1–4 mm lesion with a hyper-reflective centre and surrounding hyporeflective rim, seen when the neutrophil count returns to normal; uniformly hyporeflective; and hyper-reflective.

Malignant focal liver lesions

Hepatocellular cancer

Hepatocellular cancer is the commonest primary liver tumour. The ultrasound appearance is varied (Figs 25.107, 25.108). Fatty change within the tumour will cause it to have areas of increased reflectivity. Small (<3 cm) lesions are often hyporeflective and may demonstrate posterior acoustic enhancement. Larger tumours are often more heterogeneous (mosaic pattern) in appearance. The tumours may invade portal (Fig. 25.109) and hepatic veins. Tumour thrombus within these vessels may demonstrate neovascularity detectable on colour flow Doppler. Necrosis and haemorrhage within the tumour will add to the heterogeneous appearance. A capsule, if present, is thin and hporeflective. Most tumours will show central vascularity (Fig. 25.110). Power Doppler has been shown to be useful and more sensitive in the detection of tumour vascularity and ultrasound contrast-enhanced power Doppler may improve this further. Underlying cirrhosis or haemochromatosis should be sought.

Fibrolamellar carcinoma

Fibrolamellar carcinoma arises in a normal liver, with only 20% of patients having underlying cirrhosis. It has a better prognosis than hepatocellular carcinoma and occurs in a younger age group. The mass is usually large and hyper-reflective on ultrasound. Calcification is frequently seen.

Hepatoblastoma

Hepatoblastoma is the most common primary childhood liver tumour. A hyper-reflective mass is seen on ultrasound, with areas of calcification. Haemorrhage and necrosis may be present as areas of increased and decreased reflectivity. Neovascularity is typical, with high-frequency Doppler signals being seen.

Intrahepatic cholangiocarcinomas

Intrahepatic cholangiocarcinomas account for 10% of biliary duct cancers, with the remainder occurring at the liver hilum (Klatskin's tumour). The tumours are often large at presentation, calcification may be present, and the tumours rarely exhibit haemorrhage or necrosis, appearing homogeneous on ultrasound and usually hyporeflective.

Angiosarcoma

Angiosarcoma appears as single or multiple hyper-reflective masses that are often heterogeneous on ultrasound.

Hepatic lymphoma

Hepatic lymphoma can be primary (rare) or secondary and can be caused by Hodgkin's and non-Hodgkin's lymphoma. Liver involvement may be focal, with hypoechoic masses, or diffuse, when the liver parenchyma may appear normal or be diffusely abnormal.

Hepatic metastases

Hepatic metastases have an extremely variable appearance on ultrasound. Hyper-reflective lesions are seen from colorectal cancer and other gastrointestinal primaries. Vascular metastases, for example from carcinoid, islet cell tumours and renal cancer will also be hyper-reflective (Figs 25.111, 25.112). This is due to the many interfaces from the abnormal vessels. Hypoechoic metastases are seen in lymphoma and sarcoma. Most adenocarcinomas, such as breast, lung and pancreas, give rise to well-defined hypoechoic lesions. The bull's eye or target lesion is often seen in bronchogenic carcinoma metastases (Figs 25.113, 25.114). There is a thin, poorly defined halo around a solid liver lesion. Cystic metastases usually

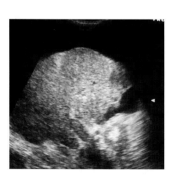

Fig. 25.109 A cirrhotic liver with multifocal hepatoma and portal vein tumour thrombus.

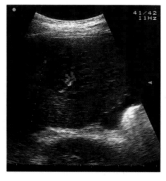

Fig. 25.110 Abnormal colour flow is seen within this focal liver lesion: a hepatoma.

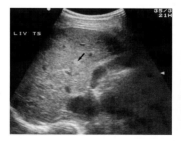

Fig. 25.111 A hyper-reflective metastasis (arrow) in a patient with carcinoid.

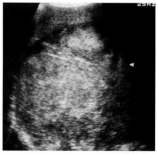

Fig. 25.112 A larger mixed but predominantly hyperreflective metastasis in a patient with a neuroendocrine pancreatic primary.

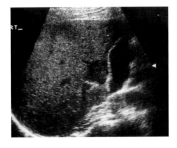

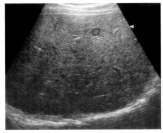

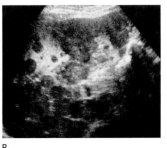

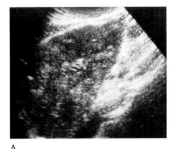

Fig. 25.113 A metastasis with an ill-defined halo (arrow) and solid centre.

Fig. 25.114 A metastasis demonstrating a better-defined target lesion from a gastrinoma.

Fig. 25.117 (A) Precontrast the liver of this patient with breast cancer has a heterogeneous echotexture. (B) After intravenous contrast (Levovist) with pulse inversion mode there is better definition of metastatic disease. (Courtesy of Shetal Patel.)

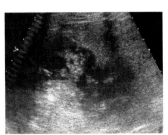

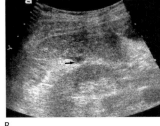

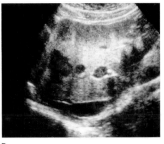

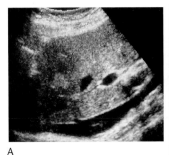

Fig. 25.115 (A) A cystic metastasis with some calcification from ovarian cancer. (B) A small subcapsular (arrow) deposit from ovarian cancer in the same patient.

Fig. 25.118 (A) Precontrast a single echogenic breast metastasis may be mistaken for a haemangioma. (B) Postcontrast (Levovist and pulse inversion mode) there is no microbubble uptake in the lesion, confirming the presence of a metastasis rather than a haemangioma.

develop in patients who have a primary lesion with a cystic component, for example ovarian cancer or cystadenocarcinoma of the pancreas (Fig. 25.115). Calcification, which may be recognised by the marked reflectivity and acoustic shadowing, is most often seen in metastases from mucinous adenocarcinoma of the colon (Fig. 25.116) but may be seen in others. As lesions increase in size, they will tend to become more heterogeneous in appearance and the presence of haemorrhage, necrosis or infection will alter the ultrasound findings. Diffuse infiltration can be difficult to recognise. Fatty infiltration can also cause problems and may be seen following chemotherapy. It may result in a deposit having apparent posterior acoustic enhancement with the metastasis attenuating the ultrasound beam less than the surrounding fatty liver (Fig. 25.80).

Ultrasound contrast agents have been used to improve the sensitivity of ultrasound for the detection of liver metastases (Fig. 25.117) and is a current area of research. Focal liver lesions have been found to have little or no signal when the liver is imaged relatively late (more than 5 min) after administration of a microbubble ultrasound contrast agent if the phenomenon of SAE is exploited. This technique has revealed metastases not visible on grey-scale images. They may have a role in lesion characterisation (Fig. 25.118). Another technique is to use ultrasound microbubble

contrast agents to measure the vascular transit through the liver by performing spectral Doppler study of a hepatic vein following bolus intravenous injection. Many patients with metastatic disease have been found to have a rapid transit time, which is thought to be due to arterialisation of the liver blood supply and to the presence of vascular shunts.

Ultrasound of the liver transplant

Improvements in immunosuppression and in the treatment of complications following transplantation have made this technique the preferred treatment for patients with non-malignant end-stage liver disease.

The use of transplantation for patients with malignant tumours, and for patients in whom the disease processes are likely to recur following transplantation, is more controversial.

Preoperative assessment

Patients are assessed prior to transplantation in order to stage any known malignancy and to detect any development of hepatocellular cancer within a cirrhotic liver, or cholangiocarcinoma in patients with sclerosing cholangitis. Malignancy beyond the liver is a contraindication to liver transplantation and should be excluded. The vascular anatomy should be delineated prior to surgery, and patency or otherwise of the portal vein, hepatic veins and IVC is assessed. The presence of any collateral vessels due to portal hypertension should be documented. The initial assessment can be carried out with ultrasound; the size of the native liver may be assessed and

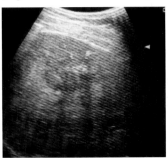

Fig. 25.116 A treated metastasis from colorectal cancer exhibiting areas of calcification and an underlying fatty liver.

focal textural abnormalities noted. It can be very difficult with ultrasound to distinguish between cirrhotic nodules and hepato-cellular cancer. If a suspicious nodule is identified, then CT or MRI is indicated.

Vessel patency is often easily assessed using ultrasound. It may be necessary to use a low-frequency probe, e.g. 2.5 MHz probe. It can be difficult with ultrasound to distinguish between a *balanced flow situation* and a portal vein thrombosis. These can usually be distinguished using either CT or MRI. Portal vein thrombosis is a relative or absolute contraindication to transplantation, depending on the level of thrombosis within the mesenteric vein.

In patients with sclerosing cholangitis, preoperative assessment should exclude significant biliary obstruction, which may be due to the presence of an occult cholangiocarcinoma. Biliary obstruction, if identified, can be further investigated with targeted biopsies or endoscopic brushings.

Vascular anastomoses

Four vascular anastomoses are performed during operation: *supra-hepatic* and *infrahepatic caval* anastomoses, the *portal venous* anastomosis and the *hepatic arterial* anastomosis. This latter anas-tomosis is technically the most difficult.

The anatomy of the arterial anastomosis varies according to the donor and recipient vessel arrangement. Knowledge of this is essen-tial when performing postoperative ultrasound assessment.

Biliary anastomosis

The preferred biliary anastomosis in patients with normal bile ducts is a choledochocholedochostomy (donor bile duct to recipient bile duct). A Roux-en-Y choledochojejunostomy is performed in patients with abnormal bile ducts, e.g. those with sclerosing cholan-gitis. In the past, other types of biliary–enteric anastomosis have been performed, including choledochoduodenostomy, cholecysto-jejunostomy, and reconstructions using the gallbladder as a conduit between the donor and recipient bile duct.

Complications

Complications following liver transplantation may be related to the vascular anastomoses, the biliary anastomosis, postoperative sepsis, and other non-technical complications such as renal dysfunction, neurological complications and systemic infections. Rejection remains a common complication.

In the early postoperative period, *hepatic arterial thrombosis* remains an important complication. It is our current practice to examine all liver transplants with ultrasound, including colour and duplex Doppler, in the first 24 h following transplantation. During this investigation, flow is confirmed within the hepatic artery, the portal vein, the IVC and hepatic veins. Liver texture, which should be homogeneous, is noted and any fluid collections identified.

Other signs of hepatic arterial thrombosis include focal lesions in the liver which may be due either to small *abscesses* (Fig. 25.119) or to small *bile leaks*. Abnormal increased reflectivity may also be seen within the biliary ducts. Extrahepatic bile leaks/collections should also be sought. Collateral vessel formation can occur after hepatic artery thrombosis. These vessels may display a lower resis-tive index and can be otherwise mistaken for the main hepatic artery.

Portal vein thrombosis is less common after adult liver transplant but portal vein *stenosis* can occur (Fig. 25.120) and give rise to the symptoms of portal hypertension. *Hepatic vein thrombosis* is more common in paediatric liver transplants where there may be difficulty in obtaining the correct size of donor organ for the recipi-ent. Cutdowns are used in this situation but, despite this, hepatic vein angulation and occlusion can occur. Significant *stenosis of the inferior vena cava* may lead to the development of ascites; this can be assessed initially with Doppler ultrasound, when high-velocity jets may be seen on colour flow and duplex Doppler. This is usually then confirmed with phlebography. Angioplasty can be used to treat it.

Bile leaks usually occur in the early postoperative period and are frequently seen as collections close to the porta hepatis. Aspiration can confirm the nature of the collection and ultrasound-guided drainage may allow stabilisation before surgery or other treatment. Other postoperative collections occur fairly commonly following liver transplantation. These are seen in the subhepatic space, the subphrenic space and posterior to the left lobe of the liver. Routine diagnostic aspiration of these collections is not advised unless infection is considered likely.

Biliary obstruction may be caused by anastomotic or non-anastomotic strictures, stones or sludge in the ducts, papillary dys-function, and cystic duct mucocoele. Non-anastomotic strictures are often intrahepatic and may be related to ischaemia, infection or pos-sibly recurrent sclerosing cholangitis. Some units have found an increased incidence with a long cold ischaemic time. Ultrasound usually demonstrates dilated ducts and may indicate the cause, but

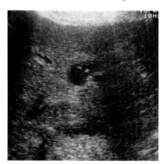

Fig. 25.119 A small abscess in a patient with hepatic artery throm-bosis after liver transplantation. Increased periportal reflectivity is also seen.

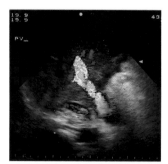

Fig. 25.120 Colour flow Doppler study of the portal vein following liver transplantation demonstrates increased flow with aliasing in the donor portal vein upstream from a mild anastomotic stenosis.

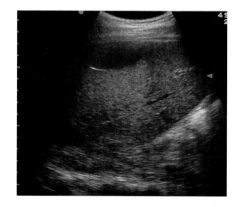

Fig. 25.121 Longitudinal scan of the right lobe of the liver performed shortly after a percutaneous liver biopsy demonstrates a subcapsular collec-tion due to haematoma.

some cases have persistent dilated ducts with no actual obstruction. A sclerosing cholangitis pattern may not be detected by ultrasound so direct cholangiography is still necessary in many cases of suspected biliary complications.

The transplant liver may be biopsied to assess the presence of rejection. *Postbiopsy complications* include subcapsular haematomas, (Fig. 25.121) and intrahepatic and perihepatic haematomas. The biopsy can also lead to the formation of fistulas between the portal tract, hepatic artery and hepatic veins. Haemobilia may be another complication caused by percutaneous liver biopsy.

Transjugular intrahepatic portosystemic shunt (TIPSS)

This has been a successful tool in the management of portal hypertension. Ultrasound is used before the procedure is performed to verify the presence of chronic liver disease and to assess the patency of portal and hepatic veins and IVC. Cavernous transformation of the portal vein or portal vein thrombosis may preclude the placement of a TIPS unless there is a large suitably-placed collateral vessel. Ultrasound is often used during the stent insertion.

Portal venous blood flow and diameter increase following successful TIPS insertion. Flow velocities are high within the shunt, with velocities of 135–200 cm/s seen in well-functioning shunts (Fig. 25.122). Ultrasound has been shown to perform well compared with angiographic studies in the follow-up of patients with TIPS. The absence of detectable flow is diagnostic of stent occlusion. A peak stent velocity of less than 60 cm/s has been said to be indicative of hepatic vein stenosis. Reversal of flow in the proximal portion of the hepatic vein can also indicate hepatic vein stenosis. Comparison of peak velocities over time has been shown to be the best detector of stenoses, ultrasound having a sensitivity of 93% and specificity of 77% if either an increase or decrease of 50 cm/s in the peak stent velocity is taken as an indicator.

The spleen

The spleen is best scanned with the patient lying in a right lateral decubitus position. Intercostal scanning is usually necessary to demonstrate the normal-sized spleen. The normal parenchyma has homogeneous reflectivity that is slightly brighter than the normal liver. The spleen can be measured using a maximum length from upper to lower pole, which should not exceed 13 cm.

Accessory spleen is congenital ectopic splenic tissue occurring in 10–30% of the population. Most are seen as small well-defined nodules of tissue of identical reflectivity to the normal spleen lying near the splenic hilum. They may be found anywhere within the abdomen or retroperitoneum, especially related to the tail of the pancreas. The accessory tissue is usually supplied by a branch of the splenic artery with venous drainage into splenic veins. Eighty-eight per cent of patients have a single focus, with 9% having two foci, and 3% having multiple foci which are usually clustered together.

Polysplenia syndrome is characterised by multiple splenic masses in patients with bilateral left-sidedness. The number of splenic masses varies from 2 to 16 and may occur in the right and left upper quadrants. *Splenosis* is autotransplantation of the spleen which usually occurs as a result of trauma.

Splenic infarction is most commonly due to embolism from cardiovascular disease followed by local thrombosis from haematological disorders. On ultrasound, infarcts tend to be hyporeflective to areflective in the acute phase and are usually wedge-shaped and peripheral in location (Fig. 25.123) but they may be rounded with well-defined or irregular margins. The delineation of the infarct from the normal spleen improves as the age of the infarct increases. Eventually infarcts appear as areas of increased reflectivity with atrophy due to scarring.

Splenic abscess is common but the frequency of this condition has grown as a result of an increasing number of immunosuppressed patients. Infection can result from metastatic infection, e.g.

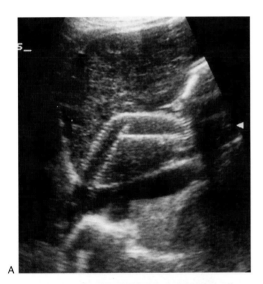

A

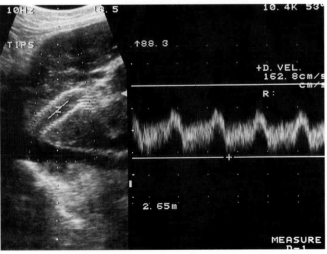

B

Fig. 25.122 (A) Longitudinal scan through the liver demonstrating a TIPSS entering the IVC via the hepatic vein. (B) Velocity measurements demonstrate a patent TIPSS with normal flow.

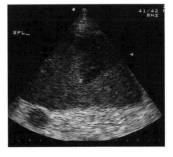

Fig. 25.123 Ultrasound of the spleen demonstrates a peripheral wedge-shaped area of low reflectivity and lack of power flow consistent with a splenic infarct in a patient with splenomegaly, portal hypertension and left upper quadrant pain.

subacute bacterial endocarditis and sepsis from infected adjacent organs, such as the kidney and pancreas, from superinfection of splenic infarcts, following trauma, and in the immunocompromised patient. The appearance of a splenic abscess on ultrasound depends upon the stage of development. Early in the course, an ill-defined mass of decreased reflectivity may be seen which will develop fluid components, debris and septation. A capsule will develop in later stages and gas within the abscess will be seen as focal areas of high reflectivity with acoustic shadowing.

There is a wide differential diagnosis for the ultrasound appearances, particularly in the early stage of development when splenic lymphoma and metastases may mimic splenic abscess. Infarction and haematoma may also have a similar appearance. Fungal microabscesses occur in immunocompromised patients. On ultrasound they appear as central areas of increased reflectivity surrounded by a rim of decreased reflectivity. If necrosis occurs centrally, the centre then becomes of decreased reflectivity and may have a 'wheel within a wheel' appearance. Fungal abscesses can alternatively appear uniformly hyper-reflective.

Infection by tuberculosis may also give rise to splenic abscesses. In the miliary form, the lesions may not be identified with ultrasound. As they increase in size, they appear as small focal or hyporeflective lesions. Healed granulomas containing calcium will be recognised by the increased reflectivity and posterior acoustic shadowing. Hyporeflective splenic lesions in patients with AIDS include lymphoma, disseminated Kaposi's sarcoma, mycobacterial, fungal and pneumocystis infection.

Pneumocystis carinii infection may give rise to *splenomegaly*, and very small highly reflective non-shadowing foci or small hyper-reflective lesions with cystic components may be seen. In the later stages of disease, ultrasound may demonstrate confluent reflective masses with acoustic shadowing. Hyporeflective masses may demonstrate reflective rims. Splenic involvement by hydatid disease is uncommon. Cystic masses with a multiloculated internal structure (the endocyst will be seen as in hepatic infestation).

Splenomegaly occurs in a significant proportion of patients with sarcoidosis. The splenic parenchyma may exhibit diffusely increased reflectivity and/or focal hyper-reflective or mixed reflectivity lesions may be present. Diffuse increased splenic reflectivity may also be seen in leukaemia, polycythaemia, tuberculosis, malaria and brucellosis.

Splenomegaly may be seen in portal hypertension from any cause. Ultrasound is an accurate means of measuring this. Splenomegaly can result from congestion, infiltrative disease, haematological disorder, inflammatory disease, rheumatic disease, cysts or tumours.

The ultrasound findings of true *splenic cysts*, i.e. those which contain a cellular lining, and false splenic cysts, i.e. those without a cellular lining, are similar. The cysts will present on ultrasound as a well-defined anechoic structure with a well-defined rounded margin and posterior acoustic enhancement. Both true and false cysts may have some low-level internal echoes. True cysts are either parasitic (echinococcal) or epidermoid in origin. False cysts are thought to be due to previous splenic infarction, infection or trauma. Splenic cysts may be mimicked by fluid collections related to pancreatitis, or by cystic metastases from melanoma, adenocarcinoma of the breast and ovary.

Malignant lesions of the spleen are much less common than those involving the liver. Lymphoma is the most common malignant tumour of the spleen. Primary splenic lymphoma without evi-

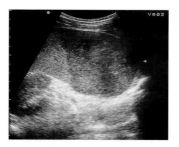

Fig. 25.124 Ultrasound of the spleen in a patient with post-transplant lymphoproliferative disorder demonstrating diffuse involvement of the tip of the spleen.

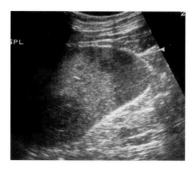

Fig. 25.125 Focal splenic deposits in a patient with chronic lymphocytic leukaemia.

dence of nodal disease is uncommon and occurs in only 1% of all cases of non-Hodgkin's lymphoma. On ultrasound, splenic lymphoma shows either a diffuse or focal hyporeflective pattern. Abnormal ultrasound of the spleen may be found in 4–15% of patients with Hodgkin's disease and non-Hodgkin's lymphoma (Figs 25.124, 25.125). Focal splenic disease occurs more commonly in AIDS-related lymphomas than in lymphomas without AIDS. Again, ultrasound will show either uniform decreased reflectivity or focal hyporeflective lesions in these patients.

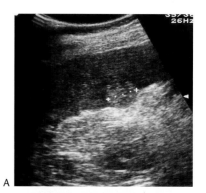

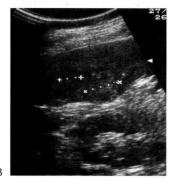

Fig. 25.126 (A, B) Mixed reflectivity splenic metastases in a patient with ovarian cancer.

Splenic involvement by *metastatic disease* is uncommon, occurring in approximately 7% of patients with malignancy at autopsy. The most likely primary tumours are breast, lung, ovary, stomach, melanoma and prostate. Splenic metastases from melanoma are often multiple, either solid or cystic. As in the liver, the ultrasound appearances of metastatic disease are extremely variable (Fig. 25.126). Other cystic splenic metastases include ovary, breast and endometrium. Direct invasion of the spleen may occur from large tumours involving adjacent organs, such as the stomach, pancreas, left kidney and adrenals. Peritoneal seedlings, most often from ovarian cancer, can also be seen around the spleen.

MAGNETIC RESONANCE IMAGING OF THE LIVER AND SPLEEN

Abdominal MRI developed more slowly than applications in the CNS, musculoskeletal system and heart for two main reasons: first, other imaging techniques are well established and effective in the investigation of upper abdominal disease; and, second, the anatomical detail available with conventional spin-echo MRI was limited by motion artefact from respiration and peristalsis. The development of breath-hold imaging techniques has largely overcome the latter problem, and the superior contrast resolution of MRI when combined with the judicious use of oral, intravenous and liver-specific contrast media has led to the emerging superiority of MRI over other techniques in many clinical applications in the upper abdomen. Specific MRI procedures can be designed to exploit differences in physicochemical and physiological properties of different tissues as well as their anatomical features. MRI characteristics include:

- *Morphology.* The size, shape, position and internal structure of the lesion, the character of its margin, and any signs of spread into adjacent structures
- *Physicochemical composition.* Water content, fat content, presence of blood and other proteinaceous fluids
- *Perfusion and local extracellular fluid volume.* The rate, pattern and persistence of enhancement after intravenous gadolinium gives a useful indication of local blood flow
- *Cellular function.* Tissue-specific contrast media are used to investigate the function of both major liver cell populations: superparamagnetic iron oxide (SPIO) particles are taken up by the reticuloendothelial cells within liver and spleen, while the presence of hepatocytes both in normal liver and in liver lesions may be identified by their uptake of gadolinium-BOPTA, gadolinium-EOB-DTPA, or manganese-DPDP.

MRI is not appropriate as a first-line routine technique as many liver imaging problems can be assessed satisfactorily using ultrasound or computed tomography (CT). However, MRI is more sensitive than CT or ultrasound in detecting small lesions, and is also more specific in the characterisation of various pathologies. Liver MRI is best used in problem cases where ultrasound or CT findings are equivocal or unexpected, and as a 'one-stop shopping' approach in patients who are surgical candidates for liver resection or transplantation.

Techniques

Choice of sequences
A basic liver examination will include images with T_1 and T_2 weighting. As in other aspects of radiology, a trade-off has to be made between spatial resolution, contrast resolution and temporal resolution. T_1-weighted images give us the greatest magnitude of signal and therefore the best information density and spatial resolution. T_2-weighted images provide high contrast between normal parenchyma and tissues with a high water content. The liver is subject to respiratory motion so breath-holding techniques should be used routinely. Flow and pulsation artefacts can be reduced by using motion compensation (e.g. gradient moment nulling) or presaturation bands above and below the liver. If available, a phased-array body surface coil should be used.

Fast spin echo
Fast spin echo (FSE), also known as turbospin echo (TSE) or RARE, uses a train of $180°$ refocusing pulses after the initial $90°$ pulse in order to obtain multiple echoes producing several different phase-encoding steps within a single repetition time. This allows considerable reduction in the acquisition time for a T_2-weighted sequence, or conversely the time saved can be used to acquire more signal averages. The effective use of a long echo train requires a much longer repetition time than with conventional spin-echo imaging, so T_1 weighting is further diminished. The signal from fat on FSE is much brighter than on conventional spin echo (CSE), due to j-coupling, so fat-suppression techniques are required. In most applications of MRI, FSE sequences are preferred to spin echo or gradient echo (GRE) for unenhanced T_2 because they give good resolution with fairly short acquisition time. In the liver, FSE T_2 is adequate for initial screening, but it is unsafe to rely on FSE sequences with a long echo train for detecting liver tumours because contrast is less with FSE than on T_2-weighted spin echo, largely due to magnetisation transfer (MT) effects, which are more marked in tumours than in the normal liver, causing liver–lesion contrast to be reduced. Further, blurring of short T_2 tissues occurs with FSE because the high spatial frequencies which define image detail are obtained late in the acquisition when the signal has decayed to a low amplitude. GRE T_2 images with SPIO are preferred for detecting small lesions. For initial screening of the liver, FSE images should be obtained with a repetition time (TR) of approximately 3000 ms and a moderate echo time (TE) of 80–100 ms. FSE-STIR sequences may be used in place of T_2W FSE. For lesion characterisation, heavily T_2W images are helpful to distinguish benign and malignant hepatic lesions. To avoid overlap between the SI characteristics on T_2W images of solid lesions (particularly hypervascular metastases) and haemangiomas, TE must be ~ 180 ms. T_2 FSE with an echo train length (ETL) of ~ 29 to facilitate breath-holding is suitable for lesion characterisation. MT effects, which cause a fall in signal intensity, occur in solid tumours and to a lesser extent in normal liver parenchyma, but not in cysts or haemangiomas. MT effects in FSE sequences increase with the ETL, so a T_2W FSE acquisition with a long ETL can be valuable in discriminating benign from malignant lesions. Single-shot fast spin-echo techniques (e.g. HASTE) are also helpful in distinguishing benign and malignant lesions. HASTE is a single-slice technique so MT effects are insignificant, but because the duration of the echo train is 600–1200 ms there is virtually no signal from solid tissues. Consequently, benign lesions exhibit a much higher SI than tumours, which may not be visible.

Fat suppression
Frequency-selective fat suppression is achieved by applying a preparatory pulse at the resonant frequency of fat, which effectively nulls out the contribution from fat protons to the signal produced by

the subsequent spin-echo sequence. Since much of the noise produced by motion artefact arises from fat, the level of noise in the subsequent images is reduced much more than the signal from water protons. Suppressing the fat signal also allows the dynamic range of the signals from the tissues of interest to be increased, so that liver–lesion contrast and gadolinium enhancement effects are magnified.

Chemical-shift imaging

For tumours which may contain fat, or in patients with a fatty liver, the combination of *in-phase* and *opposed-phase* GRE imaging provides an effective demonstration of the local pathology. The technique exploits the slightly different resonant frequencies of fat and water protons. If a single voxel contains both fat and water protons, the signal it emits during the relaxation process will contain components of two different frequencies. At a field strength of 1.5 T, fat and water are in opposite phases at a TE of 2.2 ms, while when TE = 4.4 msec they are in phase. Voxels containing fat and water components appear brighter on in-phase images because the fat and water signals are additive, and darker on opposed-phase images where the fat and water signals tend to cancel each other out. Images obtained in-phase and out-of-phase show hardly any difference in those tissues where there is normally no fat (e.g. the liver), and those tissues in which there is normally hardly any water (e.g. subcutaneous fat).

Gadolinium enhancement

A dynamic GRE T_1-weighted series following intravenous injection of a gadolinium chelate is almost always helpful for lesion characterisation, and is probably better than unenhanced T_2 imaging for the early detection of small liver lesions. As with fast CT, the advantages of intravenous contrast (gadolinium) in upper abdominal MR are most apparent when rapid sequential acquisitions are made. Hypervascular lesions are best demonstrated at the arterial phase of enhancement (the central lines of k-space should be acquired 10–15 s from the end of injection), whereas hypovascular lesions are best demonstrated 20–50 s after contrast injection. Delayed images 2–10 min after injection may be useful in lesions with a fibrous tissue component, e.g. haemangiomas and cholangiocarcinomas, and to show peripheral wash-out in malignant lesions. The shortest possible TE should be selected for dynamic imaging to facilitate the acquisition of enough slices to cover the entire liver in a breath-hold period. 3D sequences give a higher SNR and thinner effective slice thickness than 2D methods. Demonstration of portal venous anatomy in most patients is clear enough to eliminate the need for angiography in surgical liver cases and the origin of the hepatic arteries can also be demonstrated on early acquisitions, useful in liver transplant candidates.

Vascular studies

Rapid dynamic gadolinium-enhanced gradient-echo T_1 images can demonstrate the vascular structures simultaneously with the liver parenchyma and associated mass lesions. A hybrid technique using a time-of-flight (TOF) MR angiographic (MRA) method with gadolinium enhancement may have further advantages. The direction of flow in major vessels can be demonstrated by the technique of bolus tracking, which uses a series of rapid acquisitions to follow the movement of high-signal (gadolinium-labelled) blood across a presaturation band placed perpendicular to the vessel of interest.

Liver-specific contrast media
Kupffer cell agents

Superparamagnetic iron oxide (SPIO) particles in the size range of 30–200 nm are selectively taken up by the reticuloendothelial cells in the liver, spleen and bone marrow. The effect of SPIO is to produce a marked shortening of T_2^*, causing a marked reduction in signal intensity on all sequences, but particularly on proton density and T_2-weighted images. This magnifies the contrast between normal liver and intrahepatic tumours, so lesions become more conspicuous. Side-effects are few and relatively mild. The only liver neoplasm which consistently contains functioning reticuloendothelial cells is focal nodular hyperplasia, although some liver cell adenomas and well-differentiated hepatocellular carcinoma (HCC) may contain a few of these cells. A substantial drop in tumour signal intensity on T_2-weighted images after SPIO indicates a benign pathology. Because susceptibility effects are more apparent on GRE than on spin echo or FSE, the signal loss induced by SPIO is more marked on T_2W GRE than on SE sequences. Breath-hold sequences with motion compensation are essential for optimum imaging with SPIO because respiratory artefacts are eliminated and scanning time is reduced.

Hepatocyte agents

Protein-bound chelates of gadolinium (Gd) and manganese (Mn) are approximately analogous to biliary iodinated contrast media, being actively extracted from circulating blood and producing increased signal on T_1-weighted images in areas containing functioning hepatocytes. In the first few minutes after injection, the predominant effect is in the extracellular fluid space, so contrast between liver and tumours may be reduced at this stage. As blood levels fall, increasing contrast develops between normal liver tissue (high signal) and tumour (low signal). Clinical studies with *gadobenate* (Gd-BOPTA), gadoxetic acid (Gd-EOB-DTPA) and *mangafodipir* (Mn-DPDP) suggest improved visibility of mass lesions 30–60 min after injection. The contrast effect is maintained between 30 min and 4 h after injection. Cysts, haemangiomas and metastases which contain no functioning hepatocytes are all more conspicuous on postcontrast images. Focal lesions which contain hepatocytes, including hepatocellular carcinoma, focal nodular hyperplasia, and regenerating nodules in cirrhosis, may take up these agents, with some lesions becoming hyperintense to surrounding liver on delayed images, while others remain isointense. Using a slow rate of infusion there are few side-effects but, as with most liver-imaging agents, the incidence of adverse reactions is greater than it is with extracellular contrast media. With all T_1 agents, GRE images are better than SE images.

Technique summary

Basic liver technique should include axial T_2, and dynamic pre- and post-gadolinium T_1. The dynamic series is probably best obtained in the coronal right anterior oblique (RAO) position for preoperative cases and for demonstration of the portal system, although axial 3D acquisitions with voxel dimensions close to isotropic can offer an equivalent degree of anatomical detail. Unenhanced in-phase/opposed-phase T_1 is needed to detect fatty change. T_2 with extended TE may help to distinguish benign lesions from metastases. SPIO-enhanced GRE T_2 images are best for detecting small metastases and also (in combination with gadolinium-enhanced T_1) for distinguishing between benign and malignant hepatocellular lesions.

APPLICATIONS OF MRI IN LIVER DISEASE

These include the early detection and characterisation of focal lesions, the demonstration of diffuse liver disease and its vascular complications, preoperative planning for liver resection and transplantation, monitoring of treatment, and the early detection of recurrent disease.

Detection of focal lesions

MR techniques have been shown to be marginally better than contrast-enhanced helical CT in the early detection of small liver tumours, with SPIO-enhanced proton density or T_2-weighted imaging being the technique of choice.

Preoperative planning

MRI offers 'one-stop shopping' for assessing the local staging and resectability of liver tumours. Segmental localisation is largely defined by the major intrahepatic branches of the portal vein and by the hepatic veins, which are well shown on dynamic gadolinium-enhanced images. The extrahepatic portal venous system, including varices and spontaneous shunts, can be demonstrated by the same technique, or by MRA. The ability to acquire MR images in any plane facilitates the demonstration of surgical anatomy, particularly of the portal system, the extrahepatic bile ducts and the inferior vena cava. Combining gadolinium and SPIO enhancement maximises the ability to detect and characterise liver lesions.

Monitoring and detecting recurrence

The early recognition of recurrent disease remains a difficult problem in oncology generally, but the superior contrast resolution of MRI compared with CT offers advantages in some cases.

Diffuse liver disease

The combination of in-phase and opposed-phase T_1-weighted GRE images allows a demonstration of focal fatty change, focal lesions within a fatty liver, and the detection of fat elements within mass lesions. Iron deposits in the liver produce a striking reduction in signal intensity on all sequences which increases with longer TE, so that the effect is more marked on in-phase than opposed-phase images. In *dyserythropoietic haemochromatosis* the iron is mostly deposited in the hepatocytes and the spleen is unaffected until the later stages, whereas in *transfusional iron overload* the iron is stored in reticulo-endothelial cells, so both liver and spleen show marked signal loss. The liver architecture in *macronodular cirrhosis* is well shown on MR. Bands of fibrosis produce slightly increased signal on T_2 and heterogeneous early enhancement after gadolinium, while siderotic nodules in the cirrhotic liver often result in a stippled appearance with multiple foci of low signal on both T_1 and T_2 images.

Vascular disorders

Indications for MRI in portal hypertension include:

- Detecting the presence of portal hypertension, and its cause—cirrhosis, other chronic liver disorders, extrahepatic obstruction in the portal venous system, Budd–Chiari syndrome, etc.
- Demonstrating the venous anatomy—patency and direction of flow in the splenic vein, superior mesenteric vein, portal vein and its intrahepatic divisions, hepatic veins and IVC.
- Demonstrating the complications associated with portal hypertension—ascites, varices, spontaneous portosystemic shunts, flow reversal in the portal system, venous thrombosis or occlusion.
- Characterising nodules in the cirrhotic liver (see below).

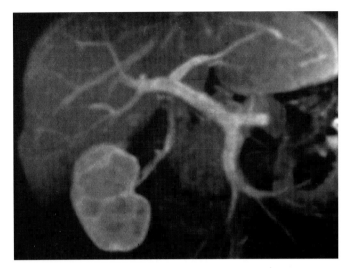

Fig. 25.127 Normal portal vein anatomy. Gd-enhanced T_1 imaging in RAO projection.

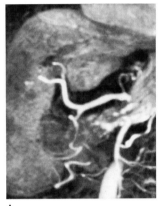 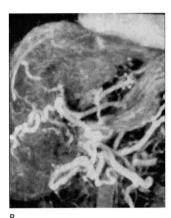

A   B

Fig. 25.128 Portal vein thrombosis. Gd-enhanced T_1 imaging in arterial and venous phases showing normal hepatic arterial supply (A) and replacement of the thrombosed portal vein by varices around the liver hilum (B).

Portal hypertension is manifest as splenomegaly and as ascites, which produces low signal on T_1 and high signal on T_2. The main vessels of the portal venous system, if patent, are brightly enhanced on postgadolinium T_1 GRE images. Demonstration of the portal vein and its branches is best achieved using the RAO plane with dynamic gadolinium-enhanced T_1 images (Figs 25.127, 25.128). This view also shows *varices* along the lesser curve of the stomach and around the porta hepatis (Fig. 25.129). The LAO view is helpful to show *perisplenic* and *peripancreatic varices*, and may also be the only non-invasive method for demonstrating *spontaneous splenorenal shunts*, which occur not infrequently in portal hypertension (Fig. 25.130). Similar results can be obtained with an axial 3D acquisition if voxel size can be reduced close to isotropic dimensions. Other common sites of varices well shown on MRI include the short gastric and right gastroepiploic veins (especially in patients with splenic vein occlusion) and the recanalised umbilical vein, which typically joins the left intrahepatic branch of the portal vein to a cluster of varices in the anterior abdominal wall.

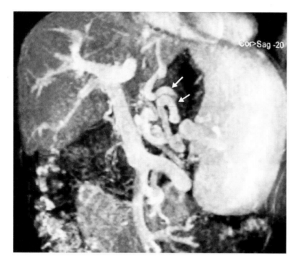

Fig. 25.129 Portal hypertension. Gd-enhanced T$_1$ imaging showing patent portal, splenic and superior mesenteric veins, but large varices along the lesser curve of the stomach (arrows).

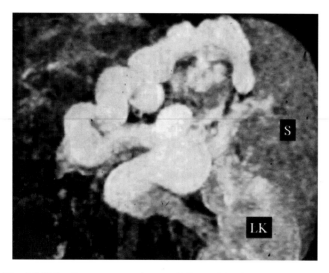

Fig. 25.130 Spontaneous splenorenal shunt. Gd-enhanced T$_1$ imaging showing huge varices draining from the hilum of the spleen to the left renal vein in a patient with portal hypertension. S = spleen; LK = left kidney.

The presence of a *TIPS shunt* is not a contraindication to MRI, although the metallic prosthesis will produce a localised area of signal drop-out on all sequences (Fig. 25.131). The *parenchymal oedema* associated with liver infarction produces low signal on T$_1$ and high signal on T$_2$ images but if *intrahepatic haemorrhage* is associated with vascular injury, patchy areas of high signal may be seen on T$_1$, as well as on T$_2$ images. The liver in *Budd–Chiari syndrome* typically shows heterogeneous perfusion with very patchy enhancement with gadolinium (Fig. 25.132). Using rapid dynamic contrast-enhanced GRE T$_1$ imaging, the thrombosed vessels may be delineated as linear areas of low signal.

Lesion characterisation

In contrast with other imaging techniques, MRI offers several different 'views' of each lesion: unenhanced T$_1$-weighted images, T$_2$-weighted images and sequential images with gadolinium enhancement. The addition of SPIO and hepatocyte-specific con-

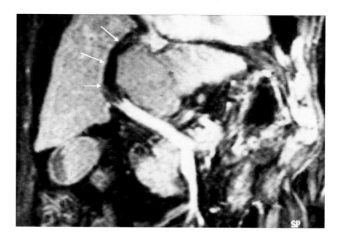

Fig. 25.131 TIPSS. Gd-enhanced T$_1$ imaging showing patent portal vein with drop-out of signal along the patent shunt (arrows).

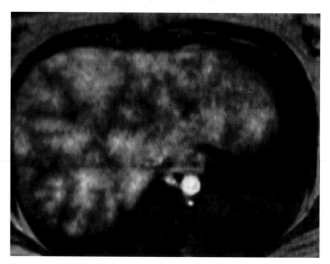

Fig. 25.132 Budd–Chiari syndrome. Gd-enhanced T$_1$ image showing typical feathery pattern of impaired perfusion.

trast media allows further discrimination of lesions containing functional liver tissue (regenerative nodules, focal nodular hyperplasia, liver cell adenoma, adenomatous hyperplasia and well-differentiated hepatocellular carcinoma) from cysts, metastases and non-functioning tumours of liver cell origin.

Cysts and cyst-like lesions

Simple liver cysts show uniform low signal on T$_1$, high signal on T$_2$, and no enhancement with gadolinium. With heavily T$_2$-weighted images (very long TE) there is little or no drop-off in signal from cysts, in contrast to metastases, which lose signal with longer TE. Small centrally placed cysts may be indistinguishable on T$_1$-weighted images from vessels seen in cross-section, so their recognition always requires a contrast-enhanced acquisition. The presence of haemorrhage or infection within a cyst will alter its signal characteristics, typically producing higher signal on T$_1$ and lower signal on T$_2$, sometimes with heterogeneity of the contents. Cystadenoma is an uncommon neoplastic lesion with an irregular cyst wall, with one or more nodules of solid tissue showing a degree of contrast enhancement (Fig. 25.133). Hydatid cysts show the morphological features well described on CT, and their proteinaceous contents typically produce high signal on both T$_1$- and

multiple cysts of various sizes. Interestingly, some patients in whom the cysts appear to be of uniform low attenuation on CT show a surprising heterogeneity of signal on T_2-weighted MR images, emphasising the greater sensitivity of MR in detecting minor differences in physicochemical composition.

Haemangioma

The typical haemangioma shows a clearly defined margin with a lobulated or geographic shape, uniform low signal on T_1 and uniform high signal on T_2. Dynamic imaging after gadolinium shows a dense peripheral discontinuous nodular blush, which begins during the arterial phase of liver perfusion and continues centripetally for several minutes so that images obtained after about 10 min often show diffuse hyperintensity of the lesion. Larger haemangiomas often contain a central core or irregular nodule of fibrous tissue which remains unenhanced even on delayed images. Small haemangiomas may show a uniform and immediate enhancement of the whole lesion. This pattern is similar to that seen with some hypervascular metastases, but these rarely become hyperintense on delayed images, and usually have lower signal on T_2 than haemangiomas. A further distinction can be made by increasing the T_2 weighting of the acquisition (using a longer TE), when haemangiomas tend to maintain a high signal while metastases lose signal. Some metastases with necrotic centres may also show centripetal

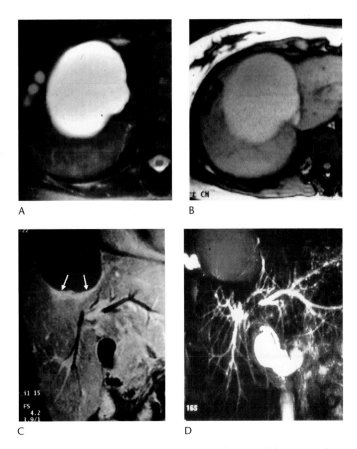

A   B

C   D

Fig. 25.133 Liver cysts and cystic tumour. Three small liver cysts show typical appearance of high signal on T_2 (A) and low signal on T_1 images (B). The large cyst appears similar on T_2, but shows high signal on T_1, indicating proteinaceous contents or haemorrhage. Gd-enhanced coronal images (C) show enhancing tumour in the wall of the large cyst (arrows). MRCP (D) shows a concurrent hilar tumour obstructing the left and right hepatic ducts.

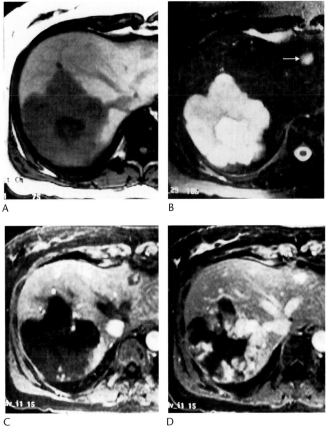

A   B

C   D

Fig. 25.135 Haemangiomas. Usual appearance of low signal on unenhanced T_1 (A) and high signal on T_2 (B) with nodular enhancement in the arterial phase (C) and more extensive enhancement in the venous phase (D). The small lesion lying close to the midline (arrow in B) shows typical features; the large right-lobe lesion contains a central core of hyalinised fibrous tissue which remains unenhanced.

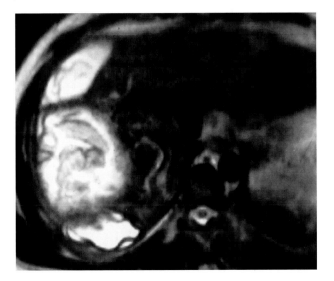

Fig. 25.134 Hydatid cysts. T_2 image shows multiple partially collapsed hydatid cysts in the right lobe producing the 'floating membrane' sign.

T_2-weighted images (Fig. 25.134). Rim enhancement with gadolinium is also characteristic. Adult polycystic disease is characterised by liver enlargement and the replacement of liver parenchyma by

enhancement after gadolinium but these lesions typically show a continuous 'rind' of enhancing tissue, rather than the nodular periphery typical of haemangiomas, and they may also show a rapid washout of contrast in the later parenchymal phase of enhancement. Atypical patterns for haemangiomas include an intense arterial-phase blush, uniform enhancement with a central vessel (central dot sign), and the presence of a large proportion of hyalinised fibrous tissue which shows little or no enhancement (Fig. 25.135).

Liver cell adenoma

This rare benign neoplasm is associated with prolonged intake of oral contraceptives or androgenic steroids, when it usually occurs as a solitary lesion. Multiple adenomas occur as a complication of glycogen storage disease. The lesions are typically heterogeneous with slightly increased signal on T_2, the signal on T_1 being hypo-, hyper- or isointense with adjacent liver (Fig. 25.136). Other features include a fibrous capsule in some cases and occasionally areas of fat within the lesion. The usual clinical presentation results from bleeding into the lesion so larger adenomas often show evidence of recent or previous haemorrhage. The lesions are well vascularised and typically show a dense but heterogeneous blush, which appears during the arterial phase of perfusion after intravenous gadolinium. Uptake of liver-specific contrast agents occurs in some cases, but is not universal.

Focal nodular hyperplasia (FNH)

FNH is much more common in both sexes than liver cell adenoma. The majority of lesions are mildly hypointense on T_1 and mildly hyperintense on T_2 but some lesions are isointense on both and can be undetectable on unenhanced images. A central scar is typically present in larger lesions. Intravenous gadolinium leads to a rapid and intense blush involving both arterial and portal inflow. The enhancement fades rapidly, leaving the tumour parenchyma close to isointense in the equilibrium phase (Fig. 25.137). Delayed enhancement of the central scar is a characteristic which results from the presence of vascularised collagenous tissue, in contrast with the central scar seen in fibrolamellar hepatoma. The signal characteristics of FNH and adenoma overlap to a large degree. The presence of a central scar favours FNH; evidence of haemorrhage or the presence of a capsule are pointers toward adenoma. SPIO uptake is typical of FNH, and the hepatocyte agents (Gd-EOB-DTPA, Gd-

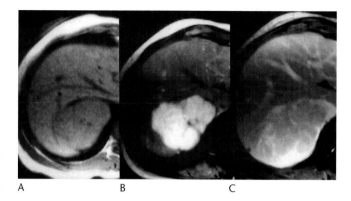

Fig. 25.137 Focal nodular hyperplasia. Unenhanced T_1 image (A) shows the lesion is slightly hypointense. Arterial phase Gd-enhanced image (B) shows a central scar with intense parenchymal enhancement, which fades during the venous phase (C), while the central scar shows delayed enhancement.

BOPTA and Mn-DPDP) may show both early uptake and prolonged retention in these lesions, owing to the presence of hepatocytes and the absence of effective bile ducts.

Hepatocellular carcinoma (HCC)

In the non-cirrhotic patient, HCC is typically solitary and large at the time of presentation. In cirrhosis, which accounts for the majority of cases, HCC may be large or small, single or multiple, rounded or irregular in shape. Unless very small, HCC is typically heterogeneous in structure. Most tumours show early (arterial phase) enhancement but a few are hypovascular (Fig. 25.138). The

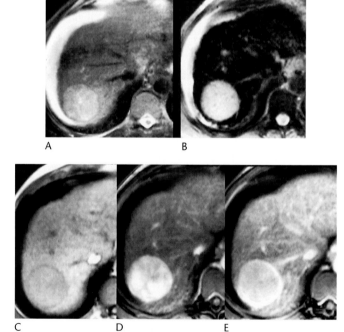

Fig. 25.138 Hepatocellular carcinoma. On unenhanced T_2 images (A) the rounded mass in the right lobe is slightly hyperintense; after SPIO enhancement (B) the lesion is much more clearly visible. Unenhanced T_1 image (C) shows a slightly hypointense lesion; Gd-enhanced images show intense vascularity in the arterial phase (D) with a peripheral capsule appearing on venous phase images (E).

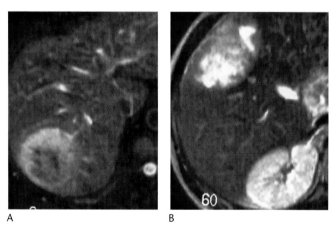

Fig. 25.136 Liver cell adenoma (two cases). T_2 images show a heterogeneous mass with predominantly high signal (A); Gd-enhanced T_1 images (B) show intense but patchy vascularity.

margin of the tumour is typically irregular and may be ill-defined on unenhanced images, but delayed images after gadolinium very often show a rim of high signal which correlates pathologically with the presence of a fibrous capsule. HCC is usually hyperintense on both T_1 and T_2, although well-differentiated lesions may be isointense on both sequences. Larger lesions may contain areas of haemorrhage, and fat-sensitive sequences may show irregular deposits of fatty change within them. Tumours of hepatocellular origin, particularly if well differentiated, may show some uptake of hepatocyte-seeking contrast agents. HCC rarely contains functioning reticuloendothelial cells, so administration of iron particles is not usually helpful in the differential diagnosis of these lesions from other malignancies, although it may improve their detection (Fig. 25.138). The most frequent difficulty in HCC diagnosis in the West is its early recognition in patients with known cirrhosis whose livers are already nodular.

Nodular lesions in the cirrhotic liver

The pathogenesis of HCC in cirrhosis involves the sequential dedifferentiation of regenerative nodules through borderline or dysplastic nodules to HCC. Regenerative nodules are commonly isointense on both T_1 and T_2 images, whereas HCC almost always shows increased signal on T_2. Dysplastic nodules usually show increased signal on T_1 and reduced signal on T_2, almost a unique appearance amongst solid liver tumours (Fig. 25.139). The explanation for the signal changes in these nodules is not clear. It is known that iron deposits may be found in some nodules in the absence of generalised liver siderosis but the finding of iron deposits in dysplastic nodules is not universal. As nodules become sequentially dedifferentiated, they show increasing loss of normal liver characteristics, first losing reticuloendothelial function so that SPIO uptake is reduced, then losing hepatocyte function so that uptake of Gd-BOPTA, Gd-EOB-DTPA and Mn-DPDP is lost. Increasing degrees of histological malignancy are associated with increasing arterialisation and loss of the normal portal supply to the nodule.

The most effective approach for detecting and characterising HCC in cirrhosis is to use a combination of SPIO and dynamic gadolinium enhancement. Regenerative nodules contain functioning liver tissue so their uptake of iron oxide is similar to that of

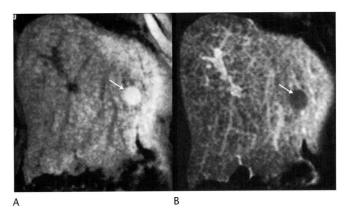

Fig. 25.140   Dysplastic nodule. Coronal unenhanced T_1 image (A) shows a finely nodular liver architecture with a larger nodule of high signal (arrow). Double-contrast technique (B) shows Gd-enhancement in vessels and perivascular fibrosis (high signal) with SPIO enhancement (low signal) in regenerative nodules and the larger dysplastic nodule (arrow).

normal liver. They do not show increased vascularity in the arterial phase with gadolinium (Fig. 25.139). Dysplastic nodules typically take up SPIO but only rarely show increased vascularity in the arterial phase of enhancement (Fig. 25.140). HCC typically shows increased arterial vascularity with gadolinium and no uptake of SPIO.

Cholangiocarcinoma

Cholangiocarcinoma may be intrahepatic or extrahepatic, both types showing reduced signal on T_1 and increased signal on T_2. Intrahepatic cholangiocarcinoma typically presents as a large liver tumour with local or widespread obstruction of the intrahepatic bile ducts. The lesions are usually solitary with ill-defined margins but often have satellite nodules. Enhancement is typically centripetal, corresponding to the pathological findings of a central fibrous component (slow persistent enhancement) and a peripheral cellular component (early hyperintense blush, fading quickly).

Extrahepatic lesions are commonly located at the liver hilum (Klatskin tumours). They are often difficult to identify on axial imaging because they may be encompassed entirely within the bile duct, but coronal oblique images often show a 1–2 cm mass at the point of ductal obstruction (Fig. 25.141). Enhancement of hilar lesions after gadolinium is of low intensity on early images, but increases over several minutes, so the lesions become hyperintense on delayed images. Vascular encasement is common and may cause focal atrophy of the obstructed liver segments, but direct invasion into the portal vein occurs less often than with HCC. Invasion of the bile ducts, with tumour growing along the lumen, is sometimes a feature. The lesions are not encapsulated. Hilar tumours spread by direct extension in perineural lymphatics, and lymph node metastases should be sought at the porta hepatis.

Carcinoma of the gallbladder

This relatively rare tumour presents either as a heterogeneous mass replacing the gallbladder or as diffuse or focal thickening of the gallbladder wall. The mass shows reduced signal on T_1 increased signal on T_2. Most patients have demonstrable gallstones and local liver invasion at the time of presentation. Intrahepatic metastases are seen in a few cases but the majority of patients will have *enlarged lymph nodes* demonstrable in the porta hepatis and upper

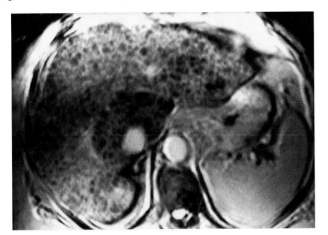

Fig. 25.139   Cirrhosis. SPIO-enhanced T_2 image illustrates the nodular architecture of the cirrhotic liver. Nodules of regenerating liver tissue show SPIO uptake giving low signal, while interstitial bands of fibrosis show relatively high signal.

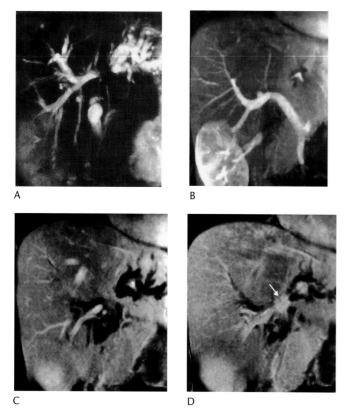

A   B

C   D

Fig. 25.141 Cholangiocarcinoma. MRCP (A) shows obstruction of the left hepatic ducts at the hilum, with less marked dilatation of the right ducts and common duct of normal calibre. Enhanced MIP image (B) shows occlusion of the left main portal vein by tumour. Early (C) and delayed (D) Gd-enhanced T_1 images show a small tumour at the site of duct obstruction, best seen on the delayed images (arrow).

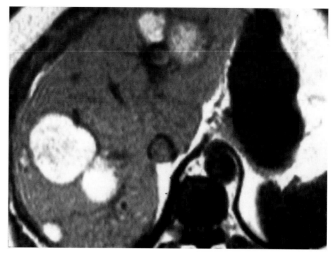

Fig. 25.142 Metastases from melanoma. Unenhanced T_1 image shows multiple lesions with high signal due to melanin content.

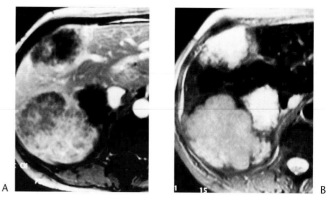

A   B

Fig. 25.143 Colorectal metastases. Typical appearance of heterogeneous enhancement on post-Gd T_1 images (A) and high signal on T_2 (B).

para-aortic regions. Direct invasion of the duodenum is a fairly common problem encountered at surgery which can be difficult to predict from axial images. Coronal views may be particularly helpful in demonstrating the relationship of the mass to the superior duodenal flexure and to the right kidney. The lesions usually show heterogeneous enhancement with gadolinium.

Metastases

Metastases from *liposarcoma* and those from *melanoma*, which may contain substantial quantities of fat and melanin, respectively, may produce increased signal on T_1 (Fig. 25.142) but in the absence of haemorrhage (rare except with trauma or bleeding diathesis) most metastatic nodules show low signal on T_1-weighted images. Metastases which are *calcified* or contain *altered blood* may produce low signal on T_2 but almost invariably the appearance is one of increased signal on T_2 (Figs 25.143, 25.144). Although some highly vascularised metastases show particularly intense signal on T_2, the correlation of signal intensity with histology has been generally unhelpful. Central necrosis occurs in a minority of metastatic lesions but when it is present the lesions are difficult to distinguish from abscesses, which may show similar signal changes. Central scars and peripheral capsules are not recognised features of liver metastases. *Enhancement patterns* of liver metastases are variable. Most lesions show less enhancement than the surrounding liver so they become more easily visible on T_1-weighted images. About 10% of colorectal metastases show increased vascularity. The

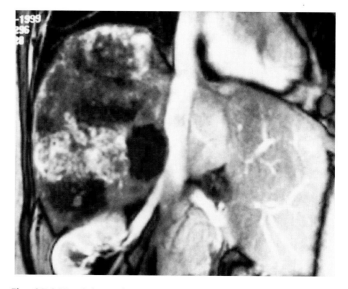

Fig. 25.144 Colorectal metastases. RAO or coronal view is helpful to show the position of metastases relative to the portal vein and IVC. The extensive tumour in this case was successfully resected.

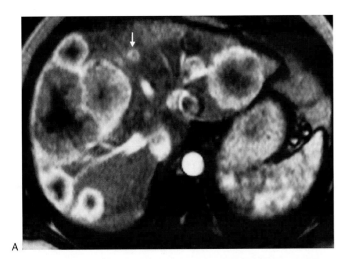

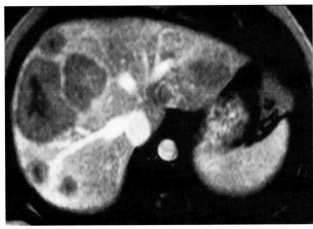

Fig. 25.145 Hypervascular metastases. Metastases from an islet cell tumour of the pancreas show intense peripheral vascularity in the arterial phase of Gd enhancement (A) which fades rapidly in the venous phase (B). Note that the small lesion arrowed in the arterial phase becomes virtually undetectable in the portal phase of enhancement.

pattern of arterial phase enhancement with fairly rapid fading of the initial blush (Fig. 25.145) is typical of metastases from *islet cell tumours* and is seen in a substantial proportion of secondaries from *phaeochromocytoma* and *carcinoid tumours*. Rapid washout of contrast from the periphery is a feature of malignant lesions, not seen with haemangiomas or benign liver cell lesions. *Renal cell cancer* and *leiomyosarcoma* may also give rise to hypervascular metastases. *Melanoma* deposits may be hyper- or hypovascular; if the former, the presence of a necrotic centre will lead to the appearance of a bright ring of enhancement.

Some specific appearances

Ringed lesions—abscess or tumour?

Although the absence of a clear-cut margin is a pointer to malignant histology, the presence of a clear-cut circumferential ring or halo is by no means confined to benign lesions. A true fibrous capsule is seen in a minority of patients with HCC and in some adenomas. Local perilesional oedema probably explains the bright halo shown around some lesions on T$_2$-weighted images. This type of halo is not a feature of benign neoplasms but it is a fairly common feature

of intrahepatic abscess as well as of liver metastases and HCC. Rim enhancement after gadolinium is seen in the majority of abscesses larger than 1.5 cm but is also a feature of metastases with necrotic centres and HCC. The continuous but ill-defined rim of enhancing tumour surrounding a necrotic core should be distinguishable from the more nodular and sharply-defined centripetal enhancement seen with haemangiomas.

Central scar

The central scar found in many cases of FNH and rarely in adenoma contains irregular blood vessels and a proportion of cellular material, in distinction to the much more densely fibrous scars found in fibrolamellar hepatoma (FLH). The central scar in FNH usually appears fairly bright on T$_2$, whereas the scar of FLH is usually hypo- or isointense. In FNH the scar shows considerable enhancement after a fairly short delay, whereas the scar of FLH typically remains unenhanced. The scars occasionally seen in HCC and the central densely fibrous areas of intrahepatic cholangiocarcinomas also show less enhancement than in FNH.

Fatty infiltration and fat within lesions

Using fat-sensitive MR techniques the presence of fat may be revealed in a substantial minority of patients with HCC and occasionally in FNH. Liver tumours containing a high proportion of fatty tissue are all rare—lipoma, angiomyolipoma and metastasis from liposarcoma. Focal fatty change is characterised by an irregular or geographic shape, peripheral location and the absence of a mass effect with normal vessels traversing the lesion. However, cases of multifocal nodular fatty infiltration simulating metastatic disease or HCC are now well recognised; focal sparing within an otherwise diffusely fatty liver is now being recognised with increasing frequency, especially in diabetic patients. Such lesions may be problematic on ultrasound or CT but will be readily diagnosed on in-phase/opposed-phase imaging.

Vascular invasion

Invasion of the major hepatic vessels by tumour is not a feature of benign neoplasms and is rarely seen with metastases except as a late phenomenon in advanced disease. Vascular invasion is relatively common with HCC and with intrahepatic cholangiocarcinoma. MRI appears to be more sensitive than CT in detecting areas of abnormal perfusion within the liver. T$_2$-weighted images may show wedge-shaped areas of increased signal (transient hepatic attenuation differences, THADs), which occur adjacent to large benign lesions or malignant lesions of any size. Similar disturbances of local perfusion are shown with dynamic contrast-enhanced imaging where locally increased enhancement in the arterial phase, equilibrating with the rest of the liver within a minute or so, occurs in some patients with malignant liver lesions, possibly caused by invasion or occlusion of intrahepatic portal vein branches.

MRI OF THE SPLEEN

The anatomy and internal architecture of the spleen are generally shown well by CT and ultrasound but MRI may provide useful additional data in a minority of cases. Compared with the normal liver, the spleen shows a lower signal on T$_1$ and a higher signal on T$_2$, probably because of its greater blood volume. The relatively greater perfusion of the spleen is illustrated by intense early enhancement after gadolinium, with capillary phase images producing the serpiginous pattern also seen on spiral CT, which coalesces to form a more uniform diffuse enhancement on equilibrium phase images. The spleen also shows moderate uptake of SPIO particles with resulting loss of signal from the normal parenchyma on T_2-weighted sequences.

In portal hypertension the spleen becomes enlarged, with no change in its signal intensities apart from the occasional finding of siderotic nodules (Gamna–Gandy bodies) producing focal areas of low signal, similar to their appearance in the liver. With transfusional haemosiderosis, the spleen shows generalised loss of signal on both T_1 and T_2 sequences, but it is less affected in primary haemochromatosis. Demonstration of splenic vein occlusion and left upper quadrant varices has been described above, and the characteristics of splenic cysts, haemangiomas, metastases and abscesses are essentially similar to those described above for the liver.

SPIO contrast agents may be used to clarify the presence of dubious mass lesions on unenhanced scans, as some tumours are isointense with normal spleen. Such lesions may also be well shown on rapid dynamic acquisitions with gadolinium enhancement. Focal lymphomas may be hyperintense on T_2, hypointense on T_1, but they also show less gadolinium enhancement than normal spleen. Inactive or treated lymphomas may show reduced signal on T_2 images. Diffuse lymphomatous involvement of the spleen usually produces no change in signal intensity but early studies with SPIO suggested that this agent may be used to differentiate the cause of enlarged spleen in patients with lymphoma. Those with diffuse splenic lymphoma show reduced uptake of SPIO, whereas those with reactive splenomegaly show normal SPIO uptake.

REFERENCES AND SUGGESTIONS FOR FURTHER READING

General, vascular, CT
Bircher, J., Benhamou, J. P., McIntyre, N. et al (1999) *Oxford Textbook of Clinical Hepatology*. Oxford: Oxford University Press.
Sherlock, S., Dooley, J. (2001) *Diseases of the Liver and Biliary System*, 11th edn. Oxford: Blackwell.

Radionuclide imaging
Kinnard, M. F., Alavi, A., Rubin, R. A., Lichtenstein, G. R. (1995) Nuclear imaging of solid hepatic masses. *Seminars in Roentgenology*, **30**, 375–395.

Ultrasound
Acalouschi, M., Badea, R., Dumitrascu, D., et al (1998) Prevalence of gall stones in liver cirrhosis—a sonographic survey. *American Journal of Gastroenterology*, **83**, 954–956.
Baker, M. K., Wenker, J. C., Cockerill, E. M., et al (1995) Focal fatty infiltration of the liver: diagnostic imaging. *Radiographics*, **5**, 923–939.
Barren, R. L., Gore, R. M. (2000) Diffuse liver disease. In: Gore, R. M., Levine, M. S. (eds) *Textbook of Gastrointestinal Radiology*, 2nd edn, vol. 2, pp. 1590–1638. Philadelphia: W. B. Saunders.
Bolondi, L., Gaiani, S., Barbara, L. (1993) The portal venous system. In: Cosgrave, D., Meire, H., Dewbury, K. (eds) *Clinical Ultrasound—A Comprehensive Text*, p. 309. Edinburgh: Churchill Livingstone.
Bolondi, L., Piscaglia, F., Valgimigli, M., Gaiani, S. (2000) Doppler ultrasound in portal hypertension. In Baert, A. L., Sartor, K., Youker, J. E. (eds) *Portal Hypertension*, pp. 57–76. Berlin: Springer.
Bromley, M. J. K., Albrecht, T., Cosgrove, D. O., et al (1998) Liver vascular transit time analyzed with dynamic hepatic venography with bolus injections of an US contrast: early experience in 7 patients with metastases. *Radiology*, **209**, 862–866.
Bromley, M. J., Albrecht, T., Cosgrove, D., et al (1999) Improved imaging of liver metastases with stimulated acoustic emission in the late phase of enhancement with the US contrast agent. SH U 508a: early experience. Feb; **201(2)**: 409–16.

Choi, B. I., Kim, T. K., Han, J. K., et al (1996) Para versus conventional colour Doppler sonography. Comparison in the depiction of vasculature in liver tumours. *Radiology*, **200**, 55–58.
Choi, B. I., Kim, T. K., Han, J. K., Kim, A. Y., Senog, C. K., Park, S. J. (2000) Vascularity of hepatocellular carcinoma: assessment with contrast-enhanced second-harmonic versus conventionl power Doppler US. *Radiology*, **214**, 381–386.
Cosgrove, D., Meire, H., Dewbury, K. (1993) *Abdominal and General Ultrasound*. Edinburgh: Churchill Livingstone.
Dodd III, G. B., Miller, W. J., Barren, R. L., et al (1992) Detection of malignant tumours in end stage cirrhotic livers: efficacy of sonography as a screening tool. *American Journal of Roentgenology*, **159**, 77–733.
Dodd III, G. B., Zajko, A. B., Orons, P. D., et al (1995) Detection of transjugular intra-hepatic porto-systemic shunt dysfunction: the value of duplex Doppler sonography. *American Journal of Roentgenology*, **164**, 1119–1124.
Feldstein, V. A., La Berge, J. M. (1994) Hepatic vein flow reversal at duplex sonography: a sign of transjugular intra-hepatic porto-systemic shunt dysfunction. *American Journal of Roentgenology*, **162**, 839–841.
Foshager, M. C., Ferral, H., Finlay, D. E., et al (1994) Colour Doppler sonography of transjugular intra-hepatic porto-systemic shunts (TIPS). *American Journal of Roentgenology*, **163**, 105–111.
Golli, M., Nhiew, J. T. V., Nathieu, D., et al (1994) Hepatocellular adenoma: colour Doppler ultrasound and pathologic correlations. *Radiology*, **190**, 741–744.
Hagen-Ansert, S. L. (1995) *Textbook of Diagnostic Ultrasonography*, 4th edn. St Louis: Mosby Year Book.
Hann, L. E., Bach, A. M., Cramer, L. D., et al (1999) Hepatic sonography: comparison of tissue harmonic and standard tissue sonography techniques. *American Journal of Roentgenology*, **173**, 201.
Kawashima, A., Urban, B., Fishman, E. (2000) Benign lesions of the spleen. In: Gore, R. M., Levine, M. (eds) *Textbook of Gastrointestinal Radiology*, 2nd edn, vol. 2, pp. 1879–1903. Philadelphia: W. B. Saunders.
Kehoe, J., Straus, D. J. (1998) Primary lymphoma of the spleen: clinical features and outcome after splenectomy. *Cancer*, **62**, 1433–1438.
Leifer, D. M., Middleton, W. D., Teefey, S. H., Menias, C. O., Leahy, J. R. (2000) Follow-up of patients at low risk for hepatic malignancy with a characteristic hemangioma at US. *Radiology*, **214**, 167–172.
Nisenbaum, H. L., Rowling, S. E. (1995) Ultrasound of focal hepatic lesions. *Seminars in Roentgenology*, **30**, 324–346.
Rengo, C., Brevetti, G., Sorrentino, G., et al (1998) Portal vein pulsitility ratio provides a measure of right heart function in chronic heart failure. *Ultrasound in Medicine and Biology*, **24**, 327–332.
Ros, P. R., Taylor, H. M., Barreda, R., Gore, R. (2000) Focal hepatic infections. In: Gore, R. M., Levine, M. (eds), *Textbook of Gastrointestinal Radiology*, 2nd edn, vol. 2, pp. 1569–1589. Philadelphia: W. B. Saunders.
Terrault, N. A., Wright, T. L. (1998) Viral hepatitis A through G. In: Seldman, M., Scharschimdt, B. F., Sleisenger, M. H. (eds) *Gastrointestinal and Liver Disease*, 6th edn, pp. 1123–1169. Philadelphia: W. B. Saunders.
Trantiano, L., Giorgio, A., De Stefano, G., et al (1997) Reverse flow in intra-hepatic portal vessels and liver function impairment in cirrhosis. *European Journal of Ultrasound*, **6**, 171–177.

MRI
Earls, J. P., Bluemke, D. A. (1999) New MR imaging contrast agents. *Magnetic Resonance Imaging Clinics of North America*, **7**, 255–273.
Krinsky, G. A., Lee, V. S., Theise, N. D. (2000) Focal lesions in the cirrhotic liver: high resolution ex vivo MRI with pathologic correlation. *Journal of Computer-Assisted Tomography*, **24**, 189–196.
Onaya, H., Itai, Y. (2000) MR imaging of hepatocellular carcinoma. *Magnetic Resonance Imaging Clinics of North America*, **8**, 757–768.
Op de Beeck, B., Luypaert, R., Dujardin, M., Osteaux, M. (1999) Benign liver lesions: differentiation by magnetic resonance. *European Journal of Radiology*, **32**, 52–60.
Robinson, P. J. A. (1996) The characterisation of liver tumours by MRI. *Clinical Radiology*, **51**, 749–761.
Robinson, P. J. (2000) Imaging liver metastases: current limitations and future prospects. *British Journal of Radiology*, **73**, 234–241.
Torres, G. M., Terry, N. L., Mergo, P. J., Ros, P. R. (1995) MR imaging of the spleen. *Magnetic Resonance Imaging Clinics of North America*, **3**, 39–50.

26

THE PANCREAS

Janet Murfitt

with contributions from Richard W. Whitehouse and Andrew R. Wright, Philip J. A. Robinson, and Paul A. Dubbins

Methods of investigation

Techniques available for the radiological assessment of the pancreas include the following:

- the plain abdominal film
- ultrasound: abdominal, endoscopic, intraoperative
- CT
- MRI
- MRCP (magnetic resonance cholangiopancreatography)
- ERCP (endoscopic retrograde cholangiopancreatography)
- fine-needle and core biopsy
- barium studies
- angiography
- percutaneous transhepatic venous sampling
- percutaneous drainage of fluid collections
- percutaneous pancreatography.

Ultrasound, CT, MRI, MRCP and ERCP, when available, are the main diagnostic tools for investigating the pancreas and are discussed in detail later. *CT* and *MRI* are considered to be the most reliable techniques for assessing the pancreas and the peripancreatic tissues, including the major blood vessels. However, small central solid pancreatic masses may be difficult to identify. *Ultrasound* has the advantage that the biliary tree is easily assessed, but the retropancreatic tissues are less well visualised, and bowel gas, particularly in the presence of an ileus accompanying acute pancreatitis, can partially or completely obscure the pancreas. *ERCP* allows assessment of the biliary tree, upper gastrointestinal tract and pancreatic ducts, as well as allowing certain therapeutic procedures, such as sphincterotomy, stone removal, stent insertion and cyst drainage, to be performed when appropriate. However, there may be a normal pancreatic duct in the presence of a small peripheral neoplasm or chronic pancreatitis. The disadvantages of ERCP are the associated morbidity, in particular iatrogenic acute pancreatitis. *MRCP* is very accurate in the diagnosis of choledocholithiasis, pancreatic duct abnormalities and pancreatic tumours and has the advantage of being non-invasive. Ultrasound-guided *percutaneous*

pancreatography with a fine needle may be undertaken if ERCP fails to demonstrate the pancreatic duct. A small volume of contrast is injected into the duct after aspiration of a similar volume of pancreatic juice to avoid overfilling and reduce the risk of pancreatitis.

Further developments in ultrasound include endoscopic and intraoperative scanning. With the advent of *intraoperative scanning* coupled with surgical palpation of the pancreas for endocrine tumours, the need for highly selective angiography and transhepatic venous sampling has diminished, even though the success rate for these techniques exceeds 90% in experienced hands. *Endoscopic ultrasound* has the advantage of visualising the pancreas from the stomach or duodenum with a high-frequency transducer without the problems of intervening bowel loops. Adjacent vessels and nodes are also seen. An accuracy exceeding 90% has been reported for the diagnosis of portal vein invasion by tumour.

Angiography has been superseded in the diagnosis and staging of pancreatic adenocarcinoma by CT and MRI but still has a place in localisation of islet cell tumours. Symptomatic metastases or inoperable primary tumours can be treated with embolisation or intra-arterial cytotoxic infusion therapy.

Radionuclide scanning of the pancreas is no longer undertaken, except for islet cell tumours (see below). *MRI* of the pancreas requires fast sequences to reduce motion artefact, with fat suppression techniques and contrast enhancement improving the diagnostic accuracy. At present MRI is considered superior to CT in the diagnosis of islet cell tumours and for assessing the pancreas following transplantation.

Percutaneous biopsy may be performed using a fine needle for aspiration cytology or fine-needle core biopsy. Complications are unusual, although seeding of tumour along the needle track has been reported.

The plain film
Up to 40% of patients with alcoholic pancreatitis develop calcification within the pancreas after 5–10 years (Fig. 26.1). The calcification lies within small intraduct calculi, which are of variable size. These are composed predominantly of crystalline carbonate with

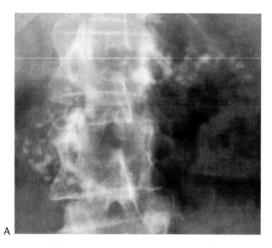
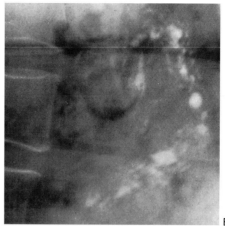

Fig. 26.1   Pancreatic calcification in a middle-aged woman. (A) AP film. (B) Lateral film.

Box 26.1   Causes of pancreatic calcification

Common
Chronic alcoholic pancreatitis

Rare
Idiopathic
Hereditary pancreatitis
Cystic fibrosis
Hyperparathyroidism
Protein malnutrition
Cystic tumours
Cavernous lymphangioma
Islet cell tumours
Haemangioma
Pseudocysts
Haematoma

small amounts of protein and polysaccharide. They form when calcium precipitates around a protein plug. Although usually distributed throughout the gland, the calculi may be focal in one-quarter of cases. This group of patients forms the majority of cases of pancreatic calcification (Box 26.1).

Idiopathic pancreatitis is an asymptomatic condition associated with a pancreatic duct stenosis with calcification developing upstream within the pancreas.

Adenocarcinomas do not calcify, whereas a sunburst pattern of calcification is seen in up to 10% of cystic tumours. Calcification within *islet cell tumours* invariably indicates malignancy. Calcified phleboliths may develop within a *haemangioma* and a *cavernous lymphangioma*. Occasionally calcification forms within the wall of a *pseudocyst* and within an area of *infarction* or a *haematoma* following pancreatic trauma.

Large pancreatic masses may be seen as soft-tissue masses displacing the gas shadows of the stomach or bowel. Plain film changes associated with acute pancreatitis are described elsewhere.

Ascites in association with pancreatic malignancy usually indicates the presence of peritoneal metastases. Occlusion of the splenic or portal veins due to tumour invasion, or thrombosis due to pancreatitis, causes splenomegaly.

Barium studies

Occasionally a tumour or pseudocyst arising in the tail of the pancreas affects the intra-abdominal oesophagus, causing elongation and straightening so that the oesophagus has a horizontal lie (Fig. 26.2). There may be tumour invasion with obstruction. Gastric varices in the fundus may develop following splenic vein occlusion.

Large pancreatic tumours or inflammatory masses displace the stomach superiorly and anteriorly, with widening of the retrogastric space as demonstrated on a recumbent film taken with a horizontal beam. Lesions in the head of the pancreas affect the pyloric antrum and duodenal loop (Fig. 26.3), whereas lesions in the body of the pancreas affect the distal duodenum, the duodenojejunal flexure and the body of the stomach. Gastric mucosal abnormalities are seen predominantly in the posterior wall. Invasion results in mucosal irregularity and ulceration, with fixation of the gastric wall resulting in abnormal peristalsis. Indentation by a mass without invasion results in splaying of the mucosal folds (Fig. 26.4). In cases of acute pancreatitis the spreading inflammation may cause oedema of the mucosal folds with spasm.

A large number of abnormalities of the duodenal loop resulting from pancreatic disease have been described, particularly with hypotonic duodenography. Changes occurring as a result of malignancy include a widened duodenal loop with mucosal irregularity

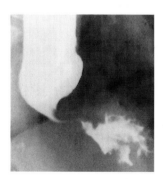

Fig. 26.2 Barium swallow. Carcinoma in the tail of the pancreas elevating the intra-abdominal oesophagus.

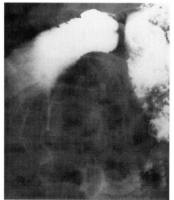

Fig. 26.3 Barium meal. Large cyst in the head of the pancreas widening and compressing the duodenal loop.

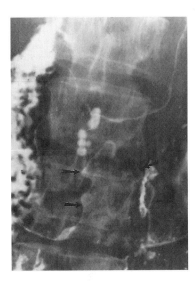

Fig. 26.4 Barium meal, supine film. Carcinoma of the body of the pancreas indenting the posterior wall of the stomach (arrows).

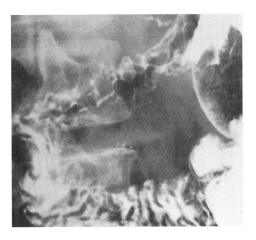

Fig. 26.5 Barium meal. Carcinoma of the head of the pancreas invading the duodenal loop with deformity of the mucosal pattern.

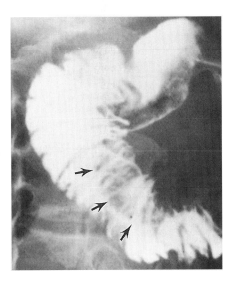

Fig. 26.6 Barium meal. A double contour (arrows) of the duodenal loop. Carcinoma of the head of the pancreas.

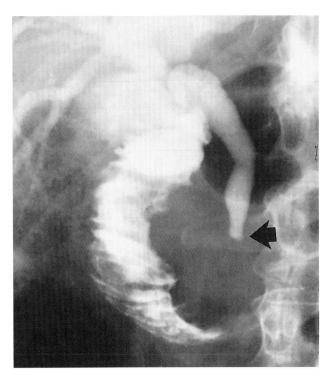

Fig. 26.7 Enlarged duodenal loop with 'reversed 3' sign of Frostberg. Earlier percutaneous transhepatic cholangiogram shows characteristic 'gloved finger' obstruction of intrapancreatic common bile duct pathognomonic of carcinoma of the pancreatic head. (Courtesy of Dr R. Dick.)

(Fig. 26.5), spiculation and nodularity of the folds, which may be blunted, or a localised stricture due to direct malignant invasion. There may be a double contour to the medial border of the loop (Fig. 26.6) due to indentation by the mass and Frostberg's 'reversed 3' sign (Fig. 26.7). An enlarged gallbladder in cases with bile duct obstruction may indent the duodenal cap.

Chronic pancreatitis may have a mass effect causing a double contour. Associated strictures have been described. Changes seen with acute pancreatitis include a widened loop with thickened folds, fold effacement, Frostberg's sign, and narrowing or dilatation of the loop.

Apart from the upper bowel, tumours may also invade the transverse and descending colon.

The inflammation of acute pancreatitis spreads along the mesentery and mesocolon, causing oedema of the folds of the small bowel and colon.

Congenital disorders

Hereditary pancreatitis is an autosomal dominant condition of variable penetrance that presents in childhood with acute and then chronic pancreatitis. Pancreatic calcification is common, with large calcified calculi containing a central lucency being characteristic. Some 20% of patients develop pancreatic malignancy.

Pancreatic insufficiency and pancreatitis are features of **cystic fibrosis** and develop due to obstruction of the ducts by inspissated secretions. Fine granular pancreatic calcification may be present, and there is an increased incidence of gallstones. In the rare **Schwachman–Diamond syndrome** there is fatty replacement of the pancreas, well demonstrated by CT, with associated skeletal abnormalities, including short stature and hypoplastic bone marrow. Inheritance is autosomal recessive.

Abnormal migration of the ventral pancreas in the embryo may result in an **annular pancreas**. This is more common in males. Fifty per cent of cases present in the neonatal period with vomiting due to duodenal obstruction caused by the pancreas encircling the duodenal loop (Figs 26.8, 26.9). The characteristic double bubble is seen on the plain abdominal film. Less commonly this condition presents in the adult with abdominal pain and vomiting. Associated abnormalities are present in 75% of cases and include congenital heart disease, Down's syndrome, imperforate anus and oesophageal atresia. ERCP is the definitive investigation, showing the duct of Wirsung encircling the duodenum, although in 15% of cases the annular segment does not drain into this duct and ERCP is unhelpful. Barium studies show eccentric narrowing of the duodenal loop.

Partial or complete **agenesis** and **aplasia** of the pancreas are extremely rare. Polysplenia is a recognised association.

Ectopic pancreatic tissue is identified in 10% of patients at postmortem. Usually there is a small nodule, which may contain functioning endocrine or exocrine tissue, with a central dimple lying submucosally within the wall of the bowel. The stomach and duodenum are the commonest sites. Large ectopic pancreatic masses may occur and there is an association with duplication cysts of the bowel.

The ducts of Wirsung and Santorini may fail to fuse during embryological development so that the smaller accessory duct drains the dorsal pancreas, which may develop pancreatitis. This

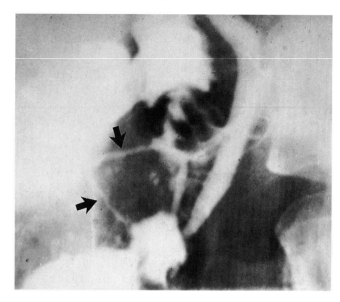

Fig. 26.9 ERCP. Duct of Wirsung (arrows) encircling gas-filled second part of duodenum. Annular pancreas. Duct of Santorini not filled. (See also Fig. 26.8.) (Courtesy of Dr R. Dick.)

condition is known as **pancreas divisum** and has a reported incidence of 0.5–11%. This is discussed later.

Pancreatitis

Acute pancreatitis

The majority of cases of acute pancreatitis can be attributed to an excessive alcohol intake or to gallstones. Other known causes include viral infections, such as mumps, cytomegalovirus and glandular fever, parasite infections, pancreas divisum, annular pancreas, abdominal trauma, surgery, ERCP, hypercalcaemia, hyperparathyroidism, hyperlipidaemia, drugs including steroids, thiazide diuretics and azathioprine, polyarteritis, and systemic lupus erythematosus (SLE). In 10–20% of cases there is no identifiable predisposing factor. The overall mortality rate is 10–15%, with 80% of cases being self-limiting.

Initially there is pancreatic oedema, which may be focal or diffuse. There may be progression due to proteolytic destruction, with resulting necrosis and haemorrhage within the pancreas and the surrounding tissues. Necrosis demonstrated on enhanced CT scanning is associated with a mortality rate of 20% and a complication rate of 80%. Complications include the formation of phlegmon (an indurated inflammatory mass), an abscess, pseudocysts, pseudoaneurysms with bleeding retroperitoneally or into the gut, fat necrosis, which may lead to hypocalcaemia, ascites, and splenic vein thrombosis. Ascites forms due to leakage of pancreatic juice from a duct damaged by surrounding necrotic tissue. It has an associated mortality of 20%; this increases threefold if the ascites becomes infected.

CT is generally considered to be the investigation of choice, particularly if there is a rapidly deteriorating clinical picture, to assess the development and progress of complications (Fig. 26.10). Ultrasound is used as the initial investigation to identify gallstones and bile duct dilatation but has the disadvantage that dilated bowel often precludes good pancreatic visualisation. In addition, the peripancreatic tissues are less well seen than with CT, and some complications, particularly vascular involvement, are less easily

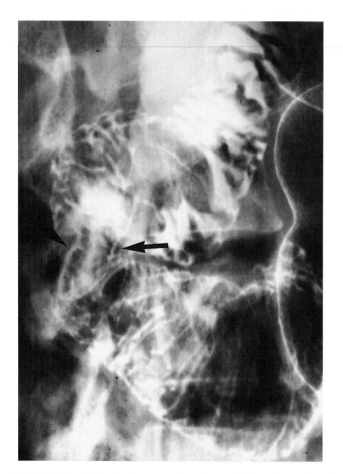

Fig. 26.8 Hypotonic duodenogram. Annular constriction of second part of the duodenum with preservation of folds (arrows). Proven annular pancreas. (Courtesy of Dr R. Dick.)

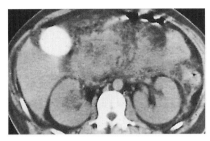

Fig. 26.10 CT scan. Acute pancreatitis. Swollen pancreas with extension of the inflammatory process into the mesentery. Some necrotic low-density areas are present in the pancreatic head.

identified. ERCP is said by many to be contraindicated in acute pancreatitis unless a gallstone is known or thought to be present in the common bile duct, in which case sphincterotomy and stone removal are indicated. Fine-needle aspiration of a cyst or phlegmon is often necessary to exclude abscess formation, in which case percutaneous drainage may be undertaken. There is a risk that needling sterile collections may introduce infection. Abscess formation is associated with a relatively poor prognosis.

Plain film changes Features associated with acute pancreatitis are well described. In the chest a left-sided pleural effusion with an elevated amylase content is characteristic. Other chest findings include splinting of the left diaphragm and basal parenchymal shadowing. Bony changes include bone infarcts, avascular necrosis, and lytic lesions due to metastatic fat necrosis.

On the abdominal film a duodenal ileus is considered to be a fairly specific finding; the duodenal folds may be thickened. Other patterns described include a gasless abdomen due to vomiting, a sentinel loop and an absent left psoas shadow (Fig. 26.11). The 'colon cut-off sign', where the dilated transverse colon becomes abruptly gasless in the region of the splenic flexure, is a less specific sign. The left kidney may be displaced downward and have a surrounding halo due to oedema. Fat necrosis appears as indistinct mottled shadowing, which is initially in the region of the pancreas but may spread throughout the abdomen (Fig. 26.12). Intrapancreatic gas suggests abscess formation or an enteric fistula. An abscess may contain a single fluid level or more commonly multiple bubbles.

Up to 10% of cases develop pseudoaneurysms, particularly of the splenic artery. There may be bleeding into the gut, biliary tree or

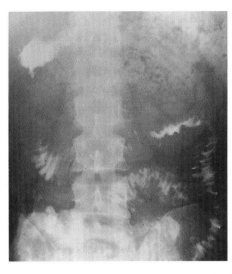

Fig. 26.12 Acute pancreatitis with fat necrosis. Multiple irregular lucencies in the left upper quadrant.

retroperitoneum and this is associated with a poor prognosis. Therapeutic embolisation may be undertaken.

Only rarely does chronic pancreatitis develop following an episode of acute pancreatitis.

Chronic pancreatitis

The 1983 Cambridge symposium classified chronic pancreatitis as a continuing inflammatory disease of the pancreas characterised by irreversible morphological change and typically causing pain and/or a permanent loss of exocrine and endocrine function.

Alcoholism is by far the commonest cause of chronic pancreatitis. There is usually a history of a heavy alcohol intake over 10 years or more. Other known associated factors include pancreas divisum, gallstones, trauma, hypercalcaemia, hyperlipidaemia, cystic fibrosis, hereditary pancreatitis and protein malnutrition. Pancreatitis can develop upstream to a mass obstructing the pancreatic duct; this is known as chronic obstructive pancreatitis. There is an associated increased risk of pancreatic adenocarcinoma.

There may be diffuse or focal enlargement of the pancreas but in the later stages size decreases and the pancreas may become atrophic with fatty infiltration. The pancreatic duct is irregularly dilated and contains calculi. Up to 10% of patients develop signs of biliary obstruction due to involvement of the intrapancreatic common bile duct, which typically has a smooth stricture (Fig. 26.13). Common bile duct occlusion is unusual with chronic pancreatitis and suggests a malignant pathology. Pseudocysts develop in 25% of patients following disruption of an acinus or the duct. Obstruction of the duodenum due to fibrosis is rare and usually involves the second part. Occasionally thrombosis of the splenic vein occurs.

Calcification is seen on the plain film in half of patients with an alcoholic aetiology (Fig. 26.14) and develops some years after the initial presentation. In addition it is a common finding with hereditary pancreatitis and hyperparathyroidism.

Using ERCP a diagnosis can be made at an earlier stage than with CT or ultrasonography, although a normal ERCP does not exclude the diagnosis. It has the added advantage of contrast delineation of the biliary tree. Pancreatic stones can be removed at ERCP, the duct can be stented or a pancreatic sphincterotomy performed to enhance pancreatic drainage.

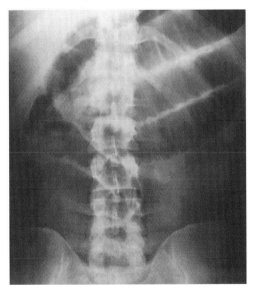

Fig. 26.11   Acute pancreatitis. Dilated duodenal and jejunal loops.

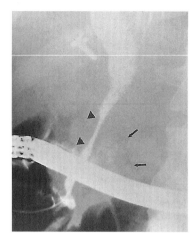

Fig. 26.13 ERCP. Chronic pancreatitis. A smooth stricture of the common bile duct (arrowheads) with calcification in the pancreatic head (arrows).

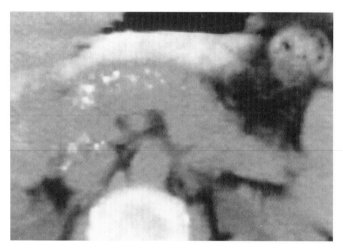

Fig. 26.14 Chronic pancreatitis. Extensive pancreatic calcification.

Pancreatic cysts

Cysts may be classified as *true cysts* (25%) or *pseudocysts* (75%). True cysts may be congenital in origin or acquired; examples include retention cysts, dermoid cysts and malignant cysts. *Congenital cysts* are usually multiple and do not communicate with the duct system. Some 10% of patients with polycystic kidneys (autosomal dominant type) have associated pancreatic cysts. In von Hippel–Lindau disease pancreatic cysts are present in over half of cases. This disease has an autosomal dominant inheritance with an increased incidence of pancreatic malignancy and haemangioblastomas of the retina and central nervous system, and cysts of multiple organs.

Pseudocysts are a feature of both acute and chronic pancreatitis. They form as a result of rupture of a pancreatic duct, and may also follow pancreatic trauma. The lesser sac is the commonest site for pseudocyst formation but they may spread throughout the abdomen and pelvis and have been described in the inguinal regions and posterior mediastinum. One-third of cysts resolve spontaneously. Persistent cysts exceeding 5 cm in diameter require drainage to prevent known complications including rupture, infection, haemorrhage and bowel obstruction. Cysts associated with chronic pancreatitis are less likely to resolve spontaneously than those which form after acute pancreatitis.

Ultrasound is useful for following their progress, although CT is the investigation of choice in the very ill or clinically deteriorating patient. At ERCP around 50% of pseudocysts are found to be in communication with the duct system.

Percutaneous drainage, CT or ultrasound guided, is indicated for infected collections and for persistent pseudocysts. These may be drained endoscopically by cystogastrostomy—insertion of a stent between the stomach and the cyst.

Non-endocrine tumours of the pancreas

The majority (75%) of pancreatic neoplasms are *ductal adenocarcinomas*. *Cystic tumours* such as the mucinous cystadenoma and microcystic adenoma are uncommon, forming less than 5% of the total.

The rare *pancreaticoblastoma* is the commonest pancreatic tumour of childhood and is of increased incidence in the Beckwith–Wiedemann syndrome. This autosomal dominant condition is associated with hemihypertrophy and a 10% incidence of malignant tumours. At presentation there is a large mass, usually situated in the pancreatic head or tail. Central cystic degeneration commonly occurs.

Peutz–Jeghers syndrome is associated with an increased incidence of pancreatic adenocarcinoma.

Other rare pancreatic tumours include sarcomas, mesenchymal tumours, lymphoma and metastases. *Metastases* are rarely apparent clinically, but are found at postmortem in one-third of patients with malignant melanoma and in 20% of cases of breast carcinoma. They may be solitary or multiple, studded on the surface or lying within the pancreas. Primary *lymphoma*, usually non-Hodgkin's, is extremely rare and usually arises in the head of the pancreas.

Adenocarcinoma of the pancreas

Some 60% of these tumours arise in the head of the pancreas, usually presenting with jaundice, anorexia and weight loss, with upper abdominal pain penetrating through to the back. Late onset diabetes mellitus may be associated. Duodenal obstruction is a late feature and usually affects the postbulbar region. Tumours arising in the body and tail of the pancreas present late as large masses, with weight loss and pain due to local tumour infiltration. Lesions in the head of the pancreas have the better prognosis, although the 5 year survival in those patients who are operable is in the region of only 5%. Any pancreatic tumour may obstruct the pancreatic duct, resulting in pancreatitis upstream, occasionally with pseudocyst formation. Peritoneal spread produces ascites. Tumour invasion of the splenic or portal veins causes splenomegaly (Fig. 26.15). Metastatic spread to the liver is common, as is spread to local nodes and throughout the peritoneum.

CT with contrast enhancement is the most effective technique for the diagnosis and staging of pancreatic carcinoma (Fig. 26.16). Ultrasound is highly accurate at determining the level of obstruction of the bile duct, and masses in the pancreatic head are often easily demonstrated. However it is less effective in assessing the body and tail and in demonstrating spread of the malignant process into the abdomen and retroperitoneal tissues. Endoscopic ultrasound overcomes some of these limitations. Percutaneous CT or ultrasound-guided biopsy can be used to confirm the diagnosis. ERCP demonstrates a stricture and obstruction of the pancreatic and common bile ducts.

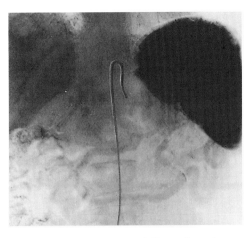

Fig. 26.15 Coeliac angiogram; delayed film to show the venous phase. Carcinoma of the pancreas. Obstructed splenic vein with multiple collaterals and splenomegaly.

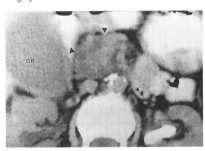

Fig. 26.16 CT scan. Carcinoma of the head of the pancreas. A large pancreatic mass (arrowheads) with a dilated gallbladder (GB). Note left renal calculus.

CT and angiography (Fig. 26.17) have similar levels of accuracy in demonstrating vascular encasement or occlusion. Adenocarcinomas are hypovascular.

On occasions there is difficulty in differentiating a carcinoma from focal pancreatitis. Bile duct occlusion or an irregular stricture favours malignancy (Fig. 26.18), whereas pancreatitis is associated with a smooth stricture. Pancreatic duct dilatation is often more marked with malignancy. Pancreatic calcification is a strong indicator of a benign condition. Pseudocysts may develop with both conditions.

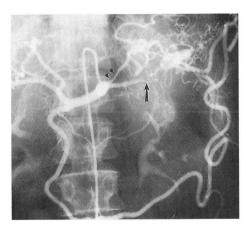

Fig. 26.17 Coeliac angiogram. Pancreatic carcinoma encasing the left gastric artery (arrowheads). The splenic artery is occluded (arrow). There is splaying of the gastroduodenal artery.

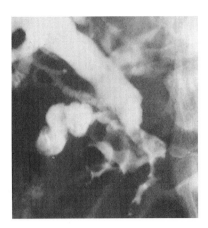

Fig. 26.18 Percutaneous transhepatic cholangiogram. Carcinoma of the head of the pancreas. A long irregular stricture of the common bile duct.

Pleomorphic adenocarcinoma

This rare and very aggressive tumour is characterised by a pancreatic mass with massive lymphadenopathy and needs to be distinguished from lymphoma.

Cystic tumours of the pancreas

The most common cystic tumours of the pancreas are serous (microcystic), mucinous (macrocystic) and papillary. Rarer cystic tumours include cystic islet cell tumours, cystic metastases, the cystic lymphangioma and cystic degeneration of adenocarcinoma and lymphoma.

1. The *serous cystadenoma*, or microcystic adenoma, is a benign tumour of elderly women, presenting with vague abdominal symptoms. A large calcified mass is often seen, with the calcification having a characteristic sunburst pattern within a central fibrotic scar. As the cysts within the tumour are microcysts, less than 2 cm in diameter, they cannot usually be identified individually at CT or ultrasound. This is a highly vascular tumour.

2. The *mucinous cystadenoma* is a very vascular premalignant or malignant mass which has single or multiple cysts containing mucin (Fig. 26.19). It commonly affects elderly females and arises predominantly in the body and tail of the pancreas. The prognosis is

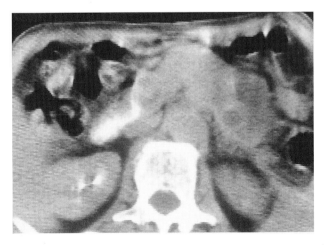

Fig. 26.19 Cystadenocarcinoma of the tail of the pancreas. (Courtesy of Dr O. Chan.)

more favourable than that of an adenocarcinoma. Dystrophic calcification is present in 10–20% of cases and may be amorphous or curvilinear. The cysts may contain septae and the wall may be irregular suggesting malignant change. However, as it is impossible to determine whether there is malignancy, and fine-needle aspiration is inadvisable because of the risk of peritoneal spillage of malignant cells, all small tumours should be resected. Differentiation from a pseudocyst may be impossible with imaging. The most reliable indicator is a past history of pancreatitis.

3. *Papillary epithelial tumours* (solid and papillary neoplasms) arise from the pancreatic ducts. They are rare tumours of low-grade malignancy, well capsulated, and can usually be resected successfully. They most often present in young black females. The tumours are solid or cystic and may contain calcium. Metastases are very rare but may be cystic.

Intraductal mucin hypersecreting tumours (intraductal papillary tumours) These are more common in males. They arise from the ducts predominantly in the pancreatic head and produce large amounts of mucin with resulting cystic dilatation of the ducts. The mucin hinders normal flow along the duct, causing low-grade pancreatitis with a slightly raised amylase level. The patient presents with recurrent upper abdominal pain.

Ampullary carcinoma

These tumours constitute 6–12% of all pancreatic malignancies, and usually present with jaundice, which may be fluctuating. The prognosis is good, with a 25% 5 year survival for resectable lesions less than 2 cm in diameter. Most tumours are diagnosed at endoscopy, but they may be picked up during a barium study as an irregular filling defect (Fig. 26.20), or as a smooth defect if the tumour is intra-ampullary. There may be duodenal invasion and barium may enter the ampulla. The differential diagnosis includes a pancreatic tumour and an oedematous ampulla due to an impacted gallstone or pancreatitis.

Islet-cell tumours of the pancreas

The islet cells are the endocrine cells of the pancreas. Pearse (1968) introduced the concept of the APUD system. Islet cells are thought to be derived from the stem cells of the neuroectoderm and have shared features of amine metabolism, Amine Precursor Uptake and Decarboxylation, with the ability to secrete multiple polypeptide

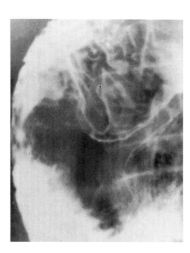

Fig. 26.20 Barium meal. Carcinoma of the ampulla producing a filling defect in the duodenum.

hormones. Not all neuroendocrine cells are now thought to fit into this system. There are four cell types.

At postmortem, islet cell adenoma has an incidence of 1–2%, although the majority are clinically silent. Between 80 and 85% of symptomatic tumours are endocrine active. Most secrete several polypeptide hormones, with one hormone having a dominant clinical effect and producing a recognisable clinical syndrome (Table 26.1). Hormones that may be secreted include insulin, gastrin, glucagon, somatostatin, vasoactive intestinal polypeptide, adrenocorticotrophin, melanocyte stimulating hormone and pancreatic polypeptides. Some islet cell tumours occur in the type I MEN (Multiple Endocrine Neoplasia) syndrome, which is characterised by hyperparathyroidism, excessive gastric secretion and pituitary tumours.

Increased hormone secretion may be due to a single adenoma, multiple adenomas, microadenosis, hyperplasia or islet cell adenocarcinoma. Although many tumours are very small at presentation, metastases are often present and these secrete the same hormone as the primary tumour. The **insulinoma** is most common, accounting for 60% of all islet cell tumours. The majority arise in elderly females. An insulinoma is usually solitary and small (less than 2 cm) at presentation and the distribution is uniform throughout the pancreas. The malignancy rate is 10%. Malignant tumours tend to be larger. Multiple tumours occur in 10% of cases and are usually less than 1 cm in size. Other tumours have a much higher malignancy rate, with the **gastrinoma** being malignant in 60% of cases. Most tumours are small at presentation, often with metastatic spread. Gastrinomas are frequently multiple. Over 90% of tumours lie in the triangle bordered by the confluence of the cystic and common hepatic ducts superiorly, the junction of the second and third parts of the duodenum inferiorly, and the head and body of the pancreas medially. Other functioning islet cell tumours predominantly arise in the body and tail of the pancreas. They are usually large at presentation and often malignant. Non-functioning islet cell

Table 26.1 Islet-cell Tumours

Hormone	Cell type	Clinical features
Glucagon	Alpha	Hyperglycaemia
		Anaemia
		Necrolytic migratory erythema
Insulin	Beta	Recurrent hypoglycaemia (early morning, before meals)
		Psychiatric symptoms
Somatostatin	Delta	Hyperglycaemia
		Low acid output
		Venous thrombosis
Pancreatic polypeptide	PP	Asymptomatic or features of another syndrome
Gastrinoma	G	Zollinger–Ellison syndrome
		Diarrhoea, malabsorption
		Peptic ulceration
VIP	Delta-1	Vipoma, Werner–Morrison syndrome or WDHA syndrome
		Watery diarrhoea, hypokalaemia
		acidosis, achlorhydria

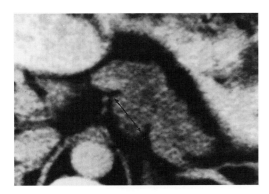

Fig. 26.21 CT scan. Insulinoma. Small mass protruding from the posterior surface of the pancreas (arrows).

tumours do not have noticeable hormonal effects even though small amounts are usually secreted. The majority are malignant and they present late, usually with jaundice or other symptoms of local invasion. *Calcification* is seen in 25% and typically has a coarse nodular pattern. Calcification invariably indicates malignancy; hepatic metastases may also calcify.

Islet cell tumours develop throughout the pancreas; insulinomas are slightly more common in the head of the pancreas, whereas other tumours have an increased tendency to arise in the tail.

Once a tumour is suspected on clinical and biochemical grounds, radiology is required to localise the lesion and to demonstrate metastatic spread. Endoscopic ultrasound and MRI are the investigations of choice. Contrast-enhanced CT (Fig. 26.21) has a higher sensitivity than transabdominal ultrasound. The advent of *intraoperative ultrasound* with high-frequency probes in conjunction with surgical palpation has resulted in successful localisation of tumours at rates of up to 100% in some series. At ultrasound an islet cell tumour is well defined, is of low echogenicity, may have an

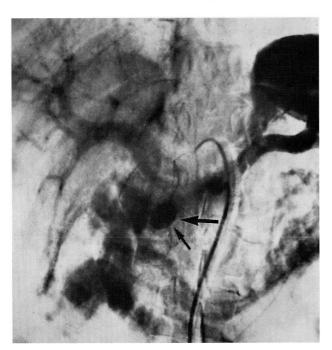

Fig. 26.22 Coeliac axis angiogram, capillary and venous phase. Subtraction film. The well-defined blush in the pancreatic head (arrowed) is an insulinoma. (Courtesy of Dr R. Dick.)

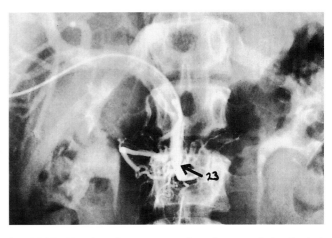

Fig. 26.23 Transhepatic venous sampling of pancreatic head vein in patient with suspected glucagonoma. ('23' is the sample number.) (Courtesy of Dr R. Dick.)

echogenic halo, and may deform the pancreatic outline. At CT the tumours are of low density with marked contrast enhancement. However, the gastrinoma is usually of low vascularity.

Angiography has a success rate of up to 90% but superselective catheterisation and multiple views may be necessary to demonstrate the typical dense tumour blush (Fig. 26.22). Very small tumours can be accurately located using *transhepatic venous sampling* (Fig. 26.23). Multiple samples are taken from the splenic vein and its pancreatic draining veins, and from the pancreaticoduodenal arcade.

Symptomatic metastases may be palliated by hepatic artery embolisation or by intra-arterial cytotoxic drug infusion. Occasionally a large primary inoperable tumour is embolised to palliate symptoms.

CT OF THE PANCREAS

Richard W. Whitehouse and Andrew R. Wright

Technical considerations

Careful attention to scanning technique is essential in order to obtain the best results in pancreatic CT, particularly in the staging of pancreatic cancer or the search for small lesions such as islet cell tumours. Water is preferred as an oral contrast agent, 500–900 ml 30 min before and 200–300 ml given immediately before the scan. Preliminary precontrast sections through the abdomen are required to establish the location of the pancreas, which may vary considerably between individuals. These plain scans are also useful for showing calcification and stones. The degree and timing of pancreatic enhancement is closely related to the amount and injection rate of the administered contrast medium. For optimal results, 150 ml of 300 mg/ml contrast medium injected at a rate of 3.5–4.0 ml/s is recommended. The exact phases and timing for pancreatic imaging depend to a degree on the scanner used. As multislice scanners can now scan larger volumes with thin slices very quickly, the different phases of contrast opacification can now be interrogated with more precision. It is generally accepted that the early arterial phase (20 s scan delay) is unsuitable for pancreatic scanning as the pancreatic parenchymal enhancement (and therefore lesion conspicuity) is poor. Optimal pancreatic enhancement and vascular opacification occurs in the so-called pancreatic parenchymal phase (40 s scan delay). The portal venous phase (65 s scan delay) gives excellent enhancement of liver parenchyma and the portal venous system. Typical slice collimation for the pancreatic phase scans would be 1.0–2.5 mm, with 2.5 mm slice width for the portal phase scans. A smaller field of view is recommended for the pancreatic phase scan, whereas the portal phase acquisition can be extended down to the pelvis with normal field of view to give an overview of the patient. When single-slice spiral scanning is used, the slice widths should be increased to give reasonable acquisition times (for example, 2.5 mm and 5.0 mm for the pancreatic and portal phases, respectively).

Normal appearances

The pancreas is an irregular or lobulated soft-tissue density organ lying in the retroperitoneum. Its body may lie at any level between L1 and L5. The long axis of the gland is usually obliquely orientated, with the head lying at an inferior level to the tail. The head lies anterior to the inferior vena cava with the second and third parts of the duodenum running around its lateral and inferior sides. Oral contrast or water opacification of the duodenal lumen is necessary for clear definition of the boundary between pancreas and bowel. The body of the pancreas lies anterior to the superior mesenteric artery and extends to the left, anterior to the left kidney and adrenal gland. Between the head and body of the gland, the neck of the pancreas is immediately anterior to the junction of the superior mesenteric and splenic veins. The tail of the pancreas extends into the splenic hilum. The uncinate process extends from the head of the gland posterior to the superior mesenteric vein, without an intervening fat plane between pancreatic tissue and the anterior, posterior and right lateral surfaces of the vein. The common bile duct can often be identified within the posterior part of the pancreatic head, adjacent to the second part of the duodenum. Normal pancreatic tissue enhances uniformly during intravenous contrast infusion. The normal pancreatic duct may be seen as a linear non-enhancing structure running along the long axis of the gland. The normal fat plane between the posterior surface of the gland and the splenic vein should not be mistaken for the duct. Reconstructions from thin section multislice scans can elegantly demonstrate the pancreatic structure and relationships in any plane (Fig. 26.24).

Clinical applications

CT is the mainstay of pancreatic imaging, able to demonstrate focal masses within the gland, calcifications, duct dilatation, cysts, abscesses and associated abnormalities in upper abdominal organs (e.g. hepatic metastases), lymph nodes and peripancreatic vascular structures. CT is a useful tool for guiding percutaneous pancreatic biopsy and cyst aspiration or drainage.

Acute pancreatitis

This is a clinical diagnosis, and the CT appearances may be unremarkable in over 25% of cases. In the rest, diffuse or focal glandular enlargement and focal areas of reduced density within the gland may be seen. Inflammation of the peripancreatic fat will produce

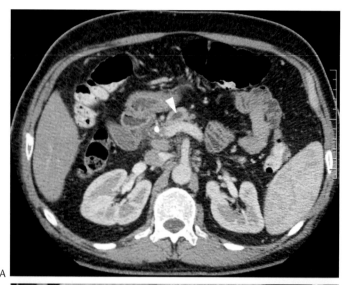

A

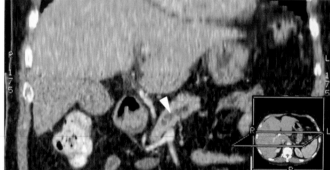

B

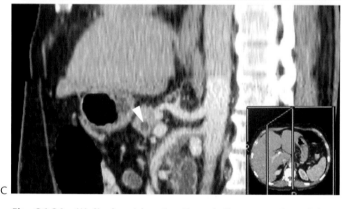

C

Fig. 26.24   (A) Single axial section through the pancreatic neck from multislice acquisition in a patient with ampullary obstruction. (B) Coronal reformat. (C) Sagittal reformat. In all images, the mildly dilated pancreatic duct can be clearly identified (arrowheads). (Courtesy of Dr H. Burnett, Hope Hospital, Salford.)

ill-defined strands of soft-tissue density within the fat ('mucky fat') (Fig. 26.25), although preservation of the fat around the superior mesenteric artery is usual. CT is useful for prognostic reasons, the degree of non-enhancement (pancreatic necrosis) seen on a dynamic contrast-enhanced study being a predictor of mortality and morbidity (Fig. 26.26). Complications of acute pancreatitis are also demonstrated—fluid collections tend to occur in the anterior pararenal spaces or lesser sac (Fig. 26.27), less commonly in the peritoneum (Fig. 26.27), and are of water density. Heterogeneous increased density collections may be due to haemorrhage, necrotic

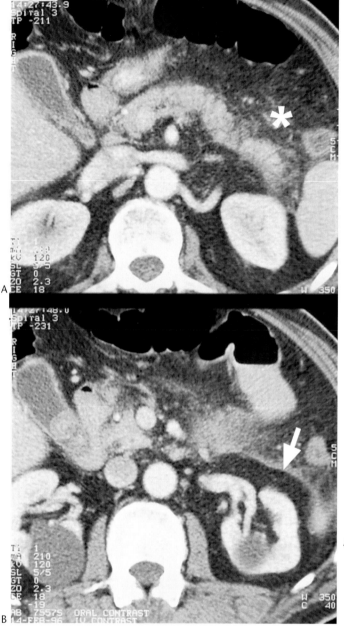

Fig. 26.25 (A,B) Acute pancreatitis. Minimal abnormality with soft-tissue density strands in the retroperitoneal fat around the tail of the pancreas (asterisk) and thickening of the anterior pararenal fascia on the left side (arrow). Note the gallstone in the gallbladder neck.

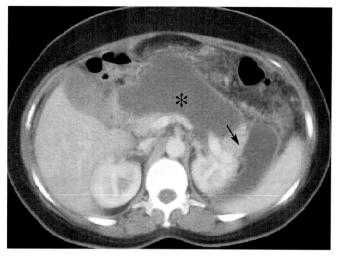

Fig. 26.26 Acute pancreatitis with necrosis and replacement of the pancreatic body by a fluid collection (asterisk). Note some persisting viable pancreatic tissue in the tail (arrow).

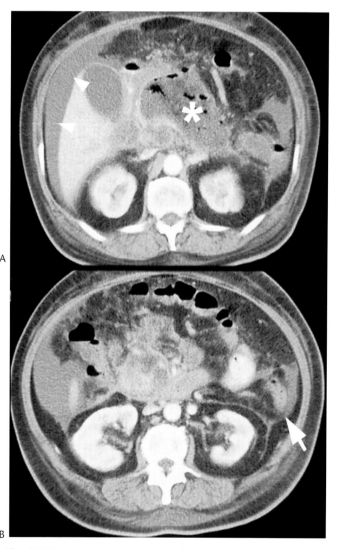

Fig. 26.27 (A,B) Acute pancreatitis with ascites (arrowheads) and focal fluid collection within the pancreas containing gas loculi (asterisk). Thickening of Gerota's fascia is evident (arrow).

tissue (pancreatic phlegmon) or secondary infection. Secondary infection to form abscesses significantly increases the mortality of acute pancreatitis. Gas in a fluid collection may indicate infection or fistula formation. Pseudoaneurysms of the gastroduodenal, splenic or other arteries may occur and can be demonstrated on contrast-enhanced CT. Fibrous encapsulation of pancreatic or peripancreatic fluid collections results in persistence of the collection as a pseudocyst. These fluid collections may persist for years. They can also become infected, and may also encase or compress adjacent vessels, particularly the portal and splenic veins, with consequent thrombosis.

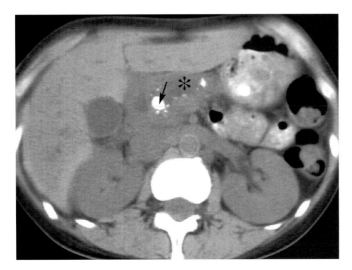

Fig. 26.28 Chronic calcific pancreatitis with a dilated pancreatic duct (asterisk) containing a calculus (arrow).

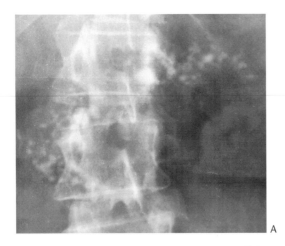

A

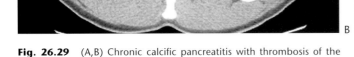

B

Fig. 26.29 (A,B) Chronic calcific pancreatitis with thrombosis of the portal vein and consequent splenic collateral veins (arrow).

Chronic pancreatitis

This may result from repeated attacks of acute pancreatitis or be an insidious progressive condition. Glandular enlargement or atrophy, irregular dilatation of the pancreatic duct ('chain of lakes' appearance), dilatation of the common bile duct, and calcifications in the pancreatic duct (Fig. 26.28) and tissue (Fig. 26.29) may all occur. Chronic pancreatitis may involve the entire gland or be focal; the latter can be difficult to distinguish from pancreatic carcinoma.

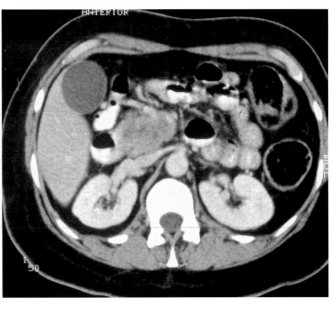

Fig. 26.30 Pancreatic carcinoma. Ill-defined poorly enhancing pancreatic mass.

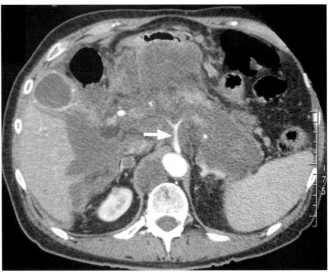

Fig. 26.31 Pancreatic carcinoma and adjacent adenopathy encasing the coeliac axis (arrow). (Courtesy of Dr H. Burnett, Hope Hospital, Salford.)

Malignant tumours

Adenocarcinoma

This accounts for over 80% of primary pancreatic neoplasms. The tumours are usually less vascular than normal pancreas, thus they produce a focal mass of lower attenuation than the adjacent gland on contrast-enhanced scans (Fig. 26.30). More than half of them occur in the pancreatic head; obstruction and dilatation of the common bile duct may be seen. Obstruction with uniform dilatation of the distal pancreatic duct in the absence of duct calculi (compared with the irregular chain of lakes of chronic pancreatitis) and atrophy of the distal gland are also characteristic CT findings. Extension beyond the gland to produce vascular encasement or obstruction can be identified on dynamic CT and is present in the majority of patients at diagnosis. It is a contraindication to surgical resection (Fig. 26.31). Metastatic disease in lymph nodes or liver may be identified, confirming the diagnosis where the differential includes chronic pancreatitis (Fig. 26.32).

Mucinous cystic tumours

Also known as *macrocystic cystadenoma* and *cystadenocarcinoma* (Fig. 26.33), these tumours are all considered to have malignant potential. They are commonest in middle-aged women, and tend to occur in the body or tail of the pancreas. Multiple large cysts with thick septa and irregular calcification are frequently seen in these lesions.

Other pancreatic neoplasms

Solid and papillary epithelial neoplasm of the pancreas is an uncommon low-grade malignant neoplasm occurring mainly in young women. At presentation the lesions may be large, and show mixed attenuation on CT with areas of haemorrhage, cystic degeneration and necrosis, fluid–debris levels and calcification in 30%. Peripheral enhancement after contrast may be present.

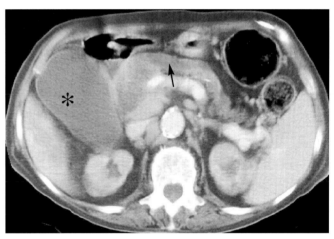

Fig. 26.33 Pancreatic cystadenocarcinoma. Ill-defined cystic mass in the pancreatic head with dilated pancreatic duct (arrow) and dilated gallbladder (asterisk) from duct obstructions.

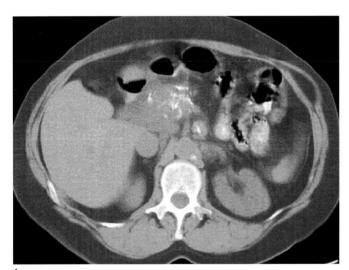

A

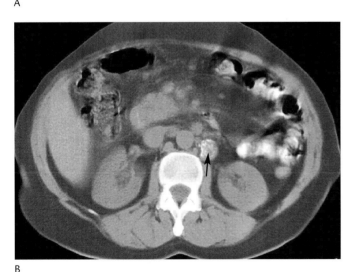

B

Fig. 26.32 (A) Calcified pancreatic carcinoma. (B) Calcification in a metastatic lymph node deposit (arrow).

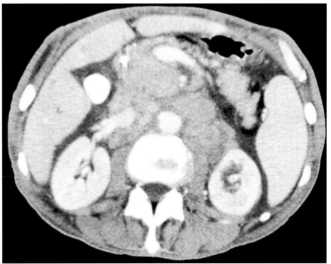

Fig. 26.34 Retroperitoneal lymphadenopathy in the region of the pancreas simulating a pancreatic mass. Note the anterior displacement of the pancreas which is marked by the position of the biliary stent.

Lymphoma in the region of the pancreas can be mistaken for a primary pancreatic tumour. In these cases, however, the pancreas is usually displaced anteriorly by the enlarged nodes (Fig. 26.34).

Benign tumours and cysts

Microcystic adenoma of the pancreas is a benign tumour most commonly found in the elderly, with a female preponderance. It may appear solid or multicystic on CT (Fig. 26.35), and any solid elements generally enhance following intravenous contrast medium. *Simple pancreatic cysts* are uncommon; they are seen in patients with von Hippel–Lindau syndrome (Fig. 26.36).

Endocrine disease

Functioning *pancreatic endocrine tumours* are rare, usually small (<2 cm) hypervascular tumours, generally found in the body or tail of the pancreas. Calcification occurs in less than a third of

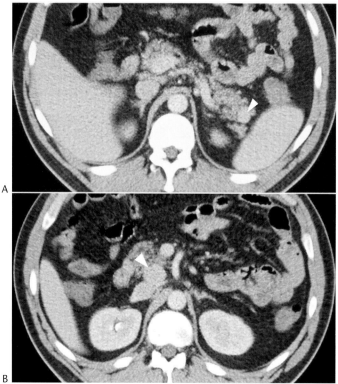

Fig. 26.37 Multifocal gastrinoma. Enhancing, hypervascular lesions are seen in the tail of the pancreas (A), and in the pancreatic head anterior to the IVC (B) (arrowheads).

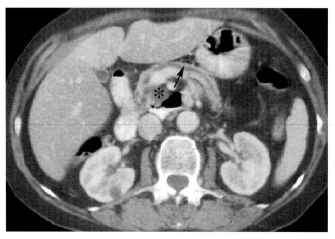

Fig. 26.35 Microcystic adenoma in the uncinate process (asterisk). Note the dilated pancreatic duct (arrow). (Courtesy of Dr S. Lee.)

lesions. The commonest of these tumours, gastrinomas and insulinomas, may be multiple (Fig. 26.37). Contrast-enhanced, thin-section spiral scanning has improved the detection of these lesions by CT. Non-functioning pancreatic endocrine tumours tend to be larger. Metastatic lesions from malignant islet cell tumours may be identified in the liver and may also show marked contrast enhancement.

Trauma

Trauma to the pancreas is uncommon and can be difficult to diagnose, but unrecognised pancreatic fracture has a mortality of 20% and causes considerable morbidity in the survivors. A high index of suspicion is necessary and dynamic or spiral contrast-enhanced scans should be performed. A fracture line, usually through the pancreas overlying the spine, focal or diffuse pancreatic swelling or haematoma, and peripancreatic or retroperitoneal fluid may be seen. Associated injury to the liver, spleen or kidneys is common.

Pancreatic transplantation

CT may be useful in assessing pancreatic transplant patients with abdominal pain or signs of sepsis, particularly in the postoperative period. The transplant is usually situated in the iliac fossa, anastamosed to the common iliac vessels. The graft duodenum may be anastamosed to the urinary bladder or directly to small bowel. On CT, the main graft vessels and degree of parenchymal enhancement can be assessed, and any perigraft fluid collections demonstrated (Fig. 26.38).

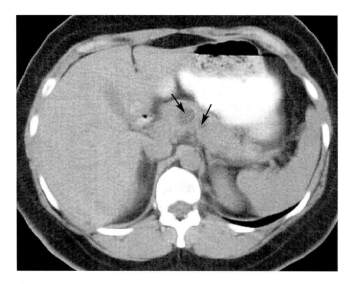

Fig. 26.36 Pancreatic cysts (arrows) in a patient with von Hippel–Lindau syndrome.

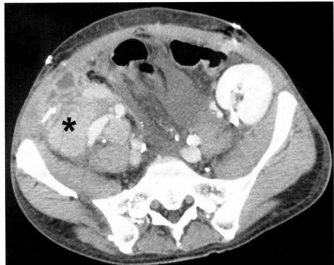

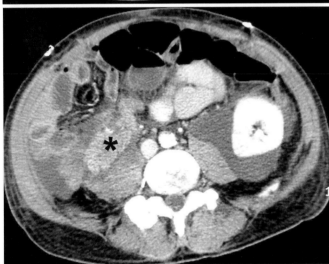

Fig. 26.38 Postoperative assessment of pancreatic transplant. (A) Good enhancement of head of right iliac fossa transplant with main vessel shown. Free fluid is present. (B) The pancreatic transplant tail is enhancing, and there is dilatation of proximal small bowel. Obstruction at the enteric anastamosis was found at laparotomy. There is a renal transplant in the left iliac fossa.

MAGNETIC RESONANCE IMAGING OF THE PANCREAS

Philip J. A. Robinson

Recent technical advances have allowed considerable improvements in the quality of pancreatic imaging by MRI. These include breath-hold acquisition using gradient-echo or long echo train fast spin-echo (FSE) sequences, dynamic studies with gadolinium enhancement, frequency-selective fat saturation, phased-array surface coils and the use of gastrointestinal and organ-specific contrast agents. MRI can now be considered to be of major value in pancreatic disease, particularly in the detection and staging of tumours, and in the preoperative demonstration of surgical anatomy. MR cholangiopancreatography (MRCP) now offers a non-invasive replacement for the diagnostic applications of endoscopic retrograde cholangiopancreatography (ERCP).

Techniques for pancreatic MRI: rationale

The parenchyma of the normal exocrine pancreas shows a characteristically bright signal on T_1-weighted images, possibly as a result of the high intracellular protein content. Pancreatic secretions (e.g. in a dilated pancreatic duct) typically show watery characteristics, with low signal on T_1 and high signal on T_2. Because of the high signal of the normal parenchyma, T_1-weighted imaging is particularly valuable in pancreatic disease. However, the fat surrounding the pancreas also produces high signal on T_1, so fat suppression is needed to define the margins of the gland. Suppressing fat from the rest of the image also has the secondary effect of expanding the dynamic range of the structures of interest, giving increased contrast between normal pancreas and areas of pathology. Breath-hold acquisitions are strongly recommended, but if non-breath-hold techniques must be used, motion correction methods such as gradient moment nulling or spatial presaturation are essential to minimise respiratory artefacts.

Technique and normal appearances

T_1-weighted imaging

On conventional spin-echo and gradient-echo T_1-weighted images, the normal pancreas is approximately isointense with the liver, or slightly hyperintense if fat suppression is used (Fig. 26.39). Pancreatic signal intensity decreases with advanced age, but with this reservation the pancreas should be considered abnormal if any part of the gland shows lower signal intensity than normal liver. A 3D breath-holding sequence (e.g. VIBE) is suitable for simultaneous display of soft tissues and vessels. With an effective slice thickness of $\simeq 2$–3 mm and a high signal/noise ratio, small (<1 cm) lesions are shown more effectively than on 2D images.

Dynamic gadolinium-enhanced imaging

Maximal enhancement of the pancreatic parenchyma occurs during the arterial and capillary phase, about 15–20 s after a bolus injection of intravenous gadolinium, and it is at this stage that carcinomas are best seen. Gastric and duodenal mucosa also show intense early enhancement. Demonstration of the anatomical relationship of tumours to the splenic, mesenteric and portal veins requires images obtained about 30 s later, but at this stage the parenchymal enhancement is already fading rapidly and many lesions will then be isointense.

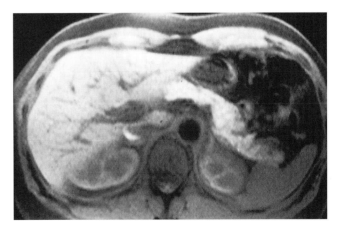

Fig. 26.39 Normal pancreas on T_1 image with fat suppression by the water excitation method. The pancreas appears slightly hyperintense to liver.

T_2-weighted imaging

The normal pancreas is moderately hyperintense on T_2 compared with the liver. T_2-weighted imaging is required for the detection of suspected islet cell tumours but is less sensitive than T_1-weighted imaging in detecting small pancreatic carcinomas. Benign lesions of the pancreas are best demonstrated on T_2-weighted images at an echo time (TE) of 90–120 msec. Because cystic lesions have a much longer T_2 than pancreatic tissue, these are best seen on heavily T_2-weighted images. In order to eliminate motion artefacts, breath-hold FSE is used. This requires a long echo train which induces magnetisation transfer in the normal pancreas, which further increases lesion–pancreas contrast. In patients with severe acute pancreatitis, T_2 imaging is particularly helpful in distinguishing between fluid and solid components of exudates and pseudocysts.

Image orientation

For the detection of either diffuse or focal pancreatic disease, transverse images are generally used (Fig. 26.40). For demonstrating the relation of tumours to the portal, splenic and superior mesenteric veins, direct coronal or coronal oblique views are helpful when used with sequential gadolinium-enhancement. 3D sequences with near-isotropic voxels provide the advantages of both axial and coronal views.

MR cholangiopancreatography (MRCP)

MRCP is a method for demonstration of the biliary and pancreatic ducts by MRI. Various sequences are used, but all rely on extreme T_2 weighting, which effectively eliminates signal from all tissues except stationary free-water protons, so that the images display only those structures containing fluid. As far as possible, gastric and duodenal contents must be excluded from the imaging volume so the pancreatic and bile ducts can be clearly seen. MRCP can be added to a conventional MRI examination of the pancreas or can be carried out as a separate study. The pancreatic duct anatomy can be shown in patients with tight strictures or total obstruction of the main duct where ERCP is unsuccessful or shows only the distal part of the duct system. MRCP is also suitable for patients in whom gastric or previous pancreatic surgery renders the endoscopic approach impractical. However, MRCP does not offer the opportu-

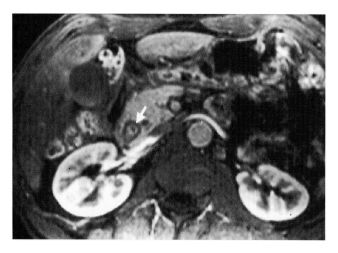

Fig. 26.40 Annular pancreas. T_1 image postgadolinium shows pancreatic tissue surrounding the second part of duodenum (arrow).

nity to carry out therapeutic manoeuvres. The sequences used are fairly resistant to artefacts arising from stents and metallic clips at the site of previous surgery.

Techniques for MRCP

Thick-slab single-shot FSE images and thin multislice HASTE images are both contributory. The thick-slab technique provides an overview of bile duct anatomy in <5 s and is suitable for imaging in different planes, while thin-slice images improve the visualisation of fine structures. Thick-slab images are obtained with a very long TE (940 msec or so) to provide complete suppression of background tissue. Careful positioning of the imaging slab will allow the slab thickness to be reduced to around 50 mm, which gives better image quality than a thicker slab. Thin slice images (4 mm) are obtained at a moderate TE of approximately 96 msec, as small calibre ducts are lost with longer TE. Thin slice images should be reviewed both as individual slices and after maximum intensity projection (MIP) reconstruction. Parallel saturation bands and fat suppression are used with both sequences. All images are acquired during breath-holding, with orientation determined by initial review of the individual anatomy of the gland—direct coronal or oblique images are often most useful.

MRI FINDINGS IN PANCREATIC DISEASE

Adenocarcinoma

The early recognition of pancreatic carcinoma remains problematic, with most tumours being unresectable at the time of diagnosis. Apart from the detection of tumours, the main role of imaging is in helping to distinguish tumours from inflammatory masses associated with chronic pancreatitis, and to determine the local extent of tumours preoperatively in those patients who are considered to be resection candidates. Adenocarcinoma is shown as an area of low signal on fat-suppressed T_1 images (Fig. 26.41). The signal intensity in the tumour is typically less than that seen in chronic pancreatitis, which is also hypointense on T_1. Carcinoma usually has more distinct margins and less enhancement with gadolinium than an inflammatory mass in chronic pancreatitis. If the remainder of the gland is normal, then the diagnosis is clear-cut, but in cases where the tumour has obstructed the main duct, causing distal pancreatitis, the distinction may be more difficult. Local staging requires visualisation of the margins of the tumour in relation to the duodenum, the posterior wall of the stomach, the main veins of the portal system, and the origin of the superior mesenteric artery. This can usually be achieved on axial images but for optimum demonstration of the relation of the pancreas to the superior mesenteric vein and the lower end of the portal vein, direct coronal or oblique coronal images are helpful. Images obtained at the peak of pancreatic enhancement, about 15–20 s after gadolinium injection, show maximum contrast between the tumour and normal tissue, while images obtained about 20–30 s later show relationships with the mesenteric and portal veins. Glandular enhancement may be already fading at this stage, so it is important to obtain sequential acquisitions to show both the tumour and the venous structures. Occlusion or circumferential involvement of the SMV or portal vein by tumour indicates that successful resection is extremely unlikely (Fig. 26.42) but if the tumour is shown to be clear of the main veins, curative resection may be feasible (Fig. 26.43). On T_2-weighted images, carcinoma may be isointense or may show signal which is slightly higher or slightly lower than that of normal pancreas.

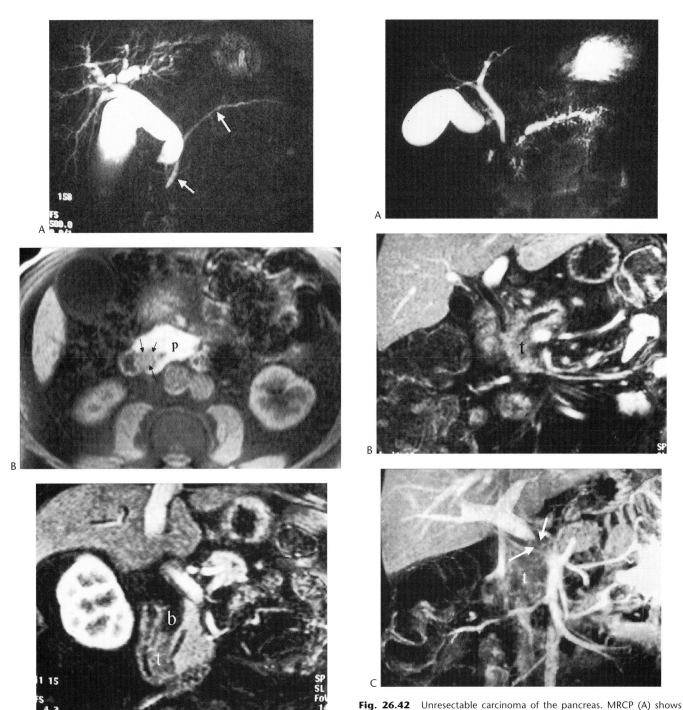

Fig. 26.41 Carcinoma of the ampulla. MRCP (A) shows grossly dilated common bile duct with mild dilatation of the pancreatic duct (arrows); fat-suppressed T_1 image (B) shows brightly enhancing normal pancreatic parenchyma (p) surrounding a small tumour with lower signal intensity (arrows); postgadolinium T_1 coronal image (C) shows the tumour (t) growing into the lower end of the common bile duct (b).

Fig. 26.42 Unresectable carcinoma of the pancreas. MRCP (A) shows obstruction of both pancreatic ducts and common bile duct; postgadolinium T_1 coronal image (B) shows the ducts are obstructed by an ill-defined tumour (t), which is slightly of lower signal intensity than adjacent pancreas; maximum intensity projection (C) shows the lower end of the portal vein to be encircled (arrows) by extension of the tumour (t) from the head of the pancreas.

Islet cell tumours

Most islet cell tumours are highly vascular and, either because of this or because of intralesional oedema, they produce marked reduction in signal on T_1 and increased signal on T_2-weighted images (Fig. 26.44). Enhancement after gadolinium is typically intense but may be either immediate or delayed, so sequential acquisitions are needed to maximise the detection of small lesions. These lesions are usually well shown on FSE T_2-weighted images, probably because of their relatively high content of free-water protons. Liver metastases from islet cell tumours are usually hypervascular, showing increased signal intensity on early post-gadolinium images.

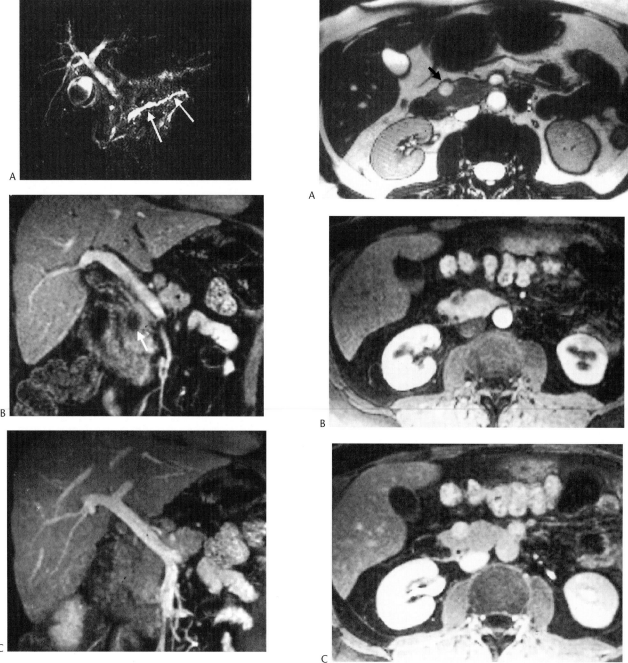

Fig. 26.43 Resectable carcinoma of the pancreas. MRCP (A) shows dilated pancreatic duct (arrows); postgadolinium T_1 coronal image (B) shows the tumour (arrow) with reduced signal intensity compared with adjacent parenchyma; maximum intensity projection image (C) shows the superior mesenteric and portal veins are not involved by the tumour.

Fig. 26.44 Insulinomas. T_2 image (A) shows a tumour as an area of high signal close to the surface of the head of pancreas and uncinate process (arrow); immediate postgadolinium T_1 image (B) shows marked enhancement in the adjacent parenchyma; delayed image 10 min after gadolinium (C) shows delayed enhancement in the lesion, while the pancreatic enhancement has faded.

Chronic pancreatitis

The anatomy of the pancreatic duct, presence of dilatation, strictures and filling defects are shown on MRCP (Figs 26.45, 26.46). The loss of functioning acinar tissue in chronic pancreatitis accounts for reduced signal intensity of the affected areas of the gland on fat-suppressed T_1-weighted images. Signal on T_2 images may be reduced or normal, while enhancement with gadolinium is less intense than in the normal pancreas. A localised inflammatory mass may be difficult to distinguish from carcinoma (Fig. 26.46) but other signs of chronic pancreatitis usually coexist. Generalised or localised dilatation of the pancreatic duct and pseudocysts either within or adjacent to the gland are shown as areas of low signal on T_1, high signal on T_2. Calcifications within the pancreas appear as areas of signal void and so are less conspicuous than 1on CT. However, the greater sensitivity of MR to detect the changes produced by fibrosis, which usually precedes calculus formation, may allow the earlier detection of structural change in chronic pancreatitis by MRI.

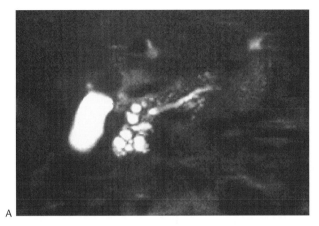

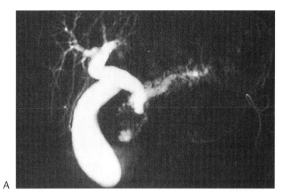

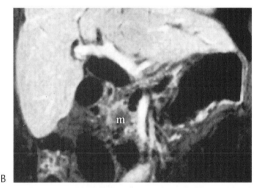

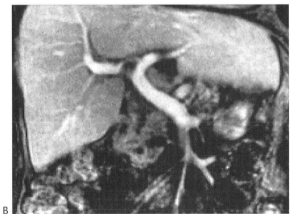

Fig. 26.45 Chronic pancreatitis. MRCP (A) shows dilated main pancreatic duct and multiple small cysts within the pancreatic head; postgadolinium coronal T$_1$ image (B) shows the pancreatic head is enlarged and heterogeneous with cystic areas of low signal.

Acute pancreatitis

Oedema of the pancreas causes diffuse signal reduction on T$_1$-weighted images and reduced enhancement after intravenous gadolinium. In more severe cases unenhanced gradient-echo T$_1$ images may show peripancreatic oedema as areas of low signal extending into the fat surrounding the gland, best seen on T$_1$ without fat suppression (Fig. 26.47). Dynamic postgadolinium acquisition is a sensitive method for demonstrating the presence and extent of pancreatic necrosis, shown as areas of diminished or absent parenchymal enhancement. Exudates and fluid collections within or around the pancreas can be seen on T$_1$ but are also well shown on T$_2$-weighted images, where they appear as areas of high signal intensity. T$_2$ images also give a clear distinction between the fluid and solid components of localised exudates and pseudocysts. This may be useful in patients who are candidates for percutaneous drainage of pancreatic collections, which often appear as areas of homogeneous low attenuation on CT even when the collection is mostly solid. Gas within the pancreas produces areas of signal void, and oral gadolinium contrast may be helpful when searching for fistulous connections with the upper gastrointestinal tract. Because of the high sensitivity of gradient-echo images to susceptibility effects produced by fresh bleeding, the presence of a haemorrhagic component in acute pancreatitis is probably detectable more readily (and over a longer time course) by MR than by CT, although the clinical value of this finding is uncertain.

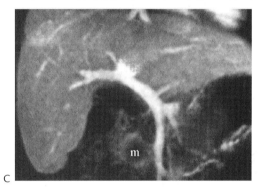

Fig. 26.46 Chronic pancreatitis with inflammatory mass. MRCP (A) shows dilated pancreatic duct, side branches and common bile duct; postgadolinium coronal T$_1$ image (B) shows a mass within the pancreatic head (m) which is obstructing the ducts; maximum intensity projection (C) shows the veins to be uninvolved.

A TECHNICAL STRATEGY FOR MRI OF THE PANCREAS

For suspected carcinoma and for islet cell tumours the examination should include transverse breath-hold T$_1$-weighted gradient-echo and T$_2$-weighted FSE images with fat suppression, and breath-hold dynamic T$_1$ after bolus injection of gadolinium. Regional tumour staging requires a series through the liver with gadolinium or superparamagnetic iron oxide (SPIO) contrast enhancement. In acute pancreatitis, pancreatic viability is assessed using gadolinium-enhanced T$_1$ images; exudates and pseudocysts also require T$_2$-weighted images. Fat-suppressed T$_1$ is probably the most useful sequence for chronic pancreatitis, with the addition of gadolinium enhancement to help distinguish between inflammatory mass and tumour. MRCP provides a demonstration of pancreatic duct anatomy in patients with chronic pancreatitis, carcinoma or pancreatic trauma.

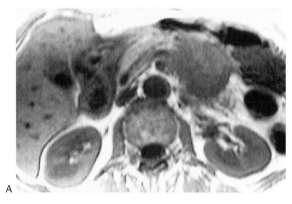

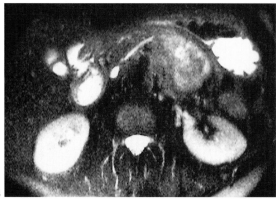

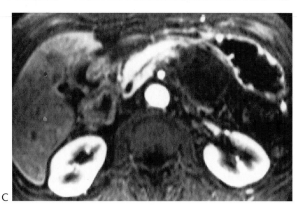

Fig. 26.47 Acute pancreatitis. Unenhanced images show the tail of the pancreas is replaced by an inflammatory mass which is hypointense on T$_1$ (A) and heterogeneously hyperintense on T$_2$ (B); postgadolinium T$_1$ image (C) shows total lack of enhancement in the mass, indicating focal necrosis.

ENDOSCOPIC RETROGRADE PANCREATOGRAPHY (ERP)

Richard Mason

The present uses of ERCP or ERP in pancreatic disease include the following:

- Further assessment of pancreatic abnormality demonstrated on ultrasound and CT, which has not been clarified by these diagnostic techniques or by fine needle aspiration or Trucut biopsy.
- Further investigation of suspected pancreatic disease where ultrasound and CT are normal or technically unsatisfactory.

- Definition of ductal anatomy in chronic pancreatitis for planning surgery (resection or drainage).
- Assessment of complications of acute pancreatitis (abscess and pseudocyst).
- Interventional—gallstone disimpaction in acute pancreatitis, pancreatic duct stone extraction, balloon dilatation of minor papilla in pancreas divisum.

The technique has a very high sensitivity for pancreatic disease but a normal ERP does not exclude either chronic pancreatitis or carcinoma.

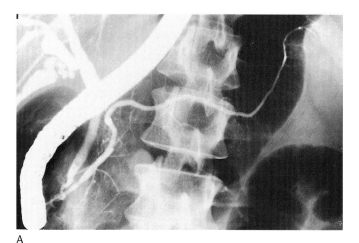

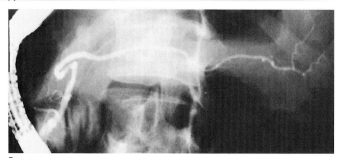

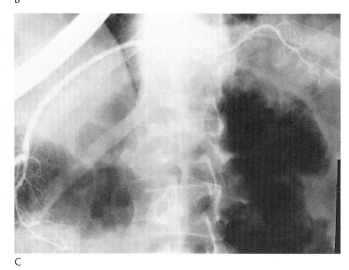

Fig. 26.48 (A–C) Normal variations in the shape of the pancreatic duct. Note complete filling of the duct system, both main and side ducts.

The normal ERP

This shows a smoothly tapering main duct. There may be a slight constriction in the duct at the junction of the head and neck as a normal variant. There are also smoothly tapered side branches distributed throughout the gland, and there is complete filling of the main duct right to the tail, which may be bifid (Fig. 26.48).

The abnormal ERP

Carcinoma

The signs of pancreatic carcinoma on the pancreatogram are, in order of frequency, main pancreatic duct abnormality, cavities, and field defects.

Main pancreatic duct abnormality

Pancreatic duct occlusion A complete block of the pancreatic duct is the commonest finding in pancreatic carcinoma (Fig. 26.49). When this occurs in the head of the gland, it is commonly accompanied by complete block of the common bile duct.

Diagnostic difficulty may arise because chronic pancreatitis may similarly produce a complete block. Reported differences in the contour of the duct stump have not proved helpful in making the distinction. Most useful is the state of the side branches downstream from the block. In pancreatic carcinoma these are usually normal, and in chronic pancreatitis usually abnormal (see below).

Pancreatic duct stricture This is an uncommon finding in carcinoma and is seen when clinical presentation occurs before the main pancreatic duct becomes completely blocked. The stricture may be from several millimetres to several centimetres in length and there may be accompanying displacement of the main and side ducts around the tumor mass.

Cavities

When the tumour is necrotic, contrast medium may enter cavities within the tumour. When irregular and multiple, this gives the pancreatogram a 'scrambled egg' appearance (Fig. 26.50).

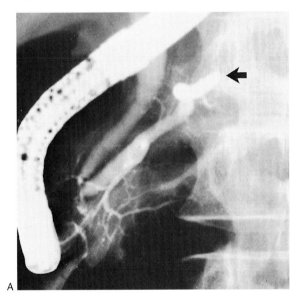

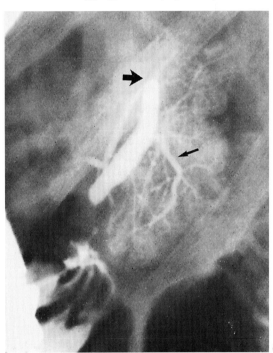

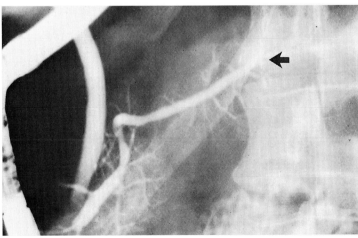

Fig. 26.49 (A,B) Pancreatic carcinoma producing complete occlusion of the main pancreatic duct (arrows). Note that the side branches downstream from the block are of normal calibre, aiding the differential diagnosis from main duct obstruction in chronic pancreatitis. (C) 'Acinarisation' has occurred because of excessive injection of contrast medium. This appearance of a block in the head of the gland must be distinguished from the ventral pancreas of pancreas divisum. The distinction can be made in this case because the main pancreatic duct is of normal calibre.

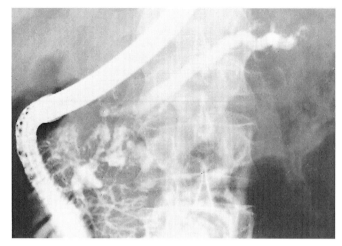

Fig. 26.50 'Scrambled egg' appearance in pancreatic carcinoma. Numerous necrotic cavities within the tumour in the head of the gland have filled with contrast medium. Note upstream dilatation of main duct and side branches resulting from obstruction.

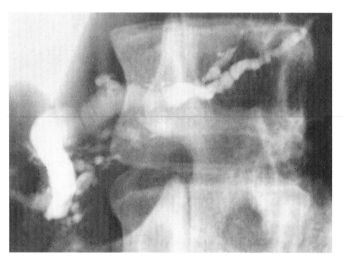

Fig. 26.51 Severe chronic pancreatitis. The main duct and the side branches are dilated and beaded.

Field defect

Destruction of part of the normal pancreas by carcinoma may simply lead to non-filling of several adjacent side branches, leaving the main pancreatic duct intact.

Chronic pancreatitis

The hallmarks of chronic pancreatitis are:

- *Dilatation and beading of the pancreatic duct and its branches* (Fig. 26.51). The changes can be classified into equivocal, mild, moderate, or severe types. In equivocal and mild chronic pancreatitis there is subtle dilatation and irregularity of some of the side branches (Fig. 26.52). In moderate and severe chronic pancreatitis, the main pancreatic duct is involved as well.
- *Block*. As in carcinoma, the block in the main pancreatic duct may be complete or incomplete.
- *Cavities*. These are variable in size but usually small and communicate with the main duct or branch ducts (Fig. 26.53).

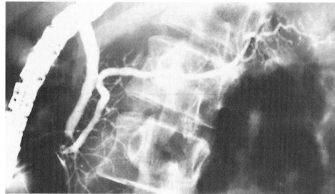

A

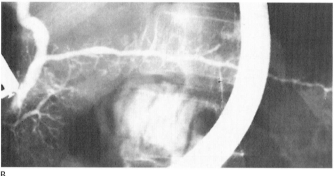

B

Fig. 26.52 Mild chronic pancreatitis. The main pancreatic duct is normal but there are subtle dilatations of some of the side branches. Note the slight narrowing of the main duct at the junction of the head and body in (A); this is a normal variant.

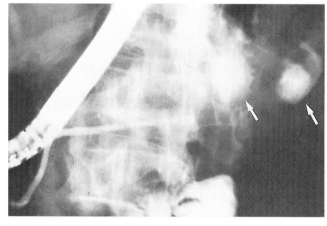

Fig. 26.53 Cavities have filled from the main duct in the tail of the gland (arrows). Chronic or recurrent pancreatitis.

- *Calculi*. Calculi are virtually pathognomonic of chronic pancreatitis. They may be single or multiple and are usually, but not always (Fig. 26.54), calcified. They may be found in a non-dilated duct system.

Pancreas divisum (*Figs 26.55, 26.56*)

In the embryo, separate dorsal and ventral pancreatic segments bud from the duodenum. The ventral segment develops in association with the bile duct, the two structures draining together through the

The clinical significance of pancreas divisum is a matter of debate. There is convincing evidence that the anomaly can lead to obstructive pancreatic pain and pancreatitis of the dorsal segment. In such cases, the dorsal duct is dilated and it is postulated that the orifice of the minor papilla is not wide enough for adequate drainage.

The pancreas divisum abnormality is diagnosed when cannulation of the major papilla at ERP outlines only a small branching duct system without communication with the main pancreatic duct. Occasionally, the ventral duct system is rudimentary or absent. No pancreatogram can be obtained via the major papilla, and the anomaly will only be detected if accessory cannulation is attempted and is successful.

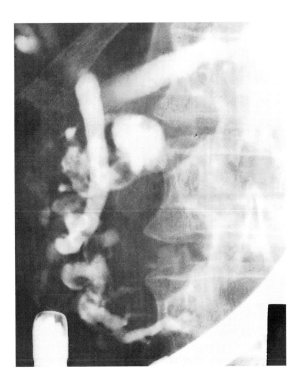

Fig. 26.54 The main pancreatic duct is dilated and contains numerous lucent stones. These findings are pathognomonic of chronic pancreatitis.

major papilla. The ventral segment rotates around the duodenum to lie below the dorsal segment and carries the bile duct with it. A communication develops between the dorsal and ventral ducts, resulting in the dorsal pancreas draining principally through the duct of the ventral pancreas. The duct of the dorsal pancreas downstream from the communication becomes relatively smaller and may disappear completely.

Sometimes the communication between the two pancreatic duct systems is not established and the embryonic state of divided pancreas persists into adult life ('pancreas divisum').

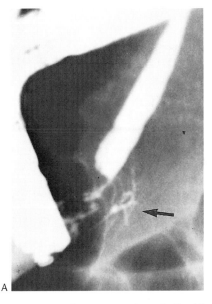

Fig. 26.55 (A) Tiny ventral component (arrow). The bile duct is also opacified.

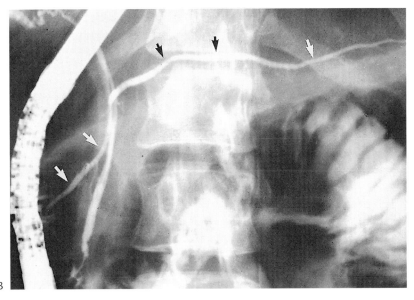

Fig. 26.55 (B) The dorsal component (in a different patient) has been filled (arrows) from the minor papilla. The bile duct terminates at the major papilla, below the minor.

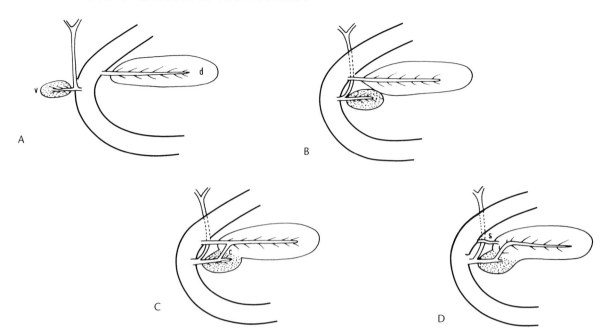

Fig. 26.56 Embryological development of the pancreas. (A) Dorsal segment (d) draining through the duct of Santorini and minor papilla. Ventral segment (v) developing in association with the bile duct and draining through the duct of Wirsung and major papilla. (B) The ventral segment has rotated with the bile duct to occupy its definitive position. This is the arrested embryological position of the adult pancreas divisum. Failure to rotate can give rise to annular pancreas (Fig. 26.9). (C) A wide communication (c) has developed between the dorsal and ventral ducts. (D) The terminal portion of the dorsal duct or duct of Santorini (s) becomes relatively smaller and may disappear completely. This is the normal adult arrangement.

ULTRASOUND OF THE PANCREAS

Techniques

Advances in equipment continue to improve visualisation of the pancreas. The pancreas is usually visualised using curved array transducers with imaging frequencies of 3–8 MHz. *Tissue harmonic imaging* has been shown to improve penetration, detail and total image quality when compared with fundamental frequency imaging but a major impediment to complete visualisation of the pancreas remains an impediment to visualisation of the entire abdomen. This is largely due to gas in the stomach and faecal matter and gas in the transverse colon. It is possible to improve visualisation by a change in patient position and the use of ingested fluid (Fig. 26.57).

Although different types of fluid have been described for optimum visualisation of the upper abdominal organs, tap water that has been allowed to settle usually suffices. Ingestion of approximately 250 mL water will act as an acoustic window and the fluid can be encouraged into the fundus, body and antrum by rotating the patient from right anterior oblique to left anterior oblique positions.

If the patient stands, the pancreas, which is retroperitoneal, remains relatively fixed in position, while liver and stomach will descend, again acting as an acoustic window. Similarly this may cause gas and faecal matter in the transverse colon to move inferiorly and afford better visualisation of the pancreas.

Optimum visualisation is afforded by a knowledge of the anatomical relations of the pancreas, particularly with respect to the origins of the coeliac axis and superior mesenteric artery. Utilising these vessels as markers in the sagittal plane, the neck of the pancreas can invariably be visualised and an axial plane achieved simply by rotating the probe through approximately 90°. It is important to recognise that the axis of the pancreas is variable. The position of the head is fixed in the duodenal loop but the tail may be at the same level as, or above or below the pancreatic head.

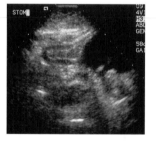

Fig. 26.57 Fluid in the fundus and body of the stomach together with some particulate matter afford visualisation of the tail of the pancreas. Harmonic imaging provides good quality images of an obese patient.

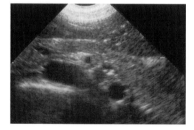

Fig. 26.58 Normal neck and body of a pancreas. Note the inferior mesenteric artery and vein situated to the left of the aorta in a slim patient.

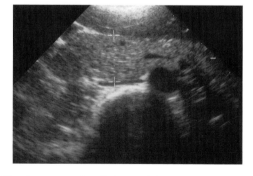

Fig. 26.59 Anteroposterior diameter of the pancreatic head. At 2.5 cm this is at the upper limit of normal.

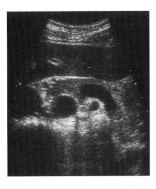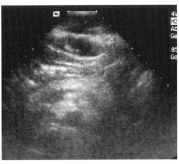

Fig. 26.60 Normal variation in the size of the pancreas. A small but normal pancreas in a 42-year-old female.

Fig. 26.61 Echogenic pancreas in an elderly obese woman. Note the poor definition of outline and poor differentiation from surrounding retroperitoneal fat, in spite of the use of tissue harmonic imaging.

Pancreatic anatomy

The pancreas is seen on ultrasound as a comma-shaped structure, draped over the anterior surface of the aorta, inferior vena cava and anterior aortic branches (Fig. 26.58). The tail extends into the splenic hilum but is frequently difficult to visualise by ultrasound, largely as a consequence of overlying bowel gas. The size of the gland has been reported to measure 25 mm, 15 mm and 20 mm in the head, body and tail, respectively, but there are significant differences between patients in the shape of the gland and significant variation in the size of the gland in individuals of different ages (Fig. 26.59). Consequently, if measurement is to be used in the assessment of the pancreas, it is important to recognise the effect that shape and age will have on these dimensions. In the child and young adult, there is a direct relationship between age and pancreatic size, whereas after the age of 40 there may be a gradual reduc-

tion in all dimensions. This change in size occurs pari passu with the changes in echogenicity that are associated with the ageing process (Fig. 26.60).

Pancreatic echogenicity

The pancreas is situated in the retroperitoneum surrounded by varying amounts of retroperitoneal fat. With ageing there is a progressive replacement of pancreatic acinar tissue by fat lobules. This process produces a gradual increase in echogenicity of the pancreas after the age of 40, as well as contributing to an increase in irregularity of the pancreatic outline, with the result that the margins are less easy to define (Fig. 26.61). Most patients over 50 years and all patients over 80 will have marked increase in echogenicity, distinctly higher than that of the liver. Similarly, obesity is associated with increase in pancreatic echogenicity. This is probably also due to replacement of the pancreas by fat lobules but may be in part due to a hardening of the ultrasound beam consequent upon sound attenuation by subcutaneous and peritoneal fat. Although the echogenicity of the pancreas changes with age and obesity, the pancreas should remain homogeneous and alterations in homogeneity are markers of pathology, whereas a uniform increase in echogenicity is rarely so. One exception to this, however, is the appearance of the ventral embryonic pancreas. It is thought that replacement by fat is less common in the ventral pancreas or uncinate process, perhaps consequent upon the different embryological origin of the ventral and dorsal pancreas. Notwithstanding the cause, the differences in fatty infiltration result in different echogenicities between ventral and dorsal pancreas. For the most part this is subtle but can occasionally be so marked as to cause a pseudomass effect. This is important since, although carcinoma of the uncinate process is rare, it may present in the absence of pancreatic or biliary duct dilatation. Variations in the echogenicity of the uncinate process are not seen prior to the age of 25 and are most common in middle-aged females with a female to male preponderance of 1.5 to 1. Thus, approxi-

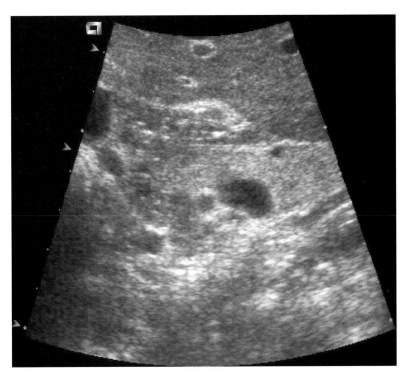

Fig. 26.62 Normal pancreas. Note the echo-poor ventral anlage.

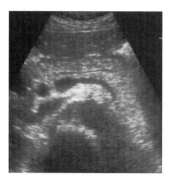

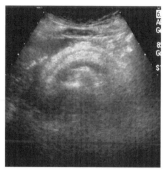

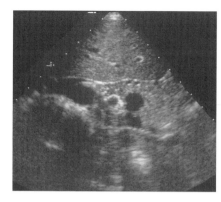

Fig. 26.65 Pancreatic head to the left of the aorta. Note the position of the superior mesenteric artery and vein.

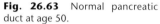

Fig. 26.63 Normal pancreatic duct at age 50.

Fig. 26.64 Echogenic pancreas in the elderly. Note the pancreatic duct.

mately 43% of women, compared with 27% of men, have an echo-poor ventral anlage (Fig. 26.62).

The technique for the examination of the pancreatic duct is critical. Evaluation of the duct should be performed during quiet respiration. In some patients, pancreatic duct diameter increases with breath-holding in inspiration. As many as 28% of lean individuals may demonstrate a diameter increase of up to 1 mm, and in a proportion of these the end-inspiration duct diameter may reach 2.5 mm.

The pancreatic duct

The normal pancreatic duct is rarely seen in its entirety in the young patient. Segments of the duct may be visualised as the duct courses in and out of the plane of scan. They appear as short segment parallel lines, usually measuring less than 1 mm in diameter. There is a gradual increase in size of the pancreatic duct with advancing years, which probably accounts for the improved visualisation as well as the greater contrast difference between an echogenic pancreas and an echo-free duct. In young patients, the mean duct diameter is 1.5 mm (18–29 years), while it is 1.9 mm between 40 and 49 years and 2.3 mm in patients over 80 years (Fig. 26.63). When visualised, the duct is seen as a linear tubular structure with highly reflective walls (Fig. 26.64). Side branches are not visualised. Because of the variation in duct size, different criteria need to be applied to different age groups in the diagnosis of dilatation of the pancreatic duct. Under the age of 50, a duct of 2 mm or greater should be considered with suspicion, while 3 mm should be so considered at any age.

Anatomical relations and vascular anatomy

The retroperitoneal location of the pancreas and the anterior relation of stomach, transverse colon and small bowel mean that these contribute very significantly not only to imaging of the pancreas but also in reflection of pancreatic pathology. Retroperitoneal fat is highly reflective but homogeneous. Consequently, abnormalities of the fat may reflect both inflammatory and neoplastic pathology.

The importance of the superior mesenteric artery and coeliac axis in pancreatic imaging has already been mentioned. Visualisation of the major branches of the coeliac axis is important in the evaluation of anatomical variations, such as accessory or replaced right hepatic artery, and in the assessment of stage of pancreatic tumour. Although anterior and posterior pancreatic arcades are rarely seen on ultrasound, nor indeed are they reliably imaged utilising colour flow Doppler, the gastroduodenal artery can be visualised. Encasement and displacement of the coeliac axis, gastroduodenal artery and/or superior mesenteric artery may be important in

staging. Furthermore, the advent of ultrasound contrast media may afford the visualisation of intrapancreatic vessels, which may be useful for differentiation of benign from malignant disease. The splenic vein which runs posterior to the body of the pancreas and forms the portal vein at the confluence with the superior mesenteric vein may similarly be involved in pancreatic pathology. In particular, splenic vein invasion can occur consequent upon pancreatic carcinoma.

Anatomical variations

Variation in the anatomy of the splanchnic arteries has already been described. It is important to recognise that the so-called normal arrangement of the coeliac axis and superior mesenteric artery are present in only 40% of the population. Although most of the anatomical variations are of little management importance, a hepatic arterial branch arising from the superior mesenteric artery may course posteriorly to the pancreatic head and occupy a posterior position within the porta hepatis, a fact that is important at the time of surgery.

The position of the pancreas within the abdomen is as stated related to the duodenal loop. However, as a consequence, the pancreas may be situated in a more cephalad or more caudad position than expected. Similarly, the head of the pancreas may not always be related to the anterior surface of the inferior vena cava, where it will normally cause a minor impression. Instead, occasionally it may be displaced to the left of the aorta. This is more commonly seen in patients who have had abdominal surgery, particularly left nephrectomy or splenectomy, but may be seen in normal individuals (Fig. 26.65).

Pancreatic neoplasms

Pancreatic carcinoma is an insidious tumour, usually presenting late. The majority arise from ductal epithelium, although adenocarcinoma and cystic pancreatic tumours also occur. Between 60 and 70% of tumours arise in the pancreatic head (Fig. 26.66), 20–30% in the pancreatic body (Fig. 26.67) and only 10% in the tail. Tumours of the pancreatic head will present with obstructive jaundice, while tumours elsewhere in the gland have a silent presentation. Unremitting epigastric pain is usually only apparent when the tumour is inoperable.

The investigation of jaundice

Ultrasound forms a central plank in the investigation of jaundice. It is highly sensitive technique for the demonstration of both intra- and extrahepatic bile duct dilatation (Fig. 26.68). The level of

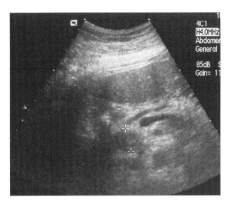

Fig. 26.66 Pancreatic carcinoma. Echo-poor rounded mass in the head of the pancreas with early dilatation of the pancreatic duct demonstrated anterior to the splenic vein.

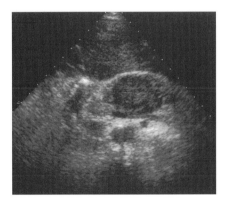

Fig. 26.67 Echo-poor tumour of the pancreatic body. Note the relatively large size of tumour prior to clinical presentation.

obstruction can be identified in the majority of patients, either by direct visualisation of the duct or by demonstration of a distended gallbladder (Fig. 26.69). Tumours greater than 1.0 cm in diameter can usually be demonstrated, although smaller periampullary tumours are frequently not directly visualised. However, the demonstration of a dilated extrahepatic bile duct, with or without intrahepatic bile duct dilatation (Fig. 26.70), in the absence of stones demonstrated within the duct by ultrasound should prompt further investigation with MRCP or spiral CT.

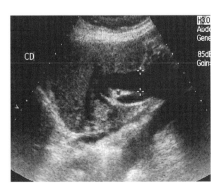

Fig. 26.68 Oblique scan through the porta hepatis demonstrating dilated common bile duct measuring 18 mm.

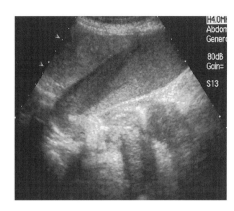

Fig. 26.69 Distended gallbladder containing partial layering sludge in a patient with a carcinoma of the pancreatic head. This is the ultrasound Courvoisier sign.

The demonstration of the 'double-duct sign', that is dilatation of the common bile duct and of the main pancreatic duct, is found in over 80% of cancers of the pancreas responsible for jaundice. It has been thought to be a pathognomonic sign for pancreatic carcinoma, although recent data would suggest that as many as 15% of patients with dilatation of both pancreatic and biliary ducts will have benign pathology. However, a high index of suspicion for neoplastic disease must be maintained in the presence of this sign (Fig. 26.71).

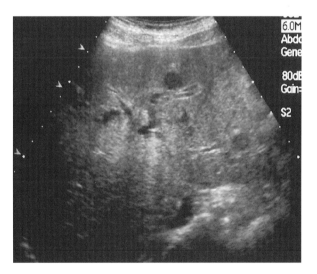

Fig. 26.70 Ultrasound of the liver. Note the dilated intrahepatic bile ducts and the small rounded echo-poor metastases.

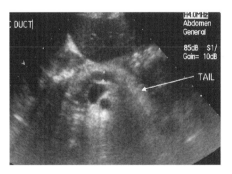

Fig. 26.71 Dilatation of the pancreatic duct in a patient with carcinoma of the head of the pancreas.

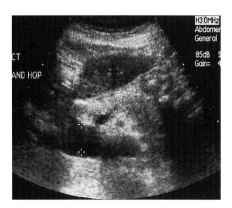

Fig. 26.72 Carcinoma of the uncinate process. An echo-poor tumour is demonstrated within the uncinate process without evidence of dilatation of the pancreatic or bile ducts.

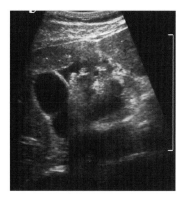

Fig. 26.73 Carcinoma associated with lymphadenopathy extending into the coeliac axis group of nodes, thickening of omentum and ascites.

Ultrasound features of the tumour

To a very large degree, CT relies upon contour alterations for the diagnosis of pancreatic tumour. By contrast, although changes in contour are important, they are less so than alterations in parenchymal texture. Although partly consequent upon absolute size, pancreatic carcinoma presents with an echogenicity that is less than that of the surrounding normal pancreas (Fig. 26.72). This sonographic contrast is less marked in younger patients when pancreatic carcinoma is rare and becomes more pronounced as the age at presentation is greater. The margins of the tumour, although irregular, are usually well defined. If ill defined, it either implies previous inflammatory disease or may suggest that the diagnosis is one of focal pancreatitis. In cases such as this, fine needle aspiration biopsy may be necessary to confirm the diagnosis. Tumours in the tail of the pancreas usually present late and may be as much as 5.0 cm in diameter by the time of presentation.

Adenocarcinoma of the pancreas is a highly malignant neoplasm that presents late and carries a dismal prognosis. Although there are no specific features that allow differentiation of the histological type, there is usually evidence of metastatic disease and/or local spread at the time of presentation.

Carcinoma of the uncinate process, although hitherto considered extremely rare, may occur in as many as 8% of cases of pancreatic carcinoma. Presentation with jaundice is rare, seen in approximately 12% of patients, and vascular involvement is frequently apparent at the time of presentation. Of particular importance is the differentiation of the different echogenicity of the ventral pancreas from a pancreatic tumour, and if in doubt fine needle biopsy should be undertaken.

Staging

Historically, patients with pancreatic carcinoma have a poor 5 year survival. It is said that in spite of a small tumour load at the time of death, most patients will present with hepatic micrometastases undetectable by any imaging methodology in the vast majority of patients. Nonetheless, local tumour staging remains important. Although most of the surgical strategies remain somewhat palliative, the feasibility of local resection should be considered. Further improvements in imaging may afford more accurate detection of hepatic metastases and prediction of successful 'curative' resection (Fig. 26.70). In this respect, tissue harmonic imaging has been shown to improve the sensitivity of detection of hepatic metastases by ultrasound and it may be that contrast-enhanced imaging, together with pulse inversion harmonics and/or other methods of enhanced visualisation of ultrasound

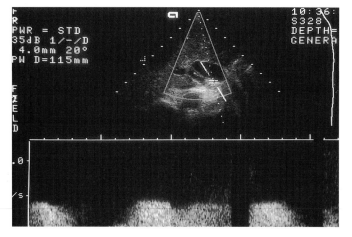

Fig. 26.74 Abnormality of flow pattern in the portal vein consequent upon invasion by tumour.

contrast will further enhance ultrasound sensitivity. In the assessment of signs of local invasion and extension, ultrasound remains of value. Although some studies would suggest that UMRI (ultrafast MRI) may display higher sensitivities, nonetheless extrapancreatic tumour extension, lymph node involvement and vascular invasion are all detected with a sensitivity approximating 80% or better. The diagnosis depends upon the demonstration of extension of irregular echo-poor tissue, for example into the root of the mesentery, enlargement of local lymph nodes or involvement and thickening of adjacent bowel wall (Fig. 26.73). Vascular involvement can be identified by distortion, encasement and straightening of vessels, together with evidence of irregularity, particularly of the splenic and portal vein wall, with intraluminal echogenic material consistent with either clot or extension of tumour. Spectral Doppler may identify significant flow disturbance (Fig. 26.74). Complete occlusion of the splenic/portal vein can be seen in up to 15% of patients (Fig. 26.75).

Differential diagnosis

The mass effect of the ventral pancreas has already been described. The major differential diagnosis for pancreatic carcinoma is focal pancreatitis. Focal pancreatitis produces similar appearances to that of a pancreatic carcinoma with an irregular echo-poor mass. As a general rule, the mass exhibits poorly defined margins and may also exhibit changes within the peripancreatic fat and the root of the mesentery consistent with inflammation (heterogeneity and coarsening of echoes). There may be other supportive signs. In particular, features of chronic pancreatitis such as calcification and irregular dilatation of the pancreatic duct may be helpful but of

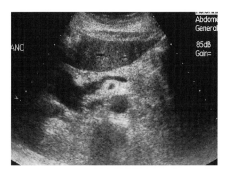

Fig. 26.75 The portal vein is filled with echogenic material. There is an irregular, partially cystic mass in the region of the head of the pancreas. Early bile duct dilatation is noted within the liver.

course pancreatic carcinoma can also occur in patients with chronic pancreatitis. The presence of a gallstone in the distal common bile duct is similarly of value but not pathognomonic. Focal chronic pancreatitis is most commonly seen in the region of the pancreatic head immediately adjacent to the common bile duct. This is called groove pancreatitis. It is possible that contrast-enhanced colour flow Doppler will contribute to the differential diagnosis of chronic pancreatitis from pancreatic carcinoma. Pancreatic carcinoma is predominantly a hypovascular tumour, whereas focal acute pancreatitis demonstrates hyperaemia. Research studies investigating the role of ultrasound have hitherto used intra-arterial injection of microbubbles (carbon dioxide) and have reported an accuracy of differentiating the two conditions as high as 95%. It is possible that some of the new generation ultrasound contrast media may achieve similar accuracies.

Cystic tumours of the pancreas

Although rare, serous and mucinous cystic tumours of the pancreas are important because of the difficulty with differentiating these from pancreatic pseudocysts. Cystic tumours are a range of tumours with varying potential for malignancy. The lesions are slow growing, usually multilocular with multiple septa which may be thick or thin. There may be solid intracystic projections but these probably occur in less than 20% of cases. Similarly, calcification is seen in a significant minority, present in more than 10%, but even utilising the features of multilocularity, tumour nodules, vascularity and calcification, probably less than half of pancreatic cystic tumours will be diagnosed prior to surgery. It is therefore critically important to consider the history prior to determining management.

The demonstration of any cystic mass within the pancreas in the absence of a history of acute or chronic pancreatitis must be considered with suspicion (Fig. 26.76). At the very least, fine needle aspiration of the cyst and assessment of the amylase content should be undertaken. However, this may be misleading if only amylase measures are made. It is important to measure serum levels of carcinoembryonic antigen and carbohydrate antigen 19-9. Whether intracystic levels of these tumour markers will be of value is not yet clear.

Other tumours

Pancreatic metastases are a late manifestation of disease and are rarely identified on ultrasound.

Benign islet cell tumours are rarely seen by ultrasound. They are usually very small and have a similar echogenicity to that of normal pancreatic tissue. They are frequently multiple and transabdominal ultrasound has very little role in their evaluation.

Insulinomas are similarly small and, although the majority are solitary, multiple lesions occur in just under a quarter. Metastases, though uncommon are characteristic, producing a studed starry-sky appearance of echogenic foci within the liver.

Gastrinomas are usually multiple and frequently malignant but are still smaller. They are rarely demonstrated by transabdominal ultrasound. Such endocrine tumours may be located by peroperative ultrasound but their size and echogenicity mean that even with this refinement the sensitivity for their detection remains low.

In countries where the prevalence of pancreatic carcinoma is high, a screening role for ultrasound has been proposed. Using this approach, tumours of less than 1 cm in diameter may be detected but the impact on outcome has not been evaluated.

Acute pancreatitis

Acute pancreatitis is a severe condition whose mortality approaches 10%. In spite of advances in intensive care, the mortality has remained unchanged for more than a decade. This may in large part be due to a failure to diagnose the condition. Up to 40% of cases may remain undetected until autopsy. The importance of imaging, therefore, as an adjunct to the assessment of serum amylase is vital. The contribution of ultrasound to achieving early diagnosis requires careful attention to technique, an understanding of the local disease process and an awareness of local and distant signs.

Acute pancreatitis is commonly accompanied by focal or generalised intestinal ileus. The sentinel loop is a characteristic finding

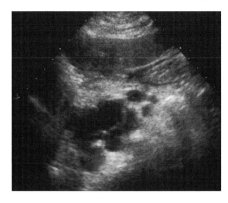

Fig. 26.76 Complex cystic mass in the head of the pancreas with adjacent lymphadenopathy. Cystadenocarcinoma.

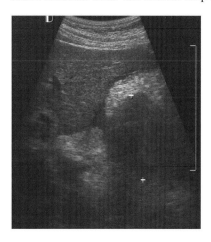

Fig. 26.77 Acute pancreatitis. Markedly enlarged and echo-poor pancreatic head is partially obscured by thickened omentum. Note the small amount of fluid beneath the liver.

on a plain abdominal X-ray. The presence of focal or diffuse gaseous distension of the bowel may seriously compromise ultrasound imaging (Fig. 26.77) In some series, as many as 40% of ultrasound examinations will be technically inadequate. Patients with acute pancreatitis will be seriously ill and consequently standard techniques for improving ultrasound visualisation, such as oral fluid or the erect position, are not possible. It is important in this situation to use both decubitus positions in order to attempt to displace gas and improve pancreatic visualisation as well as to optimise the demonstration of the gallbladder and bile ducts.

Direct findings

The appearances of the pancreas in acute pancreatitis are variable and depend upon the contribution of oedema, necrosis and haemorrhage. The gland may be diffusely or focally enlarged, is characteristically echo-poor, although if there is haemorrhagic pancreatitis or acute pancreatitis on a background of chronic pancreatitis, then the appearances may be heterogeneous with areas of increased echogenicity (Fig. 26.78). The pancreatic duct may be enlarged and this may be of particular value in the demonstration of acute pancreatitis in children, when the demonstration of a pancreatic duct

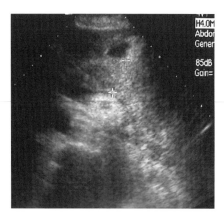

Fig. 26.78 Mild pancreatic enlargement but with significant heterogeneity of the parenchyma.

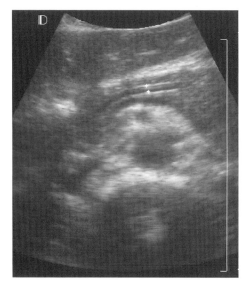

Fig. 26.79 Acute pancreatitis. Dilatation of the pancreatic duct in a 16-year-old. Note the enlargement of the pancreatic tail.

diameter of greater than 2 mm is strongly indicative of the diagnosis (Fig. 26.79). However, visualisation of the pancreatic duct may be compromised, not only by the previously described ileus, but also by reduction in the contrast between the echo-poor pancreas and the echo-free duct.

The appearances of the pancreas can change rapidly as there may be rapid clinical deterioration in patients with acute pancreatitis. Sonographic appearances may change significantly within a matter of hours. The development of peripancreatic fluid collections as well as rapid pancreatic enlargement are a particular feature of this. Demonstration of peripancreatic fluid is the precursor of pancreatic pseudocyst formation. Pancreatic phlegmon or necrosis are more readily demonstrated on CT than on ultrasound but both will show heterogeneity of the gland with irregular cyst formation.

Focal pancreatitis

Focal pancreatitis is characterised by a hypoechoic, homogeneous localised subsegmental lesion, usually situated within the pancreatic head. It may or may not cause focal enlargement of the gland. Where there is no enlargement the combination of a focal echo-poor area on ultrasound with a normal CT allows the differentiation from pancreatic tumour. Where the mass causes expansion of the gland, correlation with clinical features and clinical and imaging follow-up are vital.

In the clinical context of possible acute pancreatitis there remains difficulty with the differentiation of the normally echo-poor uncinate process and focal acute pancreatitis.

Ancillary findings

The most common aetiologies for acute pancreatitis are gallstones or alcohol abuse (Fig. 26.80). It is particularly important, therefore, to evaluate the gallbladder and biliary tract for evidence of cholecysto- and particularly choledocholithiasis. Imaging difficulties previously described remain important. Gas adjacent to the fundus of the gallbladder may predispose both over and underdiagnosis of gallstones. Consequently, although evaluation of the gallbladder and biliary tract are important during the acute attack in an attempt to identify an obstructing calculus, nonetheless sensitivities are improved by repeat examination after resolution of the attack of acute pancreatitis (Fig. 26.80). Repeat ultrasound examination prior to discharge will therefore serve two purposes. First, to re-evaluate the gallbladder and bile ducts and secondly to exclude the silent development of pancreatic pseudocyst. The appearance of gallstones and choledocholithiasis has been described elsewhere in this text. There may be gallbladder wall thickening consequent upon chronic cholecystitis or consequent upon oedema associated with acute pancreatitis.

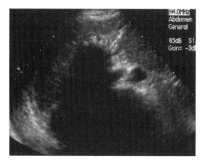

Fig. 26.80 Chronic cholecystitis. Multiple gallstones within a contracted gallbladder.

Ancillary signs and staging of acute pancreatitis

Notwithstanding the deficiencies of clinical diagnosis of acute pancreatitis, certain clinical findings have been used, such as those described by Rantzen, to provide prognostic information. Imaging correlates have been sought but with only limited success, thus the specificity of such findings in comparison with the Rantzen score is only of the order of 45%. Nonetheless, it remains appropriate to alert the surgeon to ultrasound findings, which may indicate the severity of the disease.

In clinically mild pancreatitis, the gland may be normal in up to 30% of cases and show diffuse or focal swelling in the remainder. In clinically severe acute pancreatitis the gland will always be abnormal on ultrasound after 24 h. Tissue necrosis may be seen in up to 90% of cases, with superadded infection in approximately 5%, with the subsequent potential for abscess formation. In patients with features of necrosis, consideration should be given to ultrasound-guided fine needle aspiration. The early diagnosis of pancreatic infection may be critical in improving outcome.

Other features implying severe acute pancreatitis include the demonstration of ascites, gallbladder wall thickening, pleural effusions (Figs 26.81–26.83), inflammation of mesenteric fat and vascular complications. Small amounts of peritoneal fluid can be demonstrated by careful imaging of the inferior border of the liver and the demonstration of a linear lucency between liver and adjacent bowel. Similarly, the combination of pleural fluid, particularly with evidence of focal pulmonary collapse, may be of value in determining clinical severity. Involvement of mesenteric fat is char-

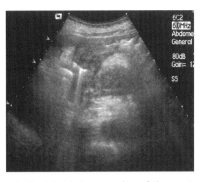

Fig. 26.83 Severe acute pancreatitis. The pancreas is markedly enlarged. There is increased reflectivity and oedema of the retroperitoneal fat and prepancreatic mesentery. There is thickening of the wall of the stomach.

acterised by heterogeneity of the root of mesentery with areas of increased echogenicity interspersed with areas of decreased echogenicity. The oedema is frequently characterised by increased attenuation of the sound beam by the echogenic fat.

Ultrasound examination of the pancreas in acute pancreatitis suggests that vascular complications may be more common than previously supposed. Colour flow Doppler may demonstrate absence of flow within the portal vein in up to 30% of patients. It is not clear whether this represents sluggish flow or true portal vein thrombosis but in approximately half of these cases portal venous collaterals are demonstrated. Arterial pseudoaneurysms are an additional complication of acute pancreatitis. Duplex and colour flow Doppler will allow the demonstration of a cystic abnormality in continuity with one of the branch vessels of the coeliac axis or superior mesenteric artery. If there is associated vascular thrombosis, the diagnosis is dependent upon demonstration of anatomical continuity, even in the absence of colour flow abnormality.

Recurrent acute pancreatitis

Recurrent acute pancreatitis is a condition associated with frequent attacks of severe epigastric pain, often over a period of many years, in association with intermittent elevation of serum amylase. Features on ultrasound may include dilatation of the pancreatic duct, occasionally with visualisation of truncated side branches, mild focal or diffuse enlargement of the gland and heterogeneity of the echo pattern. Ultrasound examination is abnormal in up to 80% of these individuals. The sensitivity of ultrasound, however, can be further improved by the use of the ultrasound secretin test. Administration of secretin (1 iu/kg) can produce persistent dilatation of the pancreatic duct 20 min after administration. This persistent dilatation correlates well with sphincter of Oddi manometry and implies sphincter dysfunction/dyskinesia or stricture formation. However, in spite of improvements in diagnosis, this group of patients remain difficult to manage. Conservative treatment is certainly appropriate in patients without demonstrable ultrasound abnormality but, even when glandular and ductal abnormalities are demonstrated, the response to treatment is frequently poor.

There may be a role for endoscopic ultrasound in the diagnosis of recurrent acute pancreatitis. The demonstration of a dilated pancreatic duct with dilated but truncated side branches is said to be characteristic.

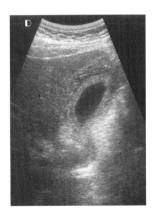

Fig. 26.81 Acute pancreatitis. Marked thickening and oedema of the gallbladder wall.

Chronic pancreatitis

Chronic pancreatitis is often silent and is consequently underdiagnosed. The incidence of chronic pancreatitis is increasing and correlates with increasing consumption of alcohol. Alcohol accounts for some 60–70% of cases of chronic pancreatitis. Other causes

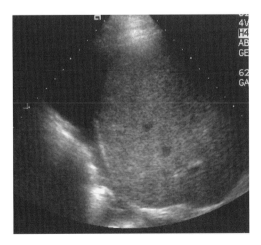

Fig. 26.82 Severe acute pancreatitis. Right pleural effusion.

include obstructive pancreatitis secondary to congenital strictures, pancreatitis and pancreas divisum, hypercalcaemia and biliary tract disease. However, in more than 20% of patients no aetiological factor is identified. This idiopathic group are often wrongly labelled as alcoholic. Chronic pancreatitis is a dynamic disease characterised by progressive destruction of the pancreatic parenchyma, with consequent change in the architecture of the gland and impairment of the pancreatic function. It is characterised by abdominal pain, steatorrhoea and weight loss. Diabetes is a relatively late manifestation of the disease, occurring usually only after the development of overt exocrine deficiency.

There is poor correlation between clinical, morphological and functional parameters, particularly in the early phase of the disease. Consequently, imaging should be used in concert with biochemical findings, such as the measurement of faecal elastase, in order to improve accuracy of diagnosis. Morphological features include enlargement of the gland and duct dilatation, as well as change in the appearance of the pancreatic parenchyma.

Size

Pancreatic enlargement is not an invariable feature of chronic pancreatitis. Indeed, in mild chronic pancreatitis, the gland is more usually of normal size. Similarly in end-stage chronic pancreatitis the pancreas may be small, consequent upon the loss of acinar tissue. Moderate pancreatitis is accompanied by an increase in size of the pancreas but this increase is usually to less than twice normal. Focal enlargement may occur in chronic pancreatitis but, when seen in a patient with evidence only of mild chronic pancreatitis, this is more likely to represent focal acute pancreatitis superimposed on chronic pancreatitis.

Change in size is also accompanied by change in outline. This is probably consequent upon fibrosis of the acinar tissue and an irregularity of the lobular outline of the pancreas. These changes are not, however, seen except in moderate to severe chronic pancreatitis and may indeed be difficult to distinguish from the lobulation of the gland that occurs consequent upon the processes of ageing and/or obesity.

Parenchyma

The echogenicity of the gland is not of significant value in the assessment of chronic pancreatitis. Increase in echogenicity is more commonly as a consequence of ageing or fatty change, rather than inflammation. Heterogeneity of the gland is a significant finding but may be difficult to characterise. However, the periductal fibrosis associated with early stages of chronic pancreatitis produces centrally placed strongly reflective foci (Fig. 26.84).

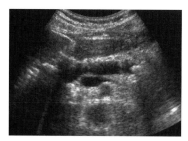

Fig. 26.85 Chronic pancreatitis. Marked dilatation of the pancreatic duct in longstanding pancreatitis. Note the intraduct calculus in the region of the tail.

Pancreatic duct

There is a subjective increase in the echogenicity of the wall of the pancreatic duct in early chronic pancreatitis. Whether this is related to wall thickening or to alteration in the contrast between the duct and the pancreatic parenchyma is not clear. Furthermore, it is a somewhat subjective sign and therefore of limited value. Dilatation of the duct, however, is much more reliably identified. In patients under 60 years old, a duct calibre of greater than 2 mm represents significant dilatation (Fig. 26.85). Irregularities in the dimension of the duct may be visualised simply as apparent discontinuities, but if the duct is markedly dilated then strictures can be demonstrated as abrupt changes in calibre. It may also be possible to demonstrate dilatation of first-order branches of the pancreatic duct.

In obstructive pancreatitis the duct dilatation may be the prominent feature in the absence of other findings.

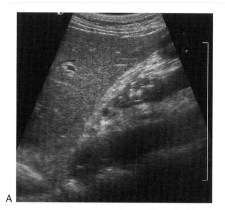

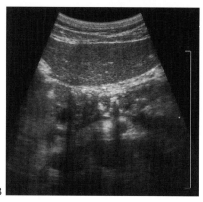

Fig. 26.86 Chronic pancreatitis. (A) Multiple bright non-shadowing foci within the head of the pancreas thought to represent protein plugs. (B) Several shadowing foci within the neck of the pancreas consistent with pancreatic calcification.

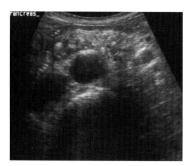

Fig. 26.84 Chronic pancreatitis. Heterogeneity of the pancreas with focal and diffuse areas of increased reflectivity.

Calculi

Pancreatic calcification usually occurs as a consequence of calcification in protein plugs within the pancreatic duct. Protein plugs are more common in alcoholic chronic pancreatitis rather than in obstructive pancreatitis and consequently calcification is also more common in this situation. Demonstration of the characteristic features of pancreatic calculi, i.e. highly reflective focus with distal acoustic shadowing, requires a finite size (Fig. 26.86). Such classical features are seen more readily with smaller and smaller calculi as the resolution and focusing of ultrasound equipment improves. Nonetheless, it may be difficult to differentiate very small calculi from periductal fibrosis.

Cysts

Small cysts of less than 5 mm in diameter probably represent dilated first-order side branches of the pancreatic duct (Fig. 26.87). Cysts greater than 10 mm in diameter usually imply severe disease. The cysts of chronic pancreatitis are usually intra- or peripancreatic. Cysts associated with acute pancreatitis are located at multiple sites within the abdomen. The classical cyst of chronic pancreatitis is usually small.

Pancreatic pseudocyst

Pseudocyst formation is a well-known complication of pancreatitis. The fluid collections may occur within the pancreatic mass, or in the peripancreatic spaces, or elsewhere within the abdomen following either acute pancreatitis or in chronic pancreatitis without any

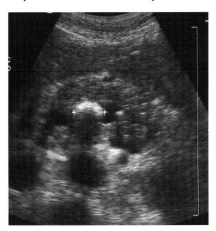

Fig. 26.87 Chronic pancreatitis. A large pancreatic calculus is demonstrated in association with two small pancreatic cysts and presumably consequent upon ductal branch ectasia.

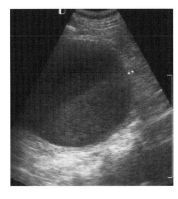

Fig. 26.88 Pancreatic pseudocyst. The large mass in the left upper quadrant adjacent to the spleen with evidence of layering debris.

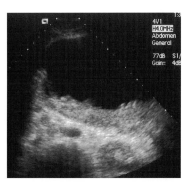

Fig. 26.89 Pancreatic pseudocyst. Large cystic mass in the midabdomen in the region of the pancreatic bed demonstrating echogenic material posteriorly, representing pancreatic necrosis.

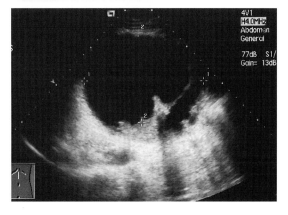

Fig. 26.90 Pancreatic pseudocyst. Large septated cystic mass in the midabdomen with nodular component. In the absence of history of pancreatitis it would be difficult to differentiate this from a cystic pancreatic tumour.

history of a previous acute episode (Figs 26.88–26.90). In acute pancreatitis, the pseudocyst contains enzyme-rich fluid and products of autodegradation of the pancreas; in chronic pancreatitis the cyst is a consequence of duct obstruction. Patients who have persistent abdominal pain or persistently elevated levels of pancreatic enzymes should be suspected of harbouring a pseudocyst. Although approximately one-third of pancreatic pseudocysts will resolve spontaneously, some will require intervention. The development of a pseudocyst may be insidious and consequently imaging of patients with acute pancreatitis should be performed prior to their discharge from hospital. It is not known how many pseudocysts in patients with chronic pancreatitis derive from a previous attack of acute pancreatitis. Some would estimate this as high as 50%, although with the greater sensitivity of imaging for the detection of smaller pseudocysts in chronic pancreatitis, this may be an overestimate. Nonetheless, the confirmation of a previous history of acute pancreatitis in a patient with chronic pancreatitis does not appear to affect the prognosis in any individual pseudocyst. Although there is no universal agreement, it appears that pseudocysts located in the head and body of the pancreas and of a diameter less than 4 cm are much more likely to resolve spontaneously than extrapancreatic pseudocysts and those larger than 4 cm in diameter (Fig. 26.91). Consequently, subject to clinical status of the patient, percutaneous drainage with ultrasound guidance should be considered in patients with pancreatic pseudocysts of 4 cm or greater, particularly when they occur outside the pancreas. Other methods of drainage, including pancreaticogastric drainage guided by endoscopy and/or ultrasound, need to be considered on merit. Utilising this approach, the requirement for surgical drainage is significantly diminished.

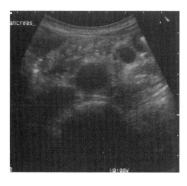

Fig. 26.91 Small pancreatic pseudocyst. A size less than 4.0 cm implies that the cyst is more likely to resolve spontaneously.

Trauma

Trauma to the pancreas is frequently occult, although the mechanism of injury is relatively characteristic. This is usually a direct frontal upper abdominal impact. Typically in a child a handlebar injury falling from a bicycle is the mechanism. Serum amylase is frequently normal or near normal at admission and consequently delay in diagnosis is common as clinical signs are also frequently subtle. Although CT is recommended as the method of choice for investigation of possible pancreatic injury, and indeed for the definitive diagnosis of all upper abdominal trauma, ultrasound is frequently used as the primary imaging modality in children and also as part of the process of triage in seriously injured patients. Sensitivity for the detection of pancreatic injury is reported to be between 70 and 100%, with appearances ranging from focal swelling and oedema through a peripancreatic fluid collection and rarely the demonstration of a pancreatic fracture. However, neither CT nor ultrasound can reliably demonstrate pancreatic duct rupture. Consequently, the management of patients with pancreatic trauma remains somewhat controversial. Many would recommend conservative management, even where trauma is significant and accompanied by the development of a pseudocyst, as in the majority these will resolve spontaneously. However, others warn that in the absence of information about the integrity of the pancreatic duct caution should be exercised if conservative management is proposed, as in those patients with pancreatic duct disruption surgical revision is inevitable.

Ultrasound guidance for pancreatic intervention

Ultrasound guidance of perabdominal needling of varying different pathologies is now widespread. The procedure can be performed either freehand, with the needle tip observed as it traverses through the ultrasound beam, or using a guidance device attached to the ultrasound probe.

Percutaneous drainage of a pancreatic pseudocyst is usually technically easy. Visualisation of a needle tip as it traverses a fluid collection is relatively straightforward. Aspiration may be used for diagnostic purposes in order to confirm the amylase content, and in the case of small cysts these can be aspirated to dryness through the fine needle. When the collection is large, however, the use of an indwelling drainage catheter is advocated. This may be inserted via a direct puncture or by guide-wire and catheter exchange technique. The catheter may be left on free drainage. Complete drainage of the pseudocyst may be achieved by this method. There remains, however, some dispute with respect to the long-term efficacy of percutaneous drainage. Since many pseudocysts will resolve sponta-

neously, it is difficult accurately to define the contribution of percutaneous drainage to an unselected population. Nonetheless, in the management of pseudocysts with severe systemic effects, catheter drainage may provide significant temporary relief from the amylase toxicity until definitive surgery can be undertaken.

Needle biopsy of the pancreas

There is now extensive worldwide experience with ultrasound-guided biopsy techniques, both with the use of fine needle aspiration (FNAB) and cutting-needle biopsies. The procedure is performed under appropriate analgesia and sedation, often a combination of midazolam and pethidine, although the specific combination of analgesia and sedation will depend upon local circumstances, the individual patient and prevailing advice, particularly about the use of intravenous sedation. Nonetheless, these patients will require significant analgesia. Pancreatic biopsy, particularly in pancreatitis or pancreatic cancer, is an extremely painful procedure and prior knowledge of this on the part of the operator is vital to ensure the procedure is undertaken with the minimum of discomfort to the patient.

The most common complication of pancreatic needle biopsy is pancreatitis followed by haemorrhage. Death following pancreatitis is reported but rare. Quoted mortality rates of 1 in 50 000 are suggested for both fine-needle biopsy and core biopsy. Different authors recommend different techniques. Some would suggest a combination of FNAB and core biopsy, whereas others use only core biopsy. Sensitivities in excess of 90% are reported for both methods, with 100% specificity.

The pancreas in specific disease disorders

Cystic fibrosis

The pathological changes of cystic fibrosis consist predominantly of glandular atrophy and fatty infiltration. This process occurs early on in the disease and consequently other predominant changes of the pancreas are of increased reflectivity, irregularity of outline and glandular atrophy. Although patients with cystic fibrosis may suffer from episodes of pancreatitis, these do not appear to be associated with pancreatic duct dilatation. Ultrasound changes are difficult to elicit but may include heterogeneity of the pancreatic parenchyma.

Similar pancreatic atrophy and increase in reflectivity are seen in other, rarer hereditary pancreatic insufficiency syndromes.

Diabetes

In diabetes the pathology affects the endocrine rather than the exocrine function of the pancreas. Nonetheless, a progressive reduction in size of the pancreas in insulin-dependent diabetics has been documented. There is an inverse correlation between the pancreatic size and the duration of insulin-dependent diabetes mellitus (IDDM). The normal process of gradual increase in reflectivity with age is accelerated in patients with IDDM, with most patients under the age of 40 exhibiting a small, highly reflective pancreas.

AIDS

Although patients with AIDS are susceptible to conditions similar to those of the general population, the pancreas is susceptible to a number of the organisms to which AIDS patients are exposed, may exhibit AIDS-specific tumours, and may be affected by some of the chemotherapeutic regimens to which AIDS patients are subjected. Specifically in this respect, infection with cytomegalovirus may result in an acute pancreatitis. The patterns of acute pancreatitis are no different from those expected in pancreatitis from other causes. However, it must be remembered that many patients with AIDS will have fatty replacement of the liver or chronic active hepatitis, and consequently the liver may be unusually echogenic and the normal pancreas in an AIDS patient may appear less echogenic than the adjacent liver parenchyma. Similarly, chemotherapeutic regimens which contain, for example, pentamidine and trimethoprim–sulfamethoxazole may result in acute pancreatitis. Pancreatic calcification may occur as a consequence of *Pneumocystis carinii* infection, which appears as multiple tiny echogenic foci distributed throughout the pancreatic parenchyma. Infection with *Cryptosporidium* sp. may produce thickening of the wall of the bile duct and sphincter stenosis at the sphincter of Oddi, with consequent dilatation of both the bile and pancreatic ducts.

Finally, 8% of patients with AIDS will develop a neoplasm. Both Kaposi's sarcoma and lymphoma may occur in the pancreas; however, these are usually subclinical but may be demonstrated in the presence of disseminated neoplastic disease elsewhere.

Endoscopic ultrasound

Since the introduction of endoscopic ultrasound there have been many reports attesting to the improved sensitivity and specificity of a wide variety of different disorders. The technique involves the use of either a radial array ultrasound scanner or a linear array attached to a flexible endoscope. Images of the pancreas are achieved by direct application of the ultrasound transducer on the endoscope to the pancreas via the wall of the stomach or the duodenum. Images are either reviewed by the endoscopist or, more frequently, by a co-operator experienced in the interpretation of ultrasound images. Greater sensitivity of diagnosis is claimed for the diagnosis of acute pancreatitis, the demonstration of vascular invasion by carcinoma of the pancreatic head and, in particular, in the diagnosis of relapsing acute pancreatitis. The technique has been claimed to be particularly important in the diagnosis of patients with neuroendocrine tumours. These are often small and, on transabdominal ultrasound, of similar reflectivity to the surrounding pancreatic parenchyma. In the best series correct localisation of neuroendocrine tumours has been achieved in 93% of patients, which is greater than that achieved by angiography. There is little doubt that, for this application, endoscopic ultrasound, perhaps combined with intraoperative ultrasound, provides the best method of tumour localisation.

The role of endoscopic ultrasound for other pancreatic pathologies has been the subject of significant re-evaluation. Although it may afford greater specificity in the diagnosis of pancreatic disease, the sensitivity may be little improved over judicious evaluation of clinical features and an imaging algorithm which starts with simple procedures such as transabdominal ultrasound.

RADIONUCLIDE IMAGING OF ISLET CELL TUMOURS

Philip J. A. Robinson

Tumours of the pancreatic islet cells, like other lesions of neuroendocrine cell origin, contain an abundance of somatostatin receptors. The somatostatin analogue, octreotide, labelled with indium [111]In-

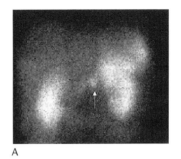
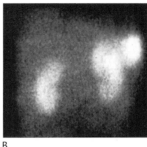

Fig. 26.92 Primary pancreatic islet cell tumour. SRS (A) shows normal uptake in liver, spleen and kidneys, but also a small focus of abnormal activity corresponding with a functioning islet cell tumour; repeat study after resection (B) shows no abnormality.

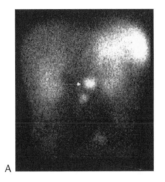
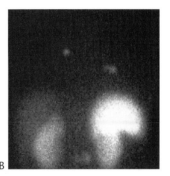

Fig. 26.93 Malignant islet cell tumour. SRS shows primary tumour (arrow) but also nodal deposits in the abdomen (A) and chest (B).

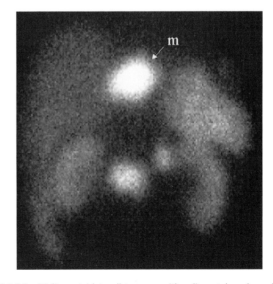

Fig. 26.94 Malignant islet cell tumour with adjacent lymph node and single liver metastasis (m) shown by SRS.

DTPA, shows a high affinity for these tumours. ^{111}In-octreotide scintigraphy is useful in the detection and localisation of islet cell tumours, and in detecting metastatic spread to other organs.

The technique of somatostatin receptor scintigraphy (SRS) is described in more detail in Chapter 20, in relation to detection of small bowel lesions and their metastases. The same method is used to detect pancreatic islet cell tumours. Anterior and posterior views of the upper abdomen are obtained 4–6 h and 24 h after injection of ^{111}In-DTPA-octreotide. Because of uptake in the normal liver, it is

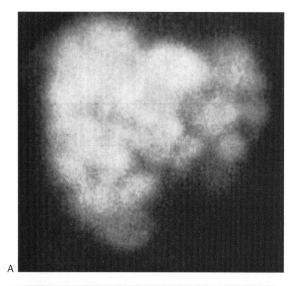

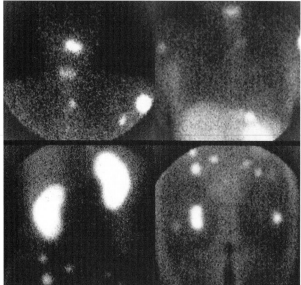

Fig. 26.95 Malignant islet cell tumour. Extensive liver replacement by functioning metastases shown on initial study (A). Six months after liver transplantation, further widespread metastases developed (B).

often helpful to obtain single-photon emission CT (SPECT) images of the upper abdomen at the second visit.

The images show activity in the normal liver tissue and more intense localisation in the spleen. Much of the tracer is excreted through the kidney, so the renal parenchyma also shows quite marked activity. A small proportion of the tracer is excreted through the biliary tract, so delayed images may show low-grade activity in the colon. Pancreatic tumours are identified as small foci of intense uptake in or around the pancreas (Figs 26.92–26.94), while liver metastases appear as high intensity lesions within a relatively lower background of normal liver uptake (Figs 26.94, 26.95). In patients with malignant lesions, metastases to lymph nodes, lung and other remote sites should be sought by obtaining views of the whole body (Fig. 26.95).

Applications and results

SRS should be used when there is biochemical evidence of a pancreatic islet cell tumour. Anatomical imaging with CT or MRI will also be needed, but occasionally SRS will be positive when the anatomical techniques are unsuccessful in locating the tumour. If one or more lesions are already found by CT/MRI, SRS is still important in helping to distinguish which of the lesions are functioning tumours, and also in identifying possible metastases in regional nodes or in the liver. SRS may also be used in follow-up to detect possible recurrence after initial surgical treatment, and to screen for distant metastasis.

The success rate for SRS in detecting glucagonomas and gastrinomas is very high—100% in some series. With insulinomas, the sensitivity of SRS is lower—probably about 60–70%—possibly because a minority of insulinomas do not exhibit somatostatin receptors.

REFERENCES AND SUGGESTIONS FOR FURTHER READING

General

Balthazar, E. J., Robinson, D. L., Megibow, A. J., et al (1990) Acute pancreatitis: value of CT in establishing prognosis. *Radiology*, **174**, 331–336.

Cotton, P. B. (1980) Congenital anomaly of pancreas divisum as cause of obstructive pain and pancreatitis. *Gut*, **21**, 105–114.

Davis, S., Parbhoo, S. P., Gibson, M. J. (1980) The plain abdominal film in acute pancreatitis. *Clinical Radiology*, **31**, 87–91.

Jones, S. N., Lees, W. R., Frost, R. A. (1988) Diagnosis and grading of chronic pancreatitis by morphological criteria derived by ultrasound and pancreatography. *Clinical Radiology*, **39**, 43–48.

King, C. P. M., Reznek, R. H., Dacie, J. E., Wass, J. A. H. (1994) Review. Imaging islet cell tumours. *Clinical Radiology*, **49**, 295–303.

Martin, D. R., Semelka, R. C. (2000) MR imaging of pancreatic masses. *Magnetic Resonance Imaging Clinics of North America*, **8(4)**, 787–812.

Meyers, M. A., Evans, J. A. (1973) Effects of pancreatitis on the small bowel and colon: spread along mesenteric planes. *American Journal of Roentgenology*, **119**, 151–156.

Millwood, S. F., Breatnach, E., Simpkins, K. C., et al (1983) Do plain films of the chest and abdomen have a role in the diagnosis of acute pancreatitis? *Clinical Radiology*, **34**, 133–137.

Pearse, A. G. E. (1968) Common cytochemical and ultrastructural characteristics of cells producing polypeptide hormones (the APUD series) and their relevance to thyroid ultimobronchial C. cells and calcitonin. *Proceedings of the Royal Society of London. Series B*, **170**, 71–80.

Sarner, M., Cotton, P. B. (1984) Classification of pancreatitis. *Gut*, **25**, 756–759.

Sarner, M., Cotton, P. B. (1984) Definitions of acute and chronic pancreatitis. *Clinical Gastoenterology*, **13**, 865.

Zeman, R. K., Cooper, C., Zeiberg, A. L., et al (1997) TNM staging of pancreatic carcinoma using helical CT. *American Journal of Roentgenology*, **169**, 459–464.

CT

Bigattini, D., Boverie, J. H., Dondelinger, R. F. (1999) CT of blunt trauma of the pancreas in adults. *European Radiology*, **9**, 244–249.

Buetow, P. C., Buck, J. L., Pantongrag-Brown, L., et al (1996) Solid and papillary epithelial neoplasm of the pancreas: imaging–pathologic correlation in 56 cases. *Radiology*, **199**, 707–711.

Council, The Royal College of Radiologists (1994) *The Use of Computed Tomography in the Initial Investigation of Common Malignancies*, p. 18. London: Royal College of Radiologists.

McNulty, N. J., Francis, I. R., Platt, J. F., et al (2001) Multi-detector row helical CT of the pancreas: effect of contrast-enhanced multiphasic imaging on enhancement of the pancreas, peripancreatic vasculature, and pancreatic adenocarcinoma. *Radiology*, **220**, 97–102.

Wegener, O. H. (1992) The pancreas. In *Whole Body Computed Tomography*, pp. 291–312. Boston, MA: Blackwell Scientific.

MRI

Mammone, J. F., Siegelman, E. S., Outwater, E. K. (1998) Magnetic resonance imaging of the pancreas and biliary tree. *Seminars in Ultrasound, CT and MR*, **19**, 35–52.

Pavone, P., Laghi, A., Catalano, C., et al (1998) MRI of the biliary and pancreatic ducts. *European Radiology*, **9**, 1513–1522.

Robinson, P. J., Sheridan, M. B. (2000) Pancreatitis: computed tomography and magnetic resonance imaging. *European Radiology*, **10**, 401–408.

Spencer, J. A., Ward, J., Guthrie, J. A., et al (1998) Assessment of resectability of pancreatic cancer with dynamic contrast-enhanced MR imaging: technique, surgical correlation and patient outcome. *European Radiology*, **8**, 23–29.

Takehara, Y. (1999) MR pancreatography. *Seminars in Ultrasound, CT and MR*, **20**, 324–339.

Ward, J., Chalmers, A. G., Guthrie, J. A., et al (1997) T_2-weighted and dynamic enhanced MRI in acute pancreatitis: comparison with contrast-enhanced CT. *Clinical Radiology*, **52**, 109–114.

Ultrasound

Abu-Yousef, M. M., El-Zein, Y. (2000) Improved ultrasound visualisation of the pancreatic tail with simethicone water and patient rotation. *Radiology*, **217**(3), 780–785.

Altobelli, E., et al (1998) Size of pancreas in children and adolescents with type I (insulin-dependent) diabetes. *Journal of Clinical Ultrasound*, **26**(8), 391–395.

Anderson, M. A., et al (2000) Endoscopic ultrasound is highly accurate and directs management in patients with neuroendocrine tumours of the pancreas. *American Journal of Gastroenterology*, **95**(9), 2271–2277.

Birk, D., et al (1998) Carcinoma of the head of the pancreas arising from the uncinate process. *British Journal of Surgery*, **85**(4), 498–501.

Boozari, B., et al (1998) 3D and colour Doppler ultrasound evaluation of cystic space-occupying lesion near the head of the pancreas. (In German.) *Ultraschall in der Medezin*, **19**(6), 280–285.

Brand, R. E., Matamoros, A. (1998) Imaging techniques in the evaluation of adenocarcinoma of the pancreas. *Digestive Diseases*, **16**(4), 242–252.

Brugge, W. R. (1995) Pancreatic cancer staging. Endoscopic ultrasonography criteria for vascular invasion. *Gastrointestinal Endoscopy Clinics of North America*, **5**(4), 741–753.

Capaccioli, L., et al (2000) Ultrasonographic study on the growth and dimensions of healthy children and adults organs. *Italian Journal of Anatomy and Embryology*, **105**(1), 1–50.

Chao, H. C., et al (2000) Sonographic evaluation of the pancreatic duct in normal children and children with pancreatitis. *Journal of Ultrasound in Medicine*, **19**(11), 757–763.

Chehter, E. Z., et al (2000) Involvement of the pancreas in AIDS: a prospective study of post-mortems. *AIDS*, **14**(13), 1879–1886.

Coulier, B. (1996) Hypoechogenic aspects of the ventral embryonic cephalic pancreas: a large prospective clinical study. (In French.) *Journal Belge de Radiologie*, **79**(3), 120–124.

Das, D. K., et al (1995) Ultrasound guided percutaneous fine needle aspiration cytology of pancreas: a review of 61 cases. *Tropical Gastroenterology*, **16**(2), 101–109.

Di Francesco, V., et al (1999) Comparison of ultrasound-secretin test and sphincter of Oddi manometry in patients with recurrent acute pancreatitis. *Digestive Diseases and Sciences*, **44**(2), 336–340.

Dorffel, T., et al (2000) Vascular complications in acute pancreatitis assessed by colour duplex ultrasonography. *Pancreas*, **21**(2), 126–133.

Feigelson, J., et al (2000) Imaging changes in the pancreas in cystic fibrosis: a retrospective evaluation of 55 cases seen over a period of 9 years. *Journal of Pediatric Gastroenterology and Nutrition*, **30**(2), 145–151.

Freeny, P. C. (ed.) (1989) Radiology of the pancreas. *Radiologic Clinics of North America*, **27**(1).

Freeny, P. C., et al (1988) Infected pancreatic fluid collections: percutaneous catheter drainage. *Radiology*, **167**, 435–441.

Galiber, A. K., et al (1988) Localisation of pancreatic insulinoma: comparison of pre and intraoperative ultrasound with CT and angiography. *Radiology*, **166**, 405–408.

Glaser, J., Stienecker, K. (2000) Pancreas and ageing: a study using ultrasonography. *Gerontology*, **46**(2), 93–96.

Gorelick, A. B., Scheiman, J. M., Fendrick, A. M. (1998) Identification of patients with resectable pancreatic cancer: at what stage are we? *American Journal of Gastroenterology*, **93**(10), 1995–1996.

Gorman, B., et al (1986) Benign pancreatic insulinoma: preoperative and intraoperative sonographic localisation. *American Journal of Roentgenology*, **147**, 929–934.

Gouyon, B., et al (1997) Predictive factors in the outcome of pseudocysts complicating alcoholic chronic pancreatitis. *Gut*, **41**(6), 821–825.

Graham, C. A., et al (2000) Pancreatic trauma in Scottish children. *Journal of the Royal College of Surgeons of Edinburgh*, **45**(4), 223–226.

Gumaste, V. V., Pitchumoni, C. S. (1996) Pancreatic pseudocyst. *Gastroenterologist*, **4**(1), 33–43.

Jones, S. N., Lees, W. R., Frost, R. A. (1988) Diagnosis and grading of chronic pancreatitis by morphological criteria derived by ultrasound and pancreatography. *Clinical Radiology*, **39**, 43–48.

Kingsnorth, A. (1998) Diagnosing acute pancreatitis: room for improvement? *Hospital Medicine*, **59**(3), 191–194.

Koito, K., et al (1997) Inflammatory pancreatic masses: differentiation from ductal carcinomas with contrast-enhanced sonography using carbon dioxide microbubbles. *American Journal of Roentgenology*, **169**(5), 1263–1267.

Kolecki, R., Schirmer, B. (1998) Intraoperative and laparoscopic ultrasound. *Surgical Clinics of North America*, **78**(2), 251–271.

Lawson, T. L. (1983) Acute pancreatitis and its complications: computed tomography and sonography. *Radiologic Clinics of North America*, **21**, 495–513.

Lorén, I., et al (1999) Abdominal radiology: new sonographic imaging observations in focal pancreatitis. *European Radiology*, **9**(5), 862–867.

Manes, G., et al (2000) Chronic pancreatitis: diagnosis and staging. *Annali Italiani Chirurgia*, **71**(1), 23–32.

Martin, I., et al (1998) Cystic tumours of the pancreas. *British Journal of Surgery*, **85**(11), 1484–1486.

Menges, M., Lerch, M. M., Zeitz, M. (2000) The double duct sign in patients with malignant and benign pancreatic lesions. *Gastrointestinal Endoscopy*, **52**(1), 74–77.

Miller, F. H., et al (1996) Pancreaticobiliary manifestations of AIDS. *American Journal of Roentgenology*, **166**(6), 1269–1274.

Mishra, G., Forsmark, C. E. (2000) Cystic neoplasms of the pancreas. *Current Treatment Options in Gastroenterology*, **3**(5), 355–362.

Neff, C. C., et al (1984) Inflammatory pancreatic masses: problems in differentiating focal pancreatitis from carcinoma. *Radiology*, **150**, 35–38.

Ooi, L. L., et al (1998) Cystic tumours of the pancreas: a diagnostic dilemma. *Australian and New Zealand Journal of Surgery*, **68**(12), 844–846.

Pandy, L., et al (1997–1998) The value of ultrasound in staging the severity of acute pancreatitis. *Acta Chirurgica Iugoslavica*, **44–45**(1–1): 63–67.

Pezzilli, R., et al (1999) Ultrasonographic evaluation of the common bile duct in biliary acute pancreatitis patients: comparison with endoscopic retrograde cholangiopancreatography. *Journal of Ultrasound in Medicine*, **18**(6), 391–394.

Rosch, T., et al (2000) Endoscopic ultrasound criteria for vascular invasion in the staging of cancer of the head of the pancreas: a blind re-evaluation of videotapes. *Gastrointestinal Endoscopy*, **52**(4), 469–477.

Rosch, T., et al (2000) Modern imaging methods versus clinical assessment in the evaluation of hospital in-patients with suspected pancreatic disease. *American Journal of Gastroenterology*, **95**(9), 2261–2670.

Shapiro, R. S., et al (1998) Tissue harmonic imaging sonography: evaluation of image quality compared with conventional sonography. *American Journal of Roentgenology*, **171**(5), 1203–1206.

Sugiyama, M., et al (1995) Diagnosis of acute pancreatitis: value of endoscopic sonography. *American Journal of Roentgenology*, **165**(4), 867–872.

Tanaka, S., et al (1996) Evaluation of routine sonography for early detection of pancreatic cancer. *Japanese Journal of Clinical Oncology*, **26**(6), 422–427.

Tomiyama, T., et al (1996) Assessment of arterial invasion in pancreatic cancer using colour Doppler ultrasonography. *American Journal of Gastroenterology*, **91**(7), 1410–1416.

Torresan, F., et al (1997) The role of ultrasound in the differential diagnosis of serous and mucinous cystic tumours of the pancreas. *European Journal of Gastroenterology and Hepatology*, **9**(2), 169–172.

Wachsberg, R. H. (2000) Respiratory variation of the diameter of the pancreatic duct sonography. *American Journal of Roentgenology*, **175**(5), 1459–1461.

Yamaguchi, K., et al (1996) 'Mass-forming' pancreatitis masquerades as pancreatic carcinoma. *International Journal of Pancreatology*, **20**(1), 27–35.

Islet cell tumours

Van Eijck, C. H., de Jong, M., Breeman, W. A., et al (1999) Somatostatin receptor imaging and therapy of pancreatic endocrine tumours. *Annals of Oncology*, **10** (suppl. 4), 177–181.

27

THE ADRENAL GLANDS

David Sutton
with a contribution from Philip J. A. Robinson

The adrenal glands are, despite their small size, among the most important and vital organs in the body. Their function was quite unknown until 1855, when Addison first described the syndrome resulting from their destruction. In 1856 Brown-Séquard showed that their removal led to death in animals. The adrenal glands lie just above the kidneys and are composed of a *cortex* and a *medulla*. The medulla has a totally different origin to the cortex, and arises with the sympathetic nervous system. Both cortex and medulla secrete hormones.

Three main groups of hormones are secreted by the adrenal *cortex*. These are all chemically related and have a similar basic chemical structure. They are:

1. *Glucocorticoids*. The secretion of these is controlled by the pituitary gland through its adrenocorticotrophic hormone (ACTH). The most important glucocorticoid is cortisol (hydrocortisone) and this is normally secreted at the rate of about 20 mg/day. The glucocorticoids have many actions, such as stimulation of protein breakdown, antagonism to the action of insulin, and the inhibition of tissue response in injury.

2. *Mineralocorticoids*. Aldosterone is the most important of these. Its secretion is mainly controlled by the renin–angiotensin system and by the level of plasma potassium. Aldosterone stimulates the reabsorption of sodium in the distal renal tubules of the kidney in exchange for potassium.

3. *Androgens*. Although they are produced in relatively large amounts, the adrenal androgens are very weak compared with testosterone.

The *medulla* also secretes hormones, mainly adrenaline (epinephrine) and noradrenaline (norepinephrine).

ANATOMY

The right adrenal gland is triangular and is closely related to the upper pole of the right kidney. The left adrenal is crescent-shaped and is related to the upper and medial part of the left kidney. The average size of the adrenals varies from 3–5 cm long by 2 or 3 cm wide and their average thickness is only about 5 mm. The average weight is 3–5 g, of which 90% is contributed by the cortex.

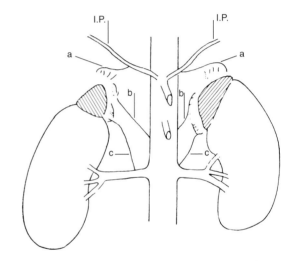

Fig. 27.1 Arterial supply of the adrenals. I.P. = inferior phrenic artery; a = superior phrenic artery; b = middle adrenal artery; c = inferior adrenal artery.

The vascular anatomy of the adrenals has been of considerable importance in radiology in the past, when both arteriography and phlebography were used for diagnostic purposes. Although now obsolete for this purpose, both techniques are still occasionally useful for special indications (see below). Anatomists describe three main arteries of supply (Fig. 27.1):

1. An inferior adrenal artery arising from the renal artery
2. A middle adrenal artery arising from the aorta
3. A superior adrenal artery arising from the inferior phrenic artery.

However, this anatomy is subject to considerable variation. Thus, the inferior phrenic artery can arise direct from the aorta or from the coeliac axis, or from other vessels. There may be arteries of supply from other adjacent large arteries. The major arteries of supply break up into numerous smaller branches before entering the gland, which thus has multiple small vessels of supply.

The venous drainage of the adrenal (Fig. 27.2) was also of considerable importance when adrenal phlebography and adrenal

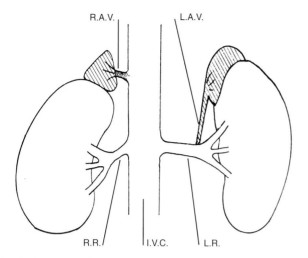

Fig. 27.2 Venous drainage of the adrenal gland. R.A.V. = right adrenal vein; L.A.V. = left adrenal vein; L.R. = left renal vein; I.V.C. = inferior vena cava; R.R. = right renal vein.

hormone assay first became established radiological techniques. There is usually a fairly large adrenal vein on the left which passes downward medial to the upper part of the kidney to join the main renal vein, and lies just lateral to the left vertebral border. This vein may also have connections with the inferior phrenic vein and veins from the kidney.

On the right side, the anatomy is quite different as the adrenal vein has only a very short trunk, which passes straight from the right adrenal into the posterolateral aspect of the inferior vena cava at a level just above the upper pole of the right kidney. Occasionally it may pass to an accessory hepatic vein before entering the inferior vena cava and, in rare cases, to the right renal vein.

The above description applies to adults, and it should be noted that the gland appears quite different in infants and small children, when its relative size is one-third of that of the kidney (Fig. 27.3).

The normal adrenal glands at axial CT or MRI With modern body scanners the normal adrenal glands can be demonstrated in all but the occasional case, usually a thin person or child with a paucity of retroperitoneal fat. In these axial cross-sections the glands appear quite different from their conventional anatomical description.

The right gland lies directly above the level of the kidney and directly behind the inferior vena cava just below its point of entry into the liver. The right lobe of the liver lies on its right lateral aspect and the right crus of the diaphragm on its medial aspect (Fig. 27.3).

The left adrenal gland is a little lower in position, its lower pole lying anteromedial to the upper pole of the left kidney. The left crus of the diaphragm is medial to it and the spleen lateral to its upper pole. Anteriorly lie the tail of the pancreas and the splenic vessels.

The right gland appears as an elongated, slightly curved structure pointing backward and laterally. It is sometimes described as having a body and two limbs. The medial elongated limb is the one easily recognisable at CT but the smaller body and lateral limb may be difficult to identify, the latter often merging with the liver shadow. The left gland is more easily identified, resembling an arrowhead pointing anteromedially (Fig. 27.4). It should be noted that, unlike the conventional anatomical descriptions, both glands

are not in direct apposition to the kidneys, but may be separated by a centimetre or more of fatty or areolar tissue. As the glands are 3–5 cm in height, they are usually seen on more than one section, particularly where contiguous narrow cuts are made. The left gland in particular may extend well down the medial surface of the kidney to just above the hilum.

PATHOLOGY

Acute infections of the adrenals, as in meningococcal or other forms of fulminating septicaemia, are of little radiological interest. *Chronic infections*, as in tuberculosis or histoplasmosis, can give rise to bilateral granulomas and are discussed below.

Adrenal haemorrhage can follow overwhelming septicaemia and can cause acute adrenal insufficiency. It may also occur in bleeding diatheses, in pregnancy and severe hypertension, following adrenal vein thrombosis or epileptic convulsions, and in patients on ACTH therapy.

Neonatal adrenal haemorrhage is one of the causes of an enlarged adrenal in infancy, the others being neuroblastoma and Wolman's disease (see below). It can result from birth trauma, coagulation disorders and acute septicaemia and may be unilateral or bilateral. Clinically, the child may be asymptomatic or present with neonatal distress, jaundice, anaemia or an abdominal mass.

Recent haemorrhage is readily characterised by CT as a high-density (50–75 HU) irregular mass. At ultrasound it appears first as anechoic but later as a complex mass becoming cystic. Calcification may develop even later.

Of greatest radiological and imaging interest are tumours of the adrenal gland and bilateral hyperplasia (Box 27.1). These lesions are discussed in detail below.

Clinical presentation Adrenal lesions may present with a wide variety of clinical signs, including several syndromes resulting from excess secretion of individual hormones or from hormone suppression. These include:

1. Addison's disease
2. Cushing's syndrome
3. Conn's syndrome (hyperaldosteronism)
4. The adrenogenital syndrome. Virilising syndrome. Feminising syndrome.
5. Adrenalism and noradrenalism (phaeochromocytoma)
6. Abdominal tumour
7. Metastases to bone or liver in childhood
8. Wolman's disease.

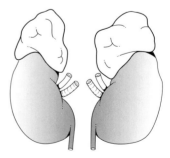

Fig. 27.3 Tracing from a photograph of neonatal kidneys and adrenals; the latter are relatively large compared with adult adrenals, being one-third the size of the kidneys.

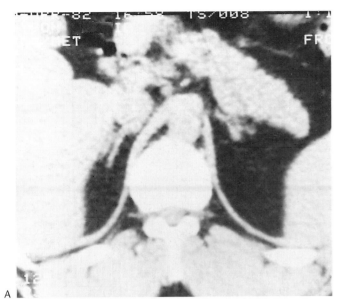

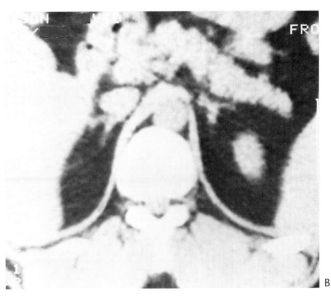

Fig. 27.4 Normal adrenals as shown by CT (see text). (A) Section just above right kidney. In this example the right adrenal has well-marked lateral and medial limbs. The top of the left adrenal is also shown behind the pancreas, although frequently it is not seen at this level (L43, W512). (B) Section including top of left kidney. The left adrenal resembling an arrowhead is well seen, as is the right adrenal, although the limbs now appear shorter (L43, W572). (C) Section at slightly lower level, including tops of both kidneys (L43, W572). Note that the adrenals are separated from the kidneys by fatty areolar tissue.

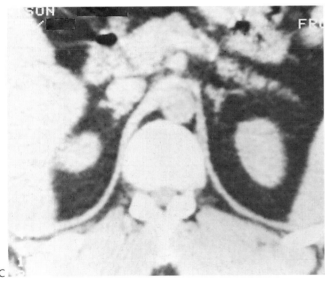

deposits, and remain symptomless while small. Benign tumours such as myelolipoma or non-secreting adenomas may also be symptomless and are only discovered accidentally during imaging for other purposes. Most patients with suspected adrenal disorder present with one or other of the syndromes or clinical manifestations listed above.

IMAGING INVESTIGATION

MR and spiral CT are now the most widely used and important imaging investigations, and are the methods of choice, except in infants and children, where ultrasound may be preferred as a simpler primary investigation. Isotope scanning, simple X-ray and needle biopsy are used less widely, but can be helpful in selected cases. Many other methods have been used in the past, but these are now obsolete or used only in special circumstances, mentioned in the text below. They included:

1. Simple X-ray and tomography
2. IVP and high-dose IVP with tomography
3. Retroperitoneal air insufflation
4. Arteriography
5. Phlebography
6. Vena caval and adrenal vein blood sampling.

Simple X-ray

As noted above CT and MR are now the imaging techniques of choice in defining adrenal tumours. However, since plain abdominal films are so widely used for other purposes, the student should be aware of the information it can provide. Thus an alert radiologist

---

Box 27.1   Adrenal tumours

A. Neoplasms
　1. Cortical
　　　Carcinoma
　　　Adenoma
　2. Medullary
　　　Neuroblastoma
　　　Phaeochromocytoma
　　　Ganglioneuroma
　3. Stromal
　　　Lipoma
　　　Myolipoma
　4. Metastases

B. Other mass lesions
　1. Granulomas
　　　Tuberculosis
　　　Histioplasmosis
　　　Blastomycosis
　2. Bilateral hyperplasia
　3. Cysts
　4. Haematoma

These clinical manifestations and syndromes are discussed in more detail below under individual lesions.

Some tumours are non-secreting. Thus about 50% of adrenal carcinomas first present with an abdominal mass or with secondary has often been the first to identify a large but symptomless non-secreting adrenal cortical carcinoma.

In adrenal lesions plain radiology of the abdomen with or without tomography may help in two ways: (i) by detecting a mass in the adrenal area; and (ii) by showing calcification in the adrenals.

Mass A mass in the adrenal area may be obvious and may be seen to be displacing the kidney. This is particularly evident with large tumours, but can occasionally be seen even with relatively small lesions, provided there is a fair amount of perinephric fat present to help contrast. In general, however, masses smaller than 5 cm in diameter are not likely to be visualised. There are several important aspects of differential diagnosis: thus, all the following structures have been known to simulate a mass in the adrenal areas and must be borne in mind:

1. Renal cysts or tumours
2. Spleen and accessory spleen
3. Pancreatic cyst or tumour
4. Liver mass
5. Para-aortic glands
6. Retroperitoneal tumour
7. Stomach mass.

Of considerable importance are the normal fluid-filled gastric fundus in the supine position, which can simulate a mass over the left kidney, and the fluid-filled antrum or duodenal bulb, which can simulate a mass over the right kidney. As long as these possibilities are borne in mind there is usually little difficulty in differential diagnosis, although occasionally erect films or even barium contrast will have to be used to exclude fluid in the stomach simulating a mass.

Calcification The second abnormality which may be seen on plain X-ray is calcification in the adrenal area. This may be seen both in tumours and in non-tumorous conditions (Box 27.2).

So-called *idiopathic calcification* may be found by chance on routine abdominal examination of patients with no relevant symptoms of adrenal disease. It is possible that such calcification may be the result of old haemorrhage or infection in infancy or childhood which has healed with no effect on function (Fig. 27.5). When tuberculosis was common in the west, involvement of the adrenals was said to be the commonest cause of *Addison's disease* and to be frequently followed by adrenal calcification. This is most clearly shown at CT (Fig. 27.6). However, tuberculosis is now rare in developed countries and most of the cases seen today are due to 'atrophy'. This atrophy is considered to be an *autoimmune disease*, as it may occur in association with such conditions as Hashimoto's thyroiditis and pernicious anaemia. Circulating antibodies to the adrenocortical tissue have been shown in the serum of such patients.

Addison's disease is not caused by primary tumours but it can very rarely be due to secondary carcinomatosis. Addison's disease may also occur with bilateral mass lesions such as granulomas or

amyloidosis. The clinical features are largely due to the resulting deficiency of glucocorticoids and mineralocorticoids. The former leads to anorexia, nausea and vomiting, and later to pyrexia, hypotension and hyperglycaemia. The latter causes sodium depletion with dehydration and hypotension. Abnormal brown pigmentation of the skin, involving, in particular, parts exposed to the sun and pressure areas, occurs. In addition, there are deposits of pigment in the mouth and conjunctival mucous membrane.

Wolman's disease (Abramov–Wolman disease) is a lipidosis which was formerly confused with Niemann–Pick disease. It is associated with hepatomegaly, splenomegaly and a characteristic calcification of the adrenal glands, which are enlarged. It was first defined in 1961 and many well-documented cases have since been reported. Most of the affected infants died in the first 6 months of life. Abdominal X-ray in these infants shows large adrenals with diffuse stippled calcification which is diagnostic, and is also well shown by CT or ultrasound (see Fig. 28.61).

Calcifying fibrous pseudotumour (CFPT) is a rare benign lesion of the pleura or soft tissues that may result from a previous inflam-

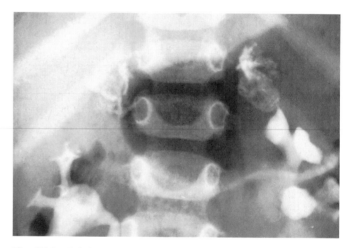

Fig. 27.5 Calcified adrenals in a child. These were a chance finding, the IVP being performed for urinary infection.

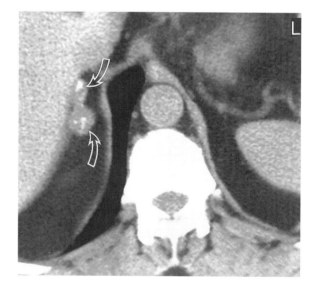

Fig. 27.6 Adrenal calcification (arrows) from tuberculosis on CT scan. (Courtesy of Dr J. P. R. Jenkins.)

Box 27.2   Adrenal calcification

1. Idiopathic
2. Neoplasm
3. Granuloma
4. Cyst
5. Old haemorrhage
6. Wolman's disease

matory focus. Cases have been described in the limbs, thorax and abdomen; including a case presenting in a child's adrenal.

Benign cysts of the adrenal, possibly of haemorrhagic origin, and in patients with no symptoms of adrenal pathology, may show arc-like marginal calcification. Similar calcification has been described in patients with *phaeochromocytomas* but is very rare.

Irregular calcification has been described in most adrenal tumours but is very uncommon except in malignant tumours. It is said to occur in about one-third of *carcinomas*, usually as faint irregular calcification. It also occurs in *neuroblastomas* in about half the cases. The calcification is usually stippled and non-homogeneous, but can occasionally be linear or curvilinear. In this respect, it is interesting that liver metastases from neuroblastomas may also calcify.

Ganglioneuromas, which may be regarded as a mature type of neurogenic tumour, also calcify frequently, the calcification being similar to that in neuroblastomas. The majority of ganglioneuromas are extra-adrenal in origin, arising from sympathetic ganglia along the sympathetic chain.

Intravenous urography

This is now little used in the investigation of suspected adrenal tumours. In the past, however, intravenous urography was often very helpful by differentiating between a mass in the upper pole of the kidney and one in the adrenal. In this respect *high-dose urography with tomography* will frequently define the kidney quite clearly and show whether it is normal. Occasionally it will accentuate a mass in the adrenal and show it more clearly. Downward displacement of an intact kidney by a large suprarenal mass is usually well shown.

Retroperitoneal air insufflation

This technique was widely practised in the 1950s for the demonstration of adrenal masses, but was replaced in the 1960s with arteriography and phlebography. The technique of air insufflation gave rise to occasional fatalities from air embolus and was not very accurate with small tumours. Some of the series reported showed a high incidence both of false-positive and false-negative results.

Arteriography

Simple flush aortography will readily show large or highly vascular adrenal masses. Small or non-vascular tumours, however, will usually require selective techniques for their demonstration, as will ectopic tumours. The method was widely used for some 20 years before the advent of the newer imaging techniques in the 1970s. It is now obsolete except in special circumstances, for example in demonstrating a renal artery involved and stenosed by an ectopic renal hilar phaeochromocytoma (see below).

Phlebography

Selective adrenal vein phlebography can be performed on both sides and has proved a most reliable method for demonstrating small tumours such as occur in primary hyperaldosteronism (see below). The adrenal veins are selectively catheterised percutaneously from the femoral vein. The right adrenal vein is the more difficult to catheterise, but, using specially designed catheters, a high success rate can be achieved on both sides. Care must be taken not to overfill the glands by using excessive doses of contrast media

or excessive injection pressures, and hand injections only are used. On the left side 5 ml of a water-soluble medium are used, and on the right side 2 ml. On both sides the volume necessary is first judged by small test doses observed while screening, as adrenal infarction has resulted from using excessive doses.

This method has been superseded by CT and MR but is still occasionally used for deliberate infarction of the adrenal or of small adrenal tumours, and for venous hormone assay.

Inferior vena cavography

This procedure has occasionally proved useful in showing the relationships of large ectopic phaeochromocytomas (Fig. 27.37), but this can now be done by non-invasive imaging. Catheterisation of the IVC is still of occasional value for hormone assay in localising an ectopic abdominal phaeochromatcytoma.

Hormone assay

Catheterisation of the vena cava can be performed for blood sampling at different sites and levels in suspected phaeochromocytomas. This is usually done when other techniques have failed to localise a suspected tumour. Samples are taken from the renal veins, and high and low in the inferior vena cava. Since phaeochromocytomas can be intrathoracic or in the pelvis, samples may also be taken from the superior vena cava and the iliac veins.

The techniques of blood sampling and hormone assay are also used in suspected Conn's tumours. Samples are taken from the adrenal veins or as near to their mouths as possible. Some consider that adrenal vein aldosterone is diagnostic in cases of Conn's tumour, even without phlebography, the value being abnormally high on the tumour side and normal on the other. In cases of bilateral hyperplasia the aldosterone level is elevated on both sides. Bilateral adrenal cortical nodularity is occasionally encountered and should be differentiated from bilateral hyperplasia. In these cases venous sampling may show a localised aldosteronoma.

Ultrasound

Large adrenal masses are readily demonstrable by ultrasound (Figs 27.7, 27.21A, 27.39), but small tumours, as with Conn's syndrome, are not easily identified by this method and can be missed. Ectopic tumours can also be easily missed. However, ultrasound should always be the investigation of first choice in infants and children, and in pregnant women.

CT scanning

The advent of high-resolution body scanners in the late 1970s revolutionised the diagnosis of adrenal tumours. A modern body scanner will demonstrate the normal adrenal glands (Fig. 37.4) in all but exceptional cases, and tumours of 1 cm diameter or less can be identified. CT will also demonstrate ectopic tumours such as phaeochromocytomas in the majority of cases where the lesion is locally ectopic in the region of the kidney. Even when the tumour lies in the pelvis or the thorax, CT can identify the lesion provided the correct area is scanned.

Although CT will demonstrate masses as small as 1 cm in diameter, it has only limited value in their characterisation. Lipomas and

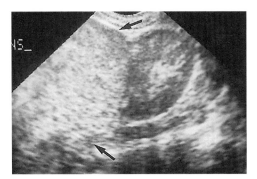

Fig. 27.7   Ultrasound scan showing echogenic suprarenal neuroblastoma (arrows). (Courtesy of Dr C. Dicks-Mireaux.)

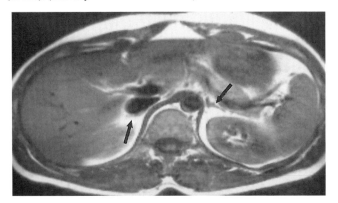

Fig. 27.8   Normal adrenal glands shown by MRI (T$_1$-weighted). (Courtesy of Professor Graham Cherryman.)

myelolipomas are readily identified by their low Hounsfield number. Adenomas also have a higher lipid content than most other masses and can be differentiated from metastases on this basis.

Staging of malignant tumours requires full CT or MR assessment. Local node involvement, spread to adjacent organs or tissues, liver or other or abdominal metastases, and IVC or renal vein spread should all be checked.

MRI

Magnetic resonance can identify the adrenals as well as CT and has the advantage of not using ionising radiation (Fig. 27.8). However, it is more costly and less freely available, so that many centres continue to use CT as the primary imaging technique in suspected adrenal tumours.

Early hopes that MRI might be able to characterise different mass lesions and differentiate benign from malignant tumours have not yet been fulfilled. Further, calcification, although resulting in foci of reduced signal, is not as easily recognised as it is by CT.

T$_1$-weighted signals show the normal adrenals well as low-signal against adjacent high-signal fat (Fig. 27.8). Most tumours show high signal on T$_2$-weighted images (Fig. 27.27) and lower signal on T$_1$-weighted studies (Fig. 27.9). Contrast-enhanced dynamic MRI has been used to differentiate types of adrenal masses; different patterns have been reported in adenomas, metastases, granulomas and phaeochromocytomas.

It is claimed that chemical shift MR can differentiate adenomas, which have a high lipid content, from metastases, which have low lipid content. Staging of malignant tumours can be performed as with CT.

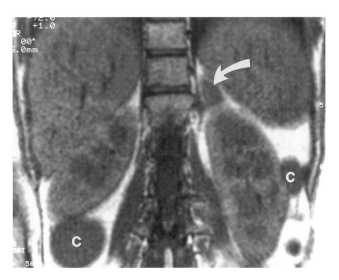

Fig. 27.9   Low-density rounded mass in left-adrenal of a 26-year-old woman with a clinical suspicion of a phaeochromocytoma (arrow) on a coronal T$_1$-weighted spin-echo (SE 560/25) image. Note the clinically unsuspected bilateral renal cysts (c)—von Hippel–Lindau disease. (Courtesy of Dr R. W. Whitehouse.)

Needle biopsy

This can be performed on adrenal masses, either with X-ray or ultrasound control when the mass is large, or under CT control with smaller lesions. The procedure is useful when an adrenal mass has been demonstrated and its nature is not at yet clinically clear. This may occur when an adrenal mass is found unexpectedly during CT of the abdomen for other causes, or when an abdominal mass in the adrenal area, but without other clinical manifestation, is under investigation. Figure 27.10 shows needling of a mass which proved positive for secondary carcinoma. Primary adrenal carcinoma frequently presents as a large mass with no other physical signs.

Complications of this procedure are rarely seen in experienced hands, but it should not be delegated to the inexperienced and junior members of the team, as pneumothorax, haemorrhage, abdominal pain and nausea have all been recorded, with an incidence of 2.5–3.5% in some reports. Most resolve spontaneously but active treatment is occasionally required for a large pneumothorax. Rarer complications reported are pancreatitis, adrenal abscess and tumour seeding along the needle track.

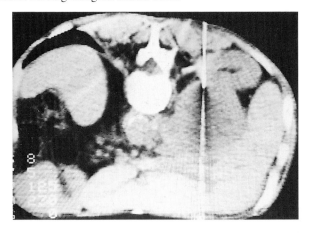

Fig. 27.10   Needle biopsy of right adrenal tumour under CT control with patient prone. Histology: adenocarcinoma from bowel (L36, W256).

RADIONUCLIDE IMAGING

Philip J. Robinson

The diagnosis of endocrine disorders caused by functioning adrenal lesions is based on clinical and biochemical findings. Ultrasound should show large masses, and smaller adrenal abnormalities can be demonstrated on CT or MRI. The usual role of scintigraphy is as a second-line test to clarify equivocal, inconclusive or unexpected results from anatomical imaging. Specifically, scintigraphy of both adrenal medulla and adrenal cortex is used:

- To demonstrate the functional status of adrenal nodules or masses shown on anatomical imaging
- To assess function in the contralateral adrenal
- To confirm bilateral disease in pituitary-driven syndromes
- To detect extra-adrenal or ectopic sites of hormone production
- To detect functioning metastases in patients with primary malignant adrenal tumours
- To detect recurrences after surgery
- In malignant phaeochromocytoma, to assess the feasibility of treatment by a therapy dose of ^{131}I-mIBG.

The investigation of adrenal cortical and adrenal medullary lesions requires individual techniques using appropriately targeted radio-pharmaceuticals.

Adrenal cortex

Radiopharmaceuticals

Labelled cholesterol analogues given intravenously are incorporated into low-density lipoproteins and concentrated by the adrenal cortex, where they join the synthetic pathway for steroid hormone production. These tracers undergo esterification, but are then stored in the intracellular lipid pool and are not further metabolised to active hormones. Only a small proportion of the injected activity reaches the adrenals, the remainder mostly being excreted in the bile, mainly as unchanged low-density lipoproteins. Because the rate of clearance and excretion of the tracers is slow, a relatively long-lived radionuclide is needed. Probably the most effective agent is ^{75}Se-labelled seleno-nor-cholesterol. This compound has a long shelf-life ($t_{1/2}$ for ^{75}Se is 120 days) and is stable in vivo. Alternatively, 19-iodo-cholesterol or preferably 6-beta-iodomethylnorcholesterol (NP59) may be used, labelled with iodine-131. Iodine binding is less resilient in vivo than selenium, so with the ^{131}I-labelled tracers, patients should undergo thyroid blockade with Lugol's solution before and after the test.

With the typical activity for an adult patient of 8 MBq of ^{75}Se-nor-cholesterol, the whole-body radiation dose is about 17 mSv. Administered activity of 37 MBq of either of the ^{131}I-labelled agents delivers a whole-body dose in the region of 10 mSv. The demonstration of autonomously functioning adrenal cortical lesions may be improved by suppressing the residual normal cortex to increase the tumour/background ration. This is achieved by giving dexamethasone, 1 mg four times daily for 7 days before the test and during the imaging period.

Imaging

Images are acquired at 5 days after injection, and again at 7 days if the diagnosis is not clear on the initial series. Earlier imaging

(3–5 days) is appropriate if dexamethasone suppression is used. The adrenals are best seen on posterior images. Anterior views are also helpful to identify activity in the gallbladder and colon, which may otherwise cause difficulty in interpretation. A useful addition to the technique is to give a small amount of ^{99}Tc-DMSA before obtaining images at the second visit, in order to show the renal outlines so as to confirm the location of suspected adrenal uptake. Normal uptake is seen in the adrenals and in the liver, with biliary excretion often outlining the gallbladder and colon. Normally-functioning adrenals are fairly symmetrical in the posterior view.

Clinical applications

In **Cushing's syndrome**, bilaterally symmetrical uptake indicates pituitary-driven hyperplasia (Fig. 27.11). Bilateral activity that is asymmetric suggests nodular hyperplasia, which may be independent of pituitary control. A functioning adrenal adenoma causing Cushing's will show increased uptake on the side of the lesion, with suppression of the contralateral gland. In the relatively rare cases of hyperfunctioning adrenal carcinoma, the most common finding is absence of uptake on both sides. This occurs because the tumours have too little uptake, relative to their size, to show a functioning focus, but produce enough steroid hormones to suppress the uninvolved gland.

In **Conn's syndrome**, unilateral uptake is seen on the side of a functioning adenoma (Fig. 27.12). However, small lesions may be masked by activity in normal adrenal tissue on both sides, as Conn's adenomas (unlike glucocorticoid-producing lesions) do not suppress ACTH production, so the contralateral adrenal remains active. For this reason, the sensitivity of scintigraphy in Conn's syndrome is improved by dexamethasone suppression, and this is adopted as routine procedure in some centres. Bilateral adrenal activity in spite of dexamethasone suppression indicates nodular hyperplasia as the cause of Conn's syndrome (Fig. 27.13). This can be difficult to distinguish from normal appearances unless quantification of adrenal activity, expressed as a proportion of the injected dose, is calculated. Also, similar bilateral uptake is seen with secondary hyperaldosteronism, so this possibility should be ruled out on biochemical and clinical criteria before embarking on scintigraphy.

Adrenal scintigraphy is not normally indicated in patients with incidentally-discovered adrenal nodules who have no biochemical

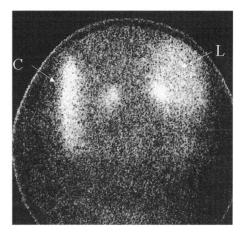

Fig. 27.11 Cushing's disease. Seleno-nor-cholesterol scintigraphy showed bilaterally symmetrical adrenal activity confirming pituitary-driven hyperplasia. CT had shown a unilateral adrenal nodule which proved to be non-functioning. L = liver; C = activity in colon.

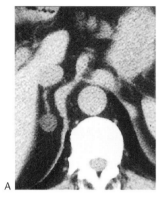

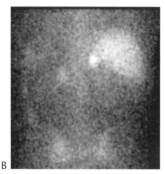

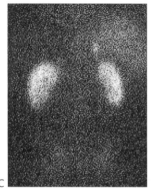

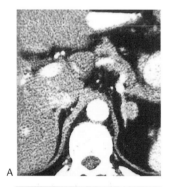

Fig. 27.12 Conn's syndrome. (A) Right-sided nodule shown at CT. (B) Seleno-nor-cholesterol scintigraphy showed a corresponding unilateral functioning adenoma (posterior view, day 7). (C) DMSA scintigraphy was used to confirm the anatomical location of the abnormal focus (posterior view, day 7).

evidence of hormonal imbalance. However, if such patients are investigated, the findings include normal appearances (small lesion not obliterating the adjacent tissue), increased unilateral function with or without contralateral suppression (adenoma functioning at low level) and non-function of the affected side (benign or malignant lesion destroying or effacing the ipsilateral adrenal tissue).

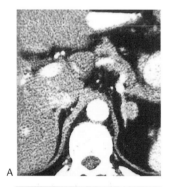

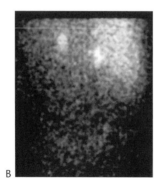

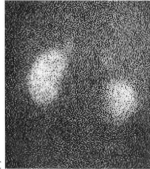

Fig. 27.13 Conn's syndrome. (A) CT revealed a left unilateral nodule. (B) Seleno-nor-cholesterol scintigraphy showed bilateral symmetrical activity (posterior view, day 7). Diagnosis: nodular hyperplasia of the adrenals. (C) DMSA scintigraphy was used to confirm the anatomical location of the adrenals (posterior view, day 7).

Adrenal medulla

Radiopharmaceuticals

Metaiodobenzylguanidine (mIBG) is a noradrenaline (norepinephrine) precursor analogue. It is concentrated in cells of neural crest origin, particularly in the adrenal medulla but also in the myocardium, salivary glands, lungs and spleen. After initial intracellular uptake, mIBG undergoes little or no further metabolism, and is gradually excreted by the kidney, with over 50% being excreted in the first 24 h, and over 80% within 4 days after injection. The major application of mIBG scintigraphy is in the detection and characterisation of phaeochromocytoma and neuroblastoma and their metastases. Apudomas, carcinoids and other neuroendocrine tumours also show mIBG uptake, but somatostatin receptor scintigraphy is usually preferred for these lesions.

The uptake of mIBG into tumours is likely to be impaired in patients who are receiving treatment with a range of drugs which affect catecholamine metabolism. This includes tricyclic antidepressants, sympathomimetic agents and compounds containing them, calcium channel blockers, various antihypertensive drugs and cocaine. A careful review of the patient's medication history must be undertaken before proceeding with an mIBG study. Drugs which are likely to interfere should be stopped or substituted 1–3 days before the study (depending on their duration of action). Thyroid blockade with Lugol's solution should also be used to cover the imaging period. Diagnostic studies are usually performed with ¹²³I-mIBG, which offers better imaging characteristics than ¹³¹I-mIBG, with less radiation dose to the patient. Typical administered activity of 150–200 MBq of ¹²³I-mIBG delivers a whole-body dose of about 8–10 mSv.

Imaging

Images of the whole body are obtained about 4 and 24 h after injection. SPECT may be helpful at the second visit to give improved detail of doubtful areas. In the normal patient, mIBG is taken up in the myocardium, lungs, liver, spleen and salivary glands, as well as in normal adrenals, which should be visible when iodine-123 is used as the tracer. Renal excretion leads to low-grade uptake in the kidney, and delayed images may show a little activity in the colon from biliary tract excretion, which accounts for a small percentage of the injected material. No uptake is seen in bone. Free iodide may result in activity in the thyroid, gastric mucosa and urinary tract.

Clinical applications

Scintigraphy with mIBG is highly accurate in the localisation of **phaeochromocytomas**, with sensitivity of over 90% for primary tumours (Figs 27.14, 27.15). False positives are rare. Specific indications for mIBG include the localisation of ectopic phaeochromocytomas, detection of recurrent disease after surgery, or of metastatic deposits (Fig. 27.16), and the characterisation of suspected phaeochromocytomas in the adrenal or elsewhere in the body, when a non-specific mass is found on anatomical imaging with ultrasound, CT or MRI. Finally, the delivery of a therapy dose of iodine-131 attached to mIBG requires prior demonstration of the avidity of uptake of mIBG into the tumour(s), which is assessed by an mIBG study using a diagnostic level of radioiodine.

The sensitivity of mIBG for detecting primary **neuroblastoma** exceeds 90%, and in finding bone metastases mIBG is probably more sensitive than bone scintigraphy. Specific indications for

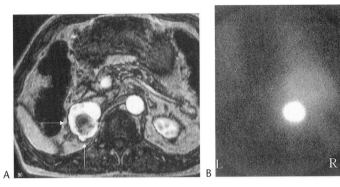

Fig. 27.14 Phaeochromocytoma. (A) Heterogeneous mass shown on MRI (arrows). (B) This was confirmed to be a highly active functioning tumour on mIBG scintigraphy.

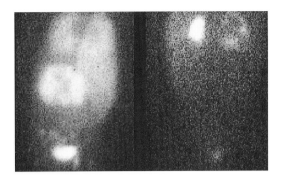

Fig. 27.17 Neuroblastoma. Posterior view mIBG appearances in two cases showing intense uptake in the tumours. (Courtesy of Dr. I. Driver).

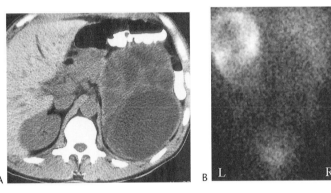

Fig. 27.15 Cystic phaeochromocytoma. (A) An atypical tumour shown on CT as a loculated cystic mass, and (B) confirmed on posterior view mIBG scintigraphy as an actively functioning tumour of the adrenal medulla.

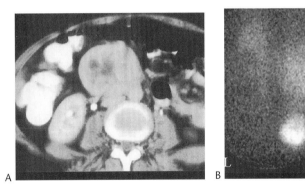

Fig. 27.18 Paraganglioma. (A) CT showed a non-specific tumour anterior to the aorta which was found to be intensely active on (B) mIBG scintigraphy.

mIBG imaging include initial tumour staging, assessment of response to treatment, and detection of residual or recurrent disease (Fig. 27.17). Tumour uptake of mIBG is typically reduced during and after chemotherapy or radiotherapy.

The results of mIBG scintigraphy with other tumours are less predictable. Somatostatin receptor scintigraphy is preferred for carcinoids, other apudomas and medullary thyroid cancers. In **paraganglioma** (Fig. 27.18) and **chemodectoma**, mIBG is often worthwhile because the initial level of uptake in the untreated lesions will determine the likely value of scintigraphy in follow-up after surgery or ablation.

CHOICE OF INVESTIGATION

It is clear from the above discussion that there is now a large battery of tests available using radiology or imaging to show adrenal tumors. On general principle, the least invasive techniques will be used first. Simple X-rays, or tomography with high-dose IVP, are relatively cheap and easily available. Of the newer imaging techniques, ultrasound is cheapest and most widely available. It is certainly the method of choice in infants and children. However, it is unlikely to be helpful with very small or ectopic lesions, and is less useful in adults, where such tumours are common.

Radionuclide scanning is useful with the small Conn's tumour and with Cushing's syndrome, but the technique is time consuming and expensive, and does not yield the immediate results possible with other techniques. The introduction of an isotope that will demonstrate phaeochromocytomas and neuroblastomas has extended the value of the method and has the advantage of including ectopic tumours and secondaries.

CT and MR have proved the most widely accepted of the newer imaging techniques, as they provide the most accurate, and yield immediate, results. They are accurate in all but the tiniest of adrenal tumours and the occasional ectopic phaeochromocytoma. They are also the best techniques for the staging of malignant tumours. The invasive techniques of arteriography and phlebography are now rarely necessary where access to modern imaging techniques is freely available. They will be reserved for the occasional problem case, such as the suspected phaeochromocytoma that other methods have failed to demonstrate.

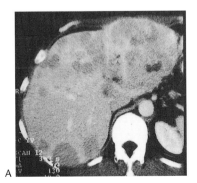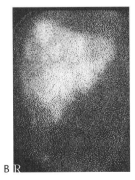

Fig. 27.16 Malignant phaeochromocytoma. (A) Non-specific appearance of liver metastases on CT, and (B) shown on mIBG scintigraphy to be functioning adrenal metastases.

SPECIFIC TUMOURS

Neuroblastoma

Characteristically these tumours occur in children and present either with an abdominal mass or with manifestations of secondary deposit. Over half of them arise in the adrenals, but 30% can arise from sympathetic tissue elsewhere in the abdomen, including the organ of Zuckerkandl; 20% arise in the thorax or neck.

Radiological investigation by plain X-rays can be very helpful. They may show an abdominal mass visible by virtue of its size, or by downward displacement of the kidney, or by the presence of calcification. Calcification has been noted to occur in over 50% of cases. An IVP may be helpful in confirming the kidney displacement, with downward drooping of the pelvis and calyces.

Sometimes it is very difficult to differentiate between a renal mass, such as a Wilms' tumour, and a suprarenal mass on simple X-ray and even on IVP. Calcification, if present, is an important point in favour of neuroblastoma, as it is uncommon in Wilms' tumour. Non-function of the affected kidney occurs in 10% of patients with Wilms' tumour and favours that diagnosis.

Ultrasound (Fig. 27.7) is now the most widely used primary investigation for abdominal masses in children (see Ch. 28). The appearances are variable, with mixed density from echogenic tumour and calcifications, and cystic areas from necrosis or haemorrhage. Major vessels such as the aorta and IVC may be surrounded and narrowed as well as elevated by the tumour mass. CT will show most of these features well and helps staging by confirming local invasion, liver metastases and spread to para-aortic nodes. Radionuclide imaging with mIBG (as noted above) can show both the primary tumour and metastases (Fig. 27.17), which can be found in bones, liver and orbits. Further discussion of neuroblastoma will be found in Chapter 28.

Ganglioneuroma

This is a mature form of neurogenic tumour. Apart from arising in the adrenal, these tumours can, like neuroblastomas, arise from the parasympathetic system elsewhere along the spine, particularly in the thorax; only some 10% arise in the adrenals.

Like neuroblastomas, they are more common in children; 60% occur before the age of 20, but a good proportion also present in adults.

Ganglioneuromas occurring in children may also show calcification, which can help in suggesting a diagnosis of neurogenic tumour. Occasionally, ganglioneuromas invade the spinal canal. In these cases there is not only an extraspinal mass but also an intraspinal component, causing neurological symptoms either from cord compression or from involvement of the cauda equina. These rare cases are often mistaken for dumb-bell neurofibromas and are best assessed by MRI (Fig. 27.19).

If the lesion presents in a child, and calcification is present in the paraspinal mass, the diagnosis of ganglioneuroma should always be considered. It is interesting that some of the recorded cases were

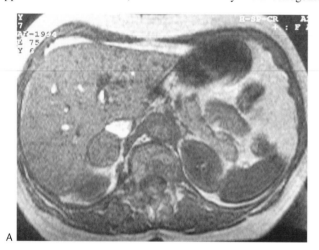

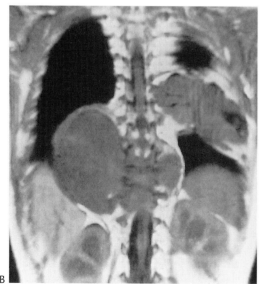

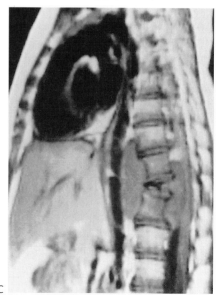

Fig. 27.19 (A) MR T$_2$-weighted axial section shows a large heterogeneous mass above the left kidney. Neuroblastoma. Sagittal (C) and coronal (B) T$_1$-weighted spin-echo (TR/TE 400/15 ms) images showing multiple ganglioneuromas. (C) A large right dumb-bell shaped paravertebral mass extends across to the left. In (B) the mass is seen to extend anterior to the spine with displacement of the aorta, and it also extends posteriorly into the spinal canal. There is destruction and collapse of the body of one of the lower thoracic vertebra. Another ganglioneuroma is present in the left intercostal region and is well shown in (C). (Courtesy of Dr C. Dicks-Mireaux.)

first reported histologically as neuroblastomas but a second and later biopsy showed ganglioneuroma. It is now well-recognised that neuroblastomas can sometimes mature into the more benign and well differentiated tumour. These tumours are best defined by CT or by MRI if there is suspicion of an intraspinal extension (Fig. 27.19).

Typical ganglioneuromas show low attenuation and punctate calcification at CT. MRI shows intermediate intensity on both T_1- and T_2-weighted images, with early enhancement and little washout on dynamic images. Some 25% of ganglioneuromas are not truly benign but contain poorly differentiated components, including ganglioneuroblastoma, neuroblastoma or malignant phaeochromocytoma. CT or MRI may suggest the presence of a malignant component by demonstrating atypical elements.

Adrenal cortical adenoma

Cortical adenomas, usually small, are said to be present in 5% of routine necropsies. The vast majority of these are presumably non-functional and symptomless during life, but the figure implies that such adenomas will occasionally be seen as purely chance findings at CT (Fig. 27.20) or at MRI investigations. CT surveys suggest an incidence of 0.6–1.5%, the figure increasing with age, for such adenomas large enough to be seen at imaging (0.8–1.0 cm in diameter or more).

Functioning adenomas may give rise to Cushing's syndrome (cortisol-secreting), Conn's syndrome (mineralocorticoid-secreting) or very rarely a virilising syndrome (androgen-secreting). These are discussed in more detail below.

Adrenal cortical carcinoma

As with adenomas, these tumours may be non-functional, and appear so in some 50% of cases. Such tumours eventually present either with metastases or with a mass in the abdomen. Like adenomas, the functioning tumours can present in different ways, depending on the type of hormone secretion—cortisol, androgens, oestrogens or aldosterone. Cushing's syndrome is the most frequent form of endocrine presentation, but a virilising syndrome, Conn's syndrome and very rarely a feminising syndrome may all occur. The left adrenal is more frequently affected than the right, although in the late stages 10% become bilateral. The sex incidence shows a slight preponderance of females over males. Although commoner in adults (the peak incidence is at 45–55 years), they are occasionally seen in children; however, malignant adrenal tumours in children are far more likely to be neuroblastomas, which outnumber adrenal cortical carcinomas by 10 to 1.

Adrenal carcinomas are often quite large at discovery, particularly when non-functioning. In one series the average diameter was about 15 cm. With such large masses, simple X-ray or IVU with tomography will often show the lesion well and there will be downward displacement of the kidney. About one-third of such carcinomas show calcification at simple X-ray, and even more do so at CT. This is usually patchy and irregular but can be nodular.

Ultrasound will readily demonstrate large adrenal masses (Fig. 27.21A) and can screen for liver metastases. It is the primary investigation of choice, particularly in childhood. The mass is usually of mixed echogenicity and may show nodules of calcification. CT is more specific in demonstrating spread to adjacent structures and will also show liver metastases and glandular involvement (Figs 27.21–27.24). Unfortunately these are present in 50% of cases

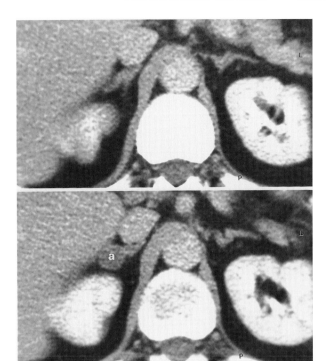

Fig. 27.20 Contiguous postcontrast CT scans showing a small right adrenal adenoma (a). Note this small adenoma is only visible on one of the adjacent scans. Normal left adrenal gland. (Courtesy of Dr J. P. R. Jenkins.)

at presentation, and the peritoneum and opposite adrenal become involved in 10%. Needle biopsy may be helpful in confirming or excluding the diagnosis with the smaller non-functioning carcinoma.

The prognosis in these cases is poor. Many are at an advanced stage when first diagnosed (stage III or IV) (Box 27.3). Few patients survive 5 years and most die within a year or two of diagnosis.

Metastases in the adrenals

The adrenal glands may be involved on one or both sides by metastases from primary carcinoma elsewhere in the body and are commonly involved in patients with bronchial and breast carcinoma. CT surveys of the liver and abdomen are frequently made in these patients, and the adrenals should always be carefully checked at such examinations (Fig. 27.25). Bilateral adrenal masses may also be seen with lymphoma (Fig. 27.26). On MRI surveys unilateral or bilateral adrenal masses can also be readily identified. They are best shown as high-signal lesions on T_2-weighted images (Fig. 27.27).

Sometimes a mass is found in the adrenal in the presence of secondaries elsewhere and no apparent primary. In such cases, or with a solitary mass in the adrenal and no clinical clue as to its nature, needle biopsy may help to establish a diagnosis (Fig. 27.10). Despite their small size the adrenal glands are a common site for metastases. At autopsy 27% of patients dying from carcinoma have adrenal deposits, a figure only exceeded by three much larger organs—lungs, liver and bone. The deposits may be unilateral or bilateral, and the commonest primary sites are lung and breast; 30–40% of these tumours will eventually metastasise to the adrenals (stage IV). Also frequently metastasising to the adrenals are melanoma (50%) and gastrointestinal and renal carcinoma

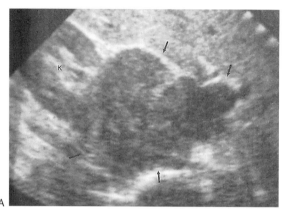

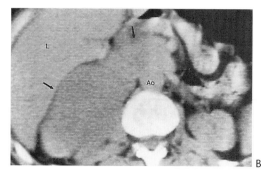

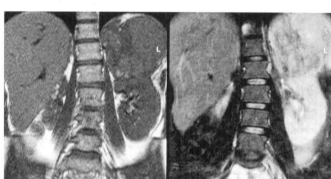

Fig. 27.21 (A) Ultrasound scan shows a large irregular mass (arrows) above the right kidney. Adrenal carcinoma. K = kidney. (B) CT shows the mass extending anteriorly and invading muscle posteriorly. Ao = aorta. (Courtesy of Dr Janet Murfitt.) (C) MR T$_2$-weighted coronal sections show a large, mainly low-density mass above the left kidney. Carcinoma of left adrenal.

tives. Thus small lesions (below 8 mm in diameter) can be missed. Needle-aspiration biopsy results suggest a figure as high as 17% for such cases. The demonstration of visible masses, even if bilateral, can be due to benign lesions such as non-functioning adenomas. As noted above, these are seen at CT in up to 1.5% of people with no relevant symptoms, the percentage increasing with age. There are also other causes of benign masses in the adrenals, listed above, which make the imaging finding non-specific for metastases, particularly with small lesions (less than 3 cm in diameter).

With adrenal metastases, the primary carcinoma is usually in lung or breast. Melanoma, kidney and gastrointestinal secondaries are also well recognised.

Lipoma and myelolipoma

These are rare non-functioning tumours of the adrenal that have been reported at autopsy in the past with an incidence of 0.1–0.2%. Although usually small, they have been recorded up to 12 cm in diameter. They are composed mainly of fat cells, but may contain focal areas of myeloid tissue. With the increasing use of CT they

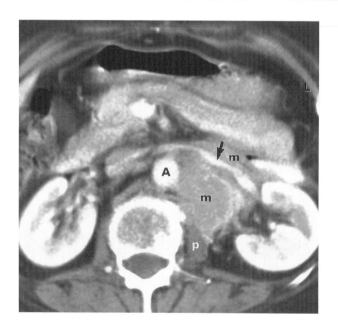

Fig. 27.22 Adrenal carcinoma (m) surrounding the left adrenal vein (arrow), abutting onto the abdominal aorta (A) and infiltrating the psoas muscle (p) on a postcontrast CT scan. (Courtesy of Dr J. P. R. Jenkins.)

(10–20% each). Secondary lymphoma can also involve the adrenals but much less frequently (Fig. 27.26), being found in only 6% of patients. Most adrenal metastases are symptomless, but cases showing hypoadrenalism have been recorded.

The demonstration of adrenal masses at cross-sectional imaging in patients with carcinoma is an important finding because it stages the patient as grade IV and affects treatment. However, imaging is not infallible and can result in both false negatives and false posi-

Box 27.3	Staging of adrenal carcinoma		
T1	Tumour <5 cm diameter	Stage I	T1N0M0
T2	Tumour 5 cm	Stage II	T2N0M0
T3	Tumour extending beyond gland but not involving adjacent organs	Stage III	T1/2N0M0
			T3N0M0
T4	Tumour extending beyond gland and involving adjacent organs	Stage IV	Any T M1
N0	No nodal involvement		
N1	Local nodes involved		
M0	No metastases		
M1	Metastases		

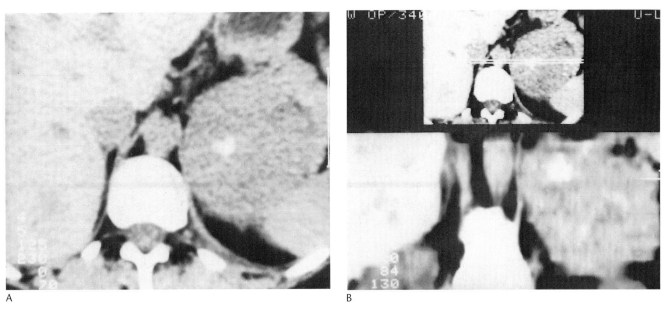

Fig. 27.23 (A) Large mass in left adrenal. Note the nodular calcification in the tumour and low-density areas in the liver. Adrenal carcinoma presenting with Cushing's syndrome (L36, W256). (B) Coronal reconstruction of tumour (L38, W128).

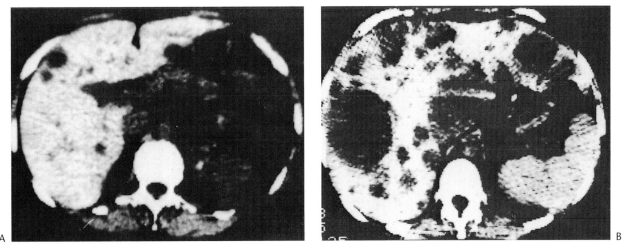

Fig. 27.24 (A) Same patient as Fig. 27.23, showing deposits in liver at narrow window (L63, W64). (B) Six months later, and following removal of adrenal tumour, deposits have increased in size (L50, W64).

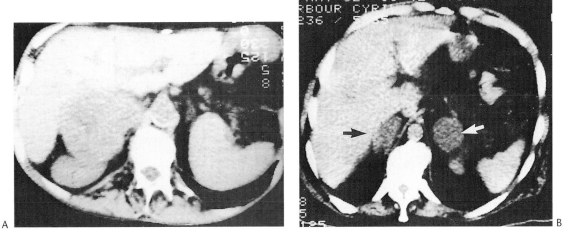

Fig. 27.25 (A) Large metastasis in right adrenal (L36, W256). (B) Bilateral metastases (arrows) in the adrenals from bronchial carcinoma (L45, W256).

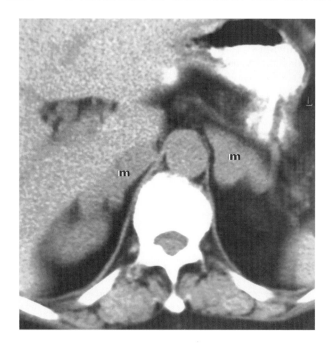

Fig. 27.26   CT scan of bilateral enlarged adrenal glands (m) from lymphomatous infiltration. (Courtesy of Dr J. P. R. Jenkins.)

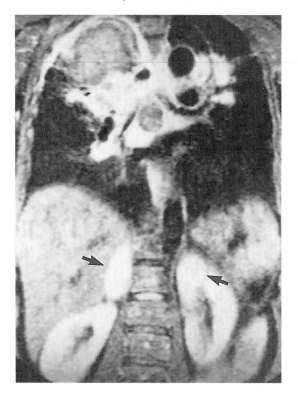

Fig. 27.27   Coronal MRI scan (T$_2$-weighted) shows bilateral adrenal metastases (arrows) as high-signal masses. Primary lung carcinoma with collapse of right upper lobe is also well shown. (Courtesy of Dr Gordon Thomson and Bristol MRI Centre.)

are now being encountered as chance findings (Fig. 27.28), when they are of fatty density, or occasionally of density suggesting mixed tissue. At ultrasound these tumours are highly echogenic, and show a diagnostic bright hyperechoic appearance.

T$_1$-weighted MRI can also be diagnostic with fat-suppression sequences and has the advantage of easy multiplanar facilities.

While these are benign tumours, some workers recommend surgery for larger tumours (over 9 cm in diameter) because there have been several such large myelolipomas reported as presenting with acute abdominal pain following tumour haemorrhage.

Calcifying fibrous pseudotumour is a well-recognised benign pathological entity occurring in the limbs, axilla, pleura and pericardium. A case has recently been described as presenting in the left adrenal of a 10-year-old girl and was 15 × 12 cm in size when diagnosed by CT. Its size and the presence of calcification led at first to a misdiagnosis of neuroblastoma.

Adrenal cysts

Kearney and Mahoney (1977) have classified adrenal cysts as:

1. Endothelial (45%)
2. Pseudocyst (39%)
3. Epithelial (9%)
4. Parasitic (hydatid).

Pseudocysts are the type clinically encountered most commonly, although endothelial cysts are more common at autopsy. Pseudocysts result from haemorrhage or necrosis and are seen in both normal glands and in tumours, varying in diameter from a few millimetres to many centimetres. Calcification may ensue in the wall of the haemorrhagic or necrotic cyst. Presentation is either in neonates or in adults, often as chance findings during imaging for other reasons (Fig. 27.29).

Neonatal adrenal haemorrhage is not uncommon in association with birth trauma or infection and often goes undiagnosed, with recovery of the child. The neonate adrenal gland is relatively huge, weighing 8 g against the adult weight of 5 g. The haemorrhage may present as an abdominal mass or as bilateral masses which can develop marginal calcification as they regress over several weeks. If clinically suspected, the diagnosis can best be confirmed by ultra-

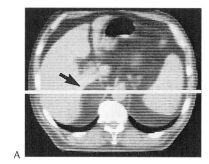

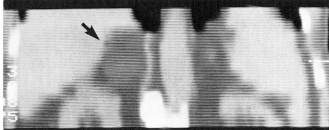

Fig. 27.28   (A,B) Right adrenal lipoma (arrow). Coronal reconstruction of low-density mass (−67 HU) (L46, 41024).

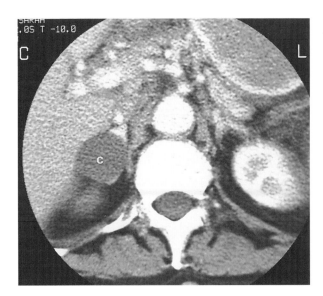

Fig. 27.29 Adrenal cyst (c) measuring 11 HU on a postcontrast CT scan. Normal enhancing left adrenal gland. (Courtesy of Dr J. P. R. Jenkins.)

sound, which should differentiate it from the more solid neuroblastoma (see Ch. 28).

Adrenal cysts in adults can occur as benign pseudocysts following haemorrhage. They may also occur following haemorrhage or necrosis in large tumours (Fig. 27.40) either benign or malignant. They are best shown by ultrasound or CT, the latter being preferred as it usually provides more information, particularly with neoplasms. Asymptomatic adrenal cysts observed as chance findings at CT and with no apparent tumour present can be treated conservatively. Marginal curvilinear or egg-shell calcification may be noted in some 20% of cases. In doubtful cases, needle aspiration of the fluid may help by cytology for malignant cells or confirming evidence of old haemorrhage.

Hormone-secreting adenomas

It has been noted above that 50% of cortical carcinomas are non-secreting. Many benign tumours are also non-secreting, but most adenomas presenting clinically do secrete hormones.

Androgen and oestrogen excess

The term 'adrenogenital syndrome' is no longer favoured by endocrinologists. Several different adrenal lesions may give rise to excess androgen or oestrogen production including *congenital adrenal hyperplasia* (CAH), adrenal adenoma and adrenal carcinoma.

CAH is a complex group of congenital disorders of adrenal steroid-synthesising enzymes with a wide spectrum of clinical presentation. These range from neonatal collapse, through intersex, to adult presentation with sex hormone disorders.

Neonates may present with ambiguous genitalia, and older children with a virilising syndrome in girls or isosexual precocity in boys. In the adult, hirsutes or masculinising features may be the presenting features.

Biochemical tests will usually establish the diagnosis and CT will clearly demonstrate CAH or an adrenal mass. In infants and children, ultrasound should be used as the primary investigation.

Cushing's syndrome

Clinically, this is characterised by a rounded 'moon-like' facies, plethora and truncal obesity. Hypertension and osteoporosis also occur, and dementia or depression may be features.

Table 27.1 summarizes the different types of spontaneous Cushing's syndrome and their approximate incidence.

Imaging findings There are many interesting simple radiological features in Cushing's syndrome. These are discussed in Chapter 42 and depend on the catabolic effect resulting in osteoporosis, which mainly affects the axial skeleton. *Vertebral collapse* is common, as are *spontaneous rib fractures*, often painless and with excessive callus formation. *Ischaemic necrosis of the femoral heads* may also occur.

In patients with suspected adrenal tumours, simple X-ray may sometimes demonstrate an adrenal mass. An adenoma may be shown by high-dose IVP with tomography. Carcinomas may contain calcification and are usually quite large at presentation. In children, ultrasound should be used as the first imaging procedure, but in adults the presence of suspected adrenal tumours is best confirmed by CT. Cortical adenomas are readily identified, being usually 3–8 cm in diameter. Carcinomas are usually larger in size and often contain calcification (Fig. 27.23). CT may also show evidence of secondaries in the liver, or glandular involvement (Fig. 27.24). *Fatty infiltration of the liver*, a recognised feature of Cushing's syndrome, may be identified at CT in some cases. Radionuclide imaging has been discussed above and can distinguish an adenoma from bilateral hyperplasia.

Pituitary-dependent cases may show clear evidence of bilateral adrenal hyperplasia (Fig. 27.30), as may cases due to ectopic ACTH production, but the adrenals usually seem normal at CT in these cases. Some of these patients with apparently normal adrenals have been operated on and moderate enlargement of the adrenals proved. It appears, therefore, that mild enlargement can be missed by CT. Bilateral nodular hyperplasia is occasionally suggested by CT or MRI and raises problems as it may be ACTH-dependent or autonomous. Adrenal venous sampling will help in assessment.

The radiologist was frequently asked to X-ray the skull in patients presenting with Cushing's syndrome, but this is rarely necessary as pituitary tumours in this condition are usually microscopic and do not produce enlargement of the sella. There are occasional exceptions to this rule; in particular, patients who have been

Table 27.1 Spontaneous Cushing's syndrome

Type		Incidence
A.	Due to excess ACTH production	
	1. Pituitary dependent	
	a. Pituitary microadenoma	Very common (80%)
	b. Alcoholic	Common
	c. Depressive psychosis	Very rare
	2. Ectopic ACTH production	
	a. Malignant tumours	Common
	b. Benign tumours	Rare
B.	Due to primary adrenal lesions	
	1. Adrenal cortical adenoma	Common (5–10%)
	2. Adrenal cortical carcinoma	Rare (1%)
	3. Micronodular dysplasia	Very rare

treated by adrenalectomy may develop large adenomas which enlarge the sella (Nelson's syndrome). MRI with enhancement is the technique most likely to show small microadenomas.

Petrosal vein sampling for raised ACTH levels has also been used to identify pituitary microadenomas. These lesions may be small and unilateral. Thus, it is vital that sampling should be bilateral, as an abnormal value may be present on one side only. Latcralisation will also be invaluable in aiding trans-sphenoidal surgery.

Patients with *ectopic ACTH production* are most commonly suffering from malignant tumour. This is most likely to be a lung carcinoma, which is the cause in 60% of such cases. Pancreatic carcinoma, malignant thymoma and medullary carcinoma of the thyroid are also well-documented causes, while isolated cases have been described with other forms of primary carcinoma. Benign tumours involved include carcinoids, benign thymomas and, very rarely, phaeochromocytomas and ganglioneuromas. In some patients with ectopic ACTH production the clinical features may give some clue as to the primary tumour. Simple X-ray of the chest may demonstrate the lesion. If not, CT may be helpful, with partic-

ular attention to the lungs, mediastinum, pancreas and upper abdomen.

Micronodular adrenal dysplasia is a rare cause of Cushing's syndrome in children. The aetiology is unknown. The adrenals are enlarged and contain multiple tiny adenomas a millimetre or so in diameter. Excess cortisol production in *alcoholism* is well recognised and, like that seen occasionally in severe *depressive psychosis*, is ACTH-dependent; however, the mechanism remains uncertain.

Primary hyperaldosteronism (Conn's syndrome)

Primary hyperaldosteronism, or Conn's syndrome, is characterised by hypokalaemia, weakness and hypertension. Excessive production of aldosterone from a function *adenoma* of the zona glomerulosa of the adrenal cortex is the cause of the syndrome in 50–80% of cases. A smaller proportion are due to *bilateral micronodular hyperplasia* and, in a few mysterious cases, the adrenals are found to be normal both macroscopically and microscopically. As noted above, a functioning adrenal *carcinoma* may also present with Conn's syndrome, in which case the tumour may be quite large.

Cross-sectional scanning by CT or MR is now routinely used as the imaging method of choice for investigating Conn's syndrome, but, as indicated below, scintigraphy may be helpful in selected cases, as may adrenal vein sampling or transvenous infarction. Both CT and MR can readily identify the small adenomas of Conn's syndrome even when only 1 cm or less in diameter (Figs. 27.32-27.35). Historically, it was the development of adrenal phlebography which first made it possible to demonstrate these small adenomas, most commonly seen in Conn's syndrome (Sutton 1968). The characteristic feature is usually an arc-like vein in the circumference of the tumour, which is relatively avascular (Fig. 27.31).

Large adenomas of the type seen in Cushing's syndrome are rare in Conn's syndrome. The average diameter is only 1–2 cm. In our material of some 30 cases, we encountered only one with a diameter over 4 cm and this proved to be malignant. A diameter of more

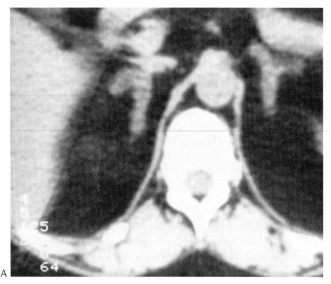

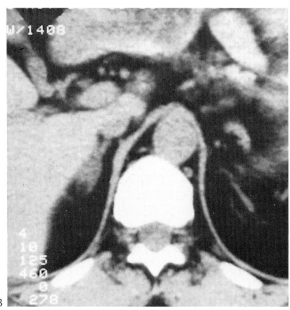

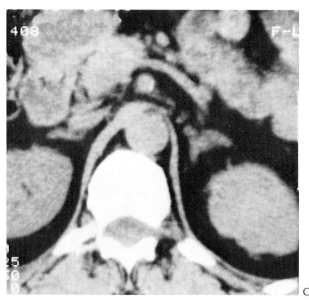

Fig. 27.30 (A) Bilateral adrenal hyperplasia (L36, W512). (B,C) Hypertrophied right and left adrenals in another patient (L36, W512).

than 4 or 5 cms should therefore raise the possibility of a functioning carcinoma.

Calcification has not been recorded in the literature in these small tumours, but was present in one unusual case reported by us. It was thought that this was in a haemorrhagic cyst in the unusually large tumour, which proved malignant.

We have noted above that small non-functioning nodules are quite common. Thus the presence of a small nodule in a patient with Conn's syndrome is not necessarily diagnostic (Figs 27.12, 27.13). Apart from isotope examination, it is also possible to prove whether the adenoma is functional by adrenal vein sampling carried out routinely at the time of phlebography. Aldosterone concentrations in relation to cortisol are measured on the two sides. In adenoma patients the concentration is increased on the affected side and suppressed on the other. In patients with hyperplasia the raised concentrations are similar on the two sides.

Functioning adenomas also have a higher lipid content than other masses and can be differentiated on this basis. A measurement of 10 HU or less is thought to be diagnostic whilst up to 20 U is suggestive.

In the latter cases the enhancement washout test is claimed by some to help confirm diagnosis. Films taken after CT enhancement and later (delayed enhancement) shows 60% or more, higher values if positive.

At T_1-Weighted MR Conn's adenomas are isodense or slightly hypodense compared to liver. It is claimed that chemical shift analysis can help differentiate functioning adenomas from non-functioning masses or metastases.

When adrenal phlebography was more widely used, occasional cases of adrenal infarction were reported. However, this was probably associated with the use of excessive doses of contrast medium or excessive injection pressures. This raised the possibility of non-surgical ablation of small tumours, and this technique has been succesfully used in practice.

Non surgical ablation of small adenomas can also be performed by the alternative technique of direct percutaneous injection of a toxic substance such as 5–11 ml of 50% Acetic acid. This can be done by the radiologist under imaging control. Both the above techniques have been successfully used in Cushing's Syndrome and in Conn's syndrome.

Phaeochromocytoma

This has proved to be the commonest adrenal tumour observed in our clinical practice. The classic clinical presentation is with attacks of paroxysmal hypertension accompanied by headache, sweating, palpitation, anxiety and tremor. The attacks may last from 15 min to an hour and may occur several times a week, or even a day. However, many cases are less typical; 50% of adult cases present with sustained hypertension.

Adrenal phaeochromocytomas secrete catecholamines in 90% of cases, giving rise to the symptoms described above, but only 50% of extra-adrenal tumours do so. They may also excrete other hormones, which can give rise to confusing endocrine symptoms; these hormones include parathyroid hormone, calcitonin, gastrin, secretin and ACTH.

Ninety per cent of these tumours arise in the adrenals but the remaining 10% may be found anywhere in the sympathetic system, from the neck to the pelvis. The majority (90%) of these *ectopic tumours* are intra-abdominal and most lie adjacent to the kidneys. We have seen such tumours at the hilum of the kidney (Fig. 27.45), medial to the inferior vena cava (Fig. 27.37) and below the kidney.

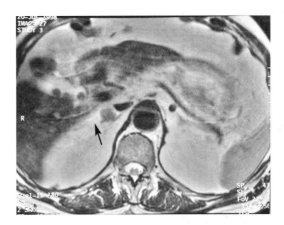

Fig. 27.32 MR study. T_2-weighted image shows a small 1 cm adenoma (arrow) behind the IVC. Right-sided Conn's tumour.

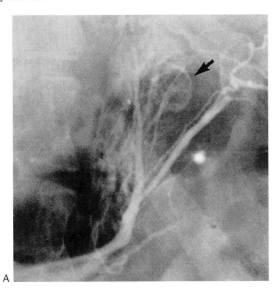

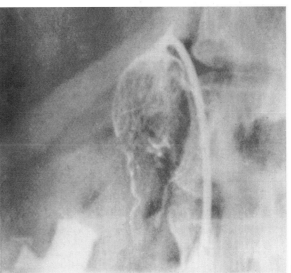

Fig. 27.31 (A) Left adrenal phlebogram showing small Conn's tumour (arrow). (B) Right adrenal phlebogram showing Conn's tumour.

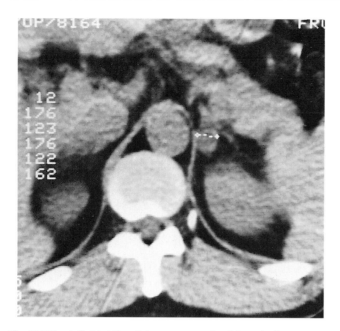

Fig. 27.33   Left-sided Conn's tumour measuring 1.2 cm in diameter.

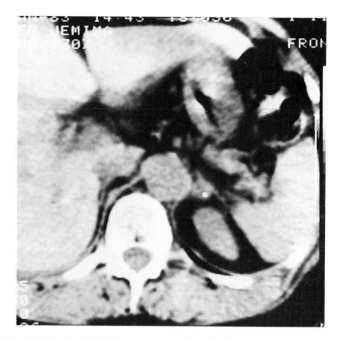

Fig. 27.35   Small left Conn's tumour 0.8 cm in diameter and marked by white dot. (Density 20 HU—L43, W512).

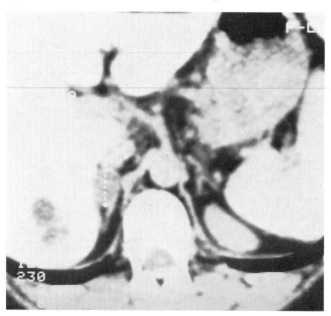

Fig. 27.34   Right-sided Conn's tumour 1.9 cm in diameter. Normal left adrenal also well shown (L36, W256).

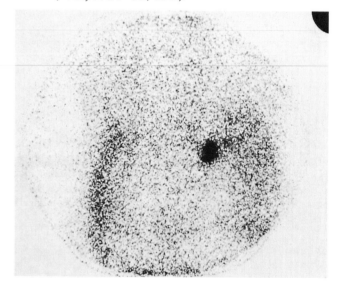

Fig. 27.36   Right-sided Conn's tumour shown by scintigraphy 7 days postinjection.

The organ of Zuckerkandl, adjacent to the aortic bifurcation, is also a recognised extra-adrenal site (1%). Other tumours have been found in the bladder wall and such patients have sometimes presented with attacks of hypertension brought on by micturition. Thoracic tumours are usually paravertebral (Fig. 27.50) but have been found in the mediastinum (Fig. 27.38). Some 10% of these tumours appear to be familial, and a similar proportion occur in children. Multiple tumours also occur in a similar percentage, as do bilateral adrenal tumours and malignant tumours. The so-called 'rule of ten' summarises this by postulating that 10% of cases are:

1. Familial
2. Bilateral adrenal
3. Multiple (other than above)
4. Extra-adrenal
5. Children
6. Malignant.

Some 5% of cases are associated with *neurofibromatosis*, but the reverse is less common, as only 1% of patients with neurofibromatosis develop phaeochromocytoma.

There are also less common, but well-recognized, associations with von Hippel–Lindau syndrome (Fig. 27.19) and with medullary carcinoma of the thyroid and hyperparathyroidism, which may be familial. This is usually referred to as multiple endocrine neoplasia (MEN) type II or Sipple's syndrome. When the medullary carcinoma of the thyroid and phaeochromocytoma are associated with

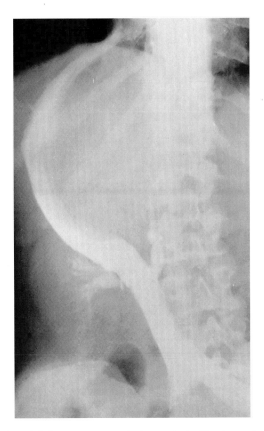

Fig. 27.37 Inferior vena cavography in a patient with a large phaeochromocytoma lying posterior and medial to the inferior vena cava.

mucosal neuromas involving conjunctiva, eyelid, mouth and sometimes gut, and with a marfanoid habitus, it is referred to as MEN type III.

Apart from the clinical aspects, the firm diagnosis of phaeochromocytoma depends on biochemical assays of catecholamines in urine or blood, or both; repeated assays may be necessary as hypersecretion may be paroxysmal.

Imaging investigation The size of the adrenal tumour at diagnosis has varied in our material from 2 or 3 cm to 20 cm in diameter, with an average of some 7 cm.

Large adrenal masses will also be quite well shown by *ultrasound* (Fig. 27.39). However, smaller and ectopic tumours will be more difficult to demonstrate by ultrasound. Very large tumours may undergo central necrosis and become cystic, a feature which is well seen at ultrasound or CT (Fig. 27.40).

Calcification is, in our experience, very rare and has only been seen once in 60 cases. In this case, as in others described in the literature, it was curvilinear and probably in the wall of a haemorrhagic cyst.

Angiography has been widely used in the past for diagnosing phaeochromocytomas and many examples are described and illustrated in previous editions of this work. Complications and the precautions against them are also well described. However, the method has been rendered obsolete with the advent of safe non-invasive methods (ultrasound, CT and MRI), although it may still occasionally prove useful to the surgeon proposing to operate on a hilar tumour stenosing or compromising a renal artery (Fig. 27.47).

CT body scanners were first used in the late 1970s and it soon became apparent that they provided an excellent non-invasive method for diagnosing phaeochromocytoma. Tumours lying in the

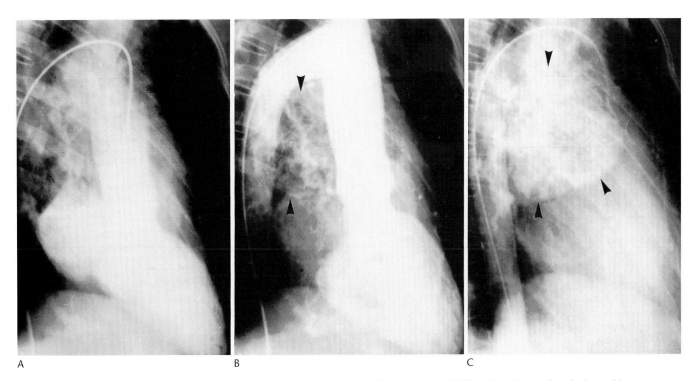

A   B   C

Fig. 27.38 Left ventricular angiocardiogram. This patient presented with mitral incompetence. (A) There is evidence of marked mitral incompetence. (B, C) Pathological vessels are shown arising from the aorta to supply a large vascular mass above the left atrium. Phaeochromocytoma removed by surgery.

adrenal gland are easily identified (Figs 27.42–27.44), as are bilateral adrenal tumours (Fig. 27.40). Locally, ectopic tumours are also easily identified if the examination covers the whole of both kidneys (Figs 27.41, 27.45). If the biochemical evidence of phaeochromocytoma is established, the demonstration of normal adrenal glands indicates that an octopic tumour is present. If there is no evidence of this in the region of the kidneys, the lower abdomen and pelvis should also be examined by CT, and simple X-rays of the thorax (Fig. 27.50) should be carefully scrutinised.

If these are negative, *scintiscanning* using mIBG should be tried. Although time-consurming and expensive, this test has been shown to demonstrate functioning phaeochromocytomas with a high degree of accuracy (Fig. 27.46), although false-positive and false-negative results have both been recorded. It is important, of course, to cover all possible sites of ectopia, including pelvis, thorax and neck. The test is particularly useful for demonstrating metastases with malignant phaochromocytomas (Fig. 27.16). Only in rare cases should it be necessary to proceed to other investigations. Then resort will be had to *venous sampling* in an attempt to localize the lesion. Samples should be obtained from the internal jugular and innominate veins on both sides, from the superior vena cava and right atrium, from the high inferior vena cava and both renal veins, from the low inferior vena cava and from both iliac veins. This should result in localization of the tumour to a confined area, which can he further assessed by CT, ultrasound or scintiscanning. Venous sampling and assay of all areas is normally possible by simple percutaneous catheterisation of a femoral vein.

It is clear from the above discussion that CT, and later MRI, became the investigation of choice for diagnosing phaeochromo-cytomas, although there is a place for ultrasound in assessing children and large tumours. The place of scintography has been discussed above. Other methods (venous sampling and arteri-ography) will occasionally be used in the search for ectopic tumours, or for other special indications.

MRI is now widely used to demonstrate adrenal masses and may eventually replace CT as the investigation of choice, as it involves no radiation and appears to be completely innocuous. To date its use in many areas of the world only remains limited by cost and availability.

Ectopic tumours at the renal hilum sometimes displace and stretch the renal arteries, giving rise to *renal artery stenosis* (see previous edition of this text). We have seen several examples where arteriography has been useful in warning the surgeon of a danger-ous situation, although MRI can now achieve the same purpose (Fig. 27.47).

Malignant phaeochromocytomas are probably less frequent than the 10% figure given in the older literature, as the diagnosis was then rarely confirmed in the atypical cases with small benign or

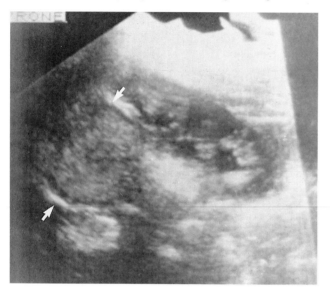

Fig. 27.39 Ultrasound scan shows large rounded tumour (arrows) above upper pole of right kidney (Same case as Fig. 27.46.)

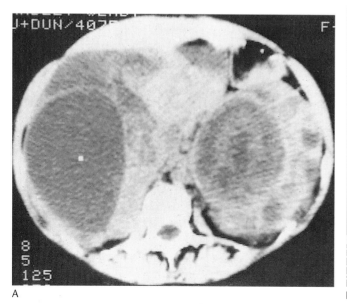

A

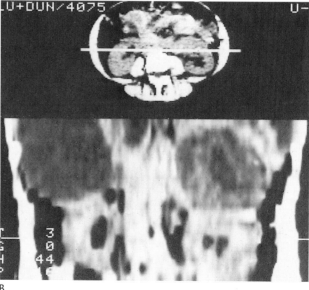

B

Fig. 27.40 (A) Giant bilateral cystic phaeochromocytomas displacing the kidneys downward and liver upward (L36, W128). (B) Coronal reconstruction through tumours and downward-displaced kidneys (L36, W64).

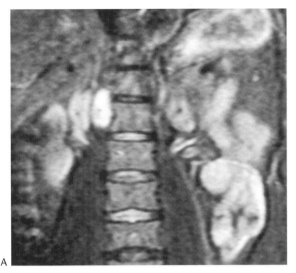

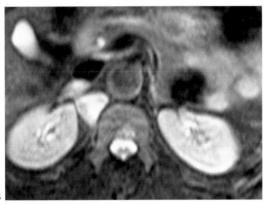

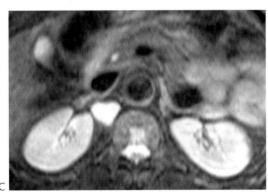

Fig. 27.41 MR T$_2$-weighted image shows bilobed high-signal tumour above the right kidney. (A) Coronal, (B,C) Axial sections. The posteromedial segment of the tumour lay behind the crus of the diaphragm and would have been missed at surgery without forewarning. (Courtesy of Dr R. Whitehouse.)

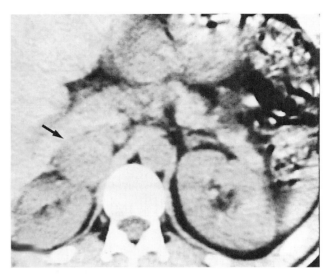

Fig. 27.42 Small phaeochromocytoma (arrow) (3 cm diameter) anterior to upper pole of right kidney (L45, W512).

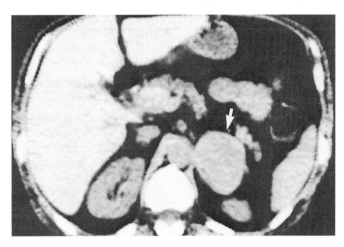

Fig. 27.43 Phaeochromocytoma (5 × 3.5 cm) in left adrenal (arrow) (L41, W256).

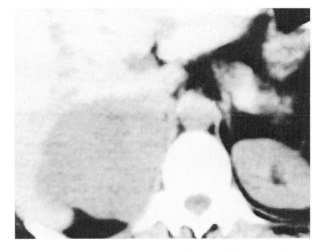

Fig. 27.44 Large phaeochromocytoma (7 × 8 cm) in right adrenal and displacing liver (L36, W256).

ectopic tumours. Metastases from malignant tumours can involve lymph glands, bone, liver and chest (Figs 27.13, 27.48, 27.49), but the tumours are usually slow growing and patients can survive for several years after surgery and careful medical treatment. Isotope scanning is particularly valuable in assessing bone and other deposits.

Phaeochromocytomas presenting in childhood are often both multiple and familial (Fig. 27.50).

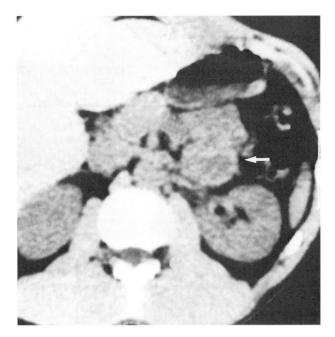

Fig. 27.45 Ectopic small phaeochromocytoma (arrow) (3 cm diameter) anterior to left hilum (L36, W256).

Other retroperitoneal tumours

Apart from renal tumours and the adrenal tumours just described, other retroperitoneal tumours are rare. Most of them are malignant, and relatively large at clinical presentation. They include, in order of frequency, sarcomas, extragonadal germ cell tumours, paragangliomas and lymphomas. Sarcomas account for 90% of these and liposarcoma is the commonest type, followed by leiomyosarcoma and malignant fibrous histiocytoma (MFH).

They present in middle-aged or elderly patients (peak incidence 40–60 years), with a soft-tissue mass in the loin or lumbar region. Leiomyosarcomas form 29% of these primary retroperitoneal malignancies. MFH is one of the commonest soft-tissue sarcomas of adults and arises in the extremities and craniofacial region as well as the retroperitoneum, where it accounts for 19% of malignancies. Malignant peripheral nerve tumours (Swannomas) are very rare and comprise only 5% of retroperitoneal malignancies.

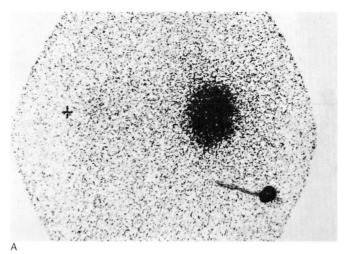

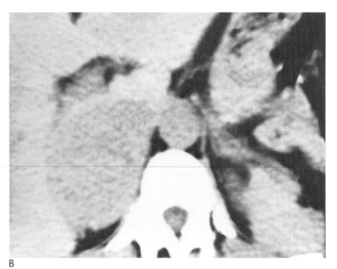

Fig. 27.46 (A) Scintiscan using mIBG shows large right phaeochromocytoma (12th rib marked). (B) CT of same patient confirms a large phaeochromocytoma (7 cm) (L45, W512). The tumour was also shown by ultrasound (Fig. 27.39).

Benign retroperitoneal tumours are seen less frequently than malignant lesions. They include lipomas, neurofibromas, Swannomas, teratomas and lymphangiomas.

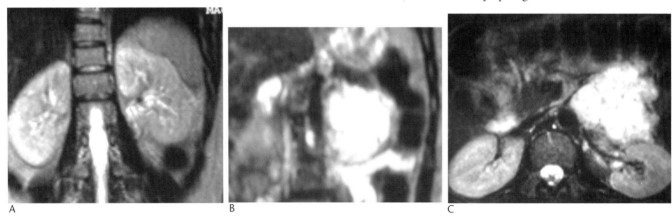

Fig. 27.47 MR T_2-weighted (A,B) coronal sections through kidneys and anterior to kidneys; (C) axial section. High-signal highly vascular tumour mass lying anterior to the hilum of the left kidney. Large drainage veins seen in (B) phaeochromocytoma. (Courtesy of Dr Philip Gishan.)

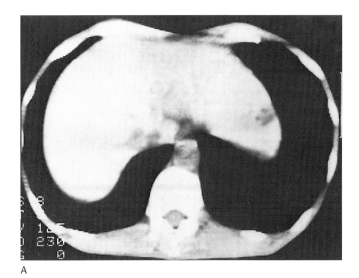

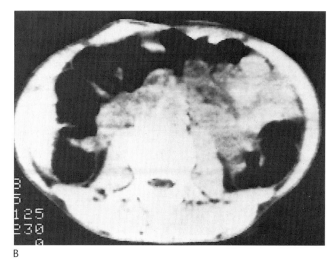

A

B

Fig. 27.48 (A) Deposits in liver (L36, W128). (B) Glandular masses around the aorta (L36, W256). The patient had a malignant phaeochromocytoma removed 6 months previously.

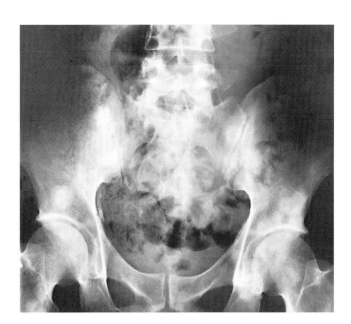

Fig. 27.49 Sclerotic bone deposits in same patient as Fig. 27.48.

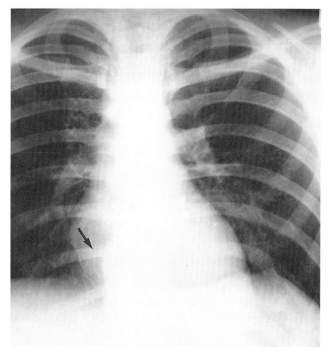

Fig. 27.50 Intrathoracic paravertebral tumour in a 12-year-old boy shown to right of lower spine (arrow). Further intra-abdominal tumours were shown. There was a familial history. (Courtesy of Dr F. Starer.)

REFERENCES AND SUGGESTIONS FOR FURTHER READING

Ackery, D. M., et al (1984) New approach to the localization of phaeochromocytoma: imaging with iodine-131-metaiodobenzylguanidine. *BMJ*, **288**, 1587–1591.

Adams, J. E., et al (1983) Computed tomography in adrenal disease. *Clinical Radiology*, **34**, 39–49.

Bernardino, M. E., Walther, M. M., Philips, V. M., et al (1985) CT guided adrenal biopsy. *American Journal of Roentgenology*, **144**, 67–69.

Birchall, D., Carney, A. S., Morse, M. H. (1995) Case report: ruptured adrenal artery aneurysm. *Clinical Radiology*, **50**, 732–733.

Doppman, J. L. (1993) Dilemmas of bilateral adrenocortical nodularity in Conn's and Cushing's syndromes. *Radiologic Clinics of North America*, **31:5**, 1039–1050.

Doppman, J. L., Oldfield, E., Krudy, A. G., et al (1984) Petrosal sinus sampling for Cushing syndrome: anatomical and technical considerations. *Radiology*, **150**, 99–103.

Dunnick, N. R., Heaston, D., Halvorsen, R., Moore, A. V., Karobkin, M. (1982) CT appearance of adrenal cortical carcinoma. *Journal of Computer Assisted Tomography*, **6**, 978–982.

Elaine, M. Casili, Korobkin, M., Francis, I. R., Cohen, R. H. (2002) Adrenal Masses: Characterization with Combined Unenhanced and Delayed Enhanced CT. *Radiology* **222**: 629–633.

Engelken, J. D., Ros, P. R. (1997) Retroperitoneal MR imaging. *Magnetic Resonance Imaging Clinics of North America*, **5**, 165–178.

Felson, B. (ed.) (1988) The adrenals. *Seminars in Roentgenology*, **23(4)**.

Fishman, E. K., Deatch, B. M., Hartman, D. S., et al (1987) Primary adrenocortical carcinoma. CT evaluation. *American Journal of Roentgenology*, **148**, 531–535.

Glazer, H. S., Weymen, P. J., Segel, S. S., Levitt, R. G., McClennan, B. L. (1982) Non-functioning adrenal masses: incidental discovery on computed tomography. *American Journal of Roentgenology*, **139**, 81–85.

Gross, M. D., Shapiro, B., Shreve, P. (1999) Radionuclide imaging of the adrenal cortex. *Quarterly Journal of Nuclear Medicine*, **43**, 224–232.

Hattner, R. S. (1993) Practical considerations in the scintigraphic evaluation of adrenal hypertension. *Radiologic Clinics of North America*, **31:5**, 1029–1038.

Huebener, K. H., Treugut, H. (1984) Adrenal cortex dysfunction. CT findings. *Radiology*, **150**, 195–199.

Husband, J., Resnik, R. (1998) *Imaging in Oncology*. Oxford: Isis.

Ichikawa, T., Ohtomo, K, Araki, T., et al (1996) Ganglineuroma, CT and MRI features. *British Journal of Radiology*, **69**, 114–121.

Ichikawa, T., Ohtomo, G., Uchiyama, H., et al (1995) Contrast-enhanced dynamic MRI of adrenal masses. *Clinical Radiology*, **50**, 295–300.

Ishikawa, H., et al. (1981) Myelolipoma of the adrenal gland. *Journal of Urology*, **126**, 777–779.

Kearney, G. P., Mahoney, E. M. (1977) Adrenal cysts. *Urologic Clinics of North America*, **4**, 305–318.

Kim, T., Murakam, T., Oi, H., et al (1996) CT and MR imaging of abdominal liposarcoma. *American Journal of Roentgenology*, **166**, 829–833.

Koh, D. M., Moskovic, E. (2000) Imaging retroperitoneal tumours. *Imaging*, **12**, 49–60.

Kornblatt, A. A., Salomon, P. (1990) ACTH induced adrenal haemorrhage. *Journal of Clinical Gastroenterology*, **12**, 371–377.

Korobkin, M., Brodeur, F. J., Yutzy, G. G., et al (1996) Differentiation of adrenal adenomas from nonadenomas using CT attenuation values. *American Journal of Roentgenology*, **166**, 531–536.

Liang, H. L., Pan, H. B., Lee, Y. H., Huang, J. S., Wu, T. D. L., Chang, C. T., Yang, C. F. (1999) Small functional Adrenal Cortical Adenoma: Treatment with CT guided Percutaneous Acetic Acid Injection. Report of Three Cases. *Radiology* **213**: 612–615.

Newhouse, J. H. (1991) Clinical use of urinary tract MRI. *Radiologic Clinics of North America*, **99**, 455–474.

Queloz, J. M., Capitanio, M. A., Kirkpatrick, I. A. (1972) Wolman's disease. Roentgen observations in three siblings. *Radiology*, **104**, 357–359.

Sisson, J. C., Shulkin, B. L. (1999) Nuclear medicine imaging of phaeochromocytoma and neuroblastoma. *Quarterly Journal of Nuclear Medicine*, **43**, 217–223.

Sohaib, S. A., Peppercorn, P. D., Allan, C., Monson, J. P., Grossman, A. B., Besser, G. M. and Reznek R. H. (2000) Primary Hyperaldosteronism (Conn Syndrome): MR Imaging Findings. *Radiology* **204**: 527–531.

Sutton, D. (1968) Diagnosis of Conn's and other adrenal tumours by left adrenal phlebography. *Lancet*, **i**, 453–455.

Wong, K. W., Lee, I. P. O., Sun, W. H. (1996) Case report: rupture and growth of adrenal myelolipoma in two patients. *British Journal of Radiology*, **69**, 873–875.

28

THE PAEDIATRIC ABDOMEN

Karen E. Thomas and Catherine M. Owens

RADIOLOGICAL TECHNIQUES IN PAEDIATRIC ABDOMINAL IMAGING

Imaging plays a pivotal role in the diagnosis, and in some cases the management, of gastrointestinal disease in the paediatric population. Multiple imaging modalities are employed with a problem-orientated approach. Many of the conditions encountered, such as malrotation, pyloric stenosis, intussusception and neonatal gastrointestinal obstruction, are largely unique to childhood. These topics will be discussed in more detail than pathologies that the general radiologist can be expected to encounter in adult practice, such as inflammatory bowel disease. The most common paediatric abdominal masses are discussed, with differential diagnoses and appropriate imaging strategies.

As in all spheres of radiology, requests for imaging must balance the risks of an examination against the potential benefits to the patient. Radiation burden to the paediatric population is particularly important and all possible measures should be taken to ensure that this is as low as possible, while maintaining examinations of diagnostic quality. Any sedation or anaesthetic procedure carries a small complication rate, and adverse reactions to contrast media, although rare, do still occur. The provision of a child-friendly environment will help reduce any emotional trauma to children undergoing unfamiliar and occasionally uncomfortable procedures. Age-appropriate booklets explaining the investigation may help alleviate a child's anxiety. Dedicated paediatric radiography and support staff are invaluable. Neonates and infants are particularly vulnerable to physiological instability. Hypothermia and fluid shifts are a very real risk in neonates requiring incubator transport to the radiology department for contrast studies. Adequate warming devices in the fluoroscopy suite and careful attention to hydration are mandatory. Some children, such as those undergoing tube oesophagrams, may be clinically unstable. Appropriate resuscitation equipment should be readily available and medical support from the clinical team present. If it is necessary to move a critically ill child from the paediatric intensive care unit to the radiology department the use of a dedicated transport team will reduce the incidence of adverse transport-related events.

Plain films
Conventional radiographs of the abdomen (AXR) probably remain the most frequently performed radiological investigation in the infant or child with acute abdominal symptoms. Diagnostic yield is highest in the assessment of suspected bowel obstruction and perforation; however, in conditions with a lower yield or frequently inconclusive radiographic findings, such as appendicitis and intussusception, ultrasound is rapidly replacing the AXR as the first-line investigation.

In UK practice a supine AXR alone is usually performed, the use of the erect radiograph having been largely discontinued in the 1990s. If free air is suspected, an erect chest radiograph is the most sensitive investigation in the infant and child. This is clearly not possible in the neonatal intensive care unit and hence lateral shoot-through or decubitus abdominal radiographs are performed. Clinically unstable older children may also require horizontal-beam abdominal films. A lateral shoot-through film may be preferred to the decubitus method as it causes minimal disturbance to an unstable and often mechanically-ventilated patient, unlike the latter method, which requires lateral decubitus positioning of the patient for a period of at least 10 min prior to exposure.

The advent of digital radiography holds potential for significant radiation dose reduction, much of which is related to a lower retake rate. Current developments in direct radiography are expected to reduce the dose of individual exposures further.

Contrast studies
Barium remains the most frequently used contrast medium for gastrointestinal studies in children. It is inexpensive, safe if used appropriately, and provides high-quality images. It is, however, contraindicated in the immediate postoperative period, following recent rectal biopsy, or any other circumstance in which an intraperitoneal or mediastinal leak could occur. It should also be avoided in patients at high risk of aspiration (Fig. 28.1), although small amounts of barium can be cleared from the tracheobronchial tree with little harm. In neonates the choice of contrast agent should be considered carefully, and in general it is advisable to use water-soluble contrast agents rather than barium for both upper and lower gastrointestinal studies.

Low osmolar water-soluble contrast agents include *iohexol* (Omnipaque 240, 300) and *iopamidol* (Niopam 200, 300). They have little adverse effect if extravasated into the peritoneum or mediastinum, or aspirated into the respiratory tract. Practice varies according to personal preference and technical considerations of the available fluoroscopic equipment but such agents are generally used

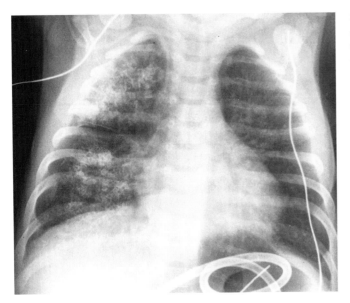

Fig. 28.1 Barium aspiration. CXR in a 2-month-old boy with congenital varicella and bulbar palsy demonstrating high-density opacities throughout the right lung secondary to aspiration during a barium meal examination performed at 2 days of age. Gastrostomy feeding was instituted.

undiluted or mildly diluted for a contrast meal and diluted approximately 1 in 2 for an enema. Earlier hyperosmolar water-soluble agents such as *meglumine/sodium* (Gastrografin) and *iothalamate meglumine* (Conray) were associated with considerable fluid shifts, drawing water into the bowel lumen with the risk of severe dehydration and haemodynamic compromise in infants. If aspirated, they may result in severe pulmonary oedema. The only remaining indication for Gastrograffin, used in dilution, is in the enema treatment of meconium ileus, as discussed later, when hyperosmolarity is beneficial.

For a *contrast meal* examination, barium or water-soluble contrast can be administered via a cup-and-straw, feeding bottle, or cautiously syringed directly into the mouth if necessary. Slightly enlarging the hole in a commercially available teat often enables a baby to swallow larger boluses and improves oesophageal distension. Using the patient's own bottle and teat may persuade a reluctant child to drink. Various flavourings are available for use in older children, but are not generally used in infants. If a nasogastric tube (8F feeding tube) has been placed in a neonate or child suspected of malrotation or high intestinal obstruction, contrast can be directly instilled into the stomach and allows greater control of contrast volume and bolus passage into the duodenal loop. The significance of gastro-oesophageal reflux occurring in the presence of a nasogastric tube should, however, be viewed with caution.

Children are generally fasted for 4 h prior to a contrast meal, or in infants, one feed is missed. A hungry child is more likely to drink barium, but if the period of fasting is too long it becomes difficult to obtain a successful examination on a fractious child. A parent should be encouraged to stay with the child during the procedure. The use of restraining devices is a matter of personal preference. They may be necessary if only remote-control fluoroscopic screening is available.

There are several differences between the paediatric contrast meal and that performed on adults; these reflect the different pathologies encountered in children. With the patient in a lateral position the swallowing mechanism and oesophageal outline and motility are assessed. A true lateral position is important in the detection of vascular impressions on the oesophagus. Turning the child to a prone right anterior oblique position, filling of the duodenal loop is observed and the patient promptly repositioned supine for documentation of the duodenojejunal junction (DJJ). The normal and abnormal positions of the DJJ are discussed later (p. 856). It is important to obtain a 'first-pass' view of the duodenal loop for confident evaluation of the DJJ. Supine views of the oesophagus can then be obtained and examination made for an hiatus hernia and gastro-oesophageal reflux. Formal reflux-eliciting manoeuvres are not necessary in paediatric practice. Reflux is most frequently observed in infants during passive relaxation and a soother may be helpful. Some practitioners gently 'jiggle' older children, others merely observe for a short period. Image-grab and pulse-fluoroscopy facilities should be used where available to reduce radiation dose.

Videofluoroscopy examination of the swallowing mechanism is performed in conjunction with a paediatric speech therapist. Various consistencies of liquid and semisolid food are tested to obtain a detailed functional study of the oral and pharyngeal phases of swallowing. A feeding plan for the patient can then be formulated.

Double-contrast barium meals can be performed in older, co-operative children and adolescents in whom there is a clinical suspicion of peptic ulcer disease. Preparation and technique are similar to adults.

The main indications for *water-soluble contrast enemas* are neonatal low gastrointestinal obstruction and suspected post-necrotising enterocolitis strictures. Occasionally a *barium enema* may be performed in an older infant or child with suspected Hirschsprung's disease or a contrast enema requested after colonic surgery. Colonoscopy has replaced the barium enema in inflammatory bowel disease, avoiding ionising radiation and allowing concurrent tissue biopsy.

In neonates, an 8F feeding tube or small Foley catheter is inserted into the rectum and taped securely to the buttocks. The catheter balloon is generally not inflated in UK practice and must not be used in cases where Hirschsprung's disease is suspected. A lateral view of the rectum and rectosigmoid junction is obtained on initial filling, with further views in the prone or supine position as the colon is opacified. Contrast may be injected manually by syringe or using gravity from a suspended source. If possible, an attempt should be made to reflux contrast into the distal ileum. However, hand injection should be cautious, as perforation of a microcolon is a well-documented risk. Paediatric enema tubes or larger Foley catheters (12–16F) are suitable for use in older children requiring enema examination.

The use of *air enemas* in intussusception reduction is now established practice. A large-bore catheter such as a 16–18F Foley catheter or similar is securely taped to the buttocks. In the UK catheter balloons are generally not inflated. Additional sealing of any potential air leak by manual compression is often helpful. Various devices, both commercially available and locally constructed, administer air at pressures of 80–120 mmHg. A pressure release valve is necessary to prevent excess pressure being delivered. An 18G needle must be accessible in the event of a tension pneumoperitoneum requiring decompression, and paediatric anaesthetic and surgical support must be available on site. Informed consent, including an explanation of complication and recurrence rates, should be obtained from the patient's parents or guardians. The procedure is discussed further on page 873.

Ultrasound

Ultrasound is the imaging modality of choice in much of paediatric radiology as it does not involve ionising radiation, is easily available, portable, rarely requires sedation and is well suited to the body habitus of children. It is now the first-line investigation in suspected pyloric stenosis, intussusception, appendicitis, abscesses and in the assessment of abdominal cystic and solid masses. It has an increasingly important role in inflammatory small- and large-bowel disease. The use of distraction devices, in particular video players above the examination couch, is remarkably effective in allowing a detailed examination of otherwise mobile children. A systematic examination of the abdominal and pelvic solid viscera is performed with a 4–7 MHz curvilinear or sector transducer, followed by examination of the bowel using a high-frequency (5–15 MHz) linear transducer. Colour flow studies and Doppler interrogation of major visceral and intraparenchymal vessels may be performed.

CT

Computed tomography is a widely available and powerful imaging modality providing high-resolution images with good tissue contrast. However, its high radiation burden must be considered and alternative non-ionising modalities used wherever possible. Ultrasound is widely available and should be the first-line abdominal cross-sectional imaging modality, except in cases of trauma. This is particularly the case in neonates, where ultrasound provides superior resolution such that the role of abdominal CT is limited. MRI can provide superior soft-tissue contrast and angiographic capabilities and should be used wherever possible, although limitations in availability restrict its use in many centres and there is a more frequent need for sedation and general anaesthesia.

Strategies to reduce the radiation dose associated with CT in children include lowering the mAs and increasing the pitch in spiral scanners. Tube currents of 60–120 mAs, depending on the age of the child, will provide high-quality images from infancy to adolescence. Pitch can be routinely increased to 1.5 and in some circumstances 2. The advent of multislice technology has enabled a considerable reduction in scanning time and is anticipated to significantly reduce the proportion of children requiring sedation or general anaesthesia for CT. However, the ability to scan larger areas with narrow collimation has raised concerns regarding the potential for radiation dose increases, of which both the radiologist and the clinician must be aware. CT technology is advancing rapidly and improved multiplanar reconstruction, surface display and rendering technology, angiographic capabilities and virtual endoscopy all hold exciting potential in paediatric imaging.

The most common uses of abdominal CT in children include diagnosis and follow-up of neoplasms, trauma, abscesses and the complications of inflammatory bowel disease. In most cases both intravenous and oral contrast are used.

MRI

Magnetic resonance imaging has many advantages in paediatric abdominal imaging. Of paramount importance, it does not involve ionising radiation and is therefore especially attractive in clinical circumstances in which serial examinations are necessary, such as tumour surveillance and follow-up. Its multiplanar imaging capability, superior tissue characterisation and the recent development of gadolinium-enhanced angiography (Fig. 28.2), MR cholangiopancreatography (MRCP) and MR urographic techniques promise an increasing role. Although scanning times are decreasing, the length

of examinations remains the major disadvantage in children, with most patients under 6–7 years requiring sedation or general anaesthesia. The abdomen and pelvis of an infant can usually be imaged well using a head coil. A body or torso coil is used in older children, reducing the field of view appropriately. Gadolinium-DTPA may be administered intravenously at a dose of 0.1 ml/kg for tissue enhancement and 0.1–0.3 ml/kg for angiography.

Radionuclide imaging

This technique can provide functional information in a variety of specific applications. The more commonly encountered investigations include Meckel's (^{99m}TcO$_4$), biliary (^{99m}Tc-HIDA), milk (^{99m}Tc-sulphur colloid), white cell (^{99m}Tc-labelled WBC), ^{131}I-MIBG and splenic (^{99m}Tc-RBC or ^{99m}Tc-sulphur colloid) scans.

THE NEONATAL GASTROINTESTINAL TRACT

Gastrointestinal obstruction

Neonatal obstruction may be due to a multitude of disorders affecting the gastrointestinal tract anywhere from the oesophagus to the anus. Clinical presentation varies with the level of obstruction, and may include inability to feed, vomiting, abdominal distension, failure to pass meconium within the first few days of life, or a visible abnormality such as an imperforate anus. Although the presence of vomiting early in the clinical course favours a high obstruction, and abdominal distension and failure to pass meconium a low obstruction, the clinical findings may not accurately predict the level of obstruction and radiological investigation is necessary.

The multiple causes of neonatal intestinal obstruction are given in Box 28.1. The more common conditions are described below.

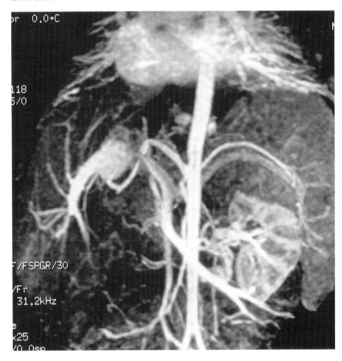

Fig. 28.2 Gadolinium-enhanced 3D MR angiogram in a 6-year-old girl following liver transplantation demonstrating stenosis of the portal venous anastomosis with poststenotic dilatation.

Box 28.1   Causes of neonatal gastrointestinal obstruction

Oesophagus
    Oesophageal atresia ± tracheo-oesophageal fistula
    Congential oesophageal stenosis, web and diverticula
    Extrinsic compression—vascular ring
                              —foregut duplication cyst
                              —neoplasm

Stomach (rare)
    Gastric atresia
    Antral web
    Duplication cyst
    Hypertrophic pyloric stenosis

Duodenum
    Duodenal atresia
    Duodenal web
    Malrotation with midgut volvulus
    Extrinsic compression—annular pancreas
                              —preduodenal portal vein

Small bowel
    Jejunal and ileal atresia/stenosis
    Meconium ileus ± meconium cyst, segmental volvulus
    Midgut volvulus
    Inguinal hernia
    Necrotising enterocolitis
    Duplication cyst

Large bowel
    Hirshsprung's disease
    Functional immaturity/hypoplastic left colon syndrome
    Colonic atresia/stenosis
    Anorectal atresia/imperforate anus
    Necrotising enterocolitis
    Duplication cyst

Oesophageal obstruction

Oesophageal atresia and tracheo-oesophageal fistula. The trachea and oesophagus arise from the common foregut. Anomalies in the separation of these two structures by the oesophagotracheal septum result in oesophageal atresia, with or without an associated tracheo-oesophageal fistula, with an incidence of 1 in 2–4000 live births. Diagnosis may be suspected on antenatal ultrasound if the gastric bubble is small or not visualised, or if a distended proximal oesophageal pouch is seen. Polyhydramnios is commonly associated. Postnatally, infants present with drooling, choking, coughing and episodes of cyanosis on feeding. When attempts to pass a nasogastric tube are made, resistance is met and a chest radiograph will show the tube coiled in a dilated air-filled proximal oesophageal pouch (Fig. 28.3).

There are five types of oesophageal atresia with or without a tracheo-oesophageal fistula. The commonest (>80%) is oesophageal atresia with a distal fistula, involving a blind-ending oesophageal pouch and a fistula between the trachea and the proximal portion of the distal oesophageal segment. Less common types are oesophageal atresia with a proximal fistula (1%), oesophageal atresia with both proximal and distal fistulas (2%), isolated oesophageal atresia (9%) and an H-type tracheo-oesophageal fistula (6%). Many infants manifest other features of the VATER (or VACTERL) association, with *V*ertebral segmentation and fusion anomalies, *A*norectal atresia, *T*racheo-o*e*sophageal fistulas, and *R*adial ray or *R*enal anomalies. Congenital heart disease, especially ventricular septal defect, patent ductus arteriosus and tetralogy of Fallot, may also be present. Isolated oesophageal atresia is associated with trisomy 21.

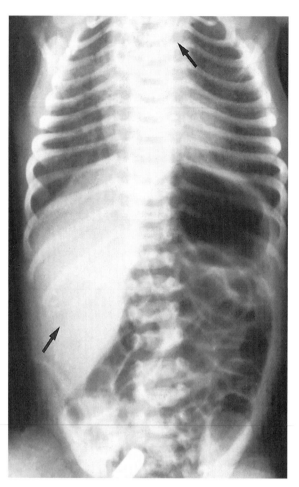

Fig. 28.3   Oesophageal atresia with tracheo-oesophageal fistula. A coiled nasogastric tube is seen in the dilated proximal oesophageal pouch (top arrow). The presence of distal air-filled bowel implies an associated tracheo-oesophageal fistula. Thirteen pairs of ribs are noted, compatible with VATER syndrome (lower arrow).

In the majority of cases, diagnosis is made on plain radiography and no further imaging is required. The presence of air-filled bowel in the abdomen indicates the presence of a tracheo-oesophageal fistula; a gasless abdomen implies an isolated oesophageal atresia. Vertebral segmentation and fusion anomalies or other features of the VATER syndrome may be seen. There is an association with hypersegmentation and 13 pairs of ribs. If a contrast study is requested, a small amount of water-soluble contrast may be instilled into the oesophageal pouch with caution, in view of the risk of aspiration.

Primary surgical anastomosis is usually possible. Following repair, patients frequently demonstrate abnormal lower oesophageal motility with a poor stripping wave. Gastro-oesophageal reflux and hiatus hernias are relatively common. Anastomotic strictures may develop. Chronic distension of the proximal pouch with pressure on the adjacent trachea in utero is believed to be responsible for the focal tracheomalacia commonly associated with oesophageal atresia. This is variable in severity but can be a cause of persistent respiratory compromise after oesophageal repair.

H-type fistulas generally present later in infancy or childhood with episodes of choking or apnoeas during feeding or recurrent lower respiratory tract infections. If suspected clinically, a 'tube oesophagram' should be performed. A nasogastric tube is passed and water-soluble contrast instilled while the tube is slowly withdrawn

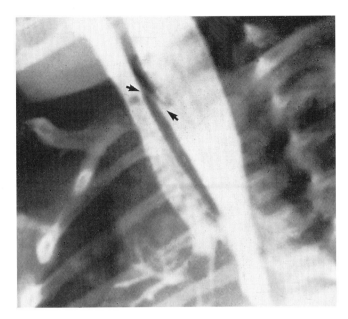

Fig. 28.4 Contrast oesophagram demonstrating oblique track (arrows) of a tracheo-oesophageal fistula with contrast filling the tracheobronchial tree.

up the oesophagus. Most fistulas involve the proximal third of the oesophagus and care should be taken to distend this segment well in order to maximise visualisation of a fistula which passes anteriorly and superiorly between the oesophagus and the trachea, in more of an 'N' than an 'H' configuration (Fig. 28.4). The examination is traditionally performed with the patient prone and utilising horizontal beam fluoroscopy. However, the difficulties of monitoring an infant, often with unstable respiratory status and liable to apnoeic attacks, strapped across the footplate of a fluoroscopy table have led some radiologists to use the lateral position, suggesting that the most important aspect of a successful examination is probably optimal distension of the oesophagus rather than the prone position per se. If C-arm fluoroscopy is available the problems of patient inaccessibility are much reduced.

Congenital oesophageal stenosis, webs and diverticula are rare causes of neonatal oesophageal obstruction. Stenoses are due to persistent tracheobronchial cartilage remnants within the oesophageal wall as a result of abnormal tracheo-oesophageal separation.

Extrinsic compression by vascular rings, foregut duplication cysts and neoplasms results in oesophageal filling defects on contrast studies. They may be an incidental finding or cause stridor and swallowing difficulties. Posterior oesophageal impressions are most commonly due to an aberrant right subclavian artery with left aortic arch, an anomaly rarely requiring treatment. The differential includes a right aortic arch with aberrant left subclavian artery and a double aortic arch. The combination of an anterior oesophageal and posterior tracheal impression with a rounded soft-tissue mass seen between these two structures on lateral chest radiograph is due to a pulmonary sling, with an aberrant left pulmonary artery arising from the right pulmonary artery and passing to the left, posterior to the trachea. The tracheobronchial tree is often abnormal with a low, horizontal carina ('inverted T') and segmental tracheomalacia or tracheal stenosis. MRI and CT are useful in further defining anomalous vascular anatomy (Fig. 28.5).

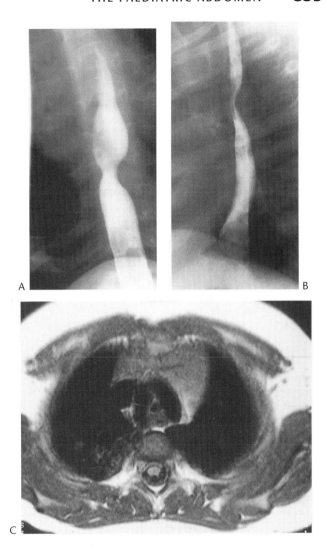

Fig. 28.5 Double aortic arch. AP barium swallow (A) demonstrating bilateral smooth extrinsic filling defects with a posterior oesophageal impression on lateral image (B). Axial T_1-weighted MRI (C) confirming double aortic arch.

Gastric obstruction

Congenital obstruction of the stomach is rare. **Microgastria** may occur alone or associated with other anomalies, especially asplenia. A small tubular stomach and dilated oesophagus are seen on contrast meal. **Antral webs** and **gastric duplication cysts** may present in the neonatal period or later in childhood. **Gastric atresia**, with complete interruption of the gastrointestinal tract at the antrum, is very rare.

Hypertrophic pyloric stenosis (HPS) is an acquired hypertrophy of the circular muscle of the pylorus, causing progressive gastric outlet obstruction. The aetiology remains largely unknown, although abnormal innervation to the circular muscle has been implicated. Peak incidence is between 2 and 8 weeks of age, although cases in infants as young as 7 days are encountered. Premature infants present at an appropriate interval after birth. There is a greater incidence in males (4:1 ratio), in Caucasians, and in those with a family history.

Clinically, infants present with increasing non-bilious vomiting, becoming projectile and leading to dehydration and a hypo-

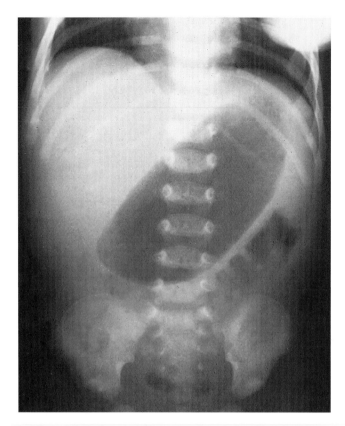

Fig. 28.6 Pyloric stenosis. AXR showing distended gastric air bubble.

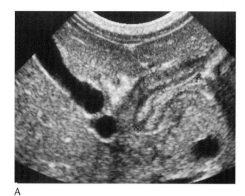

A

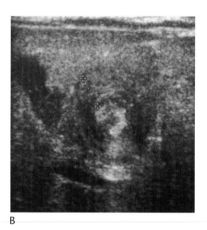

B

Fig. 28.7 Pyloric stenosis. Longitudinal US image (A) showing an elongated thickened pylorus, muscle length 17 mm and width 3.8 mm. Transverse image (B) in another patient with muscle width 6 mm. No transit of gastric contents into the duodenum was observed.

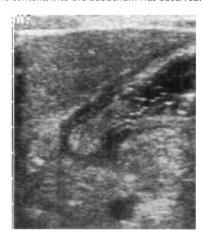

Fig. 28.8 Normal pylorus. Longitudinal US section demonstrating an open pyloric canal with transit of gastric contents observed on dynamic imaging. Wall thickness approximately 2 mm.

chloraemic alkalosis. The pylorus may be palpable as an 'olive' clinically. An abdominal radiograph shows a distended air-filled stomach with a relative paucity of bowel gas distally (Fig. 28.6).

Ultrasound has now replaced the barium meal as the first-line investigation in the infant with non-bilious vomiting in whom HPS is the most likely diagnosis. It is a safe, non-ionising investigation which, with experience, is both highly sensitive and specific. The infant is positioned in the left anterior oblique position and scanned over the right upper quadrant with a linear (>5 MHz) transducer. The gastric antrum will be fluid-filled (unless a nasogastric tube has been placed) and hyperdynamic peristaltic waves may be seen. The enlarged pylorus should be imaged in longitudinal and transverse sections. The hypertrophied muscle layer is hypoechoic to the adjacent liver, with a double line of hyperechoic mucosa seen centrally (Fig. 28.7). Measurements of the muscle width and pyloric canal length are obtained from the longitudinal section. Although over-reliance on measurement criteria should be avoided, a muscle width measurement of > 3.5 mm and a pyloric length of > 16 mm in a term infant are usually taken as diagnostic of HPS. Gastric outlet function should be observed; a hyperperistaltic antrum and the absence of gastric contents passing into the duodenum are important signs. The measurements in preterm infants may be smaller than those given above. Overdistension of the stomach can result in posterior displacement of the pylorus and difficulties in visualisation. The placement of a nasogastric tube to empty the stomach is helpful in these cases.

The normal pylorus has a muscle width of 2 mm or less (Fig. 28.8) and can be difficult to visualise directly. Intermediate measurements of 2–3 mm can be seen in pylorospasm. However, continued observation of the pylorus will usually reveal opening with the passage of gastric contents into the duodenum. The differential is early HPS and, in cases of persistent clinical suspicion, repeat scanning should be performed after a day or two.

A barium meal may be performed if ultrasound findings are equivocal, in centres with more limited ultrasound experience, or in circumstances in which the differential diagnosis is wider. Gastric emptying is markedly delayed, with eventual passage of barium into the elongated, curved pyloric canal (Fig. 28.9). The soft-tissue

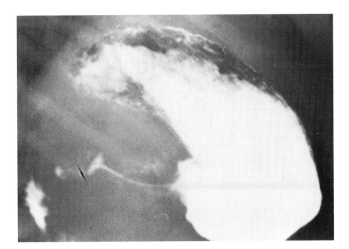

Fig. 28.9 Pyloric stenosis. Barium meal showing an elongated pyloric canal and shouldering of the antrum due to the hypertrophied pyloric muscle.

mass of hypertrophied muscle indents the antrum and the duodenal bulb (shouldering), hyperdynamic peristalsis in the antrum results in the 'pyloric tit' and a 'double-track' appearance of the pyloric canal may be seen.

Treatment is Ramstedt's pyloromyotomy following correction of any electrolyte abnormalities. Incision of the hypertrophied muscle is performed almost to the level of the mucosa. The operation has a very high success rate, but if inadequate myotomy is suspected, a barium meal examining for delayed gastric emptying is the investigation of choice, as the morphological appearances of the pylorus on ultrasound and barium studies can remain unchanged from preoperative findings for many weeks.

Duodenal obstruction

Duodenal atresia, stenosis and **webs** result from incomplete recanalisation of the duodeneum during gestational development. Atresia is commoner than stenosis or webs. Obstruction usually occurs just below the ampulla of Vater, and is not infrequently associated with anomalies of the pancreas (annular pancreas), common bile duct or a preduodenal portal vein. These may contribute towards duodenal obstruction but are rarely solely responsible. Associations include trisomy 21 (25–30% cases) and the VATER syndrome.

Abdominal radiographs demonstrate the classic 'double-bubble' sign of duodenal atresia with an absence of distal air (Fig. 28.10). If, however, a small amount of air has passed distally, the differential is wider, including duodenal stenosis and webs, duodenal atresia associated with an anomalous bifid common bile duct inserted both above and below the atresia, and, most importantly, malrotation with midgut volvulus. Neonates with partial or complete duodenal obstruction usually undergo surgery without further imaging as all possible causes require surgical treatment. However, if a delay is anticipated prior to operation, then a contrast meal may be performed in infants with distal air to exclude a midgut volvulus, which would necessitate urgent surgical intervention.

Contrast meal shows complete obstruction in cases of duodenal atresia and partial obstruction with narrowing of the second part of the duodenum in duodenal stenosis. In the neonatal period, webs are visualised as curvilinear duodenal filling defects; the wind-sock appearance often described is not usually seen until later in childhood (Fig. 28.11). After successful duodenoduodenostomy the duodenal bulb can remain dilated on contrast studies for several years.

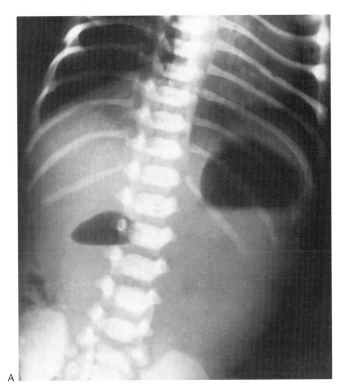

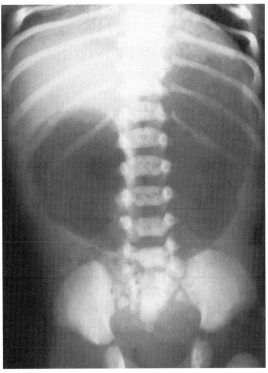

Fig. 28.10 Duodenal atresia. Erect (A) and supine (B) AXR demonstrating the 'double-bubble' sign.

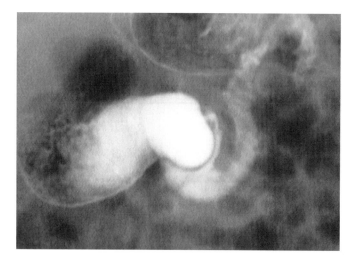

Fig. 28.11 Duodenal web. Barium meal demonstrating a curvilinear filling defect or 'wind-sock diverticulum' in the second part of the duodenum with proximal dilatation.

Malrotation and midgut volvulus is one of the major paediatric surgical emergencies and the role of radiology in its diagnosis critical. Delay in diagnosis can result in infarctive necrosis of the entire small bowel and is potentially fatal. Radiological understanding requires knowledge of the embryological development of the gastrointestinal tract. At approximately week 6 of gestation the duodenojejunal and ileocolic segments of the primitive gut herniate into the extraembryonic coelom in the umbilical cord. Both loops elongate and rotate 270° anticlockwise around the axis of the superior mesenteric artery. By the end of the third month of gestation the bowel loops are returned to their final positions in the abdominal cavity, with their mesenteries becoming fixed to the parietal peritoneum at several sites. The duodenal loop is fixed with the duodenojejunal junction (DJJ) in the left upper quadrant at the ligament of Treitz and the ileocaecal junction fixed in the right lower quadrant. The normal small bowel mesentery therefore has a broad diagonal base across the abdomen.

Any arrest in the normal 270° anticlockwise rotation occurring during physiological umbilical herniation results in malrotation and malfixation of the small bowel. The DJJ will be displaced medially and inferiorly and/or the caecum will be displaced medially and superiorly. The length of the small bowel mesentery is consequently shortened and the risk of the entire small bowel twisting on its narrow pedicle is increased. Midgut volvulus leads to small-bowel obstruction, occlusion of the superior mesenteric vessels, ischaemia and, if not recognised, complete small bowel infarction. Abnormal peritoneal bands passing from the caecum to cross the duodenum (Ladd's bands) are often present in malrotated patients. They may contribute towards partial duodenal obstruction but are rarely the sole cause.

The classic presentation of malrotation is of bilious vomiting within the first year of life, usually within the first month, but symptoms may present at any age and the diagnosis should always be considered. In older children, intermittent obstruction can occur, with chronic or recurrent abdominal pain and vomiting. Occasionally, a malabsorption syndrome results from chronic venous and lymphatic obstruction.

Abdominal radiographic findings are variable. Some cases demonstrate partial duodenal obstruction (Fig. 28.12). Occasionally duodenal obstruction is complete. Generalised dilatation of small-

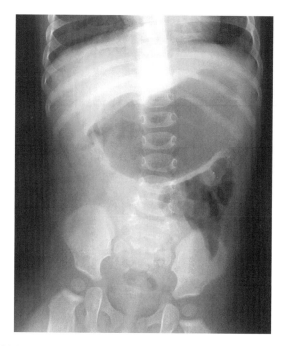

Fig. 28.12 Malrotation and volvulus. AXR in a 12-month-old boy with bilious vomiting. The stomach is distended with a relative paucity of gas distally.

bowel loops, if due to malrotation and volvulus, is generally a late sign and suspicious for small-bowel ischaemia. In many cases there is no appreciable radiographic abnormality and therefore abdominal radiography cannot exclude the diagnosis.

Clinically unstable children with signs of an acute abdomen, in whom bowel viability may be further compromised by any delay waiting for imaging, should undergo urgent surgery. A contrast meal is performed in all other cases. Views of the first pass of contrast through the duodenal loop are obtained in the right prone oblique position and then the child quickly turned to the supine position. The location of the DJJ on the supine image is the most critical element in the diagnosis of malrotation and care must be taken to ensure correct patient positioning without any degree of rotation. The stomach should not be overfilled as this can obscure the position of the DJJ. The normal DJJ lies to the left of the midline (at least over the vertebral pedicle) at the level of the pylorus. In malrotation, it is displaced medially, inferiorly or both (Fig. 28.13). The proximal jejunal loops may lie abnormally to the right. The presence of a volvulus may be indicated by partial duodenal obstruction with a dilated proximal duodenum, by the classic 'corkscrew' appearance of the duodenum and proximal jejunum twisting around its mesenteric axis or by complete obstruction of the third part of the duodenum (Fig. 28.14). However, the presence of a volvulus may not always be identified on contrast studies and malposition of the DJJ may be the only radiological abnormality. Generalised bowel distension from a variety of causes can cause mild displacement of the apparent DJJ and a false-positive diagnosis of malrotation, a phenomenon of which both radiologists and surgeons should be aware (Fig. 28.15).

Contrast enemas are less frequently performed in the investigation of potential malrotation than in the past. The caecum can be quite mobile, particularly in neonates, and its position on fluoroscopy may not accurately reflect the true site of fixation. Malrotation and volvulus have been described in children with

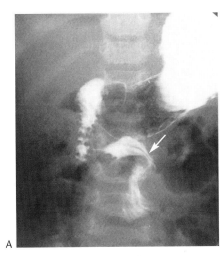
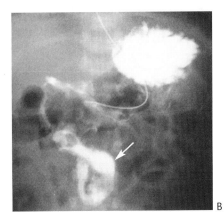

Fig. 28.13 Malrotation. Contrast meal (A) demonstrating abnormally low position of the duodenojejunal junction (DJJ) (arrow). Further case (B) demonstrating both inferior and medial displacement of the DJJ (arrow). The normal DJJ should lie to the left of the midline (over or lateral to the left vertebral pedicle) at the level of the pylorus.

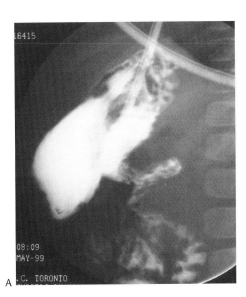
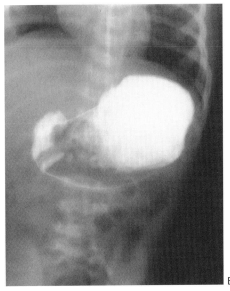

Fig. 28.14 Midgut volvulus presenting as a classic 'corkscrew' appearance of the duodenum and proximal jejunum on lateral view (A) and in a further case as complete duodenal obstruction (B). The linear filling defect is likely to represent the superior mesenteric vessels and associated mesentery.

normal caecal position but an abnormal DJJ; a normal enema cannot therefore exclude the diagnosis. However, defining the position of the caecum can sometimes be useful in providing further information in cases with equivocal or subtle findings on barium meal. The length of the small-bowel mesentery between the caecum and the DJJ, the critical factor in determining the risk of volvulus, can then be determined. A high caecum, particularly if directed medially, supports the diagnosis (Fig. 28.16).

There has been recent interest in the role of ultrasound. Approximately 70% of malrotated patients demonstrate inversion of the normal relationship of the superior mesenteric artery and vein, with the vein lying in an abnormal position anterior and to the left of the artery (Fig 28.17); however, sensitivity and specificity of this reversal sign are not sufficient to enable its use as a screening examination. Ultrasound appearances may be normal in surgically-proven malrotation, and, conversely, an abnormal relationship has been demonstrated in normal children. A more specific sign is the

'whirlpool' sign of midgut volvulus (Fig. 28.18), the ultrasound equivalent of the 'corkscrew' sign on contrast study. Twisting of the superior mesenteric vein and mesentery around the artery is a very specific sign and highly predictive of volvulus but sensitivity is lower. At present the contrast meal remains the first-line investigation of choice, and the role of ultrasound ancillary.

Chronic volvulus is a rare but recognised entity presenting in older children. Large distended mesenteric veins can be identified on ultrasound (Fig. 28.19) or CT and barium meal will confirm malrotation.

The surgical management of malrotation is the Ladd's procedure. Any volvulus is reduced and peritoneal bands are divided. The small bowel is returned to the right side of the abdomen and the large bowel to the left. Subsequent development of adhesions makes recurrent volvulus rare.

Children with congenital abnormalities of the abdominal wall (exomphalos, gastroschisis and diaphragmatic hernia) have some

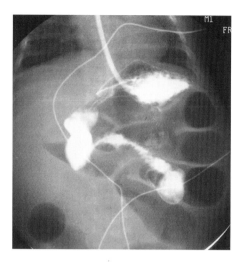

Fig. 28.15 Contrast meal showing mild inferior displacement of the duo-denojejunal junction (DJJ) in the presence of multiple dilated loops of bowel. In this case the cause of obstruction was an undiagnosed inguinal hernia. A repeat contrast meal after surgery showed a normal DJJ location.

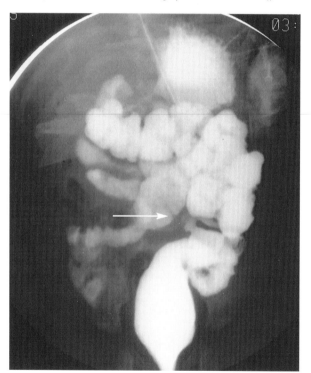

Fig. 28.16 Follow-through examination demonstrating an abnormal high and medial caecal position (arrow). Malrotation confirmed at surgery.

degree of malrotation but rarely develop clinical symptoms. There is more controversy regarding malrotation associated with visceral heterotaxy syndromes, which may require surgical intervention.

Non-rotation is an anomaly due to 90° anticlockwise rotation of the primitive midgut loop instead of the normal 270° anticlockwise movement. The duodenal loop and the entire small bowel lie on the right of the midline and the entire colon on the left. Often an incidental finding in adults, it is rarely associated with significant symptoms.

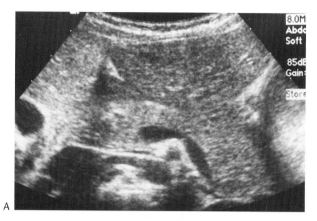

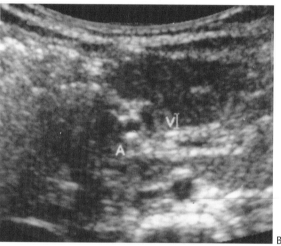

Fig. 28.17 Transverse ultrasound images of the normal superior mesenteric artery:vein relationship (A) and a malrotated child (B) in whom the SMV lies to the left of the SMA.

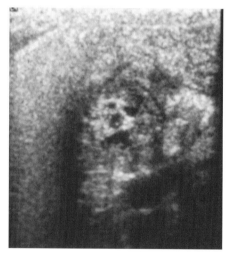

Fig. 28.18 Ultrasound 'whirlpool' sign of midgut volvulus. Twisting mesenteric vessels with concentric rings of echogenic mesentery.

High intestinal obstruction

Atresias or stenoses of the jejunum or proximal ileum present with bilious vomiting in the newborn in association with a small number of dilated bowel loops, often a 'triple bubble', on abdomi-

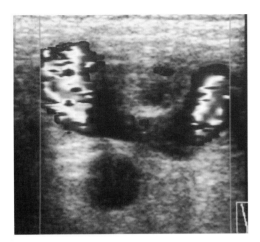

Fig. 28.19 Chronic volvulus. Doppler ultrasound showing large dilated mesenteric veins in an 8-year-old girl with a long history of intermittent abdominal pain. Barium meal confirmed malrotation, and chronic volvulus was found at laparotomy.

nal radiograph. In contrast to duodenal atresia/stenosis, they are the result of in utero vascular insults rather than failure of recanalisation. Complete atresias are more common than stenoses, and may be single or multiple. V-shaped mesenteric defects are found at surgery.

Most infants require no further imaging prior to surgery. If requested, a contrast follow-through will localise the site of obstruction. Colonic appearances depend on the gestational timing of the ischaemic injury and the level of the obstruction. The calibre of the colon is often normal or only mildly reduced in late, high (jejunal) atresias, as sufficient succus entericus is produced to stimulate near-normal colonic development. The presence of a microcolon should raise the suspicion of an earlier, more distal (ileal) atresia or the presence of further ileal atresias in addition to a proximal lesion.

Other causes of neonatal small bowel obstruction include **inguinal hernias**, **necrotising enterocolitis** and **duplication cysts** which are discussed later.

Low intestinal obstruction

Low neonatal intestinal obstruction presenting with failure to pass meconium within the first 48 h of life and multiple loops of dilated bowel on abdominal radiograph is due to one of several pathologies within the distal ileum or colon. The radiological differential diagnosis is between five conditions: meconium ileus, ileal atresia, Hirschsprung's disease, functional immaturity of the colon and, rarely, colonic atresia. Anorectal anomalies present similarly but can be diagnosed clinically. Sepsis and electrolyte abnormalities may cause a paralytic ileus that can be confused but the clinical history should be helpful. It is difficult to distinguish between dilated small and large bowel in the neonate with multiple dilated loops on abdominal radiograph (Fig. 28.20). The next investigation is a contrast enema.

Water-soluble contrast is used in preference to barium. It has a therapeutic benefit in meconium ileus and functional immaturity. Second, if perforation has occured in utero or does so during the procedure, the consequences are less severe than barium peritonitis. The aim of the study is primarily to identify the presence or

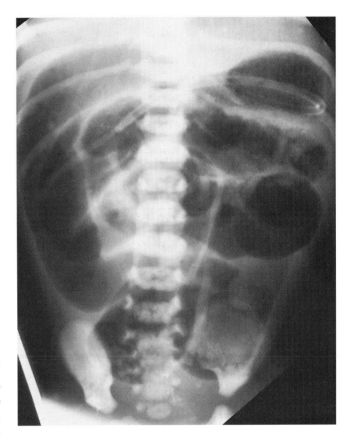

Fig. 28.20 Neonatal low gastrointestinal obstruction. Multiple loops of distended air-filled bowel.

absence of a microcolon. A microcolon implies that insufficient succus entericus has reached the colon as a result of a high-grade distal ileal obstruction. The presence of such an 'unused' colon limits the differential to meconium ileus and distal ileal atresia.

Meconium ileus is due to inspissated pellets of abnormally viscid meconium within the distal ileum and colon. Almost all cases are associated with cystic fibrosis. Conversely, 20% of children with cystic fibrosis present in this manner. It may be complicated by antenatal perforation resulting in a pseudocyst, or postnatally causing a pneumoperitoneum. Closed loop segmental volvulus may also occur perinatally.

A mottled bubbly appearance due to meconium mixed with air may be seen in the right iliac fossa on abdominal radiograph (Fig. 28.21). There may be greater dilatation of one bowel loop than of the remainder, which, in this case, represents the terminal ileum. A similar appearance is seen in ileal and colonic atresia, but the absence of fluid levels on a horizontal beam radiograph favours meconium ileus. Calcification within the wall of a pseudocyst or scattered over the peritoneum can be seen following in utero perforation, but is not specific to meconium ileus. Peritoneal calcification is more commonly associated with in utero perforation due to atresias.

Contrast enema will demonstrate a microcolon and filling of a dilated terminal ileum packed with inspissated pellets of meconium (Fig. 28.22). Non-operative treatment involves the use of hypertonic enemas to soften the impacted meconium and induce its passage. Practice varies with institution; there is no clear consensus as to the optimal composition and dilution of contrast agent, the frequency of enemas and the point at which medical management is

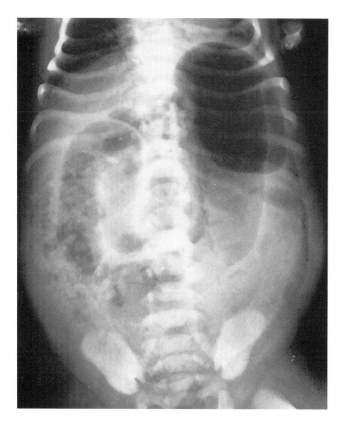

Fig. 28.21 Meconium ileus. AXR showing loops of dilated bowel with a 'bubbly' appearance of meconium mixed with air in the right side of the abdomen. Free air is seen, indicating a perforation.

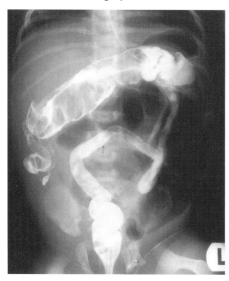

Fig. 28.22 Meconium ileus. Contrast enema demonstrating a microcolon with reflux into dilated distal ileum. Multiple filling defects of inspissated meconium are seen within the distal ileum (superimposed over the transverse colon) and the colon.

abandoned in favour of surgical intervention. In view of the risks of circulatory collapse with hyperosmolar Gastrografin, a dilute solution should be used and care should be taken to ensure adequate hydration of the baby prior to and during the procedure. Alternatively, many paediatric radiologists use low osmolar nonionic contrast media, sometimes with additional wetting agents.

Serial enemas can be performed daily provided there is evidence of some clinical improvement. It may be possible to reflux contrast further into the small bowel with successive enemas enhancing the therapeutic effect, but this should be done with caution in view of the risk of perforation. Radiological treatment is successful in approximately 60% of uncomplicated cases. Surgical intervention is required for complicated cases or if there is no significant clinical improvement after several enema attempts. Direct irrigation is performed and the appendix can be sutured to the skin to provide an irrigation channel postoperatively.

Ileal atresias are the result of in utero vascular insults. Abdominal radiographs demonstrate multiple dilated loops, sometimes with greater dilatation of one loop but, unlike meconium ileus, multiple fluid levels are common. Contrast enema will show an unused microcolon. If contrast can be refluxed into the distal ileum it will fill a non-dilated blind-ending segment (Fig. 28.23) with a persistent dilated air-filled loop seen proximally. Meconium pellets are common but fewer in number than in meconium ileus. Treatment is initial ileostomy followed by resection of the atretic segment(s) and reanastomosis.

Hirschsprung's disease is due to arrest in the normal cranial-to-caudal neural cell migration, resulting in absence of ganglion cells within the myenteric plexus of the bowel wall; 70% of cases involve the rectosigmoid region (short segment), 25% extend to the splenic flexure or transverse colon (long segment) and 5% involve the entire colon (total colonic Hirschsprung's disease). The majority of children present with failure to pass meconium within the first 48 h of life. A smaller number present with intractable constipation later in childhood and occasionally into adulthood. Enterocolitis occurs in 15% of patients and can be the initial presentation, with fever and diarrhoea. There is a male predominance (4:1) in rectosigmoid cases but an equal sex distribution in total colonic disease. Associations include trisomy 21 and neuroblastoma. Presentation in preterm infants is almost unknown.

When performing a contrast enema for potential Hirschsprung's disease, it is important to obtain a lateral rectal view during early filling. A small catheter (8–10F) is placed just inside the anus. If a Foley catheter is used the balloon should not be inflated as it may

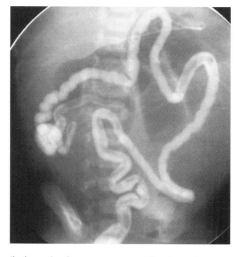

Fig. 28.23 Ileal atresia. Contrast enema with microcolon and reflux into a non-dilated distal ileal segment with abrupt convex termination. A few meconium plugs are present.

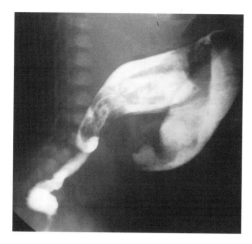

Fig. 28.24 Hirschsprung's disease. An abrupt transition zone is seen at the rectosigmoid junction on this lateral rectal view from a contrast enema performed on a 2-day-old boy with failure to pass meconium. The rectum was difficult to distend well and showed irregular contractions.

distort the rectal appearances. The normal neonatal rectum is of greater calibre than the sigmoid colon. Inversion of the rectosigmoid index, often in association with irregular contractions of the aganglionic rectum and difficulty in obtaining good rectal distension, is indicative of Hirschsprung's disease (Fig. 28.24). A discrete zone of transition with a change in calibre of the bowel is more often seen in older infants and children than in the neonatal period. Total colonic Hirschsprung's disease is particularly difficult to diagnose radiologically. Findings are subtle but the entire colon tends to be slightly short and rather featureless, with the hepatic and splenic flexures lying more medially than normal. Finally, the contrast enema may appear normal in neonatal Hirschsprung's disease and the definitive diagnostic investigation remains the rectal biopsy. Treatment involves defunctioning colostomy followed by surgical repair with the Soave, Duhamel or Swenson techniques.

Functional immaturity of the colon is known by a variety of names, including the small left colon syndrome, meconium plug syndrome and functional colonic obstruction. It is believed to be due to a relative immaturity of bowel innervation and motility in full-term infants. There is an increased incidence in infants of diabetic mothers. Contrast enema shows a dilated ascending and transverse colon with a change in calibre at the splenic flexure and a small left, descending colon. A large mucous plug may be present in the splenic flexure, but this is not invariable (Fig. 28.25). The rectosigmoid index is normal. The condition is usually self-limiting, with the contrast enema acting as a stimulus for subsequent passage of meconium and gradual improvement in clinical symptoms. The differential diagnosis includes Hirschsprung's disease with a splenic flexure transition zone. Continued clinical follow-up is required, and, if suspicion persists, a rectal biopsy should be performed.

A degree of functional immaturity of the bowel is often observed in premature infants. Contrast enema can occasionally be helpful as a therapeutic manoeuvre.

Colonic atresias are rare. Like small-bowel atresias, they have a vascular aetiology. The abdominal radiograph demonstrates low intestinal obstruction, sometimes with a very dilated proximal colon. Contrast enema demonstrates a blind-ending colon with a convex distal border at the atretic site (Fig. 28.26).

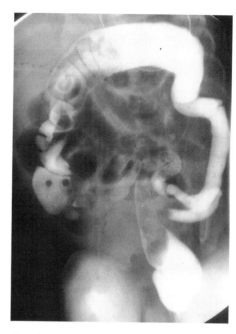

Fig. 28.25 Functional immaturity (left colon syndrome). Contrast enema in a newborn term infant showing a relatively small left colon, transition zone at the splenic flexure and a large coiled meconium plug which was dislodged from the splenic flexure to the hepatic flexure during colonic filling. The patient established a regular bowel habit over the following week and was discharged uneventfully.

Anorectal malformations are a complex spectrum of anomalies occurring with an incidence of approximately 1 in 5000 live births. They are classified into high and low anomalies, depending on whether the rectal pouch terminates above or below the level of the puborectalis sling of levator ani. There is a strong association with the VATER syndrome and with renal anomalies, including horseshoe kidney, renal agenesis, hydronephrosis and vesicoureteric reflux. Other cases are associated with spinal cord anomalies (low tethered cord) and sacral anomalies, including the caudal regression syndrome. All associated anomalies are more frequent in high than in low malformations.

Low lesions are characterised by an identifiable but anteriorly placed or stenotic anus, a perineal fistula, or, in girls, a fistula to the vaginal vestibule. Diagnosis is usually clinical and treatment involves local anoplasty or dilatations. High lesions may be blindending or associated with a urinary tract fistula (usually to the posterior urethra or bladder base) in boys or vaginal fistula in girls. Treatment involves a three-stage repair with initial defunctioning colostomy, Penna posterior sagittal anorectoplasty at 3–6 months and subsequent colostomy closure. Prognosis for faecal continence is good in low lesions but variable in high anomalies.

Abdominal radiographs demonstrate low intestinal obstruction. Occasionally, the presence of a urinary tract fistula can be inferred by air within the bladder or intraluminal calcified meconium. Further imaging is directed at excluding associated anomalies and the presence of urinary tract fistulas. Children with low anomalies should undergo renal ultrasound to exclude structural renal anomalies and micturating cystogram (MCUG) for vesicoureteric reflux. Spinal ultrasound (and, if required, MRI) is also indicated in infants with high anomalies. Fistulas to the urinary tract are demonstrated by cystogram. The fistula, usually to the posterior urethra, may be visualised directly or indirectly, implied by a kink in the posterior

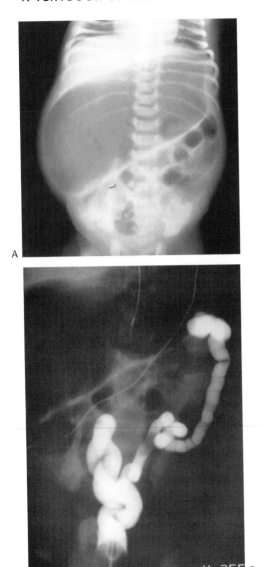

Fig. 28.26 Colonic atresia. AXR (A) showing disproportionate dilatation of one bowel loop in a neonate with abdominal distension and failure to pass meconium. Contrast enema (B) showing a blind-ending colon with a convex distal border in the splenic flexure. The dilated air-filled proximal colonic segment can be seen. An isolated colonic atresia was confirmed at surgery.

urethra at the distal insertion site of the fistula. Injection of contrast via the distal loop of the colostomy may also demonstrate a fistula, but the yield appears lower than cystography (Fig. 28.27).

Various radiological methods based on air distension of the distal rectal pouch on prone shoot-through or upside-down abdominal radiographs have been used historically to distinguish between high and low lesions They have proven unreliable and should no longer be performed. False high levels occur if air does not reach the distal pouch due to impacted meconium or if the examination is performed too rapidly after positioning the infant. The Valsalva manoeuvre during crying results in falsely low results. More recently, perineal ultrasound has been used to measure the distance from the perineum to the distal pouch (Fig. 28.28). Measurements of <10 mm indicate a low lesion and >15 mm a high lesion. Similarly, the Valsalva manoeuvre can result in falsely low measurements.

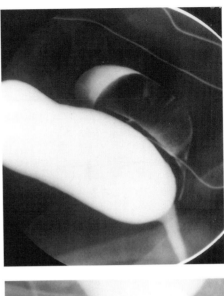

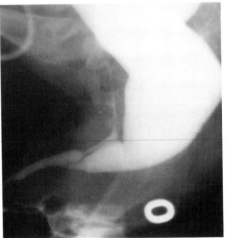

Fig. 28.27 Anorectal atresia with urethral fistula. Micturating cystogram (A) demonstrating fistula from the distal rectal pouch to the posterior urethra and distal loopogram (B) showing a fistula to the anterior urethra in two newborn boys with high anorectal malformations.

Necrotising enterocolitis

Necrotising enterocolitis (NEC) is a severe inflammatory enteritis affecting preterm infants, the majority under 2000 g. Many aetiological factors have been implicated, including sepsis, hypoxia, hypotension, early feeding and arterial umbilical lines. The common pathway appears to be via bowel ischaemia and proliferation of the intestinal flora leading to bowel necrosis and perforation. The distal ileum and ascending colon are most frequently affected, but any part of the gastrointestinal tract from oesophagus to rectum may be involved. Symptoms include abdominal distension, vomiting, diarrhoea, blood per rectum, apnoeas, metabolic acidosis and circulatory collapse.

In the early stages, abdominal radiographs are often non-specific and demonstrate generalised bowel distension. Bowel wall thickening and pneumatosis may then develop. Bubbly, rounded lucencies are believed to be due to submucosal air, linear lucencies to subserosal air. Portal venous air may be observed on radiograph or ultrasound (Fig. 28.29). In contrast to adult patients, this is not necessarily a premortem finding and does not appear to significantly

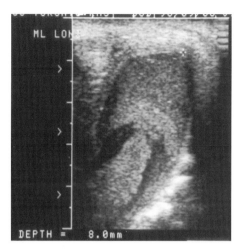

Fig. 28.28 Perineal ultrasound documenting an 8 mm rectoperineal distance consistent with a low anorectal malformation.

affect the infant's prognosis. A persistent dilated loop with no interval change on serial films is suspicious for bowel ischaemia and may precede perforation. Free air may be detected on supine radiograph by the 'football' sign, visualisation of the falciform liga-ment or Rigler's sign (Fig. 28.30). A lateral shoot-through film is more sensitive in the detection of small 'triangles' of free air between loops of bowel below the anterior abdominal wall (Fig. 28.31).

Contrast studies are not indicated acutely due to the risk of colonic perforation. Post-NEC strictures, commonly in the splenic flexure, may develop within 1–2 months, even in infants in whom the episode of NEC was not thought to be severe.

Congenital diaphragmatic hernia

Congenital diaphragmatic hernia occurs with an incidence of 1 in 2–3000 live births. Resulting from failure of division of the thoracic and abdominal cavities during the 8–10th weeks of gestation, they occur most frequently through the posterior foramen of Bochdalek (L > R), but may involve the anterior foramen of Morgagni, the diaphragmatic crura or midline defects. Most cases are now diagnosed antenatally. A smaller number present with difficulties in resuscitation at birth. Delayed presentation may be associated with neonatal strep-tococcal pneumonia, the aetiology of which remains unknown.

An infant with known congenital diaphragmatic hernia should be intubated and ventilated before the first respiratory effort and a nasogastric tube passed to decompress the stomach. Elective venti-lation and a period of stabilisation prior to surgery improves even-tual outcome. Prognosis is largely dependent on the degree of ipsilateral and contralateral pulmonary hypoplasia. The treatment of persistent pulmonary hypertension may involve the use of pulmonary vasodilators and extracorporeal membranous oxygena-tion (ECMO) (Fig. 28.32).

Initial chest radiographs demonstrate an opaque hemithorax or soft-tissue mass associated with mediastinal shift. The abdomen is gasless with a scaphoid appearance on the lateral film and on clinical exami-nation. As air is swallowed, multiple lucencies due to air-filled bowel loops can be recognised. The tip of the nasogastric tube indicates the position of the stomach; an intrathoracic location is an adverse prog-nostic factor. Ultrasound can confirm the diagnosis, identifying bowel, stomach, liver or kidney within the hernia. All patients demonstrate malrotation or malfixation on contrast meal but volvulus is rare.

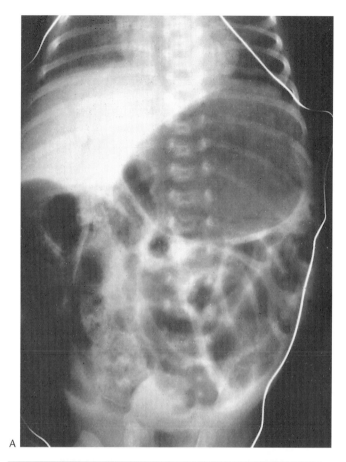

A

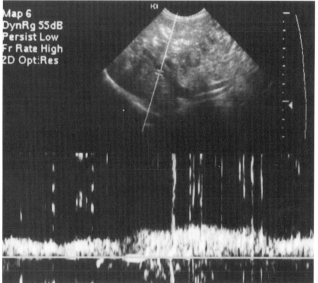

B

Fig. 28.29 Portal venous air. AXR (A) and ultrasound (B) evidence of portal venous air in a premature infant with necrotising enterocolitis.

Eventration is a focal area of thinning of the muscle of the diaphragm without communication between the thorax and the abdomen. The most common presentation is an incidental finding on chest radiograph, with a focal bulge in the diaphragmatic contour, usually on the right (Fig. 28.33). Occasionally they may cause respiratory distress requiring surgical plication.

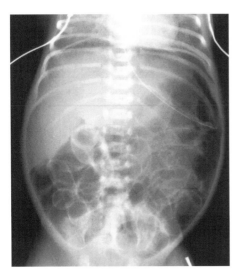

Fig. 28.30   Free intraperitoneal air in perforated necrotising enterocolitis demonstrated by lucency over the entire abdomen (football sign), subdiaphragmatic air and outlining of both sides of the bowel wall (Rigler's sign).

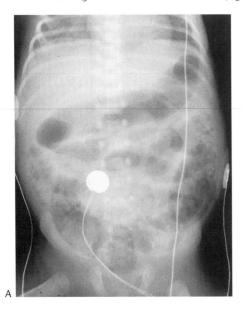

A

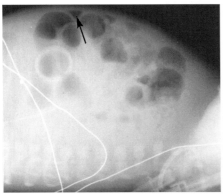

B

Fig. 28.31   Necrotising enterocolitis. Supine AXR (A) demonstrating extensive 'bubbly' pneumatosis in a 16-day-old premature infant born at 28 weeks gestation. No definite free air seen. However, lateral shoot-through radiograph (B) shows a small triangle of free air beneath the anterior abdominal wall (arrow). A localised ileal perforation was found at laparotomy.

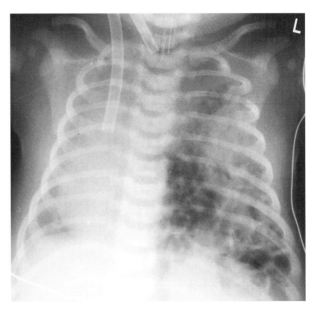

Fig. 28.32   Left congenital diaphragmatic hernia with associated mediastinal shift and pulmonary hypoplasia. The tips of the arteriovenous (AV) ECMO lines are positioned in the right atrium (radiodense dot distal to the opaque portion of the catheter) and in the origin of the right common carotid artery or aortic arch.

The anterior abdominal wall

Exomphalos (omphalocele) is due to a deficiency in the anterior abdominal wall at the umbilicus, through which bowel and other abdominal organs, covered by a sac of peritoneum and amnion, may herniate. Severe associated anomalies are common, particularly cardiac and chromosomal abnormalities, and these largely determine long-term prognosis.

Gastroschisis occurs when bowel passes through an abdominal wall defect lateral to the umbilicus (Fig. 28.34). The herniated bowel is exposed directly to amniotic fluid in utero and, after repair motility remains disordered with a slow transit time on follow-through contrast examinations. Unlike exomphalos, the incidence of associated congenital anomalies is relatively low. Both conditions are associated with some degree of malrotation but, as with congenital diaphragmatic hernia, rarely develop volvulus.

Prune-belly syndrome is an association of hypoplastic lower abdominal wall muscles, cryptorchidism and urinary tract abnormalities (including pelvicalyceal and ureteric dilatation, renal dysplasia, trabeculated bladder and various urethral anomalies) secondary to defective smooth muscle. It is found almost exclusively in males. Clinically, the abdominal wall has a wrinkled, lax appearance, with bulging of the flanks.

THE GASTROINTESTINAL TRACT IN THE OLDER CHILD

The Oesophagus

Gastro-oesophageal reflux (GOR) is commonly found in infants, and in most cases is not of pathological significance. In the first year of life, the lower oesophageal sphincter is located at the level of the diaphragm rather than inferior to it, with a less acute

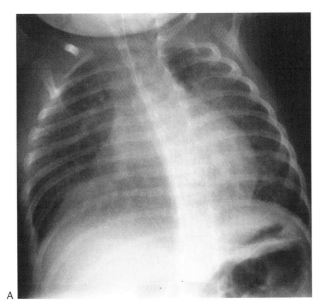

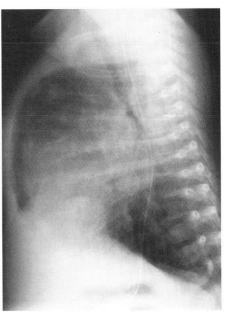

Fig. 28.33 Diaphragmatic eventration. PA (A) and lateral (B) CXR demonstrating a focal bulge in the anteromedial portion of the right hemidiaphragm. Cardiomegaly and pulmonary plethora are due to a ventricular septal defect.

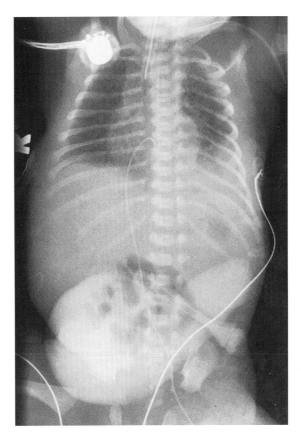

Fig. 28.34 Gastroschisis. Several air-filled extra-abdominal loops of bowel are seen in this infant of 26 weeks gestation. A small left congenital diaphragmatic hernia was also present.

oesophagocardiac angle than in adults. GOR occurs with relative ease and is considered 'physiological' in the majority of cases. After infancy the gastro-oesophageal sphincter matures and the incidence of GOR decreases. The presence of GOR is considered 'pathological' if it leads to significant clinical sequelae, including failure to thrive, aspiration pneumonitis and apnoeas in infants, or symptoms of heartburn and dysphagia in older children.

The clinical utility of the barium meal in the documentation of GOR is debatable. The majority of infants, most of whom have no attributable symptoms, will show GOR. Equally, as observations are made over a very short time period (less than 5 min), false-negative results may be obtained. The true and critical role of the barium meal is to exclude other potential causes of the patient's symptoms, including malrotation, oesophageal vascular impressions, an abnormal swallowing mechanism or oesophageal motility disorder. The presence of a hiatus hernia or a peptic stricture complicating GOR may also be documented.

Twenty-four hour pH probe monitoring is currently considered the 'gold standard' for the documentation of gastro-oesophageal reflux and allows correlation between symptoms and reflux episodes. Where clinically available, ^{99m}Tc-sulphur colloid 'milk scans' also have a high sensitivity.

Treatment is initially conservative, with feed thickeners and, if necessary, medical therapy. Rarely, persistent symptomatic reflux may require surgical intervention by Nissen's fundoplication.

Oesophageal foreign bodies are a common paediatric clinical problem. Children usually present acutely with an appropriate history from the parents, difficulty swallowing, drooling or chest pain, but presentation may be delayed.

Foreign bodies tend to impact at one of the three sites of relative narrowing in the oesophagus: the level of cricopharyngeus, the aortic arch and the gastro-oesophageal junction. If it reaches the stomach, the object will usually pass through the remainder of the gastrointestinal tract without impaction, although the ileocaecal valve may occasionally act as a site of hold-up. Impacted foreign bodies in the oesophagus may result in perforation and mediastinitis. Sharp objects such as open safety-pins may perforate at any point in the gastrointestinal tract. Identification of mercury batteries is important as these release toxic mercuric chloride and should be removed promptly.

In most cases, a 'long' PA CXR (extended to include the neck) will determine whether an object is impacted in the oesophagus and is sufficient radiological assessment (Fig. 28.35). A foreign body that has reached the stomach can then be expected to pass through the remainder of the gastrointestinal tract uneventfully. If the object is sharp, or if there are clinical signs of obstruction or peritonitis, an abdominal radiograph should also be performed.

Oesophageal foreign bodies can be removed by endoscopy or radiologically, passing an inflated Foley catheter beyond the obstruction and withdrawing it under fluoroscopic control. The latter method carries a risk of aspiration of the foreign body and is not suitable for sharp objects.

Oesophagitis and strictures. GOR is the commonest cause of oesophagitis in children. Infectious causes include candida, herpes simplex and cytomegalovirus in patients with primary or secondary immunodeficiency. Alkali caustic ingestion can result in extensive chemical injury to the oropharyngeal and oesophageal mucosa with a risk of acute perforation. The major causes of intrinsic oesophageal strictures are given in Box 28.2.

Extrinsic oesophageal compression resulting in smooth filling defects on barium swallow is associated with vascular rings or benign masses, including foregut duplication cysts (oesophageal, neuroenteric, or less commonly bronchogenic) and oesophageal leiomyoma. Malignant masses causing more aggressive appearances with irregular filling defects or oesophageal ulceration are much rarer in children.

Achalasia, due to a failure of relaxation of the lower oesophageal sphincter, is occasionally seen in children. Barium swallow shows a dilated oesophagus with a characteristic 'rat's tail' appearance at the gastro-oesophageal junction and intermittent passage of small amounts of barium into the stomach. Evidence of aspiration may be present on chest radiograph. The diagnosis is confirmed by manometry and treatment is either by serial dilatations or surgical myotomy.

Varices may be encountered in children with portal hypertension and can be demonstrated as serpiginous filling defects on barium

---

studies or a mass of prominent vessels in the region of the gastro-oesophageal junction on ultrasound in association with other features of portal hypertension.

The stomach and duodenum

Gastritis, duodenitis and **peptic ulcer disease** are rarer in children than adults. They may be primary or secondary to stress or medications, particularly non-steroidal anti-inflammatory drugs and steroids. Acute complications include perforation and gastrointestinal haemorrhage, often in the clinical setting of trauma, burns or head injury. Chronic disease presents in older children with symptoms similar to adults, including dyspepsia, nausea and vomiting, gastrointestinal bleeding and, occasionally, gastric outlet obstruction. Endoscopy is the investigation of choice. The sensitivity of single-contrast barium studies in young children is relatively low. Double-contrast studies in older children demonstrate radiological findings similar to those in adults. It is important to test for *Helicobacter pylori* and to exclude Zollinger–Ellison syndrome. Children with duodenal ulcers often have a strong family history.

Gastric bezoars are masses of ingested foreign material retained within the stomach, including trichobezoars (hair) and phytobezoars (vegetable fibre). Lactobezoars are seen in newborns due to insufficient mixing of formula milk with water. They may be identified on abdominal radiograph, barium meal or ultrasound. The intraluminal mass has a mottled appearance due to air mixed with the ingested material and is outlined by a rim of air.

Gastric volvulus is rare in children. Mesenteroaxial volvulus is more common than organoaxial volvulus, usually presenting acutely in the newborn or infant.

Duodenal haematomas are most frequently associated with blunt trauma to the abdomen, either in the setting of a road traffic accident or non-accidental injury. Associated injuries include lacerations to the left lobe of the liver and to the pancreas. Other causes include Henoch–Schönlein purpura, bleeding disorders and leukaemia. Barium meal shows thickened mucosal folds or a localised filling defect due to intramural haematoma, which may result in partial or complete intestinal obstruction. Abdominal CT performed in the assessment of acute trauma may demonstrate the haematoma directly or show abnormal duodenal enhancement. Careful inspection should be made for the presence of retroperitoneal air bubbles, indicating perforation.

Pyloric stenosis has been considered earlier (p. 851).

The small bowel

Duplication cysts may occur anywhere along the gastrointestinal tract but one-third of cases involve the distal small bowel. Due to

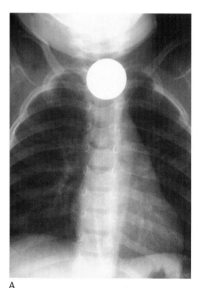
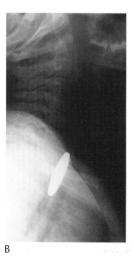

Fig. 28.35 Ingested coin. PA CXR (A) demonstrating a coin impacted in the proximal oesophagus. Coins lodged within the oesophagus are seen 'en face' on PA CXR, whereas impaction within the trachea results in 'side-on' visualisation. Lateral cervical spine X-ray (B) confirming oesophageal location of the foreign body.

A   B

incomplete recanalisation at around 8 weeks gestation, they may be spherical or tubular and are lined with gastrointestinal epithelium. This may be derived from the adjacent gastrointestinal tract, or from ectopic mucosa, usually pancreatic or gastric. Most duplications do not communicate with the adjacent bowel, although there is a higher incidence of persistent communication in tubular anomalies. Unlike neurenteric cysts, they are not usually associated with vertebral segmentation anomalies.

The most frequent sites of duplication are the ileum, then oesophagus, stomach, duodenum and jejunum. Colonic and rectal duplications are rare. Presentation depends on the site of duplication and its size. Many are detected antenatally or as an incidental ultrasound finding in the first few years of life. Large cysts, especially those associated with the stomach or duodenum, may present with abdominal pain, obstruction and vomiting. They may act as a lead point for intussusception or a source of gastrointestinal bleeding from ectopic gastric mucosa. Abdominal radiographs may show mass effect with displacement of adjacent bowel loops. Ultrasound demonstrates a simple hypoechoic cyst; if the characteristic 'gut-wall signature' of an inner echogenic mucosa and outer hypoechoic smooth muscle layer can be identified, the diagnosis can be made (Fig. 28.36). The differential diagnosis of paediatric abdominal cysts includes mesenteric, omental, choledochal, renal and ovarian cysts (Box 28.3).

Proximal oesophageal duplication cysts may be associated with tracheal compression and present with upper airway obstruction (Fig. 28.37). Distal oesophageal cysts are often relatively asymptomatic and found as an incidental chest radiograph finding. Barium meal will confirm the presence of a smooth extrinsic oesophageal filling defect and cross-sectional imaging (CT/MRI) will demonstrate its cystic nature.

Mesenteric/omental cysts (lymphangiomas) are developmental anomalies of the lymphatic system arising within the mesentery or omentum (Fig. 28.38). Presentation is similar to duplication cysts. However, ultrasound is more likely to show a multiloculated cyst with thin septations than a simple cyst. Both require surgical resection.

Meckel's diverticulum is due to persistence of the proximal part of the vitelline (omphalomesenteric) duct, resulting in a true diverticulum arising from the antimesenteric border of the distal ileum, within 60 cm of the caecum. It may contain ectopic gastric or pancreatic mucosa. With a prevalence of 2% in the population, 2% will present with complications, including acute inflammation mimicking appendicitis, gastrointestinal bleeding or as a pathological lead point within an intussusception.

Appendicitis is the most common acute surgical condition of childhood. It can occur in children as young as 1 year of age but is more frequent in older children and adolescence, with a peak incidence between 12 and 15 years. If presentation is classical, with a history of ill-defined abdominal pain moving to the right iliac fossa, accompanied by fever, vomiting, a raised white cell count and local peritoneal signs, imaging is rarely required. However, in young children presentation is often atypical and diagnosis may be delayed. Adolescent girls, in whom gynaecological causes must be considered, are also a difficult diagnostic group. Imaging is useful in these cases but surgical liaison remains essential and findings must be interpreted in conjunction with the patient's clinical status.

Plain abdominal radiographs may be normal or demonstrate non-specific findings suggesting inflammation in the right iliac fossa, such

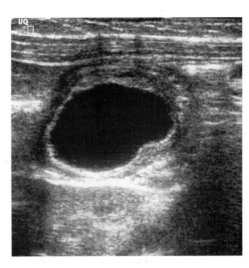

Fig. 28.36 Duplication cyst. Hypoechoic cyst with double 'gut wall signature'. In this case the adjacent segment of bowel can be seen along the superior border of the cyst, confirming its origin.

as localised dilated bowel loops or a scoliosis convex to the left. In view of their low sensitivity and specificity they are not recommended as routine in the assessment of potential appendicitis. However, in 5–10% of cases a radiodense appendicolith is identified (Fig. 28.39). In the clinical setting of a child with acute abdominal pain, this is highly predictive of acute appendicitis. Generalised bowel dilatation may indicate perforation and peritonitis.

In 1986 Julien Puylaert described the ultrasonographic appearances of acute appendicitis using the 'graded compression' technique. This has proved a highly effective diagnostic tool with a sensitivity of 80–95% and specificity of 90–95% in both adults and children.

Using a linear array transducer (5–10 MHz) and gradual compression over the right iliac fossa and the site of maximum tenderness, the landmarks of the caecum, iliac vessels and psoas muscle are identified. An inflamed appendix is demonstrated as a non-compressible blind-ending tubular structure with a diameter of 6 mm or greater (Fig. 28.40). It can often be followed back to its origin from the

---

Box 28.3   Paediatric abdominal cysts

Hepatobiliary
    Choledochal cyst
    Gallbladder hydrops

Gastrointestinal
    Duplication cyst
    Omental/mesenteric cyst

Urinary tract
    Renal/parapelvic cyst
    Severe hydronephrosis/pelviureteric junction obstruction
    Cystic Wilms' tumour (rare)
    Urachal cyst

Adrenal
    Resolving adrenal haemorrhage
    Cystic neuroblastoma/ganglioneuroma (rare)

Pancreatic
    Pancreatic pseudocyst

Pelvic
    Ovarian cyst
    Teratoma/dermoid cyst
    Anterior meningocele
    Abscess

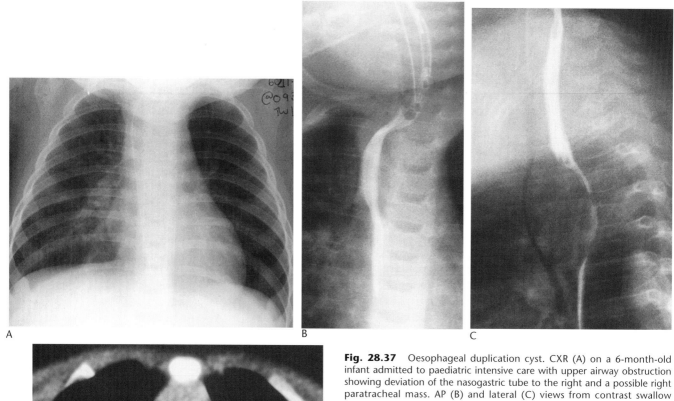

A

B

C

D

Fig. 28.37 Oesophageal duplication cyst. CXR (A) on a 6-month-old infant admitted to paediatric intensive care with upper airway obstruction showing deviation of the nasogastric tube to the right and a possible right paratracheal mass. AP (B) and lateral (C) views from contrast swallow showing smooth extrinsic compression and posterolateral deviation of the proximal oesophagus with narrowing and anterior bowing of the trachea. CT (D) confirmed the presence of a prevertebral tubular cystic mass with oesophageal and tracheal displacement. A proximal oesophageal duplication cyst was resected at thoracotomy.

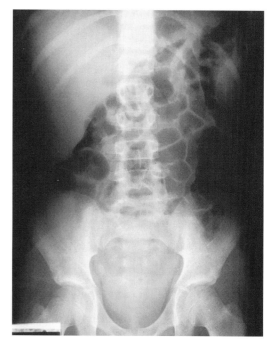

Fig. 28.38 Mesenteric cyst. CT demonstrating a large left-sided cystic abdominal mass with compression of the left kidney. Ultrasound showed multiple fine septations within the cyst (not illustrated).

Fig. 28.39 Appendicolith. Rounded calcific density projected over the right iliac fossa in a 7-year-old boy presenting with abdominal pain.

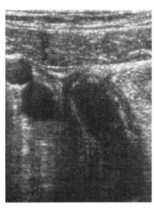

Fig. 28.40 Acute appendicitis. Transverse ultrasound image demonstrating a hypoechoic tubular structure 7 mm (markers) in diameter adjacent to the iliac vessels. It was blind-ending and non-compressible.

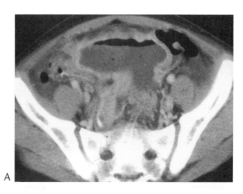

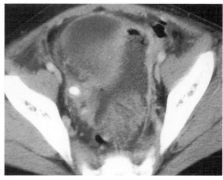

Fig. 28.42 CT pelvis (A) showing a large thick-walled pelvic abscess containing an air–fluid level in a 9-year-old girl presenting with a 10 day history of ill-defined abdominal pain and diarrhoea. An appendicolith was identified on a more superior slice (B). The patient was managed with percutaneous drainage and antibiotic therapy.

caecum, although inflammation may only be present at the tip. The appendix is usually distended with fluid and an obstructing appendicolith with acoustic shadowing may be identified. Other supporting signs include increased echogenicity of the surrounding mesenteric fat, hyperaemia of the appendix on colour Doppler examination and a small amount of free fluid. Small mesenteric lymph nodes are often noted. Periportal increased echogenicity within the liver is a nonspecific sign. Causes of potential false-negative examinations include retrocaecal appendices, severe pain preventing adequate compression and an unfavourable body habitus. Ultrasound findings should not be interpreted in isolation. Clinical correlation is important as a negative study does not preclude the diagnosis.

Ultrasound sensitivity decreases in perforated appendicitis. The appendix decompresses and is more difficult to identify. Increased echogenicity of the surrounding mesenteric fat is a useful pointer to the diagnosis. An inflammatory mass or 'phlegmon' with small pockets of fluid may contain an appendicolith (Fig. 28.41). A localised right iliac fossa or pelvic abscess may develop. Generalised peritonitis results in multiple intraperitoneal collections throughout the abdomen. Portal vein thrombosis and haematogenous spread of infection with multiple hepatic abscesses is a rarer but recognised complication.

The normal appendix is difficult to identify but with high-frequency probes and expertise it can be visualised in 5–50% of patients. Less than 6 mm in transverse diameter, it is compressible and shows no appreciable colour Doppler flow within its wall.

The differential diagnosis of acute appendicitis includes other gastrointestinal, renal and gynaecological pathologies, many of which may be diagnosed by ultrasound. Multiple enlarged mesenteric lymph nodes are seen in mesenteric adenitis but the appendix is normal. Crohn's disease and infections such as yersiniosis and campylobacteriosis cause ileal thickening. Examination of the ovaries is important to exclude ovarian torsion or cysts.

CT has an established role in 'late-presenting' appendicitis with localised or multifocal abscesses and is useful in planning radiological drainages (Fig. 28.42). More recently, it has been used in adults in the diagnosis of acute appendicitis. Its role in paediatric practice is more controversial in view of the radiation burden. While CT may have a role in equivocal cases (Fig. 28.43), ultrasound is likely to remain the initial investigation of choice in children due to its non-ionising nature and its suitability to the paediatric body habitus.

Common causes of **inflammatory and infectious small-bowel thickening** in children are given in Box 28.4. Ultrasound demonstrates hyperaemic thickened loops of bowel with a wall thickness of greater

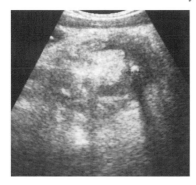

Fig. 28.41 Perforated appendicitis. Right iliac fossa mixed echogenicity inflammatory mass. A 6 mm echogenic focus with acoustic shadowing consistent with an appendicolith confirms the diagnosis.

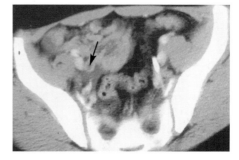

Fig. 28.43 Acute appendicitis. CT pelvis in a 12-year-old boy with a recent diagnosis of acute leukaemia and a 2 day history of abdominal pain. The appendix is identified medial to the iliac vessels (arrow). It is thick-walled and associated with a small pocket of free fluid. An acutely inflamed appendix was found at laparotomy.

Box 28.4   Causes of small-bowel thickening

Infections
  *Yersinia, E. coli, Mycobacterium tuberculosis, M. avium intracellulare,
    Campylobacter, Salmonella, Shigella, Giardia, Cryptosporidium, Ascaris*

Inflammatory
  Crohn's disease,
  Eosinophilic gastroenteritis
  Chronic granulomatous disease

Vascular
  Intramural haematoma (Henoch–Schönlein, haemophilia, idiopathic
    thrombocytopenic purpura, bleeding diathesis, trauma)
  Arterial or venous insufficiency
  Lymphatic obstruction or malformation (intestinal lymphectasia)
  Angioneurotic oedema

Metabolic
  Hypoproteinaemia
  Amyloidosis

Iatrogenic
  Graft-versus-host disease
  Radiotherapy

Neoplastic
  Lymphoma

than 3 mm. The location of abnormal loops may provide some indication of disease distribution. Proximal loops in the left upper quadrant are likely to represent jejunum, whereas pelvic or right iliac fossa loops are more likely to be ileal. If the thickened loop of bowel can be followed in continuity to the caecum, a diagnosis of terminal ileitis can be made. Barium small-bowel follow-through examination will demonstrate thickening of the bowel wall and valvulae conniventes with more accurate anatomical localisation.

Henoch–Schönlein purpura is a small vessel vasculitis of unknown aetiology, although some cases appear to be postinfectious or post-drug therapy (e.g. penicillin) in origin. Clinical features include a purpuric rash over the buttocks and legs, abdominal pain, arthritis and glomerulonephritis. The cause of the patients abdominal pain is usually recognised clinically in the presence of the characteristic rash; however, if abdominal symptoms precede the rash the radiologist may be the first to suggest the diagnosis. Oedema and haemorrhage cause bowel wall thickening, the jejunum being most frequently involved (Fig. 28.44). Transient small-bowel intussusceptions are relatively common. Echogenic kidneys suggest renal involvement.

A variety of organisms may infect the small bowel, including *Giardia*, *Campylobacter*, *Yersinia*, *Salmonella* and *Shigella* spp, *Escherichia coli* and *Mycobacterium tuberculosis*. Opportunistic infection by *Cryptosporidium* sp. and *Isospora belli* may occur in immunosuppressed patients.

Graft-versus-host disease (GVHD) is a serious complication in children who have undergone bone marrow transplantation. The small bowel is often most severely affected but the entire gastrointestinal tract may be involved (Fig. 28.45).

The terminal ileum and caecum are involved in most cases of Crohn's disease but isolated involvement of the more proximal small bowel is also described. Small-bowel thickening, strictures, inflammatory masses and fistulas may be demonstrated in addition to colonic disease.

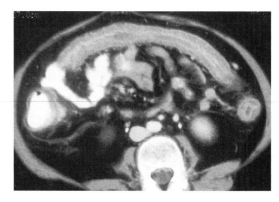

Fig. 28.45 Graft-versus-host disease. CT abdomen demonstrating extensive thickening of the bowel wall, abnormal mucosal enhancement and mesenteric stranding in pancolitis due to GVHD after bone marrow transplantation.

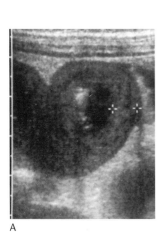

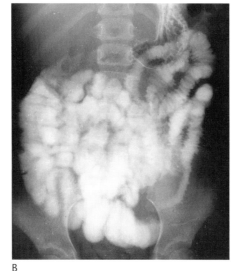

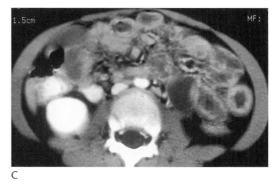

A   B   C

Fig. 28.44 Henoch–Schönlein purpura. Ultrasound (A), barium follow-through (B) and CT abdomen (C) demonstrating jejunal bowel wall thickening in a 5-year-old boy. Thickening of the valvulae conniventes can also be seen on the barium study.

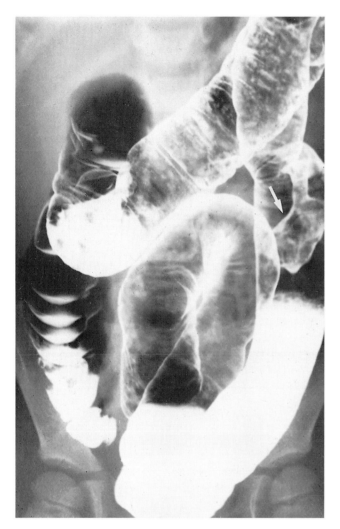

Fig. 28.46 Juvenile polyp. Barium enema demonstrating a pedunculated polyp in the descending colon (arrow).

Polyps and polyposis syndromes. *Isolated juvenile polyps* are most commonly found in the sigmoid colon and rectum. They may be single or multiple. Unlike polyps in adults, they are hamartomas rather than adenomas. Children present under 10 years of age with painless rectal bleeding which may be intermittent and insidious, leading to iron-deficiency anaemia. A pendunculated polyp, often with a long stalk, is demonstrated on double-contrast barium enema (Fig. 28.46) or endoscopy and careful examination should be made for multiple lesions. Treatment is surgical removal to prevent continued bleeding. Although the polyps are not premalignant, there are a few reports of adenomas or carcinomas arising within or simultaneously with juvenile polyps.

Juvenile polyposis, defined as the presence of five or more polyps, is associated with a higher long-term risk of colonic carcinoma. Many, although not all, children have a positive family history.

Peutz–Jeghers syndrome is an autosomal dominant condition associated with mucocutaneous pigmentation and gastrointestinal hamartomas. Polyps may occur anywhere from the stomach to the rectum, but are most numerous in the small bowel. Multiple rounded filling defects are demonstrated on small bowel follow-through examination. Intussusception around polyps is common

and usually transient, but small-bowel obstruction may occur. There is an increased risk both of gastrointestinal adenocarcinoma and of non-gastrointestinal neoplasms involving the pancreas, breast or reproductive organs.

Multiple adenomatous polyps are found in *familial polyposis coli* and *Gardner's syndrome*, both of which are dominantly inherited. Polyps are most numerous in the colon, which may be completely carpeted. In view of their high malignant potential, prophylactic proctocolectomy is usually recommended in young adulthood. *Turcot's syndrome* is a rare autosomal recessive condition in which colonic adenomas are associated with CNS gliomas.

Small-bowel malignancies are rare in childhood, the commonest being Burkitt's type non-Hodgkin's lymphoma, which most frequently involves the ileocaecal region. Presenting symptoms include abdominal pain, a palpable mass, failure to thrive, and obstruction secondary to luminal narrowing or intussusception around the tumour. Peak incidence is 5–8 years with a male predominance. Thickened hypoechoic bowel loops are seen on ultrasound, often forming adherent masses with infiltration of the adjacent omentum and mesentery. Hepatosplenomegaly and retroperitoneal lymphadenopathy support the diagnosis.

The most common causes of **small-bowel obstruction** in children beyond the neonatal period are given in Box 28.5. Previous laparotomy carries a 10% risk of subsequent adhesions, but fortunately many settle with conservative management. Intussusception and obstructed inguinal hernia are also relatively frequently encountered. **Non-obstructive paralytic ileus**, with generalised small and large bowel dilatation and absent bowel sounds, is associated with sepsis, metabolic disturbances, post-laparotomy, peritonitis, and a variety of intra-abdominal pathologies including acute appendicitis, pancreatitis and retroperitoneal infection or haemorrhage.

The large bowel

Inflammatory and infectious causes of colitis are encountered in children in many of the same conditions that affect adults (Box 28.6). Imaging features are similar. High-frequency linear array ultrasound transducers provide an excellent imaging modality in the assessment of bowel wall thickening and expertise is increasing in the accurate localisation of disease (Fig. 28.47). Sonographic features are similar irrespective of the underlying cause of colitis and the clinical history is important in arriving at the correct diagnosis. Ultrasound and CT both have a role in the imaging and therapeutic drainage of complicating collections and abscesses.

Box 28.5 Causes of small-bowel obstruction in infants and older children

Adhesions
Intussusception
Malrotation and volvulus
Appendix mass
Inguinal hernia
Congenital cysts (duplication, mesenteric/omental)
Crohn's disease
Closed loop volvulus
Ingested foreign body
Meconeum ileus equivalent/DIOS (cystic fibrosis)
Malignancy—rare (lymphoma)

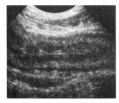

Fig. 28.47 Colitis. Ultrasound demonstrating thick-walled ascending colon, in this case due to Crohn's disease. Doppler examination showed hyperaemia of the bowel wall.

Crohn's disease may present in the prepubertal child or adolescent with rather non-specific symptoms, including weight loss, anorexia, short stature and delayed puberty. Symptoms directly attributable to the gastrointestinal tract, such as diarrhoea and abdominal pain, may be relatively less prominent. The reader is referred to the more detailed description of aetiological factors, pathology, extraintestinal manifestations and radiological features in Chapter 21. In the assessment of children with potential inflammatory bowel disease, the barium enema has been largely replaced by endoscopy, reducing radiation burden and enabling direct visualisation and biopsy. A role for the small-bowel study still remains in the identification of terminal ileal disease, small-bowel strictures and fistula. ^{99m}Tc-HMPOA leucocyte scintigraphy can provide useful information regarding the extent of active disease. CT may demonstrate transmural bowel wall thickening, 'creeping fat' within the mesentery, strictures, localised collections and evidence of fistula. Recently, MRI has also been proposed as a non-invasive non-ionising method for the assessment of disease extent (Fig. 28.48).

Childhood ulcerative colitis may present acutely, including toxic megacolon, or more insidiously with a history of bloody diarrhoea, abdominal pain and failure to thrive. Imaging features are similar to adults with contiguous disease extending proximally from the rectum. The risk of colonic carcinoma is high, approximately 20% per decade.

Typhlitis is an inflammatory condition predominantly affecting the right colon in neutropenic patients. Ultrasound demonstrates a thickened hypoechoic caecum and ascending colon with echogenic mucosa and hyperaemia. In the appropriate clinical setting, no further investigations are necessary and treatment is supportive.

Haemolytic uraemic syndrome (HUS) is the commonest cause of acute renal failure in children. Microangiopathic haemolytic anaemia, thrombocytopenia and acute renal failure follow a diarrhoeal illness caused by *E. coli* serotype 0157, recent viral infection or immunisation. The association of colonic thickening and echogenic kidneys on ultrasound is highly suggestive of the diagnosis. Unlike other causes of colitis, Doppler flow within the bowel wall is reduced in HUS, at least in the prodromal phase.

Intussusception is the invagination of a segment of bowel (the intussusceptum) into the contiguous segment (the intussuscipiens). Venous obstruction results in oedema and haemorrhage into the bowel wall, which may progress to small bowel obstruction, bowel wall necrosis and perforation if unrecognised. The ileocolic segment is most frequently involved (in approximately 90% of cases) but ileoileocolic, colocolic and ileoileal intussusception may also occur. Most cases (>90%) are associated with inflammation and enlargement of the lymphoid tissue in Peyer's patches following a viral gastroenteritis. In a small number (5–10%) there is a pathological lead point, such as Meckel's diverticulum, duplication cyst, polyp or, occasionally, lymphoma.

Peak age incidence is between 6 months and 2 years but the diagnosis should also be considered in young infants and older children. In atypical age groups, suspicion of a pathological lead point is higher. Classic presentation is with episodic abdominal pain and screaming episodes associated with the passage of blood and mucus ('red current jelly'). Considerable fluid shifts can result in haemodynamic instability. It is important to start fluid resuscitation before imaging and treatment.

The abdominal radiograph may demonstrate an absence of bowel gas in the right iliac fossa with a rounded soft-tissue mass (Fig. 28.49), a crescent of air at the apex of an intussusception, or small-bowel obstruction. However, in the majority of cases, no definite abnormality is seen. The detection of free air in the absence of clinical signs of peritonitis is rare.

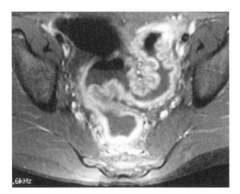

Fig. 28.48 Gadolinium-enhanced fat saturated T$_1$-weighted axial MRI pelvis showing diffuse mucosal enhancement and bowel wall thickening of the rectosigmoid colon in Crohn's disease.

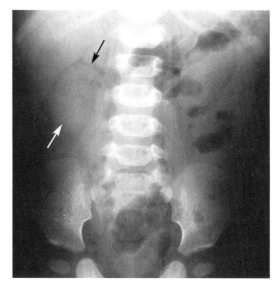

Fig. 28.49 Intussusception. Paucity of bowel gas in the right iliac fossa and a soft-tissue mass (arrows) strongly suggest intussusception in this 11-month-old child. However, in many cases, AXR shows no definite abnormality.

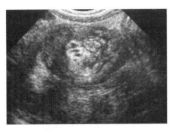

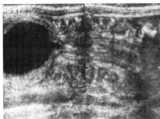

Fig. 28.50 Intussusception. Transverse ultrasound showing multiple hypoechoic concentric rings, central echogenic mesentery and a few small trapped lymph nodes.

Fig. 28.51 Pathological lead point. Composite ultrasound image showing a cystic mass at the head of an intussusception in a 3-month-old boy. A duodenal duplication cyst was found at laparotomy.

Ultrasound is a highly sensitive screening tool for intussusception. A general examination of the abdomen should be performed using a curvilinear or vector transducer followed by systematic examination of the bowel using a high-frequency linear array transducer. Most ileocolic intussusceptions can be visualised by scanning just anterior to the right kidney. Transverse sections show a mass with multiple hypoechoic concentric rings (Fig. 28.50). The identification of a central hyperechoic crescent representing mesenteric fat between the two layers of the intussusceptum confirms the diagnosis. Longitudinal images have a more reniform shape, leading to its description as a 'pseudokidney' by earlier authors. Small crescents of peritoneal fluid may be trapped between the layers of the intussusception and a small amount of free fluid is common. Colour flow within the mass suggests bowel wall viability. Small lymph nodes are frequently found within the intussusception. The presence of other soft-tissue or cystic masses suggests a pathological lead point (Fig. 28.51).

Radiological reduction is the treatment of choice, the only absolute contraindications being peritonitis and perforation. Pneumatic reduction (air enema) has now replaced the use of barium in most paediatric centres as it is cleaner and easy to use, with a higher success rate (70–90%) and without the risk of barium peritonitis. There is no consensus as to the optimal protocol and this varies with local expertise. A large (16–20F) catheter is inserted into the rectum and pneumatic pressure maintained for 1–3 min per attempt, usually starting at 80 mmHg and increasing to 110–120 mmHg. The soft-tissue mass of the intussusception is fol-

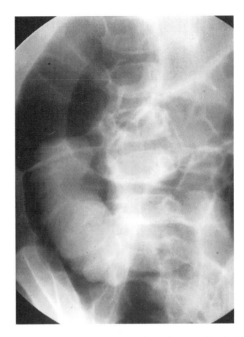

Fig. 28.52 Air enema demonstrating a large ileocaecal soft-tissue mass outlined by air. The length of the mass suggests an ileoileocolic intussusception. Radiological reduction was successful.

lowed as it moves to the ileocaecal junction (Fig. 28.52). There is often then a transitory hold-up. Successful reduction is indicated by disappearance of the mass and flooding of air into the small bowel.

Following reduction, there is a recurrence rate of 5–10%, usually within the first few days, and repeated reduction can be performed. Although most recurrent cases are not associated with a pathological lead point, an ultrasound search should be performed, especially in older children. Pneumatic reduction carries a 0.5–1% risk of inducing or uncovering a pre-existing perforation. Tension pneumoperitoneum can lead to respiratory and haemodynamic compromise requiring relief by needle puncture of the abdomen. Paediatric surgical and anaesthetic support must be available on site.

Fluoroscopic time limits for attempted radiological reduction vary between institutions but 10–15 min fluoroscopy time is a guide. If the child is clinically stable, some centres may undertake repeat attempts after an interval of 2–8 h, with careful surgical liaison and clinical monitoring. Factors associated with lower success rates and which prompt a more cautious reduction attempt include a long history, age less than 6 months or over 2 years, the presence of small-bowel

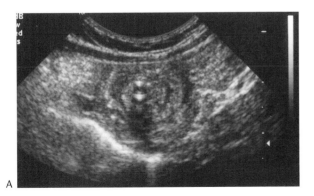

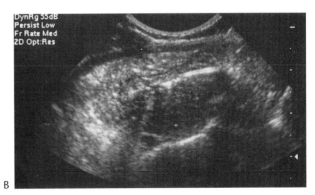

Fig. 28.53 Transverse (A) and longitudinal (B) ultrasound images demonstrating a small bowel intussusception around the tip of a gastrojejunostomy feeding tube.

obstruction, lack of colour Doppler flow and trapped peritoneal fluid within the intussusception on ultrasound.

Small-bowel intussusceptions are increasingly recognised as an incidental asymptomatic finding during abdominal ultrasound examinations. They are a well-recognised feature of Henoch–Schönlein purpura and there appears to be an increased incidence in the setting of abdominal trauma. Gastrojejunal and occasionally nasojejunal feeding tubes may act as lead points for intussusception (Fig. 28.53). These are more likely to be symptomatic, requiring manipulation or replacement of the tube.

Polyps, **polyposis syndromes** and **duplication cysts** have been discussed earlier.

PAEDIATRIC ABDOMINAL MASSES

Imaging investigation of a paediatric abdominal mass is a common clinical problem. Plain radiographs may be available, demonstrating organomegaly, mass effect on adjacent bowel, or calcification. Ultrasound is the initial investigation of choice to determine its solid or cystic nature, the organ of origin, and the presence of vascular compression or intraluminal thrombus. Further imaging and tumour staging may involve CT or MRI. Radionuclide studies have specific applications.

Renal masses

The majority of abdominal masses in childhood arise from the kidneys (Box 28.7). Pelvicalyceal dilatation, congenital lesions and renal cystic disease are discussed in Chapters xx–xx and will not be considered further.

Wilms' tumour (nephroblastoma) is the commonest renal tumour of childhood, representing approximately 10% of all childhood malignancy. Patients present under 5 years of age, with a peak incidence between 2 and 3 years. There is an increased incidence in sporadic aniridia, hemihypertrophy, Beckwith–Wiedemann syn-

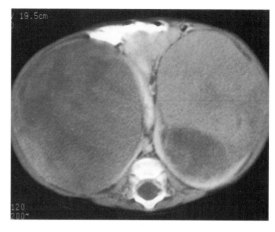

Fig. 28.54 Bilateral Wilms' tumours. CT showing bilateral large low attenuation renal masses filling the abdomen of this 5-month-old girl.

drome, Drash syndrome, horseshoe kidney and with a family history. Most children present with an asymptomatic mass but abdominal pain, haematuria, fever and hypertension secondary to renal ischaemia or increased renin production may occur.

Bilateral synchronous tumours occur in 5–10% of patients (Fig. 28.54). Nephroblastomatosis, the persistence of fetal blastema acting as a precursor to the development of Wilms' tumour, is found on histological examination in all bilateral cases and in many children with a predisposing factor. Macroscopically, it may be visualised as focal or diffuse masses within the renal cortex or medulla, hypoechoic or low attenuation on ultrasound or CT, respectively. The differentiation of Wilms' foci from nephroblastomatosis can be challenging and the tissue characterisation abilities of MRI may have a future role in this.

Wilms' tumour is usually echogenic and heterogeneous on ultrasound, with cystic areas due to haemorrhage and necrosis. The renal vein and IVC may be distended with tumour thrombus. Enlarged retroperitoneal lymph nodes may be reactive or indicate tumour spread and should be sampled at surgery. The CT 'claw sign' is useful in confirming the renal origin of the tumour (Fig. 28.55). Calcification is present in only a small proportion of cases, unlike neuroblastoma. The contralateral kidney should be examined for synchronous tumours or evidence of nephroblastomatosis and a search for lung and liver metastases made. The lung is the commonest site of distant spread.

Tumour staging is determined by imaging and surgical findings, according to the National Wilms' Tumour Study Group in the USA and the United Kingdom Children's Cancer Study Group in the UK:

Stage 1   Encapsulated tumour, completely excised
Stage 2   Extends beyond the kidney, completely excised
Stage 3   Residual tumour confined to the abdomen or nodes
Stage 4   Haematogenous metastases (lung metastases on CXR (UKCCSG) or on CT (NWTS))
Stage 5   Bilateral tumours at diagnosis

Classification into favourable and unfavourable histological groups is also important in determining prognosis. Five year survival exceeds 90% in those with early stage and favourable histology.

Other malignant renal tumours include **clear cell sarcoma** and **rhabdoid tumour**, which should be suspected in children present-

---

Box 28.7   Causes of paediatric renal masses

Congenital
    Multicystic dysplastic kidney
    Pelvi-ureteric junction obstruction
    Cystic renal disease—polylcystic kidneys (ADPCK, ARPCK), tuberous
        sclerosis, Meckel–Gruber syndrome, Zellwegger's syndrome, Jeune's
        thoracic dystrophy, Beckwith–Wiedemann syndrome, von
        Hippel–Lindau disease, trisomy 13, 18 and 21, simple cysts

Pelvicalyceal system dilatation

Infection
    Abscess
    Focal nephritis
    Xanthogranulomatous pyelonephritis

Neoplasms
    Malignant—Wilms' tumour, clear cell sarcoma, rhabdoid tumour,
        lymphoma, renal cell carcinoma (rare)
    Benign—angiomyolipoma, mesoblastic nephroma, multilocular cystic
        nephroma

Vascular
    Renal vein thrombosis
    Haematoma

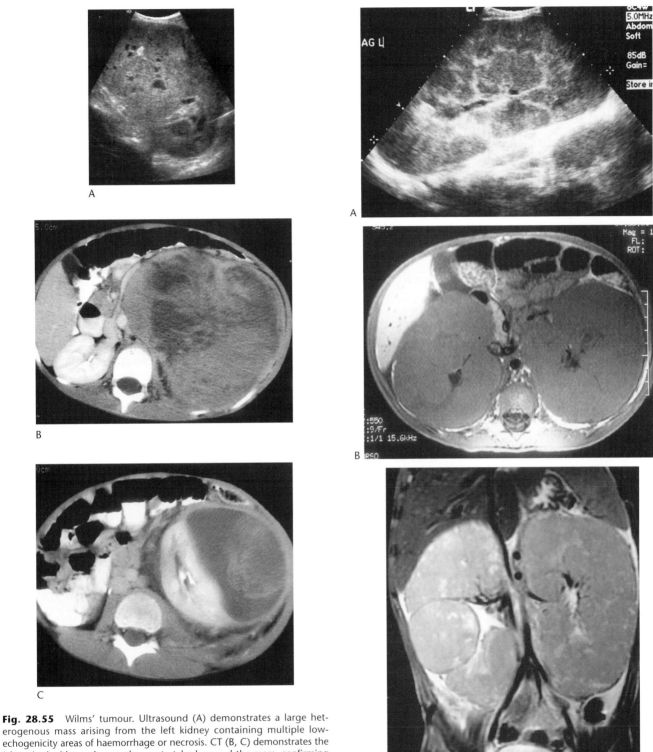

Fig. 28.55 Wilms' tumour. Ultrasound (A) demonstrates a large heterogenous mass arising from the left kidney containing multiple low-echogenicity areas of haemorrhage or necrosis. CT (B, C) demonstrates the 'claw sign' with renal parenchyma stretched around the mass, confirming its renal origin. The tumour displaces the retroperitoneal vessels without encasing them. The left renal vein lies over the anteromedial aspect of the mass. Small retroperitoneal lymph nodes are present.

Fig. 28.56 Non-Hodgkin's lymphoma of the kidneys. Londitudinal renal ultrasound (A) in a 5-year-old boy showing multiple isoechoic masses in a 17 cm kidney. Axial T_1-weighted (B) and coronal STIR MRI (C) confirming gross enlargement of both kidneys with complete loss of normal renal architecture. Differential diagnoses include lymphoma, leukaemia and nephroblastomatosis. Biopsy yielded non-Hodgkin's lymphoma.

ing with a renal mass outside of the expected age range for Wilms' tumour. Rhabdoid tumours are associated with a particularly poor prognosis. Imaging features of the primaries are similar to Wilms' tumour. However, unlike Wilms' tumour, clear cell sarcoma metastasises to bone, rather than lung. Renal rhabdoid tumour may coexist with posterior fossa rhabdoid primaries. **Renal cell carcinoma** is occasionally encountered in children, with a peak incidence of 9 years of age.

Renal involvement by **lymphoma** is more common in non-Hodgkin's lymphoma than Hodgkin's disease and most frequently manifests as multiple hypoechoic or isoechoic masses (Fig. 28.56). Direct invasion from contiguous retroperitoneal lymph nodes, solitary masses and diffuse infiltration are also described. **Leukaemic infiltration** may result in enlarged, slightly echogenic kidneys with loss of normal corticomedullary differentiation.

Benign renal masses include mesoblastic nephroma, multilocular cystic nephroma and angiomyolipomas. **Mesoblastic nephroma** is an asymptomatic solid tumour in neonates with imaging features similar to Wilms' tumour. **Multilocular cystic nephroma** has a bimodal age distribution occurring most frequently in boys under 4 years of age and young adult females. A focal mass containing multiple non-communicating cysts separated by fibrous septae is demonstrated on ultrasound and CT. The septae may contain microscopic Wilms' tumour foci and surgical resection is recommended. **Angiomyolipomas** are a common feature of tuberous sclerosis in

the older child, although renal cysts are the more frequent renal manifestation of this condition in the younger child. Ultrasound demonstrates characteristic well-defined peripheral echogenic masses (Fig. 28.57). The fat content of the lesions is well demonstrated on CT (Fig. 28.58). They may be complicated by intralesional haemorrhage.

Renal abscesses in children have similar imaging features to those described in adults. Echogenic debris and septations may be demonstrated on ultrasound within single or multiple thick-walled hypoechoic cystic lesions. Perirenal inflammatory changes may be visualised on ultrasound or CT. Occasionally **focal bacterial nephritis** may produce an ill-defined hypoechoic or hyperechoic 'pseudomass' with reduced or absent Doppler flow. Correlation with clinical presentation and follow-up imaging should exclude other focal mass lesions.

Adrenal masses

Adrenal haemorrhage is the commonest cause of an adrenal mass in the neonate. Associated with perinatal stress, hypoxia, septicaemia and hypotension, they may be unilateral or bilateral and can occur together with renal vein thrombosis. Adrenal insufficiency is rare, even in bilateral cases. Ultrasound in the first few days of life usually demonstrates an avascular heterogenous adrenal mass that becomes cystic and smaller over the following weeks as clot retraction occurs (Fig. 28.59). A hyperechoic rim may develop due to calcification, and residual calcific foci may be detected on radio-

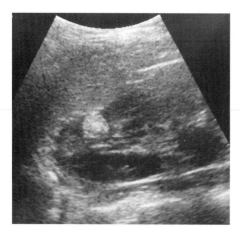

Fig. 28.57 Angiomyolipoma. Longitudinal ultrasound showing a well-circumscribed echogenic mass in the upper pole of the right kidney.

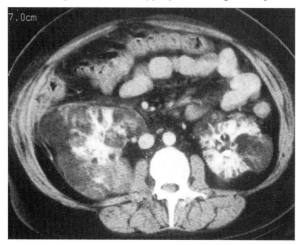

Fig. 28.58 Tuberous sclerosis. The architecture of both kidneys is distorted by multiple fat-containing angiomyolipomas. This CT was performed on a 15-year-old girl with tuberous sclerosis admitted with acute abdominal pain following haemorrhage into one of the right-sided lesions. Oedematous changes in the right abdominal wall followed removal of a percutaneous drain.

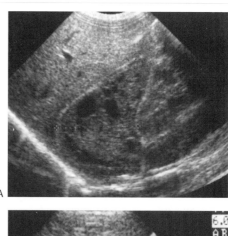

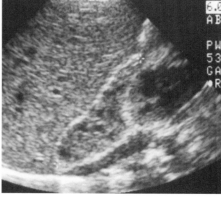

Fig. 28.59 Neonatal adrenal haemorrhage. Ultrasound of a right adrenal haemorrhage on day 2 (A) and day 10 (B) of life. Decrease in size of the mass, often with cystic change (not shown in this example) confirms the nature of the lesion.

graphs or CT later in life. The main differential diagnosis is neuroblastoma. Repeat ultrasound at 5–7 days and, if necessary, serial examinations, should be performed to document the typical course of cystic change with resolution of the haematoma. Adrenal haemorrhage associated with trauma, anticoagulation therapy and septicaemia may be encountered in older children.

Secondary infection of a neonatal adrenal haemorrhage may result in an **abscess**. Tuberculosis, histoplastomosis, and fungal infection of the adrenal glands are also described.

Neuroblastoma is the commonest extracranial solid malignant tumour in children, arising from neural crest tissue within the adrenal gland or anywhere along the sympathetic chain. Approximately 70% of tumours originate in the abdomen (of which two-thirds arise in the adrenal glands), 20% in the chest and 10% in the head and neck region. Most children present under the age of 5 years, with a median age of 22 months. Parents or carers may detect a palpable abdominal mass. Other clinical symptoms are few and non-specific (for example, anaemia and weight loss) until the tumour invades local structures, metastasises or causes a paraneoplastic syndrome. Presentations then include bone pain and marrow failure, cord compression from extradural spread and the 'dancing eyes' syndrome (myoclonic encephalopathy of infancy). Most patients have elevated urinary catecholamines (homovanillic acid and vanilylmandelic acid), although these may be normal in neonates.

Radiological investigation includes ultrasound, CT of the primary lesion and chest, MRI if intraspinal extradural extension is suspected, ^{99m}Tc-MDP and MIBG scans. Ultrasound demonstrates a hyperechoic mass in the adrenal or central retroperitoneum, often with flecks of calcification. Occasionally the tumour is cystic in neonates. CT confirms calcification within the low-attenuation mass in 90% of cases. The most characteristic imaging feature is encasement of adjacent vessels. The aorta and IVC are frequently displaced anteriorly and partially or completely encased by the mass, together with the renal vessels and origins of the mesenteric vessels (Fig. 28.60). Intraspinal extradural extension is another typical finding demonstrated on CT and MRI. Metastases are most commonly to bone cortex, bone marrow and liver. ^{99m}Tc-MDP scintigraphy is useful for the detection of bone metastases; 70% of primary tumours are also MDP-avid. MIBG scans have a role in the detection of primary disease, metastases and recurrent disease, although not all tumours will take up the isotope. Bone metastases often demonstrate characteristic periosteal sunray spiculation in association with a soft-tissue mass.

Several staging systems are used, including the Evans, International Staging and Paediatric Oncology Group systems, which involve various radiological, surgical and bone marrow aspirate criteria:

Stage I confined to organ of origin
Stage II extending beyond organ of origin, unilateral nodal disease
Stage III extending across the midline, bilateral nodal disease
Stage IV distant metastases
Stage IVs age < 1 year, localised primary (stage I or II), metastases to liver, skin and/or bone marrow

Prognostic factors include disease stage, n-*myc* amplification, the Shimada histological classification and age at presentation (favourable under 1 year). Stage I, II and IVs patients have a 75–90% survival. Stage IVS is a subgroup of infants presenting

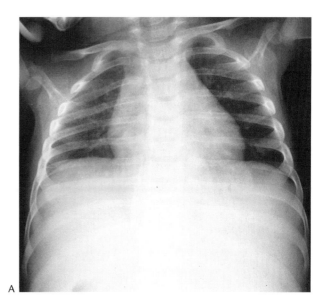

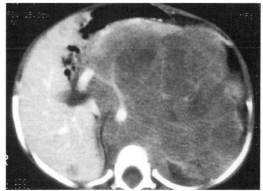

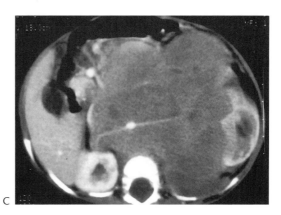

Fig. 28.60 Neuroblastoma. CXR (A) in a 7-month-old girl demonstrating a thoracoabdominal paravertebral mass. CT abdomen (B,C) showing a large retroperitoneal low-attenuation mass which extended superiorly into the posterior mediastinum on more cranial slices. The aorta is displaced anteriorly and completely encased, as are the coeliac axis and renal arteries. The IVC is compressed and adherent to the right lateral border of the mass. The left kidney was invaded directly by the tumour and liver metastases were present.

with tumours that would be classified as stage I or II but with diffuse metastatic disease involving the liver, skin and bone marrow (but not cortical bone) and has a particularly favourable prognosis. Prognosis for patients with advanced stage III or IV disease remains poor (10–30% survival).

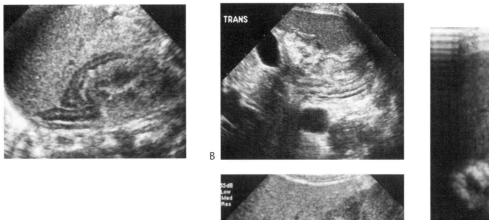

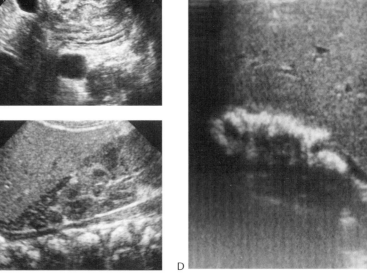

Fig. 28.61 Ultrasound of a normal neonatal right adrenal gland (A) showing the 'stripe' of hypoechoic cortex and hyperechoic medulla. Enlarged and echogenic oedematous left adrenal gland due to asphyxia (B). Enlarged 'speckled' adrenal with lobulated outline typical of congenital adrenal hyperplasia (C). Densely calcified enlarged adrenal gland in Wolman's disease (D).

Other adrenal tumours are rare in childhood. Adrenocortical tumours (carcinoma and adenoma) may occur spontaneously or be associated with the Beckwith–Wiedemann syndrome. Approximately 5% of phaeochromocytomas occur in children and present with hypertension. The 30% of bilateral or multiple tumours, often extra-adrenal in location, are usually associated with the multiple endocrine neoplasia (MEN) IIa and IIb syndromes or with the phakomatoses. MIBG scans will be positive. Lymphomatous involvement of the adrenals is described in children but other metastases are very rare.

Adrenal cysts are most frequently due to resolving adrenal haemorrhage, but can also be seen in Beckwith–Wiedemann syndrome. As mentioned previously, cystic neuroblastomas are occasionally encountered in neonates. **Enlarged adrenal glands** may be due to perinatal asphyxia, congenital adrenal hyperplasia and, rarely, Wolman's disease (Fig. 28.61).

Hepatobiliary masses

Hepatobiliary masses account for approximately 6% of all abdominal masses in childhood. Most are hepatic in origin. Two-thirds of these are malignant and one-third benign.

Hepatoblastoma is the most common malignant hepatic tumour. Children present under the age of 5 years, with the majority under 2 years. Incidence is greater in males. There is an increased risk associated with Beckwith–Wiedemann syndrome, previously affected siblings, familial polyposis coli and trisomy 18. Tumours arise in previously normal liver and there is no association with cirrhosis. Serum alpha-fetoprotein levels are elevated and can be used as a marker for disease monitoring.

Single or multiple hyperechoic masses with distortion of the adjacent hepatic vascular architecture are demonstrated on ultrasound. Heterogeneous low-attenuation lesions are seen on CT, with areas of necrosis and haemorrhage and often containing coarse calcifications (Fig. 28.62). Vascular invasion and tumour thrombus formation within adjacent hepatic veins and portal branches can be

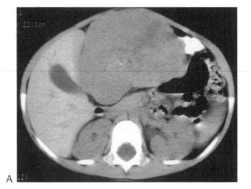

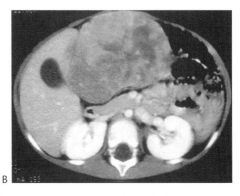

Fig. 28.62 Hepatoblastoma. Unenhanced (A) and enhanced (B) CT abdomen showing a large low-attenuation mass in the left lobe of the liver with small central calcific foci and heterogenous enhancement.

delineated on ultrasound, CT or MRI and strongly suggest malignancy. Tumour may extend into the right atrium via the intrahepatic IVC. Radiological definition of tumour extent and vascular involvement is important, as prognosis is largely determined by surgical resectability. The lung is the most frequent site of metastases. Bone, bone marrow and the brain are less common sites.

Hepatocellular carcinoma (HCC) is seen in older children (age 5–15 years) with pre-existing liver disease, including cirrhosis, hereditary tyrosinaemia, glycogen storage disease, biliary atresia and chronic hepatitis. Imaging characteristics are similar to hepatoblastoma. The rare fibrolamellar type of HCC is not associated with pre-existing liver disease. **Embryonal rhabdomyosarcoma of the biliary tree** and **undifferentiated embryonal cell sarcoma** are occasionally encountered in childhood. **Metastases** to the liver are more common than primary hepatic tumours and are most frequently associated with neuroblastoma, Wilms' tumour, lymphoma and leukaemia.

The most common hepatic mass in the newborn is the benign **infantile haemangioendothelioma**, which may be multifocal (haemangioendotheliomatosis) or solitary. Most cases present in the first month of life. Sinusoidal vascular channels lined by endothelial cells are supported by connective tissue stoma. A proliferative phase is followed by involution, during which fibrous and fatty tissue accumulates, with areas of infarction and dystrophic calcification. Arteriovenous shunting within the lesion can be considerable. Clinical presentations include hepatomegaly, high-output congestive cardiac failure, haemorrhage and consumptive coagulopathy (Kasabach–Merritt syndrome). Cutaneous haemangiomas are present in 40% of patients.

Imaging demonstrates single or multiple intraparenchymal hepatic lesions with large high-flow feeding vessels. Decrease in the calibre of the abdominal aorta below the level of the coeliac axis is characteristic in large lesions. The CT enhancement pattern is typical, with early peripheral enhancement and subsequent filling in of the mass. On MRI, lesions are low signal on T_1 imaging, high on T_2, with large vascular signal voids (Fig. 28.63). The natural history is of gradual involution. However, symptomatic control of cardiac failure, high-dose steroids and alpha-interferon may be required for a period. In refractory cases, embolisation of the feeding hepatic arterial branches may be necessary.

Mesenchymal hamartoma is a rare entity found in children under 2 years of age. Probably representing a developmental anomaly rather than a true neoplasm, it is a multicystic mass comprising mesenchyme, bile ducts, hepatocytes, inflammatory and haemopoietic cells. Other rare benign hepatic lesions include **focal nodular hyperplasia**, with imaging characteristics as described in adults, **haemangiomas**, which are often hypoechoic in contrast to the high echogenicity lesions in adults, and **hepatic adenomas**, seen in glycogen storage disease type 1, Fanconi's anaemia and galactosaemia.

Congenital hepatic cysts are rare. They may be an isolated finding or associated with autosomal dominant polycystic kidney disease or von Hippel–Lindau syndrome. Isolated cysts tend to be solitary and occur in the right lobe (Fig. 28.64). Those associated with syndromes are more likely to be multiple. Ultrasound demonstrates anechoic thin-walled cysts, sometimes with a few fine internal septations. Acquired cysts may be due to echinococcal disease, abscesses or resolving haematomas.

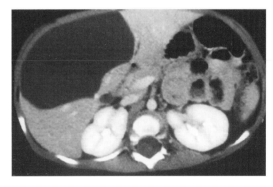

Fig. 28.64 Hepatic cyst. CT abdomen demonstrating a congenital hepatic cyst within the right lobe.

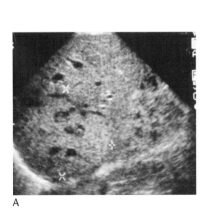

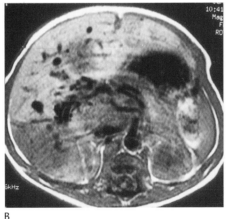

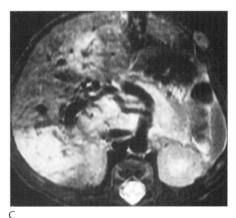

A   B   C

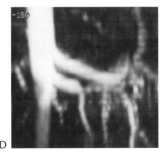

D

Fig. 28.63 Haemangioendotheliosis. Ultrasound (A) showing an ill-defined, almost isoechoic mass with multiple vascular channels in the right lobe of the liver in a newborn infant with congestive cardiac failure. Axial T_1-weighted (B) and T_2-weighted (C) MRI showing lesions within the right and left lobes (low signal on T_1, high signal on T_2) with tortuous dilated feeding vessels arising from the coeliac axis. Sagital 2D TOF MRA (D) showing large calibre proximal abdominal aorta with a reduction in calibre below the origins of the dilated coeliac axis and superior mesenteric artery.

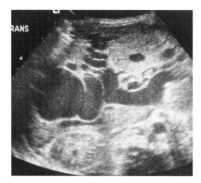

Fig. 28.65 Hepatic arteriovenous malformation. Ultrasound of the liver showing dilated portal venous and hepatic arterial vessels. Doppler spectral traces confirmed arterialisation of the portal venous system due to arterio-venous shunting. There was no associated soft-tissue mass.

Hepatic arteriovenous malformations causing significant shunting present in a similar manner to haemoangioendotheliomas with congestive cardiac failure in the neonatal period. Ultrasound demonstrates multiple large vascular channels but no solid mass component (Fig. 28.65). Vascular communication may involve two or all three of the arterial, portal venous and systemic venous systems.

Hepatic abscesses are usually haematogenous in origin, with dissemination of organisms via the portal venous or systemic circulation. Pyogenic bacteria, fungi (*Candida*, *Aspergillus*, *Cryptococcus*) or *Entamoeba histolytica* may be involved. Multiple hypoechoic or low-attenuation lesions are demonstrated on ultrasound or CT. Larger lesions may contain mobile debris, septations and occasionally air bubbles. Multiple small (<1 cm) 'target' lesions with a hypoechoic rim are typical of fungal microabscesses in the immunosuppressed patient (Fig. 28.66).

Choledochal cysts are congenital dilatations of the biliary tree. Most cause symptoms in childhood, although delayed presentation in adult life is well-described. The classic triad of episodic abdominal pain, jaundice and a right upper quadrant mass is present in approximately 20% of cases. The differential diagnosis of paediatric intra-abdominal cysts is given in Box 28.3. Complications

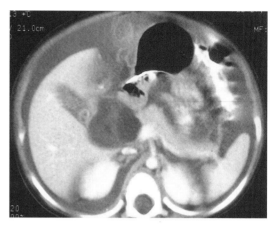

Fig. 28.67 Ruptured choledochal cyst. This 2-year-old girl presented with clinical signs of peritonitis and echogenic ascites documented on ultrasound. CT abdomen shows a right upper quadrant cyst with a 'tail' directed towards the head of the pancreas and ascites. Laparotomy confirmed the diagnosis.

include cholangitis, biliary calculi, pancreatitis and biliary cirrhosis. Spontaneous perforation of the cyst is rare (Fig. 28.67).

The aetiology of choledochal cysts remains under debate. However, both congenital stenoses and anomalies in the insertion of the distal common bile duct (CBD) into the pancreatic duct, predisposing to reflux of pancreatic enzymes and weakening of the bile duct wall, have been implicated. There are four types:

Type 1A	Fusiform dilatation of the CBD below the cystic duct
Type 1B	Fusiform dilatation of the common hepatic duct and CBD
Type 2	Eccentric diverticulum off the CBD

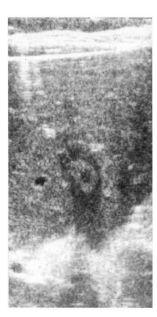

Fig. 28.66 Target lesion. Ultrasound showing a small target lesion with hypoechoic rim in the left lobe of the liver. Several other hepatic lesions were identified in this immunosuppressed patient and are highly suspicious for fungal infection in this clinical setting.

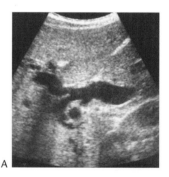

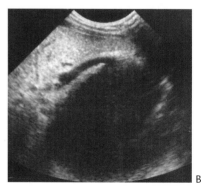

Fig. 28.68 Fusiform dilatation of the common hepatic and common bile ducts in a type 1B choledochal cyst (A) and a large saccular type 2 choledochal cyst showing connection to the common bile duct (B).

Type 3   Choledococele—dilatation of the distal intramural portion of the CBD

Type 4   Caroli's disease—saccular dilatations of the intrahepatic bile ducts

The connection of a right upper quadrant cyst to the biliary tree can usually be demonstrated on ultrasound (Fig. 28.68) or CT. ^{99m}Tc-HIDA scintigraphy will show accumulation of tracer within the cyst. Percutaneous or endoscopic cholangiography, and more recently MRCP, are helpful in preoperative planning. The cyst is excised and direct enteric loop drainage of the biliary tree is fashioned.

Acute calculous cholecystitis has similar imaging features to adults. Gallbladder calculi associated with a thickened hyperaemic gallbladder wall and pericholecystic fluid are typical. Calculi may be idiopathic, associated with gastrointestinal disease (total parenteral nutrition, short-gut syndrome, cystic fibrosis, Crohn's disease), haemolytic disorders (sickle-cell disease, thalassaemia) or diuretic therapy in premature infants (Fig. 28.69). **Acalculous cholecystitis**, in which acute inflammatory changes occur in the absence of gallstones, is encountered in the high dependency or intensive care setting, particularly associated with septicaemia or trauma (Fig. 28.70). **Gallbladder hydrops** (acute dilatation of the gallbladder with a normal wall thickness) may be a presenting feature of Kawasaki's disease.

Pancreatic masses

Pancreatic pseudocysts are the most frequently encountered cystic pancreatic mass, occurring as the sequelae of previous pancreatitis or trauma (Fig. 28.71). An unexplained pseudocyst raises the suspicion of non-accidental injury. True epithelial-lined **congenital pancreatic cysts** are less common and may be associated with von Hippel–Lindau disease, Beckwith–Wiedemann syndrome or autosomal dominant polycystic kidney disease.

Primary pancreatic tumours are rare in childhood. They include pancreaticoblastoma, with a peak incidence of 4 years, solid and papillary epithelial neoplasm, usually affecting girls in the second

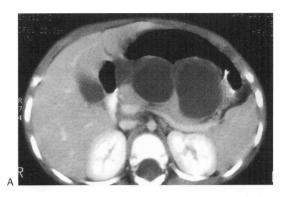
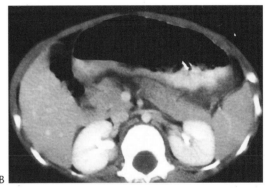

Fig. 28.71   Pancreatic pseudocyst. CT abdomen (A) showing two large pseudocysts anterior to the body of the pancreas. This 3-year-old boy had sustained a laceration to the neck of the pancreas 9 days earlier (B) following a fall from a shopping trolley.

decade of life (Fig. 28.72), and endocrine adenomas (insulinoma, gastrinoma). Burkitt's lymphoma may cause diffuse infiltration and enlargement of the gland. Local invasion by neuroblastoma is not uncommon.

Chronic fibrosing pancreatitis is a rare disease of unknown aetiology in which progressive fibrosis of the gland leads to diffuse enlargement or a localised 'pseudomass' which may mimic a tumour.

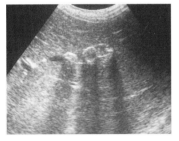

Fig. 28.69   Gallstones. Multiple calculi within a collapsed gallbladder in a 13-year-old girl with sickle-cell anaemia.

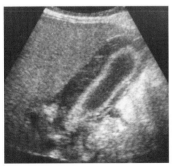

Fig. 28.70   Acalculous cholecystitis. Ultrasound demonstrating grossly thickened gallbladder wall in an 8-year-old girl admitted to paediatric intensive care with pneumonia and septicaemia.

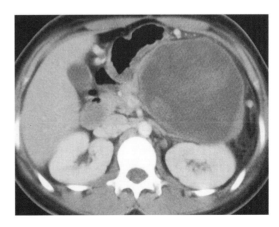

Fig. 28.72   Solid papillary tumour of the pancreas. CT abdomen with a large low-attenuation mass in the region of the tail of the pancreas in a 16-year-old girl. Ultrasound demonstrated both solid and cystic components to the mass (not illustrated).

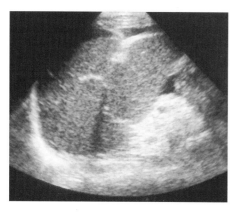

Fig. 28.73 Polysplenia. Two spleens were identified on ultrasound in this newborn infant with left isomerism.

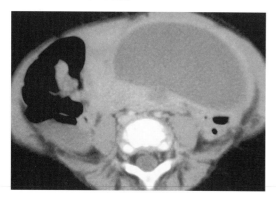

Fig. 28.74 Wandering spleen. CT abdomen in a 4-year-old boy with acute abdominal pain demonstrating a low-attenuation mass in the pelvis. No spleen identified in the left upper quadrant. The echogenicity of the mass was similar to splenic tissue on ultrasound (not illustrated) but no Doppler flow was obtained, consistent with an infarcted wandering spleen.

Box 28.8   Causes of splenomegaly

Infection—mononucleosis, tuberculosis, septicaemia, typhoid, malaria, schistosomiasis, kala-azar
Portal hypertension
Haemolytic anaemias—thalassaemia, sickle-cell disease (sequestration)
Haematological malignancies—leukaemia, lymphoma
Infiltrative disorders—Gaucher's disease, Niemann–Pick disease, Langerhans' cell histiocystosis
Collagen vascular disorders—rheumatoid arthritis
Congestive cardiac failure

Splenic masses

Asplenia and polysplenia occur as part of the heterotaxy syndrome. Asplenia is associated with right isomerism, malrotation and severe congenital cardiac defects, with the majority of infants dying in the first year of life. Polysplenia, in which multiple well-defined splenic masses are found in the left upper quadrant, is associated with left isomerism (Fig. 28.73). Gastrointestinal and vascular anomalies, most characteristically azygous continuation of the IVC, are frequent but cardiac defects are generally less severe and prognosis more favourable. Polysplenia should not be confused with **accessory splenic tissue** (or splenunculi), which are a common incidental finding in normal individuals. Ultrasound demonstrates one or more small (1–2 cm) rounded masses adjacent to the splenic hilum or inferior pole and with identical echogenicity to the main splenic bulk. A

'wandering spleen' describes a spleen found in an ectopic location outside the left upper quadrant. It is believed to be due to lax or deficient suspensory ligaments and may be complicated by torsion. Children present with acute abdominal pain, absence of a correctly-positioned spleen and an abdominal mass with splenic shape and sonographic characteristics but absent Doppler perfusion. As infarction progresses, the echogenicity of the spleen alters and it becomes more hypoattenuating on CT (Fig. 28.74).

Splenomegaly may be associated with portal hypertension, infections, haemolytic disorders and neoplastic infiltration. The main causes in children are given in Box 28.8.

Focal splenic lesions. Splenic cysts may be congenital (epithelial or epidermoid cysts) or acquired secondary to trauma, infarction or hydatid disease. Splenic abscesses may result from haematogenous spread or superinfection of a pre-existing cyst, haematoma or infarct. The interpretation of multiple small hypoechoic lesions depends on the clinical scenario. The differential diagnosis includes fungal disease in the immunosuppressed patient (*Candida, Aspergillus, Cryptococcus*), granulomatous disease, bacterial micro-abscesses (bacterial endocarditis, intravenous drug abuse), diffuse infiltrative lymphocytosis syndrome (DILS) in HIV-infected children, extramedullary haematopoiesis and, rarely, metastases (Fig. 28.75). Benign focal splenic masses include haemangiomas, lymphangiomas, arteriovenous malformations and hamartomas. Multifocal splenic masses may be a feature of lymphoproliferative disease in patients receiving long-term immunosuppressive therapy. Malignant infiltration by lymphoma or leukaemia usually results in diffuse enlargement, although focal low-attenuation lymphomatous masses may occur.

Gastrointestinal masses

Duplication cysts and mesenteric/omental cysts have been discussed earlier. **Primary bowel malignancies** are rare in childhood. The commonest malignancy is Burkitt's non-Hodgkin's lymphoma, which may present as an ill-defined mass of adherent bowel loops with infiltration of the adjacent mesentery and lymphadenopathy. Colonic carcinoma is very occasionally described in adolescents. **Inflammatory masses** are encountered more frequently. In the absence of classical symptoms, acute appendicitis may be unrecognised in children for several days after perforation has occurred and

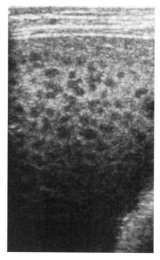

Fig. 28.75 Multiple small hypoechoic lesions within the spleen may be due to infections (fungal disease, granulomatous disease, bacterial microabscesses), diffuse infiltrative lymphocytosis syndrome in HIV-infected children (case illustrated), extramedullary haema- topoesis or, rarely, metastases.

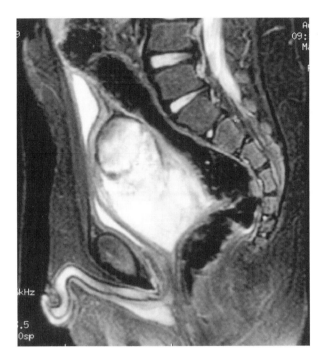

Fig. 28.76 Prostatic rhabdomyosarcoma. Sagittal fat-saturated T$_2$-weighted MRI in a 4-year-old boy demonstrating a large prerectal pelvic mass displacing the bladder anteriorly.

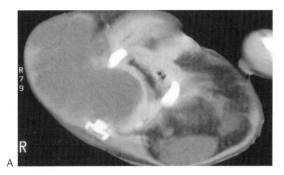

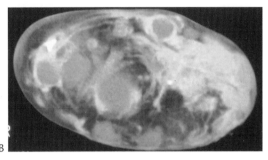

Fig. 28.77 Type II sacrococcygeal teratoma. CT pelvis (A) in a newborn girl showing a presacral mass with a large external component (B) containing soft tissue, cystic, fat and calcific elements.

may present with a right iliac fossa mass of thickened bowel loops and inflammatory phlegmon or abscess. Inflammatory bowel masses with local collections and fistulas to adjacent viscera are also seen in Crohn's disease. Tuberculous disease may present similarly, often in association with peritoneal disease, ascites and lymphadenopathy.

Pelvic masses

Rhabdomyosarcoma is the commonest paediatric soft-tissue sarcoma, accounting for 5–10% of childhood solid tumours. The pelvis is the most frequent site of origin, followed by the head and neck region. Most arise from the prostate or bladder base in boys (Fig. 28.76) and either bladder, vagina or uterus in girls. The tumour is aggressive, with invasion of adjacent viscera and pelvic side-walls and distant spread to lymph nodes, lung and bone. Age distribution is bimodal with peaks at 2–6 years and 14–16 years.

Sacrococcygeal teratomas are derived from all three germinal layers and arise from the ventral surface of the coccyx. Diagnosis is usually made at birth, with a large pelvic or gluteal mass containing solid, cystic, calcific and fat components (Fig. 28.77). Intraspinal extension may be delineated on MRI. Type I tumours are predominantly external, type II external and intrapelvic, type III extend superiorly into the abdomen, and type IV are purely intrapelvic. Almost all lesions are benign at birth but malignant transformation becomes increasingly likely with time, such that at 2 months of age over 90% contain malignant foci. It is therefore important that surgical resection is performed as early as possible. Small type IV tumours without a visible external component tend to present later in infancy or childhood with malignant elements and hence have a poorer prognosis than those diagnosed at birth. Other causes of presacral masses are listed in Box 28.9.

Ovarian masses. Simple anechoic **ovarian cysts** may be found in neonates secondary to overstimulation of normal follicular development by maternal hormones, and in pubertal girls due to failure of

---

Box 28.9   Presacral masses in childhood

Tumours
    Sacrococcygeal teratoma
    Neurogenic tumours (neuroblastoma/ganglioneuroma/neurofibroma)
    Dermoid
    Lymphoma
    Sacral chordoma

Rectal duplication cyst

Neurenteric cyst

Ectopic kidney

Anterior meningocele

Abscess

Haematoma

---

involution of a follicular or corpus luteal cyst (Fig. 28.78). Haemorrhage into the cyst can result in a more complex sonographic appearance with fine septations and internal debris. Paraovarian cysts are difficult to distinguish from ovarian cysts on imaging. Approximately 65% of **ovarian tumours** are benign and 35% malignant. Ovarian teratomas usually present at puberty and 90% are benign. CT demonstrates a well-circumscribed mixed cystic–solid mass with fat and calcific components (Fig. 28.79). There is a greater incidence of malignancy with increasing size and with a large soft-tissue component but it is not possible to determine whether a mass is benign or malignant on imaging unless evidence of local invasion or metastatic spread is present. Mucinous or serous cystadenomas may be benign or malignant. The majority of ovarian malignancies are germ cell tumours, with a smaller number of stromal sex cord tumours and epithelial carcinomas. Most are large (>15 cm) at presentation. Germ cell and stromal neoplasms disseminate by contiguous spread or lymphatic and haematogenous metastases, whereas epithelial carcinomas character-

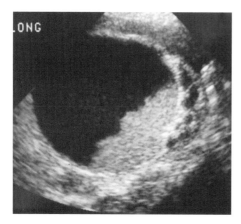

Fig. 28.78 Ovarian cyst. Ultrasound of the pelvis in a 4-week-old girl demonstrating an ovarian cyst containing mobile debris. A crescent of ovarian tissue is seen laterally and confirms the origin of the cyst.

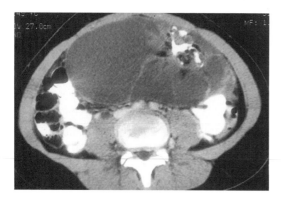

Fig. 28.79 Mature ovarian teratoma in an 11-year-old girl. CT demonstrating a large mixed solid/cystic mass arising from the pelvis and containing fat and calcification.

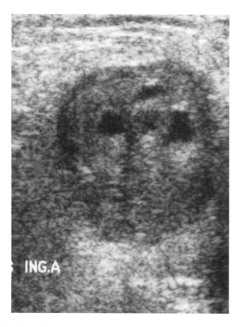

Fig. 28.80 Torted ovary. This infant girl presented with a tender left inguinal lump. Ultrasound showed a hypoechoic mass with peripheral cysts and absent Doppler flow. Surgical exploration revealed a torted left ovary that had herniated into the inguinal region.

istically seed to peritoneal surfaces and omentum. Neuroblastomas, lymphomas and leukaemia may metastasise to the ovaries.

Pelvic inflammatory disease may result in complications such as tubo-ovarian abscesses and pyosalpinx in sexually-active adolescents.

Adnexal torsion can occur at any age but is most frequent in the first two decades of life. The affected ovary may be normal or contain a cyst or tumour. Rotation of the ovary on its vascular pedicle results in venous and arterial compromise, causing congestion and resultant haemorrhagic infarction. Patients present with acute lower abdominal pain and vomiting. There is often a history of previous similar episodes of pain. Ultrasound demonstrates an enlarged swollen ovary with peripheral cysts and free fluid in the pouch of Douglas (Fig. 28.80). Doppler flow is usually absent but some signal may be obtained due to dual supply from the ovarian and uterine arteries.

Acknowledgments

With grateful thanks to the Departments of Radiology at the Hospital for Sick Children, Toronto, Canada, St Mary's Hospital, London and Great Ormond Street Hospitals, UK for the generous provision of the illustrations used in this chapter.

REFERENCES AND SUGGESTIONS FOR FURTHER READING

Babyn, P., Owens, C., Gyepes, M., et al (1995) Imaging patients with Wilms' tumor. *Hematology/Oncology Clinics of North America*, **9**, 1217–1252.

Berlin, L. (1998) Malpractice issues in radiology: reducing the intussuscepted colon. *American Journal of Roentgenology*, **170**, 1161–1163.

Berrocal, T., Lamas, M., Gutierrez, J., Torres, I., Prieto, C., del Hoyo, M. L. (1999) Congenital anomalies of the small intestine, colon and rectum. *Radiographics*, **19**, 1219–1236.

Cohen, M. D., Bugaieski, E. M., Haliloglu, M., et al (1996) Visual presentation of the staging of pediatric solid tumors. *Radiographics*, **16**, 523–545.

Daneman, A., Alton, D. J. (1996) Intussusception: issues and controversies related to diagnosis and reduction. *Radiologic Clinics of North America*, **34**, 743–756.

Donnelly, L. F., Emery, K. H., Brody, A. S., et al (2001) Minimising radiation dose for pediatric body applications of single detector helical CT—strategies at a large childrens hospital. *American Journal of Roentgenology*, **176**, 303–306.

Kirks, D. R. (ed.) (1998) Practical Pediatric Imaging, 3rd edn. Philadelphia: Lippincott-Raven.

Long, F. R., Kramer, S. S., Markowitz, R. I., Taylor, G. E. (1996) Radiographic patterns of intestinal malrotation in children. *Radiographics*, **16**, 547–556.

Paterson, A., Frush, D. P., Donnelly, L. F., et al (1999) A pattern-orientated approach to splenic imaging in infants and children. *Radiographics*, **19**, 1465–1485.

Puylaert, J. B. C. M. (1986) Acute appendicitis: ultrasound evaluation using graded compression. *Radiology*, **158**, 355–360.

Sadler, T. W. (1990) *Langman's Medical Embryology*, 6th edn, ch. 14. Baltimore: Williams and Wilkins.

Seigel, M. J. (ed.) (1996) *Pediatric Sonography*, 2nd edn. Philadelphia: Lippincott-Raven.

Seigel, M. J. (1999) *Pediatric Body CT*. Philadelphia: Lippincott Williams and Wilkins.

Shaul, D. B., Harrison, E. A. (1997) Classification of anorectal malformations—initial approach, diagnostic tests and colostomy. *Seminars in Pediatric Surgery*, **6**, 187–195.

Sivit, C. J. (1993) Diagnosis of acute appendicitis in children: spectrum of sonographic findings. *American Journal of Roentgenology*, **161**, 147–152.

Stringer, D., Babyn, P. (2000) *Pediatric Gastrointestinal Imaging and Intervention*, 2nd edn. Philadelphia: Decker B. C.

Swischuk, L. E., John, S. D. (1995) *Differential Diagnosis in Pediatric Radiology*, 2nd edn. Baltimore: Williams and Wilkins.

Vershelden, P., Filiatrault, D., Garel, L., et al (1992) Intussusception in children: reliability of ultrasound diagnosis—a prospective study. *Radiology*, **184**, 741–744.

INDEX